Sturdevant's
ART & SCIENCE OF
OPERATIVE DENTISTRY

FOURTH EDITION

EDITORS

THEODORE M. ROBERSON, DDS
Professor
Department of Operative Dentistry
University of North Carolina
School of Dentistry
Chapel Hill, North Carolina

HARALD O. HEYMANN, DDS, MEd
Professor
Department of Operative Dentistry
University of North Carolina
School of Dentistry
Chapel Hill, North Carolina

EDWARD J. SWIFT, JR., DMD, MS
Professor
Department of Operative Dentistry
University of North Carolina
School of Dentistry
Chapel Hill, North Carolina

with 2521 illustrations

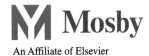 Mosby

An Affiliate of Elsevier

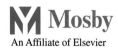
Mosby
An Affiliate of Elsevier

Publishing Director: John Schrefer
Senior Acquisitions Editor: Penny Rudolph
Developmental Editor: Kimberly Alvis
Project Manager: Catherine Jackson
Production Editor: Clay S. Broeker
Designer: Amy Buxton

FOURTH EDITION
Copyright © 2002 by Mosby

Previous editions copyrighted 1995 and 1985 by Mosby and 1968 by McGraw-Hill, Inc.

Mosby
An Affiliate of Elsevier
11830 Westline Industrial Drive
St. Louis, Missouri 63146

Printed in the United States of America

Library of Congress Cataloging in Publication Data

Sturdevant's art & science of operative dentistry.–4th ed. / editors, Theodore M. Roberson, Harald O. Heymann, Edward J. Swift, Jr.
    p. ; cm.
  Rev. ed. of: The art and science of operative dentistry / senior editor, Clifford M. Sturdevant; co-editors, Theodore M. Roberson, Harald O. Heymann, John R. Sturdevant. 3rd ed. c1995.
  Includes bibliographical references and index.
  ISBN 0-323-01087-3
  1. Dentistry, Operative. I. Title: Sturdevant's art and science of operative dentistry. II. Title: Art & science of operative dentistry. III. Roberson, Theodore M. IV. Heymann, Harald. V. Swift, Edward J. VI. Sturdevant, Clifford M. VII. Art and science of operative dentistry.
  [DLNLM: 1. Dentistry, Operative. WU 300 S9351 2001]
RK501 .A78 2001
617.6'05–dc21

                              2001045250

04 05 06 GW/ RRD-W 9 8 7 6 5 4 3

Stephen C. Bayne, MS, PhD, FADM
Professor and Section Head of Biomaterials
Department of Operative Dentistry
University of North Carolina
School of Dentistry
Chapel Hill, North Carolina

James J. Crawford, BA, MA, PhD
Professor Emeritus (Retired)
Department of Diagnostic Sciences and General
  Dentistry
University of North Carolina
School of Dentistry
Chapel Hill, North Carolina

Harald O. Heymann, DDS, MEd
Professor
Department of Operative Dentistry
University of North Carolina
School of Dentistry
Chapel Hill, North Carolina

Ralph H. Leonard, Jr., DDS, MPH
Clinical Associate Professor
Department of Diagnostic Sciences and General
  Dentistry
University of North Carolina
School of Dentistry
Chapel Hill, North Carolina

Thomas F. Lundeen, DMD
Private Practitioner
Durham, North Carolina

Kenneth N. May, Jr., DDS
Professor and Associate Dean of Administration and
  Planning
Department of Operative Dentistry
University of North Carolina
School of Dentistry
Chapel Hill, North Carolina

Jorge Perdigão, DDS, MS, PhD
Associate Professor and Director
Department of Restorative Sciences
Division of Operative Dentistry
University of Minnesota
Minneapolis, Minnesota

Patricia N.R. Pereira, DDS, PhD
Assistant Professor
Department of Operative Dentistry
University of North Carolina
School of Dentistry
Chapel Hill, North Carolina

André V. Ritter, DDS, MS
Assistant Professor and Assistant Graduate Program
  Director
Department of Operative Dentistry
University of North Carolina
School of Dentistry
Chapel Hill, North Carolina

Theodore M. Roberson, DDS
Professor
Department of Operative Dentistry
University of North Carolina
School of Dentistry
Chapel Hill, North Carolina

Daniel A. Shugars, DDS, PhD, MPH
Professor
Department of Operative Dentistry
University of North Carolina
School of Dentistry
Chapel Hill, North Carolina

Diane C. Shugars, DDS, MPH, PhD
Associate Professor
Department of Dental Ecology
University of North Carolina
School of Dentistry
Associate Professor
Department of Microbiology and Immunology
University of North Carolina
School of Medicine
Chapel Hill, North Carolina

Troy B. Sluder, Jr., DDS, MS
Professor Emeritus (Retired)
Department of Operative Dentistry
University of North Carolina
School of Dentistry
Chapel Hill, North Carolina

Gregory E. Smith, DDS, MSD
Professor
Department of Operative Dentistry
University of Florida
Gainesville, Florida

John W. Stamm, DDS, DDPH, MScD
Professor and Dean
University of North Carolina
School of Dentistry
Chapel Hill, North Carolina

Clifford M. Sturdevant, DDS
Professor Emeritus (Retired)
Department of Operative Dentistry
University of North Carolina
School of Dentistry
Chapel Hill, North Carolina

John R. Sturdevant, DDS
Associate Professor
Department of Operative Dentistry
University of North Carolina
School of Dentistry
Chapel Hill, North Carolina

Edward J. Swift, Jr., DMD, MS
Professor
Department of Operative Dentistry
University of North Carolina
School of Dentistry
Chapel Hill, North Carolina

Duane F. Taylor, BSE, MSE, PhD
Professor Emeritus (Retired)
Department of Operative Dentistry
University of North Carolina
School of Dentistry
Chapel Hill, North Carolina

Jeffrey Y. Thompson, BS, PhD
Associate Professor
Department of Operative Dentistry
University of North Carolina
School of Dentistry
Chapel Hill, North Carolina

Aldridge D. Wilder, Jr., DDS
Professor
Department of Operative Dentistry
University of North Carolina
School of Dentistry
Chapel Hill, North Carolina

We dedicate this book to the betterment of operative dentistry. The central motivating factor of the authors and editors is to provide a book that is worthy for use by our teaching colleagues. We sincerely hope that students present, past, and future will benefit from these pages.

We also dedicate this edition to the authors and editors who have preceded us. In particular, this textbook is dedicated to Dr. Cliff Sturdevant, the inspiration and driving force for the first three editions. In recognition of his contributions, we have changed the title to include his name.

We further dedicate this book to our spouses and families for their continual love, understanding, and support during this revision.

The dental sciences are undergoing enormous changes, and the field of operative dentistry is at the forefront of that transformation. No dental educator can fail to notice that various restorative dental technologies, some only 10 years old, are becoming obsolete, and that today's students and practitioners must incorporate new and enhanced concepts into provision of the care that patients require. This fourth edition textbook, now entitled *Sturdevant's Art & Science of Operative Dentistry*, is an exemplary attempt to codify the principles of operative dentistry pertinent to the education and practice of operative dentistry in the twenty-first century.

This book presents the science of operative dentistry in an evolved yet highly dynamic fashion. At the University of North Carolina, the operative dentistry discipline is constantly tested and evaluated and is forced to meet the challenge of pedagogical Darwinism. That is, the concepts that constitute operative dentistry practice are continually evaluated against the torrent of information flowing from the basic and clinical sciences that shape everything we do in the health care field. What is outdated is discarded, what remains applicable is updated, and what is new and necessary is incorporated. Only the best information and technologies survive to guide our teaching and practice of operative dentistry. In this manner, this book contributes to evidence-based dentistry.

Dental caries is not a lesion—it is a disease. This book is written with the explicit assumption that the disease of dental caries must be thoroughly understood if efforts to prevent and treat it are to improve. Molecular biology and new diagnostic technologies have so altered the field of cariology that its overview in the present volume is only cursory. The increasing ability to diagnostically measure earlier stages in the caries process is leading to a redefinition of caries and is changing contemporary approaches to caries treatment. The choice between surgical and nonsurgical caries treatment is becoming more complex.

During the last 20 years, dental caries prevalence and severity have declined in most of the industrialized world, yet significant population components have remained at high caries risk. Taking a more global perspective, it is known that dental caries prevalence is increasing in many industrializing countries. In many highly populated, mid-tier countries, caries is still a largely untreated condition. In all of these situations, the challenges of caries treatment facing dental educators, students, and practitioners are enormous and cannot be overlooked. *Sturdevant's Art & Science of Operative Dentistry* is expressly written for the dental schools and offices that represent the loci for excellence in operative dentistry in all of these settings.

Among the most illustrative examples of the continuing change facing the dental profession are the emergence of esthetic dentistry and the application of computer-aided design/computer-assisted manufacturing (CAD/CAM) in dentistry. For operative dentistry, both of these endeavors represent the pinnacle of high technology and convincingly demonstrate operative dentistry's skill in dealing with the larger issue of technology transfer into its discipline. I am particularly pleased that the fourth edition of *Sturdevant's Art & Science of Operative Dentistry* appropriately emphasizes these developments within its pages. The authors of this textbook have accumulated extensive knowledge and clinical experience pertaining to these evolving technologies, and they give an excellent account of what will surely become an increasingly important component of operative dentistry in the twenty-first century. Learn and enjoy as much as I did from this outstanding textbook.

John W. Stamm, DDS
Professor and Dean
University of North Carolina
School of Dentistry

In 1961, Dr. Doug Strickland said, "Cliff, we should write a textbook." Three days later, still trembling over the immensity of such an endeavor, we agreed to give it our best. Thus resulted the first edition, in 1968, of *The Art and Science of Operative Dentistry*.

In 1994, dental educators and private practitioners had available the third edition, which answered their earlier query, "When will we see the next edition?" The appreciation of these colleagues is a major stimulus for the talented faculty of our department to persevere under the hardships that accompany this extensive project. To have constancy in a talented, dedicated "in-house" faculty (the textbook contributors) is a blessing for any senior editor.

Dr. Theodore (Ted) Roberson is the senior editor of this fourth edition. I am confident the users of this book will value Dr. Ted's unique and blessed talents in organization, writing, vision, and leadership, as well as his hard work and long hours.

Congratulations and thanks to the editors and contributors.

Clifford (Cliff) Sturdevant
Chair, 1959-1979
Department of Operative Dentistry
University of North Carolina
School of Dentistry

Operative dentistry is a dynamic discipline. Many changes in techniques, materials, and emphasis have occurred since the third edition of this textbook. The continued development, increased use, and recognized benefit of bonding procedures are paramount and have resulted in a new emphasis on, as well as techniques for, such procedures. New information about cariology, infection control needs and procedures, diagnosis and treatment planning, and adhesive dentistry is presented in this edition, as is updated information about esthetic restorations. Throughout the book, emphasis is maintained on the importance of treating the underlying causes of the patient's problem(s), not just the restoration of the damage that has occurred.

NEW TO THIS EDITION

The fourth edition of *The Art and Science of Operative Dentistry* presents numerous changes. First, the title of the book has been changed to *Sturdevant's Art & Science of Operative Dentistry* to reflect Dr. Clifford M. Sturdevant's relationship with this book for over 30 years. Without Cliff Sturdevant, there would never have been a textbook, especially not one with this quality and reputation.

Almost all topics presented in the third edition are still included. We have added five new chapters:

Enamel and Dentin Adhesion
Preliminary Considerations for Operative Dentistry
Introduction to Composite Restorations
Introduction to Amalgam Restorations
Indirect Tooth-Colored Classes I and II Restorations.

This edition includes more than 2500 illustrations, with an increased number of color photographs and color-enhanced drawings, diagrams, tables, and boxes.

This edition also uses different terminology. The term *cavity* is used only in an historical context and is replaced by other terms such as *carious lesion* or *tooth preparation*. This change reflects the continuing evolution of operative dentistry to represent treatment necessitated by many factors, not just caries. Also, the term *composite* is used to refer to a variety of tooth-colored materials that may be designated by *composite-resin, resin-based composite,* or other terms in the literature. The term *amalgam* is used instead of *dental amalgam.*

ORGANIZATION

The fourth edition benefits from an improved organizational format. The early chapters (1 through 8) present general information necessary to understand the dynamics of operative dentistry. These chapters include introductions to operative dentistry, dental anatomy, physiology, occlusion, cariology, dental materials, enamel and dentin adhesion, tooth preparation, instruments and equipment, and infection control.

The remaining chapters (9 through 21) are specifically related to the clinical practice of operative dentistry. These chapters present composite restorations before amalgam restorations to reflect the University of North Carolina's support of composite restorations in many clinical applications. Each "technique" chapter is presented in the same format, beginning with an introduction that presents the pertinent factors about the restorative material being used; the indications, contraindications, advantages, and disadvantages of the presented procedure; and finally the tooth preparation factors and restorative factors that relate to the procedure. Common problems (with solutions) for the procedure are presented, as is a summary of the chapter.

CHAPTER SYNOPSES

Chapter 1, Introduction to Operative Dentistry, emphasizes the biologic basis of operative dentistry and presents current statistics that demonstrate the continuing need and demand for it.

Chapter 2, Clinical Significance of Dental Anatomy, Histology, Physiology, and Occlusion, is similar to the same chapter in the last edition, presenting sections on the pulp-dentin complex and occlusion. The presentation of occlusal relationships and chewing movements should aid in the assessment of occlusion and the provision of acceptable occlusion in restorations.

Chapter 3, Cariology: The Lesion, Etiology, Prevention, and Control, has a different organization but still presents the ecologic basis of caries and then deals with its management, which involves diagnosis, prevention, and treatment. The caries control restoration is also described.

Chapter 4, Dental Materials, first presents a review of materials science and biomechanics and then provides updated information about direct and indirect restorative materials, including the safety and efficacy of their use. The topics of composites, sealants, glass ionomers, and amalgam materials have been expanded.

Chapter 5, Fundamental Concepts of Enamel and Dentin Adhesion, is a new chapter authored by internationally recognized experts. Basic concepts of adhesion are presented, followed by detailed descriptions of and factors affecting enamel and dentin adhesion. Also included are sections on microleakage and biocompatibility. This chapter provides a firm scientific basis for the use of adhesives in clinical operative procedures.

Chapter 6, Fundamentals in Tooth Preparation, presents the current nomenclature related to the preparation of teeth. It should be noted again that the term *cavity preparation* has been replaced by *tooth preparation* for the reasons stated previously. Tooth preparation is still presented as a two-stage (initial and final) procedure that is divided into a number of steps. The differences in tooth preparation for composite restorations are expanded and emphasized. Current pulpal protection strategies are presented.

Chapter 7, Instruments and Equipment for Tooth Preparation, provides similar information as that in the third edition, with more emphasis and information about diamond stones.

Chapter 8, Infection Control, reviews the exposure risks associated with dental practice and presents current information for federal, state, and OSHA regulations. The chapter emphasizes the importance of appropriate infection control procedures. Expanded sections are presented on dental office water lines and handpiece sterilization.

Chapter 9, Patient Assessment, Examination and Diagnosis, and Treatment Planning, provides an excellent reference for practitioners and students. Patient assessment is presented, emphasizing the importance of a medical review that includes relevant factors of systemic and communicable diseases. Photographs of some of these oral manifestations are presented in a color insert. Factors affecting the determination of clinical treatment are covered, with special emphasis on indications for operative treatment, including the decision to replace existing restorations.

Chapter 10, Preliminary Considerations for Operative Dentistry, combines information from several chapters from the third edition. The sections on local anesthesia and isolation of the operating site have been updated. Patient and operator positioning, instrument exchange, and magnification are also part of this chapter.

Chapter 11, Introduction to Composite Restorations, is a new chapter that provides an overview of the composite restoration technique. It reviews the types of esthetic materials available, emphasizing the properties of composite. Additional information about polymerization of composites is presented. (Some of this information is also included in Chapter 6). Indications, contraindications, advantages, and disadvantages of composite restorations are detailed, often with some comparison to amalgam restorations. Expanded information is provided on the techniques of tooth preparation for composite restorations; this information recognizes the more conservative removal of tooth structure necessary for composite preparations as compared with amalgam preparations. The restorative technique necessary when using composite is reviewed in a general format. Both the tooth preparation and the restoration techniques provide the basis for the more specific information about composite restorations presented in Chapters 12 through 15. This chapter also includes sections on both the repair of composite restorations and common problems (and solutions) that may be encountered with composite restorations.

Chapter 12, Classes III, IV, and V Direct Composite and Other Tooth-Colored Restorations, presents thorough coverage of the specific rationale and technique for use of composite in these locations. There are also sections on microfill composite and glass-ionomer restorations.

Chapter 13, Classes I, II, and VI Direct Composite and Other Tooth-Colored Restorations, provides an expanded emphasis for the use of composite in posterior teeth. The rationale and technique for use of composite in Class I and II restorations is covered in more detail and a new section on the use of composite for extensive Class II and foundation restorations is included.

Chapter 14, Classes I and II Indirect Tooth-Colored Restorations, is a new chapter that presents both material formerly presented in another third-edition chapter and also new material. The chapter includes expanded coverage of the indirect techniques and the various materials and methods available. Information about indirect restorations of composite, feldspathic porcelain, pressed glass ceramics, and CAD/CAM are covered. Another section discusses common problems and solutions.

Chapter 15, Additional Conservative Esthetic Procedures, provides an excellent resource for many esthetic procedures. After reviewing the factors for artistic success, the chapter presents detailed techniques for esthetic contouring and enhancements, bleaching, veneers, splinting, and conservative bonded bridges. These procedures are well supplemented with many illustrations, most of which are in color.

Chapter 16, Introduction to Amalgam Restorations, is a new chapter that presents fundamental concepts for amalgam restorations. The material qualities of amalgam as a restorative material are identified, followed by sections on the indications, contraindications, advantages, and disadvantages for amalgam restorations. The use of amalgam is still recommended, but emphasis is placed on its use for larger restorations, especially in nonesthetic areas. Fundamental concepts of both amalgam tooth preparations and restoration techniques are included, and these are expanded upon in Chapters 17 through 19. Also included in this chapter are sections on common problems (and solutions), repairs, and controversial issues.

Chapter 17, Classes I, II, and VI Amalgam Restorations, combines several chapters from the third edition. Greater emphasis is placed on the use of amalgam in large Class I and Class II restorations, with smaller restorations recommended for the use of composite instead. However, smaller amalgam restorations are presented, primarily to serve as a method of presenting the fundamental concepts associated with larger amalgam restoration techniques. The bonding of amalgam restorations is presented in detail, and although the text does not promote the bonding of all amalgam restorations, this chapter provides the fundamental techniques of appropriate bonded amalgam restorations.

Chapter 18, Classes III and V Amalgam Restorations, presents the rationale and techniques for these restorations. The use of Class IV amalgam restorations has been deleted and the indications for Class III restorations minimized.

Chapter 19, Complex Amalgam Restorations, details the use of amalgam for very large restorations (including foundations), presenting the use of pins, slots, and bonding techniques. (Discussion of the use of slots is increased from the previous edition.)

Chapter 20, Class II Cast Metal Restorations, provides thorough coverage of the entire cast metal restoration pro-

cedure. Although similar to the chapter in the third edition, this chapter provides new information on impression, temporary, and working model procedures. The procedures are well documented, with many illustrations.

Finally, Chapter 21, Direct Gold Restorations, provides an update on gold foil restorations for Classes I, III, and V.

Theodore M. Roberson, Chair, 1979-1988
Harald O. Heymann, Chair, 1988-2000
Edward J. Swift, Jr., Chair, 2000-present
Department of Operative Dentistry
University of North Carolina
School of Dentistry

ACKNOWLEDGMENTS

In addition to teaching operative dentistry, the authors practice the principles and techniques presented in this book in a clinical setting and engage in clinical or laboratory research. Thus the restorative concepts presented here are supported by both clinical activity and research results.

The editors express special appreciation to the following:

- Warren McCollum, Director of the Learning Resources Center of the UNC School of Dentistry, and his staff for their diligence in production of illustrations.
- Marie Roberts, Paulette Pauley, and Shannon Veccia for their capable assistance in manuscript preparation. In particular, a special thanks is extended to Ms. Roberts for her vital role in organizing the revision effort and communicating with the publisher.
- Drs. Roger Barton, Tom Lundeen, Ken May, Troy Sluder, Lee Sockwell, Doug Strickland, Cliff Sturdevant, Duane Taylor, and Van Haywood, who, while inactive in this edition, have provided information still present in the fourth edition. We are grateful for their past contributions.
- Penny Rudolph and Kimberly Alvis at Harcourt Health Sciences for their constant support, encouragement, and expertise during the revision process. Their guidance and ideas provided increased professional appeal for the book, both in its appearance and its content.

CONTENTS

*These authors are inactive this edition. See the Acknowledgments.

Sturdevant's
ART & SCIENCE OF
OPERATIVE DENTISTRY

Introduction to Operative Dentistry

THEODORE M. ROBERSON

DEFINITION AND HISTORY

DEFINITION

Operative dentistry is the art and science of the diagnosis, treatment, and prognosis of defects of teeth that do not require full coverage restorations for correction. Such treatment should result in the restoration of proper tooth form, function, and esthetics while maintaining the physiologic integrity of the teeth in harmonious relationship with the adjacent hard and soft tissues, all of which should enhance the general health and welfare of the patient.

HISTORY

Although *operative dentistry was once considered to be the entirety of the clinical practice of dentistry,* today many of the areas previously included under operative dentistry have become specialty areas. As information increased and the need for other complex treatments was recognized, areas such as endodontics, prosthodontics, and orthodontics became dental specialties. However, operative dentistry is still recognized as the foundation of dentistry and the base from which most other aspects of dentistry evolved.

In the United States, dentistry originated in the seventeenth century when several "barber-dentists" were sent from England. The practice of these early dentists consisted mainly of tooth extractions because dental caries at that time was considered a "gangrene-like" disease. Many practiced dentistry while pursuing other livelihoods, and some traveled from one area to another to provide their dental services. These early dentists learned their trade by serving apprenticeships under more experienced practitioners. Later, it became known that treatment of the defective part of a tooth (the "cavity") could occur by removal of the cavity and replacement of the missing tooth structure by "filling" the cavity with some type of material. Much of the knowledge and many of the techniques for the first successful tooth restorations were developed in the United States. However, much of the practice of dentistry during the founding years of this country was not based on scientific knowledge, and disputes often arose regarding treatment techniques and materials. One such dispute concerning the use of amalgam as a restorative material played a part in the establishment of the Baltimore College of Dental Surgery in 1840,[37] which marked the official birth of formal dental education as a discipline. In 1867, Harvard University established the first university-affiliated dental program.[29]

It was in this same period in France that Louis Pasteur discovered the role of microorganisms in disease,[35] a finding that would have a significant effect on the developing dental and medical professions. Also, in the United States during this time, contributions by G.V. Black[8] became the foundation of the dental profession. *Black,* who had both honorary dental and honorary medical degrees, *related the clinical practice of dentistry to*

a scientific basis. This scientific foundation for operative dentistry was further expanded by Black's son, Arthur. Studies commissioned by the Carnegie Foundation; the Flexner report[22] in 1910; and the Gies report[25] in 1926 further identified the need for establishing dental and medical educational systems on a firm scientific foundation. The primary needs reported by these studies were relating clinical practice to the basic sciences, prescribing admissions and curriculum criteria, and promoting university-based programs.

Thus the early days of itinerant, and frequently uneducated, dentists ended. Dentists began to be educated in the basic sciences as well as clinical dentistry, resulting in practitioners who possessed and demonstrated intellectual and scientific curiosity. The heritage of operative dentistry is filled with such practitioners. In addition to the Blacks, others such as Charles E. Woodbury, E.K. Wedelstaedt, Waldon I. Ferrier, and George Hollenback made significant contributions to the early development of operative dentistry.

Although segments of what constituted early operative dentistry have now branched into dental specialties, operative dentistry continues to be a major part of most dental practices,[4,5,27,48] and the demand for it will not decrease in the foreseeable future.[48] However, the number of restorative services provided by U.S. dentists did decline from 233 million in 1979 to 202 million in 1990.[42] Also, the percentage of weekly time spent on operative procedures decreased from 38% in 1981 to 31% in 1993.[4,5] These changes have occurred because of greater emphasis by dentists to increase the number of preventive and diagnostic services,[4,5] and this increased focus on prevention and diagnosis is represented in this textbook.

The contributions of many practitioners, educators, and researchers throughout the world have resulted in operative dentistry being recognized today as a scientifically based discipline that plays an important role in enhancing dental health. No longer is operative dentistry considered only the treatment of "cavities" with "fillings." Modern operative dentistry includes the diagnosis and treatment of many problems—not just caries. Because the scope of operative dentistry has extended far beyond the treatment of caries, the term "cavity" is no longer used in this textbook to describe the preparation of a tooth to receive a restorative material. Instead, mechanical alterations to a tooth as part of a restorative procedure will be referred to as the "tooth preparation."

FACTORS AFFECTING OPERATIVE TREATMENT

INDICATIONS

The indications for operative procedures are numerous. However, they can be categorized into three primary treatment needs: (1) caries; (2) malformed, discolored, nonesthetic, or fractured teeth; and (3) restoration replacement or repair. The specific procedures associated with these treatment indicators are covered in subsequent chapters.

CONSIDERATIONS

Before any operative treatment, a number of considerations are involved, including: (1) an understanding of and appreciation for infection control to safeguard both health service personnel and patients (see Chapter 8); (2) a thorough examination of not only the affected tooth but also the oral and systemic health of the patient; (3) a diagnosis of the dental problem that recognizes the interaction of the affected area with other body tissues; (4) a treatment plan that has the potential to return the affected area to a state of health and function, thereby enhancing the overall health and well-being of the patient; (5) an understanding of the material to be used to restore the affected area to a state of health and function, including a realization of both the material's limitations and techniques involved in using it; (6) an understanding of the oral environment into which the restoration will be placed; (7) the biologic knowledge necessary to make the previously mentioned determinations; (8) an understanding of the biologic basis and function of the various tooth components and supporting tissues; (9) an appreciation for and knowledge of correct dental anatomy; and (10) the effect of the operative procedure on other dental treatments. Subsequent chapters amplify these factors in relation to specific operative procedures.

In summary, the placement of a restoration in a tooth requires the dentist to practice applied human biology and microbiology, use principles of mechanical engineering, possess highly developed technical skills, and demonstrate artistic abilities.

CONSERVATIVE APPROACH

Although tooth preparations for operative procedures originally adhered to the concept of "extension for prevention," increased knowledge of prevention methods, advanced clinical techniques, and improved restorative materials have now provided a more conservative approach to the restoration of teeth. This newer approach is a result of the reduction in caries incidence because of increased knowledge about caries, increased preventive emphasis, use of multiple fluoride applications, and proper sealant application.

Ongoing research efforts in operative dentistry have provided other benefits. For example, high-copper amalgam restorations demonstrate significant improvements in early strength, corrosion resistance, marginal integrity, and longevity than traditional amalgams. In addition, the bonding of materials to tooth structure has made possible dramatic improvements in composite, ceramic, and glass ionomer restorations and the development of expanded restorative applications of these materials.

More conservative approaches are now available for: (1) many typical restorative procedures (Classes I, II, III, IV, and V); (2) diastema closure procedure; (3) esthetic and/or functional correction of malformed, discolored, or fractured teeth; and (4) actual replacement of teeth. When compared with past treatment modalities, these newer approaches result in significantly less removal of tooth structure.

Although these are only examples, they demonstrate the current emphasis on conservation of tooth structure. *The primary results of conservative treatment are retention of more intact tooth structure and less trauma to the pulp tissue and contiguous soft tissue.* Not only will the remaining tooth structure be stronger, but the restoration should be more easily retained, offer greater esthetic potential, and cause less alteration in intra-arch and inter-arch relationships.

Efforts for the conservative restoration of teeth are ongoing. Research activity is continuing toward the development of materials and techniques to completely bond restorative materials to tooth structure, the objectives being to: (1) significantly reduce the necessity for extensive tooth preparations; (2) strengthen the remaining tooth structure; and (3) provide benefits such as less microleakage, less recurrent caries, and increased retention of the material within the tooth. These efforts will ultimately benefit the oral health of the public.

DYNAMICS OF OPERATIVE DENTISTRY

In the future, advances in treatment techniques, philosophies, and materials almost certainly will be made, just as in the past several decades, technological and scientific advances have dramatically affected the need for, demand for, and delivery of restorative services. These past (and future) developments illustrate the dynamics of operative dentistry, a constantly changing and advancing discipline.

The development of the *high-speed handpiece* played a dramatic role in the more conservative and efficient removal of tooth structure for restorative procedures. The use of high-speed instrumentation, along with the acknowledged benefits of water coolants, also led to the concept of *four-handed dentistry.* Major changes in operatory equipment design followed, resulting in a more comfortable, efficient, and productive setting for the delivery of dental care.

The mechanical bonding of restorations to tooth structure by etching enamel and dentin and the use of bonding systems has led to the development of many new composite restorative materials, as well as *conservative restorative bonding techniques.* Studies on filler composition and polymerization methodology for *composite materials* have resulted in both increased esthetic qualities and resistance to wear. Similarly, the benefits of *sealants* are becoming more widely accepted for the prevention of pit-and-fissure caries.

Increased knowledge about the carious process and the beneficial effects of multiple fluoride application has resulted in a decrease in caries incidence. Likewise, the increasing professional *emphasis on caries prevention* is as important as the recent technologic and scientific advancements. The recognition that *most dental disease is preventable* has resulted in better patient self-care and more conservative efforts by dentists in treatment.

Increased research on biomaterials has led to the introduction of *vastly improved dental materials.* Developments in impression materials and gold foil and advancements in knowledge about liners and sealers are also factors that have resulted in better care and treatment for patients. Advances in metallurgy have resulted in a variety of improved alloys that are either already available or are being developed. Corrosion-resistant amalgam alloys have been developed that will enhance the oral health of the population by providing longer-lasting restorations.

All of the factors just mentioned have played an important role in the development of operative dentistry. They have resulted in a reduction of the incidence of caries and a more conservative and effective approach toward treatment, with the ultimate result of improved oral health for all populations.

FACTORS AFFECTING THE FUTURE DEMAND FOR OPERATIVE DENTISTRY

Because of the dynamic status of operative dentistry, many future developments and advancements will undoubtedly occur. These advances in technology, science, and materials will have a significant effect on the future practice of and demand for operative dentistry. However, there are other factors that will also affect the future of operative dentistry.

To project the future demand for operative dentistry treatment, both current and projected dental health in the United States must be identified. This necessitates a projection of demographic changes, economic factors, and dental health and the effect of these on the future demand for dental services.

DEMOGRAPHICS

Between 1990 and 2050, the U.S. population is projected to increase by 146 million people (to a total of 394 million),[41] and the composition of the American population at that time will also be different; almost one half (47%) of the population will consist of minorities,[41] and the numbers of older adults will be significantly higher. These population changes will affect the entire professional lives of most of today's dental school graduates. In October 1999, the world's population reached 6 billion, which represented a 1 billion increase during the previous 12 years. During the twentieth century, the world population tripled, and by 2100, the world population is expected to reach 12 billion. While the world

birth rate in 1999 was 370,000 births each day,[52] more than 50,000 Americans also reached the age of 50 during that year.[57]

The percentage of *older adults in the population will increase* substantially in the future. This increase will occur primarily as a result of the aging of the *baby-boomer generation* (the first of whom turned 50 years old on January 1, 1996) and the increased life expectancy for U.S. residents.[23] By 2010, those 65 years old and older will represent 20% of the population;[51] that age group only amounted to 4% of the population in 1900 and 7% in 1940.[54] Those 65 years old and older (senior adults) make up the fastest growing segment of society, growing twice as fast as the general population. For example, it is projected that the group of people 85 years old and older will increase by 400% between 2000 and 2050.[6]

Because of increased life expectancy, the baby-boomer generation will grow older than the previous older adult segment of the population. Many of the baby boomers were not exposed to fluoridated water during their formative years and consequently have had extensive restorative dental care. However, this large segment of the population, as well as other age cohorts (except current older adults), has developed an appreciation for dental health and practices reasonable dental self-care. Since most of these individuals will retain more of their teeth as they age, *they will create a continuing demand for dental services* because they will not only want to keep their teeth but also will experience a standard of living that will permit a degree of discretionary income for health care expenditures.

Because of the aging of the U.S. population, emphasis will shift from the needs of the young to the concerns and demands of middle-aged people and older adults. Although the absolute numbers of children will not decrease substantially in the future, their percentage in the population and relative importance in health care policies will decrease. On the other hand, older adults will increase in both absolute number and importance.[20] Already older adults (those 65 years old and older) are receiving a much higher percentage of health care benefits than is their percentage of society. Such benefits will increase as the political and economic clout of older adults increases.

ECONOMIC FACTORS

No one can accurately project the economic future. While the U.S. economy will be part of a more global economy, the economic projections for the United States appear bright. The national deficit may not be eliminated, but it will become a lesser and lesser percentage of the Gross Domestic Product (GDP). Annual improvement of the GDP and productivity growth are projected to be at least equal to earlier periods in U.S. history that are considered "good" economic times. If inflation and unemployment continue at reasonable levels (in 1998, unemployment was only 4.3% and inflation was approximately 2%),[16] there will be more discretionary income available, and discretionary income is generally what is utilized for dental health expenditures.

Thus it appears that the economic forecast for the United States is good. With more discretionary income and more health care benefits for the adult segment of society, *the demand for future dental services should increase.*

GENERAL AND DENTAL HEALTH OF THE U.S. POPULATION

In considering the current and projected dental health of the U.S. population, a brief assessment of the general health of the population is necessary.

General Health. The general health of the U.S. population is good. The ability to prevent or cure infectious disease has led to an increase in life expectancy, and the ability to control (partially or fully) some chronic diseases is resulting in a larger proportion of older adults in the population. Life expectancy rates in 1991 were 80 years for men and 84 years for women,[9] compared to 1776 when the Declaration of Independence was signed and life expectancy was only 35 years.[53]

In 1994, Americans spent $949 billion on health care.[45] More recent projections indicate that the projected total U.S. health care expenditures of $1.1 trillion (13.5% of the GDP) in 1997 will increase to $2.2 trillion (16.2% of the GDP) by 2008.[44] However, access to and financial resources for health care are problems for some segments of society. More than 30 million Americans do not have health insurance,[34] and older adults (those over the age of 65) are responsible for four fifths of nursing home costs and one third of all health expenditures and physician fees.[58]

Dental Health. Americans generally have good dental health. Most understand the benefits of good dental health and practice good oral homecare. Except for some of current older adults, most Americans do not believe that the eventual loss of teeth is inevitable. Consequently, they are willing to invest their resources for dental health care. In 1994, $42.2 billion were spent on dental care in the United States;[45] this represented 4.4% of all health care costs for that year. Private patients paid about half of dental costs from their out-of-pocket funds. The government paid only $1.8 billion of dental costs, representing only 4.3% of dental spending for 1994. Thus the public share of dental costs was very low, while taxpayers paid 44% of the total health care costs for that year.[45] However, it is projected that dental spending will more than double between 1994 and 2008, reaching $93.1 billion by 2008. The rate of dental spending growth will be approximately double that of projected economic growth during the same period.[44]

Over 100 million Americans have dental insurance, which in 1996 covered approximately 49% of all dental care costs.[16] Dental insurance grew steadily from 1975 to 1990, then leveled off. However, because of it, dental care has become less expensive for the typical consumer of dental services.

Total real dental expenditures increased from $25.8 billion in 1970 to $47.6 billion in 1996.[3] In the early 1970s, dental spending grew at about the same rate as other personal health care spending and faster than the overall economy. In 1978, the growth rate in the dental sector flattened, and since then dental spending has increased more slowly than either personal health spending or the overall economy.[16]

In considering the future demand for operative dentistry, an assessment of the current and projected status of caries, missing teeth, and periodontal health is briefly presented here, followed by a projection of the increased numbers of teeth that will be at risk to dental disease in the future.

Caries. The incidence of caries has decreased. This reduction in caries is a result of increased usage of sealants and improved homecare efforts, but primarily it is a result of increased exposure to fluoride. Fluoridation of community water systems began in Grand Rapids, Michigan, in 1945. However, only 62% of the U.S. population on public water supplies currently receives fluoridated water;[56] this represents approximately 145 million people. Fluoridation also protects 360 million people in approximately 60 countries worldwide.[10] The expanded use of dietary fluoride supplements, school-based fluoride mouth-rinse programs, professional topical fluoride applications, and fluoride toothpastes also has contributed to this reduction.[2] For example, over one fourth of the school districts in the United States offer schoolchildren the opportunity to participate in a fluoride mouth-rinse program.[50]

Children ages 5 to 17 are experiencing less caries. In comparing the results of four U.S. surveys[12] (Table 1-1), it can be noted that the number of caries-free children is increasing and the average number of decayed, missing, and filled tooth surfaces (DMFS [for permanent teeth] or dmfs [for primary teeth]) is decreasing. In the 1971 to 1974 survey, only 26% of the children were caries-free, but by 1988 to 1991, 54.7% were caries-free. Likewise, in 1971 to 1974, children averaged 7.1 DMFS; this decreased to 2.5 in 1988 to 1991, a 65% reduction.

| TABLE 1-1 | Comparison of U.S. National Surveys |

	% OF CARIES-FREE CHILDREN (AGES 5 TO 17)	DMFS
1971-1974	26	7.1
1979-1980	36.6	4.8
1986-1987	49.9	3.1
1988-1991	54.7	2.5

From Brown LJ et al: Dental caries and sealant usage in U.S. children: 1988-1991, *J Amer Dent Assoc* 127:335-343, 1996.

However, over 45% of the total group ages 5 to 17 did have caries in the latest survey, and the percentage of caries-free children increased with age within the group. Fewer adolescents (12 to 17 years) than children (5 to 11 years) were caries-free (33% to 74%). Thus by age 17, almost three out of every four adolescents have experienced caries.

Also, of the 2.5 DMFS for the years 1988 to 1991, almost 80% were filled surfaces, with the remaining 20% primarily being decayed surfaces. The affected DMFS surfaces were: (1) occlusal, 1.4; (2) facial or lingual, 0.8; and (3) mesial and distal, 0.3.[31] This indicates that occlusal surfaces were five times more likely to be involved than proximal surfaces.[12] This also indicates that sealant usage could be a significant method to further reduce caries in children. Although the percentage of children with sealants almost doubled between the 1986 to 1987 and 1988 to 1991 surveys, only one of five children had sealants at the latter period.[12]

The decayed, missing, or filled permanent teeth (DMFT) averaged 1.6 for the 1988 to 1991 survey. Of these teeth, 21% were decayed, 78% filled, and 1% missing.[31] When comparing the ds/dfs and DS/DMFS per person, the primary tooth ratio was twice that of the permanent tooth ratio, suggesting less treatment of primary teeth.[12] All of these figures and comparisons indicate a continuing decline in caries in the permanent dentition of children.

Still, caries continues to affect millions of U.S. adolescents and adults. Almost 94% of dentate adults showed evidence of coronal caries and almost 23% showed root caries in the 1988 to 1991 survey.[43] The total DMFS for all adults was about 50, while for dentate adults it was about 40; for the latter group almost 22 of the surfaces were decayed or filled, with most of those (19) being filled surfaces.[43] Also for dentate adults, the average number of root-surface carious lesions was 1, and half of those lesions were not filled.[43] The prevalence of caries in adults increased markedly with age[28] (Table 1-2, as it relates to root caries only), and when all caries is considered, the aggregate caries increment may be higher in people over 55 years old than in children.[26,46]

Missing Teeth. During the past several decades, there has been a steady reduction in both edentulism and numbers of teeth lost per person. While these trends indicate that edentulism may be disappearing, *partial edentulism will continue*. While in 1988 to 1991, more than 9 out of 10 adults (18 years and older) were dentate, only about 30% had all of their teeth.[36] Those adults who had teeth averaged 23.5 teeth.[36] Both edentulism and the number of teeth present are strongly influenced by age. For example, the 1988 to 1991 National Health and Nutrition Examination Survey (NHANES) III revealed that 100% of the group ages 18 to 24 were dentate, while 44% of the group 75 years and older were edentulous. Likewise, the 18- to 24-year-old dentate group averaged 27.1 teeth, while the 75-years-and-older group had only 9 teeth. However, the older age groups still showed the greatest decreases in edentulism and increases in retained teeth. In a 1971 to 1974 survey, 45.6% of people ages 65 to 74 were edentulous. In the NHANES III 1988 to 1991 survey only 28.6% of this age group was edentulous, and half of those were edentulous 20 years before the survey, indicating that only about 12% of that age group had actually become edentulous in the last 20 years.[21]

Edentulism will continue to decrease, and more teeth will be retained. This will result in more teeth being at risk to dental disease, which may result in both increased need and demand for dental care.

Periodontal Status. The NHANES III survey[43] indicated, that while over 90% of those 13 years old or older had experienced some minor loss of periodontal attachment, only 25% had attachment loss of 3 to 4 mm, and only 15% had 5 mm or greater attachment loss.[11] Attachment loss (both number of affected people and severity) increased with age. Gingival recession also increased with age. While 86% of the older adults experienced some recession, only 40% of the overall population had recession.[11] More severe recession (3 mm or greater) affected half of older adults[43] (Table 1-3). Because of the increasing percentage of recession with age, there is a corresponding increased percentage of root caries.

Oral Cancer. Oral and pharyngeal cancer is the sixth most common neoplastic disease.[59] An estimated 30,750 new cases of oropharyngeal cancer are expected to be diagnosed in the United States in 1999, which will be 3% of all cancers diagnosed.[33] The mortality rate associated with oral cancer has not improved in the last 40 years. Ultimately, 50% of people who have oral cancer die as a result of the malignancy, and 8440 deaths were predicted in the United States in 1999.[33]

Teeth at Risk to Dental Disease. In 1989, Reinhardt and others[48] used some survey results in combination with other studies and Bureau of Census population projections to determine and predict how many teeth would be at risk to dental disease. Their findings reported that in 1980 2.8 billion teeth were at risk to dental disease, with expectations of 4 billion in 1990, 4.4 billion by 2000, and 5 billion by 2030.[48] Thus between 1990

TABLE 1-2	Root Caries
AGE	**%**
18-24	0
35-44	21
45-54	26
55-64	38
65-74	47
75+	56

From Hicks J, Flaitz CM, Garcia-Godoy F: Root-surface caries formation: effect of in vitro APF treatment, *J Amer Dent Assoc* 129:449-453, 1998.

TABLE 1-3	Periodontal Status/Root Caries		
AGE	% 1 MM + RECESSION	% 3 MM + RECESSION	% ROOT CARIES
18-24	11½	1	
35-44	46	12	21
45-54		26	26
55-64	78	35	38
65+	87	46	47

From National Center for Health Statistics: *Plan and operation of the Third National Health and Nutrition Examination Survey: 1988-1994* (DHHS publication number [PHS] 94-1308, series 1, no. 322), Hyattsville, Md, 1994, National Center for Health Statistics.

and 2030 there will be a projected increase of 1 billion teeth at risk to dental disease. This increase will occur because of a decreased rate of tooth loss combined with the aging of the baby boomers. Between 1990 and 2030, there will also be a projected 73% increase in people ages 45 and older and a 104% increase in senior adults, thereby resulting in 90% more teeth in the 45-and-older age group and 153% more teeth in the senior adult group.[48]

The future demand for operative dentistry care will increase. As previously noted, the population will increase, with the greatest increase occurring in the older adult component of society. Because these increased numbers of adults will retain more teeth, there will be more teeth at risk to dental disease, and many of these teeth will require operative care. In further exploring these expectations, several other factors must be addressed.

DENTAL MANPOWER

In 1996, there were 166,425 professionally active dentists in the United States.[7] Ten years earlier, there were approximately 125,000 dentists.[15] Between 1994 and 2020 the number of professionally active dentists is expected to increase by almost 13%,[7] which will be less than the expected population increase. The number of dentists per 1000 people is expected to decrease slightly between 1999 and 2020.[14] In 1990 there were 0.58 dentists per 1000 people. However, to keep that ratio, there would need to be a 58% increase in the number of dentists by 2050; because of the increasing minority percentage of the population,[41] it is thought that the greatest increase should be in the number of minority dentists.[41] This increased number of minority dentists is not likely to occur, even though between 1986 and 1996 the proportion of female dental students increased from 27% to 37% and the proportion of white male dental students decreased from 84% to 70%.[14]

While the number of first-year dental school students decreased by 28% between 1976 (5936) and 1996 (4255),[14] it is expected to increase by 36% between 1996 and 2020 (5775).[14] Likewise, the number of dental school graduates decreased by 29% between 1976 (5336) and 1996 (3810) but is expected to increase by 42% from 1996 to 2020 (5414).[14] Since 1986, six U.S. dental schools have closed and one new one has opened.[14]

Of active private dental practitioners 82% are general dentists, and 92% own their dental practice.[7] The number of hours worked per week decreased from 42.3 in 1986 to 37.1 in 1995,[15] yet the hours per week spent treating patients increased during the same period—from 77% to 90%—and more of this increased treatment time was devoted to diagnostic and preventive services.[13]

Even though the enrollment in dental schools is projected to increase, the projected increase in dentists for the next several decades will not be large. Therefore there will be fewer dentists treating more people who will have retained more teeth. This represents an effective increase in the demand for dental care.

PROJECTED NEED FOR OPERATIVE DENTISTRY

The increased *number of hours needed for operative care in the future* will be for the following operative procedures: (1) restorations for teeth with new carious lesions; (2) restorations for teeth with root caries; (3) restorations to replace existing, faulty restorations; and (4) restorations to enhance the esthetic appearance of patients.

New Caries. New caries will continue to occur. Even though almost 55% of children (ages 5 to 17) are caries-free, the remaining 45% have caries. By age 17, three out of four adolescents have experienced caries. *Adults, especially older adults, have high caries rates.* As previously mentioned, when all caries is considered, the aggregate caries increment may be higher in people over 55 years old than in children.[26,46] Less than 6% of people ages 18 to 64 have no caries.[17]

Root Caries. Root caries will increase due to the increased number of older adults who will retain more teeth and experience more gingival recession. Additionally, many older adults may have systemic problems that may directly or indirectly alter normal salivary functioning, thus increasing the potential for root caries formation. While only one fourth of all dentate adults have evidence of root caries, the prevalence increases markedly with age[17] (see Table 1-2).

Replacement Restorations. Replacement restorations will also stimulate much future demand. There is a large need for replacement dentistry. It has been estimated that 75% of all operative treatment is due to replacement of existing restorations.[32] Furthermore, 70% of all restorations per year are replacements of existing restorations.[49] The knowledge that baby boomers are reaching their older adult years, where high numbers of decayed and filled tooth surfaces often occur, documents the continuing need for future restorative care. More than 50% of the income from restorative procedures is from the replacement of restorations in patients older than 40.[38]

Esthetic Restorations. The public has come to appreciate the possibilities of esthetic enhancements from dental treatment due to publicity about bonding, publicity in the form of magazine articles, television shows, and special news programs. In 1990, it was estimated that 10% of a dentist's gross income was derived from esthetic treatment on noncarious teeth.[47] More recently it has been reported that one of every five intracoronal restorations done in the United States are tooth-colored. This same report states, "It is likely that the more esthetically pleasing materials eventually will be the predominant intracoronal and extracoronal restorative concepts."[18] With more teeth being retained, more people are likely to seek appearance enhancements, especially when most such treatments are relatively simple, noninvasive, and nonstressful.

PUBLIC'S PERCEPTION OF DENTISTRY

The public's perception of dentistry is another factor that will influence whether the increased numbers of teeth and increased need for operative services will be converted to increased demand. Fortunately, the public considers dentists and dentistry very positively. The public ranks a dentist as one of the most respected members of the community, and dentistry has the highest satisfaction rating when the public assesses the services they receive. Lastly, the public not only thinks highly of the dental profession, they also appreciate the benefits of good dental health. All of this suggests a continuing demand for operative services.

PATIENT VISITS

Because of the projected significant increase in the number of senior adults, it is important to consider their past use of dental services as well as their potential economic status. In 1970, 25.8% of senior adults visited a dentist annually; this percentage increased to 38.6% by 1983.[24] While before 1983 this group averaged only 1.5 visits to the dentist per year,[1] they increased their dental visits by 29% between 1983 and 1986.[38] Several years later they were reported to make more visits to a dentist than any other age group.[55]

The economic status of adults will affect their future dental demand. With dental expenditures considered discretionary, the availability of discretionary income will influence the amount of dental care sought. One study showed that over one half of older adults with annual incomes below $10,000 had not seen a dentist for 5 years, while only 18% of those with incomes over $35,000 had not seen a dentist during the same time period.[38] Overall, older adults (over age 65) currently have 77% of the financial assets in the United States, 68% of all money market funds, and 80% of all money in savings and loans institutions. Additionally, 75% own their own home, with 84% of the mortgages already paid off.[53] *Therefore, new older adults and future older adults will not only possess positive perceptions about dentistry and dental health but also will have the economic means to secure the dental care they need.*

For all people in the United States, less than 10% reported having unmet dental care wants.[40] This report further indicated that these individuals were more likely to: (1) be in the poorest health, (2) have chronic conditions, (3) be a head of household with minimal education, (4) have less family income, or (5) have no dental insurance. However, almost half of this group indicated that they had not tried to obtain dental care, even though almost half also indicated that their dental problems limited their activities. The predominant barrier to receipt of wanted dental care was a financial consideration.

These factors affecting the demand for operative dentistry project an *increase in operative treatment in the future.* The increased number of older adults, the increased number of teeth, the increased affluence of the population, the positive image of dentistry, and the projected increased hours of operative need all support this increased demand.

FUTURE OF OPERATIVE DENTISTRY

Many significant advancements in health care occurred in the twentieth century; included in these advancements are genetic alterations, genetic engineering, public education, vaccines, fluoridation, x-rays, computed tomography (CT) scans, magnetic resonance imaging (MRI), antibiotics, ultrasound procedures, and sanitation. During this century, life span doubled and the quality of life was greatly improved. Many of these factors had an effect on improving dental care.

"Research is the primary catalyst to professional growth and has greatly added to the understanding of the etiology, diagnosis, and treatment of dental diseases."[2] Exciting research is occurring that will have an additional effect on the future of operative dentistry, and knowledge about new developments and technologies will also affect the practice. These developments might be in the areas of molecular and cellular biology, genetics, pharmacology, radiation biology, radiation physics and technology, tomography, digital radiography, quantitative light-induced fluorescence, electrical conductivity, ultrasonography, dental materials based on polymer chemistry and ion exchange, microbiology, immunology, and behavioral science. "In terms of future scientific achievement, it is not difficult to predict startling new advances due to the application of recombinant DNA technology, the application of space age technology, and the general advancement of scientific methodology. Advances in these areas can have direct impact on dental practice through the development of new treatments and preventive modes, new biomaterials applicable to dental practice, and more sophisticated techniques to measure the health status of individuals."[19]

Research in operative dentistry is now occurring in a number of fields. The use of lasers in dentistry may lead to a new mechanism for welding dental alloys or altering tooth structure in tooth preparation. Already, lasers are used in etching enamel and making enamel more resistant to demineralization. Extended uses of bonding techniques and further developments in composite and adhesive restorative materials will lead to even more conservative restorative techniques. The beneficial use of composites in posterior teeth has become evident. Much research and clinical testing also is being done on castable or pressed ceramic materials. The introduction of computer-generated restorations has stimulated much interest, and further refinement of such technology is occurring. *Improvements in composites, adhesive systems, castable ceramics, and computer-generated restorations could result in a significant decrease in the use of metal alloy systems in operative dentistry.* Also, increasing concern about the potential toxicity of some components of current alloy systems, such as mercury and nickel, may result in decreased use of these systems in the future. Significant *environmental concerns* are surfacing regarding the disposal of certain materials used in dentistry, especially mercury.

Efforts are also being made to develop an anticaries vaccine. However, even if developed, the widespread use of such an agent may not occur in the foreseeable future in the United States because of the already documented caries reduction from multiple fluoride use, limitations imposed by regulatory agencies, and concern about possible side effects.[2] Whereas the use of such an agent in developing countries may provide greater immediate benefits, its use in the United States may be confined to high-risk patients.

Methods for adhesively bonding composite materials to dentin have improved. These developments have had dramatic effects on the practice of operative dentistry, resulting in minimal tooth preparation. "The capacity to develop relatively predictable and enduring adhesion between restorative materials and tooth structure has had the greatest impact on restorative dentistry in recent decades."[30] *Effective dentin bonding* significantly increases tooth conservation[39] while potentially reducing patient anxiety. Techniques used for such bonding procedures may also increase productivity.

Finally, the *developing concepts in cariology* may have major implications in dealing with dental caries. The increased knowledge about factors involved in the carious process has placed a greater emphasis on treating the carious lesion by means other than restorative techniques. It seems possible to foresee a time when diagnosis and treatment techniques are so refined as to preclude the necessity of tooth preparation to control some carious activity. The remineralization of a tooth surface affected by a beginning carious lesion will not only decrease the need for restorative care but also result in a tooth surface that will be more resistant to subsequent carious attacks. The development of appropriate fluoride and antimicrobial applications and techniques to produce this remineralization is now a reality. All of these developments and changes will occur in a future environment of increased need for operative treatment because of more people, especially adults, who will retain more of their teeth. *The emphasis of the profession will shift to care for the senior adult segment of the population.* This population will require significant dental care due not only to replacement needs for existing restorations but also to development of new caries, especially root caries. Increased understanding of treatment methods for older adults will be required, as will improved knowledge pertaining to their overall medical health. Dental research efforts will continue seeking treatment methods that will be more efficient and less stressful for these patients, and bonded restorations, both amalgam and composite, will provide benefits in treating this segment of the population.

SUMMARY

Many factors have been presented in this chapter, some of which will be expanded in other chapters of this book. *The objective has been to identify the factors that influence operative dentistry both today and in the future.* Certainly changes in today's society, changes in the future oral health of the U.S. population, and developments within the discipline of operative dentistry will affect future practice.

Many exciting advances have already been made, and others are expected. Important progress is being made toward the time when caries and periodontal disease will no longer be major public health problems. "As part of their professional responsibilities, dentists have an obligation to monitor the dental welfare of the public and adjust their patterns of treatment accordingly. Professional ethics dictate that dentists must embrace new and accepted dental treatment, materials and devices, and, at the same time, discard outmoded treatment and techniques in pursuit of optimal oral health for the public."[2]

Dental education should strive to produce practitioners who can think critically using the scientific method so they can be in a position to evaluate future claims related to advancing the profession. Dentistry must also continue to broaden its knowledge of the biologic basis on which it is founded. Practitioners must continually familiarize themselves with the advances being made. Increased research activity and continued practitioner adaptability will result in improved oral health of populations throughout the world.

The future of operative dentistry is good! This chapter has presented some of the reasons. The remainder of this book will present much information as it pertains to the diagnosis, prevention, and treatment of clinical operative procedures. There is emphasis on both treatment of older adults and nonsurgical treatments for caries. The use of amalgam restorations, while still promoted, is presented in more limited clinical applications. The promotion of bonding procedures is enhanced throughout the book.

REFERENCES

1. American Dental Association, Bureau of Economic Research and Statistics: *Utilization of dental services by the elderly population,* Chicago, 1980.
2. American Dental Association: Interim report of the American Dental Association's special committee on the future of dentistry: issue papers on dental research, manpower, education, practice and public and professional concerns (special report), *J Am Dent Assoc,* Sept 1982.
3. American Dental Association, Survey Center: *Consumer price index for dental services, 1960-1996.* Chicago, 1997, American Dental Association.
4. American Dental Association, Survey Center: *1994 Survey of Dental Practice.* Chicago: American Dental Association, 1995.
5. American Dental Association, Survey Center: *1982 Survey of Dental Practice,* Chicago, 1983, American Dental Association.
6. Berkey DB et al: The old-old dental patient: the challenge of clinical decision-making, *J Amer Dent Assoc* 127:321-332, 1996.
7. Berry J: The demographics of dentistry, *J Amer Dent Assoc* 127:1327-1330, 1996.
8. Black CE, Black BM: *From pioneer to scientist,* St. Paul, Minn, 1940, Brace.
9. Bowen WH: Dental caries: is it an extinct disease?, *J Am Dent Assoc* 122:49-52, Sept 1991.
10. British Fluoridation Society: *Optimal water fluoridation: status worldwide,* Liverpool, 1998, British Fluoridation Society.
11. Brown LJ, Brunelle JA, Kingman A: Periodontal status in the United States: 1988-1991. Prevalence, extent, and demographic variation, *J Dent Res* 75(Spec Iss):672-683, 1996.
12. Brown LJ et al: Dental caries and sealant usage in U.S. children: 1988-1991, *J Amer Dent Assoc* 127:335-343, 1996.
13. Brown LJ, Lazar V: Demand-side trends, *J Amer Dent Assoc* 129:1685-1691, 1998
14. Brown LJ, Lazar V: Dentist work force and educational pipeline, *J Amer Dent Assoc* 129:1700-1707, 1998.
15. Brown LJ, Lazar V: Dentists and their practices, *J Amer Dent Assoc* 129:1692-1699, 1998.
16. Brown LJ, Lazar V: The economic state of dentistry: an overview, *J Amer Dent Assoc* 129:1683-1691, 1998.
17. Brown LJ, Winn DM, White BA: Dental caries, restoration and tooth conditions in U.S. adults, 1988-1991, *J Amer Dent Assoc* 127:1315-1325, 1996.
18. Christensen GT: Intracoronal and extracoronal tooth restorations 1999, *J Amer Dent Assoc* 130:557-560, 1999.
19. DePaola DP: Application of basic and medical sciences in the dental curriculum, *J Dent Educ* 45:685, 1981.
20. Douglass CW, Furino A: Balancing dental service requirements and supplies: epidemiologic and demographic evidence, *J Am Dent Assoc* 121:587-592, Nov 1990.
21. Eklund SA, Burt BA: Risk factors for total tooth loss in the United States: longitudinal analysis of national data, *J Public Health Dent* 54:5-14, 1994.
22. Flexner A: *Medical education in the United States and Canada, a report to the Carnegie Foundation for the Advancement of Teaching,* New York, 1910, Carnegie Foundation.
23. Friend T, DeBarros A: Science finds no limit on life span (Special report), *USA Today* 5D-7D March 17, 1999.
24. Giangrego E: Dentistry and the older adult, *J Am Dent Assoc* 114:299-307, March 1987.
25. Gies WJ: *Dental education in the United States and Canada, a report to the Carnegie Foundation for the Advancement of Teaching,* New York, 1926, Carnegie Foundation.
26. Glass RL, Alman JE, Chauncey HH: A 10-year longitudinal study of caries incidence rates in a sample of male adults in the USA, *Caries Res* 21:360-367, 1987.
27. Heymann HO, Roberson TM: Operative dentistry in North Carolina: a survey, *NC Dent Gazette* 3(6):10, 1981.
28. Hicks J, Flaitz CM, Garcia-Godoy F: Root-surface caries formation: effect of in vitro APF treatment, *J Amer Dent Assoc* 129:449-453, 1998.
29. Horner HH: *Dental education today,* Chicago, 1947, University of Chicago Press.
30. Hume WR: Restorative Dentistry: current status and future directions, *J Dent Ed* 62(10):781-790, 1998.
31. Kaste LM et al: Coronal caries in the primary and permanent dentition of children and adolescents 1-17 years of age: United States, 1988-1991, *J Dent Res* 75(Spec Iss):631-641, 1996.
32. Kidd EA, Toffenetti F, Major IA: Secondary caries, *Int Dent J* 42:127-138, 1992.
33. Landis SH et al: Cancer statistics, *CA Cancer J Clin* 49:8-31, 1999.
34. Levit KR, Freeland MS: National medical care spending, *Health Aff* 7:124-136, 1988.
35. Loe H: The impact of research and technological advances on dental education, *J Dent Educ* 45:670, 1981.
36. Marcus SE et al: Tooth retention and tooth loss in the permanent dentition of adults: United States, 1988-1991, *J Dent Res* 75(Spec Iss):684-695, 1996.
37. McCluggage RW: *A history of the American Dental Association,* Chicago, 1959, American Dental Association.
38. Meskin LH et al: Economic impact of dental service utilization by older adults, *J Am Dent Assoc* 120:665-668, June 1990.
39. Mount GJ, Hume WR: *Preservation and restoration of tooth structure,* London, 1998, Mosby.
40. Mueller CD, Schur CL, Paramore LC: Access to dental care in the United States, *J Amer Dent Assoc* 129:429-437, 1998.
41. Murdock SH, Hoque MN: Current patterns and future trends in the population of the United States: implications for dentistry and the dental profession in the twenty-first century, *J Am Coll Dentists* 29-35, Winter 1998.
42. Nash KD, Bentley JE: Is restorative dentistry on its way out? *J Amer Dent Assoc* 122(9):79-80, 1991.
43. National Center for Health Statistics: *Plan and operation of the Third National Health and Nutrition Examination Survey: 1988-1994* (DHHS publication number [PHS] 94-1308, series 1, no. 322), Hyattsville, Md, 1994, National Center for Health Statistics.
44. Palmer C: Dental spending to hit $57 billion, *ADA News* 30(14):1-11, 1999.
45. Palmer C: Dental spending tops $42 billion, *ADA News* 27(12):16, 1996.
46. Papas A, Joshi A, Giunta J: Prevalence and intraoral distribution of coronal and root caries in middle-aged and older adults, *Caries Res* 26:459-465, 1992.

47. Reinhardt JW, Capilouto ML: Composite resin esthetic dentistry survey in New England, *J Am Dent Assoc* 120:541-544, May 1990.

48. Reinhardt JW, Douglass CW: The need for operative dentistry services: projecting the effects of changing disease patterns, *Oper Dent* 14:114-120, 1989.

49. Resine S, Litt M: Social and psychological theories and their use for dental practice, *Int Dent J* 43:279-287, 1993.

50. Silversin JB, Coombs JA, Drolette ME: Achievements of the seventies: self-applied fluorides, *J Public Health Dent* 40:256, 1980.

51. Slavkin HC: And we all lived happily ever after: understanding the biological controls of aging, *J Amer Dent Assoc* 129:629-633, 1998.

52. The Sun News: *Information from the United Nations Population Division*, Myrtle Beach, Oct 10, 1999.

53. Truono EJ: The aging population and its impact on the future of dentistry—a symposium, *J Am Coll Dent* 58(2):14-16, Summer 1991.

54. U.S. Bureau of the Census: Decennial census and current population, *Report Series II* 25, 1987.

55. U.S. Department of Health and Human Services: *Use of dental services and dental health, United States, 1986* (DHHS publication no. 88-1593), Washington, DC, 1988, U.S. Government Printing Office.

56. U.S. Department of Health and Human Services, Centers for Disease Control and Prevention, Division of Oral Health: *Fluoridation fact sheet* (No. FL-141), Atlanta, December 1993, Centers for Disease Control and Prevention.

57. Vatter RH: Boomers enter the golden fifties, *Stat Bull Metrop Insur Co* 79(1):2-9, 1998.

58. Waldo DR, Levit KR, Lazenby H: National health expenditures: 1985, *Health Care Financing Rev* 8:1-43, 1986.

59. Winn DM et al: Scientific progress in understanding oral and pharyngeal cancers, *J Amer Dent Assoc* 129:713-718, 1998.

2

Clinical Significance of Dental Anatomy, Histology, Physiology, and Occlusion

JOHN R. STURDEVANT

THOMAS F. LUNDEEN*

TROY B. SLUDER, JR.*

*These authors are inactive this edition. See the Acknowledgments.

Dental anatomy, histology, physiology, and occlusion are interrelated disciplines that are prerequisites for success in restorative procedures. In addition to knowledge of the instruments and materials used to prepare and restore teeth, the relationships of internal and external tooth anatomy to function and restorative procedures must be understood. A knowledge of the various structures of the teeth (enamel, dentin, cementum, and pulp) and their relationships to each other, as well as of the supporting structures, is necessary for excellence in the performance of operative dental procedures. (See Fig. 2-3 for an illustration of these structures.)

A basic understanding of proper anatomic form is essential in the restoration of either a single tooth or a group of teeth, because function depends on form. *The individual form of a tooth and the contour relationships with adjacent and opposing teeth are major determinants of function in mastication, esthetics, speech, and protection.* The protective function of tooth form applies to both the contiguous investing tissues (osseous and mucosal) and the pulp. Proper tooth form usually is a factor contributing to a healthy state of the investing tissues, with a critical balance of protection (e.g., of interproximal tissues) and stimulative massage from the passage of food during mastication (see Figs. 2-37, 2-38, and 2-39). Certainly the soft pulp is protected by the hard, overlying tooth structures of dentin, enamel, and cementum. Also, knowing the usual form of the *pulp cavity* (the pulp chamber and the pulp canal[s]), is an essential factor for determining the materials and procedures best suited to restoring the protective function of the tooth's hard tissues lost due to disease or trauma. This knowledge is helpful in maintaining the health of the pulp.

The tooth is an organ of mastication and must be treated as such in restoring it to proper form and function and preventing further insult to it and its investing tissues. A high degree of manipulative skill is required in the fabrication of a restoration to replace lost tooth structure and prevent further damage to the tooth and supporting structures. *The supporting tissue mechanism of the teeth is an important consideration in operative procedures* because the attachment apparatus must be treated with care and respect to prevent periodontal disease.

TEETH AND INVESTING TISSUES

DENTITIONS

Normally, in the human dentition, two sets of teeth erupt during the cycle from childhood to adult. The first set is the *primary dentition,* which usually consists of 10 maxillary and 10 mandibular teeth. The second set usually is referred to as the *permanent dentition* and normally consists of 16 maxillary and 16 mandibular teeth.

CLASSES OF HUMAN TEETH: FORM AND FUNCTION

Human teeth are divided into classes on the basis of form and function. Both the primary and permanent dentitions include incisor, canine, and molar classes. The fourth class, the premolar, is found only in the permanent dentition (Fig. 2-1). Tooth form predicts the function of teeth; therefore class traits are the characteristics that place teeth into functional categories. Since the diet of humans consists of both animal and vegetable foods, the human dentition is called *omnivorous.*

Incisors. The incisors are located near the entrance of the oral cavity and function as cutting or shearing instruments for food (see Fig. 2-1). From a proximal view, the crowns of these teeth have a triangular shape with a narrow incisal surface, including the incisal edge, and a broad cervical base (see Fig. 2-47, *D.*) The incisors contribute significantly in cutting actions and other functions; esthetics; and phonetics.

Canines. The canines possess the longest roots of all teeth and are located at the corners of the dental arch. They function in the seizing, piercing, and tearing of food, as well as in cutting. From a proximal view the crown also has a triangular shape with a thick incisal ridge. The stocky anatomic form of the crown and length of the root are reasons why these teeth are strong, stable abutment teeth for a fixed or removable prosthe-

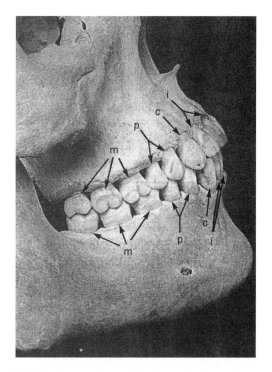

FIG. **2-1** Maxillary and mandibular teeth in maximum intercuspal position. The classes of teeth are incisors *(i),* canines *(c),* premolars *(p),* and molars *(m).* Note that cusps of mandibular teeth are one-half cusp anterior of corresponding cusps of teeth in maxillary arch.

sis. The canines serve as important guides in occlusion because of their anchorage and position in the dental arches (see Figs. 2-1 and 2-60).

Premolars. The premolars serve a dual role in function; they act like the canines in the tearing of food and are similar to molars in the grinding of food. Whereas

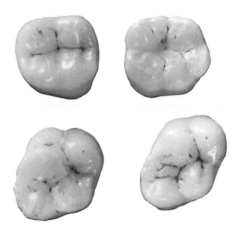

FIG. **2-2** Occlusal surfaces of maxillary and mandibular first and second molars after several years of use, showing rounded curved surfaces and minimal wear.

the first premolars are angular, with their facial cusps resembling the canines, the lingual cusps of the maxillary premolars and molars have a more rounded anatomic form (see Figs. 2-1 and 2-40). The occlusal surfaces present a series of curves in the form of concavities and convexities that should be maintained throughout life for correct occlusal contacts and function.

Molars. The molars are large, multicusped, strongly anchored teeth located nearest the temporomandibular joint (TMJ), which serves as the fulcrum during function (see Fig. 2-54). These teeth have a major role in the crushing, grinding, and chewing of food to the smallest dimensions suitable for deglutition. The occlusal surfaces of both premolars and molars act as a myriad of shears that function in the final mastication of food. The premolars and molars are also important in maintaining the vertical dimension of the face (see Figs. 2-1 and 2-2).

STRUCTURES OF THE TEETH

The teeth are composed of enamel, pulp-dentin complex, and cementum (Fig. 2-3). Each of these structures is discussed individually.

Enamel. Enamel is formed by cells called *ameloblasts*, which originate from the embryonic germ layer known

FIG. **2-3** Schematic drawing illustrating cross-section of maxillary molar and its supporting structures. *1,* enamel; *1a,* gnarled enamel; *2,* dentin; *3a,* pulp chamber; *3b,* pulp horn; *3c,* pulp canal; *4,* apical foramen; *5,* cementum; *6,* periodontal fibers in periodontal ligament; *7,* alveolar bone; *8,* maxillary sinus; *9,* mucosa; *10,* submucosa; *11,* blood vessels; *12,* gingiva; *13,* lines of Retzius. *(From Brauer JC, Richardson RE: The dental assistant, ed 3, New York, 1964, McGraw-Hill.)*

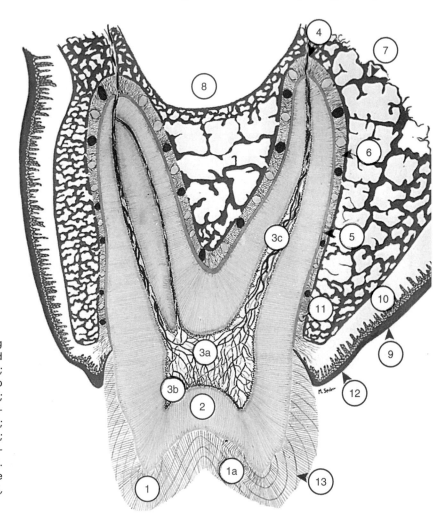

as *ectoderm*. Ameloblasts have short extensions toward the dentinoenamel junction (DEJ); these are termed *Tomes processes*. Enamel covers the anatomic crown of the tooth and varies in thickness in different areas (see Fig. 2-14). The enamel is thicker at the incisal and occlusal areas of a tooth and becomes progressively thinner until it terminates at the cementoenamel junction. The thickness also varies from one class of tooth to another, averaging 2 mm at the incisal ridges of incisors and varying from 2.3 to 2.5 mm at the cusps of premolars and 2.5 to 3 mm at the cusps of molars. Enamel usually decreases in thickness toward the junction of the developmental cuspal lobes of the posterior teeth (premolars and molars), sometimes nearing zero where the junction is fissured (noncoalesced) (see Figs. 2-12 and 2-14.)

Because enamel is mostly gray and semitranslucent, the color of a tooth depends upon the color of the underlying dentin, thickness of the enamel, and amount of stain in the enamel. The amount of *translucency* of enamel is related to variations in the degree of calcification and homogeneity. Abnormal conditions of enamel usually result in aberrant color. Enamel becomes temporarily whiter within minutes when a tooth is isolated from the moist oral environment by a rubber dam or absorbents. Thus the shade must be determined before isolation and preparation of a tooth for a tooth-colored restoration. This change in color is explained by the temporary loss of loosely bound (or exchangeable) water (less than 1% by weight).

Chemically, enamel is a highly mineralized crystalline structure containing from 95% to 98% inorganic matter by weight. *Hydroxyapatite*, in the form of a crystalline lattice, is the largest mineral constituent and is present 90% to 92% by volume. Other minerals and trace elements are contained in smaller amounts. The remaining constituents of tooth enamel are an organic content of about 1% to 2% and a water content of about 4% by weight; these total approximately 6% by volume.

Structurally, enamel is composed of millions of enamel *rods* or *prisms*, which are the largest structural components, as well as rod sheaths and a cementing inter-rod substance in some areas. Inter-rod substance, or *sheath*, may be the increased spacing between crystallites oriented differently to where the "tail" portion of one rod meets the "head" portion of another. This spacing apparently is partially organic material. The rods vary in number from approximately 5 million for a mandibular incisor to about 12 million for a maxillary molar. The rods are densely packed and intertwined in a wavy course, and each extends from the DEJ to the external surface of the tooth. In general the rods are aligned perpendicularly to both the DEJ and the tooth surface in the primary and permanent dentitions, except in the cervical region of permanent teeth where they are oriented outward in a slightly apical direction. In the primary dentition the enamel rods in the cervical and central parts of the crown are nearly perpendicular to the long axis of the tooth and are similar in their direction to the permanent teeth in the occlusal two thirds of the crown. Enamel rod diameter near the dentinal borders is about 4 μm (about 8 μm near the surface); this difference accommodates the larger outer surface of the enamel crown compared to the dentinal surface at the DEJ.

The hardest substance of the human body is enamel. Hardness may vary over the external tooth surface according to the location; also, it decreases inward, with hardness lowest at the DEJ. The density of enamel also decreases from the surface to the DEJ. Enamel is a very brittle structure with a high elastic modulus and low tensile strength, which indicates a rigid structure. However, dentin is a highly compressive tissue that acts as a cushion for the enamel. Enamel requires a base of dentin to withstand masticatory forces. Enamel rods that fail to possess a dentin base because of caries or improper preparation design are easily fractured away from neighboring rods. For maximal strength in tooth preparation, all enamel rods should be supported by dentin (Fig. 2-4).

Human enamel is composed of rods that in transverse section are shaped with a rounded head or body section

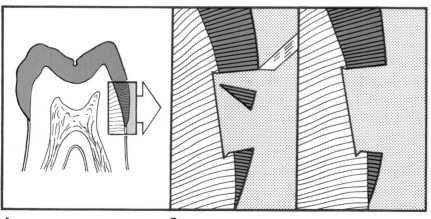

FIG. **2-4 A,** Enamel rods unsupported by dentin base are fractured away readily by pressure from hand instrument. **B,** Cervical preparation showing enamel rods supported by dentin base.

A   **B**

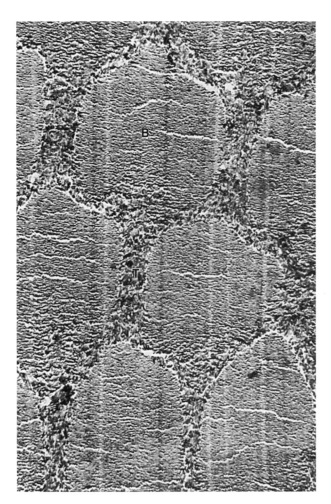

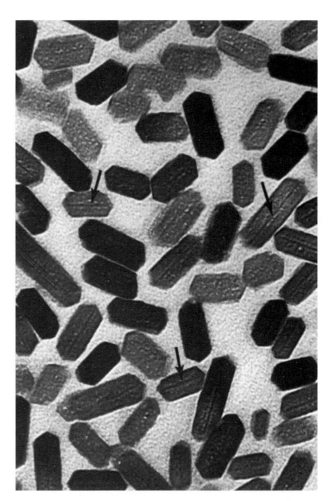

FIG. **2-5** Electron micrograph (approximately ×5000) of cross-section of rods in mature human enamel. Crystal orientation is different in "bodies" *(B)* than in "tails" *(T)*. *(From AH Meckel, WJ Griebstein, RJ Neal: Structure of mature human dental enamels observed by electron microscopy,* Arch Oral Biol, *vol 10, 1965, Pergamon.)*

FIG. **2-6** Electron micrograph (approximately ×350,000) of mature, hexagon-shaped enamel crystallites *(arrows). (From Nylen MU, Eanes ED, Omnell KA:* J Cell Biol, *vol 18, 1963, Rockefeller University Press.)*

and a tail section, which forms a repetitive series of interlocking prisms. The rounded head portion of each prism (5 μm wide) lies between the narrow tail portions (5 μm long) of two adjacent prisms (Fig. 2-5). Generally, the rounded head portion is oriented in the incisal or occlusal direction; the tail section is oriented cervically.

The structural components of the enamel prism are millions of small, elongated apatite crystallites that are variable in size and shape. The crystallites are tightly packed in a distinct pattern of orientation that gives strength and structural identity to the enamel prisms. The long axis of the apatite crystallites within the central region of the head (body) is aligned almost parallel to the rod long axis, and the crystallites incline with increasing angles (up to 65 degrees) to the prism axis in the tail region. The susceptibility of these crystallites to acid, either from an etching procedure or caries, appears to be correlated with their orientation. Whereas the dissolution process occurs more in the head regions of the

rod, the tail regions and the periphery of the head regions are relatively resistant to acid attack. The crystallites are irregular in shape, with an average length of 1600 Å and an average width of 200 to 400 Å. Each apatite crystallite is composed of thousands of unit cells that have a highly ordered arrangement of atoms. A crystallite may be 300 unit cells long, 40 cells wide, and 20 cells thick in a hexagonal configuration (Fig. 2-6).

An organic *matrix* or prism sheath also surrounds individual crystals. This appears to be an organically rich interspace rather than a structural entity.

Enamel rods follow a wavy, spiraling course, producing an alternating arrangement for each group or layer of rods as they change direction in progressing from the dentin toward the enamel surface where they end a few micrometers short of the tooth surface. Enamel rods rarely run a straight radial course because it appears there is an alternating clockwise and counterclockwise deviation of the rods from the radial course at all levels of the crown. They initially follow a curving path through one third of the enamel next to the DEJ. After that, the

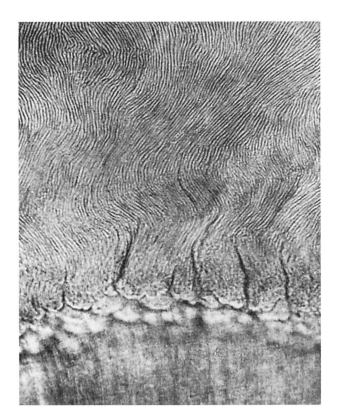

FIG. **2-7** Gnarled enamel. *(From Schour I:* H.J. Noyes' oral histology and embryology, *Philadelphia, 1960, Lea & Febiger.)*

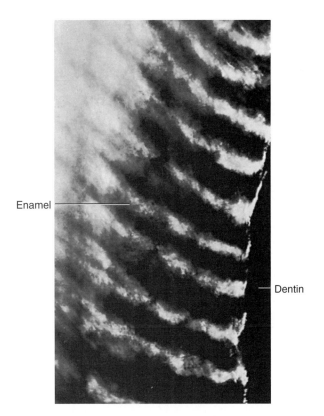

Enamel

Dentin

FIG. **2-8** Vertical ground section through enamel photographed by reflected light of Hunter-Schreger bands. *(From Yaeger JA: Enamel. In Bhaskar SN, editor:* Orban's oral histology and embryology, *ed 9, St Louis, 1980, Mosby.)*

rods usually follow a more direct path through the remaining two thirds of the enamel to the enamel surface. There are groups of enamel rods that may entwine with adjacent groups of rods, and they follow a curving irregular path toward the tooth surface. These comprise *gnarled enamel,* which occurs near the cervical regions and the incisal and occlusal areas (Fig. 2-7). Gnarled enamel is not subject to cleavage as is regular enamel. This type of enamel formation does not yield readily to the pressure of bladed, hand cutting instruments in tooth preparation.

The changes in direction of enamel prisms that minimize cleavage in the axial direction produce an optical appearance called *Hunter-Schreger bands* (Fig. 2-8). These bands appear to be composed of alternate light and dark zones of varying widths that have slightly different permeability and organic content. These bands are found in different areas of each class of teeth. Since the enamel rod orientation varies in each tooth, Hunter-Schreger bands also have a variation in the number present in each tooth. In the anterior teeth they are located near the incisal surfaces. They increase in numbers and areas of the teeth from the canines to the premolars. In the molars the bands occur from near the cervical region to the cusp tips. The orientation of the enamel rod heads and tails and the gnarling of enamel rods provide strength by resisting, distributing, and dissipating impact forces.

Enamel tufts are hypomineralized structures of enamel rods and inter-rod substance that project between adjacent groups of enamel rods from the DEJ (Fig. 2-9). These projections arise in the dentin, extend into the enamel in the direction of the long axis of the crown, and may play a role in the spread of dental caries. *Enamel lamellae* are thin, leaflike faults between enamel rod groups that extend from the enamel surface toward the DEJ, sometimes extending into the dentin (see Fig. 2-9). They contain mostly organic material, which is a weak area predisposing a tooth to the entry of bacteria and dental caries. Odontoblastic processes sometimes cross the DEJ into the enamel; these are termed *enamel spindles* when their ends are thickened (Fig. 2-10). They may serve as pain receptors, thereby explaining the enamel sensitivity experienced by some patients during tooth preparation.

Enamel rods are formed linearly by successive apposition of enamel in discrete increments. The resulting variations in structure and mineralization are called the *incremental striae of Retzius* and can be considered growth rings (see Fig. 2-3). In horizontal sections of a tooth, the striae of Retzius appear as concentric circles. In vertical sections, the lines transverse the cuspal and incisal areas in a symmetric arc pattern descending

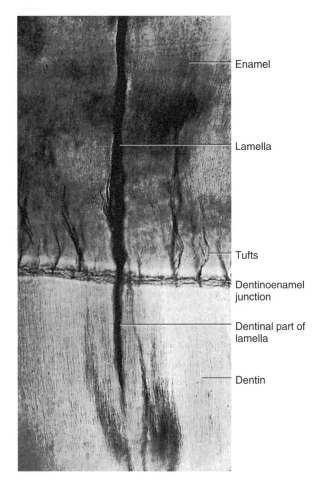

Enamel

Lamella

Tufts

Dentinoenamel
junction

Dentinal part of
lamella

Dentin

FIG. **2-9** Horizontal ground section through lamella that goes from enamel surface into dentin. Note enamel tufts. *(From Yaeger JA: Enamel. In Bhaskar SN, editor: Orban's oral histology and embryology, ed 9, St Louis, 1980, Mosby.)*

obliquely to the cervical region and terminating at the DEJ. When these circles are incomplete at the enamel surface, a series of alternating grooves, called the *imbrication lines of Pickerill*, are formed. The elevations between the grooves are called *perikymata*; these are continuous around a tooth and usually lie parallel to the cementoenamel junction and each other.

There is a structureless outer layer of enamel about 30 μm thick found most commonly toward the cervical area and less often on cusp tips. There are no prism outlines visible, and all the apatite crystals are parallel to one another and perpendicular to the striae of Retzius. It appears that this layer is more heavily mineralized. Microscopically, the enamel surface initially has circular depressions indicating where the enamel rods end. These concavities vary in depth and shape, and they may contribute to the adherence of plaque material, with a resultant caries attack, especially in young people. However, the dimpled surface anatomy of the enamel gradually wears smooth with age.

The interface of the enamel and dentin is called the *dentinoenamel junction* (Fig. 2-11). It is scalloped or wavy in outline, with the crest of the waves penetrating toward the enamel. The rounded projections of enamel fit into the shallow depressions of dentin. This interdigitation seems to contribute to a firm attachment between dentin and enamel. The DEJ is also a hypermineralized zone about 30 μm thick.

Deep invaginations occur in pit-and-fissure areas of the occlusal surfaces of premolars and molars; such invaginations decrease enamel thickness in these areas. These *fissures* act as food and bacterial traps that may predispose the tooth to dental caries (Fig. 2-12). Occlusal *grooves*, which are sound, serve an important function as

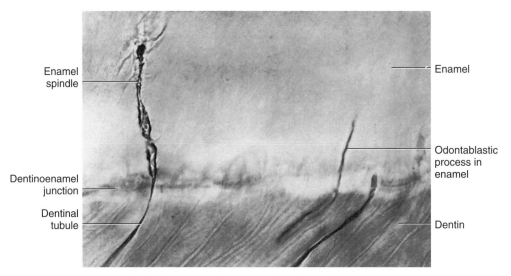

Enamel
spindle

Dentinoenamel
junction

Dentinal
tubule

Enamel

Odontablastic
process in
enamel

Dentin

FIG. **2-10** Ground section. Odontoblastic processes extend into enamel as enamel spindles. *(From Yaeger JA: Enamel. In Bhaskar SN, editor: Orban's oral histology and embryology, ed 9, St Louis, 1980, Mosby.)*

an escape path for the movement of food to the facial and lingual surfaces during mastication. A functional cusp that opposes a groove occludes on the enamel inclines on each side of the groove and not in the depth of the groove. Therefore this arrangement leaves a V-shaped escape path between the cusp and its opposing groove for the movement of food during chewing. Grooves or fissures are formed at the junction of the developmental lobes of the enamel. *Sound coalescence of the lobes results in grooves; faulty coalescence results in fissures.*

Enamel is incapable of repairing itself once destroyed because the ameloblast cell degenerates following formation of the enamel rod. The final act of the ameloblast cell is secretion of a membrane covering the end of the enamel rod. This layer is referred to as the *Nasmyth membrane,* or the *primary enamel cuticle.* This membrane covers the newly erupted tooth and is worn away by mastication and cleaning. The membrane is replaced by an organic deposit called a *pellicle,* which is a precipitate of salivary proteins. Microorganisms may invade the pellicle to form bacterial plaque, a potential precursor to dental disease.

Although enamel is a very hard, dense structure, it is permeable to certain ions and molecules, permitting both partial and complete penetration. The route of passage appears to be through structural units that are hypomineralized and rich in organic content, such as rod sheaths, enamel cracks, and other defects. Water plays an important role as a transporting medium through small intercrystalline spaces. Enamel permeability decreases with age because of changes in the enamel matrix, though basic permeability is maintained; this decrease is referred to as *enamel maturation.*

Enamel is soluble when exposed to an acid medium, but the dissolution is not uniform. Solubility of enamel increases from the enamel surface to the DEJ. When fluorides are present during enamel formation or are topically applied to the enamel surface, the solubility of surface enamel is decreased. Fluoride concentration decreases toward the DEJ. Fluoride additions can affect the chemical and physical properties of the apatite mineral and influence the hardness, chemical reactivity, and stability of enamel while preserving the apatite structures. Trace amounts of fluoride stabilize enamel by lowering acid solubility, decreasing the rate of demineralization, and enhancing the rate of remineralization. Evidence also shows that topical fluorides alter the oral bacterial flora, thereby increasing resistance to dental caries.

An established operative technique involves acid etching the enamel surface for the micromechanical "bonding" of composite restorative materials or pit-and-fissure sealants directly to the etched surface. The etchant usually is a 35% to 50% solution of phosphoric acid. This etching produces an irregular and pitted surface with numerous microscopic undercuts by an un-

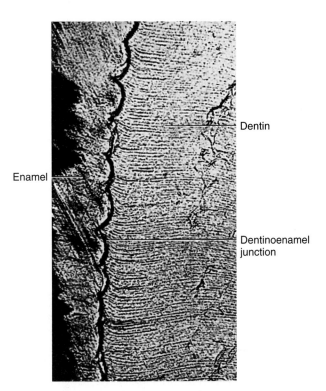

FIG. **2-11** Vertical ground section of scalloped dentinoenamel junction. *(From Yaeger JA: Enamel. In Bhaskar SN, editor: Orban's oral histology and embryology, ed 9, St Louis, 1980, Mosby.)*

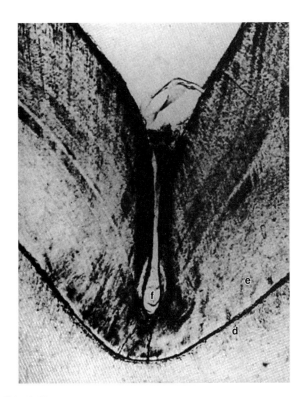

FIG. **2-12** Fissure *(f)* at junction of lobes acts as food trap predisposing tooth to dental caries. *e,* enamel; *d,* dentin. *(From Gilling B, Buonocure M: J Dent Res 40:119, Jan-Feb 1961.)*

FIG. **2-13** Odontoblastic processes (Tomes fibers), lying in dentinal tubules, extend from odontoblasts into dentin. *(From Avery JK: Dentin. In Bhaskar SN, editor:* Orban's oral histology and embryology, *ed 9, St Louis, 1980, Mosby.)*

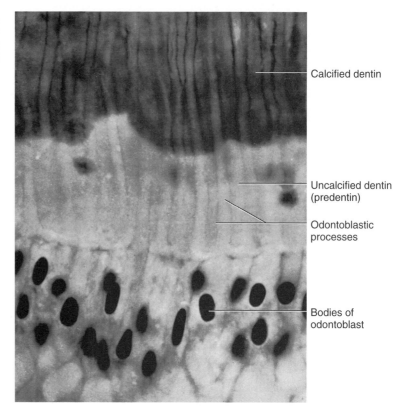

Calcified dentin

Uncalcified dentin (predentin)

Odontoblastic processes

Bodies of odontoblast

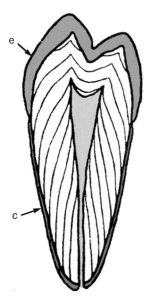

FIG. **2-14** Pattern of formation of primary dentin. This figure also shows enamel *(e)* covering the anatomic crown of the tooth and cementum *(c)* covering the anatomic root. *(From Scott JH, Symons NBB:* Introduction to dental anatomy, *ed 7, Edinburgh, 1974, Churchill Livingstone.)*

even dissolution of enamel rod heads and tails. Composite or pit-and-fissure sealant is bonded to the enamel surface by resin tags formed in the acid-etched enamel rod structures. Therefore the structure of enamel can be an asset when it is subjected to purposeful and controlled acid dissolution of the enamel rods to provide this microretention for composite or sealant.

Pulp-Dentin Complex. Dentin and pulp tissues are specialized connective tissues of mesodermal origin, formed from the dental papilla of the tooth bud. These two tissues are considered by many investigators as a single tissue, which thus form the pulp-dentin complex, with mineralized dentin comprising the mature end-product of cell differentiation and maturation. Dentin is formed by cells called *odontoblasts.* Odontoblasts are considered part of both dentin and pulp tissues because their cell bodies are in the pulp cavity but their long, slender cytoplasmic cell processes *(Tomes fibers)* extend well into the tubules in the mineralized dentin (Fig. 2-13). It is because of these odontoblastic cell processes that dentin is considered living tissue with the capability to react to physiologic and pathologic stimuli. Such stimuli can result in changes throughout the life of the tooth, such as secondary dentin, reparative dentin, sclerotic dentin, and dead tracts. Dentin and pulp are discussed separately in the following sections.

Dentin forms the largest portion of the tooth structure, extending almost the full length of the tooth. Externally, dentin is covered by enamel on the anatomic crown and cementum on the anatomic root. Internally, dentin forms the walls of the pulp cavity (pulp chamber and pulp canal[s]) (Fig. 2-14).

The odontoblasts begin dentin formation immediately before enamel formation by the ameloblasts.

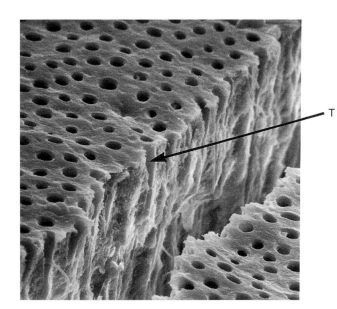

FIG. **2-15** Ground dentinal surface, acid-etched for 5 seconds with 37% phosphoric acid. The artificial crack shows part of the dentinal tubules *(T)*. The tubule apertures are opened and widened by acid application. *(From Brännström M: Dentin and pulp in restorative dentistry, London, 1982, Wolfe Medical.)*

Dentinogenesis begins with the odontoblasts laying down a collagen matrix, moving from the dentinoenamel junction inward toward the pulp. Mineralization of the collagen matrix gradually follows its secretion. The most recently formed layer of dentin is always on the pulpal surface. This unmineralized zone of dentin is immediately next to the cell bodies of the odontoblasts and is called *predentin.* Dentin formation begins at areas subadjacent to the cusp tip or incisal ridge and gradually spreads to the apex of the root (see Fig. 2-14). Unlike enamel, dentin formation continues after tooth eruption and throughout the life of the pulp. The dentin forming the initial shape of the tooth is called *primary dentin* and is usually completed 3 years after tooth eruption (for permanent teeth).

The *dentinal tubules* are small canals that extend across the entire width of dentin, from the dentinoenamel or dentinocemental junction to the pulp (Fig. 2-15 and Fig. 2-21). Each tubule contains the cytoplasmic cell process (Tomes fiber) of an odontoblast. Each dentinal tubule is lined with a layer of *peritubular dentin,* which is much more mineralized than the surrounding *intertubular dentin* (Fig. 2-16).

The surface area of dentin is much larger at the dentinoenamel or dentinocemental junction than it is on the pulp cavity side. Since the odontoblasts form dentin while progressing inward toward the pulp, the tubules are forced closer together. The number of tubules increases from 15,000 to 20,000/mm^2 at the DEJ to 45,000 to 65,000/mm^2 at the pulp.[5] The lumen of the tubules also varies from the DEJ to the pulp surface. In coronal dentin, the average diameter of tubules at the dentinoenamel junction is 0.5 to 0.9 μm, but this increases to 2 to 3 μm at the pulp (Fig. 2-17).

The course of the dentinal tubules is a slight S-curve in the tooth crown, but the tubules are straighter in the

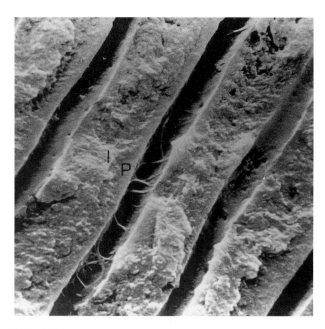

FIG. **2-16** Dentinal tubules in cross-section, 1.2 mm from pulp. Peritubular dentin *(P)* is more mineralized than intertubular dentin *(I)*. *(From Brännström M: Dentin and pulp in restorative dentistry, London, 1982, Wolfe Medical.)*

incisal ridges, cusps, and root areas (Fig. 2-18). The ends of the tubules are perpendicular to the dentinoenamel and dentinocemental junctions. Along the tubule walls are small lateral openings called *canaliculi.* As the odontoblastic process proceeds from the cell in the pulp to the DEJ, lateral secondary branches extend into the canaliculi and appear to communicate with lateral extensions of adjacent odontoblastic processes. Near the DEJ the tubules (with processes seen in young teeth) divide into several terminal branches, thus forming an intercommunicating and anastomosing network (Fig. 2-19).

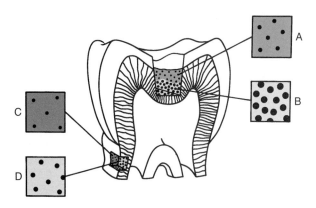

FIG. **2-17** Tubules in superficial dentin close to the dentino-enamel junction *(A)*, are smaller and more sparsely distributed compared to deep dentin *(B)*. The tubules in superficial root dentin *(C)*, and deep root dentin *(D)* are smaller and less numerous than those in comparable depths of coronal dentin. *(From Trowbridge HO:* Dentistry '82 *2:22, 1982; modified by DH Pashley.)*

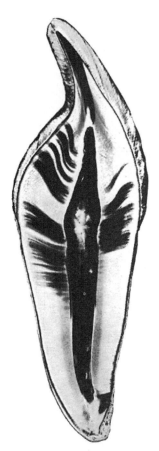

FIG. **2-18** Ground section of human incisor. Course of dentinal tubules is in a slight S-curve in the crown but rather straight at the incisal tip and in the root. *(From Avery JK: Dentin. In Bhaskar SN, editor:* Orban's oral histology snd embryology, *ed 9, St Louis, 1980, Mosby.)*

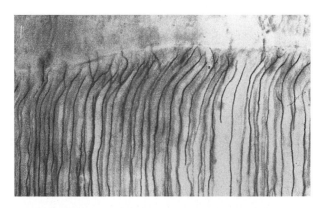

FIG. **2-19** Ground section showing dentinal tubules and their lateral branching close to the dentinoenamel junction. *(From Scott JH, Symons NBB:* Introduction to dental anatomy, *ed 7, Edinburgh, 1974, Churchill Livingstone.)*

After the primary dentin is formed, dentin deposition continues at a reduced rate even without obvious external stimuli, though the rate and amount of this physiologic *secondary dentin* varies considerably among individuals. In secondary dentin the tubules take a slightly different directional pattern in contrast to primary dentin (Fig. 2-20). Secondary dentin forms on all internal aspects of the pulp cavity, but in the pulp chamber in multirooted teeth it tends to be thicker on the roof and floor than on the side walls.[20]

Reparative dentin (tertiary dentin) is formed by replacement odontoblasts (termed *secondary odontoblasts*) in response to moderate-level irritants, such as attrition, abrasion, erosion, trauma, moderate-rate dentinal caries, and some operative procedures. It usually appears as a localized dentin deposit on the wall of the pulp cavity immediately subadjacent to the area on the tooth that has received the injury (a dentin deposit underneath the affected tubules) (Fig. 2-21). For example, reparative dentin usually is formed when teeth are mechanically prepared to within 1.5 mm of the pulp.[21] The cut fibers (odontoblastic processes) die along with the corresponding odontoblasts, leaving dead tracts (described in the next paragraph). In about 15 days new odontoblasts are differentiated from mesenchymal cells of the pulp, and these replacement odontoblasts lay down the reparative dentin. Reparative dentin is confined to the localized irritated area of the pulp cavity wall, becomes apparent microscopically about 1 month from the inception of the stimulus, is structurally and chemically different from primary and secondary dentin, and, being highly atubular, is impervious to most irritants. Reparative or tertiary dentin is a defense reaction to an area of moderate-intensity injury.

Thus when moderate-level stimuli are applied to dentin, such as moderate-rate caries or attrition, the affected odontoblastic processes may die with the associated odontoblasts. These areas of dentin are called *dead tracts* and extend from the external dentin surface to the

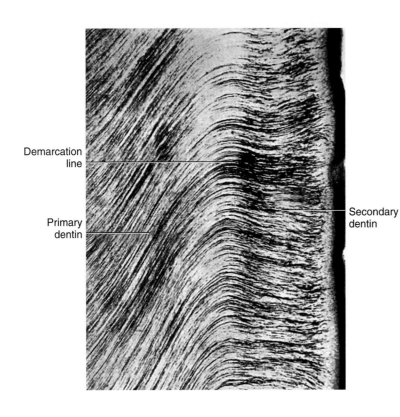

Demarcation line

Primary dentin

Secondary dentin

FIG. 2-20 Ground section of dentin with pulpal surface at right. Dentinal tubules curve sharply as they move from primary to secondary dentin. Dentinal tubules are more irregular in shape in secondary dentin. *(From Avery JK: Dentin. In Bhaskar SN, editor: Orban's oral histology and embryology, ed 9, St Louis, 1980, Mosby.)*

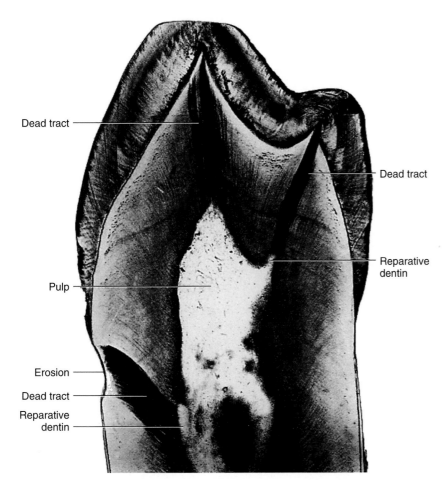

Dead tract

Dead tract

Reparative dentin

Pulp

Erosion

Dead tract

Reparative dentin

FIG. 2-21 Cross-section illustrating dead tracts and reparative dentin caused by degeneration of odontoblasts in pulpal horns and exposure of dentinal tubules to erosion on root surface, respectively. *(From Avery JK: Dentin. In Bhaskar SN, editor: Orban's oral histology and embryology, ed 9, St Louis, 1980, Mosby.)*

pulp. The tubules are empty and thus appear black when ground sections of dentin are viewed microscopically with transmitted light. Dead tracts are sealed off at the pulpal surface by reparative dentin formed by replacement odontoblasts. While dead tracts are commonly associated with areas of caries or attrition, they have occurred in unerupted incisors and teeth that show few, if any, obvious external defects. Dead tracts may be considered in some circumstances as a form of age-related change associated with the death of odontoblasts. Usually this occurs in areas of the pulp where the odontoblasts have been crowded into narrow pulp horns (see Fig. 2-21). In dried, ground sections of normal teeth the odontoblastic processes contract and may allow the tubules to fill with air, giving the appearance of a dead tract. However, a true dead tract can be distinguished by a deposit of reparative dentin on the pulpal surface.[20]

Sclerotic dentin results from aging or mild irritation (such as slowly advancing caries) and causes a change in the composition of the primary dentin. The peritubular dentin becomes wider, gradually filling the tubules with calcified material, progressing pulpally from the DEJ (Fig. 2-22). These areas are harder, denser, less sensitive, and more protective of the pulp against subsequent irritations. Sclerosis resulting from aging is *physiologic dentin sclerosis*; sclerosis resulting from a mild irritation is *reactive dentin sclerosis*. Reactive dentin sclerosis often can be seen radiographically in the form of a more radiopaque (lighter) area in the S-shape of the tubules. *Eburnated dentin* refers to the outward (exposed) portion of reactive sclerotic dentin, where slow caries has destroyed formerly overlying tooth structure, leaving a hard, darkened, cleanable surface.

The composition of human dentin is approximately 75% inorganic material, 20% organic material, and 5% water and other materials. Dentin is less mineralized than enamel but more mineralized than cementum or bone. The mineral content of dentin increases with age. This mineral phase is composed primarily of hydroxyapatite crystallites, which are arranged in a less systematic manner than enamel crystallites. Dentinal crystallites are smaller than enamel crystallites, having a length of 200 to 1000 Å and a width of about 30 Å, similar to the sizes seen in bone and cementum.[20] The organic phase of dentin consists primarily of collagen.

Dentin is significantly softer than enamel but harder than bone or cementum. The hardness of dentin averages one fifth that of enamel, and its hardness near the DEJ is about three times greater than near the pulp. Dentin becomes harder with age, primarily due to increases in mineral content. While dentin is a hard, mineralized tissue, it is somewhat flexible, with a *modulus of elasticity* of 1.67 X 10⁶ PSI. This flexibility helps support the more brittle, nonresilient enamel. Often small "craze lines" are seen in the enamel that indicate minute frac-

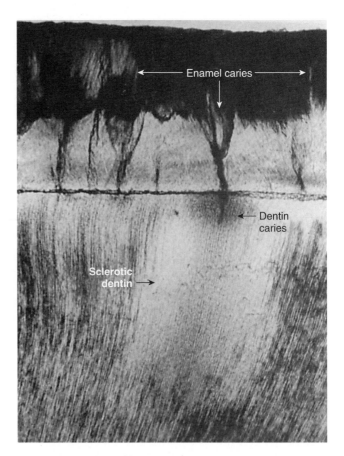

FIG. 2-22 Sclerotic dentin occurring under enamel caries with early penetration of dentin caries along enamel lamella. *(From Schour I: Noyes oral histology and embryology, Philadelphia, 1960, Lea & Febiger.)*

tures of that structure. These craze lines usually are not clinically significant unless associated with cracks in the underlying dentin. Dentin is not as prone to cleavage as is the enamel rod structure. The *tensile strength of dentin* is approximately 40 MPa (6000 PSI), which is less than cortical bone and approximately one half that of enamel. The *compressive strength of dentin* is much higher—266 MPa (40,000 PSI).[8]

During tooth preparation, dentin is usually distinguished from enamel by: (1) color, (2) reflectance, (3) hardness, and (4) sound. Dentin is normally yellow-white and slightly darker than enamel. In older patients dentin is darker, and it can become brown or black in cases where it has been exposed to oral fluids, old restorative materials, or slowly advancing caries. Dentin surfaces are more opaque and dull, being less reflective to light than similar enamel surfaces, which appear shiny. Dentin is softer than enamel and provides greater yield to the pressure of a sharp explorer tine, which tends to catch and hold in dentin. When moving an explorer tine over the tooth, enamel surfaces provide a sharper, higher-pitched sound than dentin surfaces.

Sensitivity is encountered whenever odontoblasts and their processes are stimulated during operative

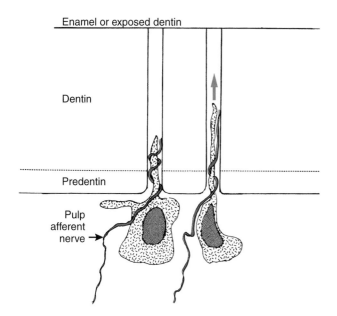

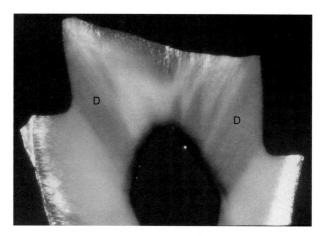

FIG. 2-24 Ground section of mesioocclusodistal (MOD) tooth preparation on third molar. Dark blue dye was placed in the pulp chamber under pressure after tooth preparation. Dark areas of dye penetration *(D)* show that dentinal tubules of axial walls are much more permeable than those of pulpal floor of preparation.

FIG. 2-23 Stimuli that induce fluid movements in dentinal tubules distort odontoblasts and afferent nerves *(arrow)*, leading to a sensation of pain. Many operative procedures such as cutting or air-drying induce such fluid movement. *(From Brännström M: Dentin and pulp in restorative dentistry, London, 1982, Wolfe Medical.)*

procedures, even though the pain receptor mechanism appears to be within the dentinal tubules near the pulp. A variety of physical, thermal, chemical, bacterial, and traumatic stimuli are transmitted through the dentinal tubules, though the precise mechanism of the transmissive elements of sensation has not been conclusively established. The most accepted theory of pain transmission is the *hydrodynamic theory*, which accounts for pain transmission through small, rapid movements of fluid that occur within the dentinal tubules.[2] Because many tubules contain mechanoreceptor nerve endings near the pulp, small fluid movements in the tubules arising from cutting, drying, pressure changes, osmotic shifts, or changes in temperature account for the majority of pain transmission (Fig. 2-23).

Dentinal tubules are normally filled with odontoblastic processes and *dentinal fluid*, a transudate of plasma. When enamel or cementum is removed during tooth preparation, the external seal of dentin is lost and the tubules become fluid-filled channels from the cut surface directly to the pulp. Fortunately, pulpal fluid has a slight positive pressure that forces fluid outward toward any breach in the external seal. Permeability studies of dentin indicate that tubules are functionally much smaller than would be indicated by their measured microscopic dimensions as a result of numerous constrictions along their paths (see Fig. 2-16).[15] Dentin permeability is not uniform throughout the tooth. Coronal dentin is much more permeable than root dentin. There are also differences within coronal dentin (Fig. 2-24).[22]

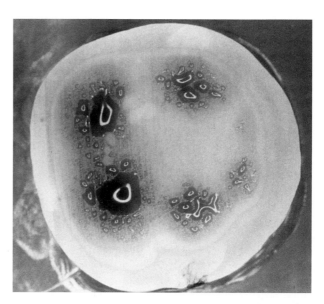

FIG. 2-25 Horizontal section in occlusal third of molar crown. Dark blue dye was placed in the pulp chamber under pressure. Deep dentin areas (over pulp horns) are much more permeable than superficial dentin. *(Reprinted from Pashley DH et al: Regional variability in the permeability of human dentin, Arch Oral Biol 32(7):519-523, 1987, with permission from Pergamon, Headington Hill Hall, Oxford OX3 0BW, UK.)*

Dentin permeability is primarily dependent on the remaining dentin thickness (i.e., length of the tubules) and the diameter of the tubules. Since the tubules are shorter, become more numerous, and increase in diameter closer to the pulp, deep dentin is a less-effective pulpal barrier than is superficial dentin near the dentinoenamel or dentinocemental junctions (Fig. 2-25).

Dentin must be treated with great care during restorative procedures to minimize damage to the odontoblasts and pulp. Air-water spray should be used whenever

Air blast

Removal of fluid = rapid outward flow due to capillary force

Aspiration of cells and nerves = stretching and/or disruption of nerves

A

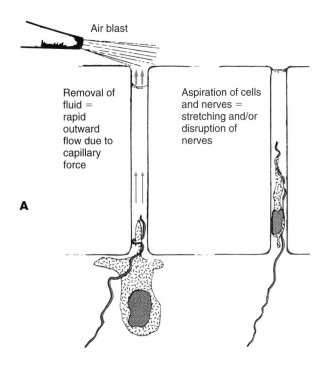

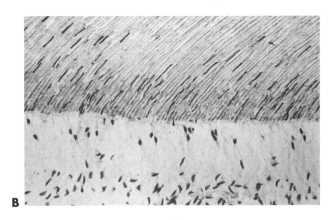

B

FIG. **2-26** **A,** Excessive drying of tooth preparations can cause odontoblasts to be aspirated into dentinal tubules. **B,** Nuclei are seen as dark rods in dentinal tubules. *(From Brännström M: Dentin and pulp in restorative dentistry, London, 1982, Wolfe Medical.)*

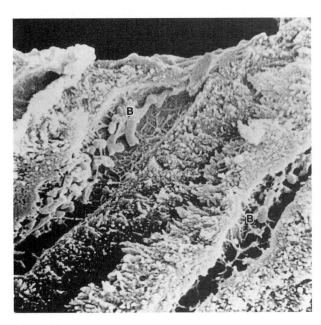

FIG. **2-27** Cross-section of dentin showing an acid-etched tooth preparation left unsealed intraorally for one week. Microorganisms *(B)* can be seen in vertically fractured, widened dentinal tubules. The peritubular zone has been removed. *(From Olgart L, Brännström M, Johnson G: Invasion of bacteria into dentinal tubules, Acta Odontol Scand 32:61-70, 1974.)*

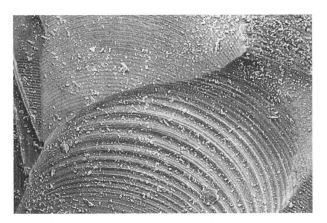

FIG. **2-28** Smear layer on cut dentin preparation surface. Swirls on surface are from end of a carbide bur. *(From Marshall GW, Marshall SJ, Bayne SC: Restorative dental materials: scanning electron microscopy and x-ray microanalysis, Scanning Microsc 2(4):2007-2028, 1988.)*

cutting with high-speed handpieces to avoid heat buildup. The dentin should not be dehydrated by compressed air blasts; it should always maintain its normal fluid content (Fig. 2-26). Protection is also provided by judicious use of liners, bases, dentin-bonding agents, and nontoxic restorative materials. Restorations must adequately seal the preparation to avoid microleakage and bacterial penetration (Fig. 2-27).

Whenever dentin has been cut or abraded, a thin altered layer is created on the surface. This *smear layer* is only a few micrometers thick and is composed of denatured collagen, hydroxyapatite, and other cutting debris (Fig. 2-28). The smear layer serves as a natural bandage over the cut dentinal surface because it occludes many of the dentinal tubules with debris called *smear plugs* (Fig. 2-29). While the smear layer is a good protective barrier, it has a relatively weak attachment to the dentin and is subject to dissolution by acids.

Reliable *dentin bonding* of composite restorations has been a difficult goal for dental manufacturers. While

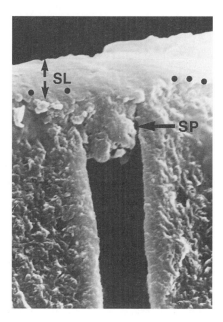

FIG. **2-29** Smear layer *(SL)* in cross-section. Smear plugs *(SP)* are formed from cutting debris forced into tubules. The smear layer and smear plugs greatly reduce the permeability of cut dentin surface. *(From Pashley DH: Dentin: a dynamic substrate,* Scanning Microsc 3(1):161-176, 1989.)

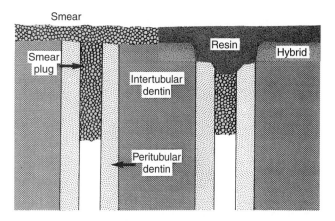

FIG. **2-31** Most dentin bonding systems remove or solubilize smear layer, allowing resins to penetrate and form "hybrid layer" with dentin structures. Ideally, smear plugs would not be removed. *(From Pashley DH: The effects of acid etching on the pulpodentin complex,* Oper Dent 17(6):229-242, 1992.)

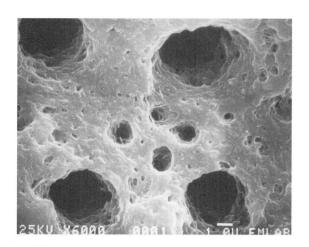

FIG. **2-30** Smear layer removed from deep human dentin with 0.5M ethylene diamine tetracetic acid (EDTA). *(Courtesy of DH Pashley.)*

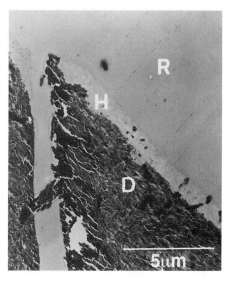

FIG. **2-32** Cross-sectional transmission electron micrograph of resin restoration bonded to dentin. Dentin-bonding agent has extensive penetration into dentin structures. The hybrid layer *(H)* is in the middle, with resin *(R)* above and dentin *(D)* below. *(From Nakabayashi N, Takarada K: Effect of HEMA on bonding to dentin,* Dent Mater 8(2):125-130, 1992.)

some manufacturers claim their products create chemical bonds to dentin, most experts agree that the primary mechanism of attachment is mechanical interlocking. Most dentin-bonding systems have acids that remove the smear layer and partially demineralize the intertubular dentin. In most systems these acidic components are weaker than the 37% phosphoric acid commonly used to etch enamel surfaces. When viewed under high magnification, dentin without a smear has many irregularities for micromechanical retention (Fig. 2-30). Ideally, such etchants remove the smear layer but leave the smear plugs because they greatly reduce

dentin permeability and sensitivity. Etchants should not excessively damage exposed collagen fibers because much of the bond strength develops from resin encapsulating these fibers.[23] After the acids, hydrophilic adhesive resins are applied that penetrate into the inherently moist dentin surfaces and copolymerize with the composite restoration.[16,17] While some of the bond forms from resin "tags" extending into the dentinal tubules, most of the bond strength develops from resin that penetrates and adapts to the demineralized intertubular dentin and exposed collagen fibers. The resultant resin interdiffusion zone is often termed the *hybrid layer* (Figs. 2-31 and 2-32).

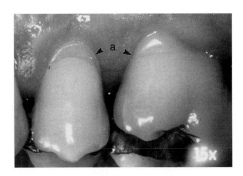

FIG. 2-33 As an alternative to restoration, sensitivity from exposed and abraded root surfaces (a) can be reduced by the application of dentin bonding agents.

While dentin bond strengths have improved, they are variable because of the dentin substrate. Bond strengths for superficial dentin close to the dentinoenamel or dentinocemental junctions are greater than those for deep dentin. In deep dentin the greater number of tubules and the larger diameter of tubules reduce the amount of intertubular dentin available for bonding.[18]

An important aspect of current dentin-bonding agents is their ability to seal cut dentinal surfaces and thus reduce permeability and microleakage. Many dentists use dentin-bonding products to seal and desensitize dentin surfaces in all tooth preparations and in unrestored Class V cervical abrasion and erosion defects (Fig. 2-33).

The *dental pulp* occupies the pulp cavity in the tooth. Each pulp organ is circumscribed by the dentin and is lined peripherally by a cellular layer of odontoblasts adjacent to the dentin. Anatomically the pulp organ is divided into: (1) coronal pulp located in the pulp chamber in the crown portion of the tooth, including the pulp horns that are directed toward the incisal ridges and cusp tips; and (2) radicular pulp located in the pulp canal(s) in the root portion of the tooth. The radicular pulp is continuous with the periapical tissues by connecting through the apical foramen or foramina of the root. Accessory canals may extend from the pulp canal(s) laterally through the root dentin to the periodontal tissues. The shape of each pulp conforms generally to the shape of each tooth (see Fig. 2-3).

The dental pulp is composed of myelinated and unmyelinated nerves, arteries, veins, lymph channels, connective tissue cells, intercellular substance, odontoblasts, fibroblasts, macrophages, collagen, and fine fibers. The central area of the pulp contains the large blood vessels and nerve trunks. The pulp is circumscribed peripherally by a specialized odontogenic area made up of the odontoblasts, the cell-free zone, and the cell-rich zone.

The pulp is a unique, specialized organ of the human body serving four functions: (1) formative or developmental, (2) nutritive, (3) sensory or protective, and (4) defensive or reparative. The formative function is the production of primary and secondary dentin by the odontoblasts. The nutritive function supplies nutriments and moisture to the dentin through the blood vascular supply to the odontoblasts and their processes. The sensory function provides sensory nerve fibers within the pulp to mediate the sensation of pain. Dentin receptors are unique because various stimuli elicit only pain as a response. The pulp usually does not differentiate between heat, touch, pressure, or chemicals. Motor fibers initiate reflexes in the muscles of the blood vessel walls for the control of circulation in the pulp. Finally, the defensive function of the pulp is related primarily to its response to irritation by mechanical, thermal, chemical, or bacterial stimuli. Such irritants can cause the degeneration and death of the affected odontoblastic processes and corresponding odontoblasts and the formation of replacement odontoblasts (from undifferentiated pulpal mesenchymal cells) that lay down irregular or reparative dentin. The deposition of reparative dentin acts as a protective barrier against caries and various other irritating factors. This is a continuous but relatively slow process, taking 100 days to form a reparative dentin layer 0.12 mm thick. In cases of severe irritation the pulp responds by an inflammatory reaction similar to that for any other soft tissue injury. However, the inflammation may become irreversible and can result in the death of the pulp because the confined, rigid structure of the dentin limits the inflammatory response and the ability of the pulp to recover.

If, however, the irritant is very mild, such as that caused by cutting the odontoblastic processes more than 1.5 mm external to the pulp at high speed with air-water coolant during tooth preparation, no replacement odontoblasts are formed; thus no reparative dentin is created, even though the processes and corresponding odontoblasts have died.[21] Therefore there is no barrier (except for the smear layer) between the dead tracts remaining and the pulp. This may explain why many teeth have pulpal problems following tooth preparation and restoration. However, newer dentin-bonding systems look promising for sealing the cut dentinal surfaces and preventing postoperative sensitivity.

A knowledge of the contour and size of the pulp cavity is essential during tooth preparation. In general, the pulp cavity is a miniature contour of the external surface of the tooth. Size varies among the various teeth in the same mouth and among individuals. With advancing age, the pulp cavity usually decreases in size. Radiographs are an invaluable aid in determining the size of the pulp cavity and any existing pathologic condition (Fig. 2-34). Also with advanced age, the pulp generally becomes more fibrous because of past episodes of various irritations, and it may contain pulp stones or denticles. The latter are nodular, calcified masses usually appearing in the pulp chamber but also in the pulp canal.

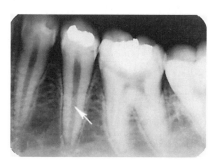

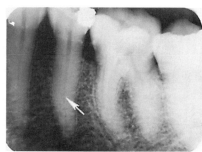

A   **B**

FIG. **2-34** Pulp cavity size. **A,** Premolar radiograph of young person. **B,** Premolar radiograph of older person. Note the difference in the size of the pulp cavity *(arrows).* *(From Shankle RJ: Clinical dental anatomy, physiology, and histology. In Sturdevant CM et al, editors:* The art and science of operative dentistry, *ed 1, New York, 1968, McGraw-Hill.)*

These may either be attached to the pulp cavity wall or free in the mass of pulp tissue.

Clinical interpretation of pain from pulpal inflammation is somewhat empiric, but it is nonetheless important to the successful practice of operative dentistry. One of the primary services rendered by the dentist is diagnosis and relief of pain of pulpal origin.

When an irritant (e.g., sugar, cold, acid from caries) first contacts dentin, the patient may be alerted by a twinge of pain. This pain is usually only momentary, ceasing if the irritant is removed. If such irritation continues or the irritant is applied repeatedly, *hyperemia* (increased blood flow and volume) and inflammation of the pulp can result, which will cause the pain elicited from the irritation to linger a few seconds. The reaction is because the pulp is contained by unyielding dentinal walls; thus drainage of the increased blood is limited by the constricted apical foramen. As long as an irritant, such as touching ice to the tooth, causes pain that lingers no more than 10 to 15 seconds after removal of the irritant, resolution of the hyperemia by immediate restorative treatment is a possibility; such hyperemia is termed *reversible pulpitis.*

When pulpal pain, either spontaneous or elicited by an irritant, lingers more than 15 seconds, infection of the pulp often has occurred and resolution by operative dentistry treatment is usually doubtful; root canal therapy is advised for this pulpal condition, termed *irreversible pulpitis,* if the tooth is to be maintained in the dentition. When this condition is untreated, suppuration and *pulpal necrosis* follows, characterized by spontaneous, continuous throbbing pain or pain elicited by heat that can be relieved by cold and later characterized by no response to any stimulus. Pulpal necrosis is treated by root canal therapy or tooth extraction.

A primary objective during operative procedures must be preservation of the health of the pulp. The successful management of the disease process by proper treatment of the pulp organ is discussed further in later chapters.

Cementum. Cementum is the hard dental tissue covering the anatomic roots of teeth and is formed by cells known as *cementoblasts,* which develop from undifferentiated mesenchymal cells in the connective tissue of the dental follicle. Cementum is slightly softer than dentin and consists of about 45% to 50% inorganic material (hydroxyapatite) by weight and 50% to 55% organic matter and water by weight. The organic portion is primarily composed of collagen and protein polysaccharides. *Sharpey's fibers* are the portions of the collagenous principal fibers of the periodontal ligament embedded in both the cementum and alveolar bone to attach the tooth to the alveolus (Fig. 2-35). Cementum is avascular.

The cementum is light yellow and slightly lighter in color than dentin. It has the highest fluoride content of all mineralized tissue. Cementum is also permeable to a variety of materials. It is formed continuously throughout life, because a new layer of cementum is deposited to keep the attachment intact as the superficial layer of cementum ages. Two kinds of cementum are formed: acellular and cellular. The *acellular layer of cementum* is living tissue that does not incorporate cells into its structure and usually predominates on the coronal half of the root; *cellular cementum* occurs more frequently on the apical half. Cementum on the root end surrounds the apical foramen and may extend slightly onto the inner wall of the pulp canal. Cementum thickness can increase on the root end to compensate for attritional wear of the occlusal/incisal surface and passive eruption of the tooth.

The cementodentinal junction is a relatively smooth area in the permanent tooth, and attachment of cementum to the dentin is firm but not understood completely. The cementum joins the enamel to form the cementoenamel junction, which is referred to as the *cervical line.* In about 10% of teeth, enamel and cementum do not meet, and this can result in a sensitive area. Abrasion, erosion, caries, scaling, and the procedures of finishing and polishing may result in denuding the dentin of its cementum covering, which can cause the dentin to be sensitive to several types of stimuli (e.g., heat, cold, sweet and sour substances). Cementum is capable of repairing itself to a limited degree and is not resorbed under normal conditions. Some resorption of the apical portion of the root often occurs during physiologic tooth movement (Fig. 2-36).

FIG. **2-35** Principal fibers of periodontal ligament continue to course into surface layer of cementum as Sharpey's fibers. *(From Armitage GC: Cementum. In Bhaskar SN, editor: Orban's oral histology and embryology, ed 9, St Louis, 1980, Mosby.)*

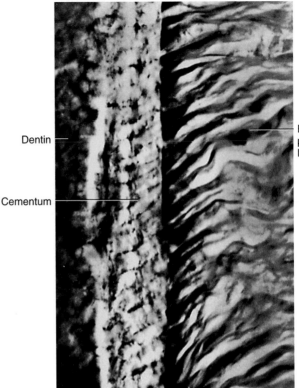

Dentin

Cementum

Fibers of periodontal ligament

PHYSIOLOGY OF TOOTH FORM

Function. The teeth serve four main functions: (1) mastication, (2) esthetics, (3) speech, and (4) protection of supporting tissues. Normal tooth form and proper alignment ensure efficiency in the incising and reduction of food with the various tooth classes—incisors, canines, premolars, and molars—performing specific functions in the masticatory process. In esthetics the form and alignment of the anterior teeth are important to a person's physical appearance. The form and alignment of both anterior and posterior teeth assist in the articulation of certain sounds that can have a significant effect on speech. Finally, the form and alignment of the teeth assist in sustaining the teeth in the dental arches by assisting in the development and protection of the gingival tissues and alveolar bone that support them.

Contours. The facial and lingual surfaces possess some degree of convexity that affords protection and stimulation of the supporting tissues during mastication. This convexity generally is located at the cervical third of the crown on the *facial surfaces* of all teeth and the *lingual surfaces* of the incisors and canines. The lingual surfaces of the posterior teeth usually have their height of contour in the middle third of the crown. *Normal tooth contours* act in deflecting food only to the extent that the passing food stimulates (by gentle massage) rather than irritates the investing tissues. If these curvatures are too great, the tissues usually receive in-

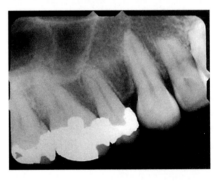

FIG. **2-36** Radiograph showing root resorption on lateral incisor following orthodontic tooth movement.

adequate stimulation by the passage of food. Too little contour may result in trauma to the attachment apparatus. These tooth contours must be considered in the performance of operative dental procedures. Improper location and degree of *facial* or *lingual convexities* can result in serious complications, as illustrated in Fig. 2-37, where the proper facial contour is disregarded in the placement of a cervical restoration on a mandibular molar. *Overcontouring is the worst offender, usually resulting in flabby, red-colored, chronically inflamed gingiva and increased plaque retention.*

Proper form of the *proximal surfaces of the teeth* is just as important to the maintenance of the periodontal tissues as proper form of the facial and lingual surfaces. The

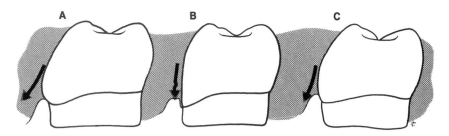

FIG. **2-37** Contours. Arrows show pathways of food passing over facial surface of mandibular molar during mastication. **A,** Overcontour deflects food from gingiva and results in understimulation of supporting tissues. **B,** Undercontour of tooth may result in irritation of soft tissues. **C,** Correct contour permits adequate stimulation for supporting tissues, resulting in healthy condition. *(From Brauer JC, Richardson RE: The dental assistant, ed 3, New York, 1964, McGraw-Hill.)*

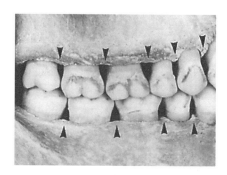

FIG. **2-38** Portion of the skull, showing triangular spaces beneath proximal contact areas. These spaces are occupied by soft tissue and bone for support of teeth

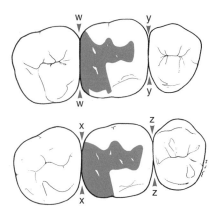

FIG. **2-39** Embrasure form. *w,* Improper embrasure form caused by overcontouring of restoration resulting in unhealthy gingiva from lack of stimulation. *x,* Good embrasure form. *y,* Frictional wear of contact area has resulted in decrease of embrasure dimension. *z,* When embrasure form is good, supporting tissues receive adequate stimulation from foods during mastication. *(From Brauer JC, Richardson RE: The dental assistant, ed 3, New York, 1964, McGraw-Hill.)*

proximal height of contour serves to provide: (1) *contacts* with the proximal surfaces of the adjacent teeth, which prevents food impaction; and (2) adequate embrasure space gingivally of the contacts for the gingival tissue, supporting bone, blood vessels, and nerves that serve the supporting structures (Fig. 2-38).

Proximal Contact Area. *Proximal contact area* denotes the area of proximal height of contour of the mesial or distal surface of a tooth that touches (contacts) its adjacent tooth in the same arch. When teeth erupt to make proximal contact with previously erupted teeth, there is initially a contact point. The contact *point* becomes an *area* because of wear of one proximal surface against another during physiologic tooth movement (Figs. 2-39 and 2-40).

The physiologic significance of properly formed and located proximal contacts cannot be overemphasized; they promote normal healthy interdental papillae filling of the interproximal spaces. Improper contacts can result in food impaction between the teeth, producing periodontal disease, carious lesions, and possible movement of the teeth. In addition, retention of food is objectionable by its physical presence and by the halitosis that results from food decomposition. Proximal contacts and interdigitation of the teeth through occlusal contacts stabilizes and maintains the integrity of the dental arches.

The proximal contact area is located in the incisal third of the approximating surfaces of the maxillary and mandibular central incisors (Fig. 2-41). It is positioned slightly facial to the center of the proximal surface faciolingually (see Fig. 2-40). Proceeding posteriorly from the incisor region through all the remaining teeth, the contact area is located near the junction of the incisal (or occlusal) and middle thirds or in the middle third. Because of these contacts being positioned progressively lower cervically (see Fig. 2-41), larger incisal or occlusal embrasures result posteriorly. Restorative procedures require maintenance of correct proximal contact relationships between teeth, which results in correct embrasures.

Embrasures. *Embrasures* are V-shaped spaces that originate at the proximal contact areas between adjacent teeth and are named for the direction toward which they radiate. These embrasures are: (1) facial, (2) lingual, (3) incisal or occlusal, and (4) gingival (see Figs. 2-40 and 2-41).

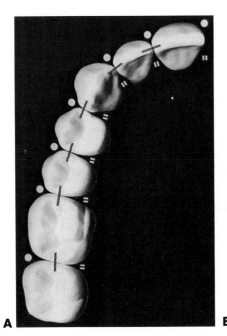
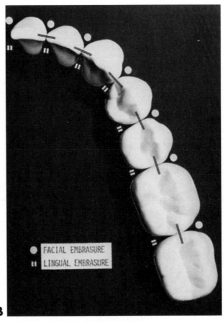

FIG. **2-40** Proximal contact area. Black lines show positions of contacts faciolingually. **A,** Maxillary teeth. **B,** Mandibular teeth. Facial and lingual embrasures are indicated.

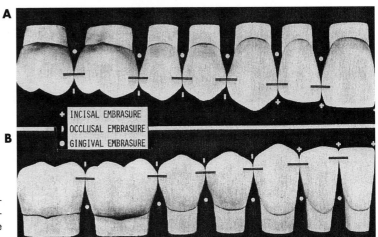

FIG. **2-41** Proximal contact area. Black lines show positions of contacts incisogingivally and occlusogingivally. Incisal, occlusal, and gingival embrasures are indicated. **A,** Maxillary teeth. **B,** Mandibular teeth.

Initially the interdental papilla fills the gingival embrasure. In a mouth where tooth form and function are ideal and optimal oral health is maintained, the interdental papilla may continue in this position throughout life. When the gingival embrasure is filled by the papilla, trapping of food in this region is prevented. In a faciolingual vertical section, the papilla may be triangular between anterior teeth, whereas in the posterior teeth the papilla may be shaped like a mountain range, with facial and lingual peaks and the *col* ("valley") lying beneath the contact area (Fig. 2-42). This col, a central faciolingual concave area beneath the contact, is more vulnerable to periodontal disease from incorrect contact and embrasure form because it is covered by nonkeratinized epithelium.

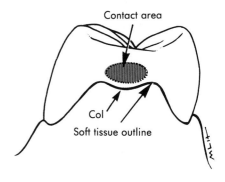

FIG. **2-42** Relationship of ideal interdental papilla to molar contact area. *(From Shankle RJ: Clinical dental anatomy, physiology, and histology. In Sturdevant CM et al, editors: The art and science of operative dentistry, ed 1, New York, 1968, McGraw-Hill.)*

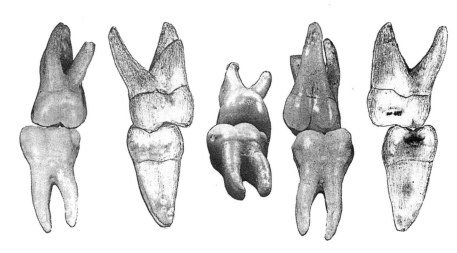

FIG. 2-43 Maxillary and mandibular first molars in centric occlusal relationship. Note the grooves for escape of food.

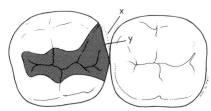

FIG. 2-44 Embrasure form. *x,* Portion of tooth that offers protection to underlying supporting tissue during mastication. *y,* Restoration fails to establish adequate contour for good embrasure form. *(From Brauer JC, Richardson RE:* The dental assistant, *ed 3, New York, 1964, McGraw-Hill.)*

The correct relationships of embrasures, cusps to sulci, marginal ridges, and grooves of adjacent and opposing teeth provide for the escape of food from the occlusal surfaces during mastication (Fig. 2-43). When an embrasure is decreased in size or absent, additional stress is created in the teeth and the supporting structures during mastication. Embrasures that are too large provide little protection to the supporting structures as food is forced into the interproximal space by an opposing cusp. A prime example is the failure to restore the distal cusp of a mandibular first molar when placing a restoration (Fig. 2-44). The lingual embrasures are usually larger than the facial embrasures to allow more food to be displaced lingually, because the tongue can return the food to the occlusal surface easier than if the food is displaced facially into the buccal vestibule (see Fig. 2-40).

The marginal ridges of adjacent posterior teeth should be at the same height to have proper contact and embrasure forms. When this relationship is absent, there is an increase in the problems associated with weak contacts and faulty embrasure form.

Preservation of the curvatures of the opposing cusps and surfaces in function maintains masticatory efficiency throughout life (see Fig. 2-2). Correct anatomic form renders the teeth more self-cleansing because of the smoothly rounded contours that are more exposed to the cleansing action of foods and fluids and the fric-

tional movement of the tongue, lips, and cheeks. Failure to understand and adhere to correct anatomic form in the performance of restorative procedures can contribute to the breakdown of the stomatognathic system (Fig. 2-45), and the importance of providing correct anatomic features in restorative dentistry cannot be overemphasized.

MAXILLA AND MANDIBLE

The human *maxilla* is formed by two bones, the maxilla proper and the premaxilla. These two bones form the bulk of the upper jaw and the major portion of the hard palate and help form the floor of the orbit and the sides and base of the nasal cavity. They initially contain the 10 maxillary primary teeth and later contain the 16 maxillary permanent teeth in the *alveolar process* (see Figs. 2-1 and 2-3, *label 7*).

The *mandible* forms the lower jaw (see Fig. 2-52, *F*). It is horseshoe shaped and relates to the skull on either side via the *temporomandibular joints* (see Fig. 2-52, *B*). The mandible is composed of a body of two horizontal portions joined at the midline symphysis mandibulae, as well as the rami, the vertical parts. The coronoid process and condyle make up the superior border of each ramus. The mandible initially contains the 10 mandibular primary teeth and later the 16 mandibular permanent teeth in the alveolar process.

The maxillary and mandibular bones consist of about 65% inorganic and 35% organic material. The inorganic portion is hydroxyapatite; the organic part is primarily collagen.

ORAL MUCOSA

The oral mucosa is the mucous membrane that covers all oral structures except the clinical crowns of the teeth. It is composed of two layers: (1) the *stratified squamous epithelium* and (2) supporting connective tissue, called the *lamina propria.* (See the lamina propria of the gingiva in Fig. 2-46, *arrow 8.*) The epithelium may be keratinized, parakeratinized, or nonkeratinized depending upon its location. The lamina propria varies in thickness

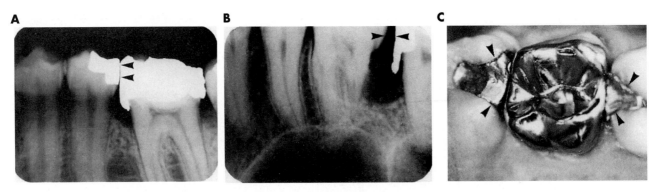

FIG. **2-45** Poor anatomic restorative form. **A,** Radiograph of flat contact and amalgam gingival excess. **B,** Radiograph of restoration with amalgam gingival excess and absence of contact resulting in trauma to supporting tissue. **C,** Poor occlusal margins.

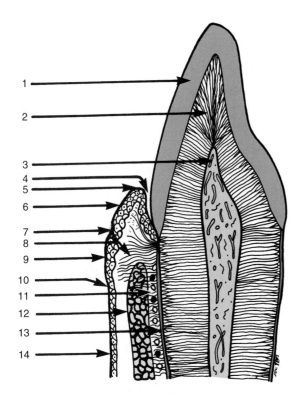

FIG. **2-46** Vertical section of maxillary incisor illustrating supporting structures: *1,* enamel; *2,* dentin; *3,* pulp; *4,* gingival sulcus; *5,* free gingival margin; *6,* free gingiva; *7,* free gingival groove; *8,* lamina propria of gingiva; *9,* attached gingiva; *10,* mucogingival junction; *11,* periodontal ligament; *12,* alveolar bone; *13,* cementum; *14,* alveolar mucosa.

and supports the epithelium. It may be attached to the periosteum of the alveolar bone, or it may be interposed over the submucosa, which may vary in different regions of the mouth (e.g., the floor of the mouth, the soft palate). The submucosa, consisting of connective tissues varying in density and thickness, attaches the mucous membrane to the underlying bony structures. The submucosa contains glands, blood vessels, nerves, and adipose tissue.

The oral mucosa may be divided into three major functional types: (1) masticatory mucosa, (2) lining or reflective mucosa, and (3) specialized mucosa.

The *masticatory mucosa* is composed of the free and attached gingiva (see Fig. 2-46, *arrows 6 and 9)* and the mucosa of the hard palate. The epithelium of these tissues is keratinized, and the lamina propria is a dense, thick, firm connective tissue containing collagenous fibers. The hard palate has a distinct submucosa except for a few narrow specific zones. The dense lamina propria of the attached gingiva is connected to the cementum and the periosteum of the bony alveolar process (see Fig. 2-46, *arrow 8).*

The *lining or reflective* mucosa covers the inside of the lips, cheek, vestibule, lateral surfaces of the alveolar process (except the mucosa of the hard palate), floor of the mouth, soft palate, and inferior surface of the tongue. Lining mucosa is a thin, movable tissue with a relatively thick, nonkeratinized epithelium and a thin lamina propria. The submucosa is composed mostly of thin, loose connective tissue with muscle and collagenous and elastic fibers, with different areas varying from one another in their structure. The junction of lining mucosa with masticatory mucosa is the *mucogingival junction,* located at the apical border of the attached gingiva facially and lingually in the mandibular arch and facially in the maxillary arch (see Fig. 2-46, *arrow 10).*

The *specialized* mucosa covers the dorsum of the tongue and the taste buds. The epithelium is nonkeratinized except for the covering of the dermal filiform papillae.

PERIODONTIUM

The *periodontium* consists of the oral hard and soft tissues that invest and support the teeth. It can be divided into: (1) the gingival unit, consisting of free and attached gingiva and the alveolar mucosa, and (2) the attachment apparatus, consisting of the cementum, periodontal ligament, and alveolar process (see Fig. 2-46). The periodontium, a connective tissue structure with its stratified squamous epithelium, attaches the teeth to the maxilla and the mandible and provides a continually adapting structure for the support of the teeth during function. The periodontium has two mineralized connective tissues, cementum and alveolar bone, and two fibrous connective tissues, the periodontal ligament and the lamina propria of the gingiva. The periodontium is attached to the jaws by alveolar bone and to the dentin of the tooth root by cementum.

Gingival Unit. As stated previously, the free and attached gingiva are masticatory mucosa. The *free gingiva* is the gingiva from the marginal crest to the level of the base of the gingival sulcus (see Fig. 2-46, *arrows 4 and 6).* The *gingival sulcus* is the space between the tooth and the free gingiva. The outer wall of the sulcus (inner wall of the free gingiva) is lined with a thin, nonkeratinized epithelium. The outer aspect of the free gingiva in each gingival embrasure is called the *gingival* or *interdental papilla.* The *free gingival groove* is a shallow groove that runs parallel to the marginal crest of the free gingiva and usually indicates the level of the base of the gingival sulcus (see Fig. 2-46, *arrow 7).*

The *attached gingiva,* a dense connective tissue with keratinized stratified squamous epithelium, extends from the depth of the gingival sulcus (free gingival groove) to the *mucogingival junction.* A dense network of collagenous fibers connects the attached gingiva firmly to the cementum and the periosteum of the alveolar process (bone).

The *alveolar mucosa* is a thin, soft tissue that is loosely attached to the underlying alveolar bone (see Fig. 2-46, *arrows 12 and 14).* It is covered by a thin, nonkeratinized epithelial layer. The underlying submucosa contains loosely arranged collagen fibers, elastic tissue, fat, and muscle tissue. The alveolar mucosa is delineated from the attached gingiva by the mucogingival junction and continues apically to the vestibular fornix and the inside of the cheek.

Attachment Apparatus. The tooth root is attached to the alveolus (bony socket) by the *periodontal ligament* (see Fig. 2-46, *arrow 11),* which is a complex, soft, connective tissue containing numerous cells, blood vessels, nerves, and an extracellular substance consisting of fibers and ground substance. The majority of the fibers are collagen, and the ground substance is composed of a variety of proteins and polysaccharides. The periodontal ligament serves the following functions: (1) attachment and support, (2) sensory, (3) nutritive, and (4) homeostatic. Bundles of the collagen fibers, known as the *principal fibers* of the ligament, serve to attach the cementum to the alveolar bone and act as a cushion to suspend and support the tooth. The portions of the principal fibers embedded in the cementum and alveolar bone are called *Sharpey's fibers.* Sensory function is provided by the nerve supply through an efficient proprioceptive

mechanism. The blood vessels supply the attachment apparatus with nutritive substances. Specialized cells of the ligament function to resorb and replace the cementum, periodontal ligament, and alveolar bone.

Cementum is a hard tissue with a calcified intercellular substance covering the anatomic roots of teeth; it has been discussed previously in this chapter.

The *alveolar process,* a part of the maxilla and mandible, forms, supports, and lines the sockets into which the roots of the teeth fit. Anatomically, no distinct boundary exists between the body of the maxilla or the mandible and the alveolar process. The tissue elements of the alveolar process are the same as for bone found elsewhere. The alveolar process is thin, compact bone with many small openings through which blood vessels, lymphatics, and nerves pass. As previously stated, both cementum and the alveolar bone contain Sharpey's fibers, the ends of the principal fibers of the periodontal ligament. The inner wall of the bony socket consists of the thin lamella of bone that surrounds the root of the tooth (and gives attachment to Sharpey's fibers). It is termed the *alveolar bone proper.* The second part of the bone is called *supporting alveolar bone,* which surrounds the alveolar bone proper and supports the socket. Supporting bone is made up of two parts: (1) the cortical plate, consisting of compact bone and forming the inner (lingual) and outer (facial) plates of the alveolar process, and (2) the spongy base that fills the area between the plates and the alveolar bone proper. Bone is composed of approximately 65% inorganic and 35% organic material. The inorganic material is hydroxyapatite; the organic material is primarily type I collagen (88% to 89%), which is surrounded by a ground substance of glycoproteins and proteoglycans.

Clinically, the level of the gingival attachment and gingival sulcus is an important factor in restorative dentistry. Soft tissue health must be maintained by the teeth having correct form and position if apical recession of the gingiva and possible abrasion and erosion of the roots are to be prevented. *The margin of a tooth preparation should not be positioned subgingivally (at levels between the marginal crest of the free gingiva and the base of the sulcus) unless dictated by caries, previous restoration, esthetics, or other preparation needs.*

OCCLUSION

Occlusion literally means "closing"; in dentistry, *occlusion* means the contact of teeth in opposing dental arches when the jaws are closed *(static occlusal relationships)* and during various jaw movements *(dynamic occlusal relationships).* The size of the jaws and arrangement of the teeth within the jaws are subject to a wide range of variation in humans. The locations of contacts between opposing teeth *(occlusal contacts)* vary as a result of differences in the size and shape of the teeth and jaws and the relative position of the jaws. A wide variety of occlusal schemes can be found in healthy individuals. Consequently, definition of an ideal occlusal scheme is fraught with difficulties.[3] Despite repeated attempts to describe an ideal occlusal scheme, descriptions are so restrictive that few individuals can be found to fit the criteria. Failing to find a single adequate definition of an ideal occlusal scheme, Carlsson et al concluded that "in the final analysis, optimal function and the absence of disease is the principal characteristic of a good occlusion."[3] The dental relationships described in this section conform to the concepts of normal or usual occlusal schemes and include common variations of tooth and jaw relationships. Fortunately, the masticatory system is highly adaptable and can function successfully over a wide range of differences in jaw size and tooth alignment. However, despite this great adaptability, many patients are highly sensitive to abrupt changes in tooth contacts, often brought about by restorative dental procedures. Some patients complain and seek correction of even very minor vertical discrepancies in occlusal contacts. Thus an operative dentist must understand the precise details of occlusion.

Occlusal contact patterns vary with the position of the mandible. Static occlusion is further defined by use of reference positions that include fully closed, terminal hinge closure, retruded, and right and left lateral extremes. The number and location of occlusal contacts between opposing teeth have important effects on the amount and direction of force applied during mastication and other mandibular clenching *(bruxing)* activities. In extreme cases, the forces can cause damage to the teeth or their supporting tissues. Forceful tooth contact occurs routinely very near the limits or borders of mandibular movement, thus showing the relevance of these reference positions.[6]

As stated previously, tooth contact during mandibular movement is termed the *dynamic occlusal relationship*. Gliding or sliding contacts occur during mastication and other mandibular movements. Gliding contacts may be advantageous or disadvantageous depending on the teeth involved and the position of the contacts. *The design of the restored tooth surface can have important effects on the number and location of occlusal contacts and must take into consideration both static and dynamic relationships.* The following sections discuss common arrangements of the teeth and masticatory system and the more common variations. Mastication and the contacting relationships of anterior and posterior teeth are described with reference to the potential restorative needs of the teeth.

GENERAL DESCRIPTION

Tooth Alignment and Dental Arches. In Fig. 2-47, *A, cusps* are drawn as blunt, rounded, or pointed projections of the crowns of the teeth. The posterior teeth have one, two, or three cusps near the facial and lingual surfaces of each tooth. Cusps are separated by distinct *developmental grooves* and sometimes have additional supplemental grooves on the cusp inclines. The facial cusps are separated from the lingual cusps by a deep groove termed the *central groove.* If a tooth has multiple facial cusps or multiple lingual cusps, the cusps are separated by facial or lingual developmental grooves, respectively. Depressions between the cusps are termed *fossae* (the singular form is *fossa).* Grooves having noncoalesced enamel are *fissures;* noncoalesced enamel in a fossa is a *pit.* Cusps in both jaws are aligned in a roughly parabolic curve. Usually the maxillary arch is larger than the mandibular arch, resulting in the maxillary cusps overlapping the mandibular cusps when the arches are in maximal occlusal contact (Fig. 2-47, *B*). In Fig. 2-47, *A,* two curved lines are drawn over the teeth to aid in the visualization of the arch form. These curved lines identify the alignment of similarly functioning cusps or fossae. On the left side of the arches, an imaginary arc connecting the row of facial cusps in the mandibular arch is drawn and labeled the *facial occlusal line.* Above that, an imaginary line connecting the maxillary central fossae is labeled the *central fossa occlusal line.* The mandibular facial occlusal line and the maxillary central fossa occlusal line coincide exactly when the mandibular arch is fully closed into the maxillary arch. On the right side of the dental arches, the maxillary lingual occlusal line and mandibular central fossa occlusal line are drawn and labeled. These lines also coincide when the mandible is fully closed.

In Fig. 2-47, *B,* the dental arches are fully interdigitated. Note again that the maxillary dental arch is larger than the mandibular arch, so the maxillary teeth overlap the mandibular teeth. The overlap of the maxillary cusps can be observed directly when the jaws are closed. *Maximum intercuspation* (MI) is the position of the mandible when the teeth are brought into full interdigitation with the maximal number of teeth contacting. Synonyms for MI include *intercuspal contact, acquired occlusion, habitual occlusion,* and *convenience occlusion.*

In Fig. 2-47, *C* (a proximal view), the mandibular facial occlusal line and the maxillary central fossa occlusal line coincide exactly. The maxillary lingual occlusal line and the mandibular central fossa occlusal line identified in Fig. 2-47, *A,* also are coincident. Cusps that contact the opposing teeth along the central fossa occlusal line are termed *supporting cusps (centric, holding,* or *stamp cusps);* the cusps that overlap the opposing teeth are termed *nonsupporting cusps (noncentric* or *nonholding cusps).* For example, the mandibular facial occlusal line identifies the mandibular supporting cusps, whereas the maxillary facial cusps are nonsupporting cusps. These terms are usually applied only to posterior teeth to distinguish the difference in function between the two rows of cusps. In some circumstances the functional role of the cusps can be reversed, as illustrated in Fig. 2-48, *C-2.*

A Dental arch cusp and fossa alignment

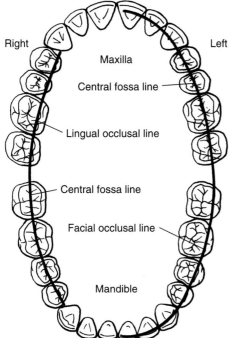

Right

Left

Maxilla

Central fossa line

Lingual occlusal line

Central fossa line

Facial occlusal line

Mandible

1. The maxillary lingual occlusal line and the mandibular central fossa line are coincident.
2. The mandibular facial occlusal line and the maxillary central fossa line are coincident.

B Maximum intercuspation (MI): the teeth in opposing arches are in maximal contact

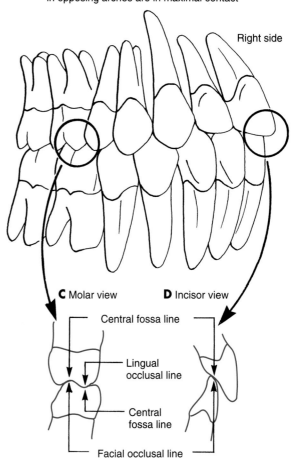

Right side

C Molar view   **D** Incisor view

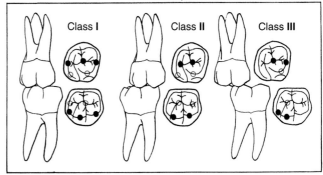

Central fossa line

Lingual occlusal line

Central fossa line

Facial occlusal line

E Facial view of anterior-posterior variations

Class **I**

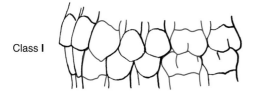

Class **II**

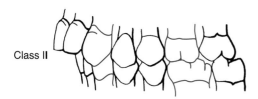

Class **III**

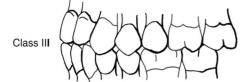

F Molar Classes **I**, **II**, and **III** relationships

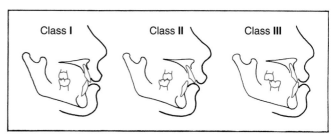

Class **I**   Class **II**   Class **III**

Class **I**   Class **II**   Class **III**

G Skeletal Classes **I**, **II**, and **III** relationships

FIG. **2-47** Dental arch relationships.

The posterior teeth are well suited to crushing food because of the mutual cusp-fossa contacts (see Fig. 2-49, *D*).

In Fig. 2-47, *D,* the anterior teeth are seen to have a different relationship in MI, but they also show the characteristic maxillary overlap. The incisor teeth are best suited to shearing food because of their overlap and the sliding contact on the lingual surface of the maxillary teeth. In MI, the mandibular incisors and canines contact the respective lingual surfaces of their maxillary opponents. *The amount of horizontal (overjet) and vertical (overbite) overlap (see Fig. 2-48, A-2) can significantly influence mandibular movement and thus influence the cusp design of restorations of posterior teeth* (discussed subsequently). Variations in growth (development) of the jaws and position of the anterior teeth result in openbite, where vertical or horizontal discrepancies prevent the teeth from contacting (see Fig. 2-48, inset *A-3*).

Anterior-Posterior Interarch Relationships. In Fig. 2-47, *E,* the cusp interdigitation pattern of the first molar teeth is used to classify anterior-posterior arch relationships using a system developed by Edward Angle.[1] During eruption of the teeth, the tooth cusps and fossae guide the teeth into maximal contact. Three interdigitated relationships of the first molars are commonly observed. (See Fig. 2-47, *F,* for an illustration of the occlusal contacts that result from different molar positions.) *The location of the mesiofacial cusp of the maxillary first molar in relation to the mandibular first molar is used as an indicator in Angle's classification.* The most common molar relationship finds the maxillary mesiofacial cusp located in the mesiofacial developmental groove of the mandibular first molar. This relationship is termed *Angle Class I.* Slight posterior positioning of the mandibular first molar results in the mesiofacial cusp of the maxillary molar settling into the facial embrasure between the mandibular first molar and the mandibular second premolar. This is termed *Class II* and occurs in approximately 20% of the U.S. population. Anterior positioning of the mandibular first molar relative to the maxillary first molar is termed *Class III* and is least common. In Class III relationships, the mesiofacial cusp of the maxillary first molar fits into the distofacial groove of the mandibular first molar. This occurs in 3% of the U.S. population. Significant differences in these percentages occur in other countries and in different racial and ethnic groups.

Although Angle classification is based on the relationship of the cusps, Fig. 2-47, *G,* illustrates that the location of the tooth roots in the alveolar bone determines the relative positions of the crowns and cusps. When the mandible is proportionally similar in size to the maxilla, a Class I molar relationship is formed; when the mandible is proportionally smaller than the maxilla, a Class II relationship is formed; and when the mandible is relatively greater than the maxilla, a Class III relationship is formed.

Interarch Tooth Relationships. Fig. 2-48 illustrates the occlusal contact relationships of individual teeth in more detail. In Fig. 2-48, *A-2, incisor overlap* is illustrated. The overlap is characterized in two dimensions, *horizontal overlap (overjet)* and *vertical overlap (overbite).* Differences in the size of the mandible and maxilla can result in clinically significant variations in incisor relationships, including: (1) openbite as a result of mandibular deficiency, (2) excessive eruption of the posterior teeth, or (3) mandibular growth excess (see Fig. 2-48, *A-3*). These variations have significant clinical effects on the contacting relationships of posterior teeth during various jaw movements, because the anterior teeth do not provide gliding contact. (See Fig. 2-58, *E* through *G,* for more details on the effects of the lack of anterior guidance.)

Fig. 2-48, *B-1,* illustrates a normal Class I occlusion in which each mandibular premolar is located one half of a tooth width anterior to its maxillary antagonist. This relationship results in the mandibular facial cusp contacting the maxillary premolar mesial marginal ridge and the maxillary premolar lingual cusp contacting the mandibular distal marginal ridge. Because only one antagonist is contacted, this is termed a *tooth-to-tooth relationship.* The most stable relationship results from the contact of the supporting cusp tips against the two marginal ridges, termed a *tooth-to-two-tooth contact.* Variations in the mesial-distal root position of the teeth will produce different relationships (see Fig. 2-48, *B-2*). When the mandible is slightly distal to the maxilla (termed a *Class II tendency*), each supporting cusp tip will occlude in a stable relationship with the opposing mesial or distal fossa; this relationship is a *cusp-fossa contact.*

Fig. 2-48, *C,* illustrates Class I molar relationships in more detail. Fig. 2-48, *C-1,* shows how cutting away the facial half of the maxillary molar reveals the mandibular facial cusp tips contacting the maxillary marginal ridges and the central fossa triangular ridges. A faciolingual longitudinal section reveals how the supporting cusps contact the opposing fossae and also shows the effect of the developmental grooves on reducing the height of the nonsupporting cusps opposite the supporting cusp tips. During lateral movements the supporting cusp can move through the facial and lingual developmental groove spaces. Faciolingual position variations are possible in molar relationships because of differences in growth of the width of the maxilla or the mandible. Fig. 2-48, *C-2,* illustrates normal molar contact position, facial crossbite, and lingual crossbite relationships. Facial crossbite in the posterior teeth is characterized by contact of the maxillary facial cusps in the opposing mandibular central fossae and the mandibular lingual cusps in the opposing maxillary central fossae. *Facial crossbite* (also termed *buccal crossbite)* results in reversal of the role of the cusps of the involved teeth. In

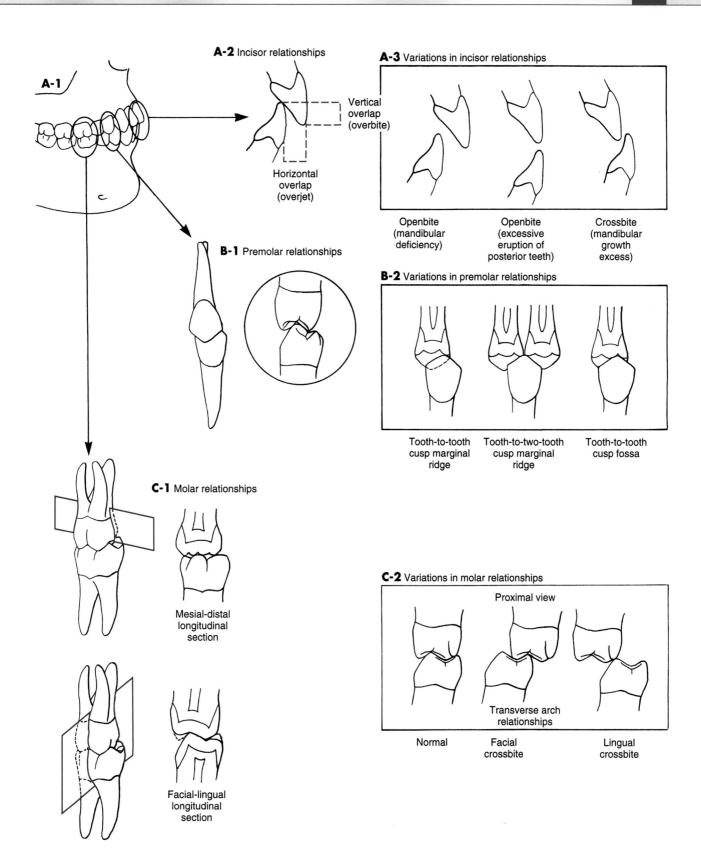

FIG. 2-48 Tooth relationships.

this reversal example, the mandibular lingual cusps and maxillary facial cusps become supporting cusps, and the maxillary lingual cusps and mandibular facial cusps become nonsupporting cusps. Lingual crossbite results in a very poor molar relationship that provides little functional contact.

Posterior Cusp Characteristics. Four *cusp ridges* can be identified as common features of all cusps. The outer incline of a cusp faces either the facial (or the lingual) surface of the tooth and is named for its respective surface. In the example using a mandibular second premolar (Fig. 2-49, *A*), the *facial cusp ridge* of the facial cusp is indicated by the line that points to the outer incline of the cusp. The inner inclines of posterior cusps face the central fossa or the central groove of the tooth. The inner incline cusp ridges are widest at the base and become narrower as they approach the cusp tip. For this reason, they are termed *triangular ridges.* The triangular ridge of the facial cusp of the mandibular premolar is indicated by the arrow to the inner incline. Triangular ridges are usually set off from the other cusp ridges by one or more supplemental groves. In Fig. 2-49, *B(1)* and *C(1)*, the outer inclines of the facial cusps of the mandibular and maxillary first molars are highlighted. In Fig. 2-49, *B(2)* and *C(2)*, the triangular ridges of the facial and lingual cusps are highlighted.

The *mesial* and *distal cusp ridges* extend from the cusp tip mesially and distally and are named for their direction. The mesial and distal cusp ridges extend downward from the cusp tips, forming the characteristic facial and lingual profiles of the cusps as viewed from the facial or lingual aspect. At the base of the cusp, the mesial or distal cusp ridge either abuts to another cusp ridge, forming a developmental groove/fissure, or the cusp ridge turns toward the center line of the tooth and fuses with the marginal ridge. *Marginal ridges* are elevated rounded ridges located on the mesial and distal edges of the tooth's occlusal surface (see Fig. 2-49, *A*). The *occlusal table* of posterior teeth is the area contained within the mesial and distal cusp ridges and marginal ridges of the tooth. The occlusal table limits are indicated in the drawings by a circumferential line connecting the highest point of curvature of these cusp ridges and marginal ridges.

Some cusps are modified to produce the characteristic form of individual posterior teeth. Mandibular first molars have longer triangular ridges on the distofacial cusps, causing a deviation of the central groove/fissure (see Fig. 2-49, *B[2]*). The mesiolingual cusp of a maxillary molar is much larger than the mesiofacial cusp. The distal cusp ridge of the maxillary first molar mesiolingual cusp curves facially to fuse with the triangular ridge of the distofacial cusp (see Fig. 2-49, *C[2]*). This junction forms the *oblique ridge*, which is characteristic of the maxillary molars. The transverse groove crosses the oblique ridge where the distal cusp ridge of the mesio-

lingual cusp meets the triangular ridge of the distofacial cusp. Textbooks on dental anatomy should be consulted for more detailed discussions of individual cusp variations.

Supporting Cusps. In Fig. 2-50, the lingual occlusal line of the maxillary teeth and the facial occlusal line of the mandibular teeth mark the locations of the *supporting cusps* (also termed *stamp cusps, centric holding cusps,* and *holding cusps*). These cusps contact the opposing teeth in their corresponding faciolingual center on a marginal ridge or a fossa. Supporting cusp–central fossa contact has been compared to a mortar and pestle because the supporting cusp cuts, crushes, and grinds fibrous food against the ridges forming the concavity of the fossa (see Fig. 2-49, *D*). Natural tooth form has multiple ridges and grooves ideally suited to aid in the reduction of the food bolus during chewing. During chewing, the highest forces and longest duration of contact occur at MI. Supporting cusps also serve to prevent drifting and passive eruption of the teeth; hence the term *holding cusp.*

Supporting cusps (see Fig. 2-50) can be identified by five characteristic features[9]:

They contact the opposing tooth in MI.
They support the vertical dimension of the face.
They are nearer the faciolingual center of the tooth than nonsupporting cusps.
Their outer incline has the potential for contact.
They have broader, more rounded cusp ridges than nonsupporting cusps.

Because the maxillary arch is larger than the mandibular arch, the supporting cusps are located on the maxillary lingual occlusal line (see Fig. 2-50, *D*), whereas the mandibular supporting cusps are located on the mandibular facial occlusal line (see Fig. 2-50, *A* and *B*). The supporting cusps of both arches are more robust and better suited to crushing food than the nonsupporting cusps. The lingual tilt of the posterior teeth increases the relative height of the supporting cusps with respect to the nonsupporting cusps (see Fig. 2-50, *C*), and the central fossa contacts of the supporting cusps are obscured by overlapping nonsupporting cusps (see Fig. 2-50, *E* and *F*). Removal of the nonsupporting cusps allows the supporting cusp–central fossa contacts to be studied (see Fig. 2-50, *G* and *H*). *During fabrication of restorations it is important that supporting cusps are not contacting the opposing teeth in a manner that results in lateral deflection of teeth. Rather, the restoration should provide contacts on plateaus or smoothly concave fossae so that masticatory forces are directed approximately parallel to the long axes of the teeth.*

Nonsupporting Cusps. Fig. 2-51 illustrates that nonsupporting cusps form a lingual occlusal line in the mandibular arch (see Fig. 2-51, *D*) and a facial occlusal line in the maxillary arch (see Fig. 2-51, *B*). *Nonsupporting cusps* (also termed *noncentric cusps* or *nonholding*

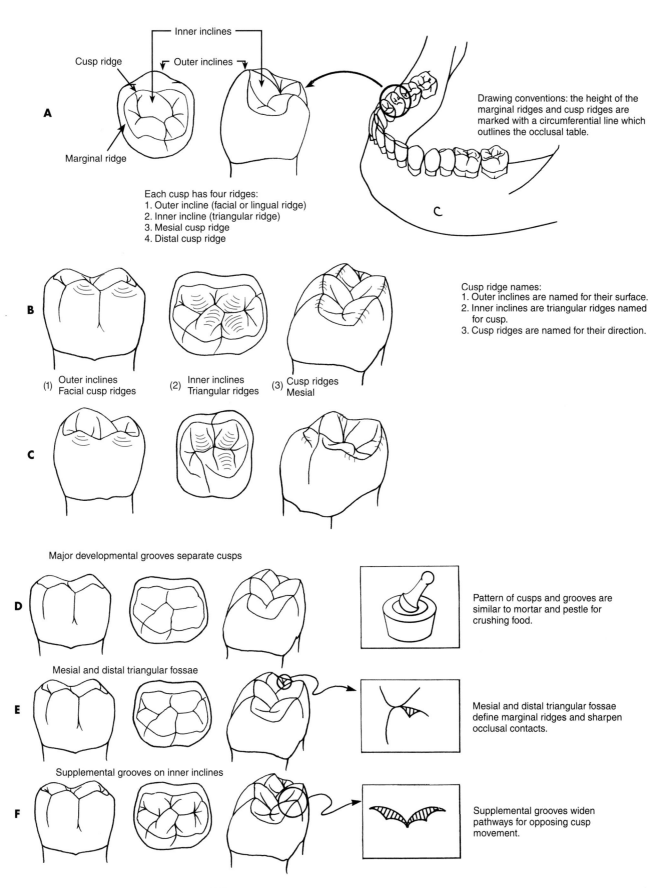

A

Inner inclines

Outer inclines

Cusp ridge

Marginal ridge

Drawing conventions: the height of the marginal ridges and cusp ridges are marked with a circumferential line which outlines the occlusal table.

C

Each cusp has four ridges:
1. Outer incline (facial or lingual ridge)
2. Inner incline (triangular ridge)
3. Mesial cusp ridge
4. Distal cusp ridge

B

(1) Outer inclines
Facial cusp ridges

(2) Inner inclines
Triangular ridges

(3) Cusp ridges
Mesial

Cusp ridge names:
1. Outer inclines are named for their surface.
2. Inner inclines are triangular ridges named for cusp.
3. Cusp ridges are named for their direction.

C

D Major developmental grooves separate cusps

Pattern of cusps and grooves are similar to mortar and pestle for crushing food.

E Mesial and distal triangular fossae

Mesial and distal triangular fossae define marginal ridges and sharpen occlusal contacts.

F Supplemental grooves on inner inclines

Supplemental grooves widen pathways for opposing cusp movement.

FIG. **2-49** Common features of all posterior teeth.

Synonyms for
supporting
cusps include:
1. Centric cusps
2. Holding cusps
3. Stamp cusps

A Mandibular arch

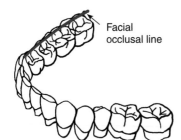

Facial
occlusal line

The mandibular arch is smaller than
the maxillary arch so the supporting
cusps are located on the facial occlusal
line. The mandibular lingual cusps that
overlap the maxillary teeth are
nonsupporting cusps.

B Mandibular right quadrant

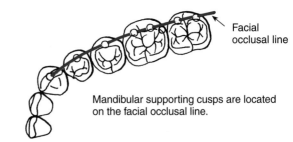

Facial
occlusal line

Mandibular supporting cusps are located
on the facial occlusal line.

C Proximal view of molar
teeth in oclusion

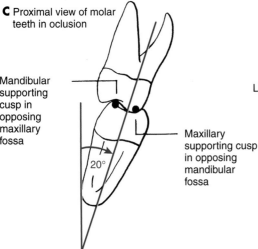

Mandibular
supporting
cusp in
opposing
maxillary
fossa

20°

Maxillary
supporting cusp
in opposing
mandibular
fossa

D Maxillary right quadrant

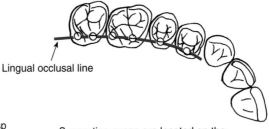

Lingual occlusal line

Supporting cusps are located on the
lingual occlusal line in maxillary arch.

E Lingual view of left dental arches in
occlusion

F Facial view of left dental arches in
occlusion

Supporting cusp features:
1. Contact opposing tooth in MI
2. Support vertical dimension
3. Nearer faciolingual center of
   tooth than nonsupporting
   cusps
4. Outer incline has potential for
   contact
5. More rounded than
   nonsupporting cusps

G Mandibular nonsupporting cusps
removed

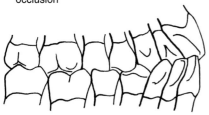

Maxillary supporting cusps occluding in
opposing fossae and on marginal ridges

H Maxillary nonsupporting cusps removed

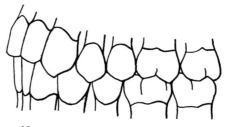

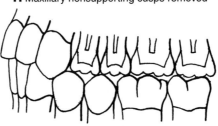

Mandibular supporting cusps occluding in
opposing fossae and on marginal ridges

FIG. **2-50** Supporting cusps.

cusps) overlap the opposing tooth without contacting the tooth. Nonsupporting cusps are located in the anterior-posterior plane in facial (lingual) embrasures or in the developmental groove of the opposing teeth, creating an alternating arrangement when the teeth are in maximum intercuspation (see Fig. 2-51, E and F). Maxillary premolar nonsupporting cusps also play an essential role in esthetics. When viewed from the occlusal, the nonsupporting cusps are farther from the faciolingual center of the tooth than supporting cusps. Nonsupporting cusps have sharper cusp ridges that apparently serve to shear food as they pass close to the supporting cusp ridges during chewing strokes. The overlap of the cusps helps keep the soft tissue of the tongue and cheeks out from the occlusal tables, preventing self-injury during chewing.

MECHANICS OF MANDIBULAR MOTION

Mandible and Temporomandibular Joints. The *mandible* articulates with a special depression in each temporal bone called the *glenoid fossa.* The joints are termed the *temporomandibular joints* because they are named for the two bones forming the articulation. The TMJs allow the mandible to move in all three planes (Fig. 2-52, A). A TMJ is similar to a ball-and-socket joint, but it differs from a true mechanical ball-and-socket in some important features. The ball part, the mandibular *condyle* (see Fig. 2-52, B), is smaller than the socket, or glenoid fossa. The space resulting from the size difference is filled by a tough, pliable, and movable stabilizer termed the *articular disk.* The disk separates the TMJ into two articulating surfaces lubricated by synovial fluid in the superior and inferior joint spaces. Rotational opening of the mandible occurs as the condyles rotate under the disks (see Fig. 2-52, C). Thus *rotational movement* occurs between the inferior surface of the disks and the condyle. During wide opening or protrusion of the mandible, the condyles move anteriorly in addition to the rotational opening (see Fig. 2-52, D and E). The disks move anteriorly with the condyles during opening and produce *sliding movement* in the superior joint space between the superior surface of the disks and the *articular eminences* (see Fig. 2-52, B). The TMJs allow free movement of the condyles in the anterior-posterior direction but resist lateral displacement. The disks are firmly attached to the medial and lateral poles of the condyles in normal, healthy TMJs (see Fig. 2-53, B). The disk-condyle arrangement of the TMJ thus allows both sliding and rotational movement in the same joint.

Because the mandible is a rigid, U-shaped bone with joints on both ends, movement of one joint will produce reciprocal movement in the other joint. The disk-condyle complex is free to move anterior-posteriorly, providing sliding movement between the disk and the glenoid fossa. One condyle may move anteriorly while the other remains in the fossa. Anterior movement of

only one condyle produces reciprocal lateral rotation in the opposite TMJ.

A TMJ cannot be expected to behave like a rigid joint as seen on *articulators* (mechanical devices used by dentists to simulate jaw movement and reference positions). Because soft tissues cover the two articulating bones and there is an intervening disk composed of soft tissue, some resilience is to be expected in the TMJs. In addition to resilience, some "play" or looseness can also be demonstrated in normal, healthy TMJs, allowing small posterior and lateral movements of the condyles. In healthy TMJs the movements are restricted to slightly less than 1 mm laterally and a few tenths of a millimeter posteriorly. This resilience and looseness can interfere with precise TMJ positioning, even in healthy joints; this is especially troublesome in diseased joints. TMJ looseness has made obsolete the concept of precise positioning of the condyle in the fossa. For this reason, the descriptive terms in this text are preferred.

When morphologic changes occur in the hard and soft tissues of a TMJ because of disease, the disk-condyle relationship is possibly altered in a number of ways, including deformation, loosening, perforation or tearing of the disk, and remodeling of the soft tissue articular surface coverings or their bony support. Diseased TMJs have unusual disk-condyle relationships, different geometry, and altered jaw movements and reference positions. Textbooks on TMJ disorders and occlusion should be consulted for information concerning evaluation of diseased joints. The remainder of this description of the movement and position of the mandible is based on normal, healthy TMJs and does not apply to diseased joints.

Mandibular Movement. Within certain limits, the mandible is free to move in three planes, providing six degrees of freedom of movement. This freedom of motion is greatest at the teeth and occurs to a lesser degree in the condyles. To describe mandibular motion, its direction and length must be specified in three mutually perpendicular planes. By convention these planes are sagittal, coronal (frontal), and transverse (horizontal) (see Fig. 2-52, A). The *midsagittal plane* is a vertical (longitudinal) plane that passes through the center of the head in an anterior-posterior direction. A vertical plane off the center line, such as a section through the TMJ, is termed a *parasagittal plane.* The *coronal plane* is a vertical plane perpendicular to the sagittal plane. The *transverse plane* is a horizontal plane that passes from anterior to posterior and is perpendicular to both the sagittal and frontal planes. Mandibular motion will be described in each of these planes.

Types of Motion. *Centric relation* (CR) is the position of the mandible when the condyles are positioned superiorly in the fossae in healthy TMJs. In this position the condyles articulate with the thinnest avascular portion of the disks and are in an anterior-superior position

A Maxillary arch

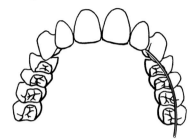

Synonyms for
nonsupporting
cusps include:
1. Noncentric cusps
2. Nonholding cusps

The maxillary arch is larger than the
mandibular arch causing the maxillary
facial line (nonsupporting cusps) to
overlap the mandibular teeth.

B Maxillary left quadrant

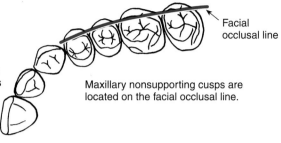

Facial
occlusal line

Maxillary nonsupporting cusps are
located on the facial occlusal line.

C Molar teeth in occlusion

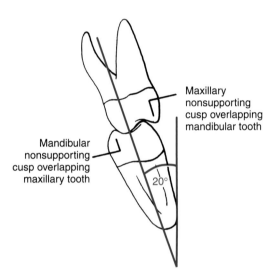

Maxillary
nonsupporting
cusp overlapping
mandibular tooth

Mandibular
nonsupporting
cusp overlapping
maxillary tooth

20°

D Mandibular left quadrant

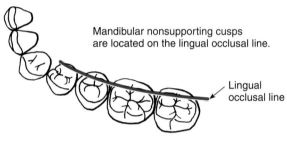

Mandibular nonsupporting cusps
are located on the lingual occlusal line.

Lingual
occlusal line

Nonsupporting cusp features:
1. Do not contact opposing tooth
   in MI
2. Keep soft tissue of tongue or
   cheek off occlusal table
3. Farther from faciolingual center
   of tooth than supporting cusps
4. Outer incline has no potential
   for contact
5. Have sharper cusp ridges than
   supporting cusps

E Views of left dental arches in occlusion
showing interdigitation of nonsupporting cusps

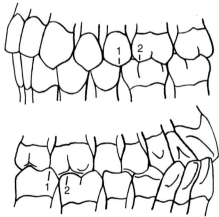

Nonsupporting cusp location:
1. Opposing embrasure
2. Opposing developmental groove

F Views of left dental arches in occlusion
showing facial and lingual occlusal lines

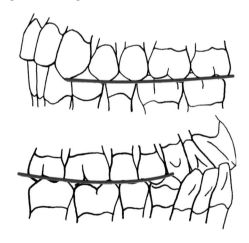

FIG. **2-51** Nonsupporting cusps.

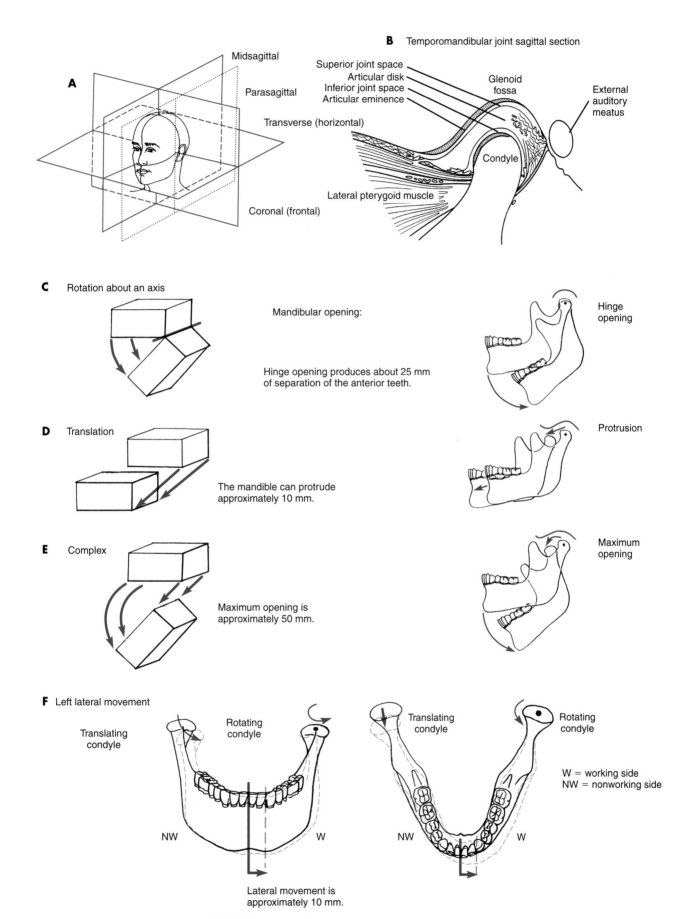

FIG. **2-52** Types and directions of motion of the mandible.

against the shapes of the articular eminences. This position is independent of tooth contacts. It has also been described as the most retruded position of the mandible from which lateral movements can be made, and the condyles are in the most posterior, unstrained position in the glenoid fossa.

Rotation is a simple motion of an object around an axis (see Fig. 2-52, *C*). The mandible is capable of rotation about an axis through centers located in the condyles. The attachments of the disks to the poles of the condyles permit the condyles to rotate under the disks. Rotation with the condyles positioned in CR is termed *terminal hinge* (TH) *movement.* TH is used in dentistry as a reference movement for construction of restorations and dentures. Initial contact between teeth during a TH closure provides a reference point, termed *centric occlusion* (CO). Many patients have a small slide from CO to MI, typically in a forward and superior direction. Maximum rotational opening in TH is limited to approximately 25 mm measured between the incisal edges of the anterior teeth.

Translation is the bodily movement of an object from one place to another (see Fig. 2-52, *D).* The mandible is capable of translation by anterior movement of the disk-condyle complex from the closed position over the articular eminence and back. Simultaneous, direct anterior movement of both condyles, or mandibular forward thrusting, is termed *protrusion.* The pathway followed by the anterior teeth during protrusion may not be smooth or straight because of contact between the anterior teeth and, sometimes, the posterior teeth. (See the superior border of Posselt's diagram in Fig. 2-53, *A.)* Protrusion is limited to approximately 10 mm by the ligamentous attachments of the masticatory muscles and the TMJs.

Fig. 2-52, *E,* illustrates *complex motion,* which combines rotation and translation in a single movement. Most mandibular movement during speech, chewing, and swallowing consists of both rotation and translation. The combination of rotation and translation allows the mandible to open 50 mm or more.

Fig. 2-52, *F,* illustrates *lateral movement* of the mandible. Left lateral movement of the mandible is illustrated. It is the result of forward translation of the right condyle and rotation of the left condyle. Right lateral movement of the mandible is the result of forward translation of the left condyle and rotation of the right condyle.

CAPACITY OF MOTION OF THE MANDIBLE

In 1952, Ulf Posselt described the capacity of motion of the mandible.[19] Using a system of clutches and flags, he was able to record the mandible's motion. The resultant diagram has been termed *Posselt's diagram* (Fig. 2-53, *A).* By necessity, the original recordings of mandibular movement were done outside of the mouth, which mag-

nified the vertical dimension but not the horizontal dimension. Modern systems using digital computer techniques can record mandibular motion in actual time and dimensions and then compute and draw the motion as it occurred at any point in the mandible and teeth.[7] This makes it possible to accurately reconstruct mandibular motion simultaneously at several points. Three of these points are particularly significant clinically— the incisor point, molar point, and condyle point (see Fig. 2-54, *A, i, m, c).*[6] The *incisor point* is located on the midline of the mandible at the junction of the facial surface of the mandibular central incisors and the incisal edge. The *molar point* is the tip of the mesiofacial cusp of the mandibular first molar on a specified side. The *condyle point* is the center of rotation of the mandibular condyle on the specified side.

Limits of Mandibular Motion: the Borders. In Fig. 2-53, *A,* the limits for movement of the incisor point are illustrated in the sagittal plane. The mandible is not drawn to scale with the drawing of the sagittal borders. Also, in this particular diagram, CO equals MI. (As mentioned, in some patients there may be a small slide from CO to MI.) The starting point for this diagram is CO, the first contact of teeth when the condyles are in CR. The posterior border of the diagram from CO to *a* in Fig. 2-53, *A,* is formed by rotation of the mandible around the condyle points. This border from CO to *a* is TH movement. *Hinge axis* is the term used to describe an imaginary line connecting the centers of rotation in the condyles (condyle points) and is useful for reference to articulators. *Hinge-axis closure* is a reference movement used in prosthetic dentistry and is only valid when the disks are properly positioned in the fossae. The inferior limit to this hinge opening occurs at approximately 25 mm and is indicated by *a* in Fig. 2-53, *A.* The superior limit of the posterior border occurs at the first tooth contact and is identified by CO. *In most healthy adults, a sliding tooth contact movement positions the mandible slightly anteriorly from CO into MI (see Fig. 2-54, B).*

Terminal hinge, centric relation, and *centric occlusion* are terms surrounded by controversy and unresolved issues.[4] Controversies include the following questions: Is CR a strained or unstrained position? Should the mandible be guided into this position by the dentist? If so, how should the mandible be grasped, shoved, or supported into position? Should only the patient's muscles be used to guide the mandible into position? Should mechanical devices such as jigs, tongue blades, or plastic shims be used to guide the mandible into position? How is CR defined in disease states such as degenerative joint disease, arthritic remodeling, or disk displacement? *It is important to remember that CR is a position determined by the condyles superiorly positioned in the glenoid fossae, independent of tooth contact. TH is rotation when the condyles are in CR. CO is the first tooth contact as the mandible closes in TH.*

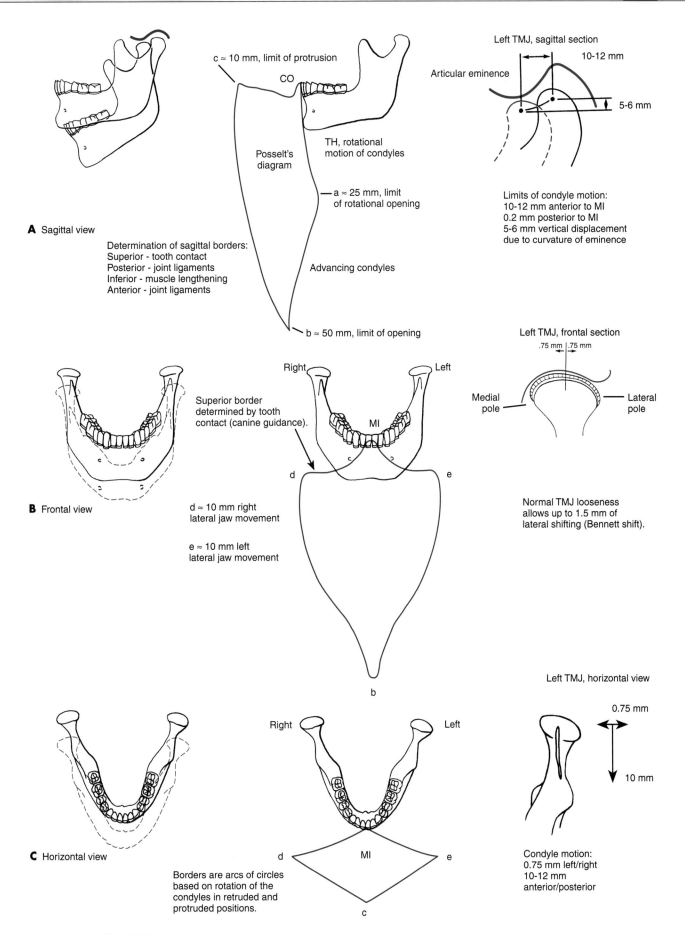

A Sagittal view

c ≈ 10 mm, limit of protrusion

CO

Posselt's diagram

TH, rotational motion of condyles

a ≈ 25 mm, limit of rotational opening

Advancing condyles

b ≈ 50 mm, limit of opening

Determination of sagittal borders:
Superior - tooth contact
Posterior - joint ligaments
Inferior - muscle lengthening
Anterior - joint ligaments

Left TMJ, sagittal section

10-12 mm

Articular eminence

5-6 mm

Limits of condyle motion:
10-12 mm anterior to MI
0.2 mm posterior to MI
5-6 mm vertical displacement
due to curvature of eminence

B Frontal view

Right   Left

MI

d   e

b

Superior border determined by tooth contact (canine guidance).

d ≈ 10 mm right lateral jaw movement

e ≈ 10 mm left lateral jaw movement

Left TMJ, frontal section

.75 mm | .75 mm

Medial pole   Lateral pole

Normal TMJ looseness allows up to 1.5 mm of lateral shifting (Bennett shift).

C Horizontal view

Right   Left

d   MI   e

c

Borders are arcs of circles based on rotation of the condyles in retruded and protruded positions.

Left TMJ, horizontal view

0.75 mm

10 mm

Condyle motion:
0.75 mm left/right
10-12 mm anterior/posterior

FIG. **2-53** Capacity of motion of the mandible. (Mandible drawings are not to scale with border diagrams.)

At point *a* in Fig. 2-53, *A,* further rotation of the condyles is impossible due to the limits of stretch of the joint capsule, ligamentous attachments to the condyles, and the mandible-opening muscles. The limit of pure rotational opening is very close to 25 mm in adults. Further opening can be achieved only by translation of the condyles anteriorly, producing the line *a-b.* Maximum opening (point *b*) in adults is approximately 50 mm. These measures are important diagnostically. For example, mandibular opening limited to 25 mm suggests blockage of condylar translation, usually the result of disk disorders. Limitation of opening in the 35 to 45 mm range is suggestive of muscular limitation. *Changes in mandibular opening are useful measures of the course of disorders involving the TMJs and the muscles of mastication.* The line *CO-a-b* represents the maximum retruded opening path. This is the *posterior border,* or the posterior limit of mandibular opening. The line *b-c* represents the *maximum protruded closure.* This is achieved by a forward thrust of the mandible that keeps the condyles in their maximum anterior positions while arcing the mandible closed.

Retrusion, or posterior movement of the mandible, results in the irregular line *c-CO.* The irregularities of the superior border are due to tooth contacts; thus the *superior border* is a tooth-determined border. *Protrusion* is a reference mandibular movement starting from *CO* and proceeding anteriorly to point *c.* Protrusive mandibular movements are used by dentists to evaluate occlusal relationships of the teeth and restorations. The complete diagram, *CO-a-b-c-CO,* represents the maximum possible motion of the incisor point in all directions in the sagittal plane. *The area of most interest to dentists is the superior border produced by tooth contact.* (Mandibular movement in the sagittal plane is illustrated in more detail in Fig. 2-54.)

The motion of the condyle point during chewing is strikingly different from the motion of the incisor point. *Motion of the condyle point is a curved line that follows the articular eminence.* The maximum protrusion of the condyle point is 10 to 12 mm anteriorly when following the downward curve of the articular eminence. *The condyle point does not drop away from the eminence during mandibular movements.* Thus chewing movements in the sagittal plane are characterized by a nearly vertical up-and-down motion of the incisor point, whereas the condyle points move anteriorly and then return posteriorly over a curved surface (see Fig. 2-54, *B*).

In the frontal view shown in Fig. 2-53, *B,* the incisor point and chin are capable of moving about 10 mm to the left or right. This lateral movement (sometimes termed an *excursion)* is indicated by the lines *MI-d* to the right and *MI-e* to the left. Points *d* and *e* indicate the limit of lateral motion of the incisor point. *Lateral movement* is often described with respect to only one side of the mandible for the purpose of defining the relative motion of the mandibular to the maxillary teeth. For example, in a left lateral movement, the left mandibular teeth move away from the midline and the right mandibular teeth move toward the midline. Mandibular pathways directed away from the midline are termed *working* (synonyms include *laterotrusion* and *function*), and mandibular pathways directed toward the midline are termed *nonworking* (synonyms include *mediotrusion, nonfunction,* and *balancing*). The terms *working* and *nonworking* are based on observations of chewing movements where the mandible is seen to shift during closure toward the side of the mouth containing the food bolus. Thus the working side is used to crush food while the nonworking side is without a food bolus.

The left lateral mandibular motion indicated by the line *MI-e* (see Fig. 2-53, *B*) is the result of rotation of the left condyle (working-side condyle) and translation of the right condyle (nonworking-side condyle) to its anterior limit (see Fig. 2-52, *F*). The translation of the nonworking condyle in a right lateral motion of the mandible can be seen in the horizontal view in Fig. 2-55, *A* and *B.* The line *e-b* in Fig. 2-53, *B,* is completed by mandibular opening that is the result of rotation of both condyles and translation of the working condyle to its maximum anterior position. Line *b-d-MI* represents similar motions on the right side.

The vertical displacement in the incisor point line from *MI* to *e* or *d,* shown in Fig. 2-53, *B,* is the result of the teeth, usually the canines, gliding over each other. Vertical displacement of the mandible due to gliding contact of the canine teeth is termed *canine guidance* and has significance for restorative procedures. *The gliding tooth contact supplied by canine guidance provides some of the vertical separation of the posterior teeth during lateral jaw movements and prevents potentially damaging collisions of their cusps.* When the canine guidance is shallow, the occlusal surface of the posterior teeth must be altered to prevent potentially damaging contacts in lateral movements. An articulator aids in evaluation of the posterior tooth relationships during construction of posterior restorations.

There is some laxity in the TMJs; consequently the condyles can move slightly to the working side during the closing stroke. This lateral shift of the condyle points, illustrated in the frontal view of a right TMJ in Fig. 2-53, *B,* is termed *Bennett shift* or *lateral shift.* This shift is variable from patient to patient and is a measure of the looseness of the TMJs (Fig. 2-55, *B* through *D*). The magnitude of the shift in normal TMJs varies from 0 to 1.5 mm and normally has little effect on the posterior teeth. Excessive lateral shift is associated with morphologic changes of the TMJs. However, excessive lateral condylar shifting coupled with shallow canine guidance poses a significant problem for restorative procedures because the resulting lateral mandibular movements are very flat; consequently,

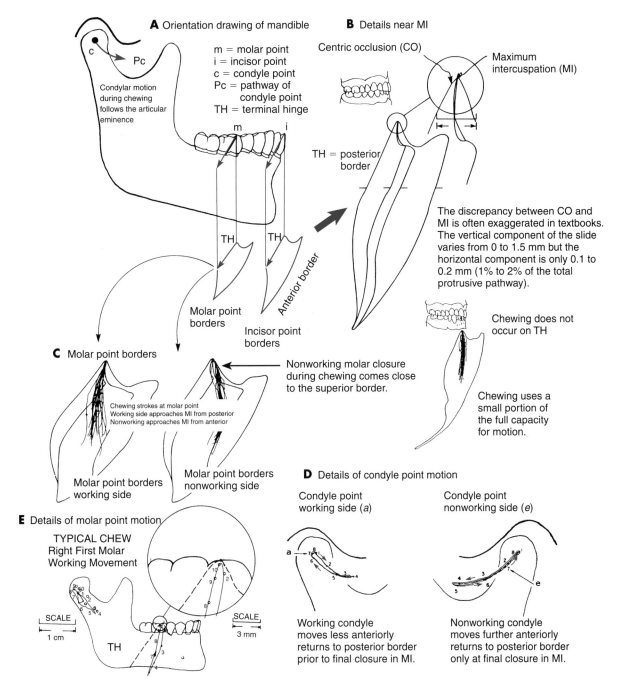

A Orientation drawing of mandible

m = molar point
i = incisor point
c = condyle point
Pc = pathway of
     condyle point
TH = terminal hinge

Condylar motion
during chewing
follows the articular
eminence

B Details near MI

Centric occlusion (CO)

Maximum
intercuspation (MI)

TH = posterior
border

The discrepancy between CO and
MI is often exaggerated in textbooks.
The vertical component of the slide
varies from 0 to 1.5 mm but the
horizontal component is only 0.1 to
0.2 mm (1% to 2% of the total
protrusive pathway).

Chewing does not
occur on TH

Chewing uses a
small portion of
the full capacity
for motion.

Molar point
borders

Incisor point
borders

Anterior border

C Molar point borders

Nonworking molar closure
during chewing comes close
to the superior border.

Chewing strokes at molar point
Working side approaches MI from posterior
Nonworking approaches MI from anterior

Molar point borders
working side

Molar point borders
nonworking side

D Details of condyle point motion

Condyle point
working side (a)

Condyle point
nonworking side (e)

Working condyle
moves less anteriorly
returns to posterior border
prior to final closure in MI.

Nonworking condyle
moves further anteriorly
returns to posterior border
only at final closure in MI.

E Details of molar point motion

TYPICAL CHEW
Right First Molar
Working Movement

SCALE
1 cm

TH

SCALE
3 mm

FIG. **2-54** Mandibular capacity for motion: sagittal view. (**B** through **D** from Gibbs CH, Lundeen HC:
Jaw movements and forces during chewing and swallowing and their clinical significance. In Lundeen HC, Gibbs CH, editors: Advances in occlusion, Bristol, 1982, John Wright PSG.)

little separation of the posterior teeth occurs (see Figs. 2-57 through 2-60).

In Fig. 2-53, *C*, the horizontal view illustrates the capability of the mandible to translate anteriorly. Extreme left lateral motion is indicated by *MI-e* produced by rotation of the left condyle (working condyle) and translation of the right condyle (nonworking condyle) to its anterior limit. From point *e,* protrusion of the left condyle moves the incisor point to *c,* the maximum protruded

position. If there is looseness in the TMJs, lateral shift of the mandible also will be seen in this view. Lateral shifting can be seen in normal chewing movements in Figs. 2-55 and 2-56.

Sagittal View. In Fig. 2-54, the drawing of the mandible is used to orient the sagittal border diagrams. Projected below the mandible are diagrams of the incisor point (*i*) and molar point (*m*) borders (see Fig. 2-54, *A*). The molar point borders are similar to the incisor

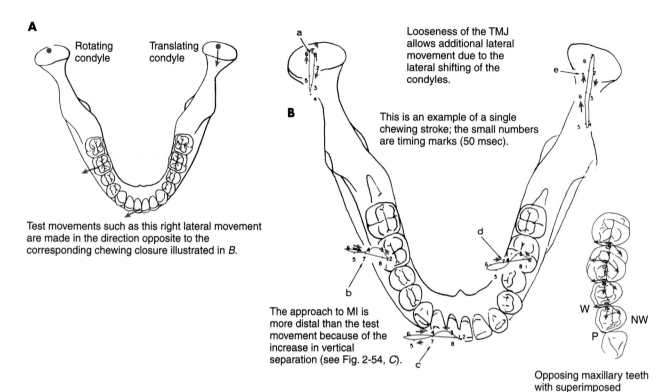

Lateral movement is produced by anterior translation of one condyle, producing rotation about the center in the opposite condyle.

A

Rotating condyle   Translating condyle

Test movements such as this right lateral movement are made in the direction opposite to the corresponding chewing closure illustrated in *B*.

Looseness of the TMJ allows additional lateral movement due to the lateral shifting of the condyles.

B

This is an example of a single chewing stroke; the small numbers are timing marks (50 msec).

The approach to MI is more distal than the test movement because of the increase in vertical separation (see Fig. 2-54, *C*).

Opposing maxillary teeth with superimposed working (W), non-working (NW), and protrusion (P) test movements.

Nonworking condyle movement:
1. Condylar translation with rotation about the center of the opposite condyle
2. Solid line indicates the change in the condylar path due to progressive shifting of the center of rotation in the opposite condyle
3. Solid line indicates the condylar path resulting from immediate shifting of the center of rotation of the opposite condyle
4. Observed motion of the condyle during chewing: note shifting as closing is initiated and the return to normal position at the end of closure

Effect of shifting at first molar:
1. Little change on working side
2. Wide lateral motion on nonworking side

Left lateral movement with shifting

D

The nonworking pathway of the maxillary mesiolingual cusp makes a wider path over the mandibular molar (compare with Fig. 2-59, *E* and *F*).

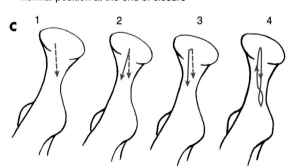

C   1   2   3   4

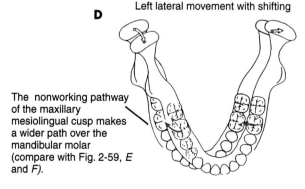

FIG. **2-55** Mandibular capacity for motion: horizontal view. (**B** *from Gibbs CH, Lundeen HC: Jaw movements and forces during chewing and swallowing and their clinical significance. In Lundeen HC, Gibbs CH, editors:* Advances in occlusion, *Bristol, 1982, John Wright PSG.)*

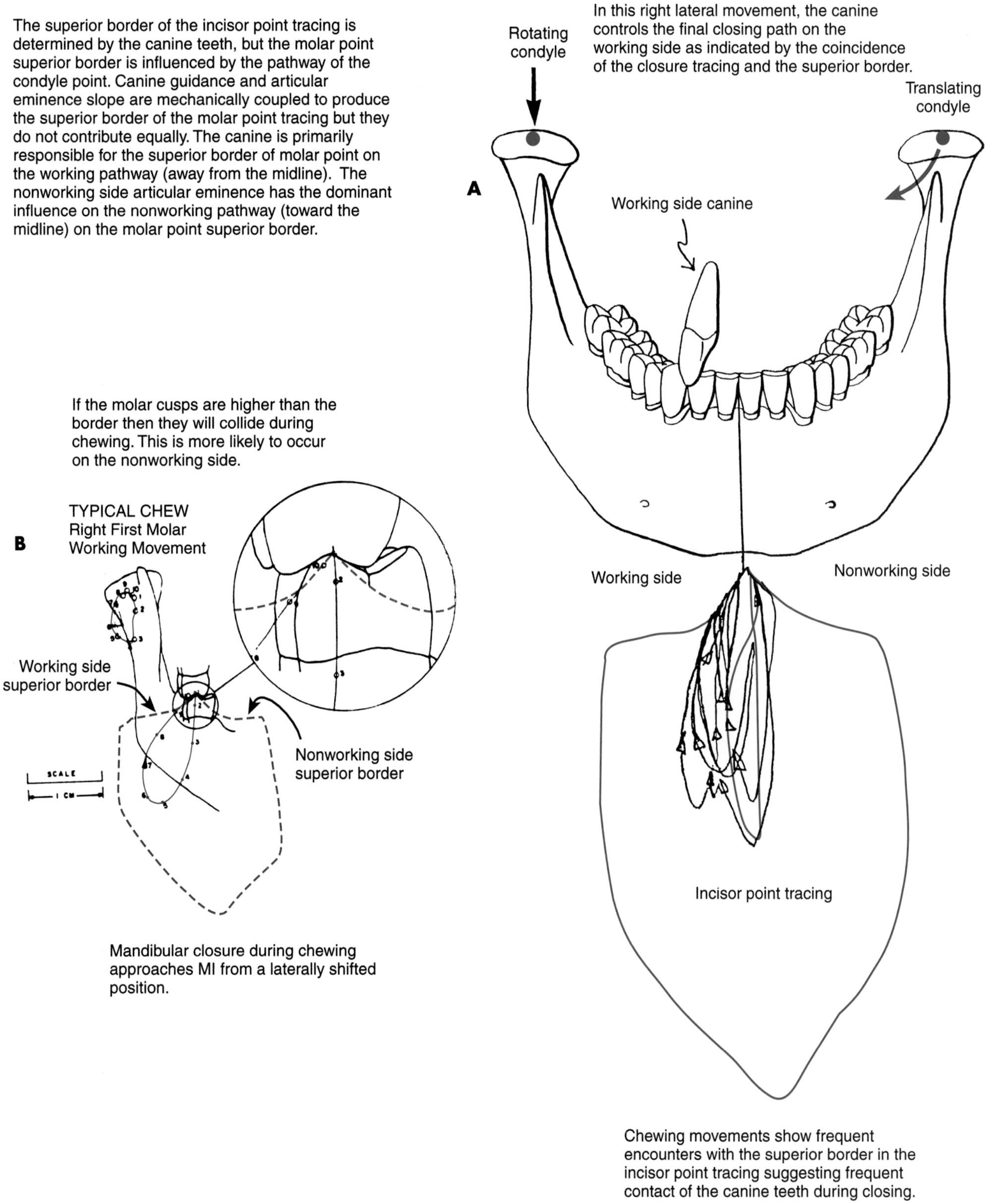

The superior border of the incisor point tracing is determined by the canine teeth, but the molar point superior border is influenced by the pathway of the condyle point. Canine guidance and articular eminence slope are mechanically coupled to produce the superior border of the molar point tracing but they do not contribute equally. The canine is primarily responsible for the superior border of molar point on the working pathway (away from the midline). The nonworking side articular eminence has the dominant influence on the nonworking pathway (toward the midline) on the molar point superior border.

In this right lateral movement, the canine controls the final closing path on the working side as indicated by the coincidence of the closure tracing and the superior border.

Rotating condyle

Translating condyle

A

Working side canine

If the molar cusps are higher than the border then they will collide during chewing. This is more likely to occur on the nonworking side.

TYPICAL CHEW
Right First Molar
Working Movement

B

Working side superior border

Nonworking side superior border

SCALE
1 CM

Mandibular closure during chewing approaches MI from a laterally shifted position.

Working side

Nonworking side

Incisor point tracing

Chewing movements show frequent encounters with the superior border in the incisor point tracing suggesting frequent contact of the canine teeth during closing.

FIG. **2-56** Mandibular capacity for motion: frontal view. (**B** *from Gibbs CH, Lundeen HC: Jaw movements and forces during chewing and swallowing and their clinical significance. In Lundeen HC, Gibbs CH, editors:* Advances in occlusion, *Bristol, 1982, John Wright PSG.)*

point diagram but are shorter in the vertical dimension because the molar point is closer to the TMJ. Closure of the jaw on the posterior border is termed *terminal hinge closure.* TH closure is a simple arc of a circle with a radius equal to the length from the incisor point to the center of the hinge axis (condyle point *c*). The area near MI is enlarged to illustrate the details of the TH closure (see Fig. 2-54, *B*). CO and MI are located in very close proximity. In the magnified view, the teeth can be seen to guide the mandible from CO to MI. The gliding (sliding) contact typically occurs on the first premolars and is 1 to 2 mm long. The horizontal component of this slide is only a few tenths of a millimeter in healthy joints. However, this has been exaggerated in many textbooks, and many dentists do not recognize that the horizontal component of the slide is much smaller than the observed diagonal slide. Traditionally, the discrepancy between CO and MI has been a source of debate in dentistry, resulting in extensive literature on the topic.[4] This CO-MI controversy is the result of misinterpretation of the inherent resiliency or looseness of normal, healthy TMJs. Failure to recognize that some patients have damaged TMJs can further add to confusion concerning the significance of the CO-MI controversy. *Damage to the TMJs as a consequence of arthritic processes or internal derangements increases the looseness of the joints and changes the relationship of CO to MI.*

Chewing movements at the incisor point involve an almost vertical opening and then a loop slightly to the posterior on closing, using only a small percentage of the total area of the sagittal border diagram. During chewing, the only border contact occurs at MI. The closing strokes never approach TH, indicating that at least one condyle (on the nonworking side) remains advanced during the closing stroke. The condyle point moves along the pathway *Pc* during all movements other than TH. In contrast to the nearly vertical closing strokes at incisor point, the sagittal closing strokes at the molar point involve an anterior component on the working side and a posterior component on the nonworking side. This difference in molar point movement is due to the deviation of the jaw to the working side during closure, illustrated by the difference in motion of the working- and nonworking-side condyles. The nonworking side closing strokes closely approach the superior border, indicating the potential for undesirable contact on the nonworking side (see Fig. 2-54, *C*).

Horizontal View. Fig. 2-55, *A,* shows a horizontal view (or occlusal view when referring to the teeth) of the mandible with superimposed incisor, molar, and condyle point test movements. Chewing movements are characterized by wide lateral movement of the mandible to the working side during closure (see Fig. 2-55, *B*). When viewed from above, the pathways of the molar and incisor points are typically in a figure-eight pattern with an S-shaped lateral opening motion and a

straight medial closing stroke. There are important differences in the directions of closure for the molar point on the working and nonworking sides. During closure on the working side (labeled *b* in Fig. 2-55, *B*), the mandibular teeth medially approach the maxillary teeth from a slightly posterior position and move slightly anteriorly into MI. On the contralateral side (the nonworking side, labeled *d* in Fig. 2-55, *B*), the mandibular molar teeth during closure approach, in a medial-to-lateral direction, the maxillary teeth from a slightly anterior position and move slightly posteriorly into MI. The closing strokes are the same pathways generated by guided (test) lateral mandibular movements used to check the occlusion, except the directions traveled are opposite (see Fig. 2-55, *B, inset*). On the inset drawing of the maxillary left teeth in Fig. 2-55, the working, nonworking, and protrusive pathways are marked *W, NW,* and *P* respectively. *These are the guided test movements employed by dentists to assess the occlusal function of the teeth.*

The horizontal, enlarged view of the mandible showing condyle point movement (working side labeled *a;* nonworking side labeled *e*) during chewing is important because it illustrates the lateral shift of the condyles during the closing stroke (see Fig. 2-55, *B*). Opening, in the typical chewing motion illustrated here, involves movement of both condyle points on the midsagittal path, producing the vertical drop in the incisor point seen in the sagittal view. Lateral opening may be seen in normal children and adults with worn and flattened teeth. As closing is initiated, the mandible shifts laterally, moving both condyle points to the working side. The nonworking condyle movement closely approaches its medial border during the closing stroke (see Fig. 2-55, *C*). During final closure, when the teeth are bought into MI, the condyle points return to their starting positions. Contact and gliding on the inclines of the teeth are responsible for bringing the mandible into its final, fully closed position (MI).

Allowance for lateral displacement of the condyles during lateral jaw movements is built into semiadjustable articulators. In older models, this usually takes the form of a Bennett angle or progressive lateral shift adjustment. The progressive lateral shift allows the condyles to shift gradually during lateral mandibular movement. As a result of mandibular movement studies, more recent articulator models have replaced the progressive lateral shift with immediate shift. (For more details on setting the medial wall of the condylar housing, see Fig. 2-59 and the later section Articulators and Mandibular Movements.) Shifting of the mandible, as depicted by the shift in the condyle points, results in a similar shift at the teeth that cannot be simulated by progressive shift (see Fig. 2-55, *C*).

Frontal View. In Fig. 2-56, *A,* lateral movement of the mandible on the superior border is controlled by three elements: the rotating condyle, the translating condyle, and the working-side canine. During chewing closures, the mandibular teeth approach the maxillary teeth from a lateral position. Frequent contact with the border occurs in the incisor and molar point tracings, indicating that lateral tooth gliding is common during chewing. This gliding contact occurs on the teeth having the highest projecting cusps that form the superior border (usually the canine teeth).

The incisor point tracing is projected below the drawing of the mandible in Fig. 2-56, *A*. The chewing strokes show the gliding contact on the border. The incisor-point superior border is shaped by the lingual surfaces of the guiding teeth, which most frequently are the maxillary canine teeth. In Fig. 2-56, *B*, the lateral side of the molar-point superior border is shaped by the working-side tooth guidance, which is usually the maxillary canine. The medial side of the molar-point superior border is predominately formed by the nonworking condyle moving over the articular eminence. The shape of the superior border at the molar point is the critical factor for determining the location and height of the molar cusps during restorative procedures. It is easy to visualize the effect of changes in cusp height when viewing the closeup of the molar teeth in the magnified inset.

ARTICULATORS AND MANDIBULAR MOVEMENTS

Figs. 2-57 to 2-60 illustrate the scientific basis for the use of articulators to aid in diagnostic evaluation of occlusion and fabrication of dental restorations. In these figures, the characteristics of chewing movements and dentist-guided test movements are compared with the characteristics of movements produced by simple articulators. This can be done by comparing the cusp movement near MI produced by the articulator with the cusp movement observed in chewing studies or guided movements. Additionally, the changes in cusp movement near MI because of variation in the adjustment of articulators are discussed with respect to their effects on dental restorations.

Fig. 2-57 illustrates the relationship between condylar movement and articulator settings. Together, the horizontal condylar guidance setting and the medial-wall setting of an articulator supply sufficient information to simulate the condyle point movement near MI. The *horizontal condylar guidance setting approximates the slope of the articular eminence; the medial-wall setting approximates the lateral shift. Collectively these two settings are referred to as the posterior guidance.*

Posterior guidance alone is not sufficient to simulate mandibular movements near MI because tooth guidance is also involved in forming the superior border. Full-arch casts mounted in the articulator supply the information concerning *anterior guidance* from the canine and the incisor teeth. The mechanical coupling of the

anterior guidance and posterior guidance settings provides sufficient information to simulate movement of the posterior teeth on the superior border. *The articulator can then be used to diagnose the need to alter the anterior guidance and to design restorations that avoid cusp collisions in mandibular movements.*

In Fig. 2-58, *horizontal condylar guidance* is used to describe the shape of the pathway of condyle point movement in the anterior-posterior direction. The condyles move in contact with the curved surface of the articular eminence. More recent designs of semiadjustable articulators have adopted curved surfaces to simulate the curvature of the articular eminence. Rotation of the condylar housing downward increases the slope of the guiding surface of the articulator. The range of adjustment of horizontal condylar inclination is well within the range of measured movements in human subjects (see Fig. 2-58, *A* and *B*).[14] Although there may be differences in the relative anterior movement of the two condyles (see Fig. 2-58, *C* and *D*), only the first few millimeters of movement have significant effects on the posterior teeth.

Horizontal condylar guidance and anterior guidance (supplied by the mounted casts) are mechanically coupled to produce separation of the posterior teeth. The combined guidance determines the amount of (or lack of) vertical separation of the posterior teeth as the mandible leaves or enters MI during protrusion and lateral movements.

Lateral mandibular movements also produce separation of the posterior teeth. Horizontal guidance of the nonworking condyle coupled with working-side canine guidance determines the amount of vertical separation of the posterior teeth on both sides as the mandible leaves or enters MI during lateral movements (see Fig. 2-56 for details). This information can be used to design restorations with the proper cusp location and height to avoid collisions during chewing and other mandibular movements.

The slope of the articular eminence varies considerably among individuals. The effect of different slopes can be evaluated by altering the horizontal condylar guidance on articulators. Increasing the horizontal condylar guidance increases the steepness of the mandibular molar movement (molar point) in protrusion. The movement of the maxillary mesiolingual cusp relative to the mandibular molar is plotted in Fig. 2-58, *E* through *G*, for 20-, 30-, and 50-degree slopes.[11] The effect of removing the anterior guidance (*a*) is also drawn on the same grid. The loss of anterior guidance has the greatest effect when the horizontal condylar guidance is shallow (20 degrees) and has the least effect when the horizontal condylar guidance is steep (50 degrees). *Anterior guidance has an additive effect on the molar pathway at all degrees of horizontal guidance. This is an important observation because anterior guidance often can be changed by*

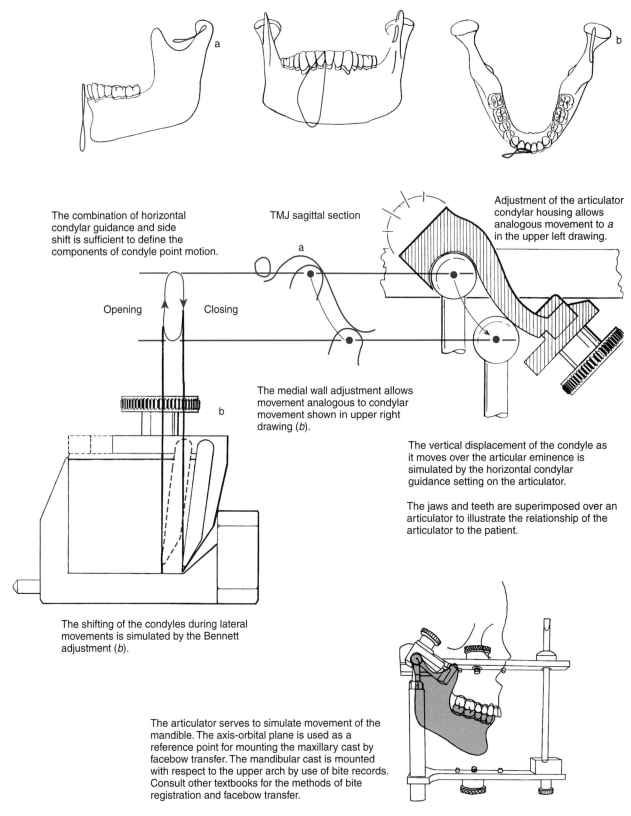

The combination of horizontal condylar guidance and side shift is sufficient to define the components of condyle point motion.

TMJ sagittal section

Adjustment of the articulator condylar housing allows analogous movement to *a* in the upper left drawing.

Opening   Closing

The medial wall adjustment allows movement analogous to condylar movement shown in upper right drawing (*b*).

The vertical displacement of the condyle as it moves over the articular eminence is simulated by the horizontal condylar guidance setting on the articulator.

The jaws and teeth are superimposed over an articulator to illustrate the relationship of the articulator to the patient.

The shifting of the condyles during lateral movements is simulated by the Bennett adjustment (*b*).

The articulator serves to simulate movement of the mandible. The axis-orbital plane is used as a reference point for mounting the maxillary cast by facebow transfer. The mandibular cast is mounted with respect to the upper arch by use of bite records. Consult other textbooks for the methods of bite registration and facebow transfer.

FIG. **2-57** The relationship between condylar motion and articulator settings.

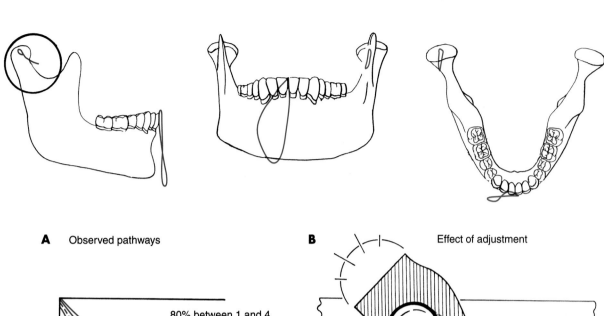

A Observed pathways

80% between 1 and 4
20% between 2 and 3

1

2

3 ← Mean

4

B Effect of adjustment

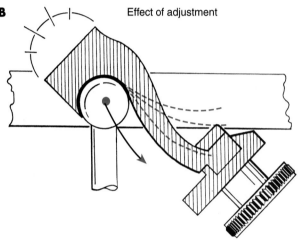

C Working
condyle point (*a*) movement

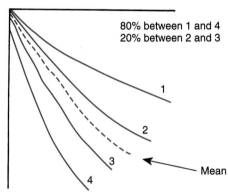

D Nonworking
condyle point (*e*) movement

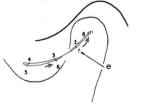

E, F, and G illustrate the combined effect of anterior and posterior guidance on the superior border of molar point. The angulation of the posterior guidance is indicated in degrees for each figure. The absence of anterior guidance is indicated by *a* and presence of anterior guidance by *b*. The tracing of the movement of the mesiolingual cusp of the maxillary molar is made on the grid in each figure. Note that the absence of anterior guidance reduces the separation of the posterior teeth, but has the greatest effect when the posterior guidance is shallow.

F

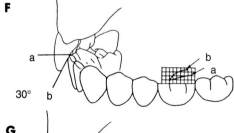

30° b

a b
a

E

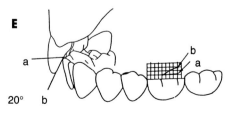

a b
a

20° b

G

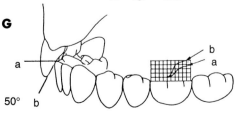

a b
a

50° b

FIG. **2-58** Horizontal condylar guidance. (**A** *modified from Lundeen HC, Wirth CG: Condylar movement patterns engraved in plastic blocks,* J Prosthet Dent *30:866-875, 1973;* **E** *through* **G** *modified from Lundeen HC, Shryock EF, Gibbs CH:* J Prosthet Dent *40:442-452, 1978.)*

the dentist. The anterior guidance can be increased by restorative or orthodontic means to facilitate separation of the posterior teeth in patients who have shallow horizontal guidance.

Fig. 2-59 *(lateral condylar guidance)* illustrates how setting the articulator simulates the looseness of the TMJs. TMJ laxity can be measured and transferred to the articulator by use of dentist-guided bite registration records, pantographic tracings, or a clutch-and-flag system. Bite registrations consistently produce lower values for the lateral shift because tooth contact tends to center the condyles.[13] A clutch-and-flag system can produce results comparable to a pantographic tracing when used to set fully adjustable articulators.[12] A series of tracings of guided movements from different patients is presented in Fig. 2-59, *A*.[14] All the tracings are parallel after the first few millimeters of movement. The difference from one patient to the next is the result of the amount of lateral shift. Fig. 2-59, *B*, illustrates simulations of arcs at different degrees of lateral shift; the similarity of lines *a, b,* and *c* to the lines similarly marked in Fig. 2-59, *A,* should be noted. One should also note that none of the tracings of lateral condylar movement exhibit the "progressive" lateral shift indicated by the dashed line *d* in Fig. 2-59, *B*. Fig. 2-59, *C*, illustrates the underside of a condylar housing of an articulator. Shifting the medial wall simulates TMJ laxity and allows movements similar to those illustrated in Fig. 2-59, *A*. Fig. 2-59, *D*, illustrates how movements *a, b,* and *c* were made for Fig. 2-59, *B*, by shifting the medial wall of the condyle box.

Increasing laxity of the TMJ, indicated by increasing lateral shift, results in significant changes in movement of the molar point near MI (see Fig. 2-59, *E*). The working-side movement is least affected because it is already a directly lateral movement. The nonworking molar-point movement is changed in both the lateral and horizontal components. The lateral pathway is extended progressively more laterally in patients with excessive lateral looseness of the TMJs. The horizontal effect is a "flattening" of the pathway by reduction of the vertical separation. These effects are illustrated by tracings of molar-point movement on an articulator as the amount of lateral shift is increased from 0 to 3.5 mm. The effect of increasing looseness is to increase the likelihood of collisions of the mesiolingual cusps of the maxillary molars with the mandibular distofacial cusps of the molars on the nonworking side (see Fig. 2-59, *E* and *F*). These types of undesirable contact between the opposing supporting cusps are termed nonworking interferences

TOOTH CONTACTS DURING MANDIBULAR MOVEMENTS

Operative dentists must design restorations capable of withstanding the forces of mastication and clenching. The choice of restorative material and the design of the restoration are frequently influenced by the need to withstand forceful contact with the opposing teeth. *Thus evaluation of the location, direction, and area of tooth contacts during various mandibular movements is an essential part of the preoperative evaluation of teeth to be restored.* The anterior teeth support gliding contacts, whereas the posterior teeth support the heavy forces applied during chewing and clenching. Fig. 2-60 shows a variety of tooth contact relationships. In Fig. 2-60, *A*, a right mandibular movement is illustrated, showing the separation of the posterior teeth on the left, or nonworking, side. This separation of the posterior teeth results from the combined effects of the canine guidance and the slope of the articular eminence on the nonworking side. The effect of the canine guidance is illustrated in the incisor point tracing in Fig. 2-60, *B*. The superior border on either side of MI is determined by the shape of the lingual surfaces of the maxillary canine teeth. Guiding contact between the right canines is illustrated in Fig. 2-60, *C*.

A variety of areas on the posterior teeth may contact the opposing tooth during mandibular movements. In Fig. 2-60, *D*, the opposing surfaces of the molar teeth are divided into five areas:

1. Inner incline of nonsupporting (noncentric) cusp. This area sometimes participates in working-side movements by contacting the outer aspect of the supporting (centric) cusp *(area 5)*.
2. Fossa or marginal ridge contact area. This is the main holding contact (or centric stop) area for the opposing supporting cusp.
3. Inner incline of the supporting (centric holding) cusp. This area has the potential for undesirable contact during nonworking movements.
4. Contact area of the supporting (centric holding) cusp. This is the main cusp contact area.
5. Outer aspect of the supporting (centric holding) cusp. This area sometimes participates in working-side movements by contacting the inner incline of the nonsupporting (noncentric) cusp *(area 1)*.

Anterior Tooth Contacts. During anterior movement of the mandible (i.e., protrusion), the lower anterior teeth glide along the lingual surfaces of the maxillary anterior teeth (see Fig. 2-60, *E* and *F*). Multiple contacts between the opposing dental arches on the anterior teeth are desirable in protrusion movements. With protrusion, multiple contacts serve to prevent excessive force on any individual pair of gliding teeth. Posterior tooth contact during protrusion is not desirable because it may overload the involved teeth. The combination of the anterior guidance (slope and vertical overlap of the anterior teeth) and the slope of the articular eminence (horizontal condylar guidance on the articulator) determines the amount of vertical separation of the posterior teeth as the mandible moves anteriorly. Some texts refer

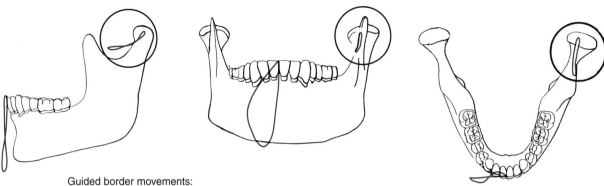

Guided border movements:
1. Follow chewing pathway in reverse direction
2. Studies of 160 subjects suggest all are similar
3. Differences are due to amount of side shift
4. Progressive side shift was not observed

Simulated movements:
1. Are arcs of circles
2. Differ by side shift
3. Are comparable to guided movements

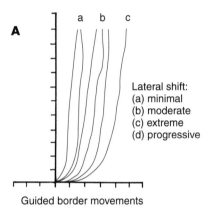

A

Lateral shift:
(a) minimal
(b) moderate
(c) extreme
(d) progressive

Guided border movements

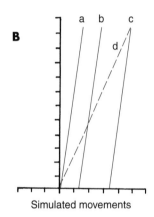

B

Simulated movements

Underside of condylar housing condylar ball movement at extreme side shift

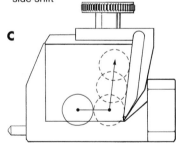

C

Adjustment of the lateral shift to produce simulated movements above

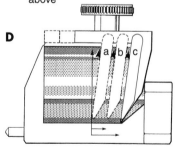

D

Maxillary molar; showing change in nonworking movement of mandibular distofacial cusp with increasing lateral shift

Mandibular molar; showing change in nonworking movement of maxillary mesiolingual cusp with increasing lateral shift

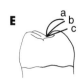

E

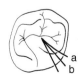

F

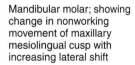

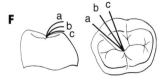

FIG. **2-59** Lateral condylar guidance: the medial wall. (**A** and **B** based on data from Lundeen HC, Wirth CG: J Prosthet Dent 30:866-875, 1973.)

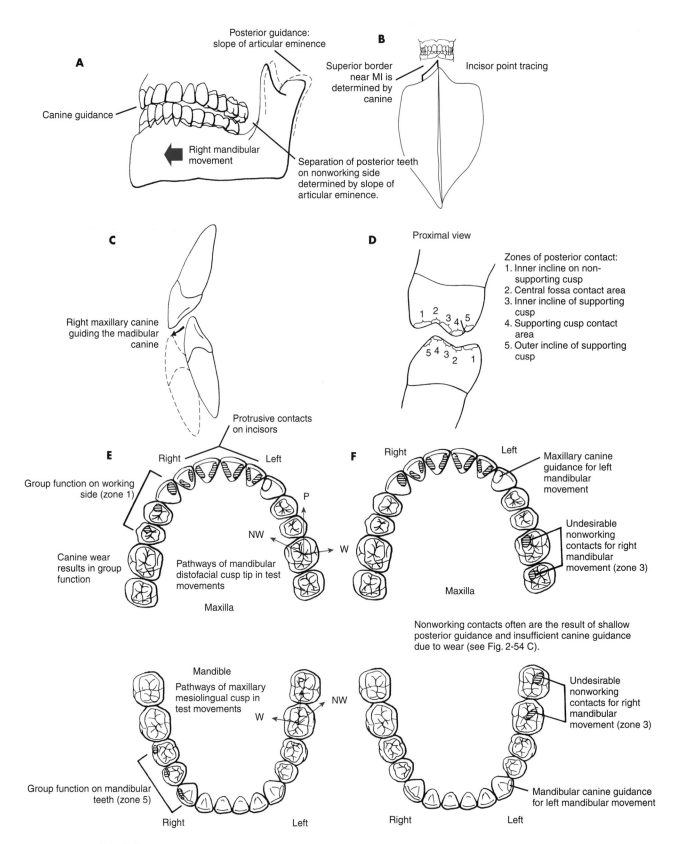

A Canine guidance

Posterior guidance: slope of articular eminence

Right mandibular movement

Separation of posterior teeth on nonworking side determined by slope of articular eminence.

B Superior border near MI is determined by canine

Incisor point tracing

C Right maxillary canine guiding the madibular canine

Protrusive contacts on incisors

D Proximal view

Zones of posterior contact:
1. Inner incline on non-supporting cusp
2. Central fossa contact area
3. Inner incline of supporting cusp
4. Supporting cusp contact area
5. Outer incline of supporting cusp

E Right   Left

Group function on working side (zone 1)

Canine wear results in group function

Pathways of mandibular distofacial cusp tip in test movements

P
NW   W

Maxilla

Mandible

Pathways of maxillary mesiolingual cusp in test movements

P
NW
W

Group function on mandibular teeth (zone 5)

Right   Left

F Right   Left

Maxillary canine guidance for left mandibular movement

Undesirable nonworking contacts for right mandibular movement (zone 3)

Maxilla

Nonworking contacts often are the result of shallow posterior guidance and insufficient canine guidance due to wear (see Fig. 2-54 C).

Undesirable nonworking contacts for right mandibular movement (zone 3)

Mandibular canine guidance for left mandibular movement

Right   Left

FIG. 2-60 Tooth contacts during mandibular movement. (*B from Gibbs CH, Lundeen HC: Jaw movements and forces during chewing and swallowing and their clinical significance. In Lundeen HC, Gibbs CH, editors: Advances in occlusion, Bristol, 1982, John Wright PSG.)*

to this separation as *disocclusion* or *disclusion* of the posterior teeth. Articulator-mounted casts can be used to assess the superior border near MI, which is the critical zone for tooth contact. This information is very useful during the fabrication of ceramic and cast metallic restorations because the position and height of the restored cusps can be evaluated and adjusted in the laboratory, which minimizes the chairside time and effort required to adjust the completed restorations.

Posterior Tooth Contacts. In idealized occlusal schemes designed for restorative dentistry, the posterior teeth should contact only in MI. Any movement of the mandible should result in separation of the posterior teeth by the combined effects of anterior guidance and the slope of the articular eminence (horizontal condylar guidance on the articulator). Forceful contact or collisions of individual posterior tooth cusps during chewing and clenching may lead to patient discomfort or damage to the teeth. Patients with shallow anterior guidance or openbite are more difficult to restore without introduction of undesirable tooth contacts. Articulator-mounted casts may be used to assess and solve restorative problems that are difficult to achieve by direct intraoral techniques.

The side of the jaw where the bolus of food is placed is termed the *working side*. *Working side* is also used in reference to the jaws or teeth when the patient is not chewing (e.g., in guided test movements directed laterally). The term can also identify a specific side of the mandible (i.e., the side toward which the mandible is moving). During chewing the working-side closures start from a lateral position and are directed medially to MI. Test movements are used by dentists to assess the occlusal contacts on the working side; for convenience, these movements are started in MI and move laterally. Thus the working-side test movement follows the same pathway as the working-side chewing closure but occurs in the opposite direction. The preferred occlusal relationship for restorative purposes is to limit the working-side contact to the canine teeth. Tooth contact posterior to the canine on the working side may occur naturally in worn dentitions. As the canine teeth are shortened by wear, separation of the posterior teeth diminishes. Lateral mandibular movements in worn dentitions successively bring into contact more posterior teeth as the height of the canines decreases. Multiple tooth contacts during lateral jaw movement are termed *group function*. Right-sided group function is illustrated in Fig. 2-60, *E*, compared with left canine guidance contact in Fig. 2-60, *F*. Because the amount of torque and wear imposed on teeth increases closer to the muscle attachments on the mandible, molar contact in group function is undesirable. Group function occurs naturally in a worn dentition; however, group function can be a therapeutic goal when the bony support of the canine teeth is compromised by periodontal disease or

when Class II occlusions where canine guidance is impossible.

The *nonworking side* is opposite the working side and normally does not contain a food bolus during chewing. During chewing closures, the mandibular teeth on the nonworking side close from a medial and anterior position and approach MI by moving laterally and posteriorly. Test movements on the nonworking side are made from MI in a medial and anterior direction. Thus the test movements and the chewing strokes are made in opposite directions along the same pathway. Voluntary lateral movements may not fully approach the borders and thus *it is recommended that the dentist guide the patient in these test movements.* Contact of the molar cusps on the nonworking side may overload the teeth or TMJs. Undesirable nonworking contacts are illustrated in Fig. 2-60, *F. Avoidance of contacts on the nonworking side is an important goal for restorative procedures on the molar teeth.*

NEUROLOGIC CORRELATES AND CONTROL OF MASTICATION

This summary of neurologic control is based on an excellent review by Lund.[10] The control of mastication is dependent on sensory feedback. Sensory feedback serves to control the coordination of the lips, tongue, and mandibular movement during manipulation of the food bolus through all stages of mastication and preparation for swallowing. Physiologists divide an individual chewing cycle into three components: opening, fast closing, and slow closing. The slow-closing segment of chewing is associated with the increased forces required for crushing food. The central nervous system receives several types of feedback from muscle spindles, periodontal receptors, and touch receptors in the skin and mucosa. This feedback controls the mandibular closing muscles during the slow-closing phase. Often sensory feedback results in inhibition of movement (e.g., because of pain). During mastication some sensory feedback from the teeth is excitatory, causing an increase in the closing force as the food bolus is crushed. However, there must be an upper limit where inhibition occurs; this prevents the buildup of excessive forces on the teeth during the occlusal stage.

A group of neurons in the brainstem produces bursts of discharges at regular intervals when excited by oral sensory stimuli. These bursts drive motor neurons to produce contractions of the masticatory muscles at regular intervals, resulting in rhythmic mandibular movement. The cluster of neurons in the brainstem that drives the rhythmic chewing is termed the *central pattern generator* (CPG). Oral sensory feedback can modify the basic CPG pattern and is essential for coordination of the lips, tongue, and mandible. Sensory input from the periodontal and mucosal receptors keeps the rhythmic chewing going. During opening, the mandibular opening muscles are contracted and the closing muscles inhibited. During closing, the mandibular closing muscles are activated but the opening muscles are not inhibited. Coactivation of the opening and closing muscles makes the mandible more rigid and probably serves to brace the condyles while the food is crushed. This coactivation of the opening and closing muscles also probably contributes to the rigidity noticed by clinicians attempting to manipulate the mandible.

The chewing cycles illustrated in Figs. 2-54 to 2-56 are due to CPG rhythms. Gliding tooth contact occurs frequently during chewing on the working side. These contacts probably cause an increase in the closing force. Working-side contacts are forceful and represent about 11% of the maximum possible bite force. The borders of mandibular function are relevant to construction of dental restorations because forceful contacts occur regularly during chewing. When the mandibular closure results in molar contact on the nonworking side, opposite the food bolus, the teeth or TMJs may be overloaded.

REFERENCES

1. Angle EH: Classification of malocclusion, *Dent Cosmos* 41:248-264, 350-357, 1899.
2. Brännström M: *Dentin and pulp in restorative dentistry,* London, 1982, Wolfe Medical.
3. Carlsson GE, Haraldson T, Mohl ND: The dentition. In Mohl ND et al, editors: *A textbook of occlusion,* Chicago, 1988, Quintessence.
4. Celenza FV, Nasedkin JN: *Occlusion the state of the art,* Chicago, 1978, Quintessence.
5. Garberoglio R, Brännström M: Scanning electron microscopic investigation of human dentinal tubules, *Arch Oral Biol* 21:355-362, 1976.
6. Gibbs CH, Lundeen HC: Jaw movements and forces during chewing and swallowing and their clinical significance. In Lundeen HC, Gibbs CH, editors: *Advances in occlusion,* Bristol, 1982, John Wright PSG.
7. Gibbs CH et al: Functional movements of the mandible, *J Prosthet Dent* 26:601-610, 1971.
8. Jordan RE, Abrams L, Kraus BS: *Kraus' dental anatomy and occlusion,* ed 2, St Louis, 1992, Mosby.
9. Kraus BS, Jordan RE, Abrams L: *Dental anatomy and occlusion,* ed 1, Baltimore, 1969, Williams & Wilkins.
10. Lund JP: Mastication and its control by the brain stem, *Crit Rev Oral Biol Med* 2:33-64, 1991.
11. Lundeen HC, Shryock EF, Gibbs CH: An evaluation of mandibular border movements: their character and significance, *J Prosthet Dent* 40:442-452, 1978.
12. Lundeen TF, Mendosa MA: Comparison of Bennett shift measured at the hinge axis and an arbitrary hinge axis position, *J Prosthet Dent* 51:407-410, 1984.
13. Lundeen TF, Mendosa MA: Comparison of two methods for measurement of immediate Bennett shift, *J Prosthet Dent* 51:243-245, 1984.
14. Lundeen HC, Wirth CG: Condylar movement patterns engraved in plastic blocks, *J Prosthet Dent* 30:866-875, 1973.
15. Michelich V, Pashley DH, Whitford GM: Dentin permeability: comparison of function versus anatomic tubular radii, *J Dent Res* 57:1019-1024, 1978.
16. Nakabayashi N, Takarada K: Effect of HEMA on bonding to dentin, *Dent Mater* 8(2):125-130, 1992.
17. Pashley DH: The effects of acid etching on the pulpodentin complex, *Oper Dent* 17(6):229-242, 1992.
18. Pashley DH: Clinical correlations of dentin structure and function, *J Prosthet Dent* 66(6):777-781, 1991.
19. Posselt U: Studies in the mobility of the mandible, *Acta Odont Scand* 10 (Suppl 10), 1952.
20. Scott JH, Symons NBB: *Introduction to dental anatomy,* ed 7, Edinburgh, 1974, Churchill Livingstone.
21. Stanley HR: *Human pulp response to operative dental procedures,* Gainesville, Fla, 1976, Sorter Printing.
22. Sturdevant JR, Pashley DH: Regional dentin permeability of Class I and II cavity preparations (abstract No. 173), *J Dent Res* 68:203, 1989.
23. Van Meerbeek M et al: Comparative SEM and TEM examination of the ultrastructure of the resin-dentin interdiffusion zone, *J Dent Res* 72(2):495-501, 1993.

Cariology: The Lesion, Etiology, Prevention, and Control

THEODORE M. ROBERSON

THOMAS F. LUNDEEN*

*This author is inactive this edition. See the Acknowledgments.

CHAPTER OUTLINE

INTRODUCTION AND DEFINITIONS

Dental caries (tooth decay) (Figs. 3-1 to 3-5) and periodontal disease are probably the most common chronic diseases in the world. Although caries has affected humans since prehistoric times, the prevalence of this disease has greatly increased in modern times on a worldwide basis, an increase strongly associated with dietary change. However, evidence now indicates that this trend peaked and began to decline in many countries in the late 1970s and early 1980s, and the decline was most notable in certain segments of the population of the United States, western Europe, New Zealand, and Australia.[28] The exact cause of the decline is unknown but is attributed to the addition of trace amounts of fluoride ion to public drinking water. Trace amounts of fluoride were discovered to have a marked limiting effect on the progression of caries lesions originating on the adjacent contacting, or proximal, surfaces of teeth. This discovery lead to widespread addition of fluoride to public water supplies in the 1950s and 1960s and the addition of fluoride to a variety of oral hygiene products, especially toothpaste. By 1984, 94% of toothpaste products contained added fluoride.[53]

The decline in caries in developed countries such as the United States has been most prominent in the upper and middle classes, while the lower socioeconomic classes and rural residents have retained a higher prevalence of tooth decay. For example, the Third National Health and Nutrition Examination Survey (NHANES III)[58] found that 80% of the caries occurred in 20% of the children, who were frequently in lower socioeconomic groups or minorities. This effect has been characterized as a "polarization" of caries, in which a limited segment of the population experiences most of the disease. A similar polarization is occurring on a worldwide basis where the prevalence of caries is declining in developed countries, is increasing in less developed countries, and is epidemic in countries with emerging economies. Thus caries is increasingly being localized in segments of populations that can least afford the necessary dental treatment.

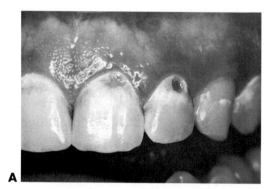
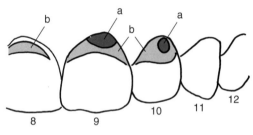

FIG. 3-1 A, A young adult with multiple active carious lesions involving teeth No. 8 to No. 12. **B,** Cavitated areas *(a)* are surrounded by areas of extensive demineralization that are chalky and opaque *(b).* Some areas of incipient caries have superficial stain.

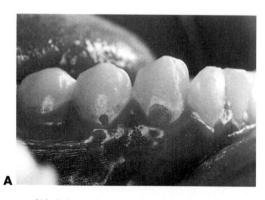
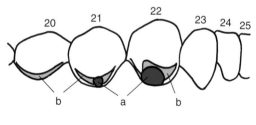

FIG. 3-2 Extensive active caries in a young adult (same patient as in Fig. 3-1). **A,** Mirror view of teeth No. 20 to No. 25. **B,** Cavitated lesions *(a)* are surrounded by extensive areas of chalky, opaque demineralized areas *(b).* The presence of smooth-surface lesions like these is associated with rampant caries. Occlusal and interproximal smooth surface caries usually occur in advance of facial smooth-surface lesions. The presence of these types of lesions should alert the dentist to the possibility of extensive caries activity elsewhere in the mouth. The interproximal gingiva is swollen red and will bleed easily upon probing. These gingival changes are the consequence of long-standing irritation from the plaque adherent to the teeth.

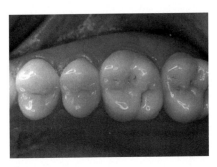

FIG. **3-3** Occlusal, mirror view of teeth No. 2 through No. 5. These healthy teeth have few suitable habitats for plaque populations. Note that many of the grooves on the occlusal surfaces are coalesced. There are some areas of stain, particularly in the distal oblique fissure (noncoalesced groove) of the first molar. This superficial stain is typically found in caries-free fissures and should not be confused with other color changes in enamel associated with caries. Compare this with Figs. 3-19 to 3-22.

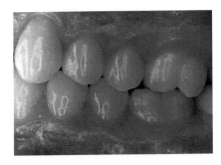

FIG. **3-4** Facial view of teeth in Fig. 3-3. Note healthy gingiva and translucent enamel, especially along the crest of the gingiva. Compare this photo to Fig. 3-2, which shows inflamed gingival tissues. Compare the enamel characteristics to Fig. 3-25.

The cost of caries to society is enormous. The bill for dental care in the United States alone was $56.6 billion in 1999.[62] This represents probably less than half the actual need, considering that only 40% to 50% of the public regularly seek dental care. This published cost represents only the direct expense of dental care services. The total indirect costs, such as loss of time from work and the training of dentists, also are substantial. Tooth loss resulting in diminished chewing ability, which can lead to nutritional disorders, is a significant problem in lower socioeconomic groups, for whom replacement may not be possible for economic reasons. In addition, caries results in other significant, although intangible, costs in the form of pain, suffering, and cosmetic defects. In 1986, Walter Loesche described caries and periodontal disease as "perhaps the most expensive infections that most individuals have to contend with during a lifetime."[47] This statement remains correct today, with perhaps the exception of human immunodeficiency virus (HIV) infection.

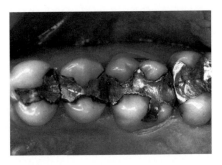

FIG. **3-5** Occlusal view of restored teeth with corroded, ditched margins. These teeth provide numerous retentive habitats for plaque communities. Note poor interproximal contours associated with broad, rough contact areas. The corrosion and breakdown at the tooth-restoration interface (margin) produces small V-shaped defects (ditches) that become new habitats for cariogenic bacteria.

Considering the magnitude and almost universal impact of caries, it is remarkable that a public-supported program for the eradication of the disease never developed as did programs against polio and smallpox. Caries eradication depends on the availability of four things: (1) a potent eradicator weapon (vaccine), (2) strong and efficient public health service support, (3) popular support for the program, and (4) an efficient surveillance system to monitor caries activity on a population level.[50] Caries eradication has not been achieved because these four basic requirements have not been met. In particular, the vaccine is not available. The single most effective population-based caries control method, public water fluoridation, is not sufficient to prevent pit-and-fissure caries of the posterior teeth. Water fluoridation and fluoride-containing dentifrices are not sufficient to prevent caries in individuals with poor dietary and oral hygiene practices. Although knowledge is not sufficient to eradicate caries on a population level, individuals under professional supervision having good dietary and oral hygiene practices can indeed live a caries-free life.

DEFINITIONS OF CARIES AND PLAQUE

Dental caries is an infectious microbiologic disease of the teeth that results in localized dissolution and destruction of the calcified tissues. It is essential to understand that cavitations in teeth (destruction of the tooth surface, creating a "cavity" or defect) are signs of bacterial infection. In clinical practice, it is possible to lose sight of this fact and focus entirely on the restorative treatment of the lesions, thereby failing to treat the underlying cause of the disease. (See Chapter 9 for a thorough discussion of clinical diagnosis of caries and treatment planning.) Although symptomatic treatment is important, failure to identify and treat the underlying cause (i.e., the infection of the tooth from odontopathic [causing disease to the teeth] bacteria) will allow the disease to continue.

The preventive section of this chapter emphasizes the components of an antibacterial treatment program that controls the infection by regulation of the oral ecologic conditions.

Caries activity, as evidenced by demineralization and loss of tooth structure, is highly variable, and therefore the course of individual lesions is not always predictable. Carious lesions only occur under a mass of bacteria capable of producing a sufficiently acidic environment to demineralize tooth structure. *A gelatinous mass of bacteria adhering to the tooth surface is termed dental plaque.* The plaque bacteria metabolize refined carbohydrates for energy and produce organic acids as a by-product. These acids may cause a carious lesion by dissolution of the tooth's crystalline structure. Carious lesions progress as a series of exacerbations and remissions as the pH at the tooth surface varies with the changes in plaque metabolism. The availability of simple carbohydrates, such as sucrose, greatly stimulates plaque metabolism. Exacerbations of caries activity are characterized by periods of high bacterial metabolic activity and low pH in the plaque near the tooth surface. During intervening episodes when few carbohydrates are available, there is little bacterial metabolic activity, and the pH rises near the surface of the tooth. Remineralization of the damaged tooth structure occurs as the local pH rises above 5.5. Saliva contains high concentrations of calcium and phosphate ions in solution that serve as a supply of raw material for the remineralization process. Acid attack on tooth surfaces continually occurs throughout an individual's life. Virtually all of the interproximal (adjacent contacting) surfaces of teeth are attacked by acid produced by plaque and are partially demineralized. Fortunately, relatively few tooth surfaces partially demineralized by plaque acids progress to cavitation. Understanding the balance between demineralization and remineralization is the key to enlightened caries management.

The evidence for the role of bacteria in the genesis of caries is overwhelming. Animal and human models have been used in an extensive series of studies, leading to the following conclusions[59]:

1. Teeth free from bacterial infection, either in germ-free animals or unerupted teeth in humans, do not develop caries.
2. Antibiotics are effective in reducing caries in animals and humans.
3. Oral bacteria can demineralize enamel in vitro and produce lesions similar to naturally occurring caries.
4. Specific bacteria can be isolated and identified from plaque over various carious lesions.

Although the role of bacterial activity in the genesis of carious lesions is well defined, establishing a cause-and-effect relationship between an individual organism in the oral flora and caries has not been completely successful. Oral bacteria do not occur as solitary colonies, but as members of a complex community of many species contained as a mass of tightly packed cells held together by the sticky matrix of polymerized glucose. Some 200 to 300 species of bacteria, yeast, and even protozoa appear to be indigenous to the human oral cavity. The metabolic activity of the complex community of bacteria that forms plaque determines the presence or absence of disease of the adjacent hard and soft tissues. Assessing the contribution of an individual species to the pathology associated with a complex plaque community has proven to be very difficult in in vivo systems. It has become clear that a relatively small group of bacteria is primarily responsible for the two major oral diseases—caries and periodontal disease.

One group of bacteria, which consists of eight *Streptococcus mutans* serotypes has been associated with caries. The serotypes have been labeled *a* through *h*. Several serotypes have been elevated to species status and given names: *Streptococcus rattus* (serotype b), *Streptococcus cricetus* (serotype a), *Streptococcus ferus* (serotype c), and *Streptoccocus sobrinus* (serotypes d, g, and h). All *S. mutans* serotypes have been demonstrated to have significant potential to cause caries, but because of their significant genetic and biochemical differences, they should not be simply referred to as the single species *S. mutans*. This text uses the term *mutans streptococci* (MS) as a collective term for all the serotypes. MS and lactobacilli can produce great amounts of acids (acidogenic), are tolerant of acidic environments (aciduric), are vigorously stimulated by sucrose, and appear to be the primary organisms associated with caries in man. *Organisms that cause caries are termed cariogenic. The degree to which a tooth is likely to become carious is described as its cariogenicity potential.* MS are present as a pandemic infection in humans; that is, MS are found in everyone regardless of race, ethnic background, or geographic origin. Normally MS exist in the mouth as an insignificantly small component of the oral flora. In patients with multiple active carious lesions, MS have become a dominant member of the plaque flora. MS are most strongly associated with the onset of caries while lactobacilli are associated with active progression of cavitated lesions.

EPIDEMIOLOGY OF CARIES

Dental caries has been studied extensively during the last 50 years in North America and Europe. These epidemiologic studies have been very useful in determining the extent of the need for and effectiveness of dental treatment. Originally, epidemiology focused on the study of epidemics, but in modern times epidemiology has expanded to cover any aspect of health needs of a population. A population consists of all individuals located in a prescribed area. The number of individuals in a population having a disease at a specific point in time is known as the *prevalence* of the disease. The number of individuals developing new cases of disease in a population over a specific period of time, usually 1 year, is the *incidence* of the disease. The length or duration of the disease has an important effect on the measures of prevalence and incidence. For short duration diseases, such as the flu, the incidence and the prevalence are nearly identical. For diseases that persist over long periods (years or decades), the prevalence is much higher than the incidence.

The most common epidemiologic measure of caries is an evaluation of the number of permanent teeth that are diseased, missing, or filled (DMF). Measures of primary teeth are reported as dmf. DMF may be reported as the number of teeth (DMFT) or surfaces affected (DMFS). This measure is cumulative because it totals the number of restorations and extractions in addition to the number of teeth having active caries. It is presumed that the restored or extracted teeth were treated because of caries at some point in time before the epidemiologic survey. Once the tooth is restored or removed, it becomes a permanent measure for the life of the patient. The M and F components are therefore historical markers of the presence of past disease and should not be confused with the D, active disease, component. Thus DMF rates are not equivalent to a true measure of caries prevalence, and in fact, they overestimate the prevalence of active caries. Having noted the problems with DMF measures of caries, it is important to recognize the importance of DMF in making decisions concerning changes in caries in populations.

Changes in caries patterns in developed countries will dramatically affect the nature of operative dentistry practiced in the near future. For example, in the United States the percentage of the population over the age of 65 doubled from 1980 to 2000 and will comprise one fifth of the population by 2030. Thus there will be more elderly people, and because of a reduced prevalence of caries, they will have retained more teeth than any preceding generation. However, this large elderly population will be at increased risk for caries, especially on exposed root surfaces. Little is known about the caries risk in adults, particularly with regard to root caries, except that the risk increases with age. It is expected that the prevalence of root caries will increase over the next several decades. Furthermore, both maintenance of teeth with existing restorations (replacement needs) and new dental disease will continue the demand for operative dentistry, despite the decline of caries in children.

The status of caries in third-world countries represents the greatest challenge to dental science. In developing economies, income for basic health care needs is minimal, including dental care. Staggering DMF increases, such as threefold to fivefold increases in children, are reported in widely diverse regions, including Uganda, Chile, Mexico, Lebanon, and Thailand.[69] It is widely believed that this increase is due to a substantial rise in dietary sucrose previously unavailable to these populations. Paradoxically, the higher social classes who have greater exposure to dietary sucrose are frequently the most affected. Unfortunately, there are many barriers to treating these populations. In addition to minimal income, social and cultural norms often do not allow ready acceptance of new oral care and hygiene procedures. The costs of fluoride toothpaste and simple materials for a school-based fluoride rinse program often are prohibitive. There usually are few trained dentists and hygienists in these countries to deliver such simple care as sealants and fluoride treatments. Public water supply fluoridation would be the best and the least expensive treatment method, but it can only be applied if public water availability is adequate and if it is culturally acceptable, and neither criterion typically is met.

HYPOTHESES CONCERNING THE ETIOLOGY OF CARIES

There are two hypotheses concerning the pathogenicity of plaque. The older hypothesis promotes the universal presence of potential pathogens in plaque and therefore assumes that all accumulations of plaque are pathogenic. The other hypothesis is based on the observation that accumulation of plaque is not always associated with disease. Under the latter hypothesis, accumulation of plaque could be regarded as normal in the absence of disease. Plaque is assumed to be pathogenic only when signs of disease are present. The difference between these two hypotheses has been clearly identified and discussed by Walter Loesche who, although studying periodontal disease, applied these concepts equally well to caries. The first hypothesis, which assumes that all plaque is pathogenic, is termed the *nonspecific plaque hypothesis*. The alternative, or *specific plaque hypothesis*, recognizes plaque as pathogenic only when signs of associated disease are present.[48]

The problem with the nonspecific plaque hypothesis is that it requires a therapeutic goal that completely eliminates plaque in all patients. This goal is unrealistic and not achievable even in the most dedicated patients. Treatment under the nonspecific plaque hypothesis requires an open-ended regimen of continuous therapy directed at total plaque elimination. Dentists trying to achieve such ambitious goals have inevitably become frustrated by repeated failure of their patients to achieve total plaque control and have abandoned such "preventive practices."

The specific plaque hypothesis provides a new scientific basis for the treatment of caries that has radically altered caries treatment (Table 3-1). Plaques can be identified as pathologic when they are associated with clinical disease. Because only a limited number of microorganisms are capable of caries production, specific plaque

TABLE 3-1 New Caries Treatment Based on the Medical Model	
Etiology	MS infection
Symptoms	Demineralization lesions in teeth
Treatment, symptomatic	Restoration of cavitated lesions
Treatment, therapeutic	Eliminate MS infection
Posttreatment assessment, symptomatic	Examine teeth for new lesions
Posttreatment assessment, therapeutic	Bacteriologic testing for MS

MS, Mutans streptococci.

hypothesis treatment is aimed at elimination of the specific pathogenic organisms, but not total plaque elimination. To quote Loesche,[47] "The goal of therapy is to suppress the cariogenic plaques and to replace them with pathogen-free plaques. This therapeutic goal may be realized if antimicrobial modalities, such as mechanical debridement and chemical agents, can be applied with sufficient intensity so as to achieve for short periods on the tooth surface some semblance of 'sterility.' If such 'sterility' can be obtained, then the newly forming plaque will be derived from organisms in the bathing saliva and will contain high proportions of *S. sanguis* and *S. mitis,* and low proportions of *S. mutans.*" The subsequent plaque, dominated by noncariogenic bacteria, will have little or no cariogenic potential.

ECOLOGIC BASIS OF CARIES

The basic premise of this chapter is that development and growth of plaque on teeth is a normal phenomenon. The plaque community structure undergoes a succession of changes during periods of unrestricted growth. These changes in the community structure consequently change the overall metabolism and other characteristics of the plaque. Community structural changes are predictable and are governed by general principles of *ecology,*[2] which is the science of interactions between organisms and their environment. Unrestricted plaque growth produces local environmental conditions that may selectively promote the accumulation of pathogenic bacterial species.

High frequency sucrose exposure may be the single most important factor in producing a cariogenic plaque. Frequent sucrose ingestion begins a series of changes in the local tooth environment that promotes the growth of highly acidogenic bacteria and eventually leads to caries. In contrast, when sucrose is severely restricted or absent, plaque growth typically does not lead to caries. Dietary sucrose plays a leading role in the development of pathogenic plaques and may be the single most important factor in disruption of the normal healthy ecology of dental plaque communities.

Multiple factors determine the characteristics of plaque. The factors that control the presence of individual species in plaque are termed *ecologic determinants.* These can be divided into several broad interrelated categories: host resistance, extent and nature of shelter for bacteria, host diet, oral hygiene, status of the dentition, and composition of the oral flora. These various factors can be viewed as links in a chain of reactions eventually leading to caries.

The decline in caries in developed countries is widely believed to be due primarily to the increased use of fluorides in public water supplies and oral hygiene products. Improvements in oral hygiene, diet, and other factors have been considered to be of much less importance to the general decline in caries worldwide. However, the mechanism of caries reduction is not entirely understood and apparently not fully explained by either the use of fluoride or a reduction in sucrose consumption. Thus, the other factors once considered to be of little importance, in fact, may have a considerable impact on caries. Whatever the cause, children in developed countries tend to have less pathogenic plaque than their parents. This is a consequence of a change in the oral ecology of these children.

ETIOLOGIC AGENT OF CARIES: PATHOGENIC BACTERIAL PLAQUE
INTRODUCTORY DESCRIPTION OF PLAQUE

As previously stated, the soft, translucent, and tenaciously adherent material accumulating on the surface of teeth is commonly called *plaque.* It is more accurately described as *bacterial plaque* because it is composed almost completely of bacteria and their by-products (Figs. 3-6 to 3-10). Plaque is neither adherent food debris, as is widely and erroneously thought, nor does it result from the haphazard collection of opportunistic microorganisms. Actually, *the accumulation of plaque on teeth is a highly organized and ordered sequence of events.* Many of the organisms found in the mouth are not found elsewhere in nature. *Survival of microorganisms in the oral environment depends on their ability to adhere to a surface.* Free-floating organisms are rapidly cleared from the mouth by salivary flow and frequent swallowing. Only a few specialized organisms, primarily streptococci, are able to adhere to oral surfaces such as the mucosa and tooth structure. These adherent bacteria have special receptors for adhesion to the tooth surface and also produce a sticky matrix that allows them to cohere to each other. This adherence and coherence allows the bacteria to successfully colonize the tooth surface. Once they are attached, these pioneering organisms proliferate and spread laterally to form a matlike covering over the tooth surface (see Fig. 3-6, *C).* Further growth of bacteria produces a vertical growth away from (external to)

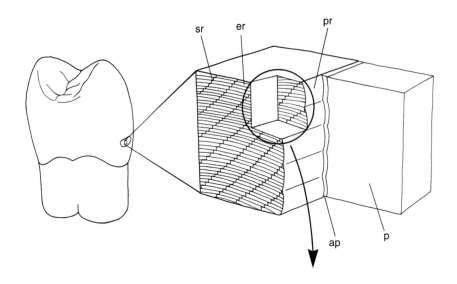

A

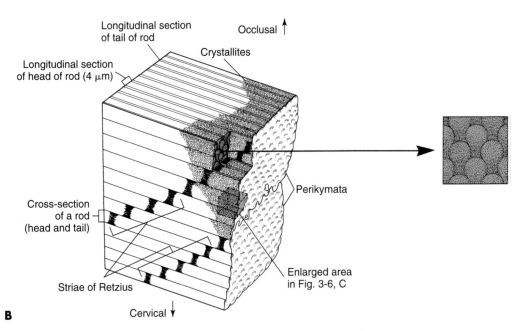

B

FIG. 3-6 For legend, see facing page.

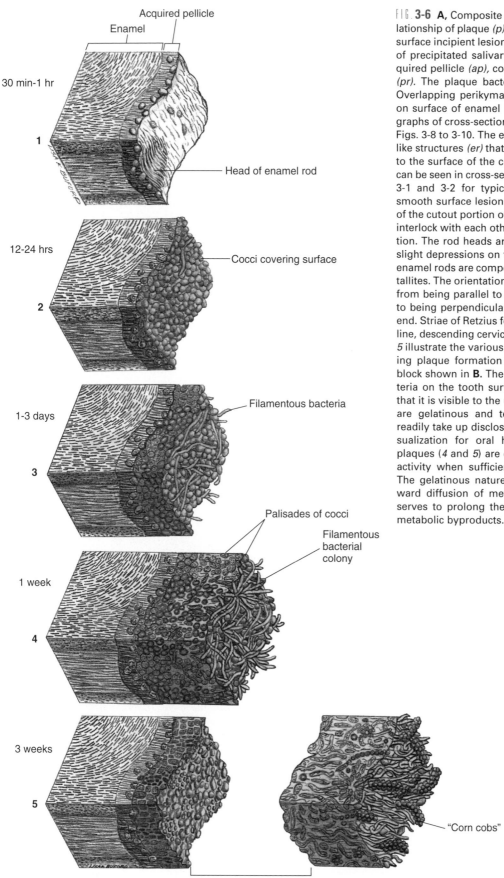

30 min-1 hr

1

12-24 hrs

2

1-3 days

3

1 week

4

3 weeks

5

C

Enamel

Acquired pellicle

Head of enamel rod

Cocci covering surface

Filamentous bacteria

Palisades of cocci

Filamentous
bacterial
colony

"Corn cobs"

Large segment removed

FIG. 3-6 **A,** Composite diagram illustrating the relationship of plaque *(p)* to the enamel in a smooth-surface incipient lesion. A relatively cell-free layer of precipitated salivary protein material, the acquired pellicle *(ap),* covers the perikymata ridges *(pr).* The plaque bacteria attach to the pellicle. Overlapping perikymata ridges *(pr)* can be seen on surface of enamel (see Fig. 3-7). Photomicrographs of cross-sections of plaque can be seen in Figs. 3-8 to 3-10. The enamel is composed of rod-like structures *(er)* that course from the inner DEJ to the surface of the crown. Striae of Retzius *(sr)* can be seen in cross-sections of enamel. (See Figs. 3-1 and 3-2 for typical incipient and cavitated smooth surface lesions.) **B,** A higher power view of the cutout portion of enamel in **A**. Enamel rods interlock with each other in a head-to-tail orientation. The rod heads are visible on the surface as slight depressions on the perikymata ridges. The enamel rods are composed of tightly packed crystallites. The orientation of the crystallites changes from being parallel to the rod in the head region to being perpendicular to the rod axis in the tail end. Striae of Retzius form a descending diagonal line, descending cervically. **C,** Drawings *1* through *5* illustrate the various stages in colonization during plaque formation upon the shaded enamel block shown in **B**. The accumulated mass of bacteria on the tooth surface may become so thick that it is visible to the unaided eye. Such plaques are gelatinous and tenaciously adherent; they readily take up disclosing dyes, aiding in their visualization for oral hygiene instruction. Thick plaques (*4* and *5*) are capable of great metabolic activity when sufficient nutrients are available. The gelatinous nature of the plaque limits outward diffusion of metabolic products and thus serves to prolong the retention of organic acid metabolic byproducts.

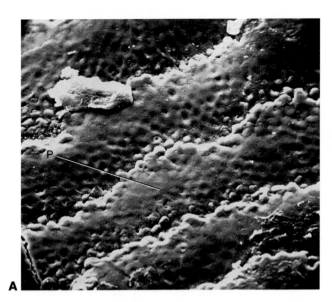
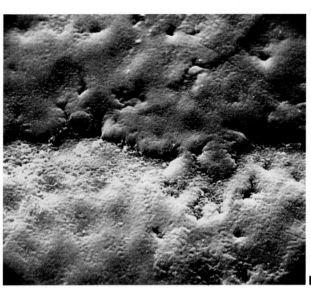

FIG. **3-7** **A,** Scanning electron microscope view (×600) of overlapping perikymata *(P)* in sound enamel from unerupted molar. **B,** Higher power view (×2300) of overlapped site rotated 180 degrees. Surface of incipient enamel lesions has "punched-out" appearance. *(From Hoffman S: Histopathology of caries lesions. In Menaker L, editor:* The biologic basis of dental caries, *New York, 1980, Harper & Row.)*

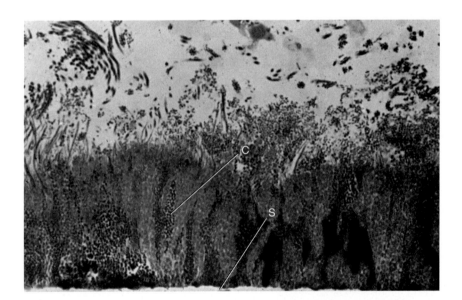

FIG. **3-8** Photomicrograph (×1350) of bacterial plaque. One-day plaque formation in patient who is a heavy plaque former. This plaque consists primarily of columnar microcolonies of cocci *(C)* growing perpendicular to crown surface *(S)*. *(From Listgarten MA, Mayo HE, Tremblay R: J Periodontol 46(1):19, 1975. Copyright 1975 Munksgaard International Publishers Ltd, Copenhagen, Denmark.)*

the tooth surface. The resulting mixed streptococcal mat allows the adherence of other organisms, such as filamentous and spiral bacteria, that otherwise are unable to adhere directly to the tooth surface (see Figs. 3-6, *C* and 3-8 to 3-10). Thus the formation of a mature plaque community involves a succession of changes (Fig. 3-11), and each change depends on the preceding

stage preparing the local environment for the next stage.

PLAQUE COMMUNITIES AND HABITATS
There are significant differences in the plaque communities found in various habitats (ecologic environments) within the oral cavity (Fig. 3-12). The oral mucosa is

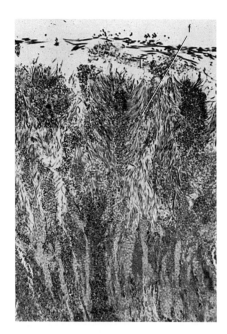

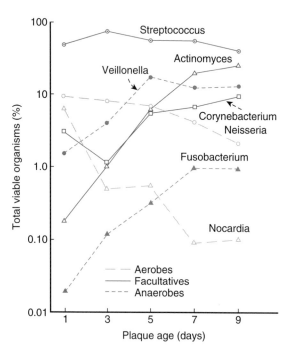

FIG. **3-9** Plaque formation at 1 week. Filamentous bacteria *(f)* appear to be invading cocci microcolonies. Plaque near gingival sulcus has fewer coccal forms and more filamentous bacteria (×860). *(From Listgarten MA, Mayo HE, Tremblay R: J Periodontol 46(1):10, 1975. Copyright 1975 Munksgaard International Publishers Ltd, Copenhagen, Denmark.)*

FIG. **3-11** Succession in plaque communities results from a shift to predominantly anaerobic conditions within the mass of plaque. Note that over a period of 9 days relative proportions of aerobic and anaerobic species change dramatically. *(From HL Ritz: Arch Oral Biol, 12, 1967, Pergamon.)*

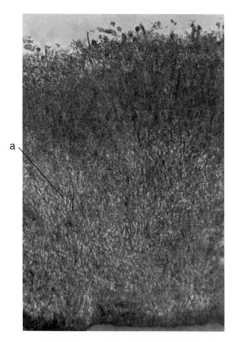

FIG. **3-10** At 3 weeks old, plaque is almost entirely composed of filamentous bacteria. Heavy plaque formers have spiral bacteria *(a)* associated with subgingival plaque (×660). *(From Listgarten MA, Mayo HE, Tremblay R: J Periodontol 46(1):10, 1975. Copyright 1975 Munksgaard International Publishers Ltd, Copenhagen, Denmark.)*

populated by organisms with receptors specialized for attachment to the surface of epithelium. The dorsum of the tongue has a plaque community dominated by *S. salivarius*. The teeth normally have a plaque community dominated by *S. sanguis* and *S. mitis*. The population size of MS on teeth is highly variable. Normally it is a very small percentage of the total plaque population, but it can be as large as one half the facultative streptococcal flora in other plaques.

Many distinct habitats may be identified on individual teeth, with each habitat containing a unique plaque community (Table 3-2). While the pits and fissures on the crown may harbor a relatively simple population of streptococci, the root surface in the gingival sulcus may harbor a very complex community dominated by filamentous and spiral bacteria. Facial and lingual smooth surfaces and proximal surfaces also may harbor vastly different plaque communities. For example, the mesial surface of a molar may be carious and have a plaque dominated by large populations of MS and lactobacilli, while the distal surface may totally lack these organisms and be caries free. Therefore, generalization about plaque communities is difficult. Nevertheless, the general activity of plaque growth and maturation is predictable and sufficiently well known to be of therapeutic importance in the prevention of caries.

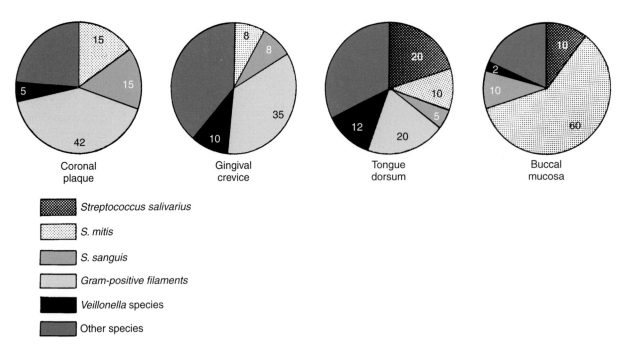

| Coronal plaque | Gingival crevice | Tongue dorsum | Buccal mucosa |

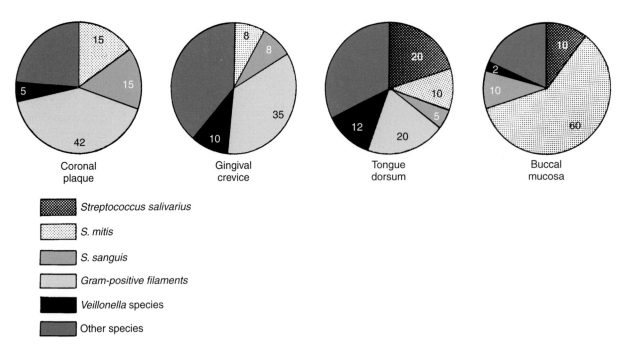

Streptococcus salivarius

S. mitis

S. sanguis

Gram-positive filaments

Veillonella species

Other species

FIG. 3-12 Approximate proportional distribution of predominant cultivable flora of four oral habitats. *(From Morhart R, Fitzgerald R: Composition and ecology of the oral flora. In Menaker L, editor:* The biologic basis of dental caries, *New York, 1980, Harper & Row.)*

TABLE 3-2   Oral Habitats*

HABITAT	PREDOMINANT SPECIES	ENVIRONMENTAL CONDITIONS WITHIN PLAQUE
Mucosa	*S. mitis* *S. sanguis* *S. salivarius*	Aerobic pH approximately 7 Oxidation-reduction potential positive
Tongue	*S. salivarius* *S. mutans* *S. sanguis*	Aerobic pH approximately 7 Oxidation-reduction potential positive
Teeth (noncarious)	*S. sanguis*	Aerobic pH 5.5 Oxidation-reduction negative
Gingival crevice	*Fusobacterium* species *Spirochaeta* species *Actinomyces* species *Veillonella* species	Anaerobic pH variable Oxidation-reduction very negative
Enamel caries	*S. mutans*	Anaerobic
Dentin caries	*S. mutans* *Lactobacillus* species	pH less than 5.5 Oxidation-reduction negative
Root caries	*Actinomyces* species	

*The microenvironmental conditions in the habitats associated with host health are generally aerobic, near neutrality in pH, and positive in oxidation-reduction potential. Significant microenvironmental changes are associated with caries and periodontal disease. The changes are the result of the plaque community metabolism.

DEVELOPMENT OF BACTERIAL PLAQUE: AN ECOLOGIC PHENOMENON

The complex and dynamic relationships among bacterial plaque, the host, and dental disease are best understood by viewing dental disease as a result of the functioning of an ecologic system that operates on widely known and accepted ecologic principles. An *ecosystem* is a circumscribed area occupied by a biologic community. The oral cavity is a well-defined ecosystem because it has recognized geographic limits and the general composition of the biologic community is known. Within the oral ecosystem are distinct habitats (see Table 3-2) such as the dorsum of the tongue; oral mucosa; gingival sulcus; and various tooth locations, including pits, fissures, and certain smooth surface areas. These habitats have unique environmental conditions and harbor significantly different communities of microorganisms (see Figs. 3-3 to 3-5). Within each habitat, special combinations of food and shelter are available to support particular species of oral bacteria. This special combination of food and shelter is termed an *ecologic niche.*

A particular niche is generally occupied by a single, best-adapted species. Thus for each habitat, a dental fissure for example, a limited number of niches are available to the oral flora. Organisms present in the greatest numbers in the saliva occupy the niches. If an organism already occupies the niches on the teeth, new opportunistic organisms will be excluded and prevented from becoming a part of the plaque. This process can prevent pathologic organisms (e.g., MS) from being established on already covered plaque surfaces. Thus plaques dominated by normal oral flora, such as *S. sanguis,* may be considered desirable because of their ability to control or prohibit the introduction of more pathogenic organisms.

As a plaque community develops on a tooth surface, eventually all the available niches will become occupied. When niche saturation occurs, only very competitive microorganisms can displace the indigenous bacteria from the community. Niche saturation provides inherent stability to plaque communities. Although large numbers of foreign organisms pass through the oral cavity, it is rare for any to become established as permanent residents. Niche saturation may be the mechanism that prevents these multitudes of exogenous organisms from becoming established in the mouth. This homeostatic mechanism has been termed *colonization resistance.* Colonization resistance can be quantified by measuring the threshold dose (number of organisms) required to establish a new resident population. MS have a very high threshold dose because they must compete with *S. sanguis* for niches. *S. sanguis* is more efficient in adhering to tooth surfaces than MS and, thus, is established more rapidly in the local community.[82] Thus the threshold dose (the total number of bacteria inoculated into the mouth) is a critical factor for establishment of an organism in plaque communities. This concept forms the basis for bacteriologic testing of saliva to determine caries risk.

In normal healthy circumstances, the oral flora capable of colonizing the teeth are not capable of causing disease. For MS to spread to other tooth surfaces, it must be present in sufficient numbers in the saliva to overcome the colonization resistance afforded by the normal oral flora. Therefore it should be noted that an active carious lesion can serve as a reservoir of MS and lactobacilli, providing the large threshold dose necessary to establish infections on other tooth surfaces. Millions of MS and lactobacilli are continually lost from the surface of active carious lesions. Consequently, it is essential to eliminate carious lesions because they may become the source for pathogenic infection of noncariogenic plaques. *Restoration of carious lesions has significant beneficial clinical effects in addition to the benefit of restoration of the damaged tooth structure and maintenance of pulpal vitality because the restorative process also effectively removes a nidus of infection.*

Some strains of MS are easier than others to establish in a host. This difference may be due in part to their ability to produce proteins called *bacteriocins,* which are lethal to closely related bacteria. Bacteriocin production is an ecologic adaptation that allows an organism to be more effective in competition with similar bacteria for the same niche.[30] Thus, bacteriocin production is an important ecologic determinant. Persistent colonization of the teeth by bacteriocin-producing MS has been demonstrated.[34,35] Bacteriocin production by itself is probably insufficient to allow MS to become a dominant plaque species. However, a combination of bacteriocin-producing MS with poor diet and oral hygiene can lead to a very extensive and persistent infection.[34,35]

The addition of another isolated and purified bacteriocin (known to inhibit MS) to the diet of rats had little effect when the availability of sucrose was good, but when sucrose was limited, the bacteriocin killed MS and related streptococci.[61] This suggests a possible therapeutic role for bacteriocins. Many oral bacteria produce bacteriocins that are effective against MS, and it is possible that some bacterial strains could give the host some immunity to caries when they are present. As already mentioned, bacteriocins effective against MS have been identified and purified.[49] Therefore an effective therapeutic treatment for caries could be the replacement of normal inhabitants of the oral cavity with strains having enhanced bacteriocin activity against the more pathogenic organisms (such as MS).[38] Some habitats on the teeth encourage caries by virtue of their physical shape. The pits and fissures of teeth are the most susceptible areas to caries and the most favorable habitat for MS. These deep recesses not only shelter bacteria residing in them but also limit access of salivary factors that attenuate and repair demineralization. Obturation of these anatomic faults by occlusal sealants or restorations prevents caries and greatly reduces the numbers of MS in the mouth. This is an excellent example of ecologic control of an undesirable plaque organism without wholesale disruption of the remainder of the oral flora. Sealing the pits and fissures eliminates a habitat of MS and is an example of disease prevention based on sound ecologic principles.

Likewise, tooth malalignment also can contribute to caries problems by providing sheltered areas for plaque retention. Correction of these problems by orthodontic or prosthodontic treatment can contribute to the overall oral health of the patient.

Plaque Growth. The growth of plaque is not the result of a random accumulation of opportunistic organisms passing through the oral cavity. Rather, an orderly sequence of replacement communities occupies the tooth surface, each community modifying the local environment of that site. The available niches, the limiting factors, and the environment conditions change as a result of the biologic activity of each plaque community. This process of mutual change of the community and its environment is called *ecologic succession* (see Fig. 3-11). Individual stages in a succession sequence are known as *seres* and the final stage of succession is a stable biologic community termed the *climax community.* Two different types of succession occur, and both can be identified in the oral cavity. In general ecology, *primary succession* occurs as the process of development of a biologic community where none previously existed. Applied to the oral cavity, primary succession is the process of normal change in the oral flora occurring over the lifetime of an individual host. *Secondary succession* is the process of restoration of the climax community after a disruption in the community structure. Secondary succession as it applies to the teeth is the process of plaque regrowth after the tooth surface is cleaned. If the environmental condi-

tions remain the same, secondary succession will result in an identical climax community. Thus a similar plaque will reform on the teeth after prophylaxis if there is no other change in the oral environmental conditions.

Primary succession occurs over the lifetime of the host. For example, a newborn's mouth is rapidly occupied by skin bacteria and *S. salivarius.* Newborns lack teeth and therefore cannot harbor organisms adapted to tooth habitats. Transient organisms, such as *Escherichia coli,* may be noted, but they fail to establish a permanent residence in the oral cavity. Major changes in the species composition of the oral cavity occur with the eruption of teeth because the teeth supply new habitats. In the adult, the general composition of a well-established oral flora remains relatively stable if there are no major changes in the health of the host. Loss of all teeth in elderly patients results in the loss of organisms specialized for tooth attachment and, consequently, the oral flora reverts to a composition similar to that of a newborn.

Plaque growth first consists of surface attachment and then lateral spreading as the attached organisms multiply (Fig. 3-13). When the entire surface is covered, growth of the colonies increases the thickness of the plaque. As the original colonizing organisms prolifer-

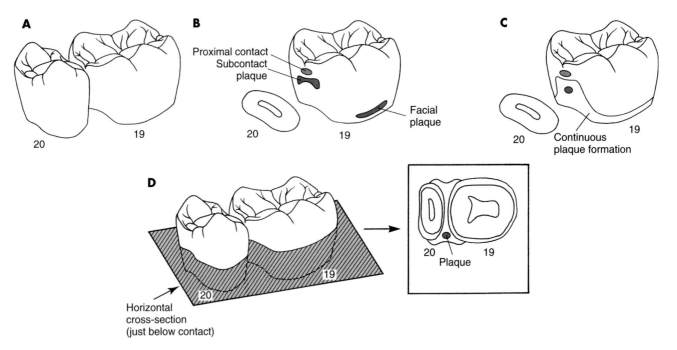

FIG. **3-13** Plaque formation on posterior teeth and associated carious lesions. **A,** Teeth No. 19 and No. 20 in contacting relationship. **B,** The crown of tooth No. 20 has been removed at the cervix. The proximal contact and subcontact plaque can be seen on the mesial surface of No. 19. A facial plaque is also illustrated. **C,** During periods of unrestricted growth, the mesial and facial plaques become part of a continuous ring of plaque around the teeth. Continuous rings of carious lesions can be seen in Fig. 3-25. **D,** A horizontal cross-section through teeth No. 19 and No. 20 with heavy plaque. The inset shows the interproximal space below the contact area filled with gelatinous plaque. This mass of interproximal plaque concentrates the effects of plaque metabolism on the adjacent tooth smooth surfaces. All interproximal surfaces are subject to plaque accumulation and acid demineralization. In patients exposed to fluoridated water, most interproximal lesions become arrested at a stage before cavitation.

ate, their progeny produce vertical columns of cells called *palisades* (see Figs. 3-6, *C* and 3-8 to 3-10). The palisades can be invaded by filamentous bacteria that otherwise could not exist on the tooth surface. Proliferation of the new, invading bacteria produce tangled masses of filaments extending upward, away from the surface of the tooth. Plaques may grow to become many thousands of cells thick, resulting in interesting plaque structures such as "corn cobs," which consist of filaments with cocci attached (see Fig. 3-6, *C, 5*). These probably indicate preferential attachment of two types of organisms that each derive some benefit from the attachment.

Early Stages of Plaque Succession. Professional tooth cleaning is a practice that is intended to control plaque and prevent disease. After professional removal of all organic material and bacteria from a tooth surface, a new coating of organic material begins to accumulate immediately. Within 2 hours a cell-free, structureless organic film, the pellicle (see Fig. 3-6, *A* and *C*), can completely cover the previously denuded area. The pellicle is formed primarily from the selective precipitation of various components of saliva. The functions of the pellicle are believed to be: (1) protect the enamel, (2) reduce friction between the teeth, and (3) possibly provide a matrix for remineralization. The pellicle is formed from salivary proteins that have apparently evolved for this function. These proteins have many basic groups and consequently adsorb to the phosphate ions while other acidic proteins adsorb to calcium ions. Among the salivary proteins isolated from the pellicle are lysozyme, albumin, and immunoglobulins A (IgA) and G (IgG). Some of these proteins are biologically active and have a significant impact on microorganisms attempting to colonize the tooth surface (Table 3-3). The strong affinity

of salivary proteins for exposed hydroxyapatite is also of critical importance in operative dentistry, because salivary contamination of a freshly etched enamel surface prevents bonding of composite restorations (see Chapters 11 to 15).

The early stages of recolonization of the cleaned tooth surface (early secondary succession) involve adhesion between the pellicle and the pioneering organisms. The number and type of organisms available, floating free in the saliva, determine how the tooth surface is colonized. Some organisms have a selective advantage due to their superior ability to attach to hydroxyapatite or to the acquired pellicle. *S. sanguis* along with *Actinomyces viscosus, Actinomyces naeslundii,* and *Peptostreptococcus* are the main pioneering species and are capable of attaching to the pellicle within 1 hour after tooth cleaning.[11] The adhesion process is very selective and requires specific organism receptors capable of binding to certain areas on the precipitated salivary proteins of the pellicle. For example, the enzyme glucosyltransferase may be of critical importance in the adherence of MS to the pellicle when sucrose is present[67] because it enhances the polymerization of the extracellular matrix that makes MS form such tenaciously adherent colonies.

Late Stages of Plaque Succession. The late stages of ecologic succession in plaque are responsible for causing either caries or periodontal disease. Early stages (seres) in a plaque succession are generally lacking in pathogenic potential because they are primarily aerobic communities and lack sufficient numbers or proper types of organisms to produce sufficient quantities of damaging metabolites. However, as the plaque matures, the production of cells and matrix slows and utilization of energy for the total community metabolism results in

TABLE 3-3 Elements of Saliva That Control Plaque Communities

NAMES	ACTION	EFFECTS ON PLAQUE COMMUNITY
SALIVARY ENZYMES		
Amylase	Cleaves—1,4 glucoside bonds	Increases availability of oligosaccharides
Lactoperoxidase	Catalyzes hydrogen peroxide–mediated oxidation; adsorbs to hydroxyapatite in active form	Lethal to many organisms: suppresses plaque formation on tooth surfaces
Lysozyme	Lyses cells by degradation of cell walls, releasing peptidoglycans; binds to hydroxyapatite in active conformation	Lethal to many organisms; peptidoglycans activate complement; suppresses plaque formation on tooth surfaces
Lipases	Hydrolysis of triglycerides to free fatty acids and partial glycerides	Free fatty acids inhibit attachment and growth of some organisms
NONENZYME PROTEINS		
Lactoferrin	Ties up free iron	Inhibits growth of some iron-dependent microbes
Secretory IgA (smaller amounts of IgM, IgG)	Agglutination of bacteria inhibits bacterial enzymes	Reduces numbers in saliva by precipitation; slows bacterial growth
Glycoproteins (mucins)	Agglutination of bacteria	Reduces numbers in saliva by precipitation

IgA, Immunoglobulin A; *IgG,* immunoglobulin G; *IgM,* immunoglobulin M.

acid production (Fig. 3-14). Since mature plaque is primarily anaerobic, it reduces the available nutrients to anaerobic metabolites, that is, fermentation products including weak organic acids, amines, and alcohol. Plots of the pH depression of plaque following a glucose or sucrose exposure illustrate this phenomenon (Fig. 3-15). Mature plaque communities rapidly metabolize sucrose through glycolytic pathways to organic acids, primarily lactic acid. In cariogenic plaque, virtually all the available sucrose is metabolized to acid, resulting in a severe and prolonged drop in pH, thereby increasing the potential for enamel demineralization. Demineralization of enamel occurs in the pH range 5.0 to 5.5. A single sucrose exposure/rinse can produce pH depression lasting up to 1 hour.[73] As discussed later, this prolonged pH fall has important implications for diet recommendations in the treatment of caries.

Plaque Community Structure. The structure and organization of the plaque community can alter greatly its pathogenic potential. Communities in dental fissures with large populations of MS are cariogenic, while similar communities dominated by *S. sanguis* are not. The mechanisms responsible for the composition of the climax community are therefore crucial factors in determining the presence of oral disease. As in any ecosystem, these determinants in their most basic form are food and shelter. In the oral cavity, the primary source of nutrition (food) for the oral flora is the host's saliva and diet. *Dietary sucrose, especially when frequently available, provides a selective advantage to the establishment of MS and thus greatly increases MS prevalence in plaque communities.*

Factors That Serve as Ecologic Determinants. *Ecologic determinants* are factors that exert ecologic control over habitats or niches and ultimately determine the characteristics of the plaque community. For example, the supragingival facial and lingual smooth surfaces of molar teeth are exposed to both saliva and the abrasive action of the tongue and cheeks. The subgingival areas immediately below them are protected from abrasion and saliva but are exposed to plasma exudate from the adjacent epithelial tissue. The two areas, supragingival and subgingival smooth surfaces, acquire different floras as a result of the effects of the local environmental ecologic determinants.

Some of the determinants that control the overall composition of the plaque community are shelter, pH, oxygen saturation, and nutrient availability. The essential factor that is least available for plaque organisms will be the one responsible for limiting the size (the limiting factor) of the population of that species. The bacterial species in plaque have a variety of growth requirements, and one factor limiting the growth of one species may not limit another. For example, a plaque organism may be unable to biosynthesize the coenzyme biotin. The food supply available to that particular organism may supply amino acids, carbohydrates, and fatty acids in excess of its needs, but they will go unused because the limited availability of biotin prevents further growth of the population. Other limiting factors important in the oral environment are vitamin K, albumins, hemins, and oxidation-reduction potentials.

The following sections discuss, in detail, important factors that serve as ecologic determinants.

Oral (Nontooth) Habitats. The oral mucosa harbors organisms that are able to attach to the surface of epithelial cells with sufficient retention to overcome the abrasive forces of food, the tongue, and teeth. The size of this flora is largely controlled by the regular replacement of

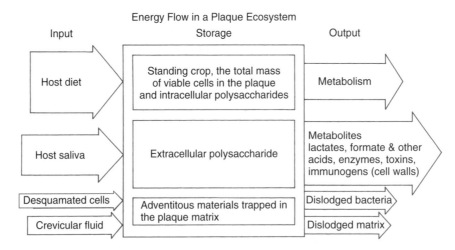

Energy Flow in a Plaque Ecosystem

FIG. **3-14** Energy flow through plaque community has important consequences to host. Some of the energy available is completely utilized, noted here as metabolism. However, because anaerobic metabolism is predominant in plaque community, many molecules are incompletely metabolized. These anaerobic by-products (metabolites) are primary agents that produce caries and periodontal disease in host.

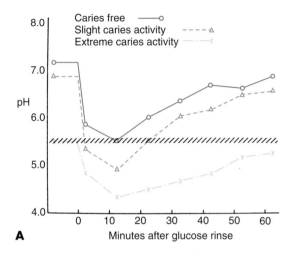

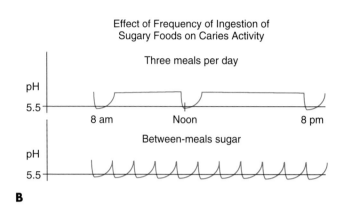

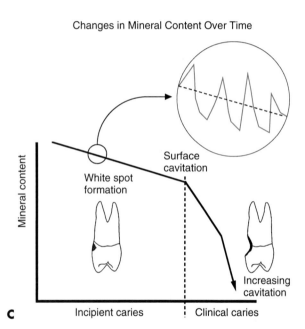

FIG. 3-15 **A,** Mature plaque communities have tremendous metabolic potential and are capable of very rapid anaerobic metabolism of any available carbohydrates. Classic studies by Stephan[72] demonstrate this metabolic potential by severe pH drops at plaque-enamel interface following glucose rinse. It is generally agreed that a pH of 5.5 is the threshold for enamel demineralization. Note that exposure to a glucose rinse for an extreme caries activity plaque results in a sustained period of demineralization (pH 5.5). Recording from a slight caries activity plaque demonstrates a much shorter period of demineralization. **B,** The frequency of sucrose exposure for cariogenic plaque greatly influences the progress of tooth demineralization. The top line illustrates pH depression, patterned after the Stephan's curves in **A**. Three meals per day results in three exposures of plaque acids, each lasting approximately 1 hour. The plaque pH depression is relatively independent of the quantity of sucrose ingested. Between-meal snacks or the use of sweetened breath mints results in many more acid attacks, as illustrated at the bottom. The effect of frequent ingestion of small quantities of sucrose results in a nearly continuous acid attack on the tooth surface. The clinical consequences of this behavior can be seen in Fig. 3-34. **C,** In active caries there is a progressive loss of mineral content subjacent to the cariogenic plaque. The inset illustrates that the loss is not a continuous process. Instead, there are alternating periods of mineral loss (demineralization) with intervening periods of remineralization. The critical event for the tooth is cavitation of the surface, marked by the vertical dashed line. This event marks an acceleration in caries destruction of the tooth and irreversible loss of tooth structure. For these reasons, restorative intervention is required. (**A** *modified from Stephan RM: J Dent Res 23(4):257, 1944.*)

the mucosal surface. To successfully survive in this habitat, the organisms (primarily streptococci) must attach, grow, multiply, then drop off the surface, and finally reattach to new cell surfaces. Because the washing effects of salivary flow cause many of these organisms to be removed from the mouth, the organisms living on the oral mucosa must reproduce in great numbers to ensure survival by reattachment.

The dorsum of the tongue presents a different oral habitat because its surface is covered with papillae. This rough topography provides additional shelter not available on the mucosal surface. *S. salivarius* and *Micrococcus mucilaginous* are two species commonly found on the tongue but rarely found on teeth.

The prevailing environmental conditions on both the mucosa and the tongue are largely determined by the saliva. Both of these habitats are aerobic, have neutral pH, and are positive in oxidation-reduction potential, and yet they harbor different communities of organisms.

Tooth Habitats for Pathogenic Plaque. The tooth surface is unique because it is not protected by the surface shedding mechanisms (continual replacement of epithelial cells) used throughout the remainder of the alimentary canal. The tooth surface is stable and covered with the pellicle of precipitated salivary glycoproteins, enzymes, and immunoglobulins. It is the ideal surface for the attachment of many oral streptococci. If left undisturbed, plaque will rapidly build up to sufficient depth to produce an anaerobic environment adjacent to the tooth surface. Tooth habitats favorable for harboring pathogenic plaque include: (1) pits and fissures; (2) the smooth enamel surfaces both immediately gingival to the proximal contacts and in the gingival one third of the facial and lingual surfaces of the clinical crown; (3) root surfaces, particularly near the cervical line; and (4) subgingival areas (see Fig. 3-16, *A* through *C*). These sites correspond to the locations where caries is most frequently encountered.

Pits and fissures. Pit-and-fissure caries has the highest prevalence of all dental caries (Figs. 3-16 to 3-22). The pits and fissures provide excellent mechanical shelter for organisms and harbor a community dominated by *S. sanguis* and other streptococci.[39] The relative proportion of MS most probably determines the cariogenic potential of the pit-and-fissure community. Complex

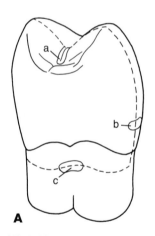 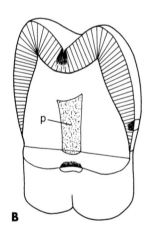 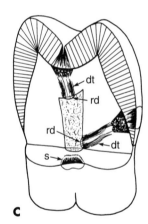

A   B   C

FIG. **3-16 A,** Caries may originate at many distinct sites: pits and fissures *(a),* smooth surface of crown *(b),* root surface *(c).* Proximal surface lesion of crown is not illustrated here because it is a special case of smooth surface lesion. Histopathology and progress of both facial (or lingual) and proximal lesions are identical. The *dotted line* indicates cut used to reveal cross-sections illustrated in Figs. 3-16, *B* and *C.* **B,** In cross-section, the three types of lesions demonstrate different rates of progression and different morphology. Lesions illustrated here are intended to be representative of each type. No particular association between three lesions is implied. Pit-and-fissure lesions have small sites of origin visible on occlusal surface but have wide base. Overall shape of pit-and-fissure lesion is inverted V. In contrast, smooth-surface lesion is V-shaped with wide area of origin and apex of V directed toward pulp *(p).* Root caries begins directly on dentin. Root-surface lesions can progress rapidly because dentin is less resistant to caries attack. **C,** Advanced carious lesions produce considerable histologic change in enamel, dentin, and pulp. Bacterial invasion of lesion results in extensive demineralization and proteolysis of the dentin. Clinically this necrotic dentin appears soft, wet, and mushy. Deeper pulpally, dentin is demineralized but not invaded by bacteria and is structurally intact. This tissue appears to be dry and leathery in texture. Two types of pulp-dentin response are illustrated. Under pit-and-fissure lesion and smooth-surface lesion, odontoblasts have died, leaving empty tubules called dead tracts *(dt).* New odontoblasts have been differentiated from pulp mesenchymal cells. These new odontoblasts have then produced reparative dentin *(rd),* which seals off dead tracts. Another type of pulp-dentin reaction is sclerosis *(s)*—occlusion of the tubules by peritubular dentin. This is illustrated under root caries lesion.

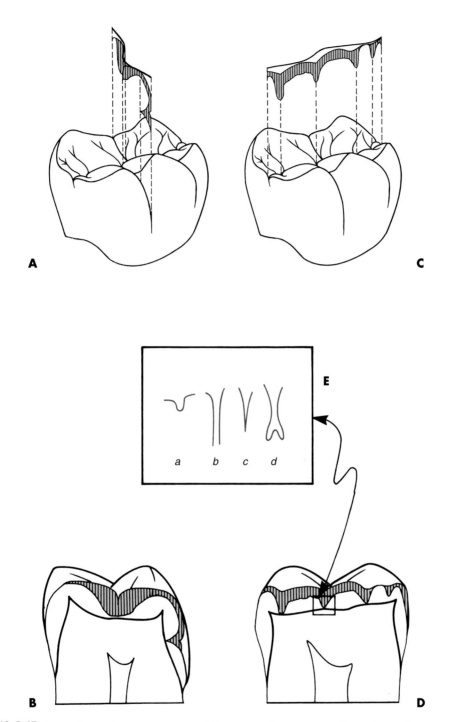

FIG. 3-17 Developmental pits, grooves, and fissures on the crowns of the teeth can have complex and varied anatomy. **A** and **B,** The facial developmental groove of the lower first molar often terminates in a pit. The depth of the groove and the pit is highly variable. **C** and **D,** The central groove extends from the mesial pit to the distal pit. Sometimes grooves extend over the marginal ridges. **E,** The termination of pits and fissures may vary from a shallow groove *(a)* to complete penetration of the enamel *(b).* The end of the fissure may end blindly *(c)* or open into an irregular chamber *(d).*

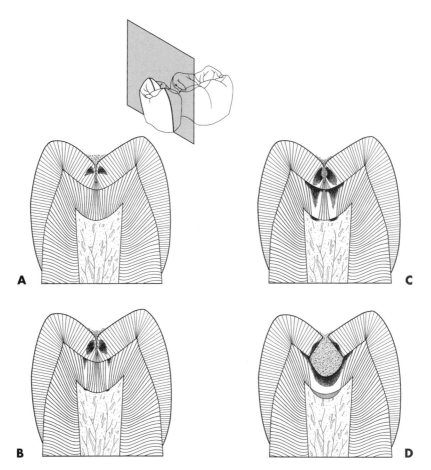

FIG. 3-18 Progression of caries in pits and fissures. A, The initial lesions develop on the lateral walls of the fissure. Demineralization follows the direction of the enamel rods, spreading laterally as it approaches the DEJ. B, Soon after the initial enamel lesion occurs, a reaction can be seen in the dentin and pulp. Forceful probing of the lesion at this stage can result in damage to the weakened porous enamel and accelerate the progression of the lesion. Clinical detection at this stage should be based on observation of discoloration and opacification of the enamel adjacent to the fissure. These changes can be observed by careful cleaning and drying of the fissure. C, Initial cavitation of the opposing walls of the fissure cannot be seen on the occlusal surface. Opacification can be seen that is similar to the previous stage. Remineralization of the enamel because of trace amounts of fluoride in the saliva may make progression of pit-and-fissure lesions more difficult to detect. D, Extensive cavitation of the dentin and undermining of the covering enamel will darken the occlusal surface (see Fig. 3-19).

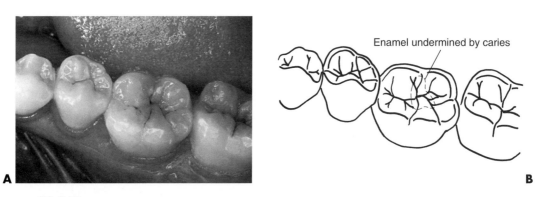

FIG. 3-19 A, Mandibular first molar has undermined discolored enamel due to extensive pit-and-fissure caries. Lesion began as illustrated in Fig. 3-18 and has progressed to stage illustrated in Fig. 3-18, D. B, Discolored enamel is outlined by broken line in the central fossa region.

communities dominated by filamentous bacteria, such as those in the gingival crevice, apparently fail to develop in the pit-and-fissure habitat.[23] The appearance of MS in pits and fissures is usually followed by caries, 6 to 24 months later. *Sealing the pits and fissures just after tooth eruption may be the single most important event in providing their resistance to caries.*

Smooth enamel surfaces. The proximal enamel surfaces immediately gingival of the contact area are the second most susceptible areas to caries (Figs. 3-23 and 3-24; also see Figs. 3-16 and 3-21). These areas are protected physically and are relatively free from the effects of mastication, tongue movement, and salivary flow. The types and numbers of organisms making up the proximal surface plaque community are variable. Important ecologic determinants for the plaque community on the proximal surfaces are the topography of the tooth surface, the size and shape of the gingival papillae, and the oral hygiene of the patient. A rough surface (caused by caries, a poor quality restoration [new or old], or a structural defect) restricts adequate plaque removal. This results in retention of a more advanced successional plaque stage, favoring the occurrence of caries or periodontal disease at the site.

In very young patients, the gingival papilla completely fills the interproximal space under a proximal contact and is termed a *col*. Thus the proximal surfaces of very young patients are in crevicular spaces that are less favorable habitats for MS. Consequently, proximal caries is less likely to develop where this favorable soft tissue architecture exists. Conversely, apical migration of the papillae creates more habitats in exposed environments for tooth surface–colonizing bacteria. Increasing the exposed surface area has a stimulating effect on the growth of MS. Therefore poor soft tissue form tends to stimulate plaque growth in the sheltered proximal areas, rendering them more susceptible to both caries and periodontal disease. More vigorous and conscientious oral hygiene practices are required to keep these open proximal regions free of disease.

Often the gingival aspect of the facial and lingual smooth enamel surface that is supragingival but gingival of the occlusogingival height of contour is neither rubbed by the bolus of food nor cleaned by the toothbrush. Therefore these surface areas are habitats for the caries-producing mature plaque. The presence of caries in these areas usually is indicative of a caries-active mouth (Fig. 3-25; also see Figs. 3-1, 3-2, and 3-39).

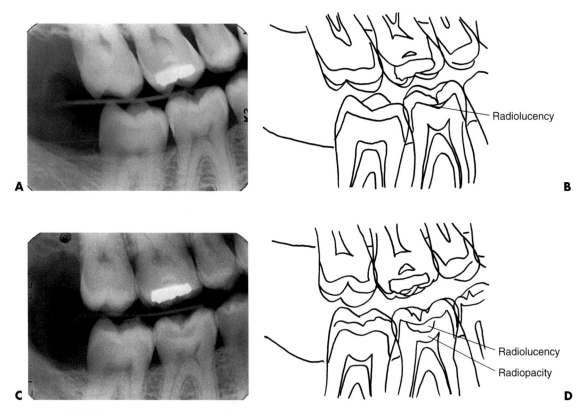

FIG. 3-20 Progression of pit-and-fissure caries. **A,** The mandibular right first molar (No. 30) was sealed. Note radiolucent areas under the occlusal enamel in **A** and **B**. The seal failed and caries progressed slowly during the next 5 years, the only symptom was occasional biting-force pain. **C** and **D,** Note the extensive radiolucency under the enamel and an area of increased radiopacity below the lesion, suggesting sclerosis.

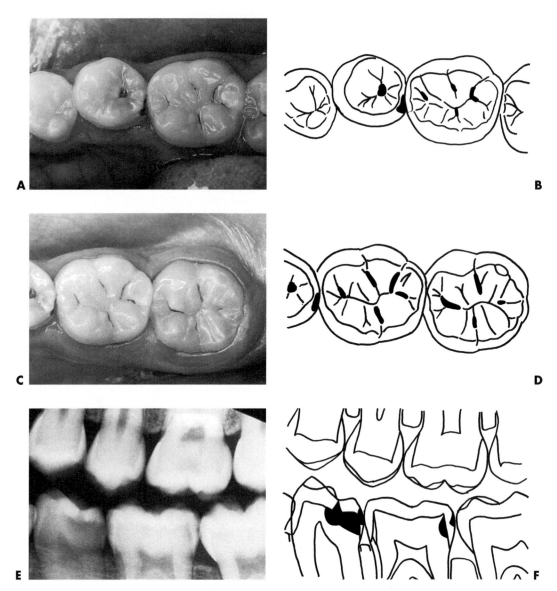

FIG. **3-21** A young patient with extensive caries. **A** and **B,** The occlusal pits of the first molar and second premolar are carious. There is an interproximal carious lesion on the second premolar. The second premolar is rotated almost 90 degrees bringing the lingual surface into contact with the mesial surface of the first molar. Normally, the lingual surfaces of the mandibular teeth are rarely attacked by caries, but here, the tooth rotation makes the lingual surface a proximal contact and, consequently, produces an interproximal habitat, which increases the susceptibility of the surface to caries. **C** and **D,** The first and second molars have extensive caries in the pits and fissures. On the bitewing radiograph (**E** and **F**), not only can the extensive nature of the caries in the second premolar be seen, but also seen is a lesion on the distal aspect of the first molar, which is not visible clinically. (Colored areas in **B, D,** and **F** indicate caries.)

Root surfaces. The proximal root surface, particularly near the cervical line, is often unaffected by the action of hygiene procedures such as flossing because it may have concave anatomic surface contours (fluting) and occasional roughness at the termination of the enamel. These conditions, when coupled with exposure to the oral environment (as a result of gingival recession), favor the formation of mature, caries-producing plaque and proximal root-surface caries. Likewise, the facial or lingual root surfaces (particularly near the cervical line), when exposed to the oral environment (because of gingival recession), are often both neglected in hygiene procedures and usually not rubbed by the bolus of food. Consequently, these root surfaces also frequently harbor caries-producing plaque. Root-surface caries is more common in older patients because of niche availability and other factors sometimes associated with senescence, such as decreased salivary flow and poor oral hygiene due to

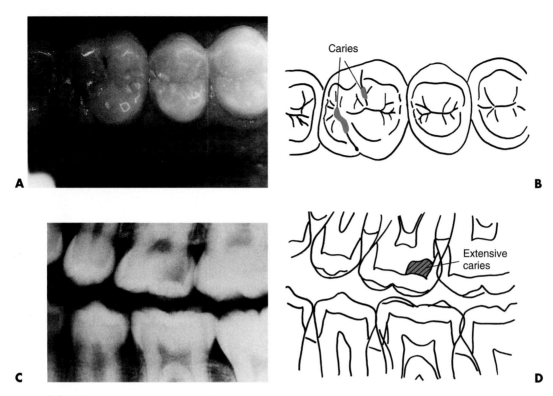

FIG. 3-22 Example of occlusal caries that is actually much more extensive than is apparent clinically. **A** and **B,** Clinical example. **C** and **D,** A bitewing radiograph further reveals an extensive area of demineralization undermining the distofacial cusp.

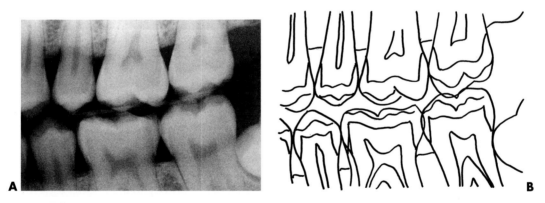

FIG. 3-23 Bitewing radiograph of normal teeth, free from caries. Note the uniform density of the enamel on the interproximal surfaces. A third molar is impacted on the distal aspect of the lower second molar. The interproximal bone levels are uniform and located slightly below the cemento-enamel junctions, suggesting a healthy periodontium.

lowered digital dexterity and decreased motivation. Caries originating on the root is alarming because: (1) it has a comparatively rapid progression, (2) it is often asymptomatic, (3) it is closer to the pulp, and (4) it is more difficult to restore.

Subgingival areas. The gingival sulcus (or crevice) habitat is unique. The initial occupants of the sulcus are merely an extension of the plaque community on the immediately adjacent surface of the tooth. Metabolites released from plaque easily penetrate the thin epithelial lining of the sulcus, inducing a strong inflammatory reaction. The capillaries dilate and become very permeable, resulting in the leakage of blood plasma into the tissue. Some metabolites have chemotactic properties that induce infiltration of white blood cells into the region. The gingival inflammatory reaction results in the sulcular tissue release of plasmalike fluid-containing immunoglobulins, polymorphonuclear leukocytes, albumins,

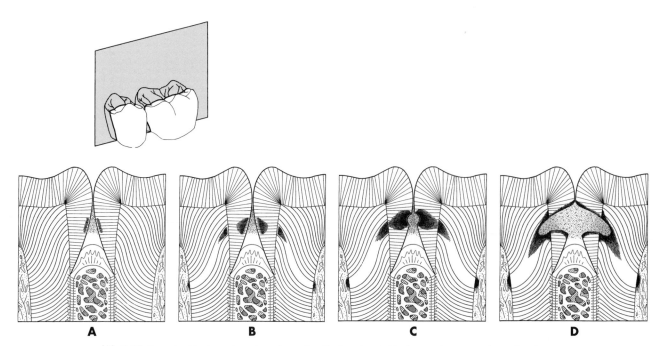

FIG. 3-24 Longitudinal sections (see *inset* for **A**) showing initiation and progression of caries on interproximal surfaces. **A,** Initial demineralization (indicated by the shading in the enamel) on the proximal surfaces is not detectable clinically or radiographically. All proximal surfaces are demineralized to some degree, but most are remineralized and become immune to further attack. The presence of small amounts of fluoride in the saliva virtually ensures that remineralization and immunity to further attack will occur. **B,** When proximal caries first becomes detectable radiographically, the enamel surface is likely to still be intact. An intact surface is essential for successful remineralization and arrest of the lesion. Demineralization of the dentin (indicated by the shading in the dentin) occurs before cavitation of the surface of the enamel. Treatment designed to promote remineralization can be effective up to this stage. **C,** Cavitation of the enamel surface is a critical event in the caries process in proximal surfaces. Cavitation is an irreversible process and requires restorative treatment/correction of the damaged tooth surface. Cavitation can only be diagnosed by clinical observation. The use of a sharp explorer to detect cavitation is problematic because excessive force in application of the explorer tip during inspection of the proximal surfaces can damage weakened enamel and accelerate the caries process by creating cavitation. Separation of the teeth can be used to provide more direct visual inspection of suspect surfaces. Fiber-optic illumination and dye absorption are also promising new evaluation procedures, but neither is specific for cavitation. **D,** Advanced cavitated lesions require prompt restorative intervention to prevent pulpal disease, limit tooth structure loss, and remove the nidus of infection of odontopathic organisms.

and hemins. These immunologic materials may change some characteristics of the adjacent plaque by removing the most susceptible organisms. New niches then become available because of the loss of some species and the availability of new nutrients. The plaque community changes progressively from masses of cocci in the supragingival plaque to a community dominated by filamentous bacteria and spirochetes in the subgingival habitat. *Bacteroides melaninogenicus* can exploit this habitat, because proteins and iron-containing compounds (hemins) are available. The establishment of a sizable population of *B. melaninogenicus* results in a very pathogenic plaque because this organism produces several enzymes capable of destroying the gingival epithelium.

Oral Hygiene. Another ecologic determinant is oral hygiene. Careful mechanical cleaning of the teeth disrupts the bacterial plaque and leaves a clean enamel surface. The recolonization of the tooth surface occurring after tooth cleaning is properly termed secondary succession. This process is much more rapid than primary succession because all normal residents of the climax community of plaque are already present in the oral cavity. The cleaning process does not actually destroy most of the oral bacteria, but merely removes them from the surfaces of the teeth. Large numbers of these bacteria are subsequently removed from the oral cavity during rinsing and swallowing after flossing and brushing, but sufficient numbers remain to recolonize the teeth. Some fastidious organisms and obligate anaerobes may in fact be killed by exposure to oxygen during tooth cleaning. However, no single species is likely to be entirely eliminated. Although all the species that make up mature plaque will continue to be present, most of these are unable to initiate colonization on the clean

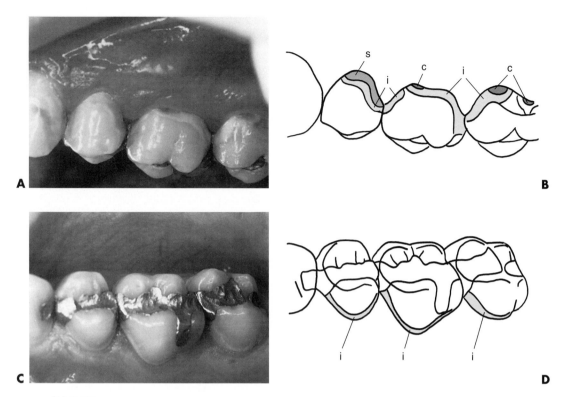

FIG. 3-25 Facial and lingual smooth-surface caries. This patient has very high caries activity with rapidly advancing caries lesions. Plaque, containing MS, extends entirely around the cervical areas of the posterior teeth. Several levels of caries involvement can be seen including: cavitation *(c)*; incipient white spot lesions *(i)*; and stained, roughened, partially remineralized incipient lesions *(s)*.

tooth surface. To return to the climax community of plaque, the tooth surface must be sequentially colonized, and the local environment must be returned to the climactic condition.

Until the environment of the climax community of plaque is restored, many of its residents are unable to grow. The pioneering organisms can have an important effect on the nature of the climax community. In experimental studies, the initial colonization of artificial fissures has been shown to depend on the relative abundance of organisms in the saliva.[75] MS and *S. sanguis* are competitive pioneering organisms. Only when MS are present in great numbers in the saliva can the organism establish itself as a significant member of the resulting mature plaque. It is of obvious benefit to the host to favor the establishment of large populations of *S. sanguis* on the teeth because MS are considerably more cariogenic than *S. sanguis*. Simple oral hygiene procedures—flossing and brushing—help achieve this desired result by frequently disrupting the plaque succession. In the absence of a high-sucrose diet, this frequent disruption favors the preferential growth of *S. sanguis* rather than MS.

Available Nutrients. The nutrients necessary for plaque growth are considered ecologic determinants. The nutritional requirements of plaque organisms can vary from simple to complex. All living organisms maintain themselves by two basic antagonistic processes: catabolic and anabolic reactions. Catabolic reactions break down complex molecules, such as carbohydrates and proteins, and release useful energy. Anabolic reactions require energy to build complex cellular molecules from simple precursors. The pioneering or initiating organisms that first colonize a tooth surface must, by necessity, have simple nutritional requirements. They must be able to catabolize almost any available energy-containing molecule. Furthermore, because they rely on the host for diet and salivary flow, they must be able to produce anabolically all necessary cellular components from relatively simple precursors. For example, MS and *S. sanguis* can produce all their amino acid needs from the metabolism of normally available salivary proteins. Organisms with complex nutritional requirements cannot occupy a tooth surface until such specific nutrients become available.

The nature and quality of the nutrient supply vary significantly from habitat to habitat. Supragingival areas on teeth characteristically have high oxygen concentrations, good carbohydrate availability, and are continually bathed in saliva. These areas are characteristically inhabited by facultative streptococci using carbohydrates as their primary energy source. Sucrose in the diet of the host strongly favors the establishment of

MS as a predominant member of the supragingival plaque. The subgingival habitat on the same tooth has low oxygen saturation, low carbohydrate availability, and few salivary components. Both hemorrhage and released sulcular tissue fluid in the subgingival habitat provide a rich variety of proteins and other complex molecules as nutrients. Thus, there is a strong selection pressure in the subgingival habitat for anaerobic bacteria that use proteins as their primary energy source. *B. melaninogenicus* is an obligate anaerobe that requires hemins and albumins for its growth and primarily depends on proteins as a source of energy. This particular organism can establish residency in a subgingival plaque only after the plaque has caused both an anaerobic interior environment and gingival bleeding. *B. melaninogenicus* produces strong proteolytic enzymes, including hyaluronidase and collagenase, and is thought to be one of the primary causative agents of periodontal disease. Its presence in plaque is largely controlled by the availability of its special nutritional requirements. Therefore, by keeping the plaque at an earlier aerobic successional stage and eliminating periodontal pockets, it is possible to prevent *B. melaninogenicus* from becoming a threat to the periodontium.

Fig. 3-14 illustrates energy flow through a hypothetical plaque ecosystem. Four sources of energy are listed. The host's diet frequently supplies the majority of the energy requirements of the plaque community in the form of fermentable carbohydrates. The plaque community also can be entirely supported by the host's saliva. Sulcular fluid and desquamated epithelial cells may play small, but important roles in supporting plaque residents such as *B. melaninogenicus*.[68]

The energy input to plaque supports a large number of organisms. The energy trapped in their cell bodies can be considered stored. Because of the inherent unreliability of the host's diet, it is expected that these plaque organisms have mechanisms to store carbohydrates intracellularly or extracellularly. The intracellular storage mechanism is the storage of glycogen-like granules that can be demonstrated by iodine staining. The extracellular storage mechanism is in the form of a variety of polysaccharides. These extracellular polysaccharides also serve other functions for the organism such as adhesion, diffusion limitation, and protection. Other energy-containing materials are trapped within the plaque matrix and make a small addition to the total stored energy.

There are four energy outputs from the plaque. First is the energy lost during metabolic processes of contained organisms. The second and largest energy output is in the production of metabolites. These are generally small molecules such as lactic, formic, and acetic acids that provide some residual energy content that the largely anaerobic plaque community is unable to metabolize. The deepest cells in the plaque may be literally starved to death and thus small amounts of large molecules such

as enzymes, cell wall components, and toxins are released from the plaque. These act as strong immunogens and can produce potent reactions from the host. The other two losses of energy include viable cells and extracellular polysaccharides that are mechanically dislodged from the plaque.

From a clinical viewpoint, the energy output side of the plaque community is of prime importance. *If the plaque community is producing large amounts of organic acids, caries will develop subjacent to the plaque.* If the output is largely toxins, proteolytic enzymes, and other antigenic materials, periodontal disease will result. This output can be controlled by regulating the input side, the habitat, or the successional stage of the plaque community.

Sulcular Fluid. In the early stages of gingival inflammation, a serous exudate is produced from the sulcular epithelium. This may occur after only 2 to 4 days of gingival tissue exposure to undisturbed plaque. This sulcular fluid contains serum proteins such as immunoglobulins, complement, fibrin, and white blood cells. Immunoglobulins of the IgG class can activate the complement system to produce several very destructive enzymes capable of lysing gram-negative bacteria and inducing phagocytosis of gram-positive bacteria. This system is therefore capable of very effective control of many microorganisms and, consequently, represents a very strong immunologic challenge to bacterial invasion of the sulcular epithelium. Actual invasion of the epithelium is only seen in acute necrotizing ulcerative gingivitis. Many organisms reside in the gingival crevice. Over long periods of residence they can produce destruction of periodontal tissues but do not normally produce caries. The effects of the immunologic controls exerted by the sulcular fluid are likely to be limited to the immediate area of the gingival crevice. Outside the crevice, the immunoglobulins and other immunologic defenses are diluted and washed away rapidly by the saliva.

Saliva. Saliva is the primary means by which the patient (host) exerts control over its oral flora (parasites). The normal oral flora is beneficial to the host. It must be recognized that the oral flora and the host have coevolved to provide a mutually satisfactory relationship. The fact that many normal residents of the oral flora do not occur naturally in any other place is strong evidence of this evolution. A parasite that rapidly destroys its host is not likely to have long-term success! However, the host can derive benefits from the parasite if that parasite occupies a niche that would otherwise be available to a more damaging parasite. The apparent result of long-term coevolution is a system in which the host cultivates a limited and specialized oral flora that, in turn, protects the host from many potential pathogens that pass through the oral cavity. The dependent relationship of the resident oral flora is demonstrated by its ability to subsist entirely on nutrients available in saliva, whereas nonresident organisms are strongly inhibited by the many antimicrobial components of saliva. Many medications are capable of reducing salivary flow and thus increasing caries risk (Table 3-4). This importance of saliva in the maintenance of the normal oral flora is dramatically illustrated by observing changes in the oral flora following therapeutic radiation to the head and neck. After radiation, the salivary glands become fibrotic and produce little or no saliva, giving the patient an extremely dry mouth, a condition termed *xerostomia*[16,19] (*xero,* dry; *stoma,* mouth). Such patients may experience near total destruction of the teeth in just a few months following radiation treatment.

Salivary protective mechanisms[51] that maintain the normal oral flora and tooth surface integrity include bacterial clearance, direct antibacterial activity, buffers, and remineralization.

Bacterial clearance. Secretions from the various salivary glands pool in the mouth to form whole or mixed saliva. The amount of saliva secreted varies greatly over time. Once secreted, saliva remains in the mouth for a short period before being swallowed. While in the mouth, saliva lubricates the oral tissues and bathes both the teeth and the plaque. The secretion rate of saliva may have a bearing on caries susceptibility and calculus formation. Adults produce 1 to 1.5 L of saliva a day, very little of which occurs during sleep. The flushing effect of this salivary flow is, by itself, adequate to remove virtually all microorganisms not adherent to an oral surface. The flushing is most effective during mastication or oral stimulation, both of which produce large volumes of saliva. Large volumes of saliva also can dilute and buffer plaque acids.

Direct antibacterial activity. Potential pathogens are continually introduced to the oral cavity from food, hands, eating utensils, or virtually anything placed in the mouth. Upon entry into the oral cavity, these organisms must first resist being washed away by the saliva. If they encounter oral surfaces, they usually find them either coated with toxic enzymes or already occupied by other organisms. Even if the new organism can survive the initial defenses and establish some adhesion to a tooth surface, it must then compete with the other oral flora organisms for nutrients. Because the normal resident oral flora is well adapted to the oral conditions and is extremely competitive, a new organism cannot successfully compete unless it is introduced in very large numbers.

Salivary glands produce an impressive array of antimicrobial products (see Table 3-3). For example, lysozyme, lactoperoxidase, lactoferrin, and agglutinins possess antibacterial activity. These salivary proteins are not part of the immune system but are part of an overall protection scheme for mucous membranes that occurs in addition to immunologic control. These protective proteins are present continuously at relatively uniform levels, have a broad spectrum of activity, and do not possess the "memory" of immunologic mechanisms. The normal resident oral flora apparently has developed resistance to most of these antibacterial mechanisms.

Although the antibacterial proteins in saliva play an important role in protection of the soft tissues in the oral cavity from infection by pathogens, they have little effect on caries because similar levels of antibacterial proteins can be found in both caries-active and caries-free individuals.[5,52] This suggests that caries susceptibility in healthy individuals is not related to saliva composition. However, *individuals with decreased salivary production (due to illness, medication, or irradiation) may have significantly higher caries susceptibility* (see Table 3-4).

Buffers. The volume and buffering capacity of saliva available to tooth surfaces have major roles in caries protection. The buffering capacity of saliva is primarily determined by the concentration of bicarbonate ion. Buffering capacity can be estimated by titration methods and may be a useful method for assessment of saliva in caries-active patients. The benefit of the buffering is to reduce the potential for acid formation.

In addition to buffers, saliva contains molecules that contribute to increasing plaque pH. These include urea and sialin, which is a tetrapeptide that contains lysine and arginine. Hydrolysis of either of these basic compounds results in production of ammonia, causing the pH to rise.

Because saliva is very important in controlling both the oral flora and the mineral content of the teeth, salivary testing should be done on patients with high caries activity. A portion of the salivary sample also may be used for bacteriologic testing.

Remineralization. Saliva and plaque fluid are supersaturated with calcium and phosphate ions. Without a means to control precipitation of these ions, the teeth

TABLE 3-4	Medications That Can Reduce Salivary Flow
MEDICATION CLASS	**EXAMPLE**
Antispasmodic	Belladonna alkaloids
Antidepressant	Amitriptyline
Antipsychotic	Chlorpromazine
Skeletal muscle relaxant	Cyclobenzaprine
Parkinsonian	Benztropine
Arrhythmia medications	Disopyramide
Antihistamine	Chlorpheniramine
Appetite depressant	Chlorphentermine
Anticonvulsant	Carbamazepine
Anxiolytic	Alprazolam
Antihypertensive	Atenolol
Diuretic	Hydrochlorothiazide
Miscellaneous	Isotretinoin

would become literally encrusted with mineral deposits. Fortunately, saliva contains statherin, a proline-rich peptide capable of stabilizing calcium and phosphate ions and thus prevents excessive deposition of these ions on the teeth.[33] This supersaturated state of the saliva provides constant opportunity for remineralizing enamel and thus can help protect the teeth in times of cariogenic challenges.

When the local pH is high enough (above 5.5) and calcium and phosphate ions are present, the demineralization of the carious process may be reversed by remineralization of the damaged enamel tooth structure. If it occurs before cavitation, the surface of the tooth may show evidence of the carious episode by the presence of discoloration (usually brownish) resulting from incorporation of exogenous pigmented material. If remineralization occurs after cavitation, the remaining exposed surface becomes harder and often becomes dark brown or black in color. Either surface is termed arrested caries and is often more resistant to future cariogenic challenge. If caries becomes arrested on a dentinal surface, it is referred to as eburnated dentin (see Figs. 9-15, C [bs] and 9-20).

PATHOPHYSIOLOGY OF CARIES

Caries causes damage by demineralization and dissolution of tooth structure, resulting from (1) a highly localized drop in the pH at the plaque-tooth interface and (2) tooth demineralization. The local pH drop occurs as the result of plaque metabolism (see Fig. 3-16), but only plaque communities with high concentrations of MS and lactobacilli can produce a sufficiently low pH to cause demineralization of teeth. A single exposure of sucrose solution to a cariogenic plaque results in rapid metabolism of the nutrients to organic acids. The organic acids (primarily lactic acid) dissociate to lower the local pH (see Fig. 3-16). Single events of lowered pH are not sufficient to produce significant changes in the mineral content of the surfaces of the teeth. However, many episodes of long-duration demineralization (lowered pH), occurring over long periods of time, will produce the characteristic lesions of caries. Frequent sucrose exposure is the single most important factor in maintaining a pH depression at the tooth surface, often resulting in demineralization.

The output (production) of acid from caries-active plaques is twice that of caries-inactive plaques per milligram wet weight of plaque.[57] The production of acid from a caries-active plaque can overcome the buffering capacity of salivary bicarbonate available at the tooth-plaque interface, causing the local pH to fall. Once the pH falls below 5.5, tooth mineral is dissolved. In caries-active individuals, the pH at the tooth surface remains below the critical pH (5.5) for 20 to 50 minutes following a single exposure to sucrose. Thus, it should be noted that sweet snacks between meals can result in almost continuous acid attack on the tooth surface.

Below the critical pH (5.5), the tooth mineral acts as a buffer and loses calcium and phosphate ions into the plaque. This buffering capacity maintains the local pH at approximately 5.0, which is responsible for the characteristic histologic form of carious lesions described in the subsequent section. At lower pH values, such as 3.0 or 4.0, the surface of enamel is etched and roughened. At a pH of 5.0, the surface remains intact while the subsurface mineral is lost. This initial carious lesion limited to the enamel is *incipient caries* and is characterized by a virtually intact surface, but a porous subsurface. The intact surface and subsurface porosity are responsible for the clinical characteristics of incipient lesions: smooth intact surfaces that become chalky white opacities when dried. When the porous body of an incipient lesion is hydrated, the lesion is not detectable clinically because the porous area remains translucent. But desiccation (drying) of the tooth with a stream of compressed air removes the subsurface water, leaving air-filled voids that render the area opaque and white. *Incipient lesions may be reversed by remineralization, restoring the enamel to a sound state. When fluoride ion is part of the remineralization process, the enamel will not only be restored to soundness but also will have increased resistance to further caries attacks.*

The intact surface over incipient lesions is critical to the process of potential remineralization because it protects the etched hydroxyapatite crystals in the enamel from being coated by salivary proteins. The etched crystal lattice remains open and can readily precipitate more hydroxyapatite when the local environmental conditions change and calcium and phosphate ions are provided to the area from saliva. Cavitation of the surface occurs when the subsurface demineralization is so extensive that the tooth structure surface collapses. Cavitation of enamel is not reversible and is usually associated with an acceleration in the process of carious destruction of the tooth. It occurs when a series of demineralization (pH drop) and remineralization (salivary ions) episodes are dominated by the demineralization process.

CLINICAL CHARACTERISTICS OF THE LESION

A plaque community of sufficient mass (thickness) to become anaerobic at the tooth surface has the potential to be cariogenic. A large population of MS virtually assures this occurrence. A sucrose-rich diet gives a selective advantage to MS and allows the organism to accumulate in large numbers in the plaque community. The sucrose-rich environment also allows MS to produce large quantities of extracellular polysaccharides (dextrans and insoluble *mutans*). These form a gelatinous material that produces a diffusion-limiting barrier in the plaque. The combination of limited diffusion and tremendous metabolic activity makes the local environment anaerobic and very acidic and, thus, an ideal environment for dissolution of the subjacent tooth surface.

Once the tooth surface becomes cavitated, a more retentive surface area is available to the plaque community. This allows filamentous bacteria that have poor adhesion abilities, such as *lactobacilli,* to become established in the lesion. In the absence of change in the host's diet and oral hygiene practices, the cavitation of the tooth surface produces a synergistic acceleration of the growth of the cariogenic plaque community and expansion of the cavitation. This results in a rapid and progressive destruction of tooth structure. Once enamel caries penetrates to the dentinoenamel junction (DEJ), rapid lateral expansion of the carious lesion takes place because dentin is much less resistant to caries attack. This sheltered, highly acidic, and anaerobic environment provides an ideal niche for lactobacilli, which were previously thought to be the primary etiologic agents of caries, but lactobacilli have no ability to adhere to the tooth surface and therefore are unlikely to be a factor in the initiation of caries. *MS are probably the most important organisms in the initiation of enamel caries, and* A. viscosus *is the most likely organism to initiate root caries.*[68] After caries initiation, *lactobacilli* then become important residents of the carious lesion, once their niche is available. Because of their acidogenic potential and aciduric lifestyle, *lactobacilli are probably very important in the progression of dentinal caries.*

CLINICAL SITES FOR CARIES INITIATION

The characteristics of a carious lesion vary with the nature of the surface on which the lesion develops. There are three distinctly different clinical sites for caries initiation: (1) the recesses of developmental pits and fissures of enamel, which is the most susceptible site; (2) smooth enamel surfaces that shelter plaque; and (3) the root surface (see Fig. 3-16, *A* through *C*).

The second site listed refers to certain areas of the smooth enamel surface where contour or tooth position protects (shelters) plaque against the rubbing action of some foods and often from being loosened by the toothbrush. These include the areas of the contacting proximal surfaces that are gingival to the contact and thereby highly susceptible to caries because of shelter afforded to plaque. (Only proper daily application of dental floss to such surfaces can disrupt the plaque's successional change.) Plaque on noncontacting proximal surfaces also may be sheltered because of tooth surface contour or position (e.g., the distal surface of the most posterior tooth). Other susceptible smooth enamel surfaces are those areas gingival to the height of contour of the facial and lingual surfaces where, again, the plaque is sheltered from the rubbing of food and often, as well, from the toothbrush because of improper brushing technique (see the later section, Oral Hygiene, for a discussion of flossing and brushing).

Each of these areas has distinct surface topography and environmental conditions. Consequently, each area has a distinct plaque population. The diagnosis, treat-ment, and prevention of these different lesion types should take into account the different etiologic factors operating at each site.

Pits and Fissures. The pits and fissures of newly erupted teeth are rapidly colonized by bacteria. These early colonizers form a "bacterial plug" that remains in the site for a long time, perhaps even the life of the tooth. The type and nature of the organisms prevalent in the oral cavity determine the type of organisms colonizing the pits and fissures and therefore are instrumental in determining the outcome of the colonization. There are large variations in the microflora found in pits and fissures, suggesting that each site can be considered a separate ecologic system. Large numbers of gram-positive cocci, especially *S. sanguis,* are found in the pits and fissures of newly erupted teeth, whereas large numbers of MS are usually found in carious pits and fissures.

The shape of the pits and fissures contributes to their high susceptibility to caries. The long narrow orifice prevents visual and tactile examination (see Fig. 3-17). There is considerable morphologic variation in these structures. Some pits and fissures end blindly, others open near the dentin, and others penetrate entirely through the enamel.

Pit-and-fissure caries expands as it penetrates into the enamel. Thus, the entry site may appear much smaller than the actual lesion, making clinical diagnosis difficult. Carious lesions of pits and fissures develop from attack on their walls (see Fig. 3-18, *A* through *C).* The progress of dissolution of the walls of a pit-or-fissure lesion is similar in principle to that of the smooth-surface lesion because there is a wide area of surface attack extending inward, paralleling the enamel rods. The occlusal enamel rods bend down and terminate on the dentin immediately below the developmental enamel fault. Thus a lesion originating in a pit or fissure affects a greater area of the DEJ than does a comparable smooth-surface lesion. In cross-section, the gross appearance of a pit-and-fissure lesion is an inverted V with a narrow entrance and a progressively wider area of involvement closer to the DEJ (see Fig. 3-18, *D).*

Smooth Enamel Surfaces. The smooth enamel surfaces of the teeth present a less favorable site for plaque attachment. Plaque usually develops only on those smooth surfaces that are near the gingiva or are under proximal contacts. The proximal surfaces are particularly susceptible to caries because of the extra shelter provided to resident plaque due to the proximal contact area immediately occlusal to the plaque. Lesions starting on smooth enamel surfaces have a broad area of origin and a conical, or pointed, extension toward the DEJ. The path of ingress of the lesion is roughly parallel to the long axes of the enamel rods in the region. A cross-section of the enamel portion of a smooth surface lesion shows a V shape with a wide area of origin and the apex of the V directed toward the DEJ. After caries penetrates the dentinoenamel junction, softening of the dentin spreads rapidly laterally and pulpally (see Fig. 3-24).

Root Surface. The root surface is rougher than enamel and readily allows plaque formation in the absence of good oral hygiene. The cementum covering the root surface is extremely thin and provides little resistance to caries attack. Root caries lesions have less well-defined margins, tend to be U-shaped in cross-section, and progress more rapidly because of the lack of protection from an enamel covering. In recent years, the prevalence of root caries has significantly increased because of the increasing number of older persons who retain more teeth, experience gingival recession, and usually have cariogenic plaque on the exposed root surfaces.

PROGRESSION OF CARIOUS LESIONS

The progression and morphology of the carious lesion is variable, depending on the site of origin and the conditions in the mouth (see Figs. 3-16, 3-18, and 3-24). *The time for progression from incipient caries to clinical caries (cavitation) on smooth surfaces is estimated to be 18 months, plus or minus 6 months.*[63] Peak rates for the incidence of new lesions occurs 3 years after the eruption of the tooth. Occlusal pit-and-fissure lesions develop in less time than smooth-surface caries. Both poor oral hygiene and frequent exposures to sucrose-containing food can produce incipient (white spot) lesions (first clinical evidence of demineralization) in as little as 3 weeks. Radiation-induced xerostomia (dry mouth) can lead to clinical caries development in as little as 3 months from the onset of the radiation. Thus, caries development in healthy individuals is usually slow in comparison to the rate possible in compromised persons.

HISTOPATHOLOGY OF CARIES
ENAMEL CARIES

Histology of Enamel. Enamel is composed of very tightly packed hydroxyapatite crystallites, organized into long columnar rods (prisms). The rods are somewhat key-shaped in cross-section as described in Chapter 2. Individual enamel rods are formed by the activity of ameloblasts. Each rod starts at the DEJ and extends as a wavy, continuous column to the surface of the crown. The mineralization process is apparently somewhat discontinuous and is characterized by alternating phases of high and low activity. Periods of low activity create "rest" lines within the rods. These rest lines, in combination with similar lines in neighboring rods, form a structure visible in mounted cross-sections of enamel and are named the striae of Retzius. The striae are regions characterized by relatively higher organic content (see Fig. 3-6, *B*). Both the striae and the inherent spaces in prism boundaries provide sufficient porosity to allow movement of water and small ions, such as hydrogen ions. Thus enamel is capable of acting as a molecular sieve by allowing free movement of small molecules and blocking the passage of larger molecules and ions. The sievelike behavior of enamel also explains why even incipient caries of enamel can produce a pulpal response before penetration of bacteria. The movement of ions through carious enamel can result in acid dissolution of the underlying dentin before actual cavitation of the enamel surface. This acid attack at the external ends of the dentinal tubules initiates a pulpal response by unknown mechanisms. Because the striae form horizontal lines of greater permeability in the enamel, they probably contribute to the lateral spread of smooth surface lesions. The decreased mineral content of the striae in incipient lesions is illustrated in Figs. 3-26

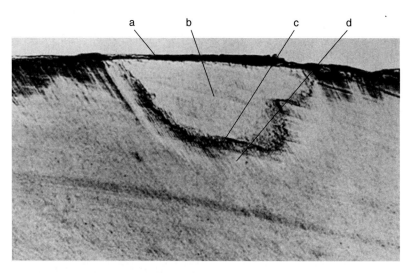

FIG. 3-26 Cross-section of small carious lesion in enamel examined in quinoline by transmitted light (×100). Surface *(a)* appears to be intact. Body of lesion *(b)* shows enhancement of striae of Retzius. Dark zone *(c)* surrounds body of lesion while translucent zone *(d)* is evident over entire advancing front of lesion. *(From Silverstone LM. In Silverstone LM et al, editors: Dental caries, London and Basingstoke, 1981, Macmillan.)*

and 3-27. Indeed, the striae appear to be accentuated in early lesions. In the occlusal enamel, the striae of Retzius and the enamel rod directions are mutually perpendicular. On the axial surfaces of the crown, the striae course diagonally and terminate on the surface as slight depressions. The surface manifestations of the striae are the imbrication lines of Pickerel that lie between the perikymata ridges (see Fig. 3-7). Caries preferentially attacks the cores of the rods and the more permeable striae of Retzius, which promotes lateral spreading and undermining of the adjacent enamel.

Clinical Characteristics of Enamel Caries: the Incipient Smooth-Surface Lesion. Caries-prone patients usually have extensive deposits of plaque on the teeth, which must be removed before clinical examination. On clean, dry teeth, the earliest evidence of caries on the smooth enamel surface of a crown is a white spot (see Figs. 3-1, 3-2, 3-25, and 9-6, *D*). These lesions are usually observed on the facial and lingual surfaces of the teeth. White spots are chalky white, opaque areas that are re-

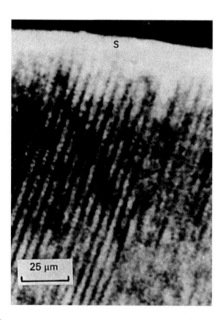

FIG. **3-27** Microradiograph (×150) of cross-section of small carious lesion in enamel. Well-mineralized surface *(s)* is evident. Alternating radiolucent and radiopaque lines indicate demineralization between enamel rods. *(From Silverstone LM. In Silverstone LM et al, editors:* Dental caries, *London and Basingstoke, 1981, Macmillan.)*

vealed only when the tooth surface is desiccated, and are termed incipient caries. These areas of enamel lose their translucency because of the extensive subsurface porosity caused by demineralization. Care must be exercised to distinguish white spots of incipient caries from developmental white spot hypocalcifications of enamel (see Fig. 9-6). Incipient caries will partially or totally disappear visually when the enamel is hydrated (wet), while hypocalcified enamel is relatively unaffected by drying and wetting (Table 3-5). Hypocalcified enamel does not represent a clinical problem except when its appearance is objectionable esthetically. The surface texture of an incipient lesion is unaltered and is undetectable by tactile examination with an explorer. A more advanced lesion develops a rough surface that is softer than the unaffected, normal enamel. Softened chalky enamel that can be chipped away with an explorer is a sign of active caries. It also should be noted that injudicious use of an explorer tip can cause actual cavitation for a previously noncavitated incipient area, thus requiring, in most cases, restorative intervention. Similar incipient lesions occur on the proximal smooth surfaces but usually are undetectable by visual or judicious tactile (explorer) examination. Incipient lesions sometimes can be seen on radiographs as a faint radiolucency, limited to the superficial enamel. When a proximal lesion is clearly visible radiographically, the lesion may have advanced significantly and histologic alteration of the underlying dentin probably has already occurred (see Fig. 3-36).

It has been shown experimentally and clinically that incipient caries of enamel can remineralize.[6,70] Tables 3-5 and 3-6 list the characteristics of enamel at various stages of demineralization. Noncavitated enamel lesions retain most of the original crystalline framework of the enamel rods and the etched crystallites serve as nucleating agents for remineralization. Calcium and phosphate ions from saliva can then penetrate the enamel surface and precipitate on the highly reactive crystalline surfaces in the enamel lesion. The supersaturation of the saliva with calcium and phosphate ions serves as the driving force for the remineralization process. Both artificial and natural carious lesions of human enamel have been shown to regress to earlier histologic stages after exposure to conditions that promote remineralization. Furthermore, the presence of trace amounts of fluoride ions during

TABLE 3-5 Clinical Characteristics of Normal and Altered Enamel

	HYDRATED	DESICCATED	SURFACE TEXTURE	SURFACE HARDNESS
Normal enamel	Translucent	Translucent	Smooth	Hard
Hypocalcified enamel	Opaque	Opaque	Smooth	Hard
Incipient caries	Translucent	Opaque	Smooth	Softened
Active caries	Opaque	Opaque	Cavitated	Very soft
Arrested caries	Opaque, dark	Opaque, dark	Roughened	Hard

this remineralization process greatly enhances the precipitation of calcium and phosphate, resulting in the remineralized enamel becoming more resistant to subsequent caries attack because of the incorporation of more acid-resistant fluorapatite (see Fig. 3-38). *Remineralized (arrested) lesions* can be observed clinically as intact, but discolored, usually brown or black spots (see Fig. 9-15, *C*). The change in color is presumably due to trapped organic debris and metallic ions within the enamel. These discolored, remineralized, arrested caries areas are intact and are more resistant to subsequent caries attack than the adjacent unaffected enamel. They should not be restored unless they are esthetically objectionable.

Zones of Incipient Lesion. Considerable research has been applied to producing caries-like lesions in simplified laboratory systems.[70,71] The first attempts to produce artificial lesions used strong organic acids. These failed because the strong acids aggressively attacked the surface of enamel, producing a damaged surface similar to that produced by the acid-etch technique now used for tooth-colored restorations. However, when acidified gels were used over a very long exposure time (10 to 12 weeks), artificial carious lesions could be produced that were histologically identical to natural incipient lesions. The success of this technique illustrates the importance of the diffusion-limiting nature of plaque described earlier (see Clinical Characteristics of the Lesion). The ability to artificially produce enamel lesions has resulted in an identification of a detailed description of the early stages of caries in enamel. Figs. 3-26 and 3-28 illustrate the four regularly observed zones in a sectioned incipient lesion: (1) the translucent zone, (2) the dark zone, (3) the body of the lesion, and (4) the surface zone.

Zone 1: Translucent Zone. The deepest zone is the translucent zone (see Fig. 3-28, *C*) and represents the advancing front of the enamel lesion. The name refers to its structureless appearance when perfused with quinoline solution and examined with polarized light. In this zone, the pores or voids form along the enamel prism (rod) boundaries, presumably because of the ease of hydrogen ion penetration during the carious process. When these boundary area voids are filled with quinoline solution, which has the same refractive index as enamel, the features of the area disappear. The pore volume of the translucent zone of enamel caries is 1%, 10 times greater than normal enamel.

Zone 2: Dark Zone. The next deepest zone is known as the dark zone because it does not transmit polarized light. This light blockage is caused by the presence of many tiny pores too small to absorb quinoline. These

TABLE 3-6	Clinical Significance of Enamel Lesions			
	PLAQUE	ENAMEL STRUCTURE	ANTIMICROBIAL TREATMENT	RESTORATIVE TREATMENT
Normal enamel	Normal	Normal	Not indicated	Not indicated
Hypocalcified enamel	Normal	Abnormal, but not weakened	Not indicated	Only for esthetics
Incipient caries	Pathogenic	Porous, weakened	Yes	Not indicated
Active caries	Pathogenic	Cavitated, very weak	Yes	Yes
Arrested caries	Normal	Remineralized, strong	Not indicated	Only for esthetics

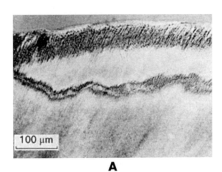
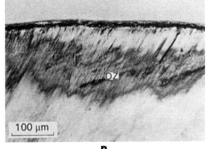
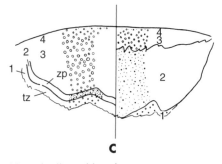

A   **B**   **C**

FIG. 3-28 **A,** Cross-section of small carious lesion in enamel examined in quinoline with polarized light (×100). Advancing front of lesion appears as dark band below body of lesion. **B,** Same section after exposure to artificial calcifying solution examined in quinoline and polarized light. Dark zone *(DZ)* covers much greater area after remineralization has occurred (×100). **C,** Schematic diagram of Fig. 3-28, *A* and *B*. Left side indicates small extent of zones 1 and 2 before remineralization. Small circles indicate relative sizes of pores in each zone. Right side indicates increase in zone 2, the dark zone, following remineralization. This micropore system must have been created where previously the pores were much larger. *(From Silverstone LM. In Silverstone LM et al, editors:* Dental caries, *London and Basingstoke, 1981, Macmillan.)*

smaller air- or vapor-filled pores make the region opaque. The total pore volume is 2% to 4%. There is some speculation that the dark zone is not really a stage in the sequence of the breakdown of enamel; rather, the dark zone may be formed by deposition of ions into an area previously only containing large pores. It must be remembered that *caries is an episodic disease with alternating phases of demineralization and remineralization.* Experimental remineralization has demonstrated increases in the size of the dark zone at the expense of the body of the lesion (see Fig. 3-28, *C*). There is also a loss of crystalline structure in the dark zone, suggestive of the process of demineralization and remineralization. The size of the dark zone is probably an indication of the amount of remineralization that has recently occurred.

Zone 3: Body of the Lesion. The body of the lesion is the largest portion of the incipient lesion while in a demineralizing phase. It has the largest pore volume, varying from 5% at the periphery to 25% at the center. The striae of Retzius are well marked in the body of the lesion, indicating preferential mineral dissolution along these areas of relatively higher porosity. The first penetration of caries enters the enamel surface via the striae of Retzius. The interprismatic areas and these cross-striations provide access to the rod (prism) cores, which are then preferentially attacked. Bacteria may be present in this zone if the pore size is large enough to permit their entry. Studies using transmission electron microscopy (TEM) and scanning electron microscopy (SEM) demonstrate the presence of bacteria invading between the enamel rods (prisms) in the body zone.[12,25]

Zone 4: Surface Zone. The surface zone is relatively unaffected by the caries attack. It has a lower pore volume than the body of the lesion (less than 5%) and a radiopacity comparable to unaffected adjacent enamel (see Fig. 3-27). The surface of normal enamel is hypermineralized by contact with saliva and has a greater concentration of fluoride ion than the immediately subjacent enamel. It has been hypothesized that hypermineralization and increased fluoride content of the superficial enamel are responsible for the relative immunity of the enamel surface. However, removal of the hypermineralized surface by polishing fails to prevent the reformation of a typical, well-mineralized surface over the carious lesion. Thus, the intact surface over incipient caries is a phenomenon of the caries demineralization process rather than any special characteristics of the superficial enamel. Nevertheless, the importance of the intact surface cannot be overemphasized, because it serves as a barrier to bacterial invasion. As the enamel lesion progresses, conical-shaped defects in the surface zone can be seen by SEM. These are probably the first sites where bacteria can gain entry into a carious lesion. Arresting the caries process at this stage results in a hard surface that may at times be rough, though cleanable (see Fig. 9-20, *C*).

DENTINAL CARIES

Histology of Dentin. Dentin is the hard portion of the tooth that is covered by enamel on the crown and cementum on the root. Dentin is the calcified product of the odontoblasts that line the inner surface of the dentin within the periphery of the external pulp tissue. Each odontoblast has an extension (termed *Tomes' fiber* in older texts) into a dentinal tubule. The tubules transverse the entire thickness of dentin from the pulp to the dentinoenamel junction (Fig. 3-29, *A*). Filling the space between the tubules is the intertubular dentin, a rigid bonelike material composed of hydroxyapatite crystals embedded in a network of collagen fibers. The walls of the tubules are lined with a smooth layer of mineral termed peritubular dentin. A thin membrane is always observed lining the tubule in normal dentin. Controversy remains concerning the nature of this lining membrane: it may be a true plasma membrane of the odontoblast or simply a limiting membrane similar to that found on the surface of bone.[84] The material within the membrane is odontoblastic cytoplasm if the membrane is part of the odontoblast, or a plasmalike exudate if the membrane is not a part of the odontoblast. In either case, the tubule allows fluid movement and ion transport necessary for remineralization of intertubular dentin, apposition of peritubular dentin, and/or perception of pain.

The dentin and the pulp are morphologically and embryologically a single unit. Teeth are formed early during development of the mandible and maxilla. A sheet of epithelial tissue grows inward and condenses with the underlying mesenchymal tissue in the developing jaws. This condensed ball of cells, called the *dental papilla*, differentiates to form dentin- and enamel-forming tissues. The surrounding epithelial cells form the enamel organ by differentiating into ameloblasts. On the inside of the bell-shaped tooth bud, the mesenchymal cells immediately adjacent to the developing ameloblasts transform into odontoblasts. The two tissues, dentin and enamel, grow away from their original junction zone to form the structure of the tooth. The DEJ is the remnant of the bell stage of the tooth bud. The odontoblasts lay down dentin and move toward the center of the tooth, while the ameloblasts lay down enamel and move outward, away from the tooth bud center. In the process of dentinogenesis (formation of dentin), the odontoblasts' cell bodies are pushed further and further inward. As they move inward, they leave a tubule behind. Thus each odontoblast is a pulp cell that is associated with a tubule extending to the external periphery of the dentin. Because of the intimate relationship between the odontoblasts and the dentin, the pulp and the dentin should be regarded as a single functional unit. More detail of the histology of dentin was presented in Chapter 2.

Clinical and Histologic Characteristics of Dentinal Caries, Acid Levels, and Reparative Responses. Progression of caries in dentin is different from progression

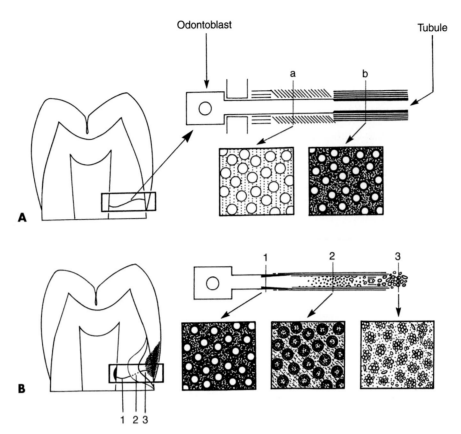

FIG. 3-29 Normal and carious dentin. Normal dentin **(A)** has characteristic tubules that follow a wavy path from the external surface of the dentin, below the enamel or cementum, to the inner surface of the dentin in the pulp tissue of the pulp chamber or pulp canal. Dentin is formed from the external surface and grows inward. As the dentin grows, the odontoblasts become increasingly compressed in the shrinking pulp chamber and the number of associated tubules becomes more concentrated per unit area. The more recently formed dentin near the pulp *(a)* has both large tubules with little or no peritubular dentin and calcified intertubular dentin filled with collagen fibers. The older dentin, closer to the external surface *(b)*, is characterized by smaller, more widely separated tubules and a greater mineral content in the intertubular dentin. The older dentin tubules are lined by a uniform layer of mineral termed peritubular dentin. These changes occur gradually from the inner surface to the external surface of the dentin. Horizontal lines indicate predentin; diagonal lines indicate increasing density of minerals; darker horizontal lines indicate densely mineralized dentin and increased thickness of peritubular dentin. The transition in mineral content is gradual as indicated in Fig. 3-28. Carious dentin **(B)** undergoes several changes. The most superficial infected zone of carious dentin *(3)* is characterized by bacteria filling the tubules, and granular material in the intertubular space. The granular material contains very little mineral and lacks characteristic cross-banding of collagen. Pulpal to (below) the infected dentin is a zone where the dentin appears transparent in mounted whole specimens. This zone *(2)* is *affected* (not infected) *carious dentin* and is characterized by loss of mineral in the intertubular and peritubular dentin. Many crystals can be detected in the lumen of the tubules in this zone. The crystals in the tubule lumen render the refractive index of the lumen similar to that of the intertubular dentin, making the zone transparent. Normal dentin *(1)* is found pulpal to (below) the transparent dentin.

in the overlying enamel because of the structural differences of dentin (Figs. 3-29 to 3-32). Dentin contains much less mineral and possesses microscopic tubules that provide a pathway for the ingress of acids and egress of mineral. The dentinoenamel junction has the least resistance to caries attack and allows rapid lateral spreading once caries has penetrated the enamel (see Figs. 3-18 and 3-24). Because of these characteristics, dentinal caries is V-shaped in cross-section with a wide base at the DEJ

and the apex directed pulpally. Caries advances more rapidly in dentin than in enamel because dentin provides much less resistance to acid attack because of less mineralized content. Caries produces a variety of responses in dentin, including pain, demineralization, and remineralization.

Often, pain is not reported even when caries invades dentin, except when deep lesions bring the bacterial infection close to the pulp. Episodes of short duration

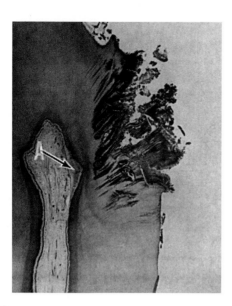

FIG. **3-30** Cross-section of demineralized specimen of advanced caries in dentin. Reparative dentin *(A)* can be seen adjacent to most advanced portion of lesion. *(From Boyle P: Kornfeld's histopathology of the teeth and their surrounding structures, Philadelphia, 1955, Lea & Febiger.)*

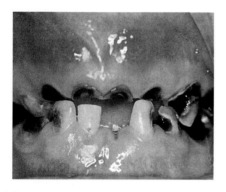

FIG. **3-31** Rampant caries in 10-year-old boy.

pain may be felt occasionally during earlier stages of dentin caries. These pains are due to stimulation of pulp tissue by movement of fluid through dentinal tubules that have been opened to the oral environment by cavitation. Once bacterial invasion of the dentin is close to the pulp, toxins and possibly even a few bacteria enter the pulp, resulting in inflammation of the pulpal tissues. Initial pulpal inflammation is thought to be evident clinically by production of sharp pains, with each pain lingering only a few seconds (10 or less) in response to a thermal stimulus. A short, painful response to cold suggests *reversible pulpitis* or pulpal *hyperemia*. Reversible pulpitis, as the name implies, is a limited inflammation of the pulp from which the tooth can recover if the caries producing the irritation is eliminated by timely operative treatment. When the pulp becomes more severely inflamed, a thermal stimulus will produce pain that continues after termination of the stimulus, typi-

cally longer than 10 seconds. This clinical pattern suggests *irreversible pulpitis,* when the pulp is unlikely to recover after removing the caries. Pulp extirpation and root canal filling usually are necessary in addition to the restorative treatment in order to save the tooth. Throbbing, continuous pain suggests partial or total pulp necrosis that is treated only by root canal therapy or extraction. Although these clinical characteristics are useful as guidelines for pulp treatment, it is emphasized that pulp symptoms can vary widely and are not always predictive of the histologic status of the tooth pulp. (See Chapter 9 for more details regarding pulpal diagnosis.)

The pulp-dentin complex reacts to caries attacks by attempting to initiate remineralization and blocking off the open tubules. These reactions result from odontoblastic activity and the physical process of demineralization and remineralization. Three levels of dentinal reaction to caries can be recognized: (1) reaction to a long-term, low-level acid demineralization associated with a slowly advancing lesion; (2) reaction to a moderate-intensity attack; and (3) reaction to severe, rapidly advancing caries characterized by very high acid levels. The dentin can react defensively (by repair) to low- and moderate-intensity caries attacks as long as the pulp remains vital and has an adequate blood circulation.

In slowly advancing caries, a vital pulp can repair demineralized dentin by remineralization of the intertubular dentin and by apposition of peritubular dentin. Early stages of caries or mild caries attacks produce long-term, low-level acid demineralization of dentin. Direct exposure of the pulp tissue to microorganisms is not a prerequisite for an inflammatory response. Toxins and other metabolic by-products, especially hydrogen ion, can penetrate via the dentinal tubules to the pulp. Even when the lesion is limited to the enamel,[8,13] the pulp can be shown to respond with inflammatory cells. Dentin responds to the stimulus of its first caries demineralization episode by deposition of crystalline material in both the lumen of the tubules and the intertubular dentin of affected dentin in front of the advancing infected dentin portion of the lesion (see Fig. 3-29, *B).* Hypermineralized areas may be seen on radiographs as zones of increased radiopacity (often S-shaped following the course of the tubules) ahead of the advancing, infected portion of the lesion. This repair only occurs if the tooth pulp is vital.

Dentin that has more mineral content than normal dentin is termed *sclerotic dentin.* Sclerotic dentin formation occurs ahead of the demineralization front of a slowly advancing lesion and may be seen under an old restoration. Sclerotic dentin is usually shiny and more darkly colored, but feels hard to the explorer tip. By comparison, normal freshly cut dentin lacks a shiny, reflective surface and allows some penetration from a sharp explorer tip. The apparent function of sclerotic dentin is to wall off a lesion by blocking (sealing) the

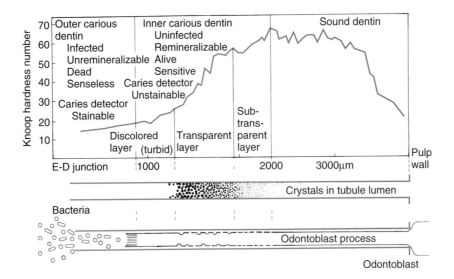

FIG. 3-32 Schematic illustration of the relationship of dentin hardness, crystal deposition, and condition of the odontoblastic process. According to Fusayama and coworkers, the odontoblastic process extends into the turbid layer but disappears before the advancing front of the bacterial invasion. Crystals are deposited in the lumen in the transparent layer and the sub-transparent layer. The area of crystal deposition corresponds to the area of damage to the odontoblast process membrane. For orientation of layers on tooth, see Fig. 3-33. (*Courtesy of Dr. T. Fusayama. Copyright Ishiyaku EuroAmerica, Inc. Tokyo, 1993.*)

tubules. The permeability of sclerotic dentin is greatly reduced in comparison to normal dentin because of the decrease in the tubule lumen diameter.[64] Therefore it may be more difficult to bond a restorative material to sclerotic dentin.

Crystalline precipitates form in the lumen of the dentinal tubules in the advancing front of a demineralization zone (affected dentin). Once these affected tubules become completely occluded by the mineral precipitate, they appear clear when a section of the tooth is evaluated. This portion of dentin has been termed the transparent zone of dentin (see next section, Zones of Dentinal Caries) and, again, is the result of both mineral loss in the intertubular dentin and precipitation of this mineral in the tubule lumen. Consequently, translucent dentin is softer than normal dentin (Fig. 3-33).[60]

The second level of dentinal response is to moderate intensity (or intermediate) irritants. More intense caries activity results in bacterial invasion of the dentin. The infected dentin contains a wide variety of pathogenic materials or irritants, including high acid levels, hydrolytic enzymes, bacteria, and bacterial cellular debris. These materials can cause the degeneration and death of the odontoblasts and their tubular extensions below the lesion, as well as a mild inflammation of the pulp. Groups of these dead, empty tubules are termed dead tracts. The pulp may be irritated sufficiently from high acid levels or bacterial enzyme production to cause the formation (from undifferentiated mesenchymal cells) of replacement odontoblasts (secondary odontoblasts). These cells produce *reparative dentin* (reactionary dentin) on the af-

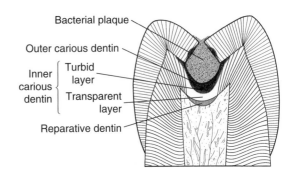

FIG. 3-33 Cross-section of occlusal caries. The occlusal enamel appears intact, with a small opening in the occlusal fissure. The enamel is darkened where it is undermined by demineralization. The surface of the enamel is unaffected. The lesion is filled with a bacterial plug containing high numbers of MS and lactobacilli. The dentin is infected below the plug. The deeper dentin is not infected but is extensively demineralized. Reparative dentin is being formed below the lesion.

fected portion of the pulp chamber wall (see Fig. 3-29, *B* and 3-33). This dentin is different from the normal dentinal apposition that occurs throughout the life of the tooth by primary (original) odontoblasts. The structure of reparative dentin can vary from well-organized tubular dentin (less often) to very irregular atubular dentin (more often), depending on the severity of the stimulus. Reparative dentin is a very effective barrier to diffusion of material through the tubules and is an important step in the repair of dentin. Severe stimuli also can result in the formation within the pulp chamber of unattached dentin, termed pulp stones, in addition to reparative dentin.

The success of dentinal reparative responses, either by remineralization of intertubular dentin and apposition of peritubular dentin or by reparative dentin, depends on the severity of the caries attack and the ability of the pulp to respond. The pulpal blood supply may be the most important limiting factor to the pulpal responses.

The third level of dentinal response is to severe irritation. Acute, rapidly advancing caries with very high levels of acid production overpowers dentinal defenses and results in infection, abscess, and death of the pulp. In comparison to other oral tissues, the pulp is poorly tolerant of inflammation. Small, localized infections in the pulp produce an inflammatory response involving capillary dilation, local edema, and stagnation of blood flow. Because the pulp is contained in a sealed chamber and its blood is supplied through very narrow root canals, any stagnation of blood flow can result in local anoxia and necrosis. The local necrosis leads to more inflammation, edema, and stagnation of blood flow in the immediately adjacent pulp tissue, which then becomes necrotic in a cascading process that rapidly spreads to involve the entire pulp.

Maintenance of pulp vitality is dependent on the adequacy of pulpal blood supply. Recently erupted teeth with large pulp chambers and short, wide canals with large apical foramina have a much more favorable prognosis for surviving pulpal inflammation than fully formed teeth with small pulp chambers and small apical foramina.

Zones of Dentinal Caries. Caries advancement in dentin proceeds through three changes: (1) weak organic acids demineralize the dentin; (2) the organic material of the dentin, particularly collagen, degenerates and dissolves; and (3) the loss of structural integrity is followed by invasion of bacteria. Five different zones have been described in carious dentin. The zones are most clearly distinguished in slowly advancing lesions. In rapidly progressing caries, the difference between the zones becomes less distinct.

Zone 1: Normal Dentin. The deepest area is normal dentin, which has tubules with odontoblastic processes that are smooth, and no crystals are in the lumens. The intertubular dentin has normal cross-banded collagen and normal dense apatite crystals. No bacteria are in the tubules. Stimulation of the dentin (e.g., by osmotic gradient [from applied sucrose or salt], a bur, a dragging instrument, or desiccation from heat or air), produces a sharp pain.

Zone 2: Subtransparent Dentin. Next is the subtransparent layer, which is a zone of demineralization of the intertubular dentin and initial formation of very fine crystals in the tubule lumen at the advancing front. Damage to the odontoblastic process is evident; however, no bacteria are found in the zone. Stimulation of the dentin produces pain, and the dentin is capable of remineralization.

Zone 3: Transparent Dentin. The transparent layer is a zone of carious dentin that is softer than normal dentin and shows further loss of mineral from the intertubular dentin and many large crystals in the lumen of the dentinal tubules. Stimulation of this region produces pain. No bacteria are present. Although organic acids attack both the mineral and organic content of the dentin, the collagen cross-linking remains intact in this zone. The intact collagen can serve as a template for remineralization of the intertubular dentin, and thus this region remains capable of self-repair provided the pulp remains vital.

Zone 4: Turbid Dentin. Turbid dentin is the zone of bacterial invasion and is marked by widening and distortion of the dentinal tubules, which are filled with bacteria. There is very little mineral present and the collagen in this zone is irreversibly denatured. The dentin in this zone will not self-repair. This zone cannot be remineralized and must be removed before restoration.

Zone 5: Infected Dentin. The outermost zone, infected dentin, consists of decomposed dentin that is teeming with bacteria. There is no recognizable structure to the dentin and collagen and mineral seem to be absent. Great numbers of bacteria are dispersed in this granular material. Removal of infected dentin is essential to sound, successful restorative procedures as well as prevention of spreading the infection.

ADVANCED CARIOUS LESIONS

Increasing demineralization of the body of the enamel lesion results in the weakening and eventual collapse of the surface covering. The resulting cavitation provides an even more protective and retentive habitat for the cariogenic plaque, thus accelerating the progression of the lesion. The DEJ provides less resistance to the carious process than either the enamel or the dentin. The resultant lateral spread of the lesion at the DEJ produces the characteristic second cone of caries activity in the dentin. Figs. 3-29 to 3-31 and Fig. 3-46 illustrate advanced lesions with infected dentin.

Necrotic dentin is recognized clinically as a wet, mushy, easily removable mass. This material is structureless or granular in histologic appearance and contains masses of bacteria. Occasionally, remnants of dentinal tubules may be seen in histologic preparations. Removal of the necrotic material uncovers deeper infected dentin (zone 4, turbid dentin), which appears dry and leathery. The leathery dentin is easily removed by hand instruments and flakes off in layers parallel to the DEJ. Microscopic examination of this material reveals distorted dentinal tubules engorged with bacteria. Clefts coursing perpendicular to the tubules also are seen in leathery dentin. Apparently these clefts represent the rest lines formed during the original deposition of the dentin and are more susceptible to caries attack. Further excavation uncovers harder and harder dentin. If the lesion is progressing slowly, there may be a zone of hard, hypermineralized sclerotic dentin that is the result of remineralization of what formerly was transparent dentin (zone 3). When sclerotic dentin is encountered, it represents the ideal final excavation depth because it is a natural barrier that blocks the penetration of toxins and acids.

Removal of the bacterial infection is an essential part of all operative procedures. Because bacteria never penetrate as far as the advancing front of the lesion, it is not necessary to remove all the dentin that has been affected by the caries process. In operative procedures, it is convenient to term dentin as either infected, and thus requires removal, or affected, which does not require removal. *Affected dentin* is softened, demineralized dentin that is not yet invaded by bacteria (zones 2 and 3). *Infected dentin* (zones 4 and 5) is both softened and contaminated with bacteria. It includes the superficial, granular necrotic tissue and the softened, dry, leathery dentin. The outer layer (infected dentin) can be selectively stained in vivo by caries detection solutions such as 1% acid red 52 (acid rhodamine B or food red 106) in propylene glycol.[26] This solution stains the irreversibly denatured collagen in the outer carious layer, but not the reversibly denatured collagen in the inner carious layer.[43] Using this staining technique clinically may provide a more conservative tooth preparation, because the boundary between two layers differentiated by this technique cannot easily be detected tactilely.

In slowly advancing lesions, it is expedient to remove softened dentin until the readily identifiable zone of sclerotic dentin is reached. In rapidly advancing lesions (see Figs. 3-34 and 3-46), there is little clinical evidence (as determined by texture or color change) to indicate the extent of the infected dentin. For very deep lesions, this lack of clinical evidence may result in an excavation that risks pulp exposure. In a tooth with a deep carious lesion, no history of spontaneous pain, normal responses to thermal stimuli, and a vital pulp (demonstrated by electric testing), a deliberate, incomplete caries excavation may be indicated. This procedure is termed *indirect pulp capping* and is characterized by placement of a thin layer of calcium hydroxide on the questionable dentin remaining over the pulp. A *direct pulp cap* is the placement of calcium hydroxide directly on exposed pulpal tissue (a pulpal exposure) and the surrounding deeply excavated dentinal area. The techniques of indirect and direct pulp capping may stimulate the formation of reparative dentin and are discussed

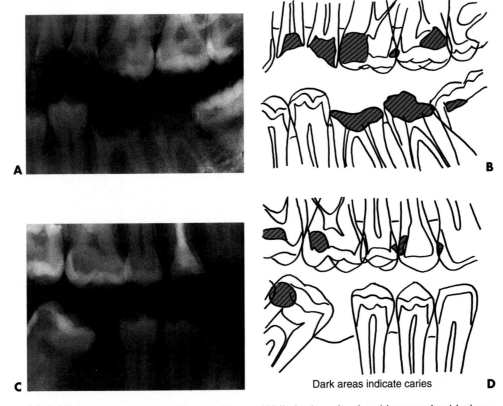

Dark areas indicate caries

FIG. **3-34** Rampant caries in a 21-year-old man. While both occlusal and interproximal lesions exist in the patient, the progress of the occlusal lesions produced the most tooth destruction. The potential for developing occlusal lesions could have been reduced by earlier application of sealants. This extensive amount of caries was the result of the patient's excessive fear of bad breath. In an attempt to keep his breath smelling fresh, he kept sugar-containing breath mints in his mouth most of the day. (Colored areas in **B** and **D** indicate caries.)

in a later section, Caries Control Restoration. However, the current use of these techniques is rapidly being replaced with another technique[78] when root canal therapy is not utilized. This newer concept results in the removal of the coronal, potentially infected area of the pulpal tissue; placement of a calcium hydroxide material over the excavated pulpal area; and then placement of a resin-modified glass-ionomer liner over the calcium hydroxide. Although not yet clear, scientific evidence seems to support this trend—the pulpal tissue appears to be disinfected and necrosed by the calcium hydroxide, and the resin-modified glass ionomer appears to adequately seal the area. Both measures may increase the success of a pulp-capping procedure.

The restorative procedures involving pulpal therapy are rapidly changing. An excellent bond and seal against microleakage can be achieved by acid-etching the dentinal (as well as enamel) walls of the tooth preparation. This treatment typically is followed by application of a suitable adhesive. Conventional bases are not required, except when thermal or mechanical (against pressure) protection of the pulp is indicated.

MANAGEMENT OF CARIES

The NHANES III of the U.S. population for 1988 to 1994[58] indicated that 45% of children (aged 5 to 17) had carious teeth. In adults, almost 94% had evidence of past or present coronal caries and of those people who had teeth, approximately 23% had root caries. Thus, caries will be of major importance for the foreseeable future.

In managing caries, the objective is to focus on the diagnosis (especially identifying those people at high risk for caries), preventive measures, and treatment modalities. Caries management must be directed, not at the tooth level (traditional or surgical treatment), but at the total patient level (medical model of treatment). It is imperative to understand that restorative treatment does not cure the carious process. Instead, identifying and eliminating the causative factors for caries must be the primary focus, in addition to the restorative repair of damage caused by caries.

For caries to occur, three factors must be present simultaneously and in the correct manner. These are: (1) cariogenic bacteria, (2) a susceptible tooth surface, and (3) available nutrients to support bacterial growth. Caries is an infectious disease caused by cariogenic plaque formation on the tooth that causes demineralization of the tooth (enamel demineralization occurs at pH of 5.5 or less), sometimes requiring restorative intervention and even extraction. As previously noted, of the over 300 species of bacteria in the oral cavity, only some of them, known as *mutans streptococci,* are caries-causing (cariogenic) organisms. MS are the primary causative agents of initial coronal caries because they (1) adhere to enamel; (2) produce and tolerate acid; (3) thrive in a sucrose-rich environment; and (4) produce bacteriocins, substances that kill off competing organisms.

Ion transfer continuously occurs at the plaque/enamel interface. The initial decalcification occurs subsurface and it may be 1 to 2 years before enough decalcification can occur to cause loss of the tooth's surface integrity (cavitation). Once enamel cavitation has occurred, the underlying dentin has already been affected by the progression of the destruction, and the lactobacillus organism then becomes the primary agent for further destruction of the dentin.

As plaque is exposed to nutrients (primarily sucrose), the plaque metabolism produces acids that cause demineralization of the tooth structure. If the nutrient or the plaque itself is removed, ions from saliva (sodium, potassium, or calcium) cause remineralization to occur, which attempts to restore the ionic component to the structure. When fluoride is present, it is picked up by the tooth structure and forms fluoroapatite in the enamel, which is even more resistant to future demineralization attacks than normal enamel.

Saliva is very important in the carious process. If sugars are the keys to success for cariogenic bacteria, then saliva is a major block barring those same bacteria. Therefore, adequate salivary functioning is critical in the defense against caries attacks. The protective mechanisms of saliva include: (1) bacterial clearance, (2) buffering actions, (3) antimicrobial actions, and (4) remineralization.

Bacterial clearance occurs because saliva has large carbohydrate-protein molecules (glycoproteins) that cause some bacteria to clump together (agglutinate) and then be swallowed as part of the normal 1.5 liters of saliva formed each day. Saliva also contains urea and other buffers that help dilute any plaque acids.

Saliva's antimicrobial actions occur because of various proteins and antibodies that discourage and even kill some bacterial growth. These include lysozyme, lactoferrin, lactoperoxidase, and Type A secretory immunoglobins. Likewise, saliva has calcium, phosphate, potassium, and sometimes fluoride ions available to assist with remineralization.

Lack of saliva significantly increases the rate of caries development.[27] Likewise, reduced salivary flow results in prolonged pH depression (decreased buffering), decreased antibacterial effects, and decreased ions for remineralization.

Frequently, the cyclic process of caries requires a long time to cause cavitation. Progression through enamel is often slow, resulting in a large percentage of enamel lesions that remain unchanged over periods of 3 to 4 years.[4] Progression rates through dentin may be comparably slow. Thus the process is lengthy, often providing the opportunity to attempt remineralization efforts that may keep cavitation from occurring.

Once the carious process is thoroughly understood, the appropriate diagnosis, prevention, and treatment of caries can occur. The following sections review the factors involved in diagnosing carious lesions and identifying those individuals at high risk for developing carious lesions; the factors and methods for trying to prevent caries from occurring; and the types of treatment that can be used for caries, including the caries-control restoration.

CARIES DIAGNOSIS

The process of caries diagnosis involves both risk assessment and the application of diagnostic criteria to determine the disease state. *The primary objectives of caries diagnosis are to identify those lesions that require surgical (restorative) treatment, those that require nonsurgical treatment, and those persons who are at high risk for developing carious lesions.* Knowing which patients are at high risk for developing caries provides an opportunity to implement specific preventive strategies that may prevent caries. These strategies are specific to high-risk individuals and are not intended for all patients (Box 3-1). For patients at low risk for caries, preventive measures may be limited to oral hygiene.

To diagnose carious lesions in patients, several factors must be considered. Some general factors are helpful in assessing a patient's risk to caries. These include patient history information and general clinical examination results. The emphasis in diagnosis must shift from detection of cavitations only to the detection of MS presence and predictions of caries progression (is the patient at high risk for caries?).

ASSESSMENT TOOLS

Patient History. Knowing certain factors pertaining to the patient's history can assist in the diagnosis of caries and identification of high-risk patients. Such factors include age, gender, fluoride exposure, smoking habits, alcohol intake, medications, dietary habits, economic and educational status, and general health. Increased smoking, alcohol consumption, use of medications, and sucrose intake result in increased risks for caries development. Children and elderly adults have increased risks, and decreased fluoride exposure, lower economic status, and lower educational attainment also increase risk. Poor general health also increases the risk. However, past caries experience is the best predictor of future caries activity.[32]

Clinical Examination. General information regarding inadequate salivary functioning, plaque accumulation, inflammation of soft tissues, poor oral hygiene, cavitated lesions, and existing restorations also are instructive in determining potential risk to caries development. The more any of these factors are present, the greater the risk. Some specific diagnostic factors are also helpful in assessing risk potential or the presence or absence of carious lesions. Assessing individual tooth surfaces for cavitation is crucial. If cavitation has occurred, usually restorative intervention is required. However, examination of tooth surfaces for cavitation must be accomplished judiciously, primarily using visual assessment of discoloration, translucency, or opacity. Injudicious use of sharp dental explorers on noncavitated, subsurface lesions could cause a cavitation.[7]

Nutritional Analyses. It must be determined if a dietary analysis should be undertaken. *Frequent exposure to sucrose increases the likelihood of plaque development by the more cariogenic MS organisms.* Although candy is not the only source of dietary sucrose, it is interesting to note that number of pounds of candy consumption per person in the United States increased from 18.4 pounds in 1986 to 20.8 pounds in 1993.[83] Sucrose intake and frequent sucrose exposures have been related to caries activity.[14]

Salivary Analyses. Analyzing saliva may provide important information about appropriateness of secretion rates and buffering capacity as well as numbers of both MS and lactobacilli. While bacterial counts may be helpful in assessing populations, they may not be accurate for an individual patient.[32] However, knowing what constitutes high values for the numbers of colony forming units (CFU) may be helpful information in identifying high-risk patients.

Radiographic Assessment. Dental radiographs provide useful information in diagnosing carious lesions. Although radiographs may show caries that is not visible clinically, the minimal depth of a detectable lesion on a radiograph is about 500 μm.[9] Although radiographs tend to underestimate the histologic extent of a carious lesion, *approximately 60% of teeth with radiographic proximal lesions in the outer half of dentin are likely to be noncavitated.*[65] Thus, many lesions evident radiographically are not cavitated and should be remineralized rather than restored. More sensitive techniques are needed for earlier detection of incipient carious lesions, allowing the increased usage of remineralizing techniques. New

---

BOX 3-1   Clinical Risk Assignment for Caries

A patient is at high risk for the development of new cavitated lesions if:

1. High MS counts are found. Bacteriologic testing MS should be done if:
   - The patient has one or more medical health history risk factors
   - The patient has undergone antimicrobial therapy
   - The patient presents with new incipient lesions
   - The patient is undergoing orthodontic care
   - The patient's treatment plan calls for extensive restorative dental work
2. Any two of the following factors are present:
   - Two or more active carious lesions
   - Large number of restorations
   - Poor dietary habits
   - Low salivary flow

techniques that may become available and useful include digital radiography, quantitative light-induced fluorescence, electrical conductivity, and ultrasonography.

Detection of carious lesions that require restoration (those that are cavitated) may be difficult. No single diagnostic technique can reliably detect precavitated carious lesions on all tooth surfaces. However, every effort should be made to pursue that detection and dentists should use the methods presented here as needed. Caries detection remains an inexact science, even though there is greater understanding of the carious process. Likewise, identification of those patients at high risk to caries is not clear, but the following factors appear to contribute to an increased risk of developing new carious lesions: (1) prior caries activity, (2) frequent sucrose intake, (3) minimal exposure to fluoride, (4) young or old age, (5) decrease in salivary functioning, (6) high numbers of cariogenic bacteria, and (7) presence of existing carious lesions.

In the past, caries diagnosis and treatment were limited primarily to the detection and restoration of cavitated lesions. This "drill and fill" approach was simply symptomatic treatment and failed to deal with the underlying etiologic factors. Undoubtedly, intact, nonrestored teeth are superior to restored teeth. Therefore, *early detection of incipient caries, limitation of caries activity before significant tooth destruction has occurred, and identification of high-risk patients are primary goals of an effective diagnosis and treatment program.* Because cavitation of the tooth surface is a late event in the carious process, it is preceded by a lengthy period of subsurface demineralization that presents the dentist an opportunity to detect the disease and start preventive measures before the advent of significant tooth damage. Various diagnostic methods are available to detect caries activity at early stages. These include: (1) identification of subsurface demineralization (inspection, radiographic, and dye uptake methods); (2) bacterial testing; and (3) assessment of environmental conditions such as pH, salivary flow, and salivary buffering. Because no single test has been developed that is 100% predictive of later development of cavitated lesions,[1,18] a concept of *caries risk* has been promoted. Once identified, patients at high risk for caries can be treated with preventive methods that reduce their likelihood of developing cavitated lesions in the future.[42]

If failure to detect caries in its earliest stage (incipient lesion) occurs, caries is diagnosed by the presence of cavitation of the tooth surface. The tooth surface is examined visually and tactilely. Visual evidence of caries includes cavitation, surface roughness, opacification, and discoloration. Tactile evidence of caries includes roughness and softness of the tooth surface. Roughness and softening have been determined by judicious probing of the suspected areas with an explorer. In the past, both penetration and resistance to removal of an explorer tip

(a "catch") have been interpreted as evidence of demineralization and weakening of tooth structure (a carious lesion). However, the use of an explorer for caries diagnosis is being replaced by visual and other diagnostic methods because injudicious use of the explorer tip may cause the actual cavitation in a previously noncavitated incipient area. Likewise, even though radiolucent areas in the proximal surfaces and below the occlusal enamel are interpreted as evidence of caries (demineralization), they do not indicate whether the surface has been cavitated.

A single test for caries diagnosis usually cannot be used alone because such tests may not be sufficient for accurate caries diagnosis. In particular, the use of the explorer is an unreliable procedure, because mechanical binding (a "catch") can be caused by factors other than the presence of caries. The use of only radiographs for caries diagnosis also is unreliable because of technical difficulties that include exposure, angulation, tooth position, the presence of restorations, and interpretation bias. Demineralization in enamel that is visible radiographically may not be indicative of active caries and is not necessarily an indication for restoration because radiolucency is visible on proximal enamel surfaces before surface cavitation. Furthermore, there are differences in caries susceptibility of persons based on age, geographic origin, ethnic background, and fluoride exposure. For example, in communities with fluoridated water supplies, susceptibility to proximal caries is greatly reduced. Therefore multiple criteria must be used, and the diagnostic criteria should be adjusted according to the patient's overall risks (age, gender, fluoride exposure history, general health, and ability to maintain good oral hygiene) (Tables 3-7 to 3-10).

TABLE **3-7**	Medical History Factors Associated With Increased Caries Risk
HISTORY FACTOR	RISK-INCREASING OBSERVATIONS
Age	Childhood, adolescence, senescence
Gender	Women at slightly greater risk
Fluoride exposure	No fluoride in public water supply
Smoking	Risk increases with amount smoked
Alcohol	Risk increases with amount consumed
General health	Chronic illness and debilitation decreases ability to give self-care
Medication	Medications that reduce salivary flow

CARIES DIAGNOSIS FOR PITS AND FISSURES

Caries cavitation is difficult to detect in pits and fissures because it is difficult to distinguish from the normal anatomic form of these features (see Table 3-9). Cavitation at the base of a pit or fissure sometimes can be detected tactilely as softness or by binding of the explorer tip. However, mechanical binding of an explorer in the pits or fissures may be due to noncarious causes, such as the shape of the fissure, sharpness of the explorer, or force of application. Thus, explorer tip binding is not, by itself, a sufficient indication to make a caries diagnosis. *Remember, injudicious use of the explorer may actually cause*

a cavitation! Discoloration of pits and grooves, limited to the depth of the fissure or pit, is almost a universal finding in normal healthy teeth of adults and, thus, as an isolated finding is not a sufficient indication for a diagnosis of caries. Because of these confounding factors, additional criteria have been developed by the U.S. Public Health Service for pit-and-fissure caries diagnosis. These factors are: (1) softening at the base of the pit or fissure; (2) opacity surrounding the pit or fissure, indicating undermining or demineralization of the enamel; and (3) softened enamel that may be flaked away by the explorer. Actual penetration of the enamel by an ex-

TABLE 3-8 Clinical Examination Findings Associated With Increased Caries Risk

CLINICAL EXAMINATION	RISK-INCREASING FINDINGS
General appearance	Appears sick, obese, or malnourished
Mental or physical disability	Patients who are unable or unwilling to comply with dietary and oral hygiene instruction
Mucosal membranes	Dry, red, glossy mucosa suggests decreased salivary flow
Active carious lesions	Cavitation and softening of enamel and dentin; circumferential chalky opacity at gingival margins
Plaque	High plaque scores
Gingiva	Puffy, swollen, and inflamed; bleeds easily
Existing restorations	Large numbers indicate past high caries rate; poor quality indicates increased habitat for cariogenic organisms

TABLE 3-9 Pit-and-Fissure Caries Treatment Decision-Making*

POSTERIOR TOOTH	CLINICAL DIAGNOSIS	PREDICTION/OBSERVATION	TREATMENT

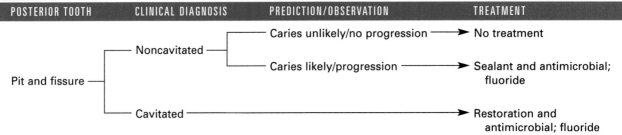

Cavitated means that extensive enamel demineralization has lead to destruction of the walls of the pit or fissure and bacterial invasion has occurred. Demineralization of the underlying dentin is usually extensive by the time the cavitation has occurred.

Noncavitated (caries-free):
- No radiolucency below occlusal enamel
- Deep grooves may be present
- Superficial staining may be present in grooves
- Mechanical binding of explorer may occur

Cavitated (diseased):
- Chalkiness of enamel on walls and base of pit or fissure
- Softening at the base of a pit or fissure
- Brown-gray discoloration under enamel adjacent to pit or fissure
- Radiolucency below occlusal enamel

*If a cavitated lesion exists in a pit or fissure, it must be restored. If the pit or fissure is not cavitated but at risk, then it should be sealed. The pits and fissures of molar teeth in children should be sealed routinely as soon as possible after eruption. Pits and fissures in adults should be sealed if the adult is found to have multiple active lesions or found to be at high risk.

plorer tip at the base of a pit or fissure suggests extensive demineralization and weakening of the enamel. Porous enamel (resulting from demineralization) appears chalky, or opaque, when dried with compressed air. Once caries penetrates to the dentin, demineralization rapidly spreads laterally through the less-resistant DEJ. Lateral-spreading caries undermines more enamel and may be seen clinically as a brown-gray discoloration that radiates away from the pit or fissure. Discolored enamel due to undermining caries is easily distinguished from superficial staining because it is more diffuse and does not affect the surface of the enamel. On bitewing radiographs, evidence of dentinal caries may be seen as a radiolucent area spreading laterally under the occlusal enamel from a pit or fissure.

CARIES DIAGNOSIS FOR SMOOTH SURFACES

Bitewing radiographs are the most typical method for evaluation of the proximal smooth surfaces for evidence of demineralization because these areas usually are not readily assessed visually or tactilely (see Table 3-10). An early lesion is detectable radiographically as a localized decrease in the density of the enamel immediately below the proximal contact, resulting in a radiolucent area on the radiograph. *Proximal radiolucencies detectable on bitewing radiographs should be examined clinically because many proximal radiolucencies are not associated with cavitation of the surface and, therefore, are not conclusive evidence of the need for restorative treatment.* A common diagnostic error concerning proximal caries diagnosis may result from an extensive superficial enamel incipient lesion that wraps around the proximal surface and extends onto the facial and lingual surfaces. Such a lesion produces a well-defined radiolucent area that appears (by overlapped images) to penetrate through the enamel, when, in fact, the lesion is only minimally extended into the enamel (Fig. 3-35).

A proximal incipient enamel lesion detectable as a faintly visible radiolucency on a bitewing radiograph is unlikely to have a cavitated surface (Fig. 3-36). Newer high-speed radiographic film and lower kV exposures provide a wide range of densities on radiographs that seem to require greater skill in interpretation than the older, higher-contrast films. Studies comparing the diagnostic information available from the two film types show them to be equal.[3] One study demonstrated a small (2%) reduction in ability to detect caries on the higher-speed film.[77] Many incipient proximal lesions in healthy patients end up as arrested lesions. Therefore, restoration of incipient proximal lesions should be delayed to allow time to observe whether or not it progresses. Arrested lesions are routinely found on proximal surfaces and are visible clinically as slightly discolored, hard spots in older persons after extraction of an adjacent tooth has occurred (see Fig. 9-15, C). However, since arrested lesions may have a decreased radiographic density that is not distinguishable from new, active caries, radiographs cannot be used solely for complete caries

| TABLE 3-10 | Proximal Caries Treatment Decision-Making* |

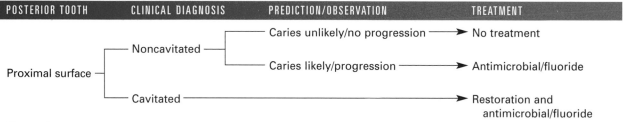

POSTERIOR TOOTH	CLINICAL DIAGNOSIS	PREDICTION/OBSERVATION	TREATMENT
Proximal surface	Noncavitated	Caries unlikely/no progression	No treatment
		Caries likely/progression	Antimicrobial/fluoride
	Cavitated		Restoration and antimicrobial/fluoride

Noncavitated:
- Surface intact; use of an explorer to judge surface must be done with caution because excessive force can cause penetration of intact surface over demineralized enamel
- Opacity of proximal enamel may be present
- Radiolucency may be present
- Marginal ridge is not discolored
- Opaque area may be seen in enamel by translumination

Cavitated:
- Surface broken, detectable visually or tactilely; temporary mechanical separation of the teeth may aid diagnosis
- Marginal ridge may be discolored
- Opaque area in dentin on translumination
- Radiolucency is present

*Proximal surfaces are difficult to judge clinically. The critical event in the caries process is surface cavitation. A cavitated surface must be restored, while a demineralized noncavitated surface can be treated only by antimicrobial and fluoride agents. Bitewing radiographs can reveal a decrease in density, but radiolucencies alone are not diagnostic of cavitation. Restoration of all radiolucent surfaces results in excessive, unnecessary restorative treatment.

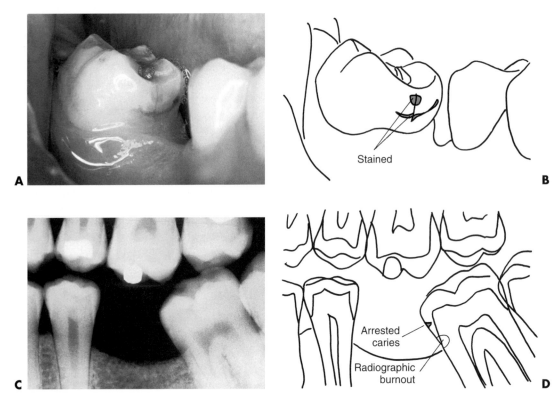

FIG. 3-35 Example of arrested caries on the mesial surface of a mandibular second molar. The area below the proximal contact (**A** and **B,** mirror view of No. 18) is partly opaque and stained. Clinically the surface is hard and intact, yet the area is more radiolucent than the enamel above or below the stain. Caries diagnosis based only on the radiograph (**C** and **D**) would lead to a false-positive diagnosis (i.e., caries present when it is not). The radiolucency is due to the broad area of subsurface demineralization that extends from the facial to the lingual line angles. The x-ray beam was directed parallel to the long axis of demineralization and consequently produced a sharply demarked zone of radiolucency in the enamel. This example illustrates the shortcomings of radiographic diagnosis. Were there not visual access to the mesial surface of the second molar, it would be very easy to incorrectly diagnose active caries and consequently restore the tooth.

diagnosis without additional clinical examination and history.

The overall accuracy (sensitivity [see Chapter 9 for a discussion of sensitivity and specificity]) of bitewing radiographs to detect caries is estimated to be 40% to 65%.[22,56] Combination of different radiographic procedures does not seem to improve the overall sensitivity. Panoramic radiographic sensitivity for caries is 18%, but is 41% when combined with bitewing radiographs. This is low when compared with a full mouth series, which has an overall sensitivity of 70%.[40] The accuracy of the diagnosis of healthy surfaces (specificity) is much better, varying from 98% to 99% from panoramic, bitewing, or full series radiographs. Thus, when radiolucencies are absent, the likelihood that caries is absent is high; however, when radiolucencies are present, the increase in the likelihood of cavitated caries being present is small. A diagnosis of cavitated caries based only on radiographs is likely to be correct between 4 (less than chance) and 7 of 10 times. When the surfaces are clear of radiolucencies, it is highly likely (98 of 100 times) that these surfaces are caries free. In clinical practice, therefore, the finding of a radiolucency should be followed by careful clinical assessment of the patient.

It is equally important to detect smooth-surface lesions on facial or lingual surfaces as soon as possible, because lesions on these surfaces are almost always seen in individuals with high caries activity. As stated earlier, incipient caries consists of opaque, chalky white areas (white spots) that appear when the tooth surface is dried. The diagnosis is confirmed when the affected area is rehydrated (wetted) and the chalky area partially or totally disappears. These incipient lesions have intact surfaces and care should be given to avoid damaging the surface with an explorer. The progress of incipient lesions can be reversed by remineralization when appropriate preventive procedures are instituted. However, once cavitation of the surface has occurred, either by natural causes or by overzealous application of an explorer tip, treatment by tooth preparation and restoration is usually advocated. Sometimes, in selected circumstances, slight surfacing/smoothing of the area by

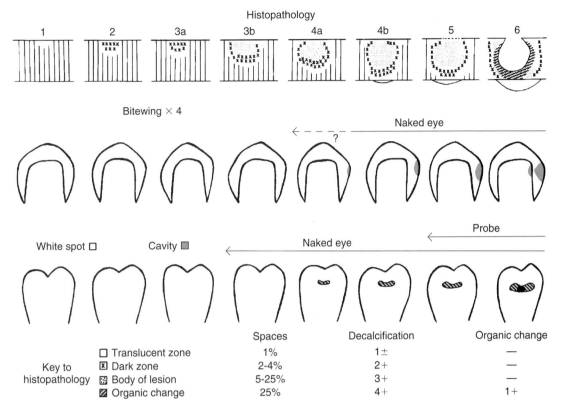

Histopathology

Bitewing × 4

Naked eye

Probe

Naked eye

White spot ☐   Cavity ■

Key to histopathology		Spaces	Decalcification	Organic change
☐ Translucent zone		1%	1±	—
☒ Dark zone		2-4%	2+	—
☒ Body of lesion		5-25%	3+	—
☒ Organic change		25%	4+	1+

FIG. 3-36 Schematic representation of developmental stages of enamel carious lesion correlated with radiographic and clinical examination. Cavitation occurs very late in development of lesion and before cavitation remineralization is possible. *(From Darling AI: Brit Dent J 107:287, 1959.)*

rotary stone or disc followed by fluoride application may be sufficient to arrest the lesion. Also acid-etching and placing an adhesive over the incipient area may seal it sufficiently to arrest the lesion.

Children and adolescents living in communities lacking fluoridated water will have much higher caries rates on smooth surfaces than their peers who have the benefit of fluoridated water. While traditional diagnostic methods for caries should continue to be used for patients living in these nonfluoridated regions, more aggressive treatment with topical fluorides, sealants, and earlier operative intervention is likely to be needed in this higher-risk group.

CARIES DIAGNOSIS FOR ROOT SURFACES

Root surfaces exposed to the oral environment, usually because of gingival recession, are at risk for caries and should be examined visually and tactilely. Discoloration of such areas is common and usually is associated with remineralization. Generally, the darker the discoloration, the greater the remineralization. On the other hand, active, progressing root caries shows little discoloration and is primarily detected by the presence of softness and cavitation.

Root caries may be caused by *Actinomyces viscusus*, although the microbiology is not fully understood. Be-

cause gingival recession is common in the population, the potential for root caries is great. The NHANES III Survey [58] indicated that 46% of elderly adults had recession 3 mm or greater and 47% of the 65- to 74-year-old group had root caries. For the entire dentate U.S. adult population, almost 23% had evidence of root caries. The DFS for root caries for U.S. adults was 1, and half of those were carious.

Root caries is usually shallow initially, spreads laterally, is light brown to yellow (although white at first), and without patient symptoms. The lesion development may be rapid because these areas have no enamel protection and the dentin is less mineralized. However, the lesion may undergo a maturation phenomenon, resulting in a remineralized area. This is probably due to the fact that this area of the tooth is exposed to the oral environment and constantly bathed with salivary ions, making the area more resistant to demineralization. Usually, after exposure of a root surface, if no caries occurs within several years, it is unlikely that root caries will develop later unless some major protective element of the patient is compromised. The arrestment or remineralization of the root caries lesion is likely because the lesion is initially shallow and therefore easier for ions to penetrate and strengthen, and dentists tend to watch rather than restore these areas because no pain usually is associated with the lesion. Presence of fluoride ion decreases root caries potential. Obviously, the potential for remineralization depends on several factors such as the degree of sclerosis of the dentinal tubules, degree of bacterial infection, degree of lesion progression, and location of the lesion.

CARIES ACTIVITY TESTS

Several caries activity tests have been developed to help detect the presence of oral conditions associated with increased risk of caries. For individual patients, currently no single caries activity test can predict caries with a high degree of confidence. Because many of these tests rely on samples of salivary bacteria, the reliability of such tests is limited because bacteria that are free floating in the saliva may not be necessarily representative of the bacteria in plaque. Other tests measure the plaque index (amount of plaque present) but also are not sufficient for complete assessment of caries risk. In his book *Caries Risk*, Krasse[42] outlines an assessment program that not only consists of microbiologic testing for the presence of MS and lactobacilli, but also is supplemented with analyses of diet and saliva. This combined approach has more promise for accuracy than any single caries activity test. Individual caries activity tests, despite their limitations, can be a useful adjunct to the clinical practitioner by guiding the clinician in making decisions concerning the need for control measures, the timing of recall appointments, the types of indicated restorative procedures and materials, and the determination of a prognosis.[59] The test results also can be used to motivate patients and to determine patient compliance with treatment regimens.

CARIES PREVENTION

A caries prevention program is a complex process involving multiple interrelated factors (Tables 3-11 and 3-12). *The primary goal of a caries prevention program should be to reduce the numbers of cariogenic bacteria.* Prevention should start with a consideration of the overall resis-

TABLE 3-11　Methods of Caries Treatment by the Medical Model

METHOD AND INDICATIONS	RATIONALE	TECHNIQUES OR MATERIAL
A. LIMIT SUBSTRATE Indications: 　Frequent sucrose exposure 　Poor quality diet	Reduce number, duration, and intensity of acid attacks Reduce selection pressure for MS	Eliminate sucrose from between-meal snacks Substantially reduce or eliminate sucrose from meals
B. MODIFY MICROFLORA Indications: 　High MS counts 　High lactobacillus counts	Intensive antimicrobial treatment to eliminate MS from mouth Select against reinfection by MS	Bactericidal mouthrinse (chlorhexidine) Topical fluoride treatments Antibiotic treatment (vancomycin, tetracycline)
C. PLAQUE DISRUPTION Indications: 　High plaque scores 　Puffy red gingiva 　High bleeding point score	Prevents plaque succession Decreases plaque mass Promotes buffering	Brushing Flossing Other oral hygiene aids as necessary
D. MODIFY TOOTH SURFACE Indications: 　Incipient lesions 　Surface roughening	Increase resistance to demineralization Decrease plaque retention	Systemic fluorides Topical fluorides Smooth surface
E. STIMULATE SALIVA FLOW Indications: 　Dry mouth with little saliva 　Red mucosa 　Medication that reduces salivary flow	Increases clearance of substrate and acids Promotes buffering	Eat noncariogenic foods that require lots of chewing Sugarless chewing gum Medications to stimulate salivary flow
F. RESTORE TOOTH SURFACES Indications: 　Cavitated lesions 　Pits and fissures at caries risk 　Defective restorations	Eliminate nidus of MS and *lactobacillus* infection Deny habitat for MS for reinfection	Restore all cavitated lesions Seal pits and fissures at caries risk Correct all defects (e.g., marginal crevices, proximal overhangs)

MS, Mutans streptococci.

tance of the patient to infection by the cariogenic bacteria. Although the general health of the patient, fluoride exposure history, and function of the immune system and salivary glands have a significant impact on the patient's caries risk, the patient may have little control over these factors. On the other hand, the patient usually is capable of controlling other factors such as diet, oral hygiene, use of antimicrobial agents, and dental care (which may include use of sealants and restorations). This section presents a variety of factors that may have an impact on the prevention of caries.

Preventive treatment methods are designed to limit tooth demineralization caused by cariogenic bacteria, thereby preventing cavitated lesions. They include: (1) limiting pathogen growth and metabolism and (2) increasing the resistance of the tooth surface to demineralization. Caries control methods are operative procedures used both to stop the advance of individual lesions and to prevent the spread of pathogenic bacteria to other tooth surfaces, and in this sense, they are preventive procedures. These operative procedures remove irreversibly damaged tooth structure and the associated pathogenic bacteria in the site. Caries control methods are most effective if all active, cavitated lesions can be treated in a very short time, even in a single appointment. Control procedures also may include pulpal therapy and restoration of the damaged tooth surface to appropriate anatomic contours and function. New restorative treatment methods have rendered the distinction between preventive and control methods less distinct. Fluoride treatment is capable of rendering tooth surfaces more acid-resistant and in some circumstances also may arrest active caries. Sealants were designed as a preventive measure, yet studies have shown that deliberately sealing active carious lesions effectively arrests the caries progress by cutting off the nutrient supply to the pathogenic plaque trapped under the sealant.[55]

Management of dental caries and its consequences remains the dominant activity of dentists. However, preventive and diagnostic service percentages of practice activity are increasing.[15] Although these activities relate to a variety of dental problems, diagnosis and prevention of caries are major parts of these increases. No longer is restoration of a carious lesion considered a cure. Rather, the practitioner must identify those patients who have active carious lesions and those at high risk for caries and institute appropriate preventive and treatment measures. This section presents some of the measures that can reduce the likelihood of a patient developing carious lesions. Depending on the risk status of the patient, the

TABLE 3-12 Treatment Strategies

EXAMINATION FINDINGS	NONRESTORATIVE TREATMENT	RESTORATIVE TREATMENT	FOLLOW-UP
Normal (no lesions)	None	None	1 year Clinical examination
Hypocalcified enamel (developmental white spot)	None for nonhereditary lesions Hereditary lesions (dentinogenesis imperfecta; may require special management)	Treatment is elective Esthetics (restore defects)	1 year Clinical examination
Incipient enamel lesions only Bitewing radiographs indicated (demineralized white spot)	Techniques *A* to *E* in Table 3-11 as indicated	Seal defective pits and fissures as indicated	3 months Evaluate: Oral flora, MS counts Progression of white spots Presence of cavitations
Possible cavitated lesions (active caries) and other incipient lesions present Bitewing radiographs indicated	Techniques *A* to *E* in Table 3-11 as indicated	Technique *F* (restorations, sealants) in Table 3-11 as indicated	3 months Evaluate: Oral flora MS counts Progression of white spots Presence of new cavitations Pulpal response
Arrested caries No active (new cavitations) or incipient lesions	None	Treatment is elective Esthetics (restore defects)	1 year Clinical examination

MS, Mutans streptococci.

dentist must decide which of these to institute. Dentistry will focus increasing effort for limiting the need for restorative treatment.

GENERAL HEALTH

The patient's general health has a significant impact on overall caries risk. Declining health signals the need for increased preventive measures, including more frequent recalls. Every patient has a very effective surveillance and destruction system for "foreign" bacteria. The effectiveness of a patient's immunologic system is highly dependent on overall health status. Patients undergoing radiation or chemotherapy treatment have significantly decreased immunocompetence and are at risk for increased caries.

Medically compromised patients should be examined for changes in the following: plaque index, salivary flow, oral mucosa, gingiva, and teeth. Early signs of increased risk include increased plaque; puffy, bleeding gingiva; dry mouth with red, glossy mucosa; and demineralization of the teeth. Decreased saliva flow is very common during acute and chronic systemic illnesses and is responsible for the dramatic increase in plaque. Ambulatory patients with chronic illnesses often take multiple medications, which individually or in combination may significantly reduce salivary flow (see Table 3-4). The saliva should be tested for both flow and buffering capacities when changes are detected from an oral examination.

FLUORIDE EXPOSURE

Fluoride in trace amounts increases the resistance of tooth structure to demineralization and is therefore a particularly important consideration for caries prevention (Fig. 3-37). When fluoride is available during cycles of tooth demineralization, it is a major factor in reduced caries activity.[14] Fluoride appears to be an essential nutrient for humans that is required only in very small quantities. Laboratory animals fed on a completely fluoride-free diet develop anemias and reduced reproduction after four generations. When available to humans, fluoride produces spectacular decreases in the

caries rate. The availability of fluoride to reduce caries risk is primarily achieved by fluoridated community water systems, but also may occur from fluoride in the diet, toothpastes, mouthrinses, and professional topical applications. The optimal fluoride level for public water supplies is about 1 part per million (ppm).[36] Approximately 62% of the U.S. population (140 million) has public fluoridated community water systems.[24] Public water fluoridation has been one of the most successful public health measures instituted in the United States. For communities that have fluoridated water systems, the annual cost averages about 50 cents per person. For every dollar spent on water fluoridation, six dollars of health savings are realized. At 0.1 ppm and below, the preventive effect is lost and the caries rate is higher for such populations lacking sufficient fluoride exposure. Excessive fluoride exposure (10 ppm or more) results in fluorosis, a brownish discoloration of enamel, termed mottled enamel.

Fluorides exert their anticaries effect by three different mechanisms. First, the presence of fluoride ion greatly enhances the precipitation into tooth structure of *fluorapatite* from calcium and phosphate ions present in saliva. This insoluble precipitate replaces the soluble salts containing manganese and carbonate that were lost because of bacterial-mediated demineralization. This exchange process results in the enamel becoming more acid-resistant (Fig. 3-38). Second, incipient, noncavitated, carious lesions are remineralized by the same process. Third, fluoride has antimicrobial activity. In low concentrations, fluoride ion inhibits the enzymatic production of glucosyltransferase. Glucosyltransferase promotes glucose to form extracellular polysaccharides, and this increases bacterial adhesion. Intracellular polysaccharide formation also is inhibited, preventing storage of carbohydrates by limiting microbial metabolism between the host's meals. Thus, the duration of caries attack is limited to periods during and immediately after eating. In high concentrations (12,000 ppm) used in topical fluoride treatments, fluoride ion is directly toxic to some oral microorganisms, including MS. Suppression of growth

FIG. **3-37** White spot lesions of enamel (stage 3 in Fig. 3-36) may remineralize, remain unchanged, or progress to cavitated lesions. In this study, done in community with fluoridated public water supply, only 9 of 72 incipient lesions became cavitated. Over one half of incipient lesions (37 of 72) actually regressed to become indistinguishable from normal enamel. *(From Baker-Dirts O: J Dent Res 45:503, 1966.)*

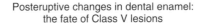

Posteruptive changes in dental enamel: the fate of Class V lesions

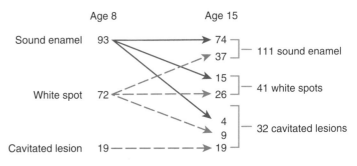

of MS following a single topical fluoride treatment may last several weeks.[76] It is possible to greatly lengthen this suppression by a change in dietary habits (especially eliminating sucrose) and by the patient's conscientious application of a good oral hygiene program.

All of the various methods for fluoride exposure (Table 3-13) are effective to some degree. The clinician's goal is to choose the most effective combination for each patient. This choice must be based on the patient's age, caries experience, general health, and oral hygiene. Children with developing permanent teeth benefit most from systemic fluoride treatments via the public water supply. In regions without adequate fluoride in the water supply, dietary supplementation of fluoride is indicated for children and sometimes for adults. The amount of fluoride supplement must be individually determined. This is of particular importance in rural areas with individual wells because the fluoride content of the well water can vary greatly over short distances.

Topical application of fluoride should be done semiannually for children and adults who are at high risk for caries development. The teeth should be cleaned free of plaque before the application of topical fluorides. Flossing and then tooth brushing are recommended for this purpose. Pumicing the teeth (professional prophylaxis) can remove a considerable amount of the fluoride-rich surface layer of enamel and therefore can be counterproductive. Acidulated phosphate fluoride (APF) is the most effective and least objectionable topical agent. APF is available in thixotropic gels

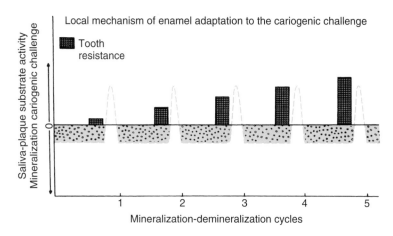

FIG. 3-38 Diagrammatic representation of enamel adaptation reaction. Enamel interacts with its fluid environment in periods of undersaturation and supersaturation, presented here as periodic cycles. Undersaturation periods dissolve most soluble mineral at the site of cariogenic attack, whereas periods of supersaturation deposit most insoluble minerals if their ionic components are present in immediate fluid environment. As a result, under favorable conditions of remineralization, each cycle could lead toward higher enamel resistance to a subsequent challenge. *(From Koulouirides T. In Menaker L, editor:* The biologic basis of dental caries, *New York, 1980, Harper & Row.)*

TABLE 3-13 Fluoride Treatment Modalities*

ROUTE	METHOD OF DELIVERY	CONCENTRATION (PPM)	CARIES REDUCTION (%)
Systemic	Public water supply	1	50 to 60
Topical	*Self-application*		
	Low-dose/high-frequency rinses (0.05% sodium fluoride daily)	225	30 to 40
	High-potency/low-frequency rinses (0.2% sodium fluoride weekly)	900	30 to 40 after 2 years
	Fluoridated dentrifices (daily)	1000	20
	Professional application		
	Acidulated phosphate fluoride gel (1.23%) annually or semiannually	12,300	40 to 50
	Sodium fluoride solution (2%)	20,000	40 to 50
	Stannous fluoride solution (8%)	80,000	40 to 50

*Caries reduction estimates for topically administered fluorides indicate their effectiveness when used individually. When they are combined with systemic fluoride treatment, they can provide some additional caries protection.

and has a long shelf life. Stannous fluoride (8% F), another option, has a very bitter, metallic taste; may burn the mucosa; and has a short shelf life. Although the tin ion in stannous fluoride may be responsible for staining the teeth, it may be beneficial for arresting root caries. Topical fluoride agents should be applied according to the manufacturer's recommendations.

Self-administered fluoride rinses have an additive effect (about 20% reduction) when used in conjunction with topical or systemic fluoride treatment. Fluoride rinses are indicated in high-risk patients and those patients exhibiting a recent increase in caries activity. Two varieties of fluoride rinses have similar effectiveness: (1) high dose/low frequency and (2) low dose/high frequency. The high-dose (0.2% F)/low-frequency rinses are best used in supervised weekly rinsing programs based in public schools. The low-dose (0.05% F)/high-frequency rinses are best used by individual patients at home. The high-risk or caries-active patient should be advised to use the rinse daily. The optimal application time is in the evening. The rinse should be forced between the teeth many times and then expectorated, not swallowed. Eating and drinking should be avoided after the rinse.

Various fluoride varnishes and gels are available and are successful in preventing caries. Varnishes provide a high uptake of the fluoride ion into enamel, yet provide a lower dosage of fluoride than gels or rinses. These are professionally applied, yet may provide the most cost-effective means of delivery of fluoride to the teeth. They are effective bacteriocidal and caries prevention agents. Fluoride varnishes were developed several decades ago in an attempt to improve fluoride application techniques and benefits. European countries have widely used fluoride varnishes for the past 20 years. Although the FDA has approved these materials for use as liners and tooth desensitizers in the United States, they have not been approved as anticaries agents. However, "numerous randomized clinical trials conducted outside the United States point to the efficacy and safety of fluoride varnishes as a caries-prevention agent."[10] The general technique for fluoride varnish use is:

1. Clinician applies a thin layer of fluoride varnish directly onto the teeth.
2. Application time is several minutes.
3. Patients are to avoid eating for several hours and then avoid brushing until the next morning.

Because the fluoride varnish sets when contacting moisture, thorough isolation of the area is not required. Furthermore, only toothbrushing, rather than prophylaxis, is necessary before application. The main disadvantage of fluoride varnish is that a temporary change in tooth color may occur.

The fluoride varnish deposits large amounts of fluoride on an enamel surface, especially on a demineralized enamel surface. Calcium fluoride precipitates on the surface and often fluorapatite is formed. The high concentration of surface fluoride also may provide a reservoir for fluoride, which promotes remineralization. Although additional research on fluoride varnishes is needed, the use of a fluoride varnish as a caries-preventive agent should be expanded because it has advantages over other topical fluoride vehicles in terms of safety, ease of application, and fluoride concentration at the enamel surface.[10]

IMMUNIZATION

Bacteria passing through the mouth into the stomach and intestines come into contact with specialized lymphoid tissue located in Peyer's patches along the intestinal walls. Certain T and B cells in Peyer's patches become sensitized to the new bacteria. The sensitized T and B cells migrate through the lymphatic system to the bloodstream and eventually settle in glandular tissues, including the salivary glands in the oral cavity. There, these sensitized cells produce IgA class immunoglobulins that are secreted in the saliva. These IgA antibodies are capable of agglutination (clumping) of oral bacteria. This prevents adherence to the teeth and other oral structures, and they are more easily cleared from the mouth by swallowing. For patients with high concentrations of MS, agglutinating IgA may have an important anticaries effect. This immunologic occurrence promotes the possibility of further vaccination against caries. Studies in rats and primates already have demonstrated the feasibility of such immunization attempts.[44,80] However, it is known that the procedure is more effective against smooth surface lesions than pit-and-fissure lesions.

Even if an anticaries vaccine were developed, concerns remain that may affect its widespread use. First, potential side effects of a vaccine must be identified. The safety of such a vaccine has not yet been demonstrated, and, in fact, there are concerns of a possible cross-reaction with human heart tissue. Second, its cost must be compared with that of public water fluoridation, which is inexpensive and already very effective at reducing caries. Vaccination may be no more effective than fluoride therapy, which has a proven safety record. However, it may be practical to use a caries vaccine when public water fluoridation is impractical or in developing third-world countries. Third, limitations imposed by governmental regulatory agencies may affect the widespread use of an anticaries vaccine.

SALIVARY FUNCTIONING

Saliva is very important in the prevention of caries. While xerostomia may occur because of aging, it is more commonly a result of a medical condition or medication. Lack of saliva greatly increases the incidence of caries. If a patient is xerostomic, consultation with the physician may be necessary to identify alternate treatments, if possible, with less salivary impact. Saliva stimulants (gums, paraffin waxes, or saliva substitutes) also may be prescribed for patients with impaired salivary functioning.

A variety of commercial salivary tests are available. These could aid the practitioner in assessing the production amount and buffering capacity of saliva, as well as assaying the numbers of microorganisms present. These results will influence the preventive regimen prescribed for high-risk patients.

ANTIMICROBIAL AGENTS

A variety of antimicrobial agents also are available to help prevent caries (Table 3-14). In rare cases, antibiotics might be considered, but the systemic effects must be considered. As already presented, fluoride has antimicrobial effects. Chlorhexidine is showing excellent results. This material was first available in the United States as a rinse and was first used for periodontal therapy. It was prescribed as a 0.12% rinse for high-risk patients for short-term use. It is used in other countries as a varnish and the most effective mode of varnish use is as a professionally applied material.[21] Chlorhexidine varnish enhances remineralization and decreases MS presence. In fact, Emilson[21] concluded that chlorhexidine varnishes provide effective reduction in MS.

Chlorhexidine is prescribed for home use at bedtime as a 30-second rinse. Used at this time, when the salivary flow rate is decreased, the agent has a better opportunity to interact with MS organisms while tenaciously adhering to oral structures. It is used for approximately 2 weeks, and results in a reduction of MS counts to below caries potential levels. This decrease is sustained for 12 to 26 weeks.

The agent also can be applied professionally once a week for several weeks, monitoring the microbial counts to determine effectiveness. This may be used in combination with other preventive measures for high-risk patients.

DIET

Dietary sucrose has two important detrimental effects on plaque. First, frequent ingestion of foods containing sucrose provides a stronger potential for colonization by MS, enhancing the caries potential of the plaque. Second, mature plaque exposed frequently to sucrose rapidly metabolizes it into organic acids, resulting in a profound and prolonged drop in plaque pH. Caries activity is most strongly stimulated by the frequency, rather than the quantity, of sucrose ingested. The message that excessive and frequent sucrose intake can cause caries has been widely disseminated and is well known by lay people. Despite this knowledge, dietary modification for the purpose of caries control has failed as a public health measure. However, for an individual patient, dietary modification can be effective if the patient is properly motivated and supervised. Evidence of new caries activity in adolescent and adult patients indicates the need for dietary counseling. *The goals of dietary counseling should be to identify the sources of sucrose in the diet and reduce the frequency of sucrose ingestion.* Minor dietary changes such as substitution of sugar-free foods for snacks are more likely to be accepted than more dramatic changes. Rampant (or acute) caries (a rapidly invading infectious process usually involving several teeth) is a sign of gross dietary inadequacy, a complete absence of oral hygiene practice, or systemic illness. The presence of rampant caries is an indication of the need for comprehensive patient evaluation. Textbooks on nutrition and medicine should be consulted.

TABLE 3-14 Antimicrobial Agents

	MECHANISM OF ACTION	SPECTRUM OF ANTIBACTERIAL ACTIVITY	PERSISTENCE IN MOUTH	SIDE EFFECTS
ANTIBIOTICS				
Vancomycin	Blocks cell-wall synthesis	Narrow	Short	Increases gram-negative flora
Kanamycin	Blocks protein synthesis	Broad	Short	Can increase caries activity
Actinobolin	Blocks protein synthesis	Streptococci	Long	Unknown
BIS BIGUANIDES				
Alexidine	Antiseptic; prevents bacterial adherence	Broad	Long	Bitter taste; stains teeth and tongue brown; mucosal irritation
Chlorhexidine	Antiseptic; prevents bacterial adherence	Broad	Long	
HALOGENS				
Iodine	Bacteriocidal	Broad	Short	Metallic taste
Fluoride	1 to 10 ppm reduces acid production; 250 ppm bacteriostatic; 1000 ppm bacterioicidal	Broad	Long	Increases enamel resistance to caries attack; fluorosis in developing teeth with chronic high doses

ORAL HYGIENE

Plaque-free tooth surfaces do not decay! Daily removal of plaque by dental flossing, tooth brushing, and rinsing is the single best measure for preventing both caries and periodontal disease (Figs. 3-39 and 3-40). Löe and others[46] have established supragingival plaque as the etiologic agent of gingivitis. Long-standing gingivitis can lead to damage of the epithelial attachment and progression to a more serious periodontal disease. Effective plaque control by oral hygiene measures results in both resolution of the gingival inflammation and remineralization of the enamel surface. Pits and fissures are not accessible to toothbrush bristles because of the small diameter of their orifices, thus these areas are highly susceptible to caries. Obturation of pits and fissures by sealants is a highly effective method for caries prevention (see Pit-and-Fissure Sealants).

Mechanical plaque removal by brushing and flossing has the advantage of not eliminating the normal oral flora. Topical antibiotics, on the other hand, could control plaque, but long-term use predisposes the host to infection by antibiotic-resistant pathogens such as *Candida albicans.* Frequent mechanical plaque removal does not engender the risk of infection of opportunistic organisms. It does change the species composition of plaque in both the selection for pioneering organisms as well as the denial of habitat to potential pathogens. Thus, the oral flora on the teeth of patients with good plaque control has a high percentage of *S. sanguis* or *S. mitis* and is much less cariogenic than older, mature plaque communities, which have a significant higher percentage of MS.

Krasse has demonstrated that a combination of oral hygiene and diet counseling is effective in children.[42] In this classic study, children in two schools were monitored for lactobacillus levels. The children in one school were given both feedback about the results of the studies and proper preventive oral hygiene and dietary instruction. After 18 months, the children in the school receiving preventive counseling had an average of 3.3 new restorations, while the control school children who received no counseling averaged 8.2 new restorations. This is an excellent demonstration that good oral hygiene and dietary improvements can be effective when using microbiologic testing as a motivational tool.

Rigid oral hygiene programs should be prescribed only to high-risk persons with evidence of active disease. Overzealous, universal application of oral hygiene training programs are frustrating to both dentists and their patients. High-risk patients should receive intensive oral hygiene training, dietary instruction, and pre-

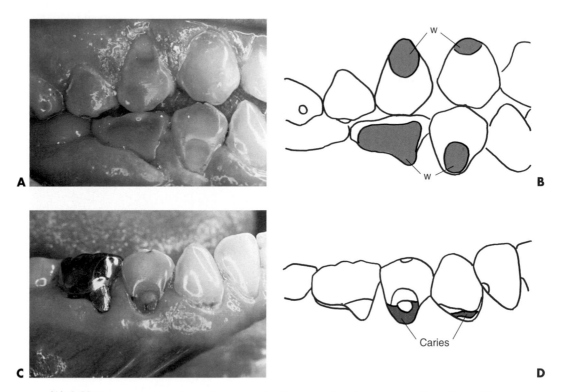

FIG. 3-39 Erosion wear and poor homecare leading to caries. A young female patient with severe wear on the facial surfaces of the posterior teeth. This patient was subsequently found to have a hiatal hernia with frequent regurgitation of stomach acids. Too vigorous brushing and acid demineralization of the teeth accelerated the loss of tooth structure (**A** and **B**). Areas of severe wear *(w)* exhibit dentin hypersensitivity. The dentin pain was the symptom that caused the patient to seek dental care. Advising the patient to reduce the vigorous tooth brushing unfortunately resulted in cessation of all brushing. Caries activity rapidly occurred (**C** and **D**).

ventive dental treatment as necessary to control the progress of the disease. Plaque removal in high-risk patients should be done frequently. Flossing, brushing, and thorough rinsing after every meal is indicated for this group. Patients without active disease do not need intensive intervention in their self-care program. However, they should still be counseled to optimize their results. Adults with a low caries experience probably only require flossing, brushing, and rinsing once a day, and the best time for this is in the evening before going to bed. During sleep, salivary flow is greatly reduced, limiting the anticaries benefits of saliva and therefore allowing unrestricted plaque metabolism and growth.

Plaque control requires a little dexterity and a lot of motivation. Some knowledge of tooth contours, embrasure form, proximal contacts, and tooth alignment is helpful to optimal plaque control. Instruction should include both the selection and use of mechanical aids, based on the patient's needs. The primary impediment to patient acceptance of flossing, as a part of routine oral hygiene procedures, is the difficulty of passing the floss through tight proximal contacts. Damage to the interproximal papilla and/or tearing or shredding of the floss are the usual reasons cited by patients for failure to use this technique.

To prepare for flossing the teeth, lightly wind one end of a 60-cm length (approximately 2 feet) of ribbon or Teflon floss twice around the ring finger of the dominant hand, anchoring this end by the second loop overlapping the first. The remaining length of floss is around the ring finger of the other hand and serves as a spool of clean floss. The section of floss remaining between the hands should be approximately 15 cm (6 inches). The middle 2 to 3 cm (½ inch) is held taut between the tips of the thumbs and first fingers (Fig. 3-41, *A*).

A braced technique is necessary for passing the floss through contacts atraumatically. The first finger of the nondominant hand is used to brace the floss in the facial embrasure adjacent to the contact to be cleaned (Fig. 3-41, *B*). With the floss pressed against the embrasure area, the free end of the floss is passed diagonally through the contact. A sliding motion helps introduce the floss into the contact area without sudden uncontrolled movement of the floss, which might injure the gingiva. Once through the contact, the floss is wrapped over a proximal surface and moved up and down to remove the adherent plaque. The adjacent proximal surfaces must be cleaned individually. Fig. 3-41, *C*, illustrates cleaning the distal surface of the approximating pair of teeth. When changing surfaces, damage to the papilla is avoided by gently lifting the floss to the underside of the contact and moving it to the adjacent proximal surface. The floss is wrapped around the opposite (mesial in this example) surface by pressing distally and moving the floss up and down

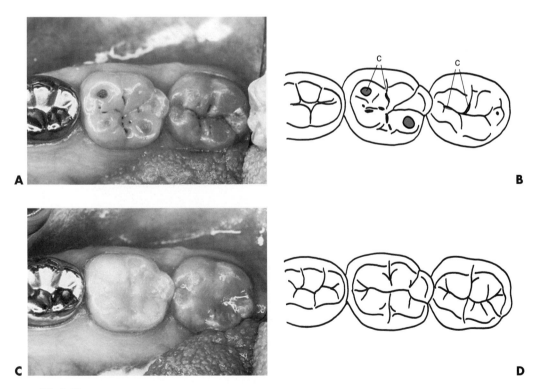

FIG. **3-40 A** and **B,** Photograph of the occlusal surfaces of the teeth illustrated in Fig. 3-39, **C.** Following cessation of oral hygiene procedures, caries *(c)* rapidly developed in the exposed dentin and fissures on the occlusal surfaces. **C** and **D,** This was conservatively treated by excavation of the softened dentin and restoration of the excavations and fissures with a highly filled light-cured composite.

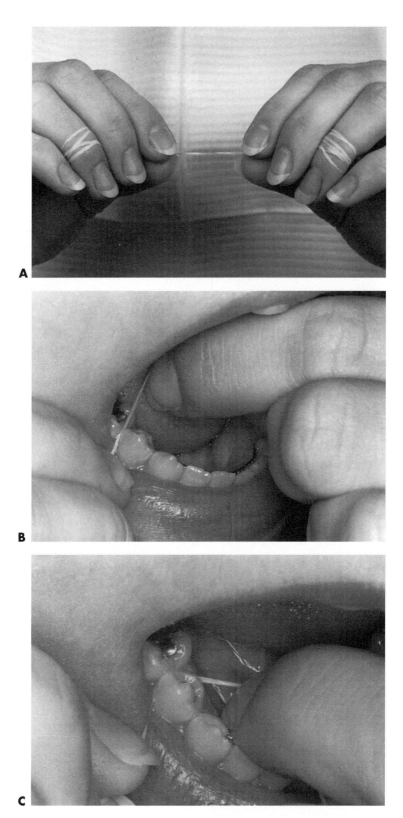

FIG 3-   Flossing. **A,** Fingers positioning the floss. **B,** The braced flossing technique prevents damage to the interproximal gingiva. The index finger braces the floss in the embrasure while the other hand presses the floss diagonally through the contact. **C,** Gentle anterior force wraps the floss around the distal surface of the more anterior tooth of the contacting pair of teeth. The floss is moved superiorly and inferiorly over the tooth surface from the inferior side of the contact to the depth of gingival sulcus.

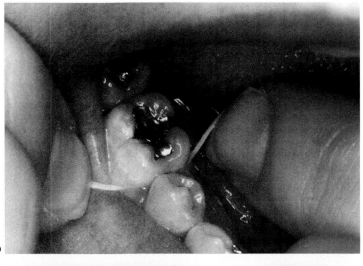

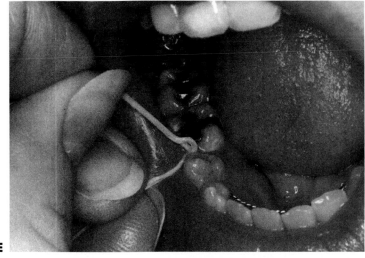

FIG. **3-41, cont'd D,** The floss is lifted over the papilla and gently positioned posteriorly to wrap over the mesial surface of the more posterior tooth of the contacting pair. The tooth surface is cleaned of plaque by the same superior-inferior motion. **E,** Removing the floss facially through contact.

Continued

(Fig. 3-41, *D*). *The purpose of routine flossing is not to remove debris from the interproximal space (although it is ideally suited for removal of fibrous food caught in contacts), but rather, it is for the removal of bacterial plaque from proximal tooth surfaces.* The floss can be removed from the interproximal space either by simultaneously pulling both ends *facially* (Fig. 3-41, *E*) or releasing one end and gently pulling the length out through the interproximal space.

With experience, satisfactory flossing can be completed in 3 or 4 minutes. Whether to use waxed or unwaxed floss is controversial, although not highly significant. The benefits are from good flossing technique rather than the choice of floss. Every effort should be made to encourage good flossing. Gingival bleeding may occur even with good flossing technique when the gingiva is inflamed. Patients should be advised that gin-

gival bleeding is a sign of gingival inflammation, not the result of damage caused by proper flossing or toothbrushing. As good oral hygiene continues, this inflammation will resolve. Within days the gingiva will change from slightly red and glossy to light pink and stippled. The healthy gingiva will become "tough" and will no longer bleed when brushed or flossed.

Each contact can be cleaned with a fresh section of the floss (Fig. 3-41, *F* through *H*) by unwinding the floss from the spool finger and taking up the increased length by winding onto the take-up finger. For flossing the distal surface of the most posterior tooth of each quadrant, it may be necessary to use the tips of the longer, middle fingers (Fig. 3-41, *I* to *K*). It is important to floss these surfaces because they are not easily reached by the toothbrush.

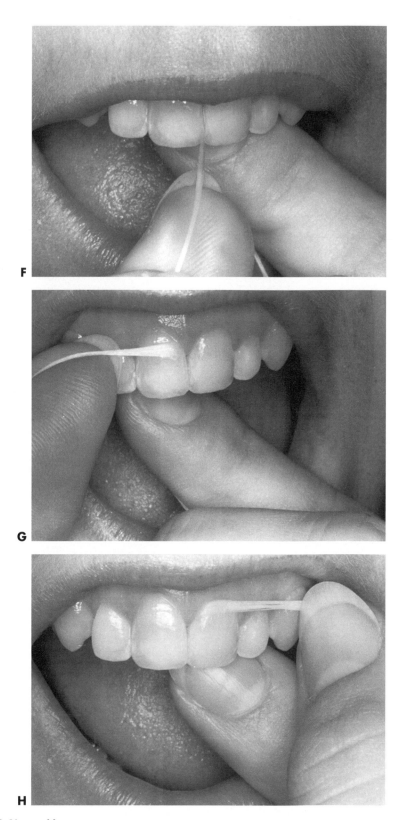

FIG. **3-41, cont'd** **F** through **H,** Passing floss through contact of maxillary central incisors (**F**) and flossing the mesial surfaces and mesial transitional angles (**G** and **H**).

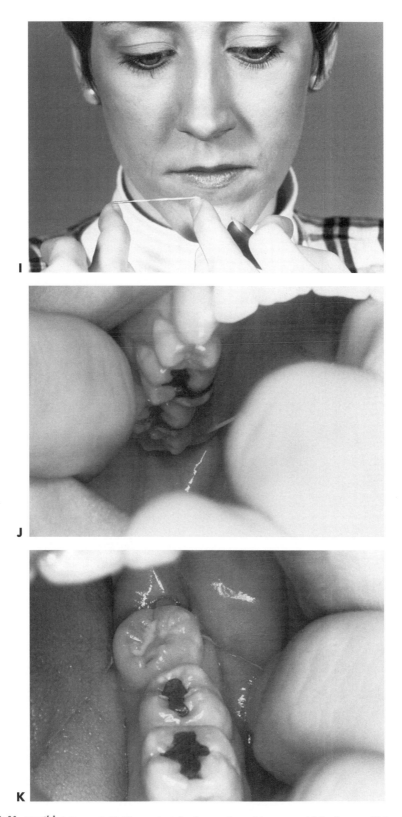

FIG. **3-41, cont'd** **I** through **K**, Floss stretched over tips of longer, middle fingers (**I**) for flossing the most posterior distal surfaces (**J** and **K**).

Flossing is followed by brushing the facial, lingual, and occlusal surfaces, as well as the most distal surfaces (Fig. 3-42, A through D). A soft toothbrush with blunt-tipped nylon bristles is applied to the teeth and gingiva with vibrating technique (see Fig. 3-42, A and B). A rapid anterior-posterior sawing motion severely abrades tooth surfaces and is not effective for interproximal plaque removal. A small amount of fluoride-containing dentifrice on the brush is useful for increasing the effectiveness of stain and plaque removal and for treating the teeth with fluoride.

The sulcular brushing technique is superior to previously advocated methods. The bristles are held at a 45-degree angle to the tooth surface and vibrated into the gingival sulcus and embrasure. The end of the brush can be applied to the lingual of the anterior teeth (Fig. 3-42, E) and the noncontacting distal surfaces (see Fig. 3-42, F). For these surfaces the toothbrush handle must be raised at a 45-degree angle (or more) to the occlusal plane. During sulcular brushing, the tips of the bristles should be forced to enter the gingival sulcus and the embrasures as far as possible. After brushing the teeth, gently brush the top (dorsal) surface of the tongue. This reduces the debris and plaque that otherwise accumulate on this rough surface.

Rinsing follows flossing and brushing. Rinse water is forced over the teeth by tongue and cheek movements while the lips are closed. Rinsing should force the water through the interproximal spaces. Rinsing is repeated until the expectorated rinse water is clear.

Professional tooth cleaning also has an important effect on caries reduction One study[41] divided grade school students into three treatment groups: control, monthly professional cleaning, and twice-a-month professional cleaning. In students with low MS levels, the once-a-month cleaning group had half as many new

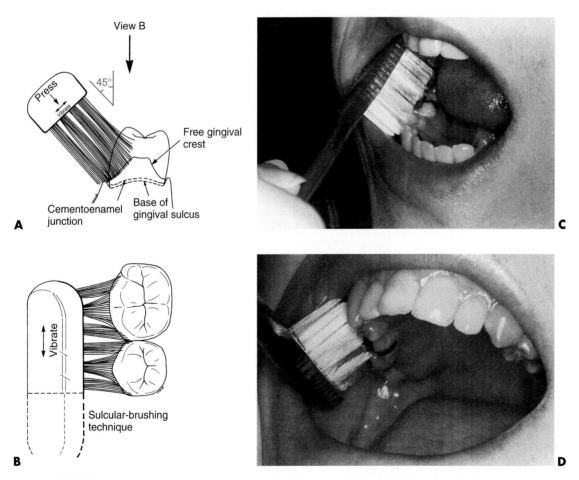

FIG. 3-42 Brushing. **A** and **B**, Sulcular-brushing technique for toothbrush applied to facial tooth surfaces with bristles directed 45 degrees gingivally (same gingival tilt of bristles when on lingual surfaces). Length of double-headed arrows indicates the short extent of vibration of brush head, causing tips of bristles to enter gingival sulci and facial embrasures (lingual embrasures when brush applied to lingual surfaces). After several seconds, move brush mesially (or distally) by one tooth (maintaining same bristle direction) and repeat the vibrating motion at each successive position until all facial and lingual surfaces are brushed. **C**, Brush applied as depicted in **A** and **B**. **D**, Sulcular vibrating the bristles on facial surfaces of maxillary posterior teeth.

carious surfaces (0.8 surfaces/student) as did the control group (1.8 surfaces/student). In the high MS group, the control group had the most new caries (2.5 surfaces/student), while the once-a-month cleaning group had similar levels (0.96 surfaces/student) to the low MS group, and the twice-a-month cleaning group had almost one-tenth the number of new lesions (0.34 surfaces/student) as the control group. This study demonstrated that professional plaque removal on grade school students, even as infrequent as once every 2 weeks, dramatically reduces the development of new carious lesions. Equal or greater reductions can be expected in patients who practice proper oral hygiene methods for plaque removal.

XYLITOL GUMS

Xylitol is a natural five-carbon sugar obtained from birch trees. It keeps the sucrose molecule from binding with MS. Furthermore, MS cannot ferment (metabolize) xylitol. Thus xylitol reduces MS by altering their metabolic pathways and enhances remineralization and helps arrest dentinal caries.[79,81] It is usually recommended that a patient chew a piece of xylitol gum after eating or snacking for 5 to 30 minutes. Chewing any sugar-free gum after meals reduces the acidogenicity of plaque because chewing stimulates salivary flow, which improves the buffering of the pH drop that occurs after eating.[20]

PIT-AND-FISSURE SEALANTS

Although fluoride treatments are most effective in preventing smooth surface caries, they are less effective in preventing pit-and-fissure caries. Although occlusal surfaces account for only 12.5% of all tooth surfaces, they account for much of the caries in school-age children. In

fact, the 1988 to 1991 NHANES III Survey[58] revealed that occlusal surfaces in children's teeth were five times more likely to be the site of caries than proximal surfaces and twice as likely as facial or lingual surfaces. Thus, a preventive measure for pit-and-fissure caries is greatly needed. Pit-and-fissure sealants (Figs. 3-43 and 3-44) were specifically designed for this purpose and have been demonstrated to be effective.[72] Sealants have three important preventive effects. First, sealants mechanically fill pits and fissures with an acid-resistant resin. Second, because the pits and fissures are filled, sealants deny MS and other cariogenic organisms their preferred habitat. Third, sealants render the pits and fissures easier to clean by toothbrushing and mastication.

A 1986 to 1987 National Institutes of Dental Research (NIDR) survey[17] indicated that an estimated 7.6% of children aged 5 to 17 had sealants on their permanent and primary teeth. The NHANES III Survey for 1988 to 1991[58] reported that about 20% of children aged 5 to 17 had sealants on their permanent or primary teeth, more than double the number in the previous survey. Yet this indicates that only 1 in 5 children had sealants! *If more children received sealants, caries prevalence would be reduced.* To date, the dental profession has been slow to accept pit-and-fissure sealants, and the procedure tends to be underutilized.[54] The reasons for this lack of professional acceptance have been concerns about the retention rate of sealants, fear of sealing caries under the sealant, and cost-effectiveness. These concerns have been addressed in various studies. For example, in a review of 15 independent clinical studies, Ripa[66] concluded that caries reductions of more than 80% after 1 year and 70% after 2 years are typical results that may be expected after a single application of sealant. One of these studies re-

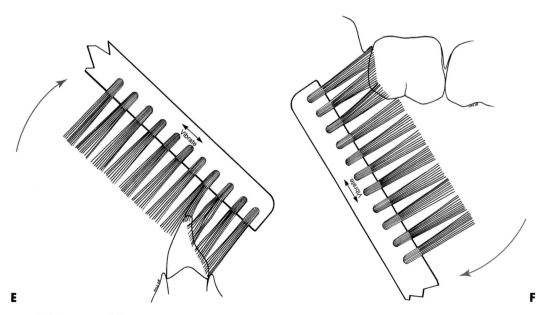

E   F

FIG. **3-42, cont'd** **E** and **F,** Sulcular-vibrating technique for lingual surfaces of mandibular anterior teeth (**E**) and a most posterior distal surface (**F**).

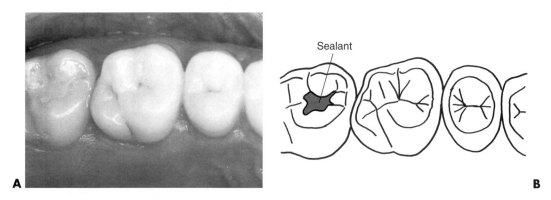

FIG. **3-43 A** and **B,** Sealant applied to the central fossa of a maxillary second molar. This tooth was treated because of the appearance of chalky enamel and softening in the central fossa. A highly filled sealant was used (see Fig. 3-44).

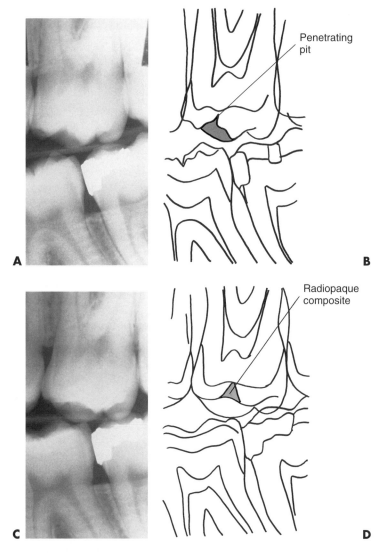

FIG. **3-44 A** and **B,** Radiograph of a maxillary first molar with a deep central fossa pit that appears to penetrate to the dentin. **C** and **D,** The central pit was sealed with a highly filled, radiopaque sealant. The sealant is readily visible on the radiograph.

ported a 37% caries reduction after 5 years.[37] Ripa also found that all studies reported a progressive loss of sealants.[66] In a 7-year-study involving 110 paired occlusal surfaces (one receiving a sealant and the other receiving an amalgam restoration), comparable effectiveness was found.[74] After the 7 years, only one sealed tooth was found to be carious while three amalgam restorations were found to have secondary caries. One half of the sealants were retained for the full 7 years, 30% required one reapplication, 10% required two reapplications, and 10% received three reapplications. The total average time required to apply the sealants was 10 minutes and 45 seconds while the average time for placement of the amalgams was 14 minutes and 26 seconds. These data demonstrate the equivalence of sealants and occlusal amalgam restorations. *Sealants, therefore, have been shown to be effective, to have long-term retention, to cause regression of active lesions, and to be superior to amalgam restoration in terms of time requirements.*

When a sealant is lost, it is most likely a result of a technical error in its application rather than a result of poor bond strength. Proper acid-etch bonding of methacrylate and resin polymers to enamel produces a bond strong enough to retain restorations, orthodontic brackets, and even prosthetic bridges. This same bond, which is used for sealants, is unlikely to fail if the sealant is applied properly. Sealing partially erupted molar teeth is a demanding technical procedure. Saliva contamination of the etched enamel results in precipitation of salivary glycoproteins that prevent the sealant polymers from bonding to the enamel. Redrying the contaminated surface will not remove the precipitated salivary proteins even though the surface will still have an etched appearance. The contaminated surface must be re-etched to remove the precipitate and properly recondition the enamel for effective bonding. Indeed, studies of sealant retention indicate the greatest loss of sealants occurs within the first 6 months of application, indicating bond failure most likely because of saliva contamination. Loss of the sealant's occlusal surface because of attrition is a less important problem. Whereas sealants lost because of bond failure leave the fissures exposed and caries-susceptible, loss of only the occlusal portion of sealants leaves the depths of the fissures still filled with sealant and therefore caries-resistant.[66] It may be impossible to clinically distinguish between these two modes of sealant loss. Therefore sealant should be replaced in patients who remain in a high-risk category.

The concern about sealing active carious lesions has been reported by other independent studies.[29,31] These studies reported that *sealed lesions fail to progress* and the number of viable bacteria that could be recovered from the lesions was progressively reduced over the period of the studies. Both reports concluded that intentional sealing of carious lesions may be an acceptable treatment modality for pit-and-fissure caries. One of these studies by Going and others[29] reported an 89% reversal from caries-active to caries-inactive after 5 years. That study further states, "There is no doubt that sealing a suspected carious pit-and-fissure area is a better clinical service than watchful waiting for an interval of six months or more."

The cost-effectiveness of sealant treatment, including replacement of lost sealant versus amalgam treatment, has been studied by Leverett and others.[45] They concluded that, although the cost of sealant treatment in caries-inactive patients was not justified, sealants were cost-effective in caries-active patients. It is recommended, therefore, that sealants not be used on patients who do not have signs of caries activity. If caries activity is noted either clinically or radiographically, strong consideration for sealing all pits and fissures should be made.

The use of sealants is an effective preventive treatment for caries. Indications for the use of sealants are presented in Table 3-15. Sealants (1) prevent caries in newly erupted teeth, (2) arrest incipient caries, (3) prevent odontopathogenic bacterial growth in sealed fissures, and (4) prevent infection of other sites. They should be used on the pits and fissures of patients at high risk for caries as an alternative to restorations. This includes the lingual pits on maxillary anterior teeth and facial pits on mandibular molars. Because caries activity is high during childhood and adolescence, the patient should receive frequent recalls and extra preventive treatment such as sealants during this time. Sealants also should be used in adults who are at high risk for developing caries, primarily on those teeth (usually molars) that have deep anatomy. Even though the occlusal portion of sealants may eventually wear off, sealants offer essential caries protection during the time of high caries risk in childhood and adolescence. Because of the well-established effectiveness of sealants, it is not acceptable clinical practice to wait for caries to develop in pits and fissures and then restore these areas. Prompt sealing of the molar teeth after eruption should be a routine practice for many children.

RESTORATIONS

The status of a patient's existing restorations may have an important bearing on the outcome of preventive measures and caries treatment. Old, corroded metallic restorations that are rough and therefore plaque-retentive could be smoothed and polished or replaced. Restoration defects, such as overhangs, open proximal contacts, and defective contours, contribute to plaque formation and retention. These defects should be corrected, usually by replacement of the defective restoration. Detection of secondary caries can be difficult around old restorations. Discoloration of the enamel adjacent to a

TABLE 3-15 Indications for Use of Sealants

CRITERIA	SEAL	DO NOT SEAL
Tooth age	Recently erupted teeth	Teeth that have remained free of caries for 4 years or longer; staining is usually present in pits/fissures
Tooth type	Molars	Premolars, except when patient is caries active
Occlusal morphology	Deep, retentive, narrow pits and fissures	Well-coalesced fossae and grooves; wide, easily cleaned grooves
Recent caries activity	Teeth showing signs of softening or opacity in pit or fissure	Teeth that have remained free of caries for 4 years or longer; staining is usually present in pits/fissures
General caries activity	Occlusal or smooth surface lesions on other teeth; no proximal cavitated lesions on tooth to be sealed	Proximal cavitated lesion on tooth to be sealed; cavitation of occlusal (tooth will require restoration)
Availability of other preventive measures	Patient receiving appropriate systemic and/or topical fluoride therapy and still caries active	Patient's water supply is fluoride-deficient; patient is not cooperating in recommended caries-preventive program (restoration of pits and fissures is preferred)

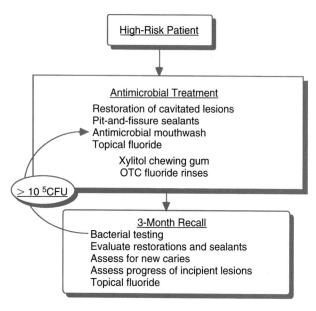

FIG. 3-45 A scheme for caries treatment based on the specific plaque hypothesis. Here caries is treated as an infectious bacteriologic disease. Signs of the disease, such as development of white spot lesions, indicate the need for antimicrobial treatment. Follow-up assessment is used to determine if the infection still persists and if new lesions are forming. Retreatment occurs if either is present. Restorative treatment in this model is an adjunct to the antimicrobial treatment, not the primary treatment. *OTC,* Over the counter.

placement unless for improvement of esthetics. Such a discoloration may be due to the amalgam itself.) Because metallic restorations are radiopaque, the radiolucency of secondary caries may be masked.

The placement of restorations is preventive only in the sense of removing large numbers of cariogenic organisms and some of the sites in which they may be protected. It should be remembered that the placement of a restoration into a cavitated carious tooth does not cure the carious process.

Strict preventive measures for caries are not necessary for all patients. Some of those measures would result in expensive treatment with few benefits for low-risk patients. Only caries-active patients and those at high risk (who will most likely benefit from preventive measures) should be treated with comprehensive regimens (Fig. 3-45). Caries activity should be viewed as a problem of oral ecology in which there is an abnormal abundance of cariogenic organisms. Preventive treatment is based on reducing the pathogen population size and increasing the resistance of the tooth to cariogenic attack. The cariogenicity of plaque can be controlled by denying the food supply, denying the habitat, using antimicrobial therapy, and stopping succession. The most successful preventive treatment combines all of these treatments in a specific program designed for an individual that considers both caries and periodontal disease.

CARIES TREATMENT

Even though diagnostic and preventive measures have been improved and are more widely used, the repair of destruction caused by the carious process will still be necessary for many patients. The treatment

restoration is suggestive of secondary caries. This appears as a localized opalescent area next to the restoration margins. (*Exception:* A bluish color of facial or lingual enamel that directly overlies an old, otherwise acceptable, amalgam restoration does not indicate re-

regimen is dictated by the patient's caries status. If the patient is at high risk for caries development, his or her treatment should consist of both restorative procedures and many of the preventive measures described previously. Then the damage done by caries can be repaired and the patient's risk status for further caries attacks reduced. Sometimes patients present with acute carious lesions in numerous teeth. Because of the jeopardy these teeth may have and the large numbers and sites of cariogenic bacteria, caries control restorative treatment may be indicated as described later in this section. This procedure rids the patient rapidly of the carious lesions, thereby providing better assessment of the pulpal responses of some teeth and greater success of the preventive measures instituted. Later, the teeth will be restored with more definitive restorations.

Important in the treatment success are the patient's education about what has caused the caries problem and what are his or her responsibilities. Having the patient understand the problem and the benefits of the recommended treatment will likely provide him or her an increased motivation to do what is necessary to obtain good oral health. Appropriate homecare is the patient's primary responsibility. This activity, which includes proper flossing and brushing as well as using prescribed adjunct treatment modalities (fluoride, chlorhexidine, xylitol gums, and so on), must be accepted by the patient. Likewise, their commitment to necessary restorative intervention also is required. Many patients will become willing partners in this approach to treatment if they understand why they have a problem and why their role is necessary.

If the patient has cavitated carious lesions, they should be restored first in the treatment regimen, sometimes using caries control restorations. By restoring the teeth first, large numbers of MS organisms and their favored and protected sites will be removed. If antimicrobial therapy is instituted first, it may disrupt the oral flora but allow the virulent cariogenic organisms in the unrestored cavitated areas to then flourish in unprotected sites. Restorations remove large masses of infectious organisms, but more importantly, they remove habitats for more bacterial adherence.

For high-risk patients, sealants should be applied to at-risk teeth while doing the necessary restorative procedures. This will better insure their caries-free status in the future. Intense, short-term use of antimicrobial agents should then be implemented. These may include various fluoride modalities, chlorhexidine, and, sometimes, antibiotics such as vancomycin or kanamycin (see Table 3-14). These antimicrobial agents will reduce the numbers of cariogenic bacteria and render tooth surfaces more prone for remineralization. The high-risk patient also should be instructed to use fluoride rinses and xylitol chewing gums regularly. After the initial phase of restorative and preventive treatment, the patient should be placed on a strict recall schedule. At recall, restorations and sealants should be evaluated, microbiologic assays done, and a careful clinical examination performed.

Many of the later chapters in this textbook focus on the techniques for restoration of tooth defects with various restorative materials. However, the following information describes the caries control type of restorative treatment.

Much success has been obtained in decreasing the incidence of caries. Research activity has been intense in developing an understanding of the carious process and, consequently, in preventing caries. However, if the carious process cannot be prevented or reversed, it must be controlled. Currently no therapeutic medicament will stop the progression of caries, and while the "arrested caries" phenomenon is recognized, it is not yet clearly understood so as to be universally applicable. Therefore the recognized control of cavitated carious lesions occurs predominantly by the clinical removal of the infected area from the tooth and the subsequent restoration of the tooth to optimal form, function, and esthetics. The specific clinical treatment depends on the extent of the destruction that has occurred, and subsequent chapters in this book relate to the definitive treatment of carious lesions.

Once caries has produced cavitation of the tooth surface, preventive measures are usually inadequate to prevent further progression of the lesion. Surgical removal of the lesion and restoration of the tooth then are required to eliminate the progression of the lesion. Currently, operative treatment constitutes the majority of all caries treatment. Restoration of carious lesions is the most effective method for control of the progression of active, cavitated lesions. The term *caries control* refers to an operative procedure in which multiple teeth with acute threatening caries are treated quickly by: (1) removing the infected tooth structure, (2) medicating the pulp, if necessary, and (3) restoring the defects with a temporary material. With this technique, most of the infecting organisms and their protecting sites are removed, limiting further acute spread of caries throughout the mouth. The caries control procedure must be accompanied by other preventive measures that reduce the likelihood of continued buildup or presence of pathogenic organisms (Table 3-16). Teeth rapidly treated by caries control procedures are subsequently treated by using routine restorative techniques, if appropriate pulpal responses are obtained. Also, the intent of caries control procedures is to make immediate, corrective intervention in advanced carious lesions to both prevent and assess pulpal disease and avoid possible sequelae such as toothache, root canal therapy, or more complex ultimate restorations.

CARIES CONTROL RESTORATION

Objectives and Indications. Although caries has declined in the general population of the United States, a significant segment of the population, including lower socioeconomic groups and minorities, continues to suffer from extensive caries. Victims of acute caries (lesions that have progressed at least half the distance from the DEJ to the pulp) typically have poor oral health care habits, minimal exposure to fluorides, a deficient or highly cariogenic diet, and poor or limited access to dental care. Missing teeth, retained roots, and periodontal and/or pulpal diseases often complicate the clinical situation (Fig. 3-46). Active, rapidly progressing caries urgently needs clinical treatment when dentin softening has progressed at least half the distance from the DEJ to the pulp. Acute caries may progress rapidly without operative intervention. Conventional restorative treatment techniques may not address acute problems with sufficient rapidity to prevent pulpal infection and/or death of the pulp. *The treatment objective for caries control is to remove the decay from all of the advanced carious lesions, place appropriate pulpal medication, and restore the lesions in the most expedient manner.* Temporary restorative materials (Intermediate Restorative Material [IRM],

Fuji IX, or amalgam) are usually the treatment materials of choice. This treatment of acute lesions will quickly remove gross infectious lesions. This will not only generate some time while many of the other associated dental problems can be treated, but also will provide a time period for pulpal assessment of the more seriously compromised teeth. These temporary restorations usually should be replaced with more permanent restorations at a later date, when the factors promoting caries formation have been controlled and the prognosis of the tooth pulp has been determined.

Caries control is an intermediate step in restorative treatment and has several other indications. Teeth with questionable pulpal prognosis should be treated with a caries control approach. In this way the progression of demineralization of the dentin is stopped, and the response of the pulp can be determined before making a commitment to permanent restoration. Another clinical situation when caries control is a useful approach occurs during an operative procedure when a tooth is unexpectedly found to have extensive caries. Caries control technique provides the busy practitioner the flexibility to respond rapidly to stop the carious process in that tooth without causing major changes in the daily time

TABLE 3-16	Caries Control Restoration as a Part of the Medical Model
Initial treatment	Thorough evaluation and documentation of lesions
	Temporization of all large cavitated lesions by caries control restorations
	Specific antimicrobial treatment (see Table 3-11, technique *B*)
	Plaque control (see Table 3-11, technique *C*)
	Dietary control (see Table 3-11, technique *A*)
Preliminary assessment	Gingival response as a marker of plaque control effectiveness
	Pulpal response of teeth with caries control restorations
	Assessment of patient compliance with medications, oral hygiene, and dietary control measures
Follow-up care	Careful clinical evaluation of teeth
	Replacement of caries control restorations with permanent restorations
	Monitoring of plaque and MS levels
	Further antimicrobial treatment and dietary reassessment as indicated by new cavitations, incipient lesions, or high MS levels

MS, Mutans streptococci.

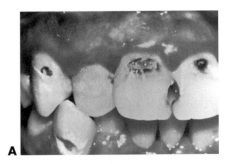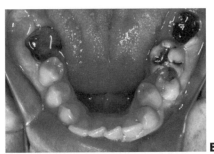

FIG. 3-46 Acute, rampant caries. **A,** Severe carious involvement in anterior teeth. **B,** Severe carious involvement in posterior teeth.

schedule. The caries control procedure allows quick removal of the caries, placement of a temporary restoration, and the rescheduling of the patient for a more time-consuming, permanent restoration. Before placement of a permanent restoration, a caries control procedure also provides a suitable delay that gives the pulp time to recover, allowing a better assessment of the pulpal status.

A caries control procedure is indicated when: (1) the caries is extensive enough that adverse pulpal sequelae are soon likely to occur, (2) the goal of treatment is to remove the nidus of caries infection in the patient's mouth, or (3) a tooth has extensive carious involvement that cannot or should not be permanently restored because of inadequate available time or questionable pulpal prognosis.

Operative Technique. When numerous acute lesions are present, the practitioner should treat these without delay in one or two appointments with the caries control procedure. Thus the rate of the carious process is significantly reduced, potential pulpal irritation is minimized, and the patient is in a healthier and more comfortable state. The following description involves only a single tooth for the sake of simplicity. Temporization of multiple teeth in a single setting is a practical clinical procedure and is simply an extension of the procedure for a single tooth. Fig. 3-47 shows a schematic representation of the caries control procedure and Fig. 3-48 provides a preoperative radiograph of the tooth described in the following sections.

Anesthesia is usually indicated for the affected area unless a test preparation for pulpal vitality is to be performed. The indications and technique for a test preparation are presented in Chapter 9. Anesthesia usually is essential for providing patient comfort, reducing saliva flow, and promoting good patient cooperation during the procedure. Because pulpal necrosis may occur when oral fluids contaminate exposure sites during excavation of advanced carious lesions, the operating site must be isolated. The rubber dam provides an excellent means of isolation and protection of the excavation site from contamination with oral fluids during the operative procedure, and therefore should be used routinely in most caries control procedures.

The primary objective of the caries control tooth preparation is to provide adequate visual and mechanical access to facilitate the removal of the infected portion of the carious dentin. The initial opening of the tooth is made with the largest carbide bur that can be used. A high-speed handpiece with an air-water spray is the most practical instrument for this procedure (Fig. 3-49).

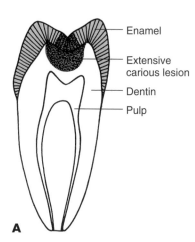

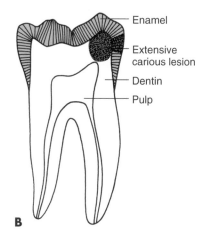

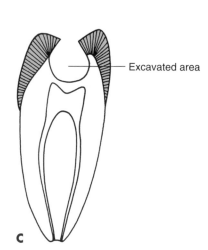

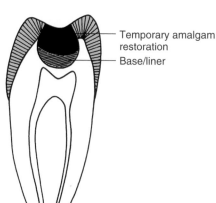

FIG. **3-47** Schematic representation of caries control procedure. Faciolingual **(A)** and mesiodistal **(B)** cross-sections of mandibular first molar showing extensive preoperative occlusal and proximal carious lesions. **C,** Tooth after excavation of extensive caries. Note remaining unsupported enamel. **D,** Temporary amalgam restoration inserted after appropriate liner/base material is applied.

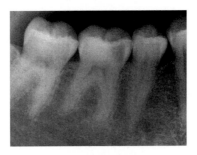

FIG. 3-48 Preoperative clinical radiograph illustrating extensive carious lesion in proximal and occlusal regions of mandibular right first molar.

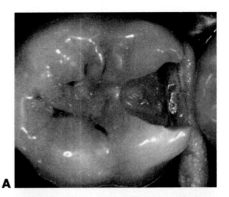

A

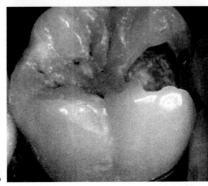

B

FIG. 3-49 Initial caries excavation of tooth in Fig. 3-48. **A,** Note remaining caries that requires further excavation. Also note wedge in place protecting rubber dam and soft tissue and that it has been lightly shaved by bur. **B,** Note remaining unsupported enamel under mesiolingual cusp.

Some steps of initial tooth preparation are modified for the caries control procedure. (See Chapter 6 for further considerations in tooth preparation.) Retaining unsupported enamel is permissible in caries control procedures because this tooth structure, even though undermined, assists in the retention of the temporary restorative material. Removal of the unsupported enamel will occur when the final restoration is placed at a later date. Retaining sound portions of old restorative material also may enhance the temporary restoration and reduce the risk of pulpal exposure. However, care must be exercised when deciding not to remove all old restorative material because it may mask residual infected dentin.

Once access has been gained, the identification and removal of caries depends primarily on the dentist's interpretation of tactile stimuli. Color differences cannot be used as a reliable index for complete caries removal, although caries-indicating solutions may provide color guides. In rapidly advancing lesions, the softened dentin shows little or no color change while more slowly advancing lesions have more discoloration. Dentin that appears leathery, peels off in small flakes, or can be judiciously penetrated by a sharp explorer should be removed.

Because fine tactile discrimination is required for complete removal of caries, the use of a high-speed handpiece at full speed is contraindicated for the removal of deep caries. Effective caries removal can be accomplished with: (1) hand instrumentation using spoon excavators, (2) a slow-speed handpiece with a large round bur, or (3) a high-speed handpiece using a round bur operated just above stall-out speed (low speed). The use of spoon excavators may result in peeling off amounts of softened dentin larger than intended and therefore result in inadvertent pulp exposure. Thus, hand excavation requires great skill and sharp instruments. Rotary instruments provide good control and require less skill. The high-speed handpiece, when running just above stalling speed, provides good control. A simple technique is to run the handpiece slowly enough that the bur stalls shortly after contacting the dentin. Repeated applications of the bur will remove dentin in small increments

and allow the operator to carefully monitor changes in both hardness and color. After removal of softened dentin, it is then helpful to carefully evaluate the excavated area with a sharp explorer to determine if the remaining dentin is hard and sound. Extreme care must be used with the explorer to prevent penetration into the pulp. Penetration of the explorer into the pulp may cause pulpal infection, increasing the possibility of pulpal death.

Usually all soft, infected dentin is removed during caries control procedures. However, in asymptomatic teeth that have deep lesions (where complete excavation of softened dentin is anticipated to produce pulpal exposure), the softened dentin nearest the pulp may be left. The deliberate retention of softened dentin near the tooth pulp and medication of the remaining dentin with calcium hydroxide is termed an *indirect pulp cap.* The goals of the caries control procedure are to prevent pulp exposure and aid pulpal recovery by medication. The portion of the remaining softened dentin is covered with a calcium hydroxide liner and the excavated area is restored with a temporary material. Calcium hydroxide promotes reparative dentin bridges over any area of frank pulpal exposure. Such repair usually occurs in 6 to 8 weeks and may be evident radiographically in 10 to 12 weeks. Success may be improved with a resin-modified glass-ionomer liner placed over the calcium hydroxide.

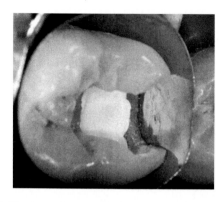

FIG. **3-50** Tooth ready for placement of temporary amalgam restoration. Carious involvement required further extension than in Fig. 3-49. Liner/base material has been applied to deepest excavated areas, and matrix, appropriately wedged, has been placed.

If the pulp is penetrated by an instrument during the operative procedure, then a decision must be made whether to proceed with root canal therapy or do a direct pulp cap. A *direct pulp cap* is a technique for treating a pulp exposure with a material that seals over the exposure site and promotes reparative dentin formation. If the exposure site is the consequence of infected dentin extending into the pulp, termed a carious pulpal exposure, infection of the pulp already has occurred and removal of the tooth pulp is indicated. If, however, the pulp exposure occurs in an area of normal dentin (usually as a result of operator error or misjudgment), termed a mechanical pulpal exposure, and bacterial contamination from salivary exposure does not occur, the potential success of the direct pulp cap procedure is enhanced. With either type of exposure, a more favorable prognosis for the pulp following direct pulp capping may be expected if:

1. The tooth has been asymptomatic (no spontaneous pain, normal response to thermal testing, and is vital) before the operative procedure.
2. The exposure is small, less than 0.5 mm in diameter.
3. The hemorrhage from the exposure site is easily controlled.
4. The exposure occurred in a clean, uncontaminated field (such as provided by rubber dam isolation).
5. The exposure was relatively atraumatic and little desiccation of the tooth occurred, with no evidence of aspiration of blood into the dentin (dentin blushing).

A deep caries excavation close to the pulp, which may result in either an undetected pulpal exposure or a visible pulpal exposure, should be covered with a calcium hydroxide liner that can stimulate formation of dentin bridges (reparative dentin) over the exposure. However, for amalgam restorations, deep excavations not encroaching on the pulp should be covered with a glass-

ionomer material that will contribute to thermal protection and provide mechanical protection from amalgam condensation forces at thicknesses of 1 to 1.5 mm or greater.

In addition to the use of calcium hydroxide materials, the use of resin bonding agents on exposed pulps may be considered, as may the technique described earlier in this chapter in the section on Advanced Carious Lesions. The choice between these approaches is controversial.

After the involved tooth has been prepared, excavated, and medicated, a suitable restorative material must be placed. The selection of a material depends on both the amount of missing tooth structure and the expected length of service anticipated for this temporary restoration. Amalgam, Fuji IX and IRM are the most frequently used materials for caries control procedures. Sometimes, a tooth-colored material (composite or glass ionomer) may be contraindicated because of difficulty in removing the esthetic material during the permanent restoration procedure.

If a long interval is anticipated between the caries control procedure and the permanent restoration, amalgam will ensure better maintenance of tooth position and proper contour. If significant portions of the proximal or occlusal surfaces are missing, an amalgam temporary restoration will maintain the adjacent and occlusal tooth contact better than other temporary restorative materials, such as IRM. The extent of the access preparation and tooth structure loss will indicate the need for a matrix application before placement of the restorative material (Fig. 3-50). Matrix choice and application are described in later chapters. Condensation and carving should be accomplished in the conventional manner. Precise anatomic form is not necessary for temporary restorations. However, proper proximal contacts and contours should be established to maintain satisfactory dimension of the embrasures to foster interdental papilla health (Fig. 3-51). Teeth lacking interproximal contacts may drift, making subsequent restoration more difficult. Also, a condensation technique that exerts less pressure (i.e., using a spheric amalgam) reduces the chance of pulpal perforation.

Controversies in Caries Control Restorative Treatment Procedures. Different opinions exist concerning various aspects of caries control technique. Some practitioners advocate removal of all caries in all teeth initially, regardless of the size of the lesion. This approach is undoubtedly the most effective for controlling the infection from dental caries. This approach, however, has disadvantages because it necessitates the excavation of all lesions, which is very laborious. Limiting caries control procedures to pulp-threatening, advanced, carious lesions is advocated in this text as a more practical procedure. The caries control restorations can be replaced after the remaining small- to moderate-sized lesions are completely restored. The interval between the caries

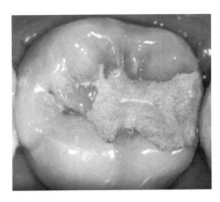

FIG. 3-51 Temporary amalgam restoration completed for caries control procedure. Caries has been eliminated, the pulp adequately protected, and interarch and intraarch positions of tooth maintained by caries control procedure.

control restoration and its replacement with a permanent restoration provides time to complete the following: assessment of the pulpal response to excavation and medication, treatment of the cariogenic infection with prescribed anticaries measures, assessment of the patient's ability to perform oral hygiene procedures, assessment of the patient's compliance with dietary changes, and assessment of caries activity elsewhere in the mouth. The outcome of these factors may have an important bearing on the choice of materials and techniques for the final restoration of the teeth. Regardless of the caries control concept endorsed, advanced carious lesions should be treated without delay to minimize the potential of adverse pulpal reaction and to provide time for assessment of the pulpal response to therapy.

Also, different opinions present regarding the indication for indirect pulp capping procedures. Some practitioners routinely remove all softened dentin even if a pulpal exposure is likely. Other practitioners routinely leave a small amount of dentin in the area of a potential pulpal exposure, regardless of the status of such dentin. Finally, some practitioners use the indirect pulp capping technique only when the status of remaining dentin in close proximity to the pulp is questionable. Data are not available to guide the final decision in this area. However, as presented in Advanced Carious Lesions, a newer concept[78] endorses the technique of deliberate removal of the coronal pulpal tissue; placement of calcium hydroxide directly on the exposed pulpal tissue; and, finally, placement of a resin-modified glass ionomer on the calcium hydroxide and surrounding dentin periphery.

Another controversial issue with the indirect pulp capping treatment is whether or not to reenter the treated tooth at a later time to determine if, in fact, the remaining dentin has remineralized, providing a sound bridge of tooth structure over the affected area. Some practitioners routinely reenter the affected area to verify this remineralization and/or to remove any caries left over the remineralized layer. Others believe that re-

mineralization will occur and any remaining bacteria become inviable; consequently, reentry into the excavated area is not practical because such a procedure may cause additional pulpal irritation. Carefully controlled studies are lacking, but the consensus is shifting against reentry procedures.

Some controversy exists concerning the medication material to place over deeply excavated areas. Although most practitioners recognize the potential for stimulating reparative dentin formation with the use of calcium hydroxide materials, this is not universally accepted. More importantly, there is controversy regarding the mechanism of action for calcium hydroxide liners. One group of practitioners supports the concept that a calcium hydroxide liner must be in direct contact with pulpal tissue to cause reparative dentin formation. Therefore these practitioners believe that the use of calcium hydroxide liners in other than a direct pulpal exposure situation will not stimulate reparative dentin formation. However, other practitioners believe that the calcium hydroxide material is soluble and therefore is transmitted by the fluid in the dentinal tubules to the pulp and, consequently, causes reparative dentin formation. Also, as mentioned earlier, the use of resin bonding agents may prove beneficial for pulp capping procedures.

Finally, there is minor controversy, or at least confusion, about the terminology related to this procedure. Although this section has termed the procedure caries control restorative treatment, other terms such as interim restoration, treatment restoration, or temporary restoration may be used. All of these descriptions have validity when applied to the technique of removing acute caries without delay and temporarily restoring the involved tooth or teeth.

SUMMARY

Diagnosis, prevention, and treatment of dental caries must be the foremost objectives of operative dentistry. Research efforts in understanding the caries process; maximizing the benefits of fluoride and chlorhexidine use; and, perhaps, developing anticaries vaccines must be continued. Patient education and motivation in the prevention and treatment of dental caries must be stressed. Finally, the clinical treatment of cavitated, carious teeth must be accomplished expeditiously, judiciously, and appropriately.

REFERENCES

1. Alaluusua S et al: Salivary caries related tests as predictors of future caries increments in teenagers: a three-year longitudinal study, *Oral Microl Immunol* 5:77-81, 1990.
2. Alexander M: *Microbial ecology,* New York, 1971, John Wiley & Sons.
3. Antoku S et al: Effect of controllable parameters on oral radiographs, *Quintessence Int* 15:71-76, 1984.
4. Anusavice KJ: Management of dental caries as a chronic infectious disease, *J Dent Educ* 62(10):791-802, 1998.

5. Arnold RR et al: Antimicrobial activity of the secretory innate defense factors lactoferrin, lactoperoxidase, and lysozyme. In Guggenheim B, editor: *Cariology Today,* Basel, 1984, Karger.

6. Backer DO: Posteruptive changes in dental enamel, *J Dent Res* 45:503, 1966.

7. Bader JD, Brown JP: Dilemmas in caries diagnosis, *J Am Dent Assoc* 123:48-50, 1993.

8. Baum LJ: Dentinal pulp conditions in relation to caries lesions, *Int Dent J* 20:309-337, 1970.

9. Beiswanger BB: The clinical validation of early caries detection methodologies. In: Stookey GK, editor: *Early detection of dental caries: Proceedings of the 1st Annual Indiana Conference.* Indianapolis, 1996, Indiana University School of Dentistry.

10. Beltrán-Aguilar ED, Goldstein JW, Lockwood SA: Fluoride varnishes—a review of their clinical use, cariostatic mechanism, efficacy, and safety, *J Am Dent Assoc* 131:589-596, 2000.

11. Bowen WH: Nature of plaque. In Meleher AH, Zarb GA, editors: Preventive dentistry: nature, pathogenicity and clinical control of plaque, *Oral Sci Rev* 9:3, 1976.

12. Brännström M, Gabroglio R: The dentinal tubules and the odontoblastic processes: a scanning electron microscopic study, *Acta Odontol Scand* 30:291-311, 1972.

13. Brännström M, Lind PO: Pulpal response to early dentinal caries, *J Dent Res* 44:1045-1050, 1965.

14. Brown JP, Lazar V: The economic state of dentistry, an overview, *J Am Dent Assoc* 129:1682-1691, 1998.

15. Brown LJ: Indicators for caries management from the patient history, *J Dent Educ* 61(11):855-60, 1997.

16. Brown LR, Dreizen S, Handler S: Effects of selected caries preventive regimens on microbial changes following radiation-induced xerostomia in cancer patients. In Stiles HM, Loesche WJ, O'Brien TC, editors: Microbial aspects of dental caries, *Microbiol Abstr Spec Suppl* 1:275, 1976.

17. Brunelle JA: Prevalence of dental sealants in U.S. schoolchildren. *J Dent Res* 68(special issue):183, 1989.

18. Disney J et al: The University of North Carolina caries risk assessment study: further developments in caries risk prediction, *Community Dent Oral Epidemiol* 20:64-75, 1992.

19. Dreizen S, Brown LR: Xerostomia and dental caries. In Stiles HM, Loesche WJ, O'Brien TC, editors: Microbial aspects of dental caries, *Microbiol Abstr Spec Suppl* 1:263, 1976.

20. Edgar WM: Saliva and dental health. Clinical implications of saliva: report of a consensus meeting, *Br Dent J* 169:96-98, 1990.

21. Emilson CG: Potential efficacy of chlorhexidine against mutans streptococci and human dental caries, *J Dent Res* 73:682-691, 1994.

22. Espelid I: Radiographic diagnosis and treatment decision on approximal caries, *Community Dent Oral Epidemiol* 14:265-270, 1986.

23. Fejerskov O et al: Plaque and caries development in experimental human fissures: structural and microbiologic features (abstract no. 457), *J Dent Res* 56(special issue), 1977.

24. *Fluoridation facts.* Chicago, 1993, American Dental Association.

25. Frank RM, Voegel JC: Ultrastructure of the human odontoblast process and its mineralization during dental caries, *Caries Res* 19:367-380, 1980.

26. Fusayama T: Two layers of carious dentin: diagnosis and treatment, *Oper Dent* 42:63, 1979.

27. Garg AK, Malo MM: Manifestations and treatment of xerostomia and associated oral effects secondary to head and neck radiation therapy, *J Am Dent Assoc* 128:1128-1133, 1997.

28. Glass RL, editor: The first international conference on the declining prevalence of dental caries, *J Dent Res* 61:1301, 1982.

29. Going RE et al: The viability of microorganisms in carious lesions five years after covering with a fissure sealant, *J Am Dent Assoc* 97:455, 1978.

30. Govan JR: In vivo significance of bacterioicins and bacteriocin receptors, *Scand J Infect Dis Suppl* 49:31-37, 1986.

31. Handleman SL: Effect of sealant placement on occlusal caries progression, *Clin Prevent Dent* 4(5):11-16, 1982.

32. Hausen H: Caries prediction—state of the art, *Community Dent Oral Epidemiol* 25:87-96, 1997.

33. Hay DI: Specific functional salivary proteins. In Guggenheim B, editor: *Cariology today,* Basel, 1984, Karger.

34. Hillman JD, Dzuback AL, Andrews SW: Colonization of the human oral cavity by a *Streptococcus mutans* mutant producing increased bacteriocin, *J Dent Res* 66(6):1092-1094, 1987.

35. Hillman JD, Yaphe BI, Johnson KP: Colonization of the human oral cavity by a strain of *Streptococcus mutans, J Dent Res* 64(11):1272-1274, 1985.

36. Hodge HC: The concentration of fluoride in drinking water to give the point of minimum caries with maximum safety, *J Am Dent Assoc* 40:436, 1950.

37. Horowitz HS, Herfetz SB, Paulsen S: Retention and effectiveness of a single application of an adhesive sealant in preventing occlusal caries: final report after five years of study in Kalespel, Montana, *J Am Dent Assoc* 95:1133, 1977.

38. Jett BD, Gilmore MS: The growth inhibitory effect of the *Enterococcus faecalis* bacteriocin encoded by pAD1 extends to the oral streptococci, *J Dent Res* 69(10):1640-1645, 1990.

39. Juhl M: Three-dimensional replicas of pit-and-fissure morphology, *Scand J Dent Res* 91(2):90, 1983.

40. Kantor ML et al: Efficacy of dental radiographic practices: opinions or image receptors, examination selection, and patient selection, *J Am Dent Assoc* 119:259-268, 1989.

41. Klock B, Krasse B: Effect of caries preventive measures in children with high numbers of *S. mutans* and lactobacilli, *Scand J Dent Res* 86:221, 1978.

42. Krasse B: *Caries risk,* Chicago, 1985, Quintessence.

43. Kuboki Y, Liu C-F, Fusayama T: Mechanism of differential staining in carious dentin, *J Dent Res* 62:713, 1983.

44. Lehner T, Challacombe SJ, Caldwell J: An immunological investigation in to the prevention of caries in deciduous teeth of rhesus monkeys, *Arch Oral Biol* 20:305, 1975.

45. Leverett JB et al: Cost effectiveness of sealants as an alternative to conventional restorations, *J Dent Res* 1143(57A):130, 1978.

46. Löe H: Human research model for the production and prevention of gingivitis, *J Dent Res* 50:256, 1971.

47. Loesche WJ: Role of *Streptococcus mutans* in human dental decay, *Microbiol Rev* 50:353-380, 1986.

48. Loesche WJ: Clinical and microbiological aspects of chemotherapeutic agents used according to the specific plaque hypothesis, *J Dent Res* 58:2404, 1979.

49. Loyola-Rodriguez JP et al: Purification and properties of extracellular mutacin, a bacteriocin from *Streptococcus sobrinus, J Gen Microbiol* 138(pt2):269-274, 1992.

50. Mandel ID: Caries prevention—a continuing need, *Int Dent J* 43:67-70, 1993.

51. Mandel ID: Salivary factors in caries prediction. In Bibby BG, Shern RJ, editors: Methods of caries prediction, *Microbiol Abstr Spec Suppl* 1978:147.

52. Mandel ID, Ellison SA: Naturally occurring defense mechanisms in saliva. In Tanzer JM, editor: *Animal models in cariology* (supplement to *Microbiology Abstracts),* Washington, DC, 1981, Information Retrieval.

53. Marketing Information Services, North Brook, Ill, 1984, A.C. Nielson.

54. Mertz-Fairhurst EJ: Guest editorial: Pit-and-fissure sealants: a global lack of science transfer? *J Dent Res* 7(80):1543-1544, 1992.

55. Mertz-Fairhurst EJ et al: Ultraconservative and cariostatic sealed restorations: results at year 10, *J Am Dent Assoc* 129:55-66, 1998.

56. Mileman P: *Radiographic caries diagnosis and restorative treatment decision making,* Gronigen, 1985, Drukkerij Vanden Deren BV.

57. Minah GE, Loesche WJ: Sucrose metabolism in resting-cell suspensions of caries-associated and non-caries–associated dental plaque, *Infect Immun* 17:43-61, 1977.

58. National Center for Health Statistics (1994). Plan and operation of the Third National Health and Nutrition Examination Survey, 1988-94 (PHS publication no. 94-1308), *Vital Health Stat* 1(32).

59. Newburn E: *Cariology,* ed 3, Chicago, 1989, Quintessence.

60. Ogawa K: The ultra structure and hardness of the transparent layer of human carious dentin, *J Dent Res* 62:7-10, 1983.

61. Ooshima T, Yasufuku Y, Izumitani A: Effect of mutacin administration on *Streptococcus mutans*-induced dental caries in rats, *Microbiol Immunol* 29(12):1163-1173, 1985.

62. Palmer C: *Dental spending to hit $57 billion. ADA News* 30(14), 1, 11, 1999.

63. Parfitt GJ: The speed of development of the carious cavity, *Br Dent J* 100:204-207, 1956.

64. Pashley DH: Clinical correlation of dentin structure and function, *J Prosthet Dent* 66:777-781, 1991.

65. Pitts NB, Rimmer PA: An in vivo comparison of radiographic and directly assessed clinical caries status of posterior approximal surfaces in primary and permanent teeth, *Caries Res* 26:146-152, 1992.

66. Ripa LW: Occlusal sealants: rationale and review of clinical trials, *Int Dent J* 30(2):127, 1980.

67. Rolla G, Ciardi JE, Schultz SA: Adsorption of glucosyltransferase to saliva coated hydroxyapatite, *Scand J Dent Res* 91(2):112, 1983.

68. Russell C, Melville TH: A review bacteria in the human mouth, *J Appl Bacteriol* 44:163, 1978.

69. Sheiham A: Dental caries in underdeveloped countries. In Guggenheim B, editor: *Cariology today,* Basel, 1984, Karger.

70. Silverstone LM: In vitro studies with special reference to the enamel surface and the enamel-resin interface. In Silverstone LM, Dogon IC, editors: *Proceedings of an international symposium on the acid etch technique,* St Paul, Minn, 1975, North Central.

71. Silverstone LM et al: *Dental caries,* New York, 1981, Macmillian.

72. Simonsen R: Cost-effectiveness of pit-and-fissure sealants at 10 years, *Quintessence Int* 20(2):75-82, 1989.

73. Stephan RM: Intra-oral hydrogen-ion concentration associated with dental caries activity, *J Dent Res* 23(4):257, 1944.

74. Straffon LH, Dennison JB: Clinical evaluation comparing sealant and amalgam after 7 years: final report, *J Am Dent Assoc* 117:751-755, 1988.

75. Svanberg M, Loesche WJ: Salivary concentration of *Streptococcus mutans* and *Streptococcus sanguis* and the colonization of artificial fissures in humans by these organisms, *Arch Oral Biol* 22:441-447, 1977.

76. Svanberg M, Westergren G: Effect of SnF2, administered as mouth rinses or topically applied, on *Streptococcus mutans, Streptococcus sanguis* and lactobacilli in dental plaque and saliva, *Scand J Dent Res* 91(2):123, 1983.

77. Svenson B: Accuracy of radiographic caries diagnosis at different kilovoltages and two film speeds, *Swed Dent J* 9:37-43, 1985.

78. Swift EJ, Trope M: Treatment options for the exposed vital pulp, *Pract Periodont Aesthet Dent* 11(6):735-739, 1999.

79. Tanzer JM: Xylitol chewing gum and dental caries, *Int Dent J* 45(Suppl 1):65-76, 1995.

80. Taubman MA, Smith DS: Effects of local immunization with glucosyltransferase fraction from *Streptococcus mutans* on dental caries in rats and hamsters, *J Immunol* 118:710, 1977.

81. Trahan L: Xylitol: a review of its action on *mutans* streptococci and dental plaque—its clinical significance. *Int Dent J* 45 (Suppl 1):77-92, 1995.

82. van Houte J: Oral bacterial colonization: mechanism and implications. In Stiles WJ, Loesche WJ, O'Bryan TC, editors: *Microbial aspects of dental caries, Microbiol Abstr Spec Suppl* 1:3, 1976.

83. Visgaitis G: How much candy we eat every year, *USA Today,* June 17, 1993, C-1.

84. Yamada T et al: The extent of the odontoblastic process in normal and carious human dentin, *Dent Res* 62:798, 1983.

4

Dental Materials

STEPHEN C. BAYNE

JEFFREY Y. THOMPSON

DUANE F. TAYLOR*

*This author is inactive this edition. See the Acknowledgments.

Dental materials science for restorative dentistry is derived from materials science. The field of materials science can be organized in terms of four categories of materials, with four categories of structural considerations governing their properties, and with four categories of general properties. For each of these, there is a rich basis of materials science definitions. This information is presented in greater depth in textbooks of dental materials, [1,11-13,19,34,51,57,59,60,83,90,99,130,147,176,178,189,193-195,202,251,262] but it is reviewed here for reference during discussions in other parts of this text.

REVIEW OF MATERIALS SCIENCE DEFINITIONS

MATERIAL CATEGORIES

The four categories of materials are metals, ceramics, polymers, and composites. Each one of these has characteristic microstructures and resulting properties. It is paramount in every situation in restorative dentistry that the structures and properties involved are known. Formal engineering definitions of each category are not practically useful. The following definitions are most often substituted instead.

Metals. A metal is based on an element that diffusely shares valence electrons among all of the atoms in the solid, instead of forming local ionic or covalent bonds. A *metal alloy* is an intentional mixture of metallic elements that occurs in a chemically intimate manner. As a result of mixing, the elements may be completely soluble (e.g., Au-Cu) or may be only partially soluble (e.g., Ag-Sn), producing more than one phase. Metallic systems are almost exclusively crystalline and most exist as polycrystalline solids. The individual crystals, or *grains*, are generally microscopic. Grains may be all the same

composition (single phase) or several different phases (multiphase). Different *phases* represent locally different chemical compositions. In metal alloys, no phase (or crystal or grain) ever represents a pure metallic element (Fig. 4-1).

The distribution of phases is influenced by the thermal and mechanical history of the solid, allowing a wide range of properties to be developed from a single overall composition. The periodic table consists mostly of metallic elements. Thus, there is a wide range of potential metallurgic systems.

Metals and metal alloys are generally prone to both chemical and electrochemical corrosion. *Chemical corrosion* occurs by direct chemical reaction on the surfaces of metallic objects of metal atoms with oxygen or other chemicals. *Electrochemical corrosion* occurs when two metallic electrodes of differing composition, structure, or local environment, while connected by a circuit and an electrolyte, produce metallic ions at the anode and an electron flow toward the cathode resulting in anodic and cathodic reactions. Most chemical reactions can proceed by both chemical and electrochemical mechanisms. Clearly, in a moist environment, such as the mouth, electrochemical reactions are very likely.

Ceramics. Ceramics are chemically intimate mixtures of metallic and nonmetallic elements, which allow ionic (K_2O) and/or covalent bonding (SiO_2) to occur. In the periodic table, only a few elements such as carbon, oxygen, nitrogen, hydrogen, and chlorine are nonmetallic. The most common ceramics in dentistry are chemical mixtures of three main metallic oxides (SiO_2, Al_2O_3, K_2O), as shown in Fig. 4-2. Ceramics also may result from corrosion of metals (Fe_2O_3, SnO, Ag_2S).

The corrosion behavior of metallic elements is classified as *active, passive,* or *immune* with respect to chemical or electrochemical reactions with other elements in their environment. Active metals corrode to form solid ceramic products or soluble products. For example, iron reacts with oxygen to form iron oxide. Passive metals

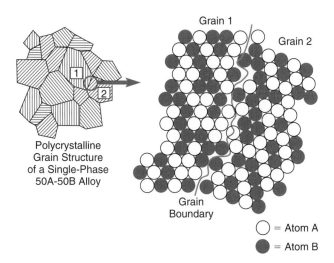

Polycrystalline Grain Structure of a Single-Phase 50A-50B Alloy

Grain 1

Grain 2

Grain Boundary

○ = Atom A

● = Atom B

FIG. **4-1** Schematic example of the microstructure of a crystalline two-phase metal alloy involving gold (clear) and copper (solid) atoms. The grain boundaries are shown as discontinuities between the individual crystals (grains).

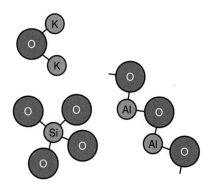

FIG. **4-2** Examples of major chemical components involved in dental ceramics.

corrode to form thin films of ceramic products that remain adherent to their surfaces and prevent further corrosion *(passivation)*. Titanium reacts with oxygen to form a titanium dioxide coating (TiO_2) that prevents further reaction and protects the surface. Immune metals, such as gold, are not reactive under normal environmental conditions. Most metals are active, and therefore ceramics are much more common than metals in the world. Most of the key ceramics used for dentistry are oxides.

Ceramics may be classified on the basis of: (1) being crystalline and/or noncrystalline, (2) being predominantly based on silica (SiO_2) and called silicates, (3) being predominantly formed by metal reactions with oxygen and called oxides, and/or (4) involving relatively simple parent structures (main structures) or highly substituted ones (derivative structures). Most ceramics are semicrystalline, silicates, oxides, and derivative structures (Fig. 4-3). Simple ceramic structures are more often ionically bonded. More complicated structures generally involve combinations of ionic and covalent bonding.

Polymers. Polymers are long molecules composed principally of nonmetallic elements (e.g., C, O, N, H) that are chemically bonded by covalent bonds. Their principal distinction from other common organic materials is their large size, and thus, molecular weight. The process of forming a polymer from identifiable subunits, *monomers*, is called *polymerization* (Fig. 4-4). *Monomer* means "one unit"; *polymer* means "many units."

A common commercial and dental example is the polymerization of methyl methacrylate monomer (100 g/mole) into methyl methacrylate polymer (typically 300,000 g/mole). Most polymers are named by adding *poly* as a prefix to the word for the major monomer in the polymer chain (e.g., polymethyl methacrylate) or

by adding *poly* to the description of the chemical links formed between monomer units (e.g., polyamide, polysaccharide, polyester, polyether, polyurethane). In other cases, the original commercial brand name has become the common name (e.g., Nylon, Teflon, Dacron, Plexiglas).

The large size and complexity of most polymers prohibits molecular scale organization that would produce crystallization. Almost all polymers under normal circumstances are noncrystalline.

Polymers may be classified in terms of the kinetics of their polymerization reaction. *Chain reaction polymerization* involves rapid monomer addition to growing chains. *Stepwise reaction polymerization* occurs slowly by random addition of monomers to any growing chain ends.

Acrylic monomers are widely used in dentistry and undergo chain reaction polymerization. The stages of chain reaction polymerization (Fig. 4-5) include: (1) activation (production of free radicals), (2) initiation (free radical combination with a monomer unit to create the beginning of a growing chain), (3) propagation (continued addition of monomer units), and (4) termination (cancellation of the growing chain end by any one of several possible events). The reaction kinetics of any step may be quite complex and may be influenced by many variables such as temperature, extent of reaction, or method of initiation. Accelerators (chemical, light, or heat) may be used to increase the rate of activation. Inhibitors or retarders (chemical) may be added to consume newly formed free radicals and prevent or postpone initiation. Once chain reaction polymerization has started, the process may proceed at extremely high speeds producing extensive release of heat. Methyl methacrylate monomers combine to form polymer as fast as 1,000,000 units per second.

Composites. Composites are physical mixtures (or blends) of metals, ceramics, and/or polymers. The goal

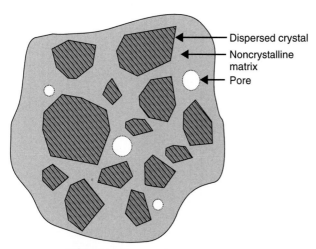

Semicrystalline ceramic

FIG. 4-3 Schematic example of the microstructure of a multiphase semicrystalline ceramic. This microstructure is typical for lab-processed feldspathic porcelins. Generally, the crystalline phase appears as islands within the noncrystalline phase. Pores are included as typical defects in these structures.

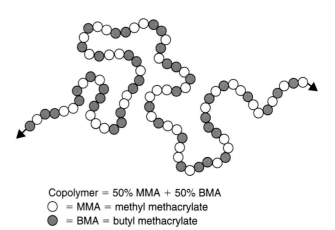

Copolymer = 50% MMA + 50% BMA
○ = MMA = methyl methacrylate
● = BMA = butyl methacrylate

FIG. 4-4 Schematic example of a portion of a copolymer molecule formed from two different types (clear and solid) of monomer units.

is to blend the properties of the parts to obtain intermediate properties and to take advantage of best properties of each phase. The classic mixture for dental restorations involves ceramic particles mixed with a polymer matrix. This is commonly called *dental composite* or *composite.*

Properties of composites can be explained readily in terms of the volume fraction of the phases being physically mixed. This principle is called the *rule-of-mixtures* and actually has wide application for all material. By knowing the phases present in the structure of any material and the interfacial interactions, it is possible to predict the overall properties fairly well.

Composites can be described as a *dispersed (filler) phase* mixed into a *continuous (matrix) phase.* The matrix phase is generally the phase that is transiently fluid during manipulation or placement of the materials. It is also the phase that tends to have the least desirable properties in the mixture. As a general rule, *minimizing the matrix of any system produces materials with more desirable clinical properties.* For a composite to distribute energy within the system to all of the phases, *it is important that the dispersed phase be bonded effectively to the continuous phase.*

MATERIAL STRUCTURE

Traditionally, a material is defined in terms of its composition. However, the composition of a material only represents one of four important categories describing its structure, and hence properties. The four *structural categories* are *atomic arrangement, bonding, composition,* and *defects. Atomic arrangement* may be crystalline (ordered) or noncrystalline (disordered, glassy, amorphous). *Primary bonding* may include metallic, ionic, and/or covalent chemical bonds. *Secondary bonding* is much weaker and may include van der Waals or hydrogen bonds. *Com-*

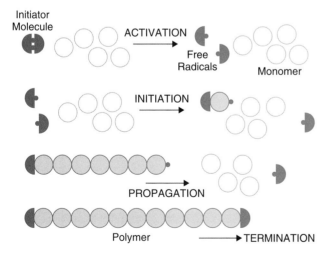

FIG. **4-5** Schematic representation of the four stages of chain reaction polymerization (activation, initiation, propagation, and termination) typical of free radical initiated acrylic systems. Each stage has different reaction kinetics. Accelerators hasten free radical formation. Retarders and inhibitors forestall initiation.

position includes the elemental components and the resulting phases that form. The *defects* encompass a wide range of imperfections from those on the atomic scale to voids or pores. *The thermal and mechanical histories strongly influence these structural categories, producing a wide range of possible properties for the same overall chemical composition.* Gold alloys will have different mechanical properties if their defect concentrations are changed. SiO_2 can be produced as a noncrystalline solid or as any of three equilibrium crystalline solids (crystobalite, tridymite, or quartz).

MATERIAL PROPERTIES

Properties are descriptions of a material's interactions with the energy in its environment. *The four common material property categories are physical, mechanical, chemical, and biologic properties. Physical properties* include mass properties, thermal properties, electrical properties, optical properties, and surface properties. *Mechanical properties* include descriptions of stresses and strains within a material as a result of an external force. *Chemical properties* include chemical and electrochemical interactions. *Biologic properties* include characterization of toxicity or sensitivity reactions during clinical use.

Physical Properties. Physical properties involve reversible interactions of a material with its environment. A few of the more common physical properties are reviewed here with respect to important dental situations.

Metals, ceramics, polymers, and composites have both different types and numbers of bonds. During temperature changes, therefore, they respond differently. During temperature increases, more frequent atomic motions stretch bonds and produce net expansion. During temperature decreases, solids undergo contraction. The relative rate of change is called the *coefficient of thermal expansion (or contraction).* If it is referenced to a single dimension, called the *linear coefficient of thermal expansion* (LCTE), symbolized by the Greek letter alpha (α). The LCTE is expressed in units of inch/inch/°F, cm/cm/ °C, or ppm/°C. Because the rate of change is small, the actual value is typically a multiple of 10^{-6} cm/cm/°C and is reduced to ppm/°C. Ceramics typically have an LCTE from 1 to 15 ppm/°C. Metals typically have values from 10 to 30 ppm/°C. Polymers typically have values from 30 to 600 ppm/°C. The LCTE of tooth structure is approximately 9 to 11 ppm/°C. It is important that the LCTE of a restorative material be as near that of tooth structure as possible. Important examples of values for dental materials are reported in Table 4-1.

One of the consequences of thermal expansion and contraction differences between a restorative material and adjacent tooth structure is percolation. This process is typified by an intracoronal amalgam restoration. During cooling, the amalgam contracts faster than tooth structure and recedes from the preparation wall, allowing the ingress of oral fluids. During subsequent expansion, the fluid is expressed. Cyclic ingress and egress of fluids at the restoration margin is called **percolation** (schematically presented in Fig. 4-6).

Other important physical properties involve *heat flow* through materials. Enamel and dentin are primarily composed of finely packed ceramic crystals (i.e., hydroxyapatite, $Ca_{10}[PO_4]_6[OH]_2$) that make those structures act as thermal insulators. If tooth structure is replaced by a metallic restoration, which tends to be a thermal conductor, then it may be important to provide thermal insulation to protect the dental pulp from rapid increases or decreases in temperature in the mouth. Generally, dental cements that may be used as bases un-

TABLE **4-1**   Linear Coefficients of Thermal Expansion

DENTAL MATERIALS/STRUCTURES	LCTE (PPM/°C)
Aluminous dental porcelain	4
Alumina	6.5-8
In-Ceram	8-10
cp-titanium	8-9
Traditional dental cements	8-10
Tooth structure	*9-11*
Stainless steel	11
PFM ceramics	14
PFM alloys	14
Gold foil	14-15
Gold casting alloys	16-18
Co-Cr alloys	18-20
Hybrid glass ionomers	20-25
Dental amalgam	25
Packable composites	28-35
Anterior and flowable composites	35-50
Composite cements	40
PMMA direct-filling resins	72-83
Dental wax	260-600

From Bayne SC, Thompson JY: *Biomaterials science,* ed 7, Chapel Hill, NC, 2000, Brightstar.
PFM, Porcelain-fused-to-metal; *PMMA,* polymethyl methacrylate.

der metallic restorations act as insulators. One of the advantages of a composite is low thermal conductivity. Composites do not need liners/bases to provide thermal insulation. Heat flow through a material is measured in terms of either the relative rate of heat conduction *(thermal conductivity)* or the amount of heat conduction per unit time *(thermal diffusivity).* Thermal diffusivity is the more important property because it determines the amount of heat flow per unit time toward the pulp through a restoration. The dental pulp can withstand small temperature changes (from 37° C up to 42° C)[19, 272,273] for relatively short periods (30 to 60 seconds) without any permanent damage. Under most circumstances, the microcirculation of the pulp transports the heat entering the pulp away to other parts of the body where it is dissipated easily. However, extreme temperature changes or extended times of exposure to high temperatures will cause pulpal changes.

Electrical conductivity is a measure of the relative rate of electron transport through a material. This is important for metallic restorations that easily conduct electricity. If a galvanic cell (electrochemical cell) is present, then electrical current may flow, and that process would stimulate nerves in the pulp. This may occur accidentally, such as when a tinfoil chewing gum wrapper contacts a cast gold restoration and produces a minor electrical shock.

Mass properties of materials involve density or specific gravity. *Density* is a material's weight (or mass) per unit volume. Most metallic materials have relatively high densities ranging from 6 to 19 g/cm³. Ceramic densities are typically 2 to 6 g/cm³. Polymer densities generally range from 0.8 to 1.2 g/cm³. Density is an important consideration for certain dental processing methods such as casting. Dense metal alloys are much easier to cast by centrifugal casting methods. Density is important in estimating the properties of mixtures of different materials (composites) because the final properties of the mixture are proportional to the volume of mixed materials (and not the weight). On occasion, the relative density (or *specific gravity*) may be reported. Relative density is the density of the material of interest compared with the

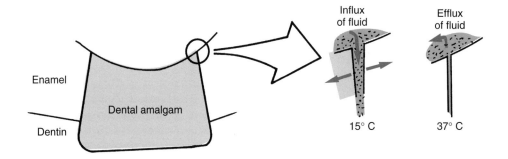

FIG. **4-6**   Percolation along the margins of an amalgam restoration due to its difference in linear coefficient of thermal expansion from tooth structure during intraoral temperature changes. Fluid influx occurs during cooling (contraction). Fluid efflux occurs during heating (expansion).

density of water under a standard set of conditions. At 25° C at 1 atmosphere of pressure, the density of water is 1 g/cm³. Therefore a specific gravity of 1.2 translates into a density of 1.2 g/cm³ under the same conditions.

Optical properties of bulk materials include interactions with electromagnetic radiation (e.g., visible light) that involve *reflection, refraction, absorption (and fluorescence),* and/or *transmission* (Fig. 4-7). The radiation typically involves different intensities for different wavelengths (or energies) over the range of interest (spectrum).

Any of these interactive events can be measured using a relative scale or an absolute scale. When the electromagnetic radiation is visible light, the amount of reflection can be measured in relative terms as *gloss,* or in absolute terms as *percent reflection.* Visible light absorption can be measured in absolute terms as *percent absorption* (or *transmission*) for every wavelength (in the visible spectrum). *Color* is a perception by an observer of the distribution of wavelengths. The same color sensation may be produced by different absorption spectra *(metamerism).* An individual's eye is capable of sensing dominant wavelength, luminous reflectance (intensity), and excitation purity. Variations among individuals' abilities to sense these characteristics give rise to varying perceptions of color.

Color measurement techniques do not measure these quantities directly. *Color* has traditionally been measured using the *Munsell color system* in terms of *hue, value,* and *chroma.* These terms correspond approximately to wavelength, intensity, and purity. The relationships of these quantities are represented schematically in Fig. 4-8. Shade guides for matching restorative dental materials to tooth structure are based on this system of describing color (see Chapter 15). The quality of color also is measured by the *Commission Internationale de l'Eclairage* (CIE) *System* as

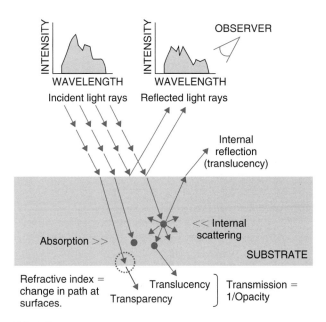

FIG. **4-7** Schematic summary of interactions of electromagnetic radiation with materials. The color perceived by the observer is the result of several interactions between substrate and incoming radiation producing reflection, internal scattering, absorption, fluorescence, and transmission.

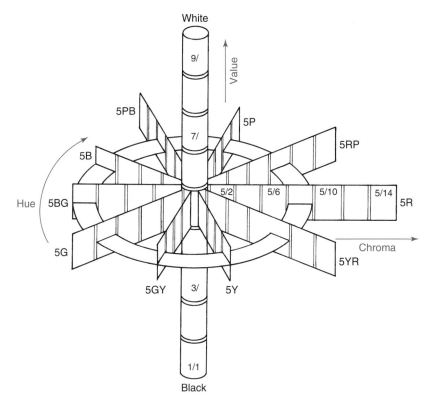

FIG. **4-8** Munsell scale of hues, values, and chromas in color space. *(Adapted from Powers JM, Capp JA, Koran A: J Dent Res 56: 112-116, 1977.)*

tristimulus values and reported as color differences (ΔL^*, Δa^*, and Δb^*) in comparison to standard conditions.

One should always remember that *color is more than a property of a material. It is coupled to the electromagnetic spectrum involved* (and the relative intensity of every wavelength in the spectrum) *and the perceptive abilities of the observer.* A practical example of the importance of the spectrum and the observer would be the appearance of anterior dental porcelain crowns in a nightclub in which the lighting involves low-level fluorescent lamps. The crowns fluoresce differently in that light and appear different from adjacent natural teeth, as compared with a very natural appearance in full-spectrum visible daylight.

Radiation of still another wavelength may be preferentially absorbed (e.g., x-rays). Composites that contain lithium, barium, strontium, or other good x-ray absorbers may appear *radiopaque* (radio-dense) in dental radiographs. Materials that are good absorbers (for whatever form of radiation) are described as *opaque.*

The appearance of a dental restoration is a combination of events of surface reflection, absorption, and internal scattering. The scattering may simply deflect the path of the radiation during transmission *(refraction),* or it may internally reflect the radiation from varying depths back out of a solid to the observer *(translucency).* Enamel naturally displays a high degree of translucency; therefore translucency is a desirable characteristic for restorative materials attempting to mimic enamel.

A wet tooth that is isolated from the wetting by saliva soon has a transient whiter appearance. Most of this shade change is due to the effect of loosely bound water lost from subsurface enamel (by dehydration) between hydroxyapatite crystals. This increases the internal scattering of light, with much of it reflected back to the observer (see internal reflection in Fig. 4-7). This probably explains why it takes 15 to 20 minutes for the isolated tooth to develop the whiter appearance, and 30 minutes or more for it to regain its original appearance after isolation is terminated. Larmas and others showed that 0.8% to 1% by weight of pulverized moist enamel is exchangeable water, and that it can be removed at 4% relative humidity and 20° C.[122] Loosely bound water also provides channels for *diffusion through enamel* of ions and molecules (see Chapter 3).

The direction of radiation may be perturbed as it crosses an interface from a medium of one type of optical character to another. *Refractive index* is the angle of changed path for a standard wavelength of light energy under standard conditions.

Another group of physical properties of great interest is *surface properties.* Surfaces are important because all restorative dental materials meet and interact with tooth structure at a surface. Also, all dental surfaces interact with intraoral constituents such as saliva and bacteria. Changing a material's surface properties can mitigate the extent of that interaction. The type of interaction between two materials at an interface is defined as the energy of interaction, and this is conveniently measured for a liquid interacting with a solid under a standard set of conditions as the *contact angle (θ).* The contact angle is the angle a drop of liquid makes with the surface on which it rests (Fig. 4-9, *A*). This angle is the result of an equilibrium between the surface tensions of the liquid-gas interface (γ_{LG}), solid-gas interface (γ_{SG}), and solid-liquid interface (γ_{SL}). These relationships can be expressed as an equation, as shown in Fig. 4-9, *A*. If the energy difference of the two materials in contact is large, then they will have a large contact angle. If the energy difference is very small, then the contact angle will be low and the liquid will appear to wet the solid by spreading. *Wetting* is a qualitative description of the contact angle. Good wetting, or spreading, represents a low contact angle. Partial (poor) wetting describes a contact angle approaching 90 degrees. Nonwetting is a contact angle approaching 180 degrees (see Fig. 4-4, *B*).

It is very important that film formers such as varnishes, liners, cements, and bonding agents (all of which are discussed later in this chapter) have good wetting on tooth preparation surfaces on which these materials may be placed, so that they adapt to the microscopic interstices of the surfaces. However, in other instances, poor wetting may be an advantage. For example, experimental posterior composites have been formulated to have high contact angles to retard water and/or bacterial interactions. In most cases, wetting can be anticipated on the basis of the *hydrophilicity* (water-loving) or *hydrophobicity* (water-hating) of materials. Hydrophilic surfaces are not wet well by hydrophobic liquids.

Mechanical Properties. The mechanical properties of a material describe its response to *loading.* Although most clinical situations involve complicated three-dimensional loading situations, it is common to simply describe the external load in terms of a single dimension (direction) as *compression, tension,* or *shear.* Combinations of these can

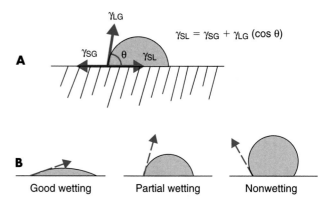

$$\gamma_{SL} = \gamma_{SG} + \gamma_{LG}(\cos\theta)$$

Good wetting   Partial wetting   Nonwetting

FIG. **4-9** Interfacial interactions of materials. **A,** Interaction quantified as contact angle (see formula). **B,** Interaction described in terms of good wetting (spreading), partial (poor) wetting, or nonwetting.

produce *torsion* (twisting) or *flexion* (transverse bending). These modes of loading are represented schematically in Fig. 4-10, with respect to a simple cylinder and a mesioocclusal (MO) amalgam restoration. For testing purposes, often it is impossible to grip and pull a specimen in tension without introducing other more complicated stresses at the same time. To circumvent problems for tensile testing of cylinders, it is possible to compress the sides of a cylinder and introduce stresses equivalent to tension. This variation of tension is called *diametral tension* (or diametral compression).

When a load is applied, the structure undergoes deformation as its bonds are compressed, stretched, or sheared. The load-deformation characteristics are only useful if the absolute size and geometry of the structure involved are known. Therefore it is typical to normalize load and deformation (in one dimension) as stress and strain. *Stress* (abbreviated, σ) is load per unit of cross-sectional area (within the material). It is expressed in units of load/area (pounds/in² = psi, or N/mm² = MPa). *Strain* (abbreviated ϵ) is deformation (ΔL) per unit of length (L). It is expressed in units of length/length (inch/inch, or cm/cm), which is a dimensionless parameter. A schematic summary is presented in Fig. 4-11. During loading, bonds are generally not compressed as easily as they are stretched. Therefore materials resist compression more readily and are said to be stronger in compression than in tension. Materials have different properties under different directions of loading. It is important to determine what the clinical direction of loading is before assessing the mechanical property of interest.

As loading continues, the structure is deformed. At first this deformation (or strain) is completely reversible *(elastic strain)*. However, increased loading finally produces some irreversible strain as well *(plastic strain)*, which causes permanent deformation. The point of onset of plastic strain is called the *elastic limit (proportional limit, yield point)*. This is indicated on the stress-strain diagram (see Fig. 4-11) as the point at which the straight line starts to become curved. Continuing plastic strain ultimately leads to failure by fracture. The highest stress before fracture is the *ultimate strength* (see Fig. 4-11, C). The total plastic tensile strain at fracture is called the *elongation.* This also may be expressed as the percent elongation. Materials that undergo extensive plastic deformation before fracture are called *ductile* (in tension) or *malleable* (in compression). Those that undergo very little plastic deformation are called *brittle.*

The slope of the linear portion (constant slope) of the stress-strain curve (from no stress up to the elastic limit) is called the *modulus, modulus of elasticity, Young's modulus,* or the *stiffness* of the material, and is abbreviated as E. It represents the amount of strain produced in response to each amount of stress. Ceramics typically have much higher modulus values (high stiffness) than polymeric materials (low stiffness). Because the slope of

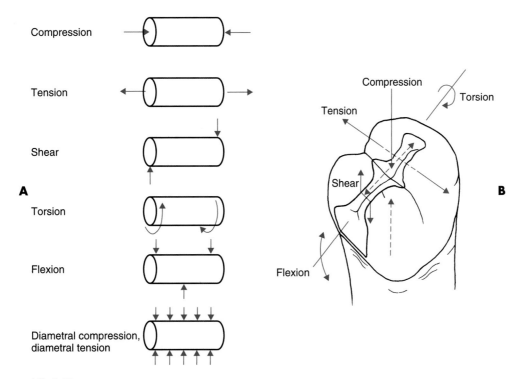

FIG. 4-10 Examples of directions of loading. **A,** Uniaxial loading of cylinder. **B,** Uniaxial loading of an MO amalgam restoration.

the line is calculated as the stress divided by the strain ($E = \sigma/\epsilon$), modulus values have the same units as stress (i.e., psi or MPa).

Two of the most useful mechanical properties are the modulus of elasticity and the elastic limit. A restorative mater-

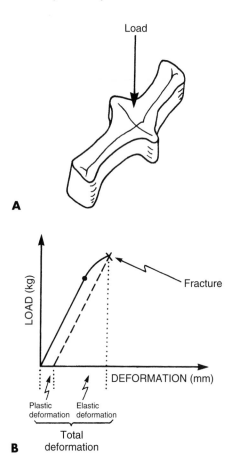

A

B

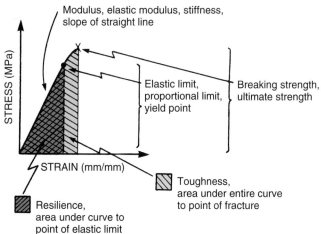

C

FIG. **4-11** Schematic summary of mechanical properties with respect to amalgam restoration in function. **A,** Occlusal loading of Class I amalgam restoration. **B,** Load/deformation curve describing behavior of amalgam. **C,** Normalization of load/deformation curve to stress-strain curve with important characteristics of curve indicated. (Mechanical responses depend on temperature and strain rate involved.)

ial generally should be very stiff so that under load, its elastic deformation will be extremely small. An exception is a Class V composite, which should be less stiff to accommodate tooth flexure (see Microfill Composites in Chapter 12). If possible, a material should be selected for an application so that the stress level during function usually will not exceed the elastic limit. If the stress exceeds the elastic limit a small amount, the associated plastic deformation will tend to be very small. If the stress is well beyond the elastic limit, then the resulting deformation is primarily plastic strain, which at some point will result in failure.

Often it is convenient to determine the elastic limit in a relative manner by comparing the onset of plastic deformation of different materials using scratch or indentation tests, called *hardness tests*. The Mohs hardness scale ranks scratch resistance of a material in comparison to a range of standard materials. The Mohs scale is presented in Table 4-2. *Rockwell, Brinell,* and *Knoop* hardness tests employ indenters instead.

The energy that a material can absorb before the onset of any plastic deformation is called its *resilience* (see Fig. 4-11, *C*), and is described as the area under the stress-strain curve up to the elastic limit. The total energy absorbed to the point of fracture is called the *toughness* and is related to the entire area under the stress-strain curve (see Fig. 4-11, *C*).

Mechanical events are both temperature and time dependent. These conditions must be carefully described for any reported mechanical property. Generally, as the temperature increases, the mechanical property values decrease. The stress-strain curve appears to move to the right and downward. The opposite occurs during cooling. As the rate of loading decreases, the mechanical properties decrease. This is described as *strain rate sensitivity* and has important clinical implications. To momentarily make a material's behavior stiffer and/or more elastic, strain it quickly. *For recording undercut areas in an elastic intraoral impression, remove it rapidly so that it will be more elastic and more accurately record the absolute dimensions of the structures.* This is an excellent example of applied materials science.

Other time-dependent responses to stress or strain also occur. Deformation over time in response to a constant stress is called *creep* (or *strain relaxation*). Materials that are relatively weak or close to their melting temperature are more susceptible to creep. Dental wax deforms (creeps) under its own weight over short periods of time. Traditional amalgam restorations are involved in intraoral creep. Deformation over time in response to a constant strain is called *stress relaxation.*

During loading, for all practical purposes, the strain below the elastic limit is all elastic strain. The amount of plastic strain is infinitesimal—so small that it is ignored. However, during multiple cycles, these very small amounts of plastic strain begin to accrue. After millions of cycles, the total plastic strain accumulated at low stress levels may be sufficient to represent the strain required to produce fracture. This process of multiple cycling at low stresses is called *fatigue* (Fig. 4-12, *A*). A standard engineering design limit for dental restorative materials is approximately 10 million cycles (or approximately 10 years of intraoral service). A rule-of-thumb is that materials on working surfaces of teeth are mechanically cycled approximately 1 million times per year on average. The curve correlating cyclic stress levels (S) to the number of cycles to failure (N) is called a *fatigue curve (S-N curve)*. These curves have only been determined for a few dental materials, because conducting the tests requires such a long period of time.[274] The compressive fatigue curves for Tytin and Dispersalloy amalgams are shown as part of Fig. 4-12, *B*.

Mechanical properties can be used to describe the behavior of liquids as well as solids. As the temperature of a solid is raised, its stress-strain curve shifts downward and to the right. At the melting point, the stress-strain curve is a horizontal line lying at zero stress along the strain axis. Rather than examining the stress-strain behavior of liquids, it is more meaningful to examine the shear stress (τ) versus shear strain rate ($\dot{\gamma}$). Well-behaved liquids (Newtonian behavior) form a straight line (Fig. 4-13). Departures may occur that produce lines curving down (pseudoplastic behavior) or curving up (dilatant behavior). In some cases, the starting point of the line is shifted up along the shear stress axis, representing a material that does not start to flow until a critical shear stress has been reached (Bingham body behavior). Pseudoplastic and Bingham body behaviors are typical for dental materials. The lines on these diagrams are described by a relatively simple equation, $\eta^n = \tau/\dot{\gamma}$ which is similar to the equation for elastic modulus, $E = \sigma/\epsilon$. The term η, or vis-

cosity, is the resistance to flow or stiffness of the liquid. As the temperature is increased above the melting point, the viscosity behavior tips down and toward the right. A 37% phosphoric acid solution gel used for etching displays pseudoplastic Bingham body behavior. It does not flow until a critical shear stress is exceeded, and as the shear stress is linearly increased, the shear strain rate increases even more rapidly producing more flow.

Chemical Properties. Chemical properties of a material are those that involve changes in primary or secondary bonding. *Primary bonding* changes occur during

TABLE 4-2 Mohs Hardness Scale

MOHS HARDNESS	REFERENCE MATERIAL	MATERIALS EXAMPLES
10	Diamond	
—		(Silicon carbide, Tungsten carbide)
9	Conundum	
—		
8	Topaz	
—		(Tool steels)
7	Quartz	
—		
6	Orthoclase	
—		(Dental enamel)
5	Apatite	
—		(Low-carbon steels)
4	Fluorite	
—		
3	Calcite	
—		
2	Gypsum	
—		
1	Talc	

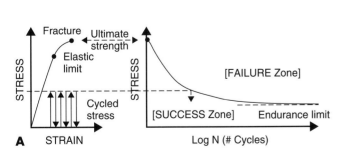

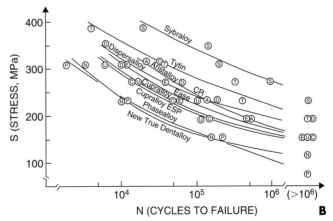

FIG. 4-12 Fatigue curves. **A,** Relationship between single-cycle stress-strain and fatigue curves. A typical fatigue curve separates characteristic regions (survival, fracture) and asymptomatically levels off at an endurance limit. **B,** Fatigue curves from compression testing for several commercial amalgams. *A,* Aristalloy; *C,* Cupralloy; *D,* Dispersalloy; *E,* Ease; *N,* New True Dentalloy; *P,* Phasealloy; *S,* Sybralloy; *T,* Tytin; *U,* Cupralloy ESP. *(From Zardiackas LD, Bayne SC:* Biomaterials *6:49-54, 1985.)*

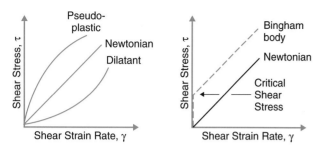

FIG. 4-13 Schematic summary of mechanical property behaviors of liquids. The curves represent typical flow behaviors described as Newtonion, pseudoplastic, dilatant, and Bingham body. *(From Bayne SC, Taylor DF, Zardiackas LD:* Biomaterials science, *ed 6, Chapel Hill, NC, 1992, Brightstar Publishing.)*

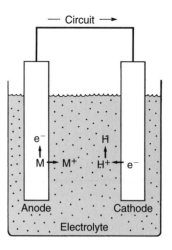

FIG. 4-14 Schematic representation of electrochemical cell. *(From Bayne SC, Taylor DF, Zardiackas LD:* Biomaterials science, *ed 6, Chapel Hill, NC, 1992, Brightstar.)*

chemical reactions and electrochemical reactions. *Secondary bonding* changes occur during processes such as adsorption and absorption.

For metallic materials in the oral environment, the principal changes in primary bonding occur as a result of *chemical corrosion (tarnish)* or *electrochemical corrosion.* Chemical corrosion involves direct reaction of species by contact in solution or at an interface. An example of this process is the sulfide tarnishing of silver in amalgams to produce a black surface film. Another example is the oxidation of very high-copper–containing casting alloys to produce a green patina.

For any material, a number of electrochemical corrosion processes may happen as well. Electrochemical corrosion involves two coupled chemical reactions (half cells) at separate sites, connected by two paths. One path (a circuit) is capable of transporting electrons, while the other path (an electrolyte) is capable of transferring metallic ions.[245] Therefore the basic components required for any *electrochemical cell* are: (1) an anode (site of corrosion), (2) a cathode, (3) a circuit, and (4) an electrolyte (Fig. 4-14).

Electrochemical corrosion occurs intraorally when these four components are present. The conditions define which of the metallic sites acts as an anode. A number of types of electrochemical cells are possible. Examples are shown schematically in Fig. 4-15.

A number of these electrochemical cells are possible in a single restorative dentistry situation. When an amalgam is in contact with a gold alloy restoration, galvanic, local galvanic, crevice, and stress corrosion are possible. *Galvanic corrosion* is associated with the presence of macroscopically different electrode sites (amalgam and gold alloy). *Local galvanic corrosion (structure-selective corrosion)* is due to the electrochemical differences of different phases in a single material (such as amalgam). Electrochemical cells may arise whenever a portion of the amalgam is covered by plaque or soft tissue. The covered area has a locally lowered oxygen and/or increased hydrogen ion concentration, making it behave more like an anode and corrode *(concentration cell corrosion).* Cracks and crevices produce similar conditions and encourage concentration cell corrosion. Both corrosion processes are commonly termed *crevice corrosion.* When the restoration is under stress, the distribution of mechanical energy is not uniform and this produces different corrosion potentials. This process is called *stress corrosion.*

Ceramics and polymers do not undergo chemical or electrochemical corrosion in the same sense. Most of their changes are related to chemical dissolution, absorption, or adsorption. *Chemical dissolution* normally occurs as a result of the solubilization created by hydrogen bonding effects of water and locally high acidity. Tooth structure is dissolved by high concentrations of lactic acid under plaque (see Chapter 3). Dental ceramics may be dissolved by very acidic fluoride solutions (acidulated phosphate fluoride [APF]) used for protecting outer layers of enamel against caries.

Sorption events include both *adsorption* (adding molecules to a surface by secondary bonding) or *absorption* (penetration of molecules into a solid by diffusion). Protein adsorption alters the behavior and reactivity of dental material surfaces. Water absorption into dental polymers affects their mechanical properties.

Biologic Properties. Biologic properties of dental materials are concerned with *toxicity* and *sensitivity* reactions that occur both locally, within the associated tissue and systemically. Most dental materials interface locally with a variety of tissues (enamel, dentin, pulp, periodontium, cheek, tongue); thus local reactions may vary. It is possible to evaluate local toxic effects on cells by clinical pulp studies or by tissue culture tests. Unset materials may release cytotoxic components. However, in clinical situations this problem is rarely evident. Two important clinical factors determining toxicity are the *exposure time* and the *concentration* of the potentially toxic substance. Generally, restorative materials harden quickly and/or are not readily soluble in tissue fluids.

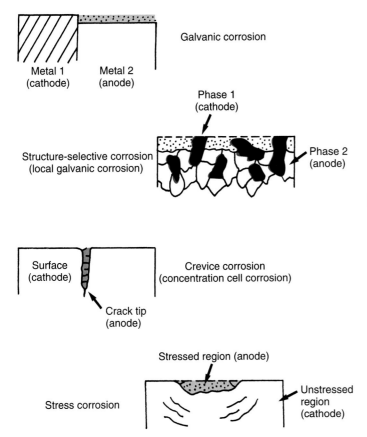

FIG. **4-15** Types of electrochemical cells. Dotted regions indicate anodic material being lost during corrosion. *(From Tomashov ND:* Theory of corrosion and protection of metals, *ed 1, New York, 1966, Macmillan.)*

Therefore potentially toxic products do not have time to diffuse into tissues. Even more importantly, *the concentration makes the poison!* Some authorities believe that if the amount of material involved is small, then the pulp or other tissues can transport and excrete it without significant biochemical damage. Others believe there is no threshold. A *threshold level* for toxicity is one below which no effect can be detected.

Systemic changes due to biomaterial interactions have been very difficult, if not impossible, to monitor. Most evidence of biocompatibility has come from long-term usage and indirect monitoring. *This is an area of increasing concern for understanding potential risks of new or alternative restorative dental materials.*

Finally, toxicology is undergoing rapid evolution. In the 1970s most toxicologic screening involved the use of the Ames test for determining mutagenicity. The inventor of that test has now withdrawn support for the conclusions derived from that screening procedure.[10,89] Therefore results from earlier screening tests of dental materials may have to be reconsidered.

BIOMECHANICS FOR RESTORATIVE DENTISTRY

Teeth are subjected to many forces during normal use. The interactions between the applied forces, the shape and structure of teeth, the supporting structures, and the mechanical properties of tooth components and restorative materials are all included in the subject of *biomechanics.* Biomechanics is the study of loads (or stresses) and deformations (or strains) occurring in biologic systems.

The biomechanical behavior of restored teeth can be studied at any level from gross to microscopic. Examples of situations of interest include the calculation of stress transfer to the margin of an amalgam restoration, from the amalgam to tooth structure, from tooth structure to the periodontal ligament, from several teeth to bone, and throughout bone. The most common analysis focuses on stress transfer at the interface between a restoration and tooth structure.

BIOMECHANICAL UNIT

The standard biomechanical unit involves the: (1) restorative material, (2) tooth structure, and (3) interface (interfacial zone) between the restoration and tooth. Different restorative procedures can involve very different interfaces. Composite/enamel interfaces are micromechanically bonded. Amalgam/enamel interfaces are weak and discontinuous unless a bonding system is used. Cemented crown/enamel interfaces are weak but are continuous. The importance of considering three structures in the biomechanical unit is to detect stresses that may cause unwanted fractures or debonding. The restorative material may be strong enough to resist fracture, but the interface or tooth structure may not be.

STRESS TRANSFER

Normal tooth structure transfers external biting loads through enamel into dentin as compression (Fig. 4-16, *A*). The concentrated external loads are distributed over a large internal volume of tooth structure and thus local stresses are lower. During this process, a small amount of dentin deformation may occur that results in tooth flexure. These deformations are discussed more carefully in the following section.

A restored tooth tends to transfer stress differently than an intact tooth. Any force on the restoration produces compression, tension, or shear along the tooth/restoration interface.[140,141] Once enamel is no longer continuous, its resistance is much lower. Therefore most restorations are designed to distribute stresses onto sound dentin, rather than to enamel (Fig. 4-16, *B*).[160] Once in dentin the stresses are resolved in a manner similar to a normal tooth. The process of stress transfer to dentin becomes more complicated when the amount of remaining dentin is thin and the restoration must bridge a significant distance to seat onto thicker dentin (see Liners and Bases).

For an amalgam restoration in a pulpally deep tooth preparation, a total of 1 to 2 mm of underlying dentin and/or other insulating material is preferred pulpal of the amalgam to provide adequate *thermal and mechanical protection of the pulp.*[194] If inadequate thickness of dentin remains, the insertion of an insulating liner or base is recommended. *However, it may be necessary sometimes to ensure that the amalgam restoration is "seated" on sound dentin at three or more widely separated areas at the level of the initial tooth preparation pulpal wall.* This provides optimal stress transfer. For a nonmetallic restoration, which has better insulating properties than a metallic one, 0.5 to 1 mm of dentin and/or liner or base is sufficient for thermal and mechanical protection.

STRAIN WITHIN TOOTH STRUCTURE (TOOTH FLEXURE)

Teeth are not rigid structures. They undergo deformation (strain) during normal loading.[210] Intraoral loads (forces) vary widely and have been reported to range from 10 to 431 N (1 N = 0.225 lb of force), with a functional load of 70 N considered clinically normal.[98] Obviously, the number of teeth, type of occlusion, and occlusal habits of patients, such as bruxism, affect the load per tooth.

The amount of strain is roughly proportional to the amount of stress. However, because tooth structure is heterogeneous and asymmetric and its properties change with time, there is no simple description of the state of stress or amount of strain. To date, increasing evidence indicates that the amount of strain and its effect on tooth structure may be very important in fatigue.

Tooth flexure has been described as either a lateral bending or an axial bending of a tooth during occlusal loading.[103] This flexure produces the maximal strain in the cervical region, and the strain appears to be resolved in tension or compression within local regions, sometimes causing the loss of bonded Class V restorations in preparations with no retention grooves (Fig. 4-17). Moreover, *one current hypothesis is that tensile or compressive strains gradually produce microfractures*[91,95,123] (called *abfractions* by some authors) in the thinnest region of enamel at the cementoenamel junction (CEJ) (Fig. 4-18). Such fractures predispose enamel to loss when subjected to toothbrush abrasion and/or chemical erosion. This process may be key in the formation of some Class V defects (Figs. 4-19 and 4-20). Additionally, in unbonded or leaking restorations, this flexure of the dentin also may produce changes in fluid flow and microleakage, leading to sensitivity and pulpal inflammation, respectively (see Chapter 2). These events are just beginning to be documented carefully.

EFFECTS OF AGING

As a tooth becomes older, it undergoes changes in structural mass and in the character of the remaining tissue. Older teeth have lost most prismless enamel along the outer surface and may have encountered numerous microfractures in cervical portions, as just discussed. In response to disease assaults, such as caries or other external stimuli, odontoblastic processes may have laid down more peritubular dentin occluding the outer zones of dentinal tubules.[85] Peritubular dentin is mostly hydroxyapatite and tends to stiffen dentin. Secondary and reparative dentin also may have been produced, replacing

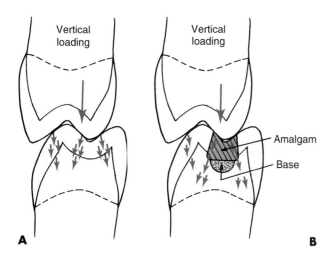

FIG. 4-16 Schmatic view of occlusal loading of amalgam restorations. **A,** Stress transfer into an unrestored tooth occurs through dental enamel into dentin. **B,** Stress transfer into a tooth restored with dental amalgam is conducted through enamel and the restoration to be distributed within dentin (and not enamel). Note the facial and lingual seats at initial cavity preparation at the pulpal wall level (before removal of remaining infected dentin and placement of base) that help transfer stresses laterally.

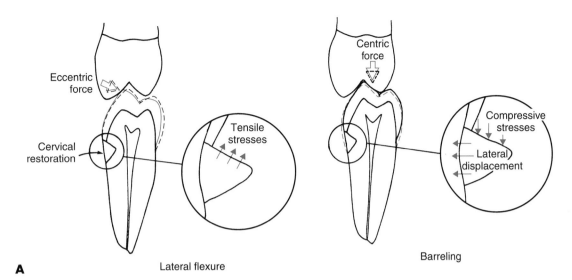

A Lateral flexure

B Barreling

F I G. **4-17** Schematic diagram of tooth flexure creating cervical stresses. **A,** Lateral flexure results from eccentric forces that produce tensile stresses at marginal interface with cervical restoration placed in facial CEJ region. **B,** Barreling results from heavy centric forces that produce compressive stresses along marginal interface with cervical restoration in entire CEJ region, resulting in lateral displacement (loss) of the restoration. *(From Heymann HO et al: J Am Dent Assoc 122:41-47, 1991.)*

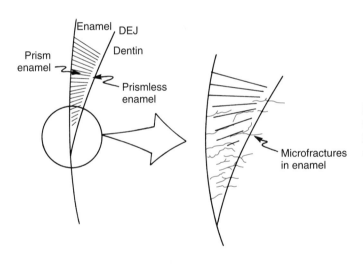

F I G. **4-18** Schematic view of microfractures developing between enamel rods in cervical enamel. The enamel near the junction of the CEJ and DEJ is prismless. *(From Lee WC, Eakle WS: J Prosthet Dent 52:374-380, 1984.)*

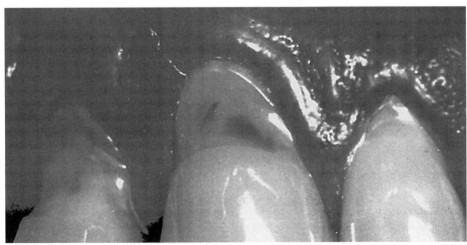

F I G. **4-19** Picture of Class V lesion suspected of arising by tooth flexure. *(Courtesy Stephen C. Bayne, School of Dentistry, University of North Carolina, Chapel Hill, NC.)*

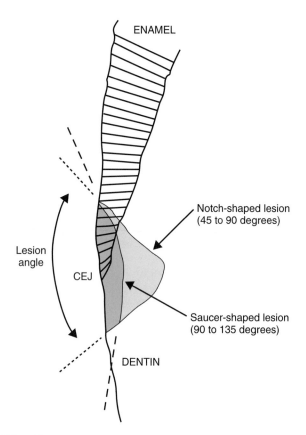

FIG. **4-20** Schematic view of Class V cervical defects comparing shallow saucer-shaped lesions to deep notch-shaped lesions. Angulation is determined by average slope of walls and not walls at perimeter of the lesion. *(From Bayne SC et al: J Dent Res 71A:314, 1992 [abstract 1669].)*

some of the pulp chamber and canals. Evidence is also strong that with aging, all type I collagen in the human body becomes more cross-linked.[270] A strong suspicion is that this process of cross-linking makes the intertubular dentin more brittle. Therefore it is logical that the modulus of teeth is observed to increase with aging (50% increase from 20 to 29 years of age, to 40 to 49 years of age) and that teeth behave in a more brittle fashion.[269] This alteration, coupled with microcracks that may have developed with fatigue, may produce large cracks or fractures in the tooth over time. Supporting bone may also undergo property changes with age.[76]

These changes produce a substrate that may not transfer stress as readily and that may no longer be well matched to the properties of a restorative material that has survived for a long time. The complete implication of these changes is not yet fully understood.

PRINCIPLES OF BIOMECHANICS

Stress transfer and the resulting deformations of structures are principally governed by (1) the elastic limit of the materials, (2) the ratio of the elastic moduli involved, and (3) the thickness of the structures. Materials with a high elastic modulus transfer stresses without

much strain. Lower modulus materials undergo dangerous strains where stresses are concentrated, unless there is adequate thickness. The resistance to strain increases approximately as the third power of the thickness of the material involved. Doubling the thickness increases the resistance to elastic strain by ninefold. If the local stress does exceed the material's elastic limit, then the capacity for plastic deformation before fracture will determine when fracture actually occurs.

These principles can be demonstrated easily using the case of a mesioocclusodistal (MOD) restoration in a first molar. A low modulus material, such as amalgam, must have sufficient thickness to resist flexural deformation that would produce fracture in this brittle material. Increased amalgam thickness improves its resistance to flexure but compromises the resistance of the remaining dentin and base floor for the restoration. However, properly prepared and condensed amalgam in a proper tooth preparation that provides the recommended occlusopulpal restoration thickness serves for many years without fracture.

DIRECT RESTORATIVE DENTAL MATERIALS

Loss of tooth structure to caries or other processes usually proceeds in a gradual way. Therefore a patient's initial encounter with a dentist often involves the restoration of a small portion of tooth structure that is defective. This can be accomplished relatively easily by designing a tooth preparation with retention features and restoring it with a pliable material that is capable of hardening in situ. While in a moldable stage, the material can be adapted to the tooth structure and shaped to re-create normal anatomic contours. This process is called *direct restorative dentistry* because it is accomplished directly in the intraoral environment. The development or selection of materials for direct application may require compromise of mechanical properties or other desired characteristics. If there is extensive loss of tooth structure, then the restorative materials must provide better stress distribution characteristics and be more carefully bonded to remaining tooth structure. In most cases, this requires the use of materials that cannot be made fluid for direct use. These materials must be fabricated into a restoration outside of the mouth and cemented or bonded in place. The procedures involved with this approach are categorized as *indirect restorative dentistry*.

AMALGAM

Terminology. *Amalgam* technically means an alloy of mercury (Hg) with any other metal. *Dental amalgam* is an alloy made by mixing mercury with a silver-tin dental amalgam alloy (Ag-Sn). In dentistry, it is common to use the term *amalgam* to mean dental amalgam.

Amalgam alloy is a silver-tin alloy to which varying amounts of copper (Cu) and small amounts of zinc (Zn)

TABLE 4-3	Composition and Classification of Dental Amalgam Alloy Powders*							
AMALGAM ALLOYS	**CLASSIFICATION**	**PARTICLE TYPE**	**AG**	**SN**	**CU**	**ZN**	**HG**	**OTHER**
New True Dentalloy	Low copper	Lathe-cut	70.8	25.8	2.4	1.0	0.0	—
Micro II	Low copper	Lathe-cut	70.1	21.0	8.6	0.3	0.0	—
Dispersalloy	High copper	Mixed	69.5	17.7	11.9	0.9	0.0	—
Tytin	High copper	Spherical	59.2	27.8	13.0	0.0	0.0	—
Sybraloy	High copper	Spherical	41.5	30.2	28.3	0.0	0.0	—
Cupralloy	High copper	Mixed	62.2	15.1	22.7	0.0	0.0	—
Aristalloy CR	High copper	Spherical	58.7	28.4	12.9	0.0	0.0	—
Indiloy	High copper	Lathe-cut	60.5	24.0	12.1	0.0	0.0	3.4 In
Valiant	High copper	Lathe-cut	49.5	30.0	20.0	0.0	0.0	0.5 Pd
Valiant PhD	High copper	Mixed	52.7	29.7	17.4	0.0	0.0	0.5 Pd

From Osborne JW et al: *J Dent Res* 57:983-988, 1978; and Vrijhoef MMA, Vermeersch AG, Spanauf AJ: *Dental amalgam,* Chicago, 1980, Quintessence.
*Elements in the composition are reported in weight percent.

have been added. *Low-copper amalgam* alloys contain 2% to 5% copper. The earliest successful amalgams were made by combining filings of such alloys with mercury. A typical modern low-copper amalgam alloy may contain 69.4% Ag, 26.2% Sn, 3.6% Cu, and 0.8% Zn (Table 4-3). Amalgams made from such low-copper alloy filings are often referred to as *conventional amalgams. High-copper amalgam* alloys contain 12% to 30% copper, and because of their higher copper content, they display significantly better corrosion resistance than low-copper amalgams. A typical high-copper amalgam alloy may contain 60% Ag, 27% Sn, 13% Cu, and 0% Zn (see Table 4-3). The particles of these alloys that are mixed with mercury may be filings, but they are often small spheres.

Amalgam is mixed for use by combining amalgam alloy particles with mercury, vigorously mixing the components *(trituration)* for a few seconds during the initial reaction, placing the plastic mass into a tooth preparation, compressing the mixture *(condensation)* to remove the excess mercury-rich phase, and then carving and finishing the hardening mass.

Because of a concern about the possible toxicity of mercury in amalgams, a number of materials have been developed as *amalgam alternatives.* Amalgam alternatives[127] comprise any materials (e.g., composite, glass ionomer, cast gold alloys) that can be used to restore a tooth instead of using amalgam. Amalgam substitutes (e.g., cast gold alloys) are materials generally considered to have equal or better properties than the amalgam restoration they replace. Most are compositions that contain some of the components of amalgam (e.g., Ag-Sn alloy particles), but they do not contain mercury. *Gallium alloys* are an example of such a substitute made with Ag-Sn particles in Ga-In.[180,232,253] Gallium melts at 28° C and can be used to produce liquid alloys at room temperature by the addition of small amounts of other elements such as indium. In this case, Ga-In has been substituted for Hg in amalgam. Other systems that use Au mixed with other noble metals to form the restoration matrix are being explored.[264]

The American Dental Association, in combination with the National Institute on Standards and Technology (ADA-NIST), has patented a *mercury-free direct-filling alloy* based on Ag-coated Ag-Sn particles that can be self-welded by compaction (hand-consolidated) to create a restoration. This approach is being proposed as an alternative to amalgam.

Other transitional approaches include redesigning amalgam to have much less initial mercury. If alloy particle sizes are judiciously chosen to pack together well, it is possible to minimize the mercury required for mixing to the 15% to 25% range. The actual clinical properties of these *low-mercury amalgams* are not yet known.

Classification. The major approaches to classification of amalgams and the amalgam alloys on which they are based are in terms of (1) *amalgam alloy particle geometry and size,* (2) *copper content,* and (3) *zinc content.* Each of these is discussed subsequently in a historical context.

In the 1830s, amalgam alloy was obtained by filing or grinding silver coins into coarse particles to mix with mercury. The compositions were inconsistent at best and the reaction conditions were quite variable. This process could not reliably produce a final amalgam with uniform properties. During the 1860s and 1870s, Townsend, Flagg, and others contributed immensely to investigations of composition versus properties. However, true amalgam science began with investigations by GV Black during the 1890s. *Traditional (or conventional) amalgam alloys* were produced by early dental manufacturers, such as S.S. White, and predominated from 1900 until 1970. The basic composition was 65% Ag, 30% Sn, 5% Cu, and less than 1% Zn.

Traditional amalgam was mixed initially by proportioning alloy and mercury components into a mortar and then grinding the mixture with a pestle. The process of manual mixing is known as *trituration.* Alloy was manufactured in bricks that were ground with a file into *filings* and mixed with mercury. A more efficient process was grinding up the ingot of alloy, typically on a lathe.

For that reason, those particles became known as *lathe-cut particles* (Fig. 4-21). Filings were irregular in shape and gradually were produced in finer and finer sizes by manufacturers to control the reaction, produce smoother mixtures, and enhance final properties. Lathe-cut particles could be purchased in regular cut, fine cut, and microfine cut versions. *Conventional amalgam alloys were commonly classified on this basis of particle size.*

Irregular powder particles pack together relatively poorly (see Fig. 4-21, *A*) and require a relatively large amount of mercury (50% to 60% by weight in the mixture) to fill in the spaces. After transfer of the mixture to the tooth preparation, it is possible to compact the mass and extrude some of the mercury-rich matrix. By eliminating the mercury-rich matrix as much as possible, the amount of reaction product matrix that forms is limited,

thereby improving the overall properties of the set amalgam. Mercury-rich mixtures, after trituration but before placement into the preparation, historically could be partially condensed by wringing the mass in a squeeze cloth. In the 1960s, Eames was the first to promote a low mercury-to-alloy mixing ratio *(Eames technique or no-squeeze-cloth technique).*[70] Later, it was demonstrated that by spherodizing the alloy particles,[67] the particles packed more efficiently (see Fig. 4-21, *B*) and required much less mercury to make a practical mixture. *Spherical particles* also increased the fluidity of the mixture by presenting less resistance to particle sliding. Using some or all spherical alloy particles, it is possible to reduce the mercury portion of the mixture to less than 50% by weight. The distinction between irregular (lathe-cut) and spherical particle geometries became the next major basis for classification of amalgam alloys. Most modern precapsulated amalgams are formulated with only 42% to 45% mercury by weight.

During the early part of the twentieth century, alloy powder and mercury were proportioned crudely and

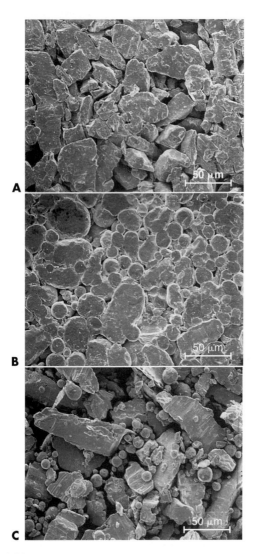

FIG. **4-21** Examples of amalgam alloy powder particles. **A,** Filings (New True Dentalloy). **B,** Spheres (Cupralloy). **C,** Mixed geometries (Dispersalloy). *(Courtesy Stephen C. Bayne, School of Dentistry, University of North Carolina, Chapel Hill, NC.)*

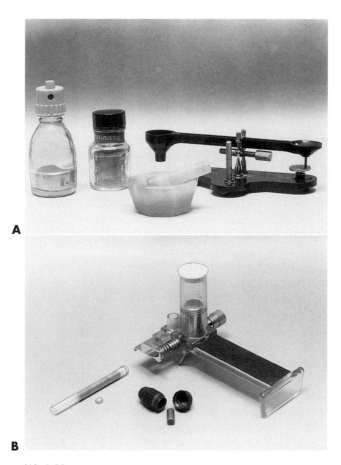

FIG. **4-22** Earlier methods of dental trituration. **A,** Equipment for hand mixing of alloy powder and mercury in mortar and pestle using excess mercury (circa 1900 to 1940). **B,** Equipment for mixing of alloy pellets and controlled mercury in reusable capsules with mechanical mixing in amalgamator (circa 1940 to 1970).

mixed manually (Fig. 4-22, *A*). To proportion and mix amalgam more carefully, manufacturers later recommended the use of alloy pellets, mercury dispensers, reusable mixing *capsules* and *pestles,* and *amalgamators* (Fig. 4-22, *B*). A typical reusable capsule (Fig. 4-23, *A*) was a hollow tube with rounded ends constructed as two pieces that could be friction-fit or screwed together. Amalgam alloy was dispensed into the capsule as a pellet of pressed powder of standard weight. Mercury was dispensed into the capsule as a standard-sized droplet from an automatic dropper bottle. A small metal or plastic pestle (Fig. 4-23, *B*) was added to the capsule and it was closed. The capsule and its contents were then automatically mixed using an amalgamator. The typical amalgamator has been designed to grasp the ends of the capsule in a claw that is oscillated in a figure-eight pattern. This accelerates the mixture toward each end of the capsule during each throw and impacts the mixture with the pestle.

To guarantee that amalgam alloy and mercury are mixed both efficiently and consistently, it is very important to periodically calibrate amalgamators. After several years of use, the bearings become worn and the mixes no longer are sufficiently triturated. On standard electric amalgamators (Fig. 4-24, *A*), the trituration speed and trituration time are manually set on the front of the equipment. Settings vary for different products. Electronic amalgamators (Fig. 4-24, *B*) have digital controls and permit programming of settings.

Modern amalgams are produced from precapsulated alloy and mercury. The components are separated in the capsule by a special diaphragm that is broken when the capsule is "activated" just before mixing (Fig. 4-25). Precapsulated *(preproportioned) amalgam* (see Fig. 4-25, *A*) provides convenience and some degree of assurance that the materials will not be contaminated before use or spilled before mixing. *Mercury hygiene* is an important consideration for safe amalgam management and is discussed later in this section.

During the 1960s, major research emphasis was placed on the benefits of increased copper contents in amalgams. It was confirmed that *increasing the copper content above 12% by weight in the amalgam alloy effectively suppressed formation of the phase (Sn-Hg), which was prone to intraoral corrosion.* A dramatic improvement in corrosion resistance led to a doubling or tripling of clinical longevity of these amalgams. Flagg originally explored the effect of copper in the 1860s, but the copper was not effectively prealloyed with silver and/or tin. Thus the effect was not demonstrated. In the 1930s, Gayler again

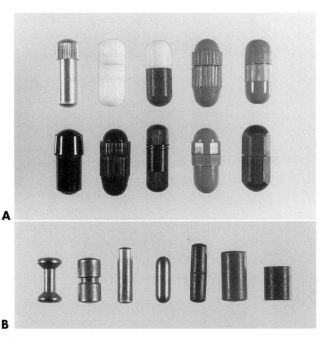

A

B

FIG. **4-23** Capsules and pestles for automatically mixing amalgam constituents using amalgamator. **A,** Reusable capsules. **B,** Magnified view of pestles.

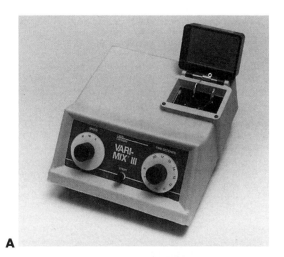

A

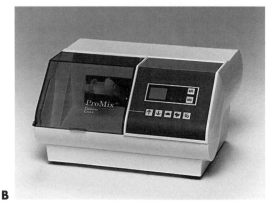

B

FIG. **4-24** Examples of dental amalgamators for automatically mixing amalgam in capsules (shown with protective cover open on equipment). **A,** Amalgamator with manually set trituration speeds and times. **B,** Amalgamator with digital controls and programming for trituration speeds and times.

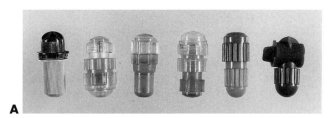

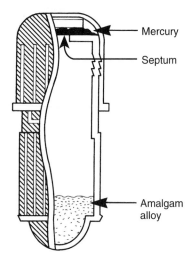

Mercury

Septum

Amalgam
alloy

A

B

FIG. **4-25** Preproportioned alloy and mercury in prepackaged capsules ("precapsulated") for mixing amalgam constituents using amalgamator. **A,** Examples of preproportioned capsule designs. **B,** Schematic of preproportioned capsule showing mercury and powder separated by septum that must be perforated before mixing. *(From Rinne VW: J Dent Res 62:116-117, 1983.)*

investigated the effect of copper and found that in the coarse filing alloys of that time, copper contents above 6% produced excessive expansion, and the corrosion-reducing effect at higher copper contents was not realized. Also in the 1930s, early pioneers were admixing copper amalgams with amalgams to produce very corrosion-resistant compositions. However, the setting times of the mixtures were slow and the compositions were quite variable. It was not until Innes and Youdelis[109] added Ag-Cu spheres to conventional amalgam alloy, with the intent of producing dispersion-hardened amalgams, that the advantageous effect of copper on corrosion resistance was clearly observed.

Classification of amalgams based on copper content is the main system in use today (see Table 4-3). High-copper amalgams can be produced from amalgam alloy particles that are irregular and/or spherical.

Another important additive to amalgam alloy is *zinc.* Originally zinc was added to conventional amalgams as a processing aid to suppress oxidation of the key elements in the alloy. Zinc tends to oxidize preferentially forming a zinc oxide film that covers the surface of liquid alloy during manufacture and suppresses oxidation of other elements. Generally, 1% or more is added to accomplish this end. However, some (0.2% to 1%) is left in the amalgam alloy at the end. A detrimental side effect

of this residual zinc was that moisture contamination before setting converted the zinc to zinc oxide and produced hydrogen gas that could expand the amalgam excessively, resulting in patient pain. Once the mechanism of *delayed expansion* was understood, care during amalgam manipulation prevented this problem. Some manufacturers also produced *nonzinc amalgams* as an alternative. These alloys often were favored where isolation was difficult. *It now seems as though zinc may have some beneficial effect on amalgam longevity.* Clinical research evidence[132,133,184] supports that zinc-containing low-copper and high-copper amalgams may last 20% to 50% longer than zinc-free ones. On the basis of this new evidence, *amalgams* continue to be produced and designated as *zinc* (zinc-containing) or *nonzinc* (zinc-free), although improved manufacturing techniques have largely eliminated the original need for zinc as a manufacturing aid.

Composition, Structure, and Properties. Examples of *compositions and structure* of amalgams of all types are summarized in Table 4-3. *The principal considerations for any amalgam are the amount of mercury in the final restoration and the types of reaction products formed.*

Conventional amalgam sets by the reaction of Ag and Sn from Ag-Sn particles with mercury to produce two reaction product phases, a Ag-Hg phase and a Sn-Hg phase. These form solids and cause the mass to harden. The metallurgic reaction is very complicated and is influenced by several variables. Schematically, the reaction is summarized in a simple way in Fig. 4-26. Because the original mixture contains a large excess of Ag-Sn alloy particles, only a minor portion of the outside of the particles is consumed during the reaction with mercury. The unreacted portion of the original amalgam alloy particles remains as residual alloy particles, reinforcing the final structure. Reaction products form a matrix surrounding the residual alloy particles. Because the residual alloy particles have physical, chemical, and mechanical properties that are significantly better than those of the reaction products, it is important to minimize the amount of matrix that forms during the reaction. Depending on the geometry and packing of the amalgam alloy particles, different amounts of mercury will be required to initially create a condensable mixture. After the reaction begins and the amalgam has been placed in the tooth preparation, it is important to compress (condense) the mixture to reduce voids in the material, adapt it closely to the tooth preparation walls, and express excess mercury-rich matrix. The mercury-rich matrix is removed from the surfaces of condensed material increments. This process ensures that the final structure is composed predominantly of reinforcing residual alloy within a minimum of reaction product matrix. This is exemplified in Fig. 4-27. The matrix phase of a well-condensed spherical dental amalgam is seen as a polished cross-section. The cracked surface can be seen only propagating through the matrix phase while following a tortuous path around the strong residual spherical alloy particles.

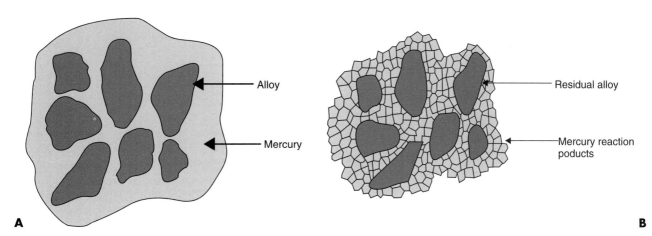

A   **B**

FIG. **4-26** Schematic summary of setting reaction of amalgam and its associated microstructure. **A,** Before reaction, alloy particles are dispersed in mercury. **B,** After reaction, residual alloy particles are embedded in matrix of crystalline reaction products. Only a small percentage of individual powder particles is required to completely react with mercury. *(Modified from Bayne SC, Barton RE. In Richardson RE, Barton RE, editors: The dental assistant, ed 6, Philadelphia, 1988, Lea & Febiger.)*

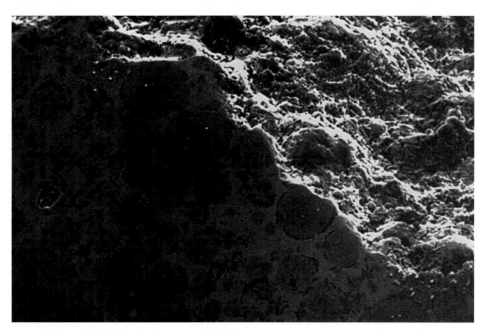

FIG. **4-27** Picture of Tytin restoration fracture surface and polished cross-section showing that fatigue failure cracks proceed through the matrix phase and around the stronger residual alloy particle phase. Greater condensation during placement reduces the amount of matrix, making the path for fatigue crack propagation more tortuous during clinical service and prolonging the service life of the restoration. *(Courtesy Stephen C. Bayne, School of Dentistry, University of North Carolina, Chapel Hill, NC.)*

The major reaction product phases of Ag-Hg and Sn-Hg are approximately Ag_2Hg_3 and $Sn_{7-8}Hg$, and are nonstoichiometric. In metallurgic terminology, the original alloy is designated as *gamma phase* (γ) and the reaction product phases are called *gamma-one* (γ_1) and *gamma-two* (γ_2), respectively.

Ag-Hg (gamma-one) crystals are generally small and equiaxed. Most of the matrix is Ag-Hg. That phase has intermediate corrosion resistance. *Sn-Hg (gamma-two)* reaction product crystals are long and bladelike, penetrating throughout the matrix. Although they con-

stitute less than 10% of the final composition, they form a penetrating matrix because of intercrystalline contacts between the blades. That image is reinforced by the scanning electron microscopy (SEM) picture of Sn-Hg crystals in Fig. 4-28. This phase is prone to corrosion in clinical restorations, a process that proceeds from the outside of the amalgam, along the crystals, connecting to new crystals at intercrystalline contacts. This produces *penetrating corrosion* that generates a porous and spongy amalgam with minimal mechanical resistance.

Two key features of this degradation process are the corrosion-prone character of the Sn-Hg phase and the connecting path formed by the bladelike geometry of the crystals. Both of these are eliminated by the use of more copper in the initial composition.

High-copper amalgams set in a manner similar to low-copper amalgams except that Sn-Hg reactions are

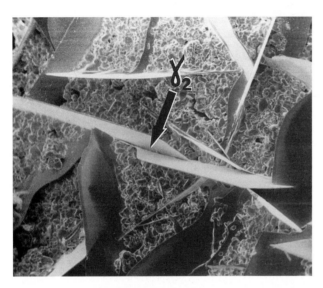

FIG. **4-28** SEM view of Sn-Hg (γ_2) crystals that occur in matrix of set low-copper amalgams. (Note the bladelike crystals that penetrate amalgam and touch each other to create continuous matrix.)

suppressed by the preferential formation of Cu-Sn phases instead. *Cu-Sn phases that are part of the set amalgam matrix are much less corrosion-prone than the Sn-Hg phase they replace.* The Cu-Sn phases are still the most corrosion-prone ones in the amalgam. However, when they corrode, penetrating corrosion does not occur because individual crystals generally are not connected.

Both low-copper and high-copper amalgams undergo two kinds of corrosion, *chemical corrosion* and *electrochemical corrosion* (Fig. 4-29 and Table 4-4). Chemical corrosion occurs most notably on the occlusal surface and produces a black Ag-S tarnish film (Fig. 4-30). This reaction is limited to the surface and does not compromise any properties, except for esthetics. Those amalgams with very high levels of copper also are capable of producing a copper oxide patina, but that is relatively uncommon. Electrochemical corrosion is an important mechanism of amalgam corrosion and has the potential to occur virtually anywhere on or within a set amalgam. Electrochemical corrosion occurs whenever chemically different sites act as an anode and cathode (see Chemical Properties). This requires that the sites be connected by an electrical circuit in the presence of an electrolyte, typically saliva. The anode corrodes, producing soluble and insoluble reaction products.

If an amalgam is in direct contact with an adjacent metallic restoration such as a gold crown, the amalgam is the anode in the circuit. This type of electrochemical corrosion is called *galvanic corrosion* and is associated with

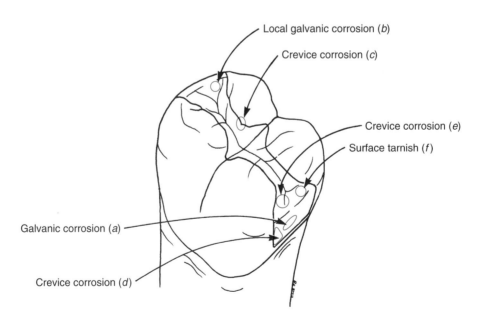

FIG. **4-29** Examples of sites susceptible to electrochemical and chemical corrosion on amalgams: galvanic corrosion *(a)* at interproximal contact with metallic restoration such as gold casting alloy; local galvanic *(b)* corrosion on occlusal surface at grain boundaries between different metallic phases; crevice corrosion *(c)* at margin due to lower pH and oxygen concentration of saliva; crevice corrosion *(d)* under retained interproximal plaque due to lower local pH; crevice corrosion *(e)* within unpolished scratches or detailed secondary anatomy; chemical corrosion *(f)* of occlusal surface with sulfide ions in saliva, producing surface tarnish.

the presence of macroscopically different electrode sites. The same process may occur microscopically (local galvanic corrosion or structure selective corrosion) because of the electrochemical differences of different phases. Residual amalgam alloy particles act as the strongest cathodes. Sn-Hg or Cu-Sn reaction product phases are the strongest anodes in low-copper and high-copper amalgams, respectively. Local electrochemical cells also may arise whenever a portion of the amalgam is covered by plaque or soft tissue. The covered area has a locally lowered oxygen and/or higher hydrogen ion concentration, making it behave more anodically and corrode. Cracks and crevices produce similar conditions and preferentially corrode (concentration cell corrosion or *crevice corrosion*). Regions within an amalgam that are under stress also display a greater propensity for corrosion *(stress corrosion)*.

TABLE 4-4 Examples of Intraoral Situations for Which Electrochemical and Chemical Corrosion (Tarnish) Would Occur

ELECTROCHEMICAL CORROSION EVENTS	
HIGH RISK	
Class I dental amalgam	• Local galvanic corrosion between amalgam phases along all surfaces of amalgam
	• Stress corrosion during occlusion with opponent tooth surfaces
	• Concentration cell corrosion within margins with tooth structure
	• Concentration cell corrosion below plaque formed on amalgam surfaces (causing pitting)
Class II dental amalgam	• Same as for Class I amalgam
	• Corrosion at interproximal contacts with adjacent metal crowns
Class III dental amalgams	• Same as for Class I amalgam
LOWER RISK	
Noble metal casting alloys for inlays, onlays, crowns, bridges, and PFM alloys	• Local galvanic corrosion between phases along all surfaces if more than a single-phase alloy
	• Stress corrosion during occlusion with opponent tooth surfaces
	• Concentration cell corrosion at margins with dental cement or tooth structure
	• Concentration cell corrosion below plaque formed on surfaces
Non-noble PFM alloys and dental implants	• Fretting corrosion where abrasion or rubbing continually removes protective passivating oxide film

PFM, Porcelain-fused-to-metal.

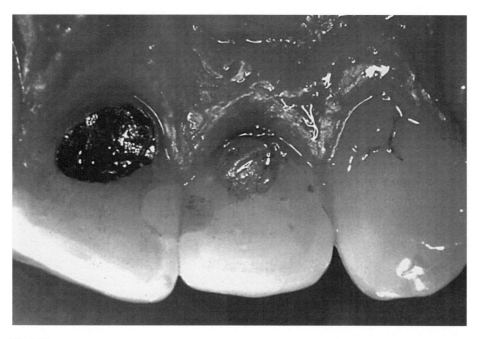

FIG. **4-30** Clinical example of tarnished occlusal surface of amalgam restoration. *(Courtesy Stephen C. Bayne, School of Dentistry, University of North Carolina, Chapel Hill, NC.)*

For an occlusal amalgam, the greatest combination of corrosion and mechanical stresses occurs along margins. Therefore most visible changes are associated with margins. These are discussed subsequently in detail.

During electrochemical corrosion of low-copper amalgams, the Sn-Hg phase is oxidized into Sn-O and/or Sn-O-Cl.[145,146] The oxychloride species is soluble. The oxide precipitates as crystals and tends to fill up the spaces occupied by the original Sn-Hg phase. Along the margins of the amalgam, Sn-O helps seal the space against microleakage (Fig. 4-31). Amalgam has a linear coefficient of thermal expansion that is 2.5 times greater than tooth structure, and it does not bond to tooth structure (unless an amalgam bonding agent is used). Therefore, during expansion and contraction, percolation could otherwise occur along the external walls (see Fig. 4-6) if corrosion products did not impede fluid ingress and egress along the margins.

Electrochemical corrosion of Sn-Hg does not appear to release free mercury into the oral environment. Rather, mercury immediately reacts with locally available Ag and Sn from residual amalgam alloy particles and is re-consumed to form more reaction products. Electrochemical corrosion of Cu-Sn in high-copper amalgams produces both copper and tin oxides and oxychlorides, but no mercury is involved in the process. *Electrochemical corrosion is not a mechanism of mercury liberation from set amalgam.*

Principal mechanical properties of amalgam are reported in Table 4-5 and include values for compressive strength, tensile strength, and creep. The compressive strengths of high-copper amalgams are greater than those of low-copper amalgams because of the presence of the copper phases. High-copper amalgams have compressive strengths that range from 380 to 550 MPa (55,000 to 80,000 psi) and are very similar to those of enamel and dentin. Therefore dental manufacturers do not place much emphasis on increasing these values. Tensile strength is important for fracture resistance. Both low- and high-copper amalgams have low tensile strengths,

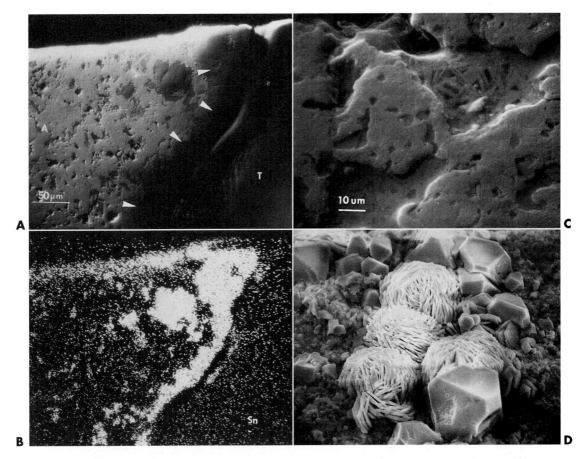

FIG. **4-31** Marginal sealing by corrosion products. **A,** SEM cross-sectional view of Sn-O corrosion products sealing amalgam (A) margin along enamel wall *(T)*. **B,** Elemental map of Sn to demonstrate high concentration of Sn (see large white areas) within amalgam near interface with tooth. **C,** Densely packed Sn-Cl crystals within pores of retrieved conventional amalgam restoration. **D,** Sn-O polyhedra and Sn-O-Cl brush-heap crystals on amalgam surface after corrosion. *(A and B, From Port RM, Marshall GW: J Am Dent Assoc 110:491-495, 1985; C, From Marshall SJ, Marshall GW, Jr: J Dent Res 59:820-823, 1980; D, From Marshall GW, Sarkar, Greener EH: J Dent Res 54:904, 1975.)*

but high-copper amalgam is lower overall. This is important because it is very likely that most intraoral loading conditions produce tensile stresses along the occlusal surface and at the margins. During direct contact by opponent teeth, cusps and/or amalgam restorations are stretched laterally, producing tension and perhaps flexion (see Fig. 4-10, *B* and *D*). Amalgams that are corroded or have inadequate bulk to distribute stresses may fracture. At margins, where amalgams are thinner, extrusion may have occurred, and corrosion may have compromised the integrity of the amalgam, fracture is even more likely.

Amalgam is generally considered a brittle material. It is not capable of much plastic deformation before fracture when stressed at moderate-to-high strain rates, such as during vigorous chewing. *Therefore traumatic stresses during chewing can produce fracture in an amalgam without sufficient bulk.* In contrast, at slow strain rates such as expansion caused by phase changes or corrosion, amalgam (particularly low-copper amalgam) is capable of clinically significant plastic deformation (*creep*), even though the stresses are well below the elastic limit.

Amalgam creep is plastic deformation principally due to very slow metallurgic phase transformations that involve diffusion-controlled reactions and produce volume increases. The associated expansion makes the amalgam protrude from the tooth preparation. Such secondary expansion can occur throughout the clinical life of a restoration. On nonocclusal surfaces, the entire amalgam restoration may appear extruded (Fig. 4-32), and this can produce unwanted esthetic problems or overhangs in some areas. On occlusal surfaces, abrasion and attrition tend to limit the overall extrusion. However, occlusal margins become fracture-susceptible ledges elevated above the natural contours of the adjacent enamel (Fig. 4-33). Extrusion at margins is promoted by electrochemical corrosion, during which mercury from Sn-Hg rereacts with Ag-Sn particles and produces further expansion during the new reaction. This mechanism, called *mercuroscopic expansion,* was originally proposed by Jorgensen[114] as an explanation for the prevalence of marginal fracture associated with occlusal amalgams. *The most common evidence of degradation of low-copper amalgams is marginal fracture.*

TABLE 4-5 | Mechanical Properties Typical of Set Dental Amalgams

AMALGAM ALLOYS	CLASSIFICATION	PARTICLE TYPE	COMPRESSIVE STRENGTH (MPa) 15 MIN	1 HR	24 HR	TENSILE STRENGTH (MPa) 15 MIN	1 HR	24 HR	CREEP % 24 HR
Velvalloy	Low copper	Lathe-cut	37	120	388	4	13	62	1.1
Spheraloy	Low copper	Spherical	40	126	392	3	11	61	1.5
Optalloy II	Low copper	Mixed	62	164	386	7	16	50	1.6
Dispersalloy	High copper	Mixed	43	154	413	4	12	48	0.25
Indiloy	High copper	Spherical	32	181	445	3	17	45	0.22
Sybraloy	High copper	Spherical	164	345	501	15	32	46	0.05
Tylin	High copper	Spherical	70	281	545	7	26	64	0.1

From Osborne JW et al: Clinical performance and physical properties of twelve amalgam alloys, *J Dent Res* 57:983-988, 1978.

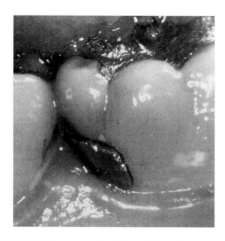

FIG. **4-32** Clinical photograph of Class V amalgam restoration being extruded by mercuroscopic expansion.

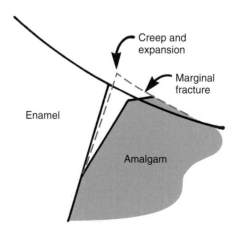

FIG. **4-33** Schematic view of Class I amalgam restoration that was extruded by mercuroscopic expansion, underwent marginal fracture, and now contains marginal ditch. *(Courtesy Stephen C. Bayne, School of Dentistry, University of North Carolina, Chapel Hill, NC.)*

Combinations of brittleness, low tensile strength, and electrochemical corrosion make occlusal amalgam susceptible to marginal fracture. Then, at some point, occlusal stress during opponent tooth contact creates local fractures that produce a *ditch* along the margin. Progression of the events to deeper or more extensive ditching has been used as visible clinical evidence of conventional amalgam deterioration (Fig. 4-34) and was the basis of the *Mahler scale*[139,142] (Fig. 4-35). Mahler ratings were established from No. 1 to No. 11 by comparing the image of the clinical restoration of interest to a series of five photographs (scale values of No. 2, No. 4, No. 6, No. 8, and No. 10) representing increasingly worse marginal breakdown. The rest of the rating scale deals with the severity of marginal ditching that is below (No. 1), intermediate (No. 3, No. 5, No. 7, and No. 9), or greater (No. 11) than the main scale images.

Unfortunately, the impression of extensive (progressive) marginal fracture (to Mahler values of 4 to 11) for low-copper amalgams has been translated as a reason to clinically intervene and replace high-copper amalgams. High-copper amalgams also undergo marginal fracture. However, despite early ditching, they do not progress to levels of extensive ditching that would place them at high risk for secondary caries. Instead, *high-copper amalgams display only modest marginal fracture (Mahler values of 3 to 5) over long periods of time.* Excellent clinical research evidence substantiates clinical half-lives for well-placed high-copper amalgam restorations of 24 to 25 years (which is addressed later in Clinical Considerations).

High-copper amalgams that are left in place may eventually fail because of bulk fracture. It is hypothesized that such bulk fracture is the result of *mechanical fatigue.* A rule-of-thumb for clinical service is that occlusal restorations are stressed an average of 1 million times per year. A 25-year service life would correspond

to 25 million cycles of mechanical stress. Typically, materials fail in the 10- to 100-million–cycle range during laboratory testing. The events contributing to mechanical fatigue affect both the restoration and the tooth structure. The stresses and strains in both must be considered together, particularly in the case of restorations bonded to tooth structure.

Mercury Management. Like all other materials in the world, mercury has the potential to be hazardous if not managed properly. Therefore it is very important that the alloying reaction of mercury with the Ag-Sn alloy go to completion to ensure that mercury does not diffuse into the oral environment. *Once the reaction is complete, only extremely minute levels of mercury can be released, and those are far below the current health standard.* Mercury is ubiquitous in the environment and is taken into the body in one form or another via water, air, and food on a daily basis.

The contribution of mercury derived from amalgam to the overall body burden has been the source of much controversy but appears to be relatively low. The important perspective is that mercury enters the body everyday no matter what restorative filling materials are present in the mouth. Under normal circumstances, that mercury is biochemically processed and excreted. As long as the levels are low, there is no threat for mercury toxicity. Although poorly understood, *mercury hypersensitivity* also at times has been claimed as a potential hazard. This is an immune system response to very low levels of mercury. However, the number of individuals identified as potentially hypersensitive is extremely low, and the sensitivity reaction is very mild and not life threatening. Mackert[137,138] and Mandel[143] have reviewed these issues in detail and scientifically refuted the hypothesized problems.

Early claims of mercury problems appeared as soon as amalgams were first used in the United States. The original amalgamation process was demonstrated by a chemist in France.[45] In 1833, two English entrepreneurs, the Crawcour brothers, realized the practical importance for dentistry, carried the idea to New York, and promoted the material as an inexpensive and convenient restoration.[158] However, no attention was given to the proper mercury-alloy ratios or the type of alloy being used. For the most part, the alloy mixed with the mercury was prepared by filing silver coins with considerably variable compositions. In many cases, the inconsistency in materials and techniques led to slow-setting amalgams that released mercury from the unset mass into unprotected dentinal tubules. Although there are no reported cases of patient deaths, there were several cases of pulp death.

A complex battle ensued *(the so-called First Amalgam War)* between dentists using traditional restorative techniques based on gold foil and those using amalgam. The dispute was based on philosophic choices as to dental

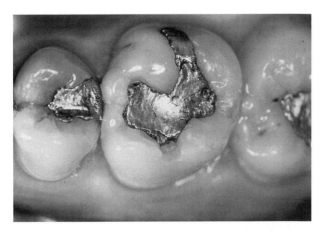

FIG. 4-34 Occlusal amalgam restoration with extensive marginal deterioration. *(Courtesy Wilder AD, School of Dentistry, University of North Carolina, Chapel Hill, NC.)*

standards and differences in points of view about the safety of amalgam. Periodically, there were calls for eliminating amalgam use because of potentially harmful mercury release. In the 1920s another series of challenges to amalgam use occurred when inferences were made that mercury was not tightly bound in amalgams.[236] The next serious controversy arose in 1980 when Dr. Hal Huggins publicly condemned amalgam. Dr. Huggins, a practicing dentist in Colorado, was convinced that mercury released from amalgam was responsible for a plethora of human diseases affecting the cardiovascular and nervous systems. Patients claimed recoveries from multiple sclerosis, Alzheimer's disease, and other afflictions as a result of removing their amalgam fillings. For almost a decade, a loyal following of patients and dentists expanded the call to ban amalgam. Research in the United States and other first world countries has since demonstrated clearly that there was no basis for any of these claims.

In 1991, the general American public was widely exposed to the controversy when it was reported by a major television program (60 Minutes). In response to numerous public questions, the profession, the National Institute of Health-National Institute for Dental Research (NIH-NIDR),[171] the Food and Drug Administration (FDA), and several other groups held forums involving world-famous scientists and clinicians to reexamine the issue. Although these experts agreed amalgam research was needed and should continue, they concluded that there was *no basis for claims that amalgam was a significant health hazard.*[171] They strictly recommended that amalgams not be removed for that reason. However, the controversy is far from being resolved. Claims of hazards continue to be published in local papers;

nonscientific journals; and occasionally, in scientific journals.[38,94,249,250,251] However, all published research demonstrates clearly that there is no cause-and-effect relationship between amalgam restorations and other health problems.[40] This controversy will probably never be resolved because there will always be a certain percentage of patients seeking a miracle cure for their problems. However, fears of amalgam are not a basis for amalgam removal.[179]

Understanding the issues related to amalgam use has been a challenging problem for dental patients. The issues are complex, and dealing with them requires some knowledge of physical chemistry and biochemical processes. It is not realistic to think that a general dentist has the time to effectively communicate this information. In addition, most dentists are perceived by patients as having a vested interest in the decision to use amalgam. Yet, clearly the public wants to know. Fortunately, very clear and concise reviews of the controversy have been published by reputable consumer affairs groups (Fig. 4-36).[150,151] *Purchased reprints from* Consumer Reports *of these reviews provide the best means of patient education.*

The health risk from amalgam use is clearly greater for members of the dental office team than for a patient. Historically a major, although rare, source of mercury contamination in dental offices was the accidental spillage of quantities of liquid mercury. Mercury was commonly purchased in bottles containing approximately 1 pound. This was then transferred to dispensers and eventually to individual capsules for mixing. Mishandling at any stage could result in mercury splashing on the bench or floor, causing it to be widely scattered as small droplets. Fortunately the current use of precapsulated amalgam has eliminated most opportunities for a

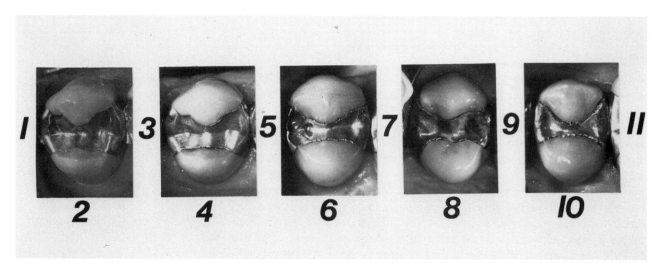

FIG. 4-35 Mahler scale showing visual levels of marginal deterioration (Rating 1 = none, rating 11 = extensive). The numbers of scale indicate ratings assigned to restoration's appearance based on comparison of an existing restoration to scale. (*Courtesy Mahler DB, School of Dentistry, Oregon Health Sciences Center, Portland, Ore.*)

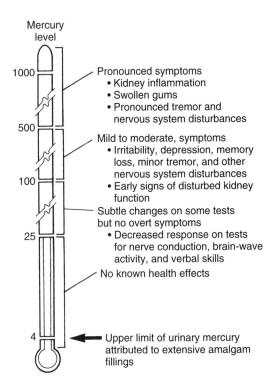

Mercury level

1000 — Pronounced symptoms
- Kidney inflammation
- Swollen gums
- Pronounced tremor and nervous system disturbances

500 — Mild to moderate, symptoms
- Irritability, depression, memory loss, minor tremor, and other nervous system disturbances
- Early signs of disturbed kidney function

100 — Subtle changes on some tests but no overt symptoms
- Decreased response on tests for nerve conduction, brain-wave activity, and verbal skills

25 — No known health effects

4 — Upper limit of urinary mercury attributed to extensive amalgam fillings

FIG 4-36 Mercury thermometer portraying different levels of mercury toxicity. Chronic exposure can be assessed by urinary mercury concentration (as micrograms of mercury per gram of creatinine. *(From The Mercury in Your Mouth, 1991, by Consumers Union of U.S., Inc., Yonkers, NY 10703-1057, a nonprofit organization. Reprinted with permission from the May 1991 issue of Consumer Reports, for educational purposes only. No commercial use or photocopying permitted. To subscribe, call 1-800-234-1645 or visit us at www.ConsumerReports.org.)*

TABLE 4-6 | **Absorption Efficiency of Mercury***

	SKIN	LUNGS	GASTROINTESTINAL TRACT
Elemental	—	80%	0.01%
Inorganic	—	80%	7%
Organic	—	—	95%-98%

*Efficiency is reported in percentage per exposure. No information is reported for some routes (e.g., skin) because the values are suspected to be very low and are not yet well established.

are passed up the food chain. *The concentration of naturally derived mercury in food is at times aggravated by the use of fungicides and pesticides containing methyl mercury. For most people, organically bound mercury in food is the primary source of mercury exposure.* Humans absorb methyl mercury from food readily, but excrete it less effectively than other forms of mercury. Once absorbed it has a tendency to concentrate in certain organs such as the liver, kidney, and brain. It is eventually all excreted, but the rate is depends on the body's ability to convert it to other forms.

It has been suggested that metallic mercury can be changed into methyl mercury by microorganisms in either the mouth or gastrointestinal tract. However, careful examination of blood mercury concentrations indicates that no biotransformation seems to occur.[44]

In the dental office, the sources of mercury exposure related to amalgam include: (1) amalgam raw materials being stored for use (usually as precapsulated packages); (2) mixed but unhardened amalgam during trituration, insertion, and intraoral hardening; (3) amalgam scrap that has insufficient alloy to completely consume the mercury present; (4) amalgam undergoing finishing and polishing operations; and (5) amalgam restorations being removed. Each of these is more carefully considered in the following paragraphs. Specific recommendations by the ADA[7,9] were recently revised[8] and are summarized in Box 4-1.

It is difficult, if not impossible, to totally contain liquid or gaseous mercury because it is very mobile, has a high diffusion rate, and penetrates through extremely fine spaces. Even in packages that include plastic blister wrapping and layers of cardboard, mercury vapor leakage is possible. Therefore mercury-containing products should not be stored in the open, but rather in closets or cabinets, to minimize local concentrations in the rest of the offices. *Storage locations should be near a vent that exhausts air out of the building.*

During amalgam trituration, small amounts of material may escape from capsules. Both reusable capsules and precapsulated designs have some leakage. Small local spills or spatters of triturated materials are best dealt with by collection with a vacuum aspirator (not a vacuum cleaner). During trituration, the high frequency of agitation can force some mercury-rich material out of the capsule and create both an aerosol of liquid drop-

major spill, but care must be maintained to avoid hazards in routine use of amalgam. Careful review of amalgam handling procedures reveals that the critical times are when metallic mercury exists in liquid or vapor form, rather than bound in a set amalgam. *As a vapor, metallic mercury can be inhaled and absorbed through the alveoli in the lungs at 80% efficiency.* This is clearly the major route of entry into the human body. Metallic mercury is poorly absorbed through the skin or via the gastrointestinal tract.[263] A summary of absorption routes is presented in Table 4-6.

In addition to metallic mercury, both inorganic and organic mercury compounds are potentially toxic. Mercury is normally mined as an inorganic sulfide (cinnabar) ore, which is heated in air to oxidize and drive off the sulfur.[200] The mercury is then collected as a liquid. Mercury can exist in a wide variety of *inorganic compounds*, in addition to the sulfide. Many of them are water-soluble and release mercury ions into solution. Some of these compounds have been used in the past as medicants. Such materials are poorly absorbed through the lungs but are easily absorbed in the gastrointestinal tract.

Mercury also can form organic compounds such as methyl mercury. Such mercury compounds are readily absorbed by many organisms and concentrated as they

BOX 4-1   Dental Mercury Hygiene Recommendations

1. Train all personnel involved in the handling of mercury or dental amalgam regarding the potential hazard of mercury vapor and the necessity of observing good mercury hygiene practices.
2. Make personnel aware of the potential sources of mercury vapor in the dental operatory (e.g., spills; open storage of amalgam scrap; open storage of used capsules; trituration of amalgam; placement, polishing, or removal of amalgam; heating of amalgam-contaminated instruments; leaky capsules or bulk mercury dispensers). Personnel should also be knowledgeable about the proper handling of amalgam waste and be aware of the environmental issues. Some state dental societies have published waste management recommendations applicable to their states.
3. Work in well-ventilated spaces with fresh air exchanges and outside exhaust. If the spaces are air-conditioned, air-conditioning filters should be replaced periodically.
4. Periodically check the dental operatory atmosphere for mercury vapor. Monitoring should be considered in case of a mercury spill or suspected spill, or when there is a reasonable concern about the concentration of mercury vapor in the operatory. Dosimeters may be used for monitoring. Mercury vapor analyzers (i.e., hand-held monitors often used by industrial hygienists), which provide rapid readouts, also are appropriate, especially for rapid assessment after a spill or cleanup. The current limit for mercury vapor established by OSHA is 50 μg/m³ (time-weighted average) in any 8-hour work shift over a 40-hour work week.
5. Use proper work area design to facilitate spill contamination and cleanup. Floor coverings should be non-absorbent, seamless, and easy to clean.
6. Use only precapsulated alloys; discontinue the use of bulk mercury and bulk alloy.
7. Use an amalgamator with a completely enclosed arm.
8. Use care in handling amalgam. Avoid skin contact with mercury or freshly mixed amalgam.
9. If possible, recap single-use capsules from precapsulated alloy after use. Properly dispose of them according to applicable waste disposal laws.
10. Use high-volume evacuation when finishing or removing amalgam. Evacuation systems should have traps or filters. Check and clean or replace traps and filters periodically to remove waste amalgam (including contact amalgam) from the waste stream.
11. Salvage and store all scrap amalgam (i.e., noncontact amalgam remaining after a procedure) in a tightly closed container, either dry or under radiographic fixer solution. Amalgam scrap should not be stored in water. If the scrap is stored dry, mercury vapor can escape into room air when the container is opened. If the scrap is stored under radiographic fixer solution, special disposal of the fixer may be necessary. Some recyclers only accept scrap amalgam that is dry.
12. When feasible, recycle amalgam scrap and waste amalgam. Otherwise, dispose of amalgam scrap and waste amalgam in accordance with applicable laws. When choosing a recycling company, it is important to check that the company has obtained all required government permits and has not been the subject of a state or federal enforcement action. Because of the nature of environmental laws, the generator of waste (e.g., the dental office) may be held legally responsible if it is improperly handled by others further down the waste stream. Dentists would be wise to check with their state or local dental society about the laws that apply to recycling and to request documentation from the recycling company that the scrap or waste has been handled properly.
13. Dispose of mercury-contaminated items in sealed bags according to applicable regulations. Consult the state or local dental society about the regulations that apply in a given area. Do not dispose of mercury-contaminated items in regulated (medical) waste containers or bags, or along with waste that will be incinerated.
14. Clean up spilled mercury properly using trap bottles, tape or freshly mixed amalgam to pick up droplets, and commercial cleanup kits. Do not use a household vacuum cleaner.
15. Remove professional clothing before leaving the workplace.

Quoted in part from the American Dental Association Council on Scientific Affairs: *J Am Dent Assoc* 130:1125-1126, 1999.
OSHA, Occupational Safety and Health Administration.

lets and a vapor that may extend 6 to 12 feet away from the triturator. To minimize this risk, small covers are mounted on mechanical triturators to contain the aerosol to the region of the triturator. This does not eliminate the hazard. These materials persist as air contaminants or as particles that may drop onto the floor and contaminate carpeting or cracks between tiles. *Air contamination is managed by ensuring that air flow is reasonably high and that fresh air is brought into the office in a path from the waiting room, through the outer office, and then into the operatories, before being expelled to the outside of the building without contaminating other building areas.*

Once small droplets of mercury-rich material contaminate the floor coverings, the only practical approach to decontaminating the area is to replace those coverings. *There is no effective treatment for removing liquid mercury from carpeting.* Mercury will react with sulfur to form a stable sulfide (cinnabar), but the reaction is slow and inefficient. Therefore sprinkling sulfur powder onto sites of mercury spills will not adequately control the problem.

During insertion of amalgam into tooth preparations, the mixture is not yet fully reacted and the high vapor pressure of mercury causes contamination of the air above the material. While the unhardened material sits in a Dappen dish for loading into an amalgam carrier, some vapor is released. This should be cleared by the air-flow system for the room. During the intraoral placement and condensation procedures some mercury vapor is released. To control the vapor, a *rubber dam* can be used to isolate the patient and *high-volume evacuation* should be used to prevent intraoral vapor from diffusing. After initial setting, the material has hardened to a solid and the vapor pressure drops several orders of magnitude.

Scrap amalgam from condensation procedures should be collected and stored under water, glycerin, or spent x-ray fixer in a tightly capped jar. The jar should be nearly filled with liquid to minimize the gas space where mercury vapor can collect. The unused amalgam will set but the mercury-rich material in the scrap does not have sufficient alloy present to become completely reacted. Spent x-ray fixer has an advantage for controlling mercury because it is a source of both silver and sulfide ions for reaction to a solid product. Periodically, this material should be recycled for profit for the office, and to minimize the amount of material being stored. *No more than a small jar of material should be present in the office at any time.* Recycling mercury, silver, and other elements is a professional job. The only known case of human death related to mercury management was due to a misinformed dental technician trying to distill mercury out of amalgam scrap in the basement of his home.

Once amalgam has solidified, the mercury is tightly bound. However, one of the reaction products, Ag_2Hg_3, has a very low melting point (127° C). It can be easily liquefied during finishing or polishing procedures that generate heat. Then, as a liquid, it has a much higher mercury vapor pressure. This situation routinely arises when dentists or dental hygienists *polish amalgams* without using adequate cooling water and slow polishing. This process is very deceptive. The Ag-Hg phase is melted producing a mercury-rich liquid phase that is easily smeared over the amalgam surface making it look bright and shiny. The operator can misinterpret this appearance as a highly polished surface.

Melting of the Ag-Hg phase also occurs during *amalgam removal.* It is common for surface temperatures to increase several hundred degrees where high-speed burs contact tooth structure.[120] This is well above the temperatures for melting the Ag-Hg phase and vaporizing mercury. Rubber dam, high volume evacuation, and water cooling can be used to control this situation.

Instruments used for inserting, finishing, polishing, or removing amalgam restorations do contain some amalgam material on their surfaces. During instrument sterilization techniques this material may be heated and can release mercury liquid or vapor.[55, 211] Therefore it is advisable to properly isolate or specially vent the air from sterilization areas.

Historically, capsules and other contaminated surfaces have not been managed very well in the operatory. *Spent capsules and mercury-contaminated cotton rolls or paper napkins should not be thrown out with regular trash.* They should be stored in a tightly capped plastic container or closed plastic bag for separate disposal. In most locations, these materials can be placed into a sanitary landfill, but those regulations may change in the future.

A summary of all of the potential mercury management problems is presented in Fig. 4-37. In addition to materials storage and materials recycling, there are routine precautions for exposure. By using a rubber dam and high-volume evacuation, the patient is well protected from even minor, transient exposure to mercury vapor. These precautions are easy to provide and also effectively protect the dentist, assistant, and hygienist from the same vapor. Mercury vapor that may escape into the room air is not effectively removed by infection control masks. Masks may catch particulate debris above 1 μm in size and catch droplets or sprays in the air, but they will not filter mercury vapor from the air. Routine exposures can be monitored with *exposure badges (dosimeters)* worn by individuals in the office[136] or positioned within dental operatories near working areas.

In the dental office, the dentist, assistant, hygienist, and other staff are at more risk of mercury toxicity than patients because of their long-term contact with mercury vapor. ADA monitoring of mercury levels in dentists has shown that they are in safe ranges despite the fact that the levels are almost twice the national average for nondentists. As a group, dentists actually show better-than-average survival rates. The inference is that if dentists are exposed and survive better than most individuals, then there does not seem to be any basis for the perceived problem.

Much of the confusion about mercury effects is related to inadequate understanding of mercury processing by the human body. Mercury that is absorbed into the circulatory system may be deposited in any tissue. Higher-than-average accumulations occur in the brain, liver, and kidneys. Mercury ions (Hg^{+2}) circulate readily in the blood but pass the membrane barriers of the brain and placenta only with difficulty. In contrast, nonionized mercury (Hg^0) is capable of crossing through lipid layers at these barriers and, if subsequently oxidized within these tissues, is removed only slowly. This fact has become the basis for many claims of neuromuscular problems in patients with amalgams. However, this mercury is not uniquely from amalgam, the levels are low, and removing amalgam restorations does not eliminate exposure to mercury. Mercury does not collect irreversibly in human tissues. There is an *average half-life of 55 days for transport through the body to the point of excretion.*

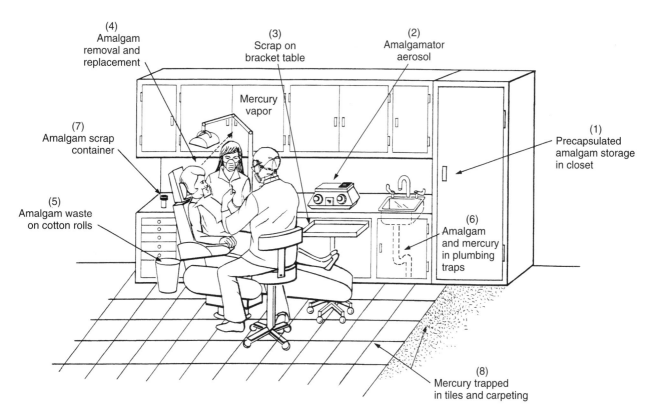

FIG. **4-37** Sources of mercury hazards in dental operatory include: (1) some mercury vapor released from stored materials; (2) small losses from capsules during trituration; (3) spillage during maipulation for tooth restorations; (4) some vapor exposures to dentist, assistant, and patient during removal, placement, or finishing and/or polishing of amalgam; (5) contamination of cotton rolls; (6) collection of debris via vacuum suction into plumbing system and sewer system; (7) collection of remnants in jar for recycling; and (8) mercury trapped in small cracks between floor tiles and/or in carpet fibers.

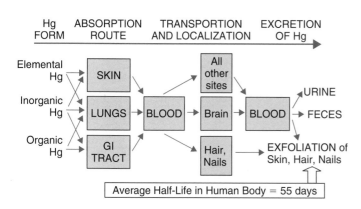

FIG. **4-38** Summary of events occurring during mercury absorption, transportation, and excretion in the body.

Thus, mercury that came into the body years ago, is no longer present in the body. The variety of events involved in mercury absorption and elimination are summarized in Fig. 4-38.

Various events mitigate the conversion of mercury into ions and affect the conversion of the ions to other compounds. For example, ethyl alcohol is known to interrupt some of the biochemical steps required for blood-brain transport, thereby facilitating its rapid excretion.

The placental barrier is less effective than the blood-brain barrier, and some mercury ions are capable of placental transfer, as is about anything else in the circulatory system. Fetal mercury contents, although elevated, are lower than brain concentrations in the mother. *Effects on fetal development* are not fully known. All of the contemporary evidence from surveys and posthoc surveys indicates that female dentists, assistants, and hygienists who are pregnant are at no higher risk of miscarriage or fetal misdevelopment. Even so, it seems to be judicious to minimize any exposure of these individuals to any potential hazard such as mercury during pregnancy.

In philosophic terms, the threat that may someday eliminate amalgam use as a restorative material is not a question of human toxicity, but rather of environmental protection.[23] It is now well known that improper disposal of contaminated waste greatly affects the environment. There are federal regulations to control large-scale industries that pollute. However, there has not yet been a wide-ranging focus on small-scale polluters, which could include local hospitals and dental offices. Although the relative contributions are small, the local community problems may mandate that either dental offices control all mercury effluent or cease using amalgam.

Human beings are constantly exposed to mercury in their environments from a multitude of sources as a result of both natural emissions and human pollution. These exposures include the breathed air, consumed water, ingested food, and medical or dental products.

Typical concentrations of mercury in air vary considerably (pure air contains $0.002 \, \mu g/m^3$; urban air contains $0.05 \, \mu g/m^3$; air near industrial parks contains $3 \, \mu g/m^3$; air in mercury mines contains $300 \, \mu g/m^3$). *The generally accepted threshold limit value (TLV) for exposure to mercury vapor for a 40-hour work week is $50 \, \mu g/m^3$.*[263]

It is key to remember that the body is constantly excreting mercury from these exposures. *Therefore the actual body burden at any time is a function of both the dosage and time of exposure.* Under almost all circumstances, the dosages are low and infrequent, and thus, the body bur-

den poses no health risk. Even if the exposure occasionally is above the TLV, active excretion quickly reduces the body burden to normally low levels. In this scenario, any very small contributions from amalgam restorations are very low compared to other naturally occurring exposures, and the material is naturally excreted.

Mercury also occurs naturally in a wide range of foods but not necessarily in the same chemical form in all cases. The greatest source of naturally occurring mercury, other than the ore, is as mercury vapor released during volcanic eruptions. This vapor gradually is deposited in the world's oceans and accounts for the largest portion of dissolved mercury in water. Material is absorbed by small organisms such as plankton at the start of the food chain. It becomes more concentrated in larger fish higher in the food chain. Swordfish and tuna have essential no natural enemies and are considered at the top of the ocean food chain. Within them, the concentration of mercury is typically $1000 \, \mu g/kg$ of mass. Therefore, eating large amounts of tuna or swordfish can increase dramatically an individual's body burden. Since methyl mercury compounds are routinely used as fungicides and herbicides to coat seeds used to plant farm fields, these compounds are invariably incorporated into growing vegetables, fruits, and grains. Then, mercury is concentrated within the land-based animal food chain. The levels are typically $160 \, \mu g/kg$ in cattle and $25 \, \mu g/kg$ in humans.

Only under very rare circumstances have the symptoms of mercury toxicity been observed in human beings (industrial pollution in Minamata Bay; inadvertent contaminated grain consumption in New Mexico and

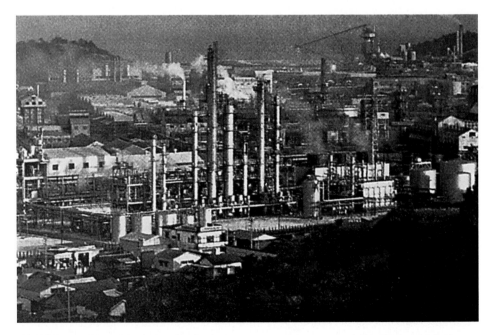

FIG. 4-39 Landscape of Minamata Bay, Japan (seen in background) in relation to the Chisso Corporation, that was responsible for Hg contamination of the bay during discharges of pollutants.[200] *(Courtesy National Geographic.)*

in Iraq). The Minamata Bay incident in Japan in 1952 is the most infamous (Fig. 4-39).[200] A local chemical plant (Chisso Corporation) disposed of its methyl mercury waste into the nearby bay, contaminating the shellfish, and causing toxic levels of mercury in the fish eaten by the local population.[96] By the time the source was identified, 52 individuals had died and 202 others were stricken by mercury poisoning. Since this time, mercury poisoning of this kind is known as Minamata disease. The symptoms of mercury poisoning identified during this incident were: (1) ataxic gait, (2) convulsions, (3) numbness in mouth and limbs, (4) constriction in the visual field, and/or (5) difficulty in speaking. Unfortunately, none of this symptomatology is particularly unique to mercury poisoning. Therefore it is very difficult to diagnose the problem without some special knowledge of an individual's risk to environmental exposure. Similar symptoms are typical of a wide range of other medical problems. Therefore it is easy for antiamalgamists to improperly associate diseases such as multiple sclerosis with the intraoral presence of amalgam restorations.

Amalgam Waste Management. Whereas the use of mercury in amalgam restorations represents an almost insignificant risk to patients, the management of the unused or recovered material in dental offices is a much more complicated situation. The path of mercury from the purchase of an amalgam product to the end of the clinical lifetime of a restoration has been monitored (Fig. 4-40).[14] Concerns about mercury management form the primary basis for the challenge to dentistry to continue to use amalgam restorations.

As individual political entities (countries, states or provinces, counties, towns) examine their own pollution problems, they will adopt restrictions that intend to limit future contributions of toxic metallic and organic wastes to the environment. The problem of pollution is less one of the concentration or amount of individual disposal, but rather one of accumulation of waste within a relatively closed system.

Small amounts of mercury, silver, lead, or other toxic heavy metals are accumulated as part of an ever-increasing load to the local environment. This is

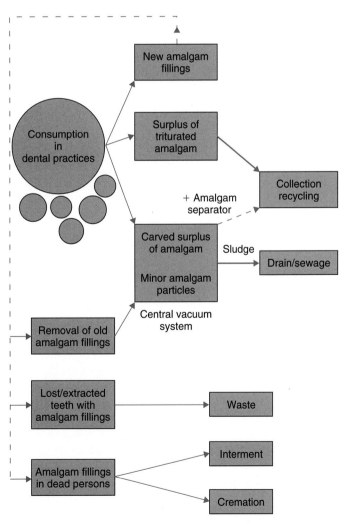

F I G. **4-40** Cycle of mercury in dentistry in dental amalgam.[14,107] *(From Hoersted-Bindslev P et al: Dental amalgam—a health hazard? Copenhagen, Denmark, 1991, Munksgaard.)*

Total Mercury Burden in Sludge (1988) (kg)

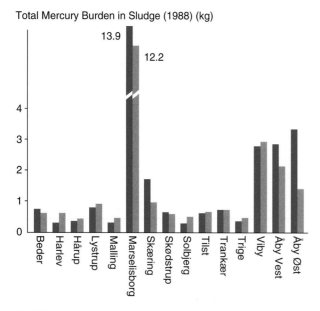

FIG. 4-41 Contributions of mercury from dental offices in Denmark to wastewater in sewage systems compared to the total wastewater levels.[14,107] Black bars indicate dental contributions. Gray bars indicate total levels. *(From Hoersted-Bindslev P et al: Dental amalgam—a health hazard? Copenhagen, Denmark, 1991, Munksgaard.)*

exemplified in the case of amalgam. Scrap from amalgam replacement procedures or from the removal of failed restorations is typically disposed into the local sewer system (Fig. 4-41) from a dental office. Amalgam debris may include large particles ($\sim$ 70% $\geq$ 100 μm), medium-sized particles ($\sim$ 20% = 10 to 100 μm), and fine material ($\sim$ 10% < 10 μm) particles, liquid mercury, or mercury dissolved in water).

Some of this material (large particles) can be trapped with chairside filters in dental offices. Typically the medium- and small-sized debris escapes into the sewer system. Because the materials are relatively dense, they settle out in virtually all regions of the system. Within the office, amalgam waste collects in corrugations of the flexible tubing connected to the intraoral suction devices, in plumbing traps, in plumbing lines along the side walls, and in all piping that connects to the local sewer line. Materials also collect along the entire path of the community sewer system up to the sewage treatment plant.

Materials arriving at the sewage treatment plant are extracted and become part of the waste *sludge*. This material, besides containing heavy metal wastes, also is rich in nitrogen and phosphate. Because quantities of waste sludge are large, municipal wastewater treatment facilities are anxious to dispose of it as quickly as possible. Often the material is claimed by local farmers for the nitrogen and phosphate as fertilizer. Other times the material is burned. In either case, the probability that the solid or vapor will end up on local farming fields and be reincorporated into the food supply is very high.

It is this "closed system" problem that represents the real challenge to dentistry. Unless amalgam waste can be recaptured efficiently, the dental contribution will be viewed as a significant form of pollution.

In the mid-1980s, Sweden was the first country to draw specific attention to potential contributions of dental mercury to the environment. As part of their overall mercury pollution management plan, the Swedish National Board of Health and Welfare in 1992 recommended the phase-out of amalgam use. For various similar reasons, countries such as Finland, Norway, Denmark, Switzerland, and Germany began to adopt a strict view on the potential impact of amalgam waste. These decisions simply fueled the amalgam debates occurring in the United States and Canada during the early 1990s. While the European concerns were environmental ones, the antiamalgamists conveniently reinterpreted these rulings as evidence of the hazard of amalgam use for restorations.

The real volume of amalgam waste in sewer systems is quite low. However, since most other industries have been heavily regulated in this regard for many years, their contributions are extremely low. Analyses of industrial levels in Denmark revealed that approximately 90% of all mercury-containing waste arriving at wastewater treatment plants could be traced to contributions from dental offices.[107] *Mercury waste in sewage systems is primarily from commercial or industrial sources, with smaller amounts from residential sources.*

Recent intraoffice *recapture systems* have helped dramatically lower the actual contributions to the sewage system from dental practices. However, these have only been installed on a limited basis. They represent an initial investment to modify the plumbing and vacuum system of the office, and require continual maintenance. Although these can be relatively inexpensive, the process of recapture certainly does increase the true cost of using and managing amalgam restorations.

Early recapture systems appeared in Europe in the 1990s and involved sedimentation or centrifugation of wastewater in advance of the local sewer connection. Systems were relatively inefficient and rarely exceeded 75% recovery. Newer systems (using medium particle-size filters[16] and/or mercury plating approaches[68]), in combination with chair-side filters, provide much more efficiency (>92% and >98%, respectively). These can be installed quickly and without much problem in new dental practices. However, in older practices there may be a large number of complicating factors. Existing plumbing often is highly contaminated and may need to be removed. Cleaning products are advertised that remove adherent solids from plumbing, but there is no evidence of their effectiveness.

Newer and potentially much more efficient wastewater treatment systems are being investigated such as blue-green algae racks in small tanks that would actively concentrate mercury waste. Other bioactive approaches for individual dental offices are under consideration as well.

Unfortunately for the dental profession, even if a practitioner ceased to use amalgam as a restorative material, there are still millions of amalgams remaining in service in the United States alone. Because these restorations will need repair or replacement at some point in time, the challenge of managing amalgam recapture exists for every dentist. Phasing out of all amalgam restorations currently in service might take 25 to 35 years. Sewer systems themselves are contaminated from historical disposals of mercury- and silver-containing waste. Because the materials are heavy and slow to dissolve, it has been estimated that it might require 25 to 35 years to effectively flush out the sewer lines. Therefore the problem of amalgam recapture and disposal will remain for many more years, despite any new rules and philosophies governing amalgam use.

Regulations concerning amalgam waste disposal are not uniform by region or by permitted levels. Amalgam waste products are part of the: (1) routine solid trash from a dental office, (2) air within the operatory, and (3) wastewater or sewage. The regulations are different for all situations.

Historically, dental personnel have not managed well the amalgam capsules and other contaminated surfaces in the operatory. Spent capsules and mercury-contaminated cotton rolls or paper napkins have been thrown directly into the regular trash. They may be disposed with that trash but should be isolated to limit the vaporization of unreacted mercury into the office air. In most locations that material can be placed into a sanitary landfill, but the restrictions might change in the future. The materials should not be incinerated. Do not place mercury-contaminated materials in medical waste bags because these will be burned and mercury will be vaporized. Do not burn office waste locally because that also would release mercury into the air.

Air within the dental office contains some mercury vapor. Adequate fresh air should be mixed into the existing office air to produce a relatively rapid air turnover. Do not mix office air into a large system that could permit contaminated air to enter other offices in a larger office building unless it can be established that no risk exists in this regard.

Regulations for amalgam waste disposal are quite variable. In general, the hierarchy is that regulations are stricter as one progresses from the federal, to state, to county, and finally to city levels. The United States Environmental Protection Agency (US EPA) regulations govern discharges onto land or into water that are not part of a sewage reprocessing system. Local EPA regulations are focused primarily on statewide water protection, registration of large or small-scale polluters, assays of problems, and leverage of fines. County regulations, if they exist at all, are generally more intolerant and have stringent pollution levels, but generally rely on state support for assays. Cities are increasingly involved in setting standards, assessing local pollution levels, and levying fines to protect their local wastewater treatment facilities from unacceptable discharge burdens. At the same time, cities and counties are under some legal burden to respond to environmentalist groups that may bring lawsuits against them for perceived pollution of streams and recreational areas.

Three important problems for regulators of all waste discharges are: (1) proper technical protocols to detect the chemical of interest, (2) appropriate assay procedures to define the average discharge, and (3) meaningful limits for discharges. In some cases, the equipment is itself a source of mercury for the samples being tested. Many protocols have error levels greater than the detection limits. In other cases, collected samples do not appropriately represent the operating conditions of the wastewater source. A dental office should not be surveyed at 8 AM on Monday. The regulated limits should represent the risk. *Dental mercury wastewater contributions should be measured in terms of volumes and not in terms of concentrations.* Running twice as much water through the system would halve the effective concentration. The wastewater treatment plant, and ultimately the environmental impact, is a function of the quantity of material and not the aqueous dilution at the time of discharge.

Actual effluent from dental offices into a wastewater sewer has been strictly limited in some localities. The detection limit for mercury in water is ~ 0.02 $\mu g/L$. Typical regulatory limits enforced by some cities are 0.0002 mg/L = 0.2 $\mu g/L$ = 0.2 ppb. A new dental office with fully functional recapture systems will pass this level. An older dental office with limited recapture activities may not. Rural dental offices may not be connected to wastewater treatment systems at all, using either direct disposal, a septic tank, or a drainage field. Drainage fields most likely will be prohibited as paths for dental office disposal because the probability of groundwater contamination is high.

These important environmental considerations, combined with evidence that: (1) current amalgams last 3 to 5 times longer than low-copper amalgams, (2) caries rates are lower because of fluoridation effects, (3) anterior restorations are now exclusively made from tooth-colored materials, and (4) many posterior restorations are now made from tooth-colored materials, has resulted in a *dramatic reduction overall in amalgam use.* Recent ADA surveys indicate that amalgam use decreased 45% from 1979 to 1990 alone.[168] If this trend continues, the amount of amalgam used for new restorations by the year 2010 may be almost insignificant. This pattern, however, does not eliminate the profession's problem of mercury containment during amalgam removal.

As a response to environmental issues connected to amalgam and because of the increasing patient demand for more esthetic restorative materials, there has been great pressure from 1995 to 2000 to provide alternatives to amalgam. For all practical purposes, use of amalgam for anterior restorations has disappeared since 1970 because of widespread use of composite, glass ionomers, and all-ceramic restorations. Amalgam's primary indication is for large intracoronal restorations on molar teeth or as foundations for crowns. For these situations, three types of alternatives to amalgam have arisen: metal alloys (gallium alloys; condensable self-welding metal alloy powders), modified composites (packable composites; laboratory-processed composite inlays; fiber-reinforced composite inlays, onlays, or crowns), and all-ceramic restorations (milled restorations; castable or pressable ceramics; high-strength ceramics). None of these has yet displaced amalgam.

Gallium alloys are currently being placed as amalgam alternatives but are not accepted by the ADA for use in the United States. These alloys generally have mechanical properties similar to that of amalgam.[73,267,268,275] Clinical trials with these materials,[116,172,186,187] have indicated problems with mixing[159] and with early moisture sensitivity leading to excessive expansion.[248] Additionally, unidentified and potentially toxic corrosion products accumulate on the intraoral surfaces.[100] Although the microstructures of gallium-based restorations are similar to those for high-copper amalgams, it may be even more complex. Gallium alloy powder particles that are triturated with 65% Ga–19% In–15% Sn produce a set material with phases of Ag_2Ga, $CuPdGa_2$, β-Sn, Ag-Sn, and unreacted alloy.[101]

Clinical Considerations. Clinical longevity is a primary concern for selecting any restorative dental material. *Clinical longevity* is the median age for a "group" of related or similar restorations at which 50% of the restorations have been replaced because of clinical failure. Clinical longevity is determined by monitoring many restorations for clinical failure over a long period of time (longitudinal clinical research study) or by collecting information on random failures over a short period of time (cross-sectional clinical study).

Clinical failure is the point at which the restoration is no longer serviceable or at which time the restoration poses other severe risks if it is not replaced. Amalgam restoration–related failures include: (1) bulk fracture of the restoration, (2) corrosion and excessive marginal fracture, (3) sensitivity or pain, (4) secondary caries, and (5) fracture of tooth structure forming the restorative tooth preparation wall(s). The incidence of different failure modes depends on a large number of factors. Restorations in caries-prone individuals may fail more often as a result of secondary caries. Restorations in caries-free individuals generally survive much longer, to the point that either fatigue results in bulk fracture of the restoration or the remaining tooth structure fractures from masticatory force.

In many cases, amalgam restorations are not permitted to reach the point of clinical failure. They are replaced before that time in anticipation of failure (*clinical replacement*). An example would be the replacement of a functionally sound restoration because of unacceptable esthetics. Restorations also have been replaced rather than being routinely maintained, depending on the government or private insurance coverage policy provisions. Therefore the clinical failure time is often longer than the clinical replacement time (Fig. 4-42).[18] For any single restoration, clinical failure or replacement may be shorter or longer than the average clinical longevity value describing a group of restorations.

Failure or replacement times may vary from a few months to as many as 45 to 50 years. This distribution is

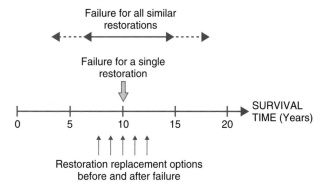

FIG. **4-42** Timeline to compare clinical failure, actual clinical replacement, and options for clinical replacement. Clinical failure and clinical replacement refer to individual restoration that may not reflect average condition for the larger group of similar restorations. Clinical longevity refers to the average time for replacement for a group of similar restorations being studied.

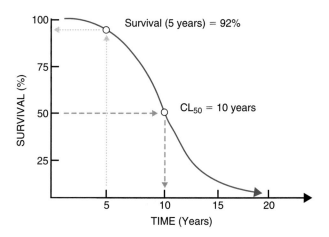

FIG. **4-43** Distribution of clinical failures (survival or failure rate) for dental restorations. Survival curves can be described in terms of the clinical longevity in years for 50% of the restorations, or the surviving population of restorations in percentage at a particular time. *(Courtesy Stephen C. Bayne, School of Dentistry, University of North Carolina, Chapel Hill, NC.)*

typified by the curve in Fig. 4-43. This average has been designated the CL_{50} (clinical longevity for 50% of the restorations) value.[28]

Many clinical failures of amalgam restorations occur because of some combination of electrochemical corrosion and mechanical stress. The combination produces continual marginal breakdown that creates conditions for more frequent failure due to secondary caries. In anticipation of this failure, amalgams with advanced marginal breakdown are often replaced. The average replacement age of conventional (low-copper) amalgams in clinical practice is in the range of 5 to 8 years (Table 4-7). There is much less corrosion and marginal fracture in high-copper amalgams. They more commonly fail because of *bulk fracture,* presumably related to fatigue. In recent years evidence has been mounting that high-copper amalgams, regardless of initial compositional differences, have a CL_{50} of 24 to 25 years. High-copper amalgams not containing zinc do not last quite as long.

Normally, early failure of amalgams is uncommon, but when it does occur it is related to bulk fracture, improper preparation design factors, or postoperative sensitivity. Conventional amalgams initially have very low tensile strength because of slow overall setting reactions. Therefore they must be protected from high stresses during the first few hours after placement. Spherical high-copper amalgams develop strength more rapidly and are relatively immune to early fracture from loading. However, if the final amalgam does not have adequate depth and/or width at the narrowest portion of its bulk, then it is possible for intraoral loads to produce high resolved stresses causing fracture in the isthmus of the restoration. This is true of all amalgams.

During setting, most amalgams undergo very little dimensional change. Improperly manipulated and/or improperly condensed amalgams, however, might undergo increased expansion. This could produce stresses on tooth structure and create unusual postoperative sensitivity or pain. However, it should not be confused with slight sensitivity, related to the fact that an amalgam is a metallic restoration that may conduct heat or become electrochemically coupled, producing a minor current that may induce pulpal sensitivity for a few hours. After that time, corrosion products eliminate the problem. Until initial corrosion occurs, some oral fluid penetration may occur along the walls of the tooth preparation. If the dentin is not adequately sealed, then fluid flow in the tubules may be induced and sensitivity could result. This should not occur with adequately sealed dentin surfaces. The normal resolution of the problem of persistent sensitivity is replacement of the restoration.

There are occasional reports of high incidences of amalgam sensitivity with some spherical alloys, but there is no careful documentation of any cause and effect. Complaints arise only sporadically and are certainly not universal. No investigation has been able to identify the causes or solutions to this problem. The prevalence of this type of sensitivity is presumed to be very low.

TABLE 4-7 Lifetimes Reported for Dental Amalgams in Use in General Clinical Practices*

CITATION, YEAR	STUDY TYPE	AMALGAM TYPE	RESTORATIONS	SURVIVAL LEVEL	50% LONGEVITY
Robinson, 1971	(Cross-sectional)	Low-copper	145	25% at 20 yr	10 yr
Allan, 1977	(Cross-sectional)	Low-copper	241	10% at 15-20 yr	5-8 yr
Crabb, 1981	(Cross-sectional)	(Low-copper)	1061		7-8 yr
Elderton, 1983	(Cross-sectional)	(Low-copper)	1206	52% at 4.5 yr	
Patterson, 1984	(Cross-sectional)	(Low-copper)	2344		7.5 yr
Bentley, Drake, 1986	(Longitudinal)	(Low- and high-copper)	433	71%-92% at 10 yr	
Mjor, 1981	(Cross-sectional)	Low- and high-copper	3527	40% at >10 yr	
Smales, 1991	Longitudinal	Low- and high-copper	1042	>70% at 10 yr	
Smales et al, 1991	Longitudinal	Low- and high-copper	1801	75% at 10.9 yr	
Smales et al, 1992	Longitudinal	Low- and high-copper	1813	70% at 20 yr	20-24 yr (est.)
Dawson, Smales, 1992	(Longitudinal)	Low- and high-copper	1345	75% at 6.6 yr	14.4 yr
Letzel et al, 1982	Longitudinal	Low- and high-copper	360	73.6% at 7 yr	
Letzel et al, 1990	Longitudinal	High-copper		83%-91% at 10 yr	24 yr (est.)

*Parentheses indicate that information not stated definitively in reference.
References may be found in References list.

External surfaces on amalgams should be relatively smooth. This discourages the formation of crevice sites for electrochemical corrosion or for stress concentration during mechanical loading. The general rule for carving an amalgam is to produce only surfaces and grooves that can be made smooth. Detailed secondary tooth anatomy, which can be carved into amalgam surfaces, is usually more of a liability to longevity than an esthetic advantage.

For many years, the smoothness of the restoration surface as a means of reducing corrosion sites has been a concern. Until 1985, it was standard procedure to wait for more than 24 hours and then to polish the amalgam at a subsequent visit. Polishing has been replaced by burnishing the surface at the time of placement (see Chapters 16 to 19). Polishing amalgams occurs only when the surfaces are not smooth when inspected. Clinical studies have shown no detectable clinical advantage for polished restorations compared with initially smooth restorations.[50,129]

Amalgam repair is possible to a limited extent. If secondary caries or fracture involves only a portion of an amalgam restoration, it is possible to leave the unaffected portion and prepare a tooth preparation that includes part of the old restoration as one of its external walls. Differences in amalgam compositions and corrosion behaviors will contribute to corrosion, but the effect appears to be insignificant.

At sites where support for remaining tooth structure is compromised, amalgam bonding systems have been proposed to increase retention and strengthen weak tooth structure. There are no long-term clinical research results for the success of bonded amalgam restorations, but some increases in retention and resistance forms usually occur. However, when used, the bonded amalgam tooth preparation also should utilize conventional secondary retention and resistance form features (see Chapters 17 and 19). Amalgam bonding agents (see Bonding Systems) also are effective in sealing tooth preparations, bonding new to old amalgam, and/or repairing marginal defects.

LINERS AND BASES

Many restorative dental materials that provide excellent properties for the bulk of a dental restoration may not protect the dental pulp during setting or during cyclic thermal or mechanical stressing. *Pulpal protection* requires consideration of (1) *chemical protection*, (2) *electrical protection*, (3) *thermal protection*, (4) *pulpal medication*, and (5) *mechanical protection* (Fig. 4-44). These concerns become more important as the tooth preparation extends closer to the pulp. *Liners* and *bases* are materials placed between dentin (and sometimes pulp) and the restoration to provide pulpal protection or pulpal response. Protective needs for a restoration vary depending on the extent and location of the preparation and the restorative material to be used. The characteristics of the liner or base selected are largely determined by the purpose it is expected to serve. Because they share similar objectives, liners and bases are not fully distinguishable in all cases, but some generalizations can be made.

Terminology and Classification. *Liners* are relatively thin layers of material used primarily to provide a barrier to protect the dentin from residual reactants diffusing out of a restoration and/or oral fluids that may penetrate leaky tooth-restoration interfaces. They also contribute initial electrical insulation; generate some thermal protection; and, in some formulations, provide pulpal treatment as well (Fig. 4-45). The need for liners is greatest with pulpally extended metallic restorations that are not well bonded to tooth structure and that are not insulating, such as amalgam and cast gold, or with other indirect restorations. Direct composite restorations, indirect composite or ceramic restorations, and resin-modified glass-ionomer restorations routinely are bonded to tooth structure. *The insulating nature of these tooth-colored materials and the sealing effects of the bonding agents preclude the need for traditional liners and bases unless*

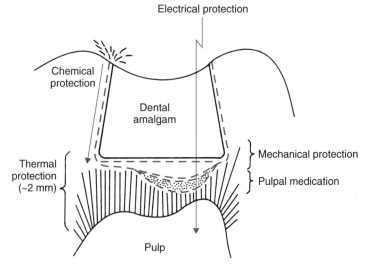

FIG. **4-44** Schematic view of needs for pulpal protection below metallic restoration. Varnishes, liners, and/or bases may be added to tooth preparation under amalgam for purposes of chemical, electrical, thermal, or mechanical protection, and/or pulpal medication. *(From Bayne SC, Barton RE. In Richardson RE, Barton RE, editors:* The dental assistant, *ed 6, Philadelphia, 1988, Lea & Febiger.)*

the tooth preparation is extremely close to the pulp and pulpal medication becomes a concern. This situation is described in more depth later in discussions of bonding agents (see Bonding Agents). Thin film liners (1 to 50 μm) can be subdivided into *solution liners* (varnishes, 2 to 5 μm) and *suspension liners* (typically 20 to 25 μm). Thicker liners (200 to 1000 μm = 0.2 to 1 mm), selected primarily for pulpal medication and thermal protection, are sometimes identified as *cement liners.*

Bases (cement bases, typically 1 to 2 mm) are used to provide thermal protection for the pulp and to supplement mechanical support for the restoration by distributing local stresses from the restoration across the underlying dentin surface. This mechanical support provides resistance against disruption of thin dentin over the pulp during amalgam condensation procedures or cementation procedures of indirect restorations. Metallic restorations may benefit from seating (resting) on sound dentin peripheral to the lined and/or based regions that result from excavating infected dentin (see Fig. 4-45). These seats may help distribute stresses laterally to sound dentin and away from weaker underlying structures. Various liners and bases may be combined in a single preparation, and the *dimension between restoration and pulp may be a combination of natural dentin, liner, and base.*

Objectives for Pulpal Protection. To understand the actions of these agents, it is extremely important to recall the anatomy and physiology of dentin presented in Chapter 2. Normal coronal dentin includes dentinal tubules that contain cellular extensions (odontoblastic processes) of the cells (odontoblasts) that originally laid down dentin during dentinogenesis. These columnar cells remain as a layer along the periphery of the dental pulp, partially embedded in poorly mineralized dentin (predentin), and with processes extending outward into dentinal tubules. The processes are surrounded by

dentinal fluid when they do not contact the walls of the tubules. In response to mild, long-term chemical or mechanical insults, the processes slowly recede toward the pulp while occluding the tubules with peritubular dentin by depositing hydroxyapatite crystals (see Chapter 2). If the insult is strong and/or near to the pulp, the odontoblastic processes are retracted more rapidly from that region and a thin local bridge of hydroxyapatite is created across the affected tubules. Both of these responses are natural defense mechanisms to insulate the pulp from chemical, thermal, mechanical, or biologic challenges.

If the insult produces fluid flow, in or out of the dentinal tubules, the pressure change is sensed by mechanoreceptors within the pulp, and the patient experiences sensitivity. If leakage of chemical irritants from dental materials or bacteria occurs, then the pulp complex can become inflamed. To protect against these events, it is paramount to seal the outer ends of the tubules along the dentinal tooth preparation wall.

Tooth preparation with rotary instruments generates cutting debris, some of which is compacted unavoidably into a layer on the cut surface. That layer of material is called a *smear layer* and is typical of any cut surface, dental or otherwise. Enamel and dentin smear layers are left in place for unbonded amalgam restorations. The dentin smear layer (Fig. 4-46) produces some degree of dentinal tubule sealing, although it is 25% to 30% porous. Flow or microleakage in or out of tubules is proportional to the fourth power of the diameter of the opening (Fig. 4-47). Halving the diameter of the opening produces a sixteenfold reduction in flow. Therefore the smear layer is a very effective barrier. However, because it is partially porous, it cannot prevent slow long-term diffusion. Therefore, for amalgam restorations that can leak along their enamel margins, the smear layer should

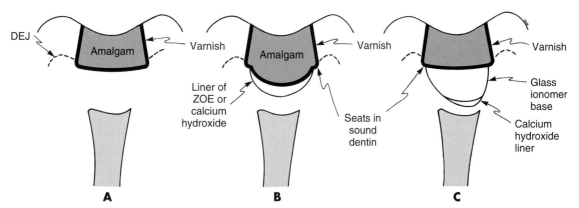

FIG. **4-45** Schematic examples of use of liners and bases for amalgam restorations. **A,** For shallow amalgam tooth preparations, varnish or sealer is applied to walls of preparation before insertion of restoration. **B,** For moderate depth tooth preparations, liners may be placed for thermal protection and pulpal medication. (Note seats in sound dentin for amalgam restoration.) **C,** In very deep preparation, light-cured calcium hydroxide is placed in deepest region in which infected dentin was excavated, and then base of glass ionomer is inserted. Amalgam bonding systems are being advocated as a substitute for liner and varnish, except for calcium hydroxide liner in the deepest region (judged to be within 0.5 mm of pulp).

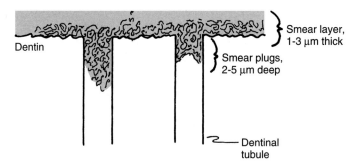

Smear layer,
1-3 μm thick

Dentin

Smear plugs,
2-5 μm deep

Dentinal
tubule

FIG. **4-46** Schematic view of dentin smear layer.

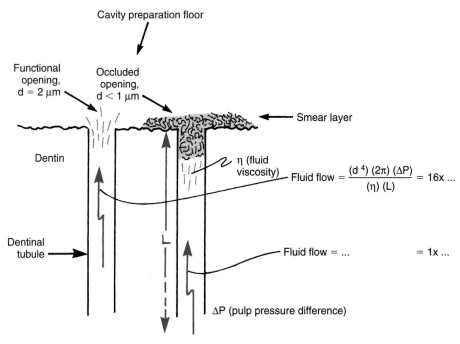

Cavity preparation floor

Functional
opening,
d = 2 μm

Occluded
opening,
d < 1 μm

Smear layer

Dentin

η (fluid
viscosity)

$$\text{Fluid flow} = \frac{(d^4)\,(2\pi)\,(\Delta P)}{(\eta)\,(L)} = 16x\;...$$

Fluid flow = ...   = 1x ...

Dentinal
tubule

L

ΔP (pulp pressure difference)

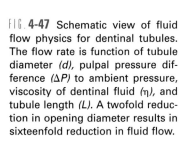

FIG. **4-47** Schematic view of fluid flow physics for dentinal tubules. The flow rate is function of tubule diameter *(d)*, pulpal pressure difference *(ΔP)* to ambient pressure, viscosity of dentinal fluid *(η)*, and tubule length *(L)*. A twofold reduction in opening diameter results in sixteenfold reduction in fluid flow.

be sealed to produce chemical protection. *Traditional liners may be used, but dentin and amalgam bonding systems, discussed later in this chapter, can produce the same or better effect and are becoming substitutes for liners.*

To produce a thin film liner, liner ingredients are dissolved in a volatile nonaqueous solvent. The solution is applied to tooth structure and dries to generate a thin film. Any liner based on nonaqueous solvents that rely on evaporation for hardening is designated as a *solution liner* (or varnish). Liners based on water have many of the constituents suspended instead of dissolved and are called *suspension liners*. Liners are also intended to provide thermal protection and need to be thicker in dimension.

Most varnish coatings are produced by drying solutions of copal or other resin dissolved in a volatile solvent. Copalite (HJ Bosworth) has been used more widely than most other varnishes and contains 10% copal resin in a combination of ether, alcohol, and acetone. The resin content is kept intentionally low to produce a thin film on drying. Thin films work best because they are flexible and dry rapidly. Thick films tend to trap solvent during

rapid superficial drying and become brittle when they finally dry. Most solvent loss occurs in 8 to 10 seconds and does not require forced air assistance. A thin film of 2 to 5 μm is formed over smear layers along the tooth preparation wall. Because some moisture is in the smear layer and varnishes are hydrophobic, the film does not wet the surfaces well. A single coat effectively covers only 55% of the surface (Fig. 4-48). A second thin layer is recommended to produce sealing of 80% to 85% of the surface. However, because of the use of bonding systems or desensitizing systems (discussed later in this chapter) with amalgams, the use of varnishes has decreased considerably in the late 1990s.

Suspension liners can produce the same effect, but dry more slowly and produce thicker films. The typical film thickness is 20 to 25 μm in contrast to the 2 to 5 μm film produced by solution liners (varnishes). Both types of liner are often extended out over the cavosurface margins of the preparation. Excess material on external surfaces is not necessary but is difficult to avoid. It is easily abraded off. The primary purpose of the liners is to provide a protective seal on the exposed dentin surface. The liner layer at the restoration enamel interface also provides a means of electrically isolating metallic restorations from external electrical circuits with restorations in adjacent teeth. Otherwise amalgam restorations may produce small electrical currents during the first few days that cause patient pain or discomfort. This sensitivity rapidly disappears as electrochemical corrosion and/or tarnish modify the surfaces of the amalgam.

A key function of enamel and dentin is thermal insulation of the pulp. Most restorative materials are not as insulating as dentin and therefore thermal insults may occur during intraoral temperature changes. The need for insulation is greatest for metallic restorations. Thermal insulation is proportional to the thickness of the insulating material. Approximately 2 mm of dentin, or an equivalent thickness of material, should exist to protect the pulp (see Fig. 4-45). This thickness is not always possible, but 1 to 1.5 mm of insulation is accepted as a practical thickness. As the tooth preparation extends closer to the pulp, a thick liner or a base is used to augment dentin to the proper thickness range. Such a liner or base cannot harden by evaporation of solvent or water because it would not dry effectively. Material used for this purpose hardens by a chemical reaction or is light-cured.

In addition to thermal protection, liners are formulated to provide pulpal medication whenever possible. Two important aspects of pulpal medication are the relief of pulpal inflammation and facilitation of dentinal bridging for physiologic protection. The materials (eugenol and calcium hydroxide) most commonly used to provide these two functions are not mutually compatible and cannot be used in the same formulation.

Eugenol is used to alleviate discomfort resulting from mild-to-moderate pulpal inflammation. Eugenol is a parasubstituted phenolic compound that is slightly acidic and produces palliative or obtundent actions on the pulp when used in very low concentrations. High concentrations can be chemically irritating. Several eugenol-containing dental materials are based on the reaction of eugenol with zinc oxide (zinc oxide–eugenol [ZOE]) to produce liners, bases, or cements. In the liner compositions, small amounts of eugenol are released during setting and over several days. For this reason, these liners were used in the past in those sites where tooth preparations were moderately deep. Currently, moderate-depth needs for a liner or base are met with the use of a resin-modified glass ionomer, as described later.

In the deepest portions of the preparation or when a microscopic pulp exposure is suspected, it is more important to encourage dentinal bridging by using *calcium hydroxide* compositions. Calcium hydroxide in saturated solutions (suspensions) is extremely caustic (pH >11), but when ionized in low concentrations it stimulates the formation of reparative dentin. Traditionally, calcium

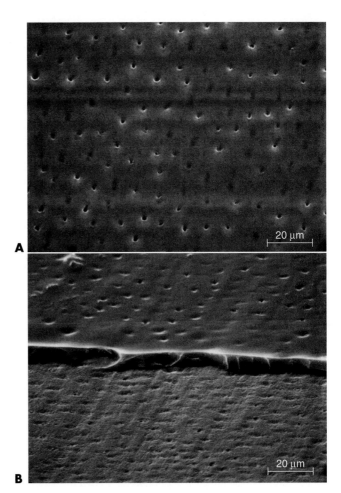

FIG. **4-48** Copalite varnish partially occluding dentinal tubules. **A,** SEM of one layer of Copalite varnish over smear layer that seals approximately 55% of the tubules. **B,** SEM of two layers of Copalite varnish adjacent to region protected only by smear layer. *(SEM micrographs courtesy Stephen C. Bayne, School of Dentistry, University of North Carolina, Chapel Hill, NC.)*

hydroxide liners are formulated to undergo a chemical setting reaction, but allow minor amounts of calcium hydroxide to be released from the liner surface to produce the desired effect. Calcium hydroxide liners generally are based on the reaction of calcium ions from calcium hydroxide particles with phenolic moieties on monofunctional or multifunctional molecules. Excess calcium hydroxide is in the composition, so that some is always available as a source of calcium and hydroxyl ions. Unfortunately, these liners may degrade severely over long periods of time, to an extent that they no longer provide mechanical support for the overlying restoration.

Water is an important component for the chemical setting of both eugenol- and calcium-based liners. The setting reaction of ZOE is accelerated by moisture. Most formulations contain reaction modifiers to produce setting in a reliable way, but moisture does not interfere with the reaction. For calcium hydroxide–based liners, the setting reaction involves calcium ions. To start the reaction,

TABLE 4-8 Composition, Structure, and Properties of a Typical Solution Liner (Varnish)*	COPAL RESIN VARNISH (COPALITE)
COMPONENTS	
Solid	10% copal resin
Solvent	90% ether, acetone, alcohol
Setting reaction	Physical (by solvent evaporation)
STRUCTURE	
Arrangement	Amorphous film
Bonding	Covalently bonded organic material
Composition (phases)	Single phase
Defects	Pores and cracks
PHYSICAL PROPERTIES	
Thermal	[Insulator]
Electrical	[Insulator]
LCTE (ppm/° C)	[High]
Wetting	[Poor on hydrophilic surfaces]
CHEMICAL PROPERTIES	
Solubility (% in water)	[Low]
MECHANICAL PROPERTIES	
Tensile strength (MPa)	< 1
Elongation (%)	< 0.1%
BIOLOGIC PROPERTIES	
Toxicity	[None, if solvent eliminated safely]

*Relative properties are reported in brackets.
LCTE, Linear coefficient of thermal expansion.

some calcium hydroxide must be dissociated by moisture from air or from moist dental surfaces. If the site has been dried excessively, a moist cotton pledget may have to be introduced to make the liner set correctly.

Eugenol and calcium hydroxide cannot be incorporated into the same formulation because eugenol rapidly chelates calcium ions in a strongly exothermic reaction. Therefore the choice of a eugenol-based versus calcium hydroxide–based liner is based on the relative depth of the tooth preparation.

Newer liners place less emphasis on pulpal medication and focus more on chemical protection by sealing, adhesion, and mechanical protection. Sealing may prove to be the most important property overall. As long as restorations are primarily ceramic and/or polymeric materials, they will provide excellent thermal insulation. Newer compositions rely on mechanically strong acrylic resin matrices, and that choice makes the release of eugenol or calcium hydroxide ions from the composition much more difficult or impossible.

Historically, restorative material bases have been generated by mixing dental cements at higher-than-normal powder-to-liquid ratios to increase the final compressive strength and reduce the concentration of potentially irritating liquids. (The thick mixes of some materials are sticky and at times lead to problems with adaptation to the preparation walls and with control of the amount and contour of base material.)

Zinc phosphate cement and resin-reinforced ZOE cement were widely used for bases before the 1960s. Polycarboxylate cement bases gained popularity starting in 1970. Glass-ionomer cement became more popular from 1985 to 1994. Highly modified forms of glass-ionomer cement (light-cured resin-modified glass ionomers or compomers) provide chemical adhesion, good mechanical strength, potential fluoride release, well-controlled setting, and rapid achievement of strength.

Before the development of modified glass ionomers, the functions of liners and bases were relatively distinct, but have since begun to converge. Previously, in a deep preparation, a calcium hydroxide liner would be placed first. Then a base would be added to provide mechanical support and stress distribution. The base would be covered with varnish at the same time the tooth structure walls were varnished (except that when using zinc phosphate cement the varnish would be applied before the cement), and the amalgam would be placed. Currently, light-cured calcium hydroxide and glass-ionomer materials are being used to both line and base relatively deep preparations (see Fig. 4-45, C).

For indirect restorations, provisions must be made to prevent dislodgment of the base during impression-taking or removal of a temporary restoration. Mechanical undercuts or bonding of the base material to prepared dentin is used depending on the type of base material (see Fig. 20-11).

Composition, Structure, and Properties. Representative examples of the composition, structure, and important properties of solution liners (varnishes), liners, and bases are reported in Tables 4-8, 4-9, and 4-10, respectively.

Clinical Considerations. Clinical judgments about the need for specific liners and bases are linked to the amount of *remaining dentin thickness* (RDT), considerations of adhesive materials, and the type of restorative material being used. A summary of recommendations for various restorative procedures is presented in Table 4-11. As discussed later in this chapter (see Dental Adhesion: Dentin Sealers), dentin sealers are being used more frequently instead of dentin bonding systems or varnishes to seal amalgam tooth preparations. Except in the deepest portions of preparations for composite restorations, only dentin bonding systems are being used.

In a shallow tooth excavation, which includes 1.5 to 2 mm or more of RDT, there is no need for pulpal pro-

TABLE 4-9 Composition, Structure, and Properties of Typical Liners*

	CALCIUM HYDROXIDE (VLC DYCAL)	TRADITIONAL GLASS LINOMER (FUJI LINING LC)	REINFORCED ZOE IONOMER (IRM)
COMPONENTS			
Components 1 and 2	Paste (with Ca(OH)$_2$; LC resin, and polyphenolics)	Powder (Al-silicate glass); liquid (polyalkenoate acid, LC resin)	Paste (with ZnO); paste (with Eugenol)
P/L or paste/paste ratio	(1 component)	1.4/1.0 by weight	6.0/1.0 by weight
Setting reaction	Acid-base reaction	Acid-base reaction	Acid-base reaction
STRUCTURE			
Arrangement	Amorphous matrix Crystalline fillers	Amorphous matrix Crystalline fillers	Crystalline matrix Crystalline fillers
Bonding	Covalent; ionic	Covalent; ionic	Covalent; ionic
Composition (phases)	Multiphase	Multiphase	Multiphase
Defects	Pores; cracks	Pores; cracks	Pores; cracks
PHYSICAL PROPERTIES			
LCTE (ppm/°C)	[Low]	[Low]	[Low]
Thermal conductivity	[Insulator]	[Insulator]	[Insulator]
Electrical conductivity	[Insulator]	[Insulator]	[Insulator]
Radiopacity (mm Al)	—	4	—
CHEMICAL PROPERTIES			
Solubility (% in water)	0.3-0.5 [high])	0.08 [low]	[Modest]
Shrinkage on setting (μm/mm)	—	24 [low]	—
MECHANICAL PROPERTIES			
Elastic modulus (MPa)	588	1820	—
Hardness (KHN$_{100}$)	—	—	—
Elongation (%)	—	—	—
Compressive strength, > 24 hr (MPa)	138	128	71
Diametral tensile strength (MPa)	—	24	—
Flexural strength (MPa)	—	46	—
Shear bond strength to dentin (MPa)	—	5.8	—
BIOLOGIC PROPERTIES			
Biocompatibility	[Acceptable]	[Acceptable]	[Acceptable]

*Relative properties are shown in brackets. The values reported are from a variety of published sources from 1988-2000, including manufacturer's product bulletins. Comparisons should be made only in terms of the overall application requirements and not in terms of any single property. *LCTE*, Linear coefficient of thermal expansion; *ZOE*, zinc oxide–eugenol.

tection other than in terms of chemical protection. For an amalgam restoration, the preparation is coated with two thin coats of a varnish, a single coat of dentin sealer, or a dentin bonding system, and then restored. In most cases a dentin sealer is the material of choice. For a composite restoration, the preparation is treated with a bonding system (etched, primed, coated bonding agent) and then restored. Both the sealer for amalgams and the bonding system for composites provide chemical protection. To provide any adhesion of amalgams to the surfaces of the tooth preparation, amalgam bonding systems must be used instead.

In a moderately deep tooth excavation for amalgam that includes some extension of the preparation toward the pulp so that a region includes less-than-ideal dentin protection, it may be judicious to apply a liner only at that site using ZOE or calcium hydroxide. Either one may provide pulpal medication, but the effects will be different. ZOE cement will release minor quantities of eugenol to act as an obtundent to the pulp. It also will provide thermal insulation. However, in a composite tooth preparation, *eugenol has the potential to inhibit polymerization of layers of bonding agent or composite* in contact with it. Therefore calcium

TABLE 4-10 Composition, Structure, and Properties of Typical Bases*

	ZINC PHOSPHATE CEMENT (MODERN TENACIN)	POLYCARBOXYLATE CEMENT (DURELON)	GLASS IONOMER CEMENT (KETAC-CEM)
COMPONENTS			
Component 1	ZnO powder	ZnO powder H$_2$O	F-Al-Si glass powder
Component 2	H$_3$PO$_4$/H$_2$O	Polyacrylic acid/H$_2$O	Polyacrylic acid/H$_2$O
P/L ratio	[High]	[High]	[High]
Setting reaction	Acid-base reaction	Acid-base reaction	Acid-base reaction
STRUCTURE			
Arrangement	Crystalline matrix Crystalline fillers	Amorphous matrix Crystalline fillers	Amorphous matrix Crystalline fillers
Bonding	Ionic	Covalent; ionic	Covalent; ionic
Composition (phases)	Multiphase	Multiphase	Multiphase
Defects	Pores and cracks	Pores and cracks	Pores and cracks
PHYSICAL PROPERTIES			
Thermal	[Insulator]	[Insulator]	[Insulator]
Electrical	[Insulator]	[Insulator]	[Insulator]
LCTE (ppm/°C)	[Low]	[Low]	10 [Low]
CHEMICAL PROPERTIES			
Solubility (% in water)	0.10 [Low]	[Low]	0.10 [Low]
MECHANICAL PROPERTIES			
Modulus (MPa)	—	—	—
Hardness (KHN$_{100}$)	—	—	—
Percent elongation (%)	—	—	—
Compressive strength (MPa)	77	[100]	120
Diametral tensile strength (MPa)	—	[17]	—
BIOLOGIC PROPERTIES			
Safety	[Acceptable]	[Acceptable]	[Acceptable]

*Relative or estimated properties are shown in brackets.
LCTE, Linear coefficient of thermal expansion.

TABLE 4-11 Summary of Pupal Protection Procedures (Medicament/Liner/Sealer)

	SHALLOW EXCAVATION (RDT >2mm)	MODERATE EXCAVATION (RDT 0.5-2mm)	DEEP EXCAVATION (RDT <0.5mm)
Amalgam	No/No/Sealer	No/Base/Sealer	CH/Base/Sealer
Composite	No/No/DBS	No/No/DBS	CH/No/DBS
Gold inlays and onlays	No/No/ Cement	No/Base/ Cement	CH/Base/ Cement
Ceramic, PR, FRP	No/No/DBS, CC	No/No/DBS, CC	CH/No/DBS, CC

Note: Pulpal protection includes pulpal medication, dentin sealing, thermal insulation, electrical insulation, and mechanical protection.
Sealer = Gluma or Hurriseal; base = Vitremer or Durelon cement; cement = Luting cement (e.g., resin-modified glass ionomer).
CC, Composite cement (e.g., Rely X Luting Cement); *CH,* Dycal liner; *DBS,* Dentin bonding system; *FRP,* fiber-reinforced prosthesis; *PR,* processed resin; *RDT,* remaining dentin thickness.

hydroxide is normally used, if a liner is indicated. If the RDT is very small or if pulp exposure is a potential problem, then calcium hydroxide is used to stimulate reparative dentin for any restorative material. A thickness of 0.5 to 1 mm of set calcium hydroxide liner is sufficient to treat a near or actual pulp exposure and provide adequate resistance for amalgam condensation forces. Under these circumstances (when a minimum thickness of material is protecting the pulp), for an amalgam restoration, a spherical amalgam type is recommended for use because less condensation pressure is required. A sealer is then applied before placing a final amalgam restoration. In the case of a composite procedure, a bonding system is used.

If extensive dentin is lost because of caries and the tooth excavation extends close to the pulp, then a cement base should be applied over the already-placed calcium hydroxide liner. If an adhesive cement base is chosen (i.e., polycarboxylate cement or resin-modified glass-ionomer cement) for amalgam or composite restorations, then the adhesive cement base should be applied over the liner and tooth structure to permit chemical adhesion to occur. Sealer or bonding agent is not applied until after the base is in place.

In indirect restorative procedures requiring multiple appointments, any necessary base must be placed, with its own retentive features ensured either by mechanical preparation features or bonding. This guarantees that it will not be displaced during impression procedures or during the removal of temporary restorations.

Survival of liners and bases under restorations has never been well understood. Even during restoration removal, it is difficult to completely remove the restorative materials and to assess the acceptability of the liners and bases. Solution liners (varnishes) are relatively brittle and thin and may only provide chemical protection for a matter of days to weeks. However, that should be sufficient for their purpose. Sealers maintain their integrity much better than varnishes. Bonding agents may survive years. Liners and bases may be sufficiently intact to limit the extent of tooth repreparation to only the outline necessary for removal of the old restorative material. Traditional calcium hydroxide liners are suspected to continue to dissolve and may lose 10% to 30% of their volume over 10 or more years.[203] Radiolucent lines often are observed in dental radiographs at the border of liners. Thus, liners may need to be replaced or augmented if such changes are obvious when the restoration is replaced. Long-term changes in both cement liners and cement bases are not well characterized. It may be judicious under these circumstances to remove most liners and bases during the rerestoration procedure.

DENTAL ADHESION

Terminology. *Adhesion* is a process of solid and/or liquid interaction of one material (*adhesive* or *adherent*) with another (*adherend*) at a single interface.[42] Most instances of *dental adhesion* also are called *dental bonding*. Adhesive bond strength is evaluated by debonding the system.

Most situations involving dental adhesion really involve adhesive joints. An *adhesive joint* is the result of interactions of a layer of intermediate material (*adhesive* or *adherent*) with two surfaces (*adherends*) producing two adhesive interfaces (Fig. 4-49). Examples of the classification of different dental uses are presented in Fig. 4-50.

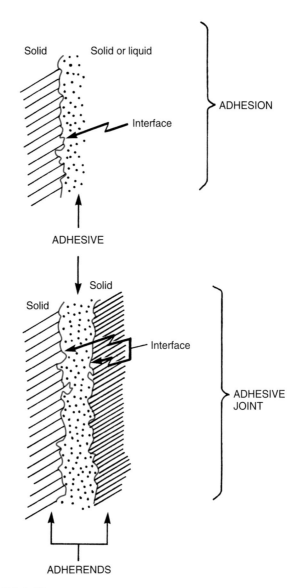

FIG. **4-49** Schematic summary of dental adhesion and dental adhesive joint.

A pit-and-fissure sealant bonded to etched enamel is an illustration of dental adhesion. An enamel bonding agent that bonds together etched enamel with composite is a classic dental adhesive joint.

Bond strength is calculated as the initial mechanical load that generates final fracture divided by the simple, geometrically defined, cross-sectional area of the bond. In most cases, the true contact area between the materials involved may be much greater because of a mechanically rough interface. However, the roughness is not considered in the calculation. The type of bond strength test is categorized in terms of the initial mechanical loading direction and not the resolved loading direction. Almost all bond strength tests are categorized as *tensile* or *shear bond strengths* (Fig. 4-51). Samples that have dimensions similar to dental restoration sizes are considered macrotests. In a practical sense, most macrotensile

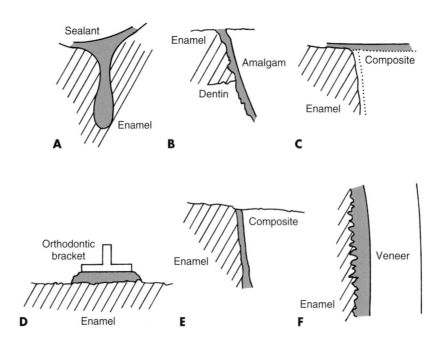

FIG. **4-50** Examples of classification of dental adhesion (**A** to **C**) and dental adhesive joints (**D** to **F**). **A,** Fissure sealant. **B,** Varnished wall of amalgam preparation. **C,** Surface sealer on composite restoration. **D,** Orthodontic bracket bonding resin. **E,** Enamel bonding system for a composite restoration. **F,** Bonded porcelain veneer.

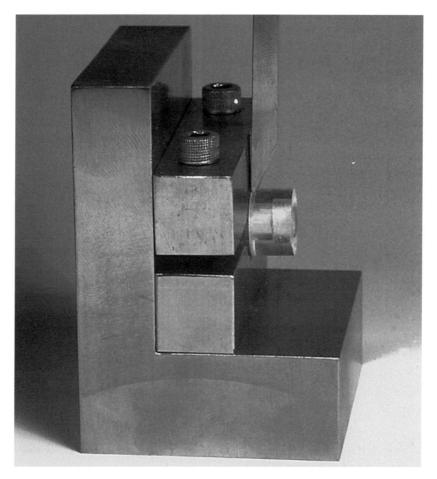

FIG. **4-51** Example of macroshear bond strength testing of bonded dentin samples. A knife-edged wedge is moved parallel to the bonded surface (dentin) and used to load the composite attached with a bonding system over a 4-mm diameter bonded area (12.4 mm²) to the point of failure.

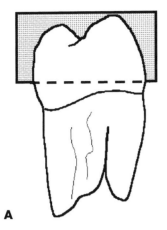 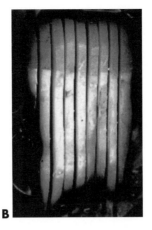 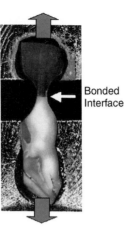

A   B   C

Bonded
Interface

FIG. **4-52** Example of production of microtensile bond strength samples for dentin-bonding system testing. **A,** The crown is removed to create a surface in dentin parallel to the occlusal surface of the tooth. The crown is then replaced with composite bonded to detin. **B,** The tooth is sectioned through the width and breadth of the crown to produce longitudinal sections containing composite, bonding system, and dentin. **C,** The longitudinal section is ground to produce a neck in the region of bonded interface with a small cross-sectional area (e.g., 0.1 mm²). The elongated test sample is bonded at its broad ends to the test apparatus and pulled in tension to the point of faliure. *(Courtesy Bruno Rosa, Londrina-PR, Brazil.)*

bond strengths are often only approximately half of the value of shear bond strengths. Samples that have much smaller test area dimensions are referred to as microtests. Microtests, such as microtensile bond strength tests (Fig. 4-52), usually produce strengths two to three times larger than in macrotests. This occurs because the microsamples have a much lower flaw concentration, and during bond strength testing, almost all fractures occur by crack propagation from flaws in the neighborhood of the adhesive. Any comparison of bond strengths should be in terms of equivalent testing conditions.[233]

Classification. The local interactions that occur at the interface are classified in terms of the types of atomic interactions that may be involved. Adhesion is classified as physical, chemical, and/or mechanical bonding. *Physical bonding* involves van der Waals or other electrostatic interactions that are relatively weak (Fig. 4-53). It may be the only type of bonding if surfaces are smooth and chemically dissimilar. *Chemical bonding* involves bonds between atoms formed across the interface from the adhesive to the adherend. Because the materials are often dissimilar, the extent to which this bonding is possible is limited, and the overall contribution to bond strength is normally quite low. *Mechanical bonding* is the result of an interface that involves undercuts and other irregularities that produce interlocking of the materials. The microscopic degree to which this occurs dictates the magnitude of the bonding. *Almost every case of dental adhesion is based primarily on mechanical bonding.* Chemical bonding may occur as well, but generally makes a limited contribution to the overall bond strength.

The common method for producing surface roughness for better mechanical bonding is to grind or etch the surface. *Grinding* produces gross mechanical roughness but leaves a *smear layer* of hydroxyapatite crystals

and denatured collagen that is approximately 1 to 3 μm thick. *Acid etching* (or conditioning) dissolves this layer and produces microscopic relief with undercuts on the surface to create an opportunity for mechanical bonding.[41] If the mechanical roughness produces a microscopically interlocked adhesive and adherend with dimensions of less than approximately 10 μm, then the situation is described as *micromechanical bonding (micromechanical retention or microretention).*

Requirements for Adhesion. To develop good adhesion (good bonding) it is necessary to form a microscopically intimate interface. The adhesive must be able to approach the molecules of the substrate within a few nanometers. Forming the interface is described in terms of the adhesive *wetting* the adherend.

To produce good bonding, there must be good wetting. Wetting is a measure of the energy of interaction of the materials (see Fig. 4-9, *B*). Materials that interact significantly, producing chemical bonds and reducing their total energy, are said to wet one another. A liquid that wets a solid spreads readily onto the solid surface. If a state of complete wetting occurs, the contact angle approaches zero degrees.

A second requirement for adhesion is that the surfaces being joined are clean. Quite often this is a difficult situation to produce and maintain. Clean surfaces are at a high energy state and rapidly absorb contaminants from the air, such as moisture or dust. If contaminants are not excluded, then the adhesive interface will be weak. A standard process for cleaning any surface is the application of solvents or acids to dissolve or dislodge contaminants.

Bonding Strengths. Most often the bond strengths of materials are measured by shearing the adhesive or adhesive joint to produce fracture. Bond strength is measured as a single cycle stress to fracture. However, in the

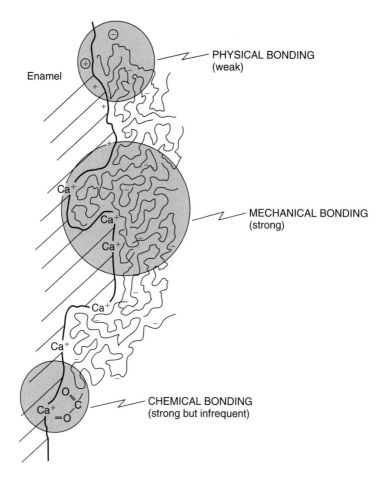

FIG. **4-53** Schematic summary of contribution of physical, mechanical, and chemical bonding to interfacial adhesion. Physical bonding occurs when negative and positive sites on polymer and on tooth structure are attracted electrostatically. Mechanical bonding occurs when bonding agent is mechanically interlocked into microundercuts on tooth surfaces. Chemical bonding occurs as reactive sites on polymer form primary bonds with surfaces of tooth structure.

clinical situation, fatigue may be much more important than single-cycle loading. Currently, fatigue is too complex to be simulated by laboratory bond strength tests. The fracture strength measured depends on the path of the fracture. For an adhesive joint, such as composite bonded to dentin with a dentin bonding agent, the bulk materials' strengths control the fracture path. Dentin is stronger than composite, which is stronger than the dentin bonding agent. If the interfaces are well bonded, then the fracture occurs within the dentin bonding agent or is driven into the adherends. If one or both of the interfaces is not well bonded, then the fracture occurs along the weakest interface.

If the dentin bonding agent is chemically matched to the composite, it will be wet well by the composite, chemically intermix with it, and produce true chemical bonding that will create a very strong interface. Bond strengths for the interface of bonding systems with dentin depend on the degree to which wetting occurs. Cut dentin contains a smear layer, is moist, and is not necessarily micromechanically rough. Selective etching removes some or all of the smear layer, locally controls the wetness, and

produces a micromechanically rough surface. However, dentin is still *hydrophilic* (water loving). Therefore the dentin bonding agent must be designed to be hydrophilic. This quality produces a chemically intimate and micromechanically well-bonded interface. Most current dentin bonding systems have been designed with etching, priming, and bonding steps to accomplish this.

As the interfacial bond strength of an adhesive joint becomes stronger, the bulk strength of the adhesive becomes the limiting factor to adhesive joint strength. One way of improving the bond strength is to decrease the adhesive thickness to the point that a fracture cannot propagate through it in a practical sense. If the adhesive is thin and/or tortuous in geometry, then any crack is constantly driven into one or the other adherends. Thus the joint begins to behave more like the simple adhesion of the two materials on either side of the adhesive. This is the status for current dentin bonding agents. By impregnating a finely etched dentin surface, the final thickness of the dentin bonding agent approaches 1 μm. Fractures are now diverted into dentin, and bond strengths of 25 to 40 MPa are common.

TABLE 4-12	Summary and Comparison of Macroshear Bond Strengths for Different Materials and Systems Involved With Dental Adhesion*

ADHEREND/(ADHESIVE)/(ADHEREND)	MACROSHEAR STRENGTH (MPA)
Enamel	90-200
Dentin	170
Composite	30-120
Traditional glass ionomer	—
Resin-modified glass ionomer	—
Dental amalgam	[125]
Enamel/enamel SL	4-6
Dentin/dentin SL	4-6
Enamel/EBS/composite	18-22
Enamel/ABS/composite	10-12
Enamel/ABS/amalgam	2-22
Enamel/no SL/traditional glass ionomer	8-12
Enamel/EBS/orthodontic bracket	18-20
Enamel/composite cement/Maryland bridge	—
Dentin/DBS/composite	22-35
Dentin/SL/traditional glass ionomer	[6]
Dentin/no SL/resin-modified glass ionomer	10-12
Composite/EBS/resurfacing composite	10-27

* Estimated values are shown in brackets. The combination of adherend, adhesive, and/or overlying adherend is indicated in the left column.
ABS, Amalgam bonding system; *DBS,* dentin bonding system; *EBS,* enamel bonding system; *SL,* smear layer.

An alternative approach to improve bonding is to increase considerably the thickness of the bonding system (50 to 100 μm) by applying numerous coats of the bonding material. This appears to work by behaving like a stress-relieving liner and increasing the toughness of the system. Clinical trials with systems based on this approach have been very successful over at least 3 years.[30]

The problem for dentistry is that different clinical situations may require different chemical characteristics for an adhesive to achieve good wetting. Materials that are good dentin or enamel bonding systems may not necessarily be good porcelain-bonded-to-metal repair bonding agents or amalgam bonding agents.

A number of dental adhesion or adhesive joint situations are tabulated in Table 4-12 with examples of bond strengths. These situations are described in the following paragraphs.

Bonding Systems. In dentistry, the agents producing adhesive dental joints are referred to as *bonding systems* and generally have been classified on the basis of the primary adherend.

Enamel Bonding Systems. Enamel bonding systems (or dental bonding systems that also produce enamel bonding) most often consist of an unfilled (or lightly filled) liquid acrylic monomer mixture placed onto acid-etched enamel. The monomer flows into interstices between and within enamel rods.

Enamel bonding depends on *resin tags* becoming interlocked with the surface irregularities created by etching. Resin tags that form between enamel rod peripheries are called *macrotags* (Figs. 4-54 and 4-55).[31] A much finer network of thousands of smaller tags form across the end of each rod where individual hydroxyapatite crystals have been dissolved, leaving crypts outlined by residual organic material. These fine tags are called *microtags.* Macrotags and microtags are the basis for enamel micromechanical bonding. Microtags are probably more important because of their large number and great surface area of contact. During the 1970s and 1980s, before these details were known, bonding studies concentrated more on the length of macrotags and the patterns of etching (Type I = core etching, Type II = periphery etching, Type III = mixed patterns).[222] Macrotag length is unimportant because fracture occurs in the neck of the tag. Most macrotags are only 2 to 5 μm in length. Rod etching patterns also are generally not important to the resulting bond strength.

The bonding system copolymerizes with the matrix phase of the composite, producing strong chemical bonding. The macroshear bond strength for the joint is 18 to 22 MPa and is affected by both the film thickness of the bonding system and the shear strength of adjacent enamel rods. The theoretic upper limit for joint strength is probably approximately 50 MPa. The current bond strengths of approximately 20 MPa appear to be acceptable clinically. More than 20 years of clinical monitoring has not revealed any significant degradation of the mechanical bonds due to fatigue.

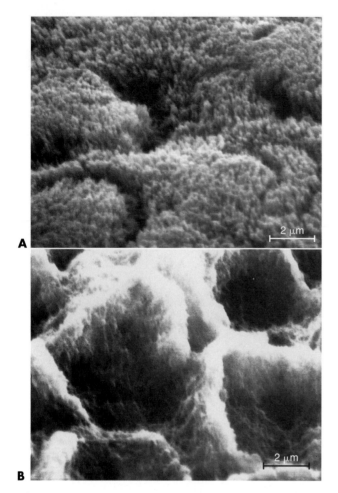

FIG. **4-54** Micromechanical retention of bonding systems to dental enamel. **A,** SEM view of etched enamel showing relief between enamel rods and within their ends. **B,** SEM view of enamel bonding agent, from which etched enamel has been removed, with cup-shaped macrotags and thousands of fine microtags on each one. *(Courtesy Stephen C. Bayne, School of Dentistry, University of North Carolina, Chapel Hill, NC.)*

Dentin Bonding Systems. Dentin bonding systems involve an unfilled (or lightly filled), liquid acrylic monomer mixture placed onto an acid-etched and primed dentin surface. The bonding primer depends on *hydrophilic monomers,* such as 2-hydroxyethyl methacrylate *(2-HEMA or HEMA),* to easily wet hydrophilic dentin surfaces that contain some moisture. Although primer and/or bonding agent may flow into dentinal tubules, the bond strength is primarily achieved by micromechanical bonding to the *intertubular dentin* (between tubules) along the cut dentin surface (see Chapter 5). Despite the fact that many dentin bonding systems have been formulated to allow chemical reactions to take place with dentin, this has had little or no apparent contribution on the final bond strength.[235] Generally, 90% or more of dentin bond strength is presumed to be due to mechanical bonding. Mechanisms of bonding and the effectiveness of current systems are presented in detail in Chapter 5.

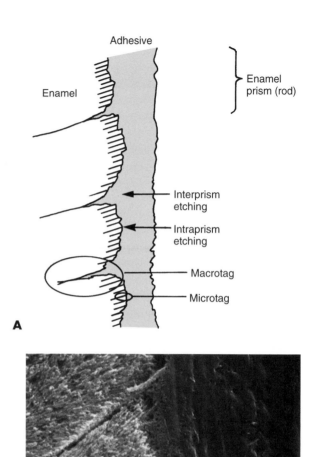

FIG. **4-55** Cross-sectional views of micromechanical retention of enamel bonding systems. **A,** Schematic view of macrotags and microtags. **B,** SEM cross-sectional view of interface of enamel bonding agent with enamel revealing microtags between macrotags. *(Courtesy Stephen C. Bayne, School of Dentistry, University of North Carolina, NC.)*

As noted earlier, mechanical preparation of dentin leaves behind a highly distorted debris layer (smear layer) that covers the surface and conceals the underlying structures (Fig. 4-56, *A*). Early dentin bonding systems were hydrophobic and were bonded directly to the dentin smear layer. Therefore macroshear bond strengths were found to be less than 6 MPa, because that is the strength of the bond of the smear layer to sound dentin. Initial dentin etching processes removed the smear layer, but tended to overetch dentin (Fig. 4-56, *B*). Bond strengths of 10 to 12 MPa were produced, and were not significantly increased until bonding systems were chemically modified to become more hydrophilic (18 to 20 MPa). Careful dentin etching produced micromechanical relief for bonding between tubules (intertubular dentin) without excessive demineralization of peritubular dentin. Coupled with hydrophilic primers, bond strengths increased to 22 to 35 MPa. The theoretic limit for dentin bonding system strength may actually be higher (80 to 100 MPa) than that for enamel, because dentin is more resistant to shear fracture. The clinically important limit for dentin bonding is not yet known. However, because of the presence of more water in dentin than enamel, *the clinical longevity of dentin bonding may not be as long as that of enamel.*

As portrayed in Fig. 4-57, the priming action in dentin bonding systems is designed to penetrate through any remnant smear layer and into the intertubular dentin and to fill the spaces left by dissolved hydroxyapatite crystals.[247] This allows acrylic monomers to form an interpenetrating network around dentin collagen. Once polymerized, this layer produces what Nakabayashi[167] referred to as the *hybrid zone (interdiffusion zone or interpenetration zone).* Depending on the particular chemistry of a bonding system, the hybrid layer may vary from 0.1 to 5 μm deep. Unfortunately, excessive etching may decalcify dentin from 1 to 10 μm deep. If this decalcified dentin zone is not filled (bonded) by bonding system, it may act as a weakened layer or zone contributing to fracture (see Chapter 5). In addition, the extent of the etching effect on the strength of the collagen fibers is not yet known. However, these systems demonstrate that stronger dentin bonding is possible and portend a bright future for bonding systems.

The key ingredient for priming in many dentin bonding systems is hydroxyethyl methacrylate (HEMA; Fig. 4-58, *A*). This molecule is an analog to methyl methacrylate, except that the pendant methyl ester is replaced by an ethoxy ester group to make it hydrophilic. Importantly, it is relatively volatile and has some tendency to produce mild sensitivity.[47,87,88,201,271] Dentists and assistants should be aware that it is very mobile, can diffuse through rubber gloves,[165] and will cause skin dryness and cracking in many individuals. *Therefore during the use of primers and bonding agents, high-volume evacuation should be used to minimize HEMA vapor contact.*

Bonding normally has been conducted in three steps (*three-component systems*). During the late 1990s, the number of stages (etching, priming, bonding) was reduced by combining the actions of various steps. *Two-component systems* were devised that either employed etching with priming/bonding or etching/priming with bonding. In the latter case, the term *self-etching primer* was used to describe the first component of the system. This is most often achieved by employing acidic monomers that dissolve or disrupt the smear layer, dissolve hydroxyapatite in the intertubular zone and tubules, and then polymerize to generate a hybrid zone. Despite the approach to designing two-component systems, they generally required significant solvent to cosolubilize the

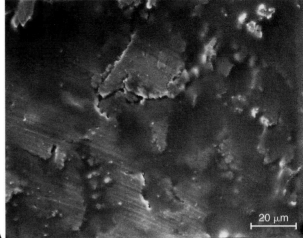

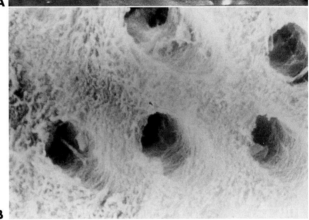

FIG. 4-56 SEM views of dentin in various stages of etching. **A,** Unetched dentin with smear layer. **B,** Overetched dentin revealing intertubular spaces and enlarged dentin tubule openings. (**A,** *Courtesy Stephen C. Bayne, School of Dentistry, University of North Carolina, Chapel Hill, NC;* **B,** *Courtesy Bruggers K, School of Dentistry, University of North Carolina, Chapel Hill, NC.)*

modifying material. Solvent levels among systems vary considerably but are generally in the range of 65% to 90% solvent.[32] Choices for solvent systems, based on acetone or ethanol with water, do affect the wetting efficiency (see Chapter 5).

For bonding systems to efficiently produce a hybrid layer, it is extremely important to keep the dentin hydrated. Quite often, the rinsing and drying of dentin that follows tooth preparation or specific etching steps, results in dehydrated superficial layers of dentin. Etched dentin no longer contains hydroxyapatite crystals between collagen fibers. It consists only of the remaining collagen and water. Dehydration, whether intentional or not, causes the remaining collagen sponge to collapse with collagen molecules forming a mat and excluding monomers necessary for hybrid layer formation. Therefore etched dentin either must be kept moist or be intentionally rehydrated. Rehydration can be accomplished with a moist cotton pledget or applicator tip in contact

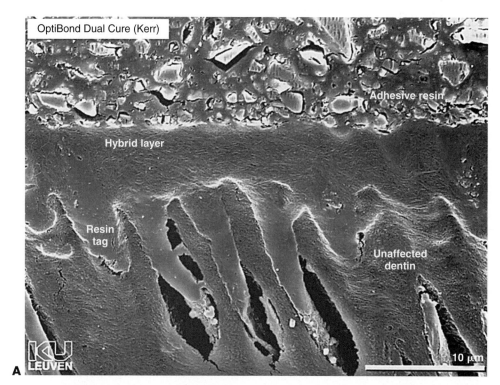

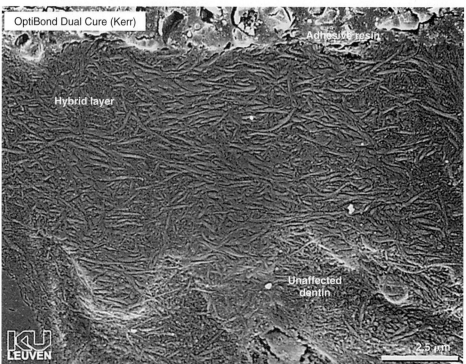

FIG. **4-57** Cross-sectional views of micromechanical retention of dentin bonding system. **A,** Schematic view of composite, hybrid layer with microtags, and tubules with resin microtags after dentin dissolution. **B,** Schematic view of resin-impregnation phase, which is responsible for most adhesion, showing the microtags within intertubular dentin as resin wrapped around collagen fibers. *(Courtesy Bart Van Meerbeek, Department of Operative Dentistry and Dental Materials, Catholic University of Leuven, Kapucijnenvoer 7, B-30000 Leuven, Belgium.)*

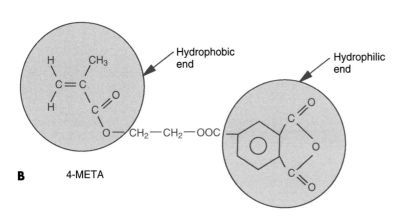

FIG. **4-58** Examples of acrylic monomers used in bonding systems because of their hydrophilicity. **A,** HEMA. **B,** 4-META.

with the surfaces for approximately 10 seconds or by the use of *rewetting agents.* If dentin moisture is inadequate, then the hybrid layer will not form, and the bonding system will fail to seal and bond. It is suspected that inadequate precautions in this regard in many bonding instructions during the early 1990s may have contributed to the premature failure of many dentin bonding systems.

The latest dentin bonding systems combine all three stages of dentin bonding into a single component (*one-component system*). This approach provides a much simpler procedure for bonding to enamel and dentin, but is not necessarily well designed to wet and bond onto other substrates such as ceramic, composite, or amalgam. Therefore, three-component systems, which allow procedural modifications to accommodate for differences in substrate properties (*multipurpose bonding systems*), may continue to be used. It is extremely challenging to create a truly universal one-component bonding system that performs well in all possible bonding situations.

Amalgam Bonding Systems. Amalgam bonding systems may be used to seal underlying tooth structure and bond amalgam to enamel and dentin. They require dual characteristics to achieve optimal wetting. Amalgam is strongly hydrophobic, whereas enamel and dentin are hydrophilic. Therefore the bonding system must be modified with a wetting agent (comonomer) that has the capacity to wet both hydrophobic or hydrophilic surfaces. Typical dentin bonding systems may be used, but special *4-methyloxy ethyl trimellitic anhydride*

(4-META)-based systems are used frequently. This monomer molecule contains both hydrophobic and hydrophilic ends (Fig. 4-58, *B*).

Macroshear bond strengths for joining amalgam to dentin are relatively low (2 to 6 MPa). Although good bonding occurs to tooth structure, micromechanical bonding at the interface of the amalgam with the bonding system is poor. Most debonding occurs by fracture along this interface. Since no chemical bonding occurs at this interface, it is important to develop micromechanical bonding. To accomplish this, the bonding system is applied in much thicker layers (10 to 50 μm), so that amalgam being condensed against the resin adhesive layer will force fluid components of the amalgam to squeeze into the unset bonding adhesive layer and produce micromechanical laminations of the two materials (Fig. 4-59). Thicker bonding agent films can be produced by adding thickening agents to the unset bonding materials or by applying many (five to eight) applications of bonding material.

The primary advantages for amalgam bonding agents in most clinical situations are the dentin sealing and improved resistance form, but the increase in retention form is not significant. Adhesion of amalgam to tooth structure is not necessary in clinical circumstances when satisfactory retention and resistance forms of tooth preparation already exist. Primary indication for amalgam bonding is when weakened tooth structure remains and bonding may improve the overall resistance form of the restored tooth.

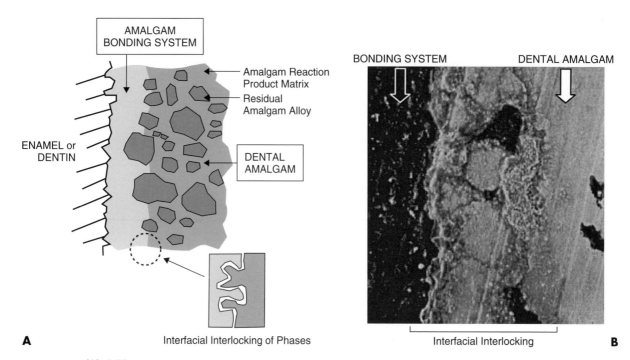

AMALGAM
BONDING SYSTEM

Amalgam Reaction
Product Matrix

Residual
Amalgam Alloy

ENAMEL or
DENTIN

DENTAL
AMALGAM

A   Interfacial Interlocking of Phases

BONDING SYSTEM   DENTAL AMALGAM

Interfacial Interlocking   B

FIG. 4-59 **A,** Schematic view of the adhesive joint created with amalgam bonding system. Micromechanical bonding holds bonding agent to the surface of etched and primed tooth structure. Thick unset bonding agent becomes interdigitated along the interface with residual amalgam alloy particles and amalgam matrix to create micromechanical interlocking. **B,** Cross-section of set amalgam *(right)* intermixed with set bonding agent *(left)* to create micromechanical bonding. *(**A,** Courtesy Stephen C. Bayne, School of Dentistry, University of North Carolina, Chapel Hill, NC. **B,** Courtesy Jorge Perdigão, Division of Operative Dentistry, University of Minnesota, Minneapolis, Minn.)*

If sealing amalgam preparations is the sole purpose for bonding, then an alternative is the use of *dentin sealers.* The earliest version of such a system (Gluma 2, Bayer Dental Products) was actually the primer component of a dentin bonding system. Since the introduction of that product, several others have been developed that are essentially primer monomers and/or polymers dissolved in solvent that penetrate the surfaces of the preparation and dry or are cured as a polymer film. The action of this film is very similar to that of varnish, except the film has much better wetting characteristics and produces a completely impervious layer. The film actually covers enamel as well as dentin but is still categorized as a dentin sealer. Because the same material may be used over open dentin tubules on exposed root surfaces to eliminate fluid flow and desensitize dentin, dentin sealers are also known as *dentin desensitizers.* However, an expansive list of other products also may be called dentin desensitizers, but they are not routinely used to seal dentin under amalgam restorations.

Bonding systems used below insulating restorations, such as composite, do not utilize traditional liners and bases except when the tooth excavation is extremely close to the pulp (RDT <0.5 mm). In that case, a traditional calcium hydroxide liner is used for pulpal medication, to stimulate reparative dentin (see Fig. 4-45).

Porcelain and Ceramic Repair Systems. Fractured regions on porcelain-fused-to-metal or all-ceramic restorations may be repaired by etching the surface with hydrofluoric (HF) acid, silanating the etched ceramic material, applying bonding agent, and adding composite to replace the missing material. This is not a long-term solution to the problem but does provide an immediate alternative rather than complete replacement of the original restoration. Wetting of ceramic materials by bonding materials is different than for dentin and may not work well with all bonding systems. If the substrate being repaired includes exposed metal alloy on a portion of a porcelain-fused-to-metal restoration, then the metal should be sandblasted and etched to enhance retention.

Cast Restoration Bonding/Luting Systems. Cast restorations are retained in teeth by appropriate preparation design and by dental cements, whose structure and properties are detailed later in this chapter. The adhesion process involves cement adaptation to surface irregularities *(dental luting cement)* in a way that helps prevent the restoration's withdrawal along the original path of insertion. Cements may be chemically adhesive (polycarboxylate or glass ionomer), but most of the bond strength results from mechanical adhesion. The limits to bond strength in these situations relate to: (1) the relatively poor wetting characteristics of viscous luting cements and (2) the relative thickness of luting cement. Both of these features contribute to low bond strength. If the cement does not wet the substrate well, then fractures propagate easily along the interface, typically with dentin. If the cement is more hydrophilic and wets dentin well, then fractures propagate within the weakest solid in the joint, which is the dental cement. *The adhesive joint bond strength is improved by using the strongest cements (composite or resin cements), roughening and etching both the casting surfaces and dentin surfaces, using composite materials that contain wetting agents, and attempting to reduce the cement thickness in the adhesive joint.* All of these features are in the section on cements used for Maryland bridges (see Chapter 15).

These same principles also apply to all other situations involving adhesion in dentistry, such as sealants, bonded orthodontic brackets, denture adhesives, porcelain-to-metal bonding, and osseointegration of implants. In some cases, adhesion involves several interfaces and is complex.

PIT-AND-FISSURE SEALANTS

Terminology. Pit-and-fissure *sealants* were first proposed for dentistry in the late 1960s. They prevent tooth preparation and restoration techniques for the elimination of caries-prone pits-and-fissures on occlusal surfaces of teeth. Pits-and-fissures that are not self-cleansing are considered caries-prone (see Figs. 3-17, 9-5, *B,* and 13-3, *A*). Normally, they accumulate organic debris and oral bacteria, providing an ideal site for the development of caries. The objectives of pit-and-fissure sealants are simply to eliminate the geometry that harbors bacteria and to prevent nutrients reaching bacteria in the base of the pit or fissure. Sealants are used to occlude portions of these sites that are not self-cleansing. Any material placed to seal these sites tends to overfill the area. Because sealant has only modest wear resistance, contact area wear and food abrasion may quickly wear it away from naturally self-cleansing areas where it is not needed. However, key areas remain occluded, resulting in continued benefits.

The principal feature of a sealant required for success is *adequate retention.* Most pits and fissures have some degree of macroretention but debris may be in the fault, access may be inadequate, or fluidity of the sealant may be insufficient to allow its penetration to the deepest recesses of these sites. Therefore micromechanical retention is required. Sealant is applied only after gross debridement, isolation, and acid etching of the surfaces. Sealant cannot be applied so precisely that there is no excess extending onto self-cleansing areas of occlusal surfaces. Therefore it is important that the material be adjusted as needed following placement (see Chapter 13 for the technique) so that it does not interfere with normal occlusal contacts or disrupt occlusal paths. Once it has been removed from self-

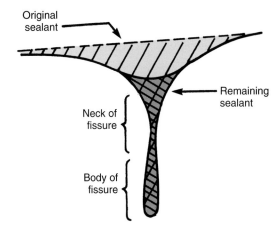

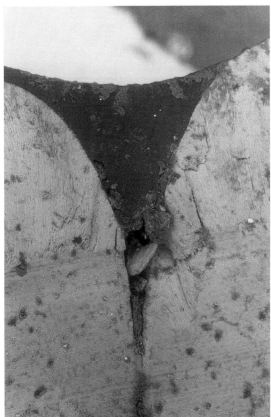

FIG. 4-60 Fissure sealants. **A,** Schematic view of idealized fissure after sealing and after loss of excess sealant. **B,** SEM cross-section of sealed fissure. Sealant does not penetrate into entire fissure. Excess sealant on occlusal surface has been mostly worn away to boundary of self-cleansing zone. (**A,** *From Bayne SC, Barton RE. In Richardson RE, Barton RE, editors:* The dental assistant, *ed 6, Philadelphia, 1988, Lea & Febiger;* **B,** *Courtesy Mitchell S, School of Dentistry, University of North Carolina, Chapel Hill, NC.*)

cleansing areas, the remaining sealant blocks bacterial accumulation occurring in otherwise non–self-cleansing locations (Fig. 4-60).

Classification. The division of sealants into classification categories is trivial. Sealants are categorized in terms of polymerization method, as *self-curing* or *visible-light–*

curing. Early sealants were based on methyl methacrylate or cyanoacrylate cements. Most contemporary compositions are unfilled (or only lightly filled) and based on difunctional monomers such as those used for the matrix of composites. The principal monomer in these systems (e.g., BIS-GM; see the section in this chapter on Historical Development) has largely been replaced by BIS-GMA analogues for political reasons during the late 1990s. This issue is discussed shortly. The principal monomer may be diluted with lower molecular weight species (e.g., triethylene glycol dimethacrylate [TEGDMA, also abbreviated TEGDM]) to reduce the viscosity. Small amounts of colorant, such as TiO_2, may be added to make the appearance slightly different from occlusal enamel. Otherwise the sealant is clear and often difficult to locate during clinical inspection on recall. Self-curing compositions have the advantage of curing quickly enough that they are retained in sites whose orientation may encourage flow away from the area. Self-curing materials have to be applied when they are fluid enough to penetrate the pit or fissure and so that they begin to cure before running away from the site. This combination of characteristics sometimes causes problems in obtaining adequate penetration. If occlusal surfaces are appropriately oriented during the procedure to control flow, then light-curing materials are actually simpler to use. They can be applied and allowed to flow for a convenient time before exposure to a visible light source for curing.

Composition, Structure, and Properties. Because the primary clinical property is flow into small access spaces, a *penetration coefficient* is normally calculated for comparison of products. It describes the relative rate of flow in a standard sized orifice. Penetration is a function of both capillary action and viscosity. If the site is well cleaned, etched, rinsed, and dried, then acrylic monomers such as BIS-GMA tend to wet the surface reasonably well. Even if the opening in the pit or fissure is small, if there is good wetting, then capillary action will

tend to draw the material into the orifice. The viscosity must be low enough, for a long enough time, for the material to penetrate into the defect site. Penetration coefficients for first generation sealants are reported in Table 4-13.

Complete penetration of sealant is not absolutely critical. It is possible to occlude only the neck region of a fissure and produce clinically acceptable results. An example of a fissure is shown in Fig. 4-60, *A*. An example of a typical cross-sectional view is shown in Fig. 4-60, *B*. Quite often, the local geometry creates a defect with a wide orifice.

Glass-ionomer sealants were explored for pit-and-fissure applications. However, they lacked sufficient abrasion resistance and were easily lost. In addition, they were brittle and prone to fracture, exposing the underlying portions of unfilled pits or fissures to the intraoral environment.

Traditional composites, by themselves, are not good sealants because they do not penetrate into pits and fissures readily because of their comparatively high viscosity. However, they may be involved in treating pit-and-fissure caries, especially when used with a bonding adhesive, because the bonding system adhesive is very similar to a sealant material. *If a fissure is minimally carious, then excavation of the caries and restoration with a very small composite provides conservative management of the defective enamel region* (see Chapter 13).

Newer low-viscosity versions of composites, flowable composites (see Composites later in this chapter), have been advocated for a wide range of applications including pit-and-fissure sealants. They have good wetting, sufficient flow, adequate abrasion resistance, and good fracture resistance. In fact, one of the earliest flowable composites was a pit-and-fissure sealant, to which a modest amount of filler had been added.

The properties of sealants are essentially those of the resin matrix component of composite materials. There is no evidence that water absorption, chemical degradation, or other events observed with composites, detract from the longevity of these materials. However, there has been a controversy concerning the BIS-GMA monomers in sealants. In 1994, a single report suggested that BIS-GMA (produced from bisphenol-A and glycidyl methacrylate reaction) could be decomposed into its constituents releasing *bisphenol-A* (BPA). BPA is known to be an estrogenic material.[181,199,217] Further investigation revealed a number of scientific problems with this report, such as the misidentification of TEGDMA as BPA. However, to avoid political controversy over the safety of these materials, manufacturers quickly switched to alternative monomers that did not include BPA as a precursor. Another problem with the original report was that measured levels of monomer released from sealants seemed unusually high. Unfortunately, it was not noted during the sampling procedure that the air-

TABLE **4-13**	Penetration Coefficients for Typical Pit-and-Fissure Sealants and Surface Sealers	
SEALANT SYSTEM	**PENETRATION COEFFICIENT**
Adaptic bonding agent	12.80 cm/s
Delton pit-and-fissure sealant	7.22 cm/s
	10.00 cm/s
Concise enamel bond	6.40 cm/s
	4.80 cm/s
Nuva Seal	3.00 cm/s
Concise white sealant	2.43 cm/s
Adaptic glaze	0.62 cm/s

Adapted from Retief DH, Mallory WP: *Pediatr Dent* 3:12-16, 1981; O'Brien WJ, Fan PL, Apostolides A: *Oper Dent* 3:51-56, 1978; and Fan PL, O'Brien WJ, Craig RG: *Oper Dent* 4:100-103, 1979.

inhibited superficial layer (see Composites later in this chapter) of resin had not been removed by wiping with a cotton roll before sampling the sealants. This small layer is generally wiped away or quickly lost during the first few chewing strokes. This material is not representative of the actual cured sealant material below. Even so, sealants are not totally innoccuous. Some of the diluent monomer (TEDGMA) remains unreacted (residual monomer) and is slowly diffused out of the sealant. However, both the small amount and the very long time period of release (see Biocompatibility earlier in this chapter) suggest that only minimal health risk would ever be involved.

Clinical Considerations. During the early 1970s a large number of clinical studies were initiated to determine both the relative reduction in caries possible with sealant use as well as the clinical longevity of sealants. Simonsen[225] has reported excellent clinical success after 15 years with teeth sealed only with a single application of sealant. Prevention of occlusal caries at defects depends simply on the exclusion of bacteria or their nutrients (Fig. 4-61). Numerous clinical investigations have demonstrated that as long as pits-and-fissures remain completely sealed, there is 100% prevention of caries at those sites.[170,207] As long as the sealant is retained, it will achieve this end. Sealant types differ in both short- and long-term retention.[152]

Absolutely no evidence indicates that sealant ever completely wears away. If the sealant is lost or leaks, then the site is once again at risk to caries. It may be lost because of failure of the acid-etching or the micromechanical retention to the acid-etched surface. It is common for saliva or moist air contamination to interfere with the effects of acid-etching. However, loss of sealant from areas that are not self-cleansing is minimal.

The ideal time to apply sealants is soon after occlusal surfaces erupt into the oral environment. However, at that time, very little of the tooth has erupted and it is difficult or impossible to use a rubber dam for moisture control. Therefore cotton rolls and/or absorbent wedges may be used instead. Without special care, it is common for some contamination of the acid-etched enamel to occur. This contamination prevents resin penetration into micromechanical spaces and leads to premature failure. During recalls, if the sealant has been lost, then it can be reapplied. With careful management and repair of sealed surfaces it is possible to achieve 100% reduction in occlusal caries in those areas.

Sealants also have been applied to smooth-surface tooth structure to try to eliminate caries. For smooth surfaces, however, fluoridated water is very effective in reducing caries prevalence. Sealants that have been applied to smooth surfaces are abraded by food and/or toothbrushes and may be lost at relatively rapid rates. Because toothbrush bristles are large, they do not affect sealants in pits-and-fissures.

Fluoride-containing sealants have been investigated. The contribution of fluoride in these circumstances may be very small at best. Clinical studies in which sealants were used to seal fissures that were minimally carious, produced complete inhibition of the caries process. Therefore fluoride modification of the enamel would not seem to be very beneficial. Although not proven, there is strong suspicion that any retained sealants do not leak along their margins. Those that are poorly bonded are lost almost immediately. In those circumstances, the limited time for diffusion of fluoride from the sealant to the underlying tooth structure would probably not provide sufficient fluoride to completely discourage caries.

Another important consideration for sealant use is the degree to which children and adolescents are susceptible to caries. Strong evidence supports that there are two categories of young patients, one with a much greater caries predisposition (see Chapter 1 and 3). This latter category of patients would benefit the most from the use of pit-and-fissure sealants. One sure indication of apparent caries susceptibility is a dental history of caries on the occlusal surfaces of primary teeth.[17,69,218] If

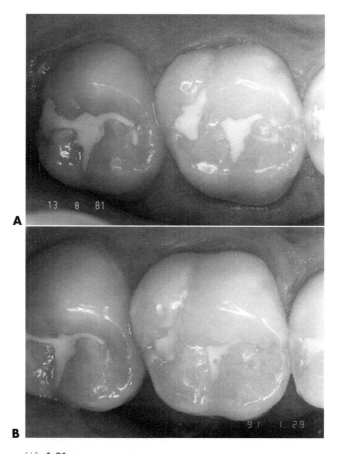

FIG. **4-61** Example of function of sealant on first molar after (**A**) 5 years and (**B**) 15 years of clinical service. Some abrasion of sealant has occurred in occlusal areas that appear self-cleansing. *(From Simonsen RJ: J Am Dent Assoc 122(11):34-42, 1992.)*

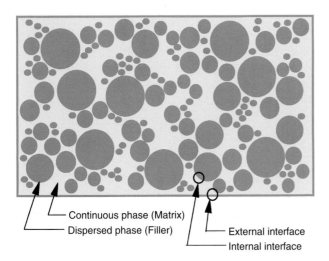

Continuous phase (Matrix)
Dispersed phase (Filler)
External interface
Internal interface

FIG. **4-62** Key components of composites. Schematic view of generalized composite showing continuous phase, dispersed phase, internal interfaces, and external interface.

all individuals were routinely being examined by a dentist, then their record would provide simple evidence for the choice of whether to apply sealants to the permanent teeth. Older patients with reduced saliva flow are at increased risk to caries and also should be considered candidates for sealants.

Sealants also are used to repair or seal leaking or failing dental restorations.[152] Sealants have demonstrated great usefulness in sealing poor margins of amalgam restorations for up to 15 years.[153] In some cases, sealants also have been used to successfully seal surfaces of incipient carious lesions adjacent to existing restorations.

Despite the enormous long-term benefit for patients with sealed pits-and-fissures, this prevention method was used routinely by only approximately 16% of dental practices in the United States in 1992. This low level of usage reflects several influences. When the first sealants were placed several decades ago, a high level of technical difficulty led to early failure. For many years, some dentists have expressed limited enthusiasm for prevention. Frustration was associated with delayed commitment by insurance carriers to reimburse dental practices for these procedures. It is now accepted that *sealants provide outstanding service, when done properly, for very low costs. In societies committed to dental care, this is a core strategy for early management of caries.*

An interesting adjunct preventive technique has been the use of fluoride varnishes.[118,191] Fluoride varnishes first appeared in clinical practice in the late 1960s in Europe, about the same time as pit-and-fissure sealants, but were not adopted for use in the United States[20] until the late 1990s. Due to the fluoride-releasing levels of these materials, they are treated as medical devices and strictly regulated by the Food and Drug Administration (FDA). Clinical trials[192] on effectiveness have been exclusively conducted in children to date, demonstrating ex-

cellent effectiveness. The only clinical disadvantage is the temporary discoloration of the teeth.

Fluoride-containing varnishes (e.g., Duraphat [Colgate], Durafluor [Pharmascience], Fluor Protector [Ivoclar-Vivadent]) are intended only as temporary films on teeth that extend the contact of fluoride with existing tooth structure.[35] They remain on tooth structure for many hours, affording more opportunity to produce fluoride-modified hydroxyapatite that is more acid resistant (i.e., more caries resistant) and accelerating the remineralization of early carious lesions. These are generally considered as effective as or more effective than topical fluoride treatments. These varnishes contain a film-forming agent (e.g., as ethyl cellulose or collodion), releasable fluoride, solvents, and wetting agents. They are applied to teeth with a brush, cotton-tip applicator, or syringe-type applicator in just a couple of minutes during which time they dry to coat tooth surfaces. To maintain the fluoride effect, these should be reapplied approximately every 6 months. *The main cariostatic effect of fluoride varnishes is the remineralization of early carious lesions.*

COMPOSITES

Terminology. A *composite* is a physical mixture of materials. The parts of the mixture generally are chosen with the purpose of averaging the properties of the parts to achieve intermediate properties. Quite often a single material does not have the appropriate properties for a specific dental application.

A schematic view of a generalized composite is presented in Fig. 4-62. Composites typically involve a *dispersed phase* of *filler particles* distributed within a *continuous phase (matrix phase).* In most cases, the matrix phase is fluid at some point during the manufacture or fabrication of a composite system.

A *dental composite* has traditionally indicated a mixture of silicate glass particles within an acrylic monomer that is polymerized during the application. The silicate particles provide mechanical reinforcement of the mixture (reinforcing fillers) and produce light transmission and light scattering that adds enamel-like translucency to the material. The acrylic monomers make the initial mixture fluid and moldable for placement into a tooth preparation. The matrix flows to adapt to tooth preparation walls and penetrate into micromechanical spaces on etched enamel or dentin surfaces.

Because the flow of uncured composite is quite limited, most composite manufacturers provide a *bonding system*. Bonding systems are primarily unfilled acrylic monomer mixtures, similar to the matrix of the composite, that are preplaced onto etched tooth surfaces to form a 1- to 5-μm film. It micromechanically interlocks with the etched surfaces, seals the walls of the preparation, and copolymerizes with the composite restorative material that fills the tooth preparation. Dentin and/or enamel

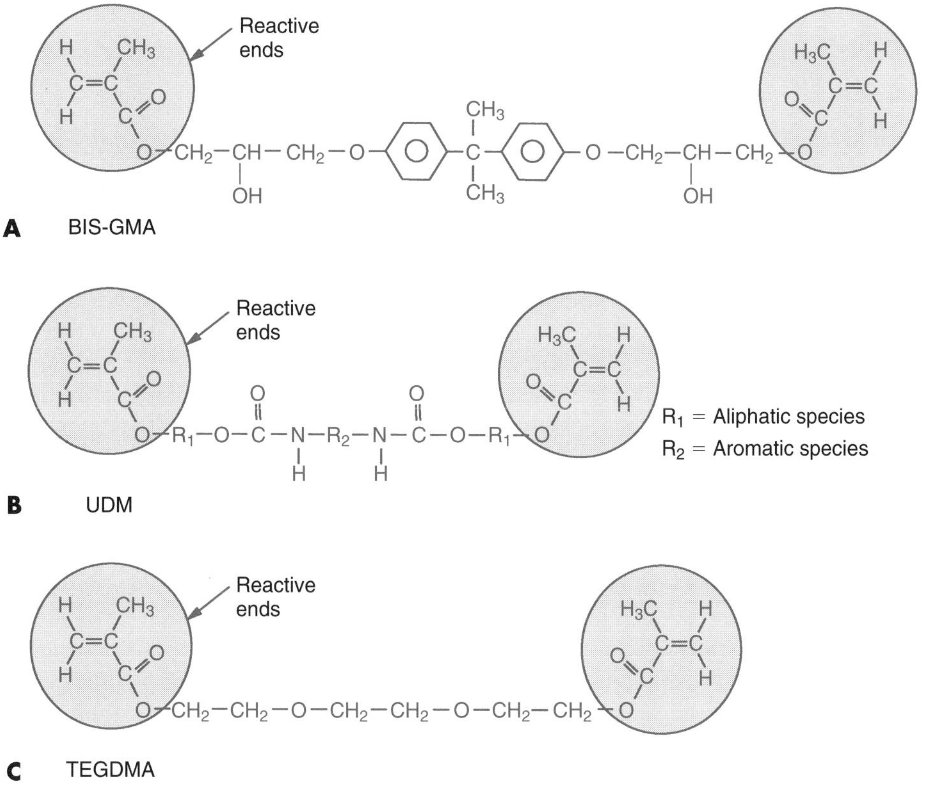

FIG. 4-63 Chemical formulas of difunctional monomers commonly used in composites. **A,** BIS-GMA monomer. **B,** UDM monomer. **C,** TEGDMA monomer.

bonding systems, or universal bonding systems, may be provided as part of the composite product package.

Although "dental composite" or "composite" is the technically correct term for these materials, various terms have been widely accepted as well. Composites often have been called *composite restorative materials, filled resins, composite resins, resin composites, resin-based composites,* or *filled composites.*

These alternative terms become more confusing as the field of dental polymers becomes more sophisticated and simultaneously more complex. In this textbook, the term *composite* is used. Most dental materials are composites of some type. If these compositions are modified to include special polymer phases, then they may be called resin-containing composites. For example, glass-ionomer cements have been modified with both polymer-containing fillers and monomer-containing matrices. They are classified as *hybrid* or *resin-modified glass ionomers* but could equally well be described as modified composites.

Historical Development. Early attempts at esthetic filling materials that predated acrylic resins and composites were based on silicate cements. These cements resulted from reactions of phosphoric acid with acid-soluble glass particles to form a silica gel matrix containing residual glass particles. Solubility problems with these materials led to the introduction of unfilled acrylic systems based on polymethyl methacrylate (PMMA).

Methyl methacrylate (MMA) monomer contracted excessively during polymerization, permitting subsequent marginal leakage. Also, PMMA was not strong enough to support occlusal loads. Therefore reinforcing ceramic fillers, principally containing silica, were added to the composition. Retrospectively, the original PMMA materials now are called *unfilled acrylics.* (If the amount of filler or fillerlike phase added to a resin matrix is small, the overall composition is considered unfilled. Therefore 1% to 2% filler-modified sealant compositions are still classified as unfilled.)

MMA-based matrices were supplanted by *BIS-GMA* (alternatively Bis-GMA). BIS-GMA is a difunctional monomer originally produced as the reaction product of bisphenol-A and glycidyl methacrylate (Fig. 4-63, *A*).[37] Several analogues of that structure have been investigated (modified BIS-GMA). Another very similar difunctional molecule used in composites is *urethane dimethacrylate (UDMA).* UDMA replaces the bisphenol-A backbone with a linear isocyanate one (see Fig. 4-63, *B*). Both BIS-GMA and UDMA are extremely viscous. For practical reasons, they are diluted with another difunctional monomer with an aliphatic backbone, *TEGDMA,* of much lower viscosity (see Fig. 4-63, *C*).

To gain the full advantage of a composite formulation, it is very important to provide interfacial bonding between the phases. In modern composites, silica particles are precoated with monomolecular films of *silane coupling agents.* These molecules are difunctional. One end is capable of bonding to hydroxyl groups, which exist along the surface of the silica particles, and the other end is capable of copolymerizing with double bonds of monomers in the matrix phase. Coupling agents work best with silica particles. Therefore all composites have been based on silica-containing fillers.

Filler compositions often are modified with other ions to produce desirable changes in properties. Lithium (Li) and aluminum (Al) ions make the glass easier to crush to generate small particles. Barium (Ba), zinc (Zn), boron (B), zirconium (Zr), and yttrium (Y) ions have been used to produce *radiopacity* in the filler particles. Excessive modification (by replacement of the silicon in the structure) however, can reduce the efficacy of silane coupling agents.

Pure silica occurs in several crystalline forms (such as crystobalite, tridymite, or quartz) and in a noncrystalline form (glass). Crystalline forms are stronger and harder, but when used, result in composites that are difficult to finish and polish (Fig. 4-64). Therefore most composites are now produced using silicate glass. Barium, zinc, and yttrium-modified silicate glasses are currently the most popular fillers.

The *fluidity* of a mixture of filler and matrix monomer is affected by the fluidity of the monomer and the amount of filler incorporated. The friction between the filler particle surfaces and the monomer is a principal factor controlling the fluidity. As the filler surface area increases, the fluidity decreases. Large filler particles have a relatively small amount of particle surface area per unit of filler particle volume. As an equivalent volume of smaller filler particles is used to replace larger ones, the surface area increases rapidly. For example, when filler particles with diameters that are one tenth as large are substituted, the surface area increases by a factor of 10. The situation is further exacerbated for microfiller particles made from SiO_2, which tend to agglomerate into chains.

Placement of composites cannot be accomplished so precisely that adjustments to anatomic contours will not be needed after curing. Typically, the restoration is produced by intentionally overfilling the tooth preparation a small amount. The anatomic contours are accomplished by gross cutting (*grinding*), fine cutting (*finishing*), and then smoothing (*polishing*) the material after polymerization.

Particle sizes in composites affect other properties as well as fluidity. For example, filler particle size has a direct effect on the surface roughness of the ground, finished, or polished composite. Filler particles are harder than the matrix. Thus during finishing, some particles may be left protruding from the surface, while others are stripped out of the surface leaving holes. If the particles are very small, then the resulting surface rough-

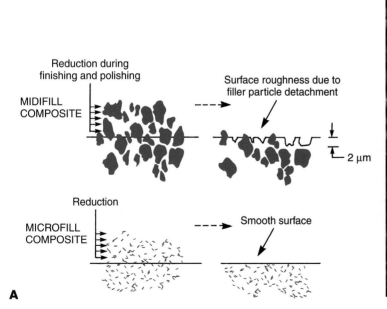

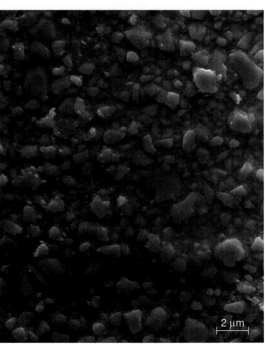

A   **B**

FIG. **4-64** Effect of particle size on surface finish of composite. **A,** Schematic illustration of finishing midifill versus microfill composite surfaces. **B,** SEM view of coarsely finished midifill composite surface. (*Courtesy Stephen C. Bayne, School of Dentistry, University of North Carolina, Chapel Hill, NC.*)

ness is of little concern. This effect is illustrated schematically in Fig. 4-64. Otherwise, the rough areas may contribute to light scattering and collection of organic debris or stain.

Effectiveness of restoration finishing and polishing procedures depends on careful use of successively finer abrasive materials to eliminate larger scratches or defects and replace them with smaller ones. This process is schematically summarized in Fig. 4-65. Final finish of the composite surface is a result of the combination of filler particle size effects and finishing scratches. Average roughness of the surface is recorded in terms of the extent of hills and valleys measured on surface profiles. The measurements can be collected with profilometers (e.g., Surfanalyzer) or atomic force microscopes (AFM). An example of an AFM image and the calculated *surface roughness*, Ra, is demonstrated in Fig. 4-66. Surfaces

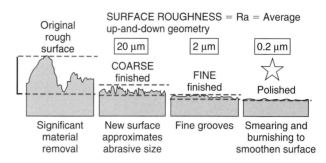

FIG. **4-65** Schematic summary of the microscopic events during finishing and polishing operations. Rough surface is gradually cut away by finer and finer abrasives (coarse and fine finishing). Polishing produces very little cutting but does tend to smear material (burnishing) from remaining high spots into low spots and create a smooth surface. The final surface finish is measured as the average up-and-down surface roughness remaining (Ra) by profiling select areas of the surface.

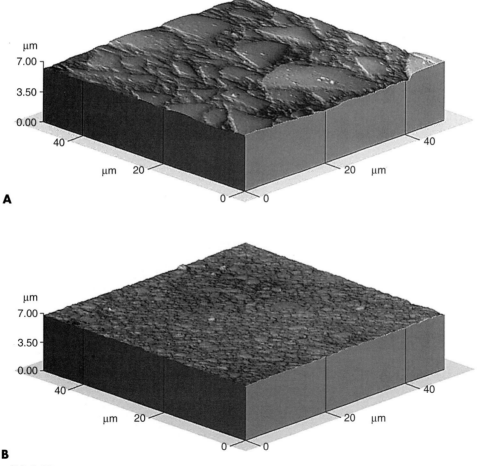

FIG. **4-66** AFM view of a surface with an average roughness (Ra) corresponding to 0.2 μm. **A,** AFM image of finely finished midifill composite (note the relief of filler particle margins produced by the finishing process). **B,** AFM image of finely finished minifill composte. *(Courtesy Thompson JY, School of Dentistry, University of North Carolina, Chapel Hill, NC.)*

TABLE 4-14	Examples of Filler Level Ranges for Typical Composites in Terms of Weight and Volume Percent*		
WEIGHT %	**VOLUME %**	**COMPOSITES**
0	0	[Unfilled resin, bonding agents, pit-and-fissure sealants]
	10	[Sealants filled with colorants]
	20	
50	30	Homogenous microfills
	40	Flowables (low filler content)
75	50	Macrofills, midifills
	60	Hybrid midifills, heterogenous microfills, flowables (high filler content)
85	70	Hybrid minifills, packable composites
	80	
	90	[ENAMEL]
100	100	

*The composites are reported using a classification system based on filler particle sizes. Systems that are not dental composites are reported in brackets. Volume percent filler is always less in amount than weight percent filler for the same composition because the glass filler is denser than the resin matrix. Typically, 75 weight percent filler is equal to 50 volume percent filler, as shown on the table.

with average roughness values of less than 1 μm are considered, clinically, very smooth. It is common to be able to achieve surface smoothness in the range of 0.2 to 0.6 μm using submicron polishing pastes on materials that include submicron filler phases.

Classification. Composites generally are classified with respect to the components, amounts, properties of their filler or matrix phases, or by their handling properties. The most common classification method is based on filler content (weight or volume percent), filler particle size, and method of filler addition. Composites also could be defined on the basis of the matrix composition (*BIS-GMA or UDMA*) or polymerization method (*self-curing, ultraviolet light-curing, visible light–curing, dual curing, or staged curing*), but these do not communicate as much information about the properties.

Almost all important properties of composites are improved by using higher filler levels. The only practical problem is that, as the filler level is increased, the fluidity decreases. Highly filled compositions typically contain large filler particles, but as previously stated, this composition results in a rougher finished surface. Smaller filler particles are used to guarantee that composites have a relatively smooth finished surface; however, this choice compromises the filler level possible and therefore the material's properties.

The degree of filler addition is represented in terms of the weight percent or volume percent of filler. Because silica fillers are approximately three times as dense as acrylic monomer (or polymer), 75 weight percent filler is equivalent to approximately 50 volume percent filler. Properties of composites are proportional to the volume percent of the phases involved. But, it is much easier to both measure and formulate composites using weight percentages rather than volume percentages and, in dentistry, the weight percent is much more commonly reported. A conversion of *filler levels* and cor-

responding classifications of composites is presented in Table 4-14.

Filler particle sizes for the earliest composites averaged 10 to 20 μm in diameter, with many of the larger particles as large as 50 μm (Figs. 4-67 and 4-68). At first, there was no need to distinguish the particle size range or ranges of composites because all commercial products were in approximately the same range. During the evolution of formulations toward better finishing characteristics and greater resistance to wear, smaller and smaller filler particles were used. Because the early filler particles were relatively large, composites based on those large fillers became known as *macrofill* materials. The terms macrofill or macrofiller are preferred to macrofilled because they properly describe the filler particle size and not the method of producing the mixture. During the course of composite evolution, nomenclatures and classification systems have been neither consistent nor uniform.[33,58,121,135,212,246,259] In the following sections, composites are classified either in terms of their particle size range or comparative finishing characteristics. Each classification is presented.

Classification of composites based on the range of filler particle size range has been partially developed by several authors.[58,110,112,121,135,212,246,258,259] That system is extended here to include the particle size by order of magnitude, acknowledging mixed ranges of particle sizes, and distinguishing precured composite pieces as special filler. Composite filler particles are called *macrofillers* in the range of 10 to 100 μm, *midifillers* from 1 to 10 μm, *minifillers* from 0.1 to 1 μm, and *microfillers* from 0.01 to 0.1 μm. Very large individual filler particles, called *megafillers*, also have been used in special circumstances. New ultrasmall fillers are being investigated that are from 0.005 to 0.01 μm in diameter and are called *nanofillers*. Accordingly, composites are classified by particle size as *megafill, macrofill, midifill, minifill, microfill,* and

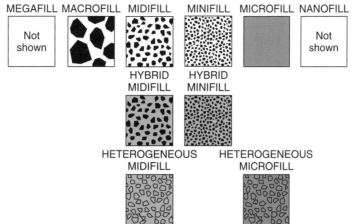

FIG. **4-67** Summary of filler particle size-based classification system for dental composites. Composites are grouped on the basis of: (1) primary particle size, (2) whether they are hybrids because of particle size mixing, (3) whether composite is a homogeneous mixture of filler and resin or includes precured composite (heterogeneous), and (4) whether chopped fiber is added to composite (not shown).

nanofill. Composites with mixed ranges of particle sizes are called *hybrids,* and the largest particle size range is used to define the hybrid type (e.g., minifill hybrid) because microfillers are normally the second part of the mixture. If the composite simply consists of filler and uncured matrix material, it is classified as *homogeneous.* If it includes precured composite or other unusual filler, it is called *heterogeneous.* If it includes novel filler modifications in addition to conventional fillers, then it is called *modified,* such as *fiber-modified homogeneous minifill.*

After the early macrofill composites, the next generation had fillers that were 8 to 10 μm in average size (midifillers) and were originally designated *fine particle* composites to imply their improved finishing characteristics. These new materials quickly became popular and were used primarily for anterior restorations in place of silicate cements and direct-filling resins. The category soon became known as *traditional* or *conventional* composites, but that designation has become confusing as newer composites continue to evolve with even smaller particle size ranges. The next step in composite evolution was to utilize 0.02- to 0.04-μm diameter particles to produce *microfill* composites. The term microfiller was already in common use for these particles in nondental applications. Microfill composites also were called *fine finishing* composites. The small filler particle size produced high viscosities in the uncured mixes of BIS-GMA with TEGDMA and requires the addition of greater amounts of monomer diluents, along with a reduced overall filler content to maintain workable consistencies.

To circumvent part of the viscosity problem, two strategies were developed. The first was to blend precured microfill composite with uncured material. Precured particles were generated by grinding cured composites to a 1- to 20-μm sized powder. The precured

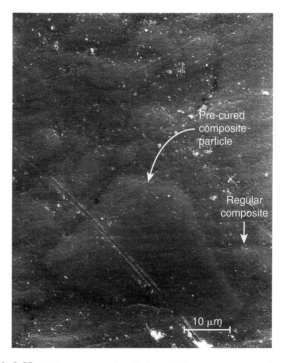

FIG. **4-68** SEM cross-sectional view of heterogeneous microfill composite. *(Courtesy Stephen C. Bayne and Duane F. Taylor, School of Dentistry, University of North Carolina, Chapel Hill, NC.)*

particles become chemically bonded to the new material, provide islands with better properties, and can be finely finished. These variants are known as *heterogeneous microfills* (or *organic filler* composites). An example is shown schematically in Fig. 4-67 and in a scanning electron micrograph in Fig. 4-68. Unmodified microfills are called *homogeneous microfills.* A second approach has been to sinter small filler particles into large but porous filler particles, impregnate them with monomer, and add the new particles to a microfill composite. Within the local region of the sintered filler particle, the material is highly filled and yet capable of being polished.

After it was realized that highly filled microfills were difficult to use, composites were formulated with mixtures of particles in the microfiller range and 2 to 5 μm range. These bimodal distributions allowed higher filler levels and still permitted good finishing. All types of mixtures are known collectively as *hybrid* composites. Currently, the principal particle size for newer materials is in the 0.1 to 1 μm range. These composites might be called *minihybrids*.

New composites are being developed with nanofillers that range in size from 0.005 to 0.01 μm, which is below the wavelength range for visible light (0.02 to 2 μm).[72] Because these particles do not interact with visible light, they do not produce scattering or significant absorption. Nonsilicate-based compositions can be used for nanofillers because they are effectively invisible. Nonsilicate fillers do not tend to agglomerate in chains like typical silica-based fillers. Nanofillers are so small that they fit between several polymer chains. These characteristics permit the opportunity to achieve very high filler loading levels in composites while still maintaining workable consistencies. Consideration of nanofillers, particularly of compositions other than silica, complicates the classification system for composites even further. Potentially, the composition will have to be stated along with the particle size range in order to identify the material structure.

Although the vast preponderance of filler in composite is equiaxed rough particles, there is increasing interest in fiber-reinforced systems. The main advantage of fibers is that they have excellent strength in the primary fiber direction. Unfortunately, it is difficult to efficiently pack the fibers or orient their direction. Small additions of fibers to regular fillers are effective in improving properties. The limiting factor is that fibers only may be used with dimensions greater than 1 μm because of the concerns for carcinogenicity of submicron fibers such as asbestos. Most current fibers have diameters of 5 to 10 μm and effective lengths of 20 to 40 μm.

Single crystals generally have symmetric shapes and are commonly long plates, behaving like fibers. Their singular advantage is that they are much stronger than noncrystalline or polycrystalline fibers. The strongest example of a crystal-modified composite is an experimental composition that employs SiC single crystals.[265,266] Unfortunately the crystals are colored and not well suited for esthetic compositions. However, in clinical uses in which esthetics are not important, these crystal-modified composites could be very valuable.

Another consequence of advances in the control of filler particle size, particle size distribution, particle morphology, and monomer technology has been the introduction of composites with specific handling characteristics. These include *flowable composites* and *packable composites*. Flowable composites are a class of low-

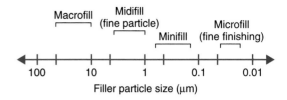

FIG. **4-69** Composite filler ranges versus particle size (shown on a logarithmic scale).

viscosity materials that possess particle sizes and particles size distributions similar to those of hybrid composites, but with reduced filler content, which allows the increased amount of resin to decrease the viscosity of the mixture. Because flowable composites were developed with specific handling characteristics in mind, their range of advertised clinical uses is quite varied. Within the range of materials classified as flowable composites, those with lower filler content are intended for uses such as pit-and-fissure sealants or small anterior restorations. Those with higher filler content have been suggested for use in Classes I, II, III, IV, and V restorations, although they are better suited only for very conservative restorative procedures. In general, the mechanical properties of flowable composites are inferior to those of standard hybrid composites.[26,257]

Packable composites, also referred to as *condensable composites*, were developed in a direct effort to produce a composite with handling characteristics similar to amalgam, thus the moniker of "packable" or "condensable." These "amalgam alternatives" are intended primarily for Class I and Class II restorations. The composition and properties reported for early examples of this class of composites suggest that they represent little or no improvement over traditional hybrid composites.[126,213] The distinguishing characteristics of packable composites are less stickiness and higher viscosity (stiffness) than traditional hybrid composites, which allows them to be placed in a manner that somewhat resembles amalgam placement, although they do not truly undergo condensation like amalgam. Because of this, "packable composite" is a more appropriate description of this class of composites.

Examples of the filled composite designations are shown in Fig. 4-67. Mean filler particle sizes of those designations are shown in Fig. 4-69. Mean filler particle sizes may often not correspond to any actual particle size because of polydisperse distributions. Fig. 4-70 shows examples of the particle size distributions for several composites. There is no practical limitation on the complexity of filler particle compositions or particle size distributions. New composites may be better described simply as polydisperse.

In addition to inorganic or composite fillers, it is possible to add *crystalline polymer fillers*. Some newer composites include crystalline polymer to supplement traditional fillers. Crystalline polymer is not nearly as strong as inorganic filler, but it is stronger than amorphous polymer material.

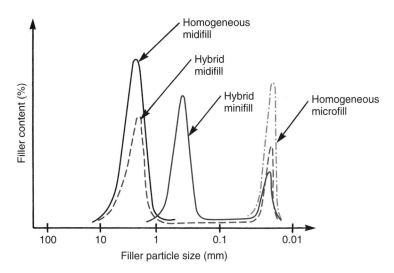

FIG. **4-70** Schematic of particle size distributions for homogeneous midifill, hybrid midifill, hybrid minifill, and homogeneous microfill composites.

Microfill and hybrid composites utilize microfillers of SiO_2 that can be produced in a variety of ways and therefore are designated with different names. Two basic forms are used in dental compositions. *Colloidal silica* is chemically precipitated from a liquid solution as amorphous silica particles. *Pyrogenic silica* is precipitated from a gaseous phase as amorphous particles.[108] The actual properties of each form are slightly different, but the differences have not yet been shown to produce different clinical properties for composites.

For posterior composite restorations, it is also possible to place one or two large glass inserts (0.5- to 2-mm particles) into composites at points of occlusal contact or high wear. These pieces of glass are referred to as *inserts* (or *megafillers*). Although they have demonstrated improved wear resistance to contact area wear, the techniques are more complicated and do not totally eliminate contact-free area (CFA) wear. Furthermore, the bonding of the composite to the insert is questionable.

Matrix monomers for composites used in the United States traditionally have been based on BIS-GMA as the primary monomer. UDMA has been more popular in European composites. Initially, better adhesion and/or resistance to color change was predicted for the UDMA formulations, but clinical studies have not been able to document these advantages.

Matrix monomers can be polymerized in a variety of ways. The original composites adopted self-curing chemistry that was typical of dental denture base compositions. These composites have been called *self-cured, chemically cured,* or *two-component systems.* Amine accelerators that were used to increase polymerization rates, however, contributed to discoloration after 3 to 5 years of intraoral service. An alternative system was introduced that used *ultraviolet light (UV light-cured)* to initiate polymerization. The curing units required were of limited reliability and presented some safety problems. They, in turn, were replaced with *visible light–cured* (VLC) or *light-cured* (LC) systems.

LC composites are the most popular today, but their

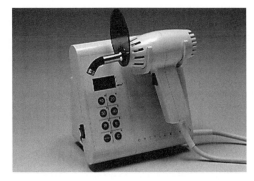

FIG. **4-71** Example of visible light–curing unit for use with composites, bonding agents, and other light-curing materials. The main power supply is connected to a pistol-grip light gun that generates a beam that is passed through the fiber-optic tube. A shield is supplied to protect against direct observation of high-intensity light at the tip *(Courtesy Kerr-Sybron, Orange, Calif.).*

success depends on the access of high-intensity light to cure the matrix material (Fig. 4-71). If the composite thickness exceeds 1.5 to 2 mm, then the light intensity can be inadequate to produce complete curing, especially with darker shades of composite. Filler particles and coloring agents tend to scatter or absorb the curing light in the first 1 to 2 mm of material. Darker shades and microfills are more difficult to cure. Access to interproximal areas is limited and may require a special technique to guarantee adequate light-curing energy. Because of these problems, more and more composite compositions are *dual cured*, combining self-curing and light-curing. The self-curing rate is slow and is designed to cure only those portions not adequately light-cured. Another approach is to provide *staged curing*. In some instances, composite finishing can be complicated by relatively hard, fully cured material. By filtering the light from the curing unit during an initial cure, it is possible to produce a soft, partially cured material that can be easily finished. Afterwards, the filter is removed and the composite curing is completed with full spectrum visible light.

Light-Curing Variables. A key consideration for *light-curing* in dentistry is the plethora of variables associated with the operation. Light-curing can be accomplished with *quartz-tungsten-halogen* (QTH) curing units, *plasma arc* curing (PAC) units, *laser* curing units, and *light-emitting diode* (LED) curing units. Examples of each are shown in Fig. 4-72. Each has different operational characteristics but acts as a source of visible light energy. The spectral output (intensity versus wavelength; Fig. 4-73) of different types of lights or different commercial units may vary, but each one attempts to maximize the light in the absorption range of the photoinitiator within the composite being cured. The vast majority of current composites employ camphoroquinone as the photoinitiator, and it absorbs photons of light energy, predominantly at 474 nm.

The challenge to effectively cure light-cured dental materials is illustrated by the large number of variables shown in Fig. 4-74. Light-curing variables are logically grouped in terms of those associated with the: (1) curing equipment, (2) clinical manipulation of the curing light, and (3) restoration effects on curing light absorption. Each of these is considered separately in the following paragraphs.

Different categories of curing lights produce a spectrum of light in different ways. The problems of all are illustrated by considering QTH light-curing systems. Within the light-curing unit is a power supply that heats a tungsten filament in a quartz bulb containing a halogen gas. The output of the bulb depends on the voltage control and operational characteristics of the bulb. New bulbs are not necessarily equivalent. Older curing units often demonstrate voltage variations. A typical QTH bulb is rated for 80 to 100 hours (approximately 2½ years of average clinical practice use) but may last two to three times as long under ideal conditions. Within the light-curing unit, the light from the bulb is collected by reflecting it from a silverized mirror behind the bulb toward the path down the fiber-optic chain to the tip. It is extremely important that the mirror surface be kept clean. This surface becomes heated during the operation of the light and then cools down between uses. It often condenses vapors from mercury, bonding system solvents, or moisture in the operatory air onto its surface, dulling or clouding its surface. It is possible to routinely clean this surface with alcohol or methyl ethyl ketone solvents on cotton swabs to renew its reflection effectiveness. The reflector is parabolic in geometry (Fig. 4-75), rather than being hemispherical, in order to focus the light toward a small fiber-optic entry. Of the light produced, less than 0.5% is suitable for curing, and most is converted at some point into heat. To minimize any heating that might occur during light-curing, two filters are inserted in the path of the light just before the fiber-optic system. The ultraviolet and infrared bandpass filters eliminate significant amounts of unnecessary light

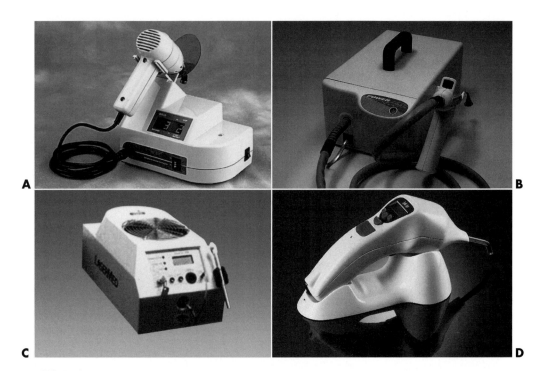

FIG. **4-72** Examples of four types of visible light–curing units used to polymerize composite materials. **A,** QTH curing unit; **B,** plasma arc curing (PAC) unit; **C,** laser curing unit; **D,** light-emitting diode (LED) curing unit. (**A,** *Courtesy Bisco, 1100 Irving Park Road, Schaumburg, Ill.* **B,** *Courtesy DMD Dental/Medical Diagnostic Systems, Inc., 6416 Variel Avenue, Woodland Hills, Calif.* **C,** *Courtesy LaserMed, West Jordan, Utah.* **D,** *Courtesy DMD Dental/Medical Diagnostic Systems, Inc., 6416 Variel Avenue, Woodland Hills, Calif.*)

and convert it into heat within the unit. A small fan is used to dissipate unwanted heat from the filters and reflector. Bandpass filters can be made from special glass or plastic coatings on clear glass. Filters may degrade as they become fatigued by numerous heating and cooling cycles.

Light passed through the fiber-optic bundle is emitted from the tip of the curing unit. Some light intensity is lost through the fiber-optic system. The output characteristics of the tip are generally not uniform, with high intensity light observed in the center of the bundle. Resin contamination on the curing unit tip tends to scatter the light, reducing the effective output quite a bit. Therefore the tip should be cleaned of cured resin, when necessary, using an appropriate rubber wheel on a slow-speed handpiece.

The curing light output can be monitored directly with a built-in or portable radiometer or by trial-curing of some composite material. However, the former approach is much more sensitive to curing problems. Most modern curing lights include a convenient radiometer as part of the unit that measures the number of photons per unit of area per unit of time. Unfortunately, it does not discriminate the light energy that is matched to the photoinitiator. It measures all light energy. Thus, the real value of the measurement is limited. Generally, QTH curing lights functioning in the normal range have outputs from 400 to 800 mW/cm². *A good rule of thumb is that the minimum output should never drop below 300 mW/cm2.* A radiometer is designed to measure the photon level per unit time through a standard 11 mm diameter window. Therefore smaller or larger curing unit tips cannot be effectively tested. Light energy entering into a fiber-optic bundle is diffused or concentrated depend-

ing on whether the curing unit tip is larger or smaller, respectively. Shifting from a standard 11-mm diameter tip to a small 3 mm diameter has the effect of increasing the light output eightfold. This increases the chance that heat produced in the curing procedure will raise the temperature of the restoration and surrounding dentin to much more dangerous levels. Increases in pulpal temperatures of more than 5° to 8° C easily cause cell death.[272,273]

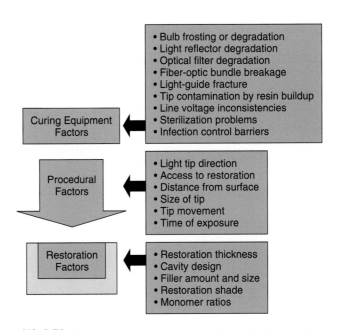

FIG. 4-74 List of variables associated with visible light–curing linked to the equipment, manipulation procedure, and restorative material.

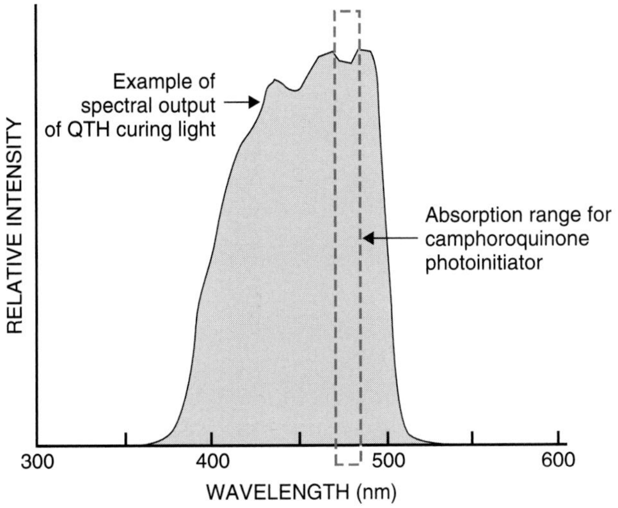

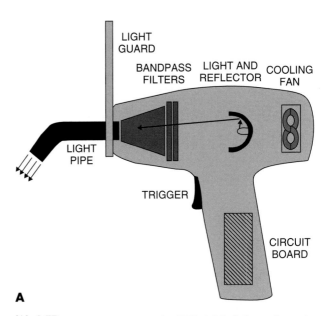

FIG. 4-73 Example of spectral output of QTH light-curing unit compared to absorption range for camphoroquinone photoinitiator, which is in most bonding agents and composites that are light-cured. Unabsorbed light is principally converted into heat energy.

FIG. 4-75 Internal operation of a QTH visible light–curing unit. **A,** Schematic of a typical pistol grip handle attached to the power supply for the unit.

Continued

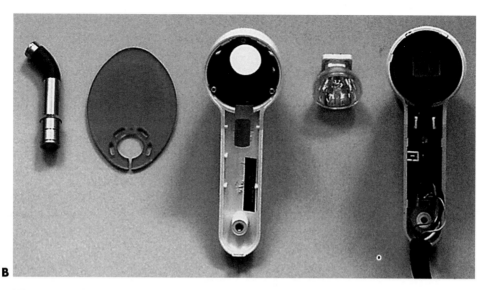

FIG. **4-75, cont'd** **B,** Picture of a dissembled pistol grip of unit (Demetron, Kerr Dental Products) showing light pipe (*left*), shield to prevent operator from directly viewing light tip, filters in light path, light bulb and reflector, light socket, cooling fan (*behind socket*), trigger, circuit board, and wired connection to power supply. (**B,** *Courtesy Kerr Dental Products, Orange, Calif.*)

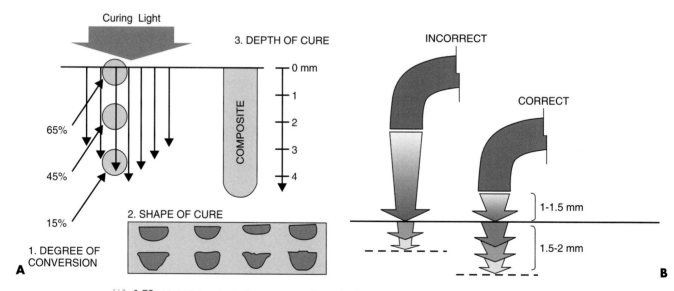

FIG. **4-76** Light intensity influences on polymerization zone. **A,** Varying light intensity with width and depth affects the degree-of-conversion of monomer-to-polymer, shape-of-cure, and depth-of-cure. **B,** Proximity of curing light to the surface affects the depth of penetration of light into the surface.

Light emanating from the tip of a curing unit does not maintain its intensity, but is scattered by molecules in the air on the path to the restoration. Ideally the fiber-optic tip should be adjacent to the surface being cured, but this would most likely cause the tip to be contaminated by the material being cured. The intensity of light striking the composite is inversely proportional to the distance from the tip of the fiber-optic bundle of the curing light to the composite surface. Ideally, *the tip should be within 2 mm of the composite* to be effective (Fig. 4-76).

This is not possible in many dental procedures because the anatomy of a tooth or the distance into the preparation extensions create geometric interference. Distances of 5 to 6 mm often are encountered. At distances beyond 6 mm for QTH lights, the output may be less than one third that at the tip. To permit closer approximation of the curing light to the composite, *light-transmitting wedges* have been promoted for interproximal curing, and *light-focusing tips* have become available for access into proximal boxes.[75] Smaller tips are very useful to overcome this problem but require many more light-curing cycles to cover the same amount of cured area. Certain walls containing bonding systems to be cured within complex preparation extensions such as Class II restorations, may not be oriented ideally to the curing light direction and may still be undercured.

The composite itself also affects the light-curing process. Filler particles tend to scatter the light, and darker colorants tend to absorb the light. Therefore it is generally *recommended that no more than 1.5- to 2-mm increments be light-cured at a time.*[54,149] Smaller filler particles, in the range of 0.1 to 1 μm, interfere most with the light and maximize scattering. That particle size corresponds to the wavelength range for the photoinitiator used for curing.

Within a composite, the pattern of curing varies as a function of curing tip radius and light penetration depth into the material. The intensity of the tip output generally falls off from the center to the edges. Therefore, bulk curing of composite produces a bullet-shaped *curing pattern.* This may lead to inadequate curing in regions such as the proximal box line angles of Class II restorations. The *degree-of-conversion* (or degree-of-cure) is related to both the intensity of light and duration of exposure. It decreases considerably with depth into a composite material. Restorative materials based on BIS-GMA–like restorative matrices generally can only be converted to 65% because of technical problems with steric hindrance of the reacting molecules. Therefore, 65% would be considered a good degree of conversion. A curing light may only produce a 55% degree of cure at 1 mm into a composite and even less at greater depths. Clinically, it is impossible to distinguish differences in the degree of cure. One can only detect the start of uncured material. The boundary between somewhat cured and uncured material is called the *depth of cure* and is often as much as 5 mm for light Vita shades (A2 or A3) of material, in which the tip is close to the composite. However, in cases of poor access or darker shades it is recommended that materials be placed and cured in increments of 1.5 to 2 mm. For the darkest shades, increments should be limited to 1 mm of thickness. Problems of light penetration are only slightly overcome by increasing curing times.

Most light-curing requires a minimum of 20 seconds for adequate curing under optimal conditions of access. To guarantee adequate curing has occurred, it has become common practice to postcure for 20 to 60 seconds. There is some evidence that *postcuring* (curing again after completion of the recommended curing procedure) may slightly improve the surface layer properties such as *wear resistance.*

Typical curing cycles of 20 seconds are laborious and interest in much shorter ones is strong. It has been estimated that for a standard restorative practice during the course of a normal year that as many as 40 hours (typical work week) may be consumed solely with light-curing. Therefore, more intense curing units have been developed to hasten the curing cycles. PAC lights and laser curing units are advertised with curing times of 3 to 10 seconds.

High-intensity light-curing involves a combination of increased light output and a narrowed wavelength range for the output, using more discriminating band pass filters or other means. This process works well only if the photoinitiator is coincident with the wavelength range of the light source. However, some composites use slightly different photoinitiators and those wavelengths may have been excluded by the high-intensity light filters. Heat is also an important problem for these systems. Therefore a wide range of wavelengths that might cover all available photoinitiators is not practical.

Under ideal curing conditions, improvement is observed, but there are accompanying risks as well. High-intensity lights also generate much more intense heat with tissues. High-intensity lights do not necessarily produce the same type of polymer network during curing. Rapid polymerization may produce excessive polymerization stresses and weaken the bonding system layer against tooth structure. The physics of polymerization is much more complex than has yet been considered.

As noted earlier (see Materials Structure), acrylic resin monomers used in dentistry undergo polymerization in stages named activation, initiation, propagation, and termination. Activation involves the production of free radicals. Initiation is the step in which free radicals react with monomer units to create the initial end of a polymer chain. Propagation is the addition of monomer to the growing chain. Termination is the conclusion of the process as a result of steric hindrance, lack of monomer, or other problems. Light-curing influences the initiation process. Increased light intensity increases the amount of effective activation and the subsequent number of chains started. However, there is a practical point at which it is no longer useful to encourage activation. The stages in polymerization occur quickly already. Activation and initiation occur in less than a second. Early propagation rates are extremely fast (100,000 to 1,000,000 reactions per second). *Therefore increased light intensity is useful only to push the degree of conversion to high levels deeper within a material.*

However, the amount of unreacted material that remains is still of concern. If the degree of conversion is 65% in systems with difunctional or polyfunctional molecules, then this will include monomer that has at least one site reacted to tie it into the polymer network and some monomer that is totally unreacted. The unreacted materials may diffuse out of the system. Current composites are complex mixtures that generally include two or more principal monomers and these do not coreact equally. Evidence is increasing that TEGDMA constitutes most of the unreacted monomer in the system. This is apparently influenced by the activation step as well.

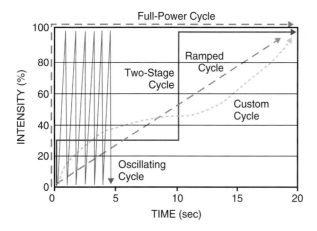

FIG. 4-77 Examples of the variety of duty cycles (intensity versus time) available with different types of light-curing units.

curing) has been explored. There is some evidence that this approach to achieve "soft-start" polymerization works for certain composites cured by specific curing lights, but evidence is also strong that this is not a universal response for all systems.

The original stepped curing system was possible with the Elipar Highlight (ESPE) in 1997. It produced a 100 mW/cm² output for 10 seconds, followed by an immediate jump to 600 mW/cm² output for 30 seconds. The presumption was that lower curing energy allowed the newly forming polymer network to stress-relax and eliminate strains before completion of the curing process. A wide range of soft-start polymerization approaches are possible (Fig. 4-77). Curing cycles may involve variable light intensities and variations in on-and-off periods during the cycle. Although there seems to be newly discovered interest to understand these effects, all of the curing cycles are complicated by the problems mentioned earlier such as light tip sizes, tip orientations, material thickness, and material composition.

Alternatives to the wide range of challenges with light-curing systems are few. One approach is to consider LED technology to generate the appropriate wavelength and curing cycle. This eliminates many of the current equipment problems. However, it does not solve manipulation and restoration curing problems. Other polymerization mechanisms also are being considered that do not include traditional acrylic monomers. Whatever the final solution, it is extremely important that light-curing in general practice will be economical, simple-to-manage, and extremely reliable.

Composition, Structure, and Properties. Composites originally were designed for restoration of Classes

Rapid polymerization also affects the mechanical properties of the polymer network that is forming. As the first polymerization occurs, only some monomer is consumed and the system is still principally a viscous liquid. During conversion from monomer to polymer, the formation of new monomer-to-monomer bonds causes shrinkage, decreasing the net volume of the system. As long as the system is a liquid, it deforms quickly. However, as the degree of conversion approaches 10% to 20% the network is extensive enough to create a gel. Beyond the *gel point*, polymerization shrinkage creates strain on the network and the attachment area to the bonding system. Built-in stresses are relieved ultimately but are considered deleterious at the time of curing because of potential effects on restoration marginal walls. To decrease or eliminate this problem, quite a range of altered curing cycles (*staged*

TABLE 4-15 Comparison of Properties of Representative Composites*

	MACROFILL	MIDIFILL	MICROFILL	HYBRID	FLOWABLE	PACKABLE
Material	Adaptic	Concise	A110	Prodigy	Æliteflo	Surefil
Manufacturer	J&J	3M	3M-ESPE	Kerr	Bisco	Dentsply
Filler level (weight %)	78	81	—	79	56	77
Filler level (volume %)	64	68	40	66	37	58
Depth of cure (mm)	—	—	5.0	6.1	5.6	5.5
Flexural modulus (GPa)	—	—	4.4	9.5	5.4	10.3
3-pt. flexure strength (MPa)	100	111	52	124	—	91
Biaxial flexure strength (MPa)	—	—	—	183	113	—
Compressive strength (MPa)	236	262	219	285	203	256
Diametral tensile strength (MPa)	—	—	24	42	34	34
Fracture toughness (MPa·m$^{1/2}$)	[Poor]	[Poor]	—	2.05	1.36	—
Diamond pyramid hardness (kg/mm²)	—	—	45	68	—	96
In vitro wear (μm/100K cycles)	—	—	—	5	28	2

From Bayne SC et al: *J Am Dent Assoc* 129:567-577, 1998; Leinfelder KF, Bayne SC, Swift EJ: *J Esthet Dent* 11:234-249, 1999; Ruddell DE et al: *J Dent Res* 78:156, 1999 (abstract 407); and Wilkerson MD et al: *J Dent Res* 77: 203, 1998 (abstract 779).

*Relative properties are shown in brackets. The values reported are from a variety of sources from 1963-2000, including manufacturer's product bulletins. Comparisons should be made only in terms of general application requirements, and not in terms of any single property.

III, IV, and V tooth preparations, but now are used in modified forms for most other restorative dental uses. Based on their intended application, they can be used in all classes (I to VI) of restorations, cements, bases, cores, veneers, or repair materials.

A summary of the composition, structure, and properties of five composite compositions is provided in Table 4-15 as examples of commercially available materials. It should be noted that *as the overall filler content increases, the physical, chemical, and mechanical properties generally improve.*

A physical property of historical concern has been the LCTE. Tooth structure expands and contracts at a linear rate of approximately 9 to 11 ppm/°C (see Materials Properties). Unfilled acrylics (such as PMMA) have linear rates of 72 ppm/°C. The LCTE for composites (28 to 45 ppm/°C) may be almost twice as much as the value for amalgam (25 ppm/°C) and three to four times greater than that for tooth structure. Thus, during extreme intraoral temperature changes and times, significant stresses may be generated at the tooth/restoration interfaces where composites are micromechanically bonded. If the interfacial bond fails, microleakage may produce unesthetic staining, pulpal sensitivity due to dentinal fluid flow, pulpal irritation due to diffusion of bacterial endotoxins, and/or predisposition toward recurrent caries. Thermal changes alone do not produce significant thermal expansion problems. Polymeric and ceramic materials are insulators, have low thermal diffusivities, and only change in temperature at relatively slow rates. Intraoral temperature changes of 20° to 30°C that involve only 20 to 30 seconds may be insufficient to produce any significant temperature change in either the tooth structure or the composite. For this reason, much of the thermal cycling information from laboratory experiments may be of little or no value in predicting clinical performance of composite margins.

Well-cured composites are very resistant to chemical change. However, *most compositions only can be practically cured to levels of 55% to 65% degree of conversion of the reactive monomer sites.* During conversion of monomer to polymer, a composite undergoes polymerization shrinkage. In the early stages of conversion, there are only a limited number of polymer chains and they are not well connected (cross-linked). However, in the range of approximately 20% conversion, the polymer network is sufficient to create a gel. At this point, the system changes from behaving like a liquid that can flow, to a solid that has increasingly stronger mechanical properties. Therefore, during the first 20% or so of chemical reaction, the accompanying polymerization shrinkage is accommodated by fluid changes in the dimension of the system. However, after the gel point, polymerization shrinkage produces both internal stresses within the network and stresses along all the surfaces of the system. Bounded surfaces of enamel and dentin may undergo some local

stress, which could reduce the strength of the recently formed bonding layer. Unbounded surfaces will distort, when possible, to accommodate the stress.

In the 1980s, when composites were less highly filled and bonding systems were not as reliable or strong, it was quite possible that shrinkage stresses from composite curing actually dislocated the newly bonded surfaces and created marginal openings. The consequences of this process were first analyzed by Feilzer and others[63,81] and described in terms of the ratio (*configuration-factor*, or *C-factor*) of surface area of fixed walls bounding a tooth preparation versus unbounded walls. C-factors for dental restorations typically range from 0.1 to 5.0 with higher values (> 1.5) indicating more likelihood of high interfacial stresses (Fig. 4-78). Bulk-cured heterogeneous microfill systems in Class I situations were projected to generate preparation wall shrinkage stresses that exceeded 8 MPa. A key effect on actual stress is the complexity of a dental tooth preparation.[79] The effect of tooth structure deformation to accommodate potential stress is unknown. Light-cured composites develop higher stress than auto-cured analogues,[80,117] and higher energy curing lights further exacerbate the situation.[65,82] Surprisingly, more highly filled composites produce larger bulk polymerization stress.[52] Contraction stresses in thin films are much higher and decrease with increasing film thickness.[3,4,46,64] Margin analysis in clinical situations has shown evidence of disruption,[183] but parallel studies have not confirmed microleakage associated with this problem.[182] Glass ionomers set more slowly and seem to develop less interfacial stress.[62]

Because of its simplicity, this theory has been an attractive explanation for potential clinical problems. However, the real importance of these effects for current clinical systems may be much less. Many composites are highly filled, placed incrementally, and less well cured

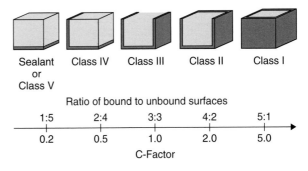

FIG. 4-78 C-factors associated with polymerization shrinkage for different situations using dental restorative materials.[81] C-factors are the ratio of bound-to-unbound surface areas on restorations and are shown in the figure as calculated using average estimates of dimensions of tooth preparations. C-factors may be estimated as the ratio of the number of bound-to-unbound preparation surfaces and those are reported as well, but do not necessarily produce the same numbers or order on the scale.

with visible light than self-cured materials. Newer bonding systems are much more well bonded. Some newer dentin bonding systems are designed thicker to be stress relieving. Therefore typical wall stresses during curing may actually be only 1 to 2 MPa, well within acceptable ranges. The effects of wall stresses on postoperative sensitivity are not known. Stresses both within the cured composite and along the walls appear to be relieved quickly in a few hours. That process is accelerated by the absorption of water.[78]

There has always been interest in eliminating the shrinkage of composites. Early investigations centered on the use of ring-opening reactions with spiro-orthocarbonates to produce expansion that would counteract normal shrinkage.[244] However, these materials were easily combined with existing composite monomers. Recently, there has been a strong interest in oxirane and oxitane chemistry as a method of designing controlled-shrinkage composites that undergo very little curing shrinkage compared to traditional composites.

Water absorption swells the polymer portion of the composite and promotes diffusion and desorption of any unbound monomer. Water and other small molecules can plasticize the composite and chemically degrade the matrix into monomer or other derivatives.[188] Beef or cholesterol esterase has been shown to produce chemical decomposition of polymer matrices into formaldehyde and/or low molecular monomer species.[84,]

[165,216] The consequences for the properties of the composite are obvious. The biologic consequences of small releases of these materials are not known, although it has been hypothesized that unreacted leachable monomer components, such as bisphenol-A, could act as estrogenic agents in the body. However, initial studies in this area concluded that this is not likely to be a significant concern.[15,86,169,174]

There is no clear relationship of clinical performance to any single mechanical property. However, most investigators agree that stronger composites should resist intraoral occlusal stresses better in most situations. Therefore, there is a general consensus that filler contents should be maximized. The material's elastic modulus is of concern as well. There is now evidence that teeth deform more than previously suspected.[103] Composites with high elastic moduli may not be able to accommodate some changes in tooth shape that are associated with flexural forces. This limitation could then result in debonding of the composite restoration from enamel or dentin. This situation is more critical for cervical restorations on facial surfaces where flexural stresses may produce large deformations (see Fig. 4-17). *Flexible restorations (low elastic modulus) would be clinically more retentive because of improved accommodation to flexural forces. The opposite requirement would be true for large MOD restorations. Composites in those cases should be very rigid and thus minimize tooth flexure of remaining cusps.*

Wear resistance of composites on occlusal surfaces of posterior restorations has received considerable attention in clinical studies.[39,102,105,125,175,256] At least five types (Fig. 4-79) of composite wear events are based on the location on the restoration surface: (1) wear by food (*contact-free area, or CFA wear*), (2) impact by tooth contact in centric (*occlusal contact area, or OCA wear*), (3) sliding by tooth contact in function (*functional contact area, or FCA wear*), (4) rubbing by tooth contact interproximally

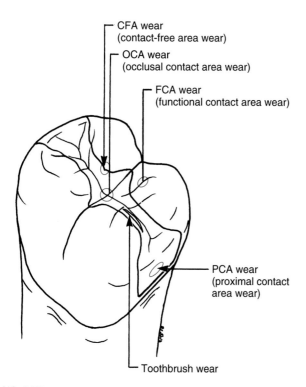

CFA wear
(contact-free area wear)

OCA wear
(occlusal contact area wear)

FCA wear
(functional contact area wear)

PCA wear
(proximal contact area wear)

Toothbrush wear

FIG. **4-79** Locations of different types of wear on posterior composite restorations.

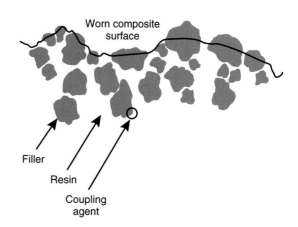

Worn composite surface

Filler

Resin

Coupling agent

FIG. **4-80** Schematic view of wear of composite restoration. *(From Bayne SC, Taylor DF, Heymann HO: Dent Mater 8:305-309, 1992.)*

(*proximal contact area*, or *PCA wear*), and (5) wear from oral prophylaxis methods (*toothbrush or dentifrice abrasion*). The relative contributions of these processes are poorly understood.

Several mechanisms of wear are hypothesized on the basis of clinical information for CFA wear on relatively small posterior occlusal restorations. Mechanisms of wear are associated with failure of composite components (Fig. 4-80). The *microfracture theory* proposes that high modulus filler particles are compressed onto the adjacent matrix during occlusal loading and this creates microfractures in the weaker matrix.[124] With the passage of time, these microfractures become connected, and surface layers of the composite are exfoliated. The *hydrolysis theory*[234] purports that the silane bond between the resin matrix and filler particle is hydrolytically unstable and becomes debonded. This bond failure allows surface filler particles to be lost. The *chemical degradation theory*[264] supposes that materials from food and saliva are absorbed into the matrix, causing matrix degradation and sloughing from the surface. Finally, the *protection theory*[33,115] proposes that the weak matrix is eroded between the particles.

If a posterior occlusal restoration is narrow enough, occlusal contact wear is significantly reduced or eliminated, and wear is due almost entirely to food bolus contact (CFA wear [see Fig. 4-81, *A*]). It now appears that CFA wear resistance is not related to composite mechanical strength, but rather to filler spacing. Filler particles are much harder than the polymer matrix, and thus resist wear very well. If filler particles are closely spaced, then they shelter the intervening matrix polymer. This is called *microprotection* (see Fig. 4-81, *B*). In microfill composites the particles are very small, and thus the interparticle spacing is very small.[33] As a result,

microfills, even with their low filler contents, show very good CFA resistance. However, if their strengths are low, then they do not resist direct tooth contact wear forces very well. Composite restorations with relatively narrow tooth preparations minimize food bolus contact and provide sheltering of the restoration. This process is called *macroprotection* (see Fig. 4-81, *A*). The size of the anticipated restoration is a good indication for the discretionary use of posterior composite materials. *If the tooth preparation is narrow, then composites can be used with little concern about wear. If the tooth preparation is wide, and/or is located in a molar tooth (which is most frequently involved in masticating the food bolus), then the restoration will be more susceptible to wear.*

Large, extensive posterior composites that include total occlusal contact coverage are more prone to failure because of impact (OCA wear) and fatigue (FCA wear).[134,212] If the opponent teeth contact only the composite restoration, then undesirable composite wear usually occurs at those contacts. *However, this process is restricted if centric contacts remain on enamel elsewhere in the restored tooth.*

Wear resistance of posterior composites has been evaluated extensively in longitudinal clinical studies at the University of North Carolina[28,105,208,238,240,254,256] and the University of Alabama[125] over 20 years. Results of this research have demonstrated that *microfill composites are the most wear-resistant formulations*, although as of the year 2000, most commercially available restorative composites (microfills, hybrids, packables) display extremely low in vitro and in vivo wear rates. Numerous in vitro wear simulators have been investigated over more than 30 years to try to duplicate the complicated combination of intraoral wear events. Only one device[128] (Leinfelder wear tester) has demonstrated excellent correlation with a wide range of clinical results.

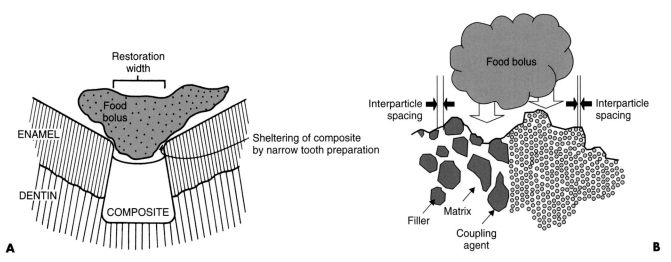

FIG. 4-81 Protection theory of CFA wear. **A,** Macroprotection of composite by sheltering effect of narrow tooth preparation. **B,** Microprotection of matrix resin from small abrasive particles in a food bolus is created by close interparticle spacing of filler particles. Interparticle spacing is reduced from midifill composites (*left*) to minifill composites (*right*). (*From Bayne SC, Taylor DF, Heymann HO: Dent Mater 8:305-309, 1992.*)

Several other devices are used routinely to measure in vitro wear (Krejci wear simulator[119]; Ferracane wear simulator[53])

Toothbrush (and toothpaste) abrasion of composites is poorly understood. There is no direct evidence from anterior composites that this process occurs other than at very low rates. Still, some intuitive thinking suggests that aggressive tooth brushing may produce significant abrasion. Recent studies on flowable composites demonstrate that they wear more than sealants.[219]

Clinical Considerations. Composites are monitored in clinical studies by using United States Public Health Service (USPHS) categories[61,215] of interest: color matching, interfacial staining, secondary caries, anatomic form (wear), and marginal integrity.

Color matching not only depends on proper initial color match, but also on the relative changes that occur with time. Both the restoration and tooth structure are known to change in color with age. The assessment is made with the tooth structure properly hydrated. Temporarily drying the tooth structure makes it appear lighter and whiter in color because of dehydration of enamel (refer to the discussion of optical properties in Materials Properties). With time, chemical changes in the matrix polymer may cause the composite to appear more yellow. This process is accelerated by exposure to UV light, oxidation, and moisture. Anterior restorative materials with high matrix contents that are self-cured are more likely to undergo yellowing.[255] Newer systems that are visible light–cured, contain higher filler contents, and are modified with UV absorbers and antioxidants are more resistant to color change.

Even if a composite is relatively color stable, tooth structure undergoes a change in its appearance over time because of dentin darkening from aging. Aged tooth structure appears more opaque and darker yellow. The clinical challenge is to match the rate and type of color change of the restoration with the tooth structure. A color mismatch that appears after several years is difficult to avoid. Dentin is likely to change color most rapidly during middle age (35 to 60 years old).

Bleaching of teeth (see Chapter 15) has become extremely popular (both in-office and home bleaching). This complicates the process of trying to establish and maintain good color match of an anterior restoration to adjacent tooth structure. If bleaching occurs as a treatment of fixed duration, restorative procedures should be postponed until after teeth have assumed a stable lighter shade. However, continual bleaching or on-and-off bleaching ("data bleaching" or "weekend bleaching") generally makes it impossible for the restoration shade to perfectly match tooth color. Newer whitening toothpastes and continual bleaching may have some effect on restoration surfaces as well, but these are not known.

Another important consideration for esthetics is a gradual transition in color and translucency between the restoration and tooth structure. This goal is accomplished in two ways. *Beveling* the enamel tends to blend any color difference associated with the margin over approximately 0.5 to 1 mm (depending on the preparation size and requirements for bevel width), rather than making it abrupt. This step is particularly beneficial for anterior restorations. It also produces more surface area for a well-bonded margin that does not leak. Marginal leakage leads to the accumulation of subsurface *interfacial staining* that is difficult or impossible to remove and creates a marked boundary for the restoration appearance. Restorations that have been properly acid-etched should be well bonded for years. The longevity of micromechanical enamel retention is unknown. Likewise the effects of fatigue stresses or other intraoral events are unknown. However, clinical studies as long as 14 years indicate relatively good resistance to interfacial staining.

As long as margins are well bonded and no marginal fractures occur, resistance to secondary caries should be good. Although not well documented, *most secondary caries seems to occur along proximal or cervical margins* where enamel is thin, less well-oriented for bonding, difficult to access during the restorative procedure, and potentially subject to flexural stresses as well. Only rarely is secondary caries observed along margins on occlusal surfaces or noncervical aspects of other surfaces.[156] The incidence of caries is quite variable, depending largely on the degree of technical excellence during composite placement. *Clinical research studies indicate that for well-controlled insertion techniques the incidence of secondary caries after 10 years can be as low as 3%.*[24] Under these circumstances, the primary reason for composite failure is poor esthetics or excessive wear. Cross-sectional studies of dental practices that did not strictly conform to recommended techniques indicate that caries levels as high as 25% to 30% have been observed after 10 years for composites placed during the 1970s and early 1980s.

The principal concern for posterior composites has been that occlusal *wear* could occur at a high rate and continue over long periods of time, exposing underlying dentin and leading to secondary caries or sensitivity. Excellent evidence from clinical research studies for small- to medium-width restorations now indicates the rate of occlusal wear tends to decrease over time, with total wear approaching an average limiting value of approximately 250 μm over approximately 5 years (Fig. 4-82). Wear-resistant composites still wear but take longer to reach that level of wear. Evidence that composites actually wear to the point of exposing underlying dentin is only minimal. Morever, after many years of clinical service, worn restorations can be repaired simply by rebonding a new surface onto the old composite to replace a worn or discolored surface.

Wear of posterior composite restorations has been compared in references to that for amalgams, but this comparison may be misleading. Occlusal amalgams do wear but the wear is gradually compensated by continuing expansion of the restoration. Therefore the amalgam restoration appears to have the same occlusal contour. Although this expansion may be a functional advantage, the biologic effects of the wear of the amalgam are not known.

Marginal integrity of composites is very good under most circumstances. Clinical appearance is affected by the nature of the margin. Butt joint margins emphasize composite wear more than beveled margins. Butt joint margins of well-bonded restorations wear more slowly and create a meniscus appearance against the enamel. However, as beveled composite margins wear, thinner edges of material are produced that are more prone to fracture.

Bulk fracture of posterior composite restorations is rare. Although there has been a persistent rumor that microfill composites are more subject to fracture at OCAs, there is no published evidence of that fact, except for a few restorations.[105] Whereas bulk fracture may be the most prevalent failure mechanism for high-copper amalgam restorations, it is only rarely observed for intracoronal composite restorations.

Another clinical concern for all restorative material procedures has been the occurrence of *postoperative sensitivity*. Actual causes of this event are poorly researched but are hypothesized to be due to either: (1) marginal diffusion of species that induce fluid flow within dentin or (2) dimensional changes of the restoration itself. Contraction resulting from polymerization shrinkage and/or expansion from water sorption can cause flexure of bonded cusps and produce pain. The incidence of postoperative sensitivity for posterior composite restorations is relatively low.[113] In most cases, it occurs within the first 6 months to 1 year of the procedure and subsides within 6 months of initial onset. Only rarely must a posterior composite be removed to manage the problem.[22]

There are only limited problems of *biocompatibility* for most composites with the dental pulp. Although the unpolymerized materials are potentially cytotoxic and may even have been classified as carcinogenic, they are very poorly soluble in water and are polymerized into a bound state before there is significant time for dissolution and diffusion. Monomers that do not polymerize may diffuse slowly out of the restoration, but the concentration of released monomer at any given time is so low that the materials do not appear to represent any practical risk. As noted with mercury migration from amalgam restorations, concentration and time are the key factors in assessing biohazards. However, these events still need to be examined more closely. *From long-term clinical studies there is no evidence of any clinical problems resulting in pulp death or soft tissue changes with the use of composite.*

GLASS IONOMERS

Terminology and Classification. Glass ionomers are materials consisting of ion-cross-linked polymer ma-

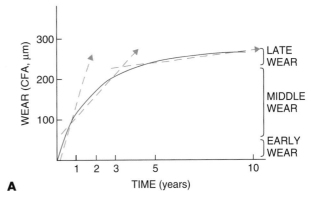

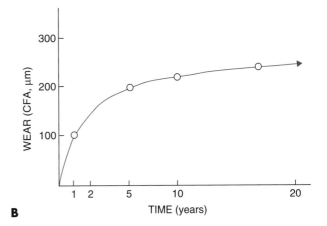

FIG. **4-82** Clinical wear curves for posterior composite restorations. **A,** Continually decreasing wearrate until the wear almost stops as a result of sheltering from occlusal preparation margins of small-to-moderate–sized posterior restorations. **B,** Pooled average of clinical wear for several types of UV-cured posterior composte restorations monitored over 17 years. *(From Wilder AD Jr et al: Seventeen-year clinical study of ultraviolet-cured posterior composite Class I and II restorations,* J Esthet Dent *11:135-42, 1999.)*

trices surrounding glass-reinforcing filler particles. The earliest glass-ionomer materials for restorations were based on a solution of polyacrylic acid liquid that was mixed with a complex alumino-silicate powder containing calcium and fluoride. The acidic liquid solution (pH = 1.0) dissolves portions of the periphery of the silicate glass particle, releasing calcium, aluminum, fluoride, silicon, and other ions. Divalent calcium ions are quickly chelated by ionized carboxyl side groups on polyacrylic acid polymer chains, cross-linking the chains and producing an amorphous polymer gel. During the next 24 to 72 hours, the calcium ions are replaced by more slowly reacting aluminum ions to produce a more highly cross-linked matrix that is now mechanically stronger.[261] It is now believed that during the maturation involving aluminum ion cross-linking, silicon ions and unbound water participate in producing an inorganic comatrix best described as a hydrated silicate.[173]

The same carboxylic acid side groups also are capable of chelating surface ions on the glass particles, or calcium ions from the tooth structure. This process generates true chemical bonds at all internal and external interfaces when the reaction conditions are correct. Set materials have modest properties compared with composites but have relatively good adhesion and the ability to release fluoride ions from the matrix for incorporation into neighboring tooth structure to suppress caries. The perceived advantages of adhesion and fluoride *release* have driven more than 30 years of intense research to improve glass-ionomer products to the point of being competitive with other restorative materials options.

Historical Development. The design of the original glass-ionomer cements was a hybrid formulation of silicate and polycarboxylate cements. Glass ionomers used the aluminosilicate powder from silicates and the polyacrylic acid liquid of polycarboxylates. The earliest commercial product was named using the acronym for this

hybrid formulation and was called aluminosilicate polyacrylic acid (ASPA). The different types of compositions and certain variables that have been explored are summarized in Box 4-2. A schematic of the various chemical reactions involved in the setting and adhesion of glass-ionomer compositions is shown in Fig. 4-83.

A significant number of liquid and powder modifications were soon incorporated to improve the physical, chemical, and mechanical properties. Despite these changes, however, early materials were very technique sensitive. Mixing, placement, and early intraoral conditions were critical to the properties achieved.[163,164]

The original polyacrylic acid in the liquid component was modified by copolymerization with different amounts of maleic acid, itaconic acid, and/or tartaric acid to increase the stability of the liquid and modify its reactivity. Powder particles were reduced in size and modified by incorporating additional types of powder particles for reinforcement. Ag-Sn particles (amalgam alloy particles) were admixed in some formulations to produce an amalgam substitute. This combination[224] became known as the "miracle mixture" because it was initially introduced during the early 1980s at the time when the mercury controversy was increasing dentists' questions about the safety of amalgams. However, the prop-

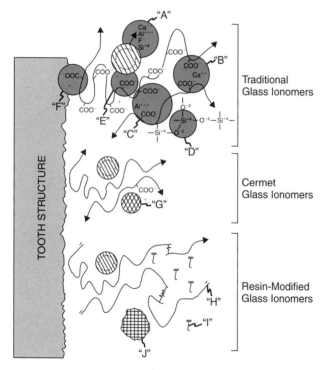

FIG. **4-83** Schematic view of setting and adhesion reactions for a variety of glass ionomer compositions. Traditional glass ionomers: *A,* Ions released from periphery of alumino-silicate glass particle by acid. *B,* Divalent Ca ions initially cross-link adjacent carboxyl ions on polymer chains to cause setting. *C,* Trivalent Al ions gradually replace divalent Ca ions and form tighter network of cross-links between polymer chains. *D,* Si ions react with available water and form covalent silicate network. *E,* Pendant carboxyl groups on polymer chains chelate surface ions on powder particles to produce internal bonding. *F,* Pendant carboxyl groups on polymer chains chelate surface ions on tooth structure to produce chemical bonding. Glass ionomers that are metal-modified for mechanical reinforcement. *G,* Cermet filler particles with ceramic coatings are bonded to pendant carboxyl groups on polymer chains. Hybrid or resin-modified glass ionomers. *H,* Acrylic functional modifications of polymer allow light-curing to cause initial cross-linking. *I,* Water soluble monomers added for polymerization during light-curing reactions. *J,* Resin, silica, or composite filler particles added as modifiers.

BOX 4-2   Variety of Compositions and Changes in the Evolution of Glass Ionomer Materials

1. Traditional glass ionomers (liners, bases, cements)
   Modified by adding comonomers to polyacrylic acid
   Smaller powder particle size
   Experimentation with dehydrated liquid component
2. Metal-modified glass ionomers (filling materials, bases, cores)
   Miracle mixtures (with amalgam alloy admixed with cement)
   Cermet-particle reinforced
3. Light-cured glass ionomers (liners, bases)
   HEMA added to liquid component; monomers in liquid modified with acrylic functional groups
   Other powder particles mixed with alumino-silicate glass
4. Hybrid (resin-modified) glass ionomers (cements, restorative filling materials, cores)
   HEMA and other monomers added to liquid component
   Polymers and other phases added to powder component
   Silicate glass of composites substituted for some of the powder component
   Precured glass ionomer blended into composites
5. Polyacid-modified resin composites (compomers) (cements, restorative filling materials, cores)
   Methacrylate monomers with multiple carboxylic groups; addition of ion-leachable glass (as in a conventional glass ionomer)

HEMA, Hydroxyethyl methacrylate.

erties of miracle mixtures were far inferior to amalgam, and it was not well received as a restorative material. In part, the problem with the admixture was that the matrix would not strongly adhere to the Ag-Sn alloy particles.

To circumvent this difficulty, silver-palladium (Ag-Pd) was substituted. Ag-Pd generates a passivating oxide film of PdO that is chemically reactive by chelation with polyacrylic acid. These mixtures, termed ceramic-metal (*cermets*) mixtures (see Fig. 4-83, *B*), were much stronger than unmodified glass-ionomer cements, but had poor esthetics and could not be highly modified, or else they would not set as well.

In the face of limited success with these modifications, glass-ionomer compositions were promoted for less demanding applications, such as liners, bases, cements, cores, and root canal filling materials, rather than as restorative materials. During the 1980s the utilization of glass ionomers for such applications increased. However, glass ionomers were plagued by technique sensitivities due to mixing requirements, potential problems with postoperative sensitivity, and the need for moisture protection to prevent surface degradation before the secondary setting reaction was completed. With careful attention to procedural details, glass ionomers have proven clinically successful in many applications.[163] However, in restorative filling applications, glass ionomers have never been as esthetic as composites.

In the early 1990s reformulated ionomer-based materials were introduced. The modified materials are based on modifications that replace part of the original glass-ionomer formulation with alternative filler particles and/or matrix setting reactions to make them more composite-like (see Fig. 4-83, *H* to *J*).[155] These materials are categorized as *hybrid* or *resin-modified glass ionomers. They are usually light-cured, less technique sensitive, and may be finished at the time of placement.* Although more composite-like in composition and structure, resin-modified glass ionomers still undergo acid-base reactions during setting and retain much of the chemical behavior of traditional glass-ionomer materials. Because resin-modified glass ionomers are significantly stronger than traditional glass ionomers, they are recommended for Class V restorations and can be used for Class I and Class II restorations in primary teeth.

The most recent evolution of glass-ionomer chemistry is the class of materials known *as polyacid-modified resin composites* or *compomers.*[93,149,154,214,231] These materials are similar to resin-modified glass ionomers in that they contain all the major components of both polymer-based composites and glass ionomers, with the exception of water. Water is excluded to prevent premature setting of the material and also to ensure that setting occurs only through a polymerization reaction. Limited acid-base reactions are believed to occur once the material is exposed to, and absorbs, water. Although the name compomer implies that the material possesses a combination of characteristics of both composites and glass ionomers, these materials are essentially polymer-based composites that have been slightly modified to take advantage of the potential fluoride-releasing behavior of

TABLE 4-16 Comparison of Compositions, Structures, and Properties of Typical Examples of Three Broad Classes of Glass Ionomers

		CONVENTIONAL GLASS IONOMER	RESIN-MODIFIED GLASS IONOMER	POLYACID GLASS IONOMER RESIN COMPOSITE (COMPOMER)
Abbreviation		GI	RMGI	CM
Commercial Name		Fuji II	Vitremer	Dyract
Manufacturer		GC	3M-ESPE	Dentsply
Applications		Liner, base, cement	Cement, restorative	Restorative
Acid-base setting reaction		Yes	Yes	No
Polymerization setting reaction		No	Yes	Yes
Properties				
VLC depth of cure (mm)		NA	2.7	4.7
Water absorption (µg/mm³)	7d	236	—	—
	180d	—	174	26
Radiopacity (mm of Al)		2.5	1.8	3.0
Fluoride release (µg/cm²)	7d	25.9	21.2	7.8
	22d	9.3	8.8	7.8
Flexural modulus (GPa)	Dry	12.9	9.6	7.6
	Wet	5.5	—	7.5
3-Pt. flexure strength (MPa)	Dry	20	68	96
	Wet	4	—	—

Adapted from McCabe JF: *Biomaterials* 19:521-527, 1998; Meyer JM, Cattani-Lorente MA, Dupuis V: *Biomaterials* 19:529-539, 1998; and Smith DC: *Biomaterials* 19:467-478, 1998. *NA,* Not applicable, *VLC,* visible light-cured.

glass ionomers. The mechanical properties of polyacid-modified resin composites are superior to those of traditional glass ionomers and resin-modified glass ionomers, and in some cases, are equivalent to those of contemporary polymer-based composites.

Composition, Structure, and Properties. Examples of a traditional glass-ionomer cements, resin-modified glass ionomers, and polyacid-modified resin composites (compomers) are listed in Table 4-16 along with certain key properties.

Clinical Considerations. The mainstay arguments for glass ionomer use are chemical adhesion and fluoride release. Despite intuitive belief in benefits due to these properties, little clinical evidence indicates that these systems produce better restorations than systems based on composites. Relative advantages of these two factors and other considerations are discussed in this section.

Adhesion of conventional glass ionomers (not resin-modified) to enamel and/or dentin only produces macroshear bond strengths in the range of 6 to 12 MPa. By comparison, dentin bonding agents now can produce bond strengths of 22 to 35 MPa. Most glass ionomers are aqueous systems (before setting) and wet tooth structure very well because they are hydrophilic. However, glass ionomers tend to have relatively high viscosities and therefore do not flow and adapt to micromechanical spaces very readily. In contrast, bonding agents are hydrophobic, but have been formulated for use with hydrophilic primers to facilitate wetting, flow, and bonding. Bonding of glass ionomers is achieved in part by mechanical retention and in part by chemical chelation. Although there always has been enchantment with chemical bonding for dental systems, the bond density per unit area of retentive interface is actually higher for mechanical bonding than for chemical bonding. Excel-

lent bonding cannot be achieved by chemical bonding alone. In most cases, *good mechanical bonding is much more important than chemical bonding.* Thus, the potential of glass ionomers for chemical bonding is only an advantage in situations in which it is difficult or impossible to produce effective micromechanical retention.

Historically, widespread evidence indicates that little secondary caries is associated with fluoride-containing silicate cement restorations, despite significant marginal disintegration during restoration solubilization. That same success is expected with glass ionomers, but the pattern has never been directly demonstrated. Two factors limit the influence of fluoride ion release. First, fluoride ion release is proportional to the concentration available to diffuse from the matrix and/or residual silicate particles through to the restoration surface. Generally, fluoride ion release is relatively high during the first few days but that rate of release falls as fluoride concentration is depleted in the matrix (Fig. 4-84). *A critical level of fluoride release over time never has been defined clinically.* The second and more important factor is that the absence of significant secondary caries is not evidence of a fluoride ion effect. As noted in the clinical considerations section for posterior composites, for appropriately placed restorations, the incidence of secondary caries can be less than 3% at 10 years even in the absence of fluoride release. No clinical evidence indicates that glass-ionomer restorative materials can produce comparable or better results. Esthetic problems with glass ionomers have resulted in replacement or repair in much less than 10 years after placement. Therefore fluoride release from restorations may not be a major advantage if other factors do not favor long-term service.

Nonetheless, fluoride release from restorative materials such as glass ionomers may have therapeutic effects

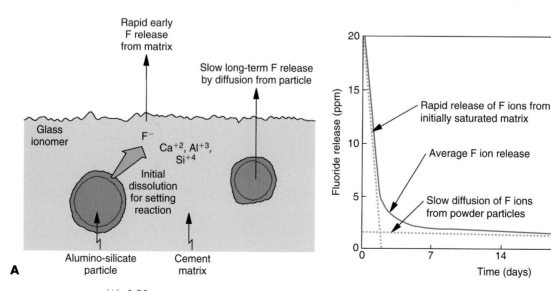

A

B

FIG. 4-84   Fluoride release. **A,** Possible sources of fluoride within set cements. **B,** Examples of fluoride release rates from glass ionomer cements versus time.

that have yet to be demonstrated. Glass-ionomer restorations seem very well suited for situations that involve high-caries risks. These include patients who are known to be more susceptible to caries, patients with reduced or no saliva flow, or patients with oral diseases that accelerate the pathogenic activities associated with caries. In some cases, when bonding composite to gingival areas with little or no enamel, a glass-ionomer liner extended just short of the margins has been suggested as a way to reduce caries risks if microleakage occurs.

Around 1990, a special form of temporary filling material was fabricated from glass ionomer with the objective of maximum fluoride release for use in the *atraumatic restorative treatment* (ART) technique. In locations, such as rural regions of underdeveloped countries, in which treatment was not accessible or routine treatment was not possible, untrained dental personnel could use ART to halt or lessen the progression of frank carious lesions[229] until the patient could access dental facilities. An ART technique restoration is based on a self-cured version of resin-modified glass ionomer that is mixed as powder with liquid and is capable of a relatively high fluoride release. A frank lesion is excavated using a simple plastic scoop. The temporary restoration is mixed by rubbing the materials together between the tips of the thumb and forefinger and inserted into the tooth excavation. Biting onto the restoration, the patient creates some gross anatomy and occlusal adjustment. Since their development, these materials also have been adapted as good temporary restorations for indirect restoration techniques in dental offices.

Fluoride release from glass ionomer and other compositions is diffusion limited and affected by the concentrations in both the matrix and the particles (see Fig. 4-84, *A*). For glass ionomers, the initially high burst of fluoride release is due to the high concentration of fluoride that exists in the matrix immediately after the setting reaction is complete. During the initial acid dissolution of powder particle edges, a large amount of fluoride becomes part of the reaction product matrix. This fluoride diffuses quickly from the matrix exposed on the surface of the material and is only slowly replaced by fluoride diffusing from greater distances in the matrix below the surface or by fluoride diffusing from the particles into the matrix for the first time. Therefore the long-term release of fluoride is at much lower rates (see Fig. 4-84, *B*).

Biocompatibility of traditional glass-ionomer cements has been a clinical concern. Traditional glass ionomers are very acidic at the time of initial mixing and have the potential to produce postoperative sensitivity and pulpal irritation. As the reaction proceeds, the pH increases from initial values near 1 to a range of 4 to 5. As the setting reaction nears completion, the final pH value reaches 6.7 to 7. Because the acid groups are attached to polymer molecules that have limited diffusibility, the potential pulpal effects of the low initial pH are limited to areas immediately adjacent to the material. *If the RDT is less than 0.5 mm, it may be necessary to protect dentin surfaces from direct contact with unset glass-ionomer materials by using a calcium hydroxide liner.* When fluid-filled dentinal tubules are in direct contact with setting cement, two problems occur. High ionic concentrations in the unset glass ionomer cause dentinal fluid to rapidly diffuse outward into the cement. This phenomenon produces a change sensed by pressure receptors near pulpal odontoblasts and causes pulpal sensitivity or pain. At the same time, unset components, such as hydrogen ions, may move into tubules and toward the pulp. This may cause chemical irritation when RDT is inadequate. Tubule fluid contents will be inadequate to buffer the acid before it can diffuse to the pulp. The key to successful use of these materials is strict attention to specific techniques. The risks for postoperative sensitivity with resin-modified glass ionomers and compomers seem to be much lower.

To increase mechanical strength, glass-ionomer materials for use as restorations are mixed at higher powder-to-liquid (or filler-to-matrix) levels than materials used for luting. The reduced matrix content decreases the risks of postoperative sensitivity or pulpal problems. In addition, tooth preparations may be lined with calcium hydroxide that provides a barrier to the diffusion of unset glass-ionomer components while the material is curing.

DIRECT-FILLING GOLD

Gold is extremely malleable and may be welded to itself under pressure at room temperature if the surfaces being joined are clean. This makes gold a candidate for a direct restoration. Although it has been used this way for more than a century, the process is tedious, demanding, and relatively expensive for the patient. These reasons, in addition to the fact that the restoration is not esthetic nor trouble free, has resulted in disuse of this technique by most general practitioners.

Terminology and Classification. Gold for direct-filling restorations may be classified on the basis of (1) the geometric form in which it is supplied, (2) the surface condition of the piece, and (3) the microstructure of the piece. It may be supplied as *ropes, sheets, strips,* or *pellets* (see Chapter 21). The surface condition is described as *cohesive* (clean) or *noncohesive* (containing adsorbed gas). To prevent unwanted adsorption of hard-to-remove gases, the gold piece may be intentionally protected by ammonia gas adsorption. At the time of use, the ammonia layer is removed easily by properly heating the piece, making it cohesive once again. Different microstructural conditions are possible in forms referred to as *gold foil, mat gold,* or *powdered gold.*

Composition, Structure, and Properties. Direct gold is essentially 100% gold. Pre-alloying with other elements would reduce the weldability and malleability at

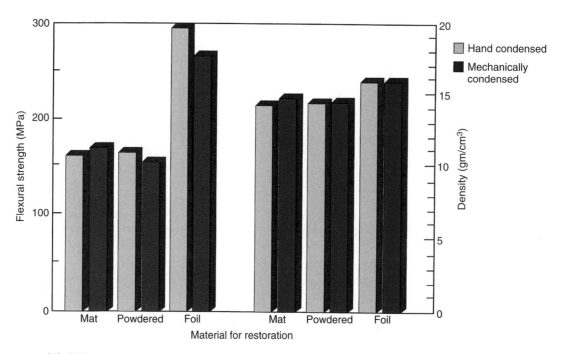

FIG. **4-85** Bar graph comparing the flexural strengths and densities of different direct filling golds for conditions of hand condensing versus mechanical condensing for cold welding. *(Data from Anusavice K: Phillips' science of dental materials, ed 10, Philadelphia, 1996, WB Saunders.)*

room temperature. However, other elements may be incorporated (platinum or calcium) indirectly into the final structure by layering them onto the gold in forms such as gold foils.

During cold welding, much greater compaction pressures are required to remove pores or spaces in mat gold and powdered golds than in gold foil. However, these other forms are often used because they reduce the time required to build up a restoration. Restorations of mat or powdered golds are never quite as dense as those made from gold foil, and thus the former have lower flexural strengths. The theoretic density for defect-free pure gold is 19.3 g/cm^3, but as can be seen by reference to Fig. 4-85, final restorations range from 14.3 to 15.9 g/cm^3.

Clinical Considerations. The LCTE of gold is 16.2 ppm/°C, which is closer to tooth structure (9 to 11 ppm/°C) than all other currently available direct restorative materials except for traditional glassionomer cement. There is very little differential expansion at the margins of the restoration and percolation is not a problem.

Placing a liner or base may result in compaction and welding problems. Gold foil is not indicated for restoring extensive lesions. Sometimes there is pulpal sensitivity to a thermal stimulus because of gold's high conductivity. However, this usually ceases after several months.

Direct-filling gold restorations have transverse strength significantly lower than that for cast alloys (five to six times lower) and less than that for tooth structure (two times lower). Because direct gold has a low elastic limit, large restorations cannot adequately distribute occlusal stresses without plastic deformation.

Another major disadvantage is that direct-filling gold restorations are not adhesive to tooth structure. Therefore they cannot function to reinforce tooth structure in a manner similar to that for strong, properly bonded composites or bonded ceramic restorations.

Finally, gold foil cannot be considered an esthetic restorative material. Most patients are less than pleased by its appearance.

INDIRECT RESTORATIVE DENTAL MATERIALS

Traditional stages of fabricating dental restorations by indirect restorative techniques involve impressions, dies, wax patterns, investing, casting or molding, finishing and polishing, and cementing. CAD/CAM approaches are possible as well, and are discussed in a later section, Machined Restorations. Because of the multiple stages of these techniques, errors that enter into the procedures at any point tend to be compounded and carried into the next stage. It is important to strictly adhere to the procedural details throughout the techniques, or else the final restoration will not fit. Those clinical procedures that involve impression materials, choice of restorative materials, and cementing of restorations are discussed in Chapters 14, 15, and 20. The rationale for these procedural choices is discussed in this section in a limited way.

IMPRESSION MATERIALS

Terminology and Classification. Impression materials are used to record the surface topography and detail of hard and soft tissues, and thereby produce a mold for making a replica (cast) of those structures. Nine types of

TABLE 4-17 Classification of Dental Impression Materials

TYPE (AND SYNONYMS)	MECHANICAL BEHAVIOR	SETTING REACTIONS	SPECIAL VERSIONS
Impression plaster	Rigid	Chemical (irreversible)	
Impression compound	Rigid	Physical (reversible)	
ZOE	Rigid	Chemical (irreversible)	
Alginate	Flexible	Chemical (irreversible)	
Agar-agar	Flexible	Physical (reversible)	
Polysulfide (rubber base, Thiokol rubber)	Flexible	Chemical (irreversible)	
Silicone (conventional or condensation silicone)	Flexible	Chemical (irreversible)	
Polyether	Flexible	Chemical (irreversible)	Hydrophilic
Polyvinal siloxane (vinyl polysiloxane, additional silicone)	Flexible	Chemical (irreversible)	Hydrophilic

ZOE, Zinc oxide–eugenol

impression materials have been used historically in dentistry. Their generic compositions, common names, and key clinical properties are summarized in Table 4-17.

Plaster, impression compound, and *ZOE* are rigid solids incapable of being removed directly from undercut areas of hard or soft tissues. Therefore they have limited use for dentulous patients. *Alginate (irreversible hydrocolloid)* and *reversible hydrocolloid (agar-agar)* are elastic and have the advantage of wetting intraoral surfaces well, but have very limited dimensional stability because they include as much as 85% water in their composition. *Polysulfide (rubber base, Thiokol rubber), silicone (condensation silicone, conventional silicone), polyether,* and *polyvinyl siloxane (vinyl polysiloxane, addition silicone, addition polydimethyl siloxane)* are nonaqueous polymer-based rubber impression materials that have good elasticity (see Table 4-17). They are listed in order of development. Polyvinyl siloxane is the most widely used.

Composition, Structure, and Properties. To be totally effective, an impression material must be fluid before setting, hydrophilic to wet intraoral surfaces, highly elastic to prevent permanent distortion during removal, sterilizable, dimensionally stable, compatible with the cast material, and must undergo complete conversion to an elastic solid. To meet these mechanical requirements, the most common formulation for an impression material is a mixture of nonreactive filler with a flexible polymer matrix.

Elastomeric polymer matrices are produced by polymerizing fluid monomer and/or oligomer mixtures either by stepwise polymerization or chain reaction polymerization reactions. Polysulfide, condensation silicones, and polyether impression materials involve *stepwise polymerization.*

Stepwise reactions are relatively slow and do not go to completion for several hours. Approximately 65% to 85% conversion occurs within 6 to 8 minutes during initial setting before a dental impression is removed from the mouth. As long as the impression is in the mouth,

the shrinkage is confined to noncritical areas because the intraoral surfaces restrain the impression material. After removal, the impression experiences more shrinkage as the polymerization continues. Although these materials are elastic, the elastic recovery is viscoelastic and requires 20 to 30 minutes to reach a point of accurately returning to the intraoral dimensions being duplicated. During this pause for elastic recovery, continued polymerization can distort the impression size and shape. To minimize these effects, high levels of fillers are incorporated in the matrix. Filler levels vary between 15 and 60 weight percent and are chosen on the basis of compatiblity with the matrix material and expense.

Portions of the impression that must record fine details of the tooth structure are normally impressed with the least-filled formulations (light-bodied material) so that there is maximal flow and adaptation to intraoral structure before curing. However, the bulk of the impression is the highly filled material (heavy bodied material), which minimizes shrinkage contributions and greatly reduces inaccuracy. Examples of the relative degree of dimensional change versus filler content and material types are reported in Fig. 4-86.

Polyvinyl siloxane undergoes a chain reaction polymerization (which is also an addition reaction) during setting that is fast, goes almost to completion, and does not generate condensation by-products. This characteristic provides a major advantage for these materials compared with other elastic impression materials. Once the impression is removed, it is dimensionally stable, and the casts that will be fabricated from the impression can be produced at any time. In the case of the other rubber elastic impression materials, the impression should be poured immediately after pausing 20 to 30 minutes for viscoelastic recovery.

Polyvinyl siloxanes commonly use exotic curing systems based on chloroplatinic acid (a platinum catalyst). During the reaction, the acid decomposes and generates small amounts of hydrogen gas as a by-product. Early

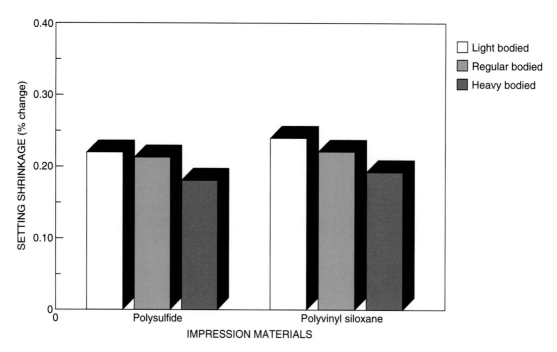

FIG. **4-86** Examples of setting shrinkage of polysulfide and polyvinyl siloxane impression materials for light-, regular-, and heavy-bodied consistencies. *(Data from Eames et al: J Prosthet Dent 42:159-162, 1979.)*

versions of polyvinyl siloxane were plagued by gas bubble formation that ruined casts poured in the impressions unless 24 to 48 hours were permitted for out-gassing. However, newer materials contain hydrogen scavengers that react with, and tie up, the hydrogen by-products.

Another recent modification to many commercial polyvinyl siloxane impression materials is the addition of surfactant to increase the hydrophilic nature of the material. Although this appears to have a favorable effect on the ease with which these new "hydrophilic" siloxane materials can be poured up with gypsum products, there is no conclusive evidence that these newer materials wet tooth structure better than unmodified (no surfactant added) siloxane materials.[43,144,239]

Clinical Considerations. The most significant clinical consideration when using an elastic impression material is the *rate of removal* of the initially set impression. All polymer-based materials are strain-rate sensitive. If they are stressed quickly, they behave as though they are stronger and more elastic than if stressed slowly. Therefore elastic impression materials should be removed from intraoral surfaces with a relatively rapid motion. The objective is to minimize the time that the impression is distorted. This approach prevents conversion of mechanical energy into plastic, rather than elastic, deformation. Teasing or slowly deforming an impression produces unwanted plastic deformation and introduces inaccuracies into both the final impression and resulting cast.

Properties of impression materials not only influence clinical techniques, but also preparation of casts

and dies. Hydrophobic impressions are not wet well by water-based cast and die materials. Wetting agents are used to avert air entrapment in detailed areas under these conditions. A final mechanical property of the impression material dictates ease of cast removal. The stiffness of impressions (e.g., polyether material) can cause breakage of thin "teeth" of the cast.

The impression must remain accurate while being disinfected. Chapter 8 provides information for infection control of the impression and related items.

CAST METAL RESTORATIONS

Creation of a cast metal restoration involves a chain of procedures from waxing a pattern of the intended final restoration on a die, investing the pattern to create a mold space for casting, casting the restoration, finishing and polishing the casting, and cementing the restoration intraorally. Because of the complexity of this sequence, properties desirable for a casting alloy are as much governed by technique limitations as by the final intraoral service considerations. Each of these is addressed in the following paragraphs.

Terminology. *Cast metal alloys* may be used to form the entire restoration, or may be designed as a substructure and veneered with porcelain to create a tooth-colored restoration. Those that are veneered with porcelain may be described generically as *porcelain-bonded-to-metal* (PBM), *ceramic-bonded-to-metal* (CBM) or *porcelain-fused-to-metal* (PFM) restorations. For successful porcelain application, the metal alloy must have a relatively high melting point to tolerate the high porcelain firing temperatures with-

TABLE 4-18 Objectives for Allying the Components of Gold Casting Alloys

ALLOYING ELEMENT (CHEMICAL SYMBOL)	MAJOR CONTRIBUTION TO CASTING ALLOY	DENSITY (GM/CM³)	MELTING POINT (°C)	CORROSION BEHAVIOR
Gold (Au)	Corrosion resistance	19.28	1063	Immune
Copper (Cu)	Solution hardening	8.93	1083	Active
Silver (Ag)	Counteract orange color of copper	10.50	961	Active
Palladium (Pd)	Increase hardness; elevate melting range	12.02	1552	Immune
Platinum (Pt)	Elevate melting range	21.45	1769	Immune
Zinc (Zn)	Scavenge oxygen during processing	7.14	420	Active

out sagging or melting. The melting temperature of restorations that are all metal (without porcelain) can be any temperature that can be conveniently processed.

Classification. *Corrosion resistance* is an essential characteristic of dental casting alloys. These alloys are categorized in terms of their: (1) mechanism of corrosion resistance and (2) main elements in the composition affecting the corrosion resistance (see the next section, Composition, Structure, and Properties of Gold Castings). Corrosion resistance is achieved with either immune or passivating alloy systems. For dentistry, immune systems are divided into gold systems and gold substitute systems. Passivating systems are divided into nickel-chromium (Ni-Cr), cobalt-chromium (Co-Cr), iron-chromium (Fe-Cr), and titanium (Ti) systems.

Many of the terms relating to corrosion resistance have very special meanings. *Noble metal alloys* are very resistant to both corrosion and electrochemical corrosion. These systems are based on gold, platinum, palladium, rhodium, iridium, ruthenium, and/or osmium. *Precious metal alloys* contain metals of high economic value and, as a group, traditionally include all of the noble metals and silver. *Low-gold alloys* contain only 3 to 50 weight percent gold or other noble metal elements. If less than half (75 weight percent) of the atoms in a gold alloy are corrosion-resistant (gold [Au], platinum [Pt], or palladium [Pd]), the overall corrosion resistance decreases dramatically. Low-gold alloys are attempts at producing lower cost alloys that still retain some of the qualities of premium-priced gold-based alloys. However, the actual quantity of gold may be deceptively low.

Gold substitute alloys are precious metal alloys that do not contain gold. The best examples are Ag-Pd systems and other Pd alloys.

Base metal alloys are based on active metallic elements that corrode but develop corrosion resistance via surface oxidation that produces a thin, tightly adherent film that inhibits further corrosion. Alloys are formulated with 18% to 28% by weight Cr that produces films of Cr_2O_3 that passivate the surface. The films are brittle and may be ruptured, but reform immediately if suffi-

cient Cr remains locally in the composition. Oxidation of other elements, such as Ni and Co, also produce superficial oxides, but Cr_2O_3 is principally responsible for the corrosion resistance. Ti (and Ti-6Al-4V) alloy is widely used in dentistry for implant systems, because it passivates by forming TiO_2, is biocompatible, and permits osseointegration with bone.

Composition, Structure, and Properties of Gold Castings. Cast restorations are constructed traditionally from gold alloys because of their potentially excellent corrosion resistance. In the nineteenth century, gold coins had been used as the source of alloy for casting restorations. Standardization of casting materials occurred in the 1930s. Dental gold casting alloys were defined in terms of their relative noble metal concentration, physical properties (fusion temperature), and mechanical properties (hardness, elongation, and yield point). The original *ADA classification system* defined Types A, B, and C gold alloys.[241] This specification was then revised and extended to include four types (I, II, III, IV) of alloys. Types I, II, and III corresponded to the original Types A, B, and C, while Type IV included higher strength alloys.[6] These four alloy types contain approximately 83%, 78%, 78%, and 75% noble metal elements, respectively, of which gold is the principal one. Types I and II alloys are not capable of being heat treated, while Types III and IV alloys are. *Type I* compositions are intended for small inlays that do not involve significant occlusal loads. *Type II* alloys are for inlays and onlays. *Type III* alloys are for onlays and crowns. *Type IV* alloys are for crowns, bridges, and removable partial dentures.

The major elemental components of gold casting alloys are listed in Table 4-18 for several commercial products. Gold is primarily responsible for producing corrosion resistance, but it also is relatively soft and requires other alloying element additions to solution-harden the composition. *Copper* is the primary alloying element that increases the hardness of the material. However, copper also tends to make the color less yellow and more orange. *Silver* is added to offset the color contributions of copper. *Palladium* is added to increase the hardness of the alloy and has a strong whitening effect. Both palladium and *platinum* tend to raise the melting range for the alloy. Finally, *zinc* is added as a processing aid to scavenge oxygen at the surface of a melt and prevent oxidation and loss of other key elements during the casting procedure.

In recent years, the relatively high cost of gold has prompted increased use of low-gold, gold substitute, and *base metal alloys* for dental castings.[97] Cast partial dentures are almost exclusively made of base metal alloy. Many full crowns and fixed bridges are made of palladium-based *gold substitute alloys,* but the mechanical properties of these materials make them difficult to fabricate into inlays and onlays. However, gradual improvement in the materials has made the *low-gold alloys* acceptable for selective use for these applications. *A number of products containing approximately 50 weight percent of gold are available that exhibit acceptable tarnish resistance and adequate properties if extensive marginal burnishing is not required.*

Key properties for casting alloys are reported in Table 4-19. A low melting range is desirable for simplified heating and casting procedures. Moderately high density is advantageous, because most dental alloys are normally cast by centrifugal force casting machines. High density helps force the alloy quickly into the intricate details of the pattern within the casting mold before cooling solidifies the material. Gold-based alloys are much better in this regard than most other alloys. Finally, a low coefficient of thermal expansion helps reduce the shrinkage that occurs from the solidus temperature down to room temperature. Because cooling produces shrinkage, there must be some expansion somewhere else in the technique sequence to compensate for dimensional changes upon cooling. Alloys with low coefficients of thermal contraction and that possess low melting temperatures can be controlled more easily.

Certainly the primary chemical property of concern is corrosion resistance. To achieve this quality it is desirable that the entire alloy be a single-phase composition. Two-phase compositions are prone to local galvanic (structure-selective) corrosion. Types I, II, and III compositions are single-phase alloys. Type IV compositions may include two phases. There is a mechanical advantage with a second phase because of a hardening effect, but that benefit must be weighed against the loss of some corrosion resistance. Contamination or improper

TABLE 4-19 Properties of Typical Gold Casting Alloys*

REPRESENTATIVE ALLOY (SUPPLIER)	PENTRON I (PENTRON)	MODULAY (JELENKO)	FIRMALAY (JELENKO)	STERNGOLD 100 (STERNGOLD)
COMPOSITION (WEIGHT %)				
Au	84.0	77.0	74.5	60.0
Cu	Balance	Balance	Balance	Balance
Ag	12.0	14.0	11.0	19.0
Pt	—	—	—	—
Pd	1.0	1.0	3.5	4.0
Zn	< 1	< 1	< 1	< 1
CLASSIFICATION				
Gold content	High gold	High gold	High gold	High gold
ADA type	I	II	III	IV
PHYSICAL PROPERTIES				
Color	Gold	Gold	Gold	Gold
LCTE (ppm/°C)	[14-18]	[14-18]	[14-18]	[14-18]
Density (gm/cm³)	16.60	15.90	15.50	13.90
CHEMICAL PROPERTIES				
Corrosion resistance	[Excellent]	[Excellent]	[Excellent]	[Excellent]
Tarnish resistance	[Good]	[Good]	[Good]	[Good]
MECHANICAL PROPERTIES				
Modulus (MPa)	—	—	—	—
Elongation (%)	0-22	0-38	19-39	4-25
Hardness (BHN, soft/hard)	68/—	101/—	110/165	150/257
Compressive strength (MPa)	—	—	—	—
Tensile strength (MPa)	—	—	—	—
BIOLOGIC PROPERTIES				
Biocompatibility	[Acceptable]	[Acceptable]	[Acceptable]	[Acceptable]

*Relative properties are shown in brackets.
ADA, American Dental Association; *BHN,* Brinell hardness number; *LCTE,* linear coefficient of thermal expansion.

casting of gold-based alloys can produce unwanted phases that compromise both the mechanical properties and the corrosion resistance.

The *primary mechanical properties of interest for the final cast restoration are a high modulus of elasticity (stiffness) and a high elastic limit (hardness) to resist deformation in service.* However, high values are not necessarily desirable properties during the fabrication of the restoration. Laboratory procedures such as finishing, polishing, and burnishing are more complicated if the restoration has a high resistance to plastic deformation (high hardness). During these processes, it is important for the casting metal near the margins to be adapted closely to the die (but without damaging the die), by minimal mechanical deformation *(burnishing).* Marginal gaps that exceed 0.1 mm should not be burnished. Rather the casting should be remade. Alloys with a high percentage elongation and a low yield point (low hardness) facilitate burnishing. After these procedures are complete, it is desirable to increase the overall hardness to high levels for clinical service. This goal can be accomplished with Types III and IV ADA gold alloys, which are heat-treatable. The heat treatment produces disorder-order and/or spinodal hardening processes.

Cast alloys should not produce toxic reaction products or release toxic elements from their surfaces. Immune and passive alloys appear to have excellent biologic properties. However, some casting alloys are active and generate soluble corrosion products. Although the restorations look unchanged, toxic soluble products can be released.

Clinical Considerations. The three principal clinical considerations for long-term success of cast restorations are *close fit, corrosion resistance, and retention.* Sturdevant and others[237] and Morris[162] have shown that gold-based alloys demonstrate excellent corrosion resistance for at least 10 years. *If the cemented restorations have a close fit (within 20 μm) and the tooth preparations are adequately designed, then the conventional dental cements resist degradation and provide excellent retention and service for 20 to 40 years.*

Retention and service life of cast restorations are produced by a combination of factors, such as the taper of the tooth preparation, stress distribution design of the tooth preparation to protect remaining tooth structure against fracture (see Chapter 20), the cement type, surface roughness on the internal aspects of the restoration, and potential micromechanical or chemical bonding of cement with the restoration and tooth structure. Under most circumstances the restoration surface for gold-based alloys is not well suited to cement adhesion. The gold alloy surfaces are not wet well with cements and do not have the potential to be chemically bonded by existing formulations. However, *if the internal surfaces are sandblasted, then sufficient micromechanical irregularities are produced to permit excellent luting.* Tin or other metal plating also can be used as a surface modification that is chemically reactive toward some cements.

In some cases, such as Maryland bridges, the retention of the casting is dependent on well-developed micromechanical spaces along the bonded surfaces of enamel and the casting. The retentive surface of the casting is accomplished by choosing a two-phase dental casting alloy. The metal surface to be bonded is then relieved by chemical or electrolytic etching of one phase in preference to the other. The relieved surface is micromechanically interlocked with composite cement onto etched tooth structure.

DENTAL CEMENTS

Traditional dental cements are based on reactions between acidic liquids and basic powders to produce reaction product salts that form a solid matrix surrounding residual powder particles (Fig. 4-87). Microscopically, these cements are classic examples of filler and matrix microstructures. Newer cements are formulated as modified versions of materials originally developed as composite restorative materials. In all cements, the properties of interest are governed by the extent to which the matrix is minimized in the final material.

Terminology and Classification. Traditional dental cements are listed in Table 4-20, along with identification of the major powder and liquid components and the reaction products. *ZOE, reinforced ZOE, ZOE-EBA, silicate,* and *zinc silicophosphate cements* are no longer routinely used to permanently cement restorations. *Zinc phosphate* cement has been extensively replaced by *poly-carboxylate* or *glass-ionomer cements.*[48,49] The latter two are based on ion-cross-linked polyacrylic acid matrices that

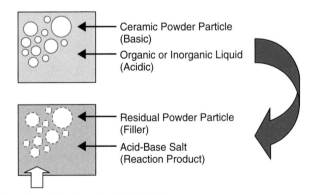

Powder reinforces set cement matrix

F I G. **4-87** Schematic representation of all dental cement components and microstructures. An acid-functional liquid is mixed with a basic powder. Reaction of the periphery of the powder consumes the acid groups of the liquid, producing a reaction product matrix that surrounds residual powder particles. The microstructure is a classic composite-like one with residual powder particles reinforcing the weaker matrix. *(Courtesy Stephen C. Bayne SC, School of Dentistry, University of North Carolina, Chapel Hill, NC.)*

TABLE 4-20 Summary of Dental Cement Classifications, Abbreviations, Reactants, and Reaction Products				
CLASSIFICATION	ABBREVIATION	LIQUID COMPONENTS	POWDER COMPONENTS	REACTION PRODUCT MATRIX
ZINC OXIDE–EUGENOL				
Unmodified	ZOE	Eugenol	ZnO	Crystalline zinc eugenolate
Resin reinforced	R-ZOE	Eugenol	ZnO, polymer, rosin	Crystalline zinc eugenolate
EBA-modified	ZOE-EBA	Eugenol, EBA	ZnO, Al_2O_3, polymer	Crystalline zinc eugenolate, crystalline zinc ethoxybenzoate
ZINC PHOSPHATE SILICATE	ZP	H_3PO_4, H_2O	ZnO	Tertiary zinc phosphate
Unmodified	SC	H_3PO_4, H_2O	F-Al-Silicate glass	Amorphous silicophosphate
Zinc silicophosphate	ZSP	H_3PO_4, H_2O	F-Al-Silicate glass, ZnO	Amorphous silicophosphate, zinc phosphate
POLYCARBOXYLATE GLASS IONOMER	PC	PAA, H_2O	ZnO	Zinc-polyacrylate gel
Conventional	GI	PAA, H_2O	F-Al-Silicate glass	Aluminum-polyacrylate gel
Resin-modified	RMGI	PAA, H_2O, water-soluble monomers	F-Al-Silicate glass	Aluminum-polyacrylate gel, Cross-linked polymer
Compomer	CM	Water-soluble monomers	F-Al-Silicate glass, pre-reacted GI resin	Cross-linked polymer, aluminum-polyacrylate gel
Composite (or Resin)	CP	Monomers	Silicate glass	Cross-linked polymer

*Relative properties are shown in brackets.
ADA, American Dental Association; *BHN,* Brinell hardness number; *EBA,* ethoxybenzoic acid; *LCTE,* linear coefficient of thermal expansion; *PAA,* polyacrylic acid.

have the potential to react chemically with residual powder particles and surface tooth structure.

Zinc phosphate cement was originally developed more than 100 years ago, and was extremely popular during most of the twentieth century. For that reason it is often referred to as the "gold standard" for all dental cements, despite the fact that its laboratory properties are generally inferior to those of most other currently used cements. The powder component is 90% zinc oxide powder with 10% magnesium oxide added. The liquid is 50% phosphoric acid in water, and is buffered with aluminum and zinc salts to control the pH. Components are mixed typically 2:1 (powder-to-liquid by weight) on a chilled glass slab using controlled additions of powder to the liquid. These precautions are necessary to reduce reaction speed, alter the pH in a controlled manner, dissipate heat from the exothermic reaction, and provide sufficient working time. During setting, phosphoric acid ions react with zinc ions to produce a successive series of hydrated zinc phosphate salts. Ultimately, tertiary zinc phosphate crystals are produced that form a matrix around residual zinc oxide particles. Of all the contemporary dental cements, zinc phosphate is the only one with a crystalline

reaction product matrix. Intercrystalline spaces within the matrix more readily allow diffusion or leakage of small molecules than other cement systems. Zinc phosphate also tends to be more brittle than other cements that have amorphous matrices instead.

Polycarboxylate cement was developed in the 1960s by Dennis Smith in an effort to circumvent potential pulpal problems associated with the low pH of traditional cements (e.g., zinc phosphate cement) and biocompatibility problems related to the mobility of small acidic ions. By choosing an acid-functional polymer as a substitute for phosphoric acid in forming the matrix, it also was possible to produce cements that could adhere via chelation to dental surfaces. The original acid-functional polymer was polyacrylic acid. However, current commercial products include two or more monomers in the polymer; thus it is technically more correct to refer to the final polymer as a *polyalkenoate.* Cements based on solutions of these polymers (i.e., polycarboxylate or glass-ionomer cements) may be called *polyalkenoic cements.*

Glass-ionomer cements are hybrids of silicate and polycarboxylate cements designed to combine the optical and fluoride-releasing properties of silicate particles with

TABLE 4-21	Characteristic Properties of Categories of Luting Dental Cements*						
	R-ZOE	EBA	ZP	PC	GI	RMGI	COMP
WORKING CHARACTERISTICS							
P/L ratio	[Low]	[Low]	[Low]	[Low]	[Low]	1.2-1.6	
Film thickness (μm, ADA flow test)	32	—	18	21	24	—	10-60
Setting-time range (minutes)	6-8	—	5-7	2-3	3-5	2-3	—
PHYSICAL PROPERTIES							
LCTE (ppm/°C)	[Low]	[Low]	[Low]	—	—	[Low]	50
Thermal conductivity	[Low]	[Low]	[Low]	[Low]	[Low]	[Low]	[Low]
CHEMICAL PROPERTIES							
Solubility/disintegration (%, ADA test)	0.08	0.05	0.06	0.60	1.25	—	0.01
MECHANICAL PROPERTIES							
Compressive strength (MPa)	48	65	160	70	120	148-180	170-190
Diametral tensile strength (MPa)	4	7	10	10	12	30-35	30-35
BIOLOGIC PROPERTIES							
Pulpal response	[Mild]	[Mild]	[Moderate]	[Moderate]	[Mild]	[Mild]	—

*Relative values are shown in brackets. These values are representative of a wide range of possible values. *ADA,* American Dental Association; *LCTE,* linear coefficient of thermal expansion; *P/L,* powder-to-liquid ratio. (See Table 4-20 for abbreviations for cement.)

the chemically adhesive, and more biocompatible, characteristics of the polyacrylic acid matrix compared with the extremely acidic matrix of silicate cement.

Composite cements (or resin cements or composite resin cements) have the same general components as composite restorative materials (see Composites earlier in this chapter), but generally have lower concentrations of filler particles. These materials are reserved almost exclusively for use with all ceramic restorations and are discussed later (see Milled Ceramics), although they are suitable for use with all indirect restorative materials. These materials have the best laboratory properties of all cements, but require more complicated clinical procedures and generally include bonding systems for dentin, enamel, and the restoration.

Although dental cements are most often used for *luting* indirect restorations, they also may be used as bases. As *luting agents, the most important clinical requirements are flow, wetting, and film thickness.* To enhance flow, the materials are mixed at relatively low powder-to-liquid ratios. To guarantee that a film thickness of less than 25 μm can be produced, cement particles of 5 μm or less in diameter should be used. The actual film thickness that is achieved ranges from 20 to 100 μm and depends on (1) the viscosity of the mixture and (2) the availability of space for displacement of the cement (as discussed in the next section). Although low powder-to-liquid ratios produce low viscosities for luting agents, cements used for bases should be mechanically stronger and are mixed with the maximum powder content manageable.

Composition, Structure, and Properties. Final properties of dental cements depend on the powder-to-liquid ratios used during mixing. Higher powder-to-liquid ratios not only increase the mechanical strength, but also increase the viscosity and reduce wetting and flow. The final matrices of the set cement are indicated in Table 4-20. Details of the cementing procedures are presented in Chapters 14, 15, and 20. A brief summary of dental cement properties is provided in Table 4-21.

Cements are routinely evaluated for their solubility and disintegration in laboratory tests. Unfortunately, no laboratory tests or pseudoclinical tests of cements have ever been correlated with clinical performance categories, such as retention. At the same time, only limited long-term clinical trials of cements have ever been reported. A unique clinical research study was performed in the 1970s at the University of Michigan, by Silvey and Myers,[223] to compare zinc phosphate, reinforced ZOE, and polycarboxylate cements for retention of crowns and bridges over 7 years. There was practically no difference in failure rates (ZP = 2%, ZOE-EBA = 8%, PC = 5%) and no differences were statistically significant.

Mechanisms of failure for these materials are not well understood. Because most cements are brittle, it is presumed that fatigue loading produces cracks at internal defects, propagates the cracks into a network, and causes cement loss or microleakage at the margins, which is accompanied by sensitivity or secondary caries. Cemented crowns and bridges transfer most stresses from occlusal loading laterally, through the restoration and onto the margins, rather than directly onto the underlying coronal structure. Cement at the margins is in the most critical region. The greatest portion of cement is involved in retention. Although cements most likely undergo long-term changes in composition and properties, loss of retention is generally much less of a problem, than problems at margins.

Clinical Considerations. Zinc phosphate cements have the potential during setting to release components from the acid-rich matrix into dentin and irritate the pulp. Therefore, when using zinc phosphate cement, dentin is routinely protected with varnish or dentin sealer. However, other cements that can chemically bond to dentin must be allowed to come into direct contact with that surface. *Thus, varnishes or sealers should not be used to coat dentin if a polycarboxylate or conventional glass ionomer cement is to be used for chemical adhesion.* When bonding composite or ceramic restorations, the dentin should not be varnished or sealed, but, instead, the entire preparation should be treated with the bonding system used (see Chapters 11 to 15).

Cement displacement is a key factor for successfully cementing restorations. The process is a *hydraulic* (liquid in motion) one, dependent on rapid flow and escape of excess cement between the restoration and tooth preparation during cementation. The *seating* of the restoration must be completed within a few seconds while the cement is sufficiently fluid. One way to increase the potential of maximum seating is to make channels large enough (larger if they are longer) to permit rapid escape of cement that otherwise would be entrapped. For metal cast-

ings, the channels could be created internally in the wax pattern or cut in the casting, extending gingivally from the occlusal (pulpal wall) aspect of the preparation (casting) to a point approximately 0.5 mm short of the restoration margins. *Inlay and onlay preparations have short enough external walls so that the castings do not usually require escape channels* (see Chapter 20), but crowns may require them if considerable axial length is present. Channels allow seating with 330 N load (75 lb), the recognized possible masticatory pressure achievable in the molar region (see Cementation in Chapter 20). To further produce cement flow, *loading* (forces placed on the restoration being seated) must be applied rapidly, at sufficiently high levels, and steadily maintained until the cement has initially set. The final result ideally is a restoration so well-seated that its preparation-side surface is in intimate contact with the tooth preparation, particularly along the margins, resulting in a cement film thickness no greater than 25 μm.

MACHINED RESTORATIONS

Until 1988, indirect ceramic dental restorations were fabricated exclusively by casting and/or sintering techniques. Neither technique is capable of consistently producing pore-free restorations. Cooling shrinkage distortions and residual stresses can initiate fractures at residual pores in ceramics. However, pore-free restora-

TABLE 4-22 Examples of CAD/CAM and Copy Milling Systems in Dentistry (Circa 1999)

SYSTEM	DEVELOPER/MANUFACTURER	APPLICATIONS	COMMERCIAL INTRODUCTION
CAD/CAM SYSTEM			
Automill	Alldent (Liechtenstein)	Crown, bridge	1994
CAP	Nikon (Japan)	Inlay, onlay, crown	—
Cerec 1/2/3	Seimans/Sirona (Germany)	Inlay, onlay, crown	1988/1994/1999
Cicero	Elephant (Netherlands)	Inlay, onlay, crown, bridge	—
COMET	Steinbichler Optotechnik (Germany)	Crown, bridge	—
DENStech	Microdenta (Germany)	Inlay, onlay, crown, bridge	—
DentiCAD	Bego (Germany/USA)	Inlay, onlay, crown, bridge	—
DCS-President	DCS/Girrbach (Germany)	Crown, bridge	1991
Inlac	Ritter (Germany)	Inlay, onlay	—
Nissan	Nissan (Japan)	Inlay, onlay, crown	—
Sopha-Duret	Sopha Biomedical/NIMS (France)	Inlay, onlay, crown, bridge	1991
COPY MILLING SYSTEM			
Celay	Mikrona (Switzerland)	Inlay, onlay, crown, bridge	1991
Ceramatic	Askim (Sweden)	Inlay, onlay, crown, bridge	1994
DCP	Ivoclar-Vivadent (Liechtenstein)	Inlay, onlay	—
DCS-Titan	Gim-Alldent (Germany)	Crown, bridge	1996
DFE	Krupp (Germany)	Inlay, onlay, crown, bridge	1995
Erosonic	ESPE (Germany)	Inlay, onlay, crown	—
PRO-CAM	IntraTech (USA)	Crown	1996
Procera	Nobel Biocare (Sweden)	Inlay, onlay, crown, bridge	1994

Adapted from Hickel R et al: *Inter Dent J* 47:247-258, 1997; Preston JD, Duret F: *Oral Health* 87:17-27, 1997; and Willer J, Rossbach A, Weber H: *J Prosthet Dent* 80:346-353, 1998. *CAD,* Computer-aided design; *CAM,* computer-assisted manufacturing.

tions can be produced by machining blocks of commercially fabricated pore-free ceramic or composite.

Terminology and Classification. The two principal *machining approaches* for dental restorations are: (1) copy milling and (2) CAD/CAM milling. Examples of commercial systems are indicated in Table 4-22.

Copy milling uses a replica (e.g., wax, plastic, stone, or metal) of the desired form as a guide for a milling machine. The surface of the replica is traced by turning the pattern and touching the pattern's surface with a finger stylus. The positions of the pattern and stylus are used to adjust the positions of a block of machinable material and a milling tool cutting the block, respectively. This procedure is represented schematically in Fig. 4-88.

A wide variety of material types can be used in conjunction with copy milling systems, including materials difficult to process using other methods. For example, titanium, which has a very high melting temperature, is difficult to cast. However, it can be copy milled easily and inexpensively. Composite and ceramic materials are being used for copy milling. The choice of material depends in large part, on the type of margin required for the restoration. Virtually any geometry and size can be copy milled as long as there is direct access of the finger guide and cutting tool to the surfaces involved.

CAD/CAM milling uses digital information about the tooth preparation (computerized surface digitization [CSD]), or a pattern of the restoration to provide a computer-aided design (CAD) on the video monitor for inspection and modification. The image is the reference for designing a restoration on the video monitor. Once the three-dimensional image for the restoration design is accepted, the computer translates the image into a set of instructions to guide a milling tool (computer-assisted manufacturing [CAM]) in cutting the restoration from a block of material (Fig. 4-89).

Stages of Fabrication. A number of approaches to CAD/CAM for restorative dentistry have evolved, but all systems ideally involve five basic stages: (1) computerized surface digitization, (2) computer-aided design, (3) computer-assisted manufacturing, (4) computer-aided esthetics, and (5) computer-aided finishing.[21,24] The last two stages are very difficult and have not yet been included in commercial systems. Various computerized surface digitization techniques have been explored. Examples of different approaches are listed in Box 4-3. Laser (optical) techniques and contact digitization are the most promising approaches from the point of view of cost and accuracy.

The *Ceramic Reconstruction System* (CEREC) (Siemens, Germany) was the first commercially available CAD/CAM system used in dentistry. An intraoral video camera images the tooth preparation and the adjacent tooth surfaces. Elevations of the imaged surfaces are calculated by Moiré fringe displacement. Features of the tooth preparation are used to define the limits of the restoration. External surfaces of the restoration are estimated as distances to adjacent tooth structure in the computer view. Occlusal surfaces are more highly refined later by the operator intraorally after cementing the CEREC restoration. Other CAD/CAM systems have become available during the 1990s, including improved versions of the CEREC System (see Table 4-22).[106,198,260]

Composition, Structure, and Properties of Machined Materials. Restorations can be machined from metals, ceramics, or composites. Ceramics are generally

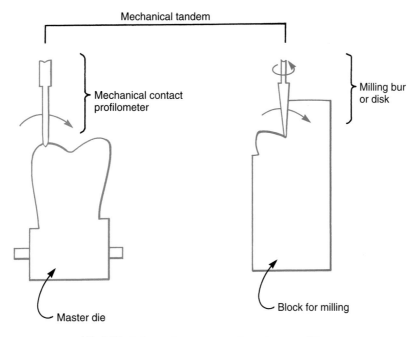

FIG. **4-88** Schematic representation of copy milling.

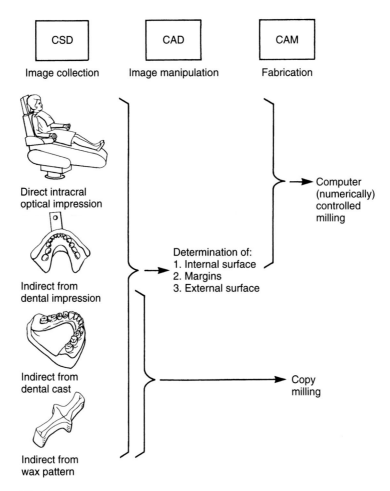

FIG. 4-89 Schematic summary of CAD/CAM and copy milling operations.

BOX 4-3 Computerized Surface Digitatization Techniques

1. Photogrammetry
2. Moiré
3. Laser scanning
4. CT scanning
5. MRI
6. Ultrasound
7. Contact profilometry

CT, Computed tomography; *MRI,* magnetic resonance imaging.

---

preferred because of their superior esthetics and biocompatibility. The machinable ceramics used are generally either some form of *modified feldspathic porcelain* or *special fluoro-alumino-silicate glass-ceramics* with excellent *fracture and wear resistance.* In addition, partially sintered high strength ceramic compositions of alumina, spinel, and zirconia can be machined for use as copings. The porcelain and glass-ceramic materials being machined are *pore-free* and generally have both crystalline and noncrystalline phases. A two-phase composition permits differential etching of internal restoration walls for mi-

cromechanical retention using bonding agents and/or luting cements. Table 4-23 summarizes the typical properties of machinable ceramic materials in clinical use.[220, 221,242] Fig. 4-90 shows an example of the phases, revealed by etching for bonding of a machinable glass-ceramic material.

Bonding of ceramic CAD/CAM restoration is a critical step in achieving good long-term results. Ceramic restorations are bonded to tooth structure by: (1) etching enamel to increase the bondable surface area; (2) etching, priming, and applying the bonding agent to dentin (when appropriate); (3) etching (by *HF acid*) and then priming *(silanating)* the restoration; and (4) cementing the restoration with composite cement. This situation is schematically summarized in Fig. 4-91.

CAD/CAM systems for fabricating restorations are not currently designed to produce esthetics comparable to the characterization possible in a dental laboratory. Most CAD/CAM systems use uniform color (monolithic) materials for the entire restoration. Despite the fact that increased shades of ceramic are becoming available for use with CAD/CAM and copy milling systems, the final esthetics depend on a combination of color match

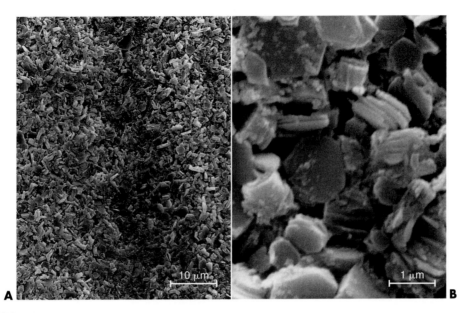

FIG. **4-90** Ammonium bifluoride acid-etched machinable glass ceramic inlay (Dicor MGC, Dentsply International, York, Pennsylvania) in preparation for cementation. Approximately 65% of glass ceramic is fluoromica crystals embedded in an amorphous matrix. The matrix at its surface is partially dissolved by etching. **A,** Etching partially reveals crystals that are 1 to 5 μm in size. **B,** Higher magnification view of fluoromica crystals that provide micromechanical interlocking for bonding. *(Courtesy Stephen C. Bayne, School of Dentistry, University of North Carolina, Chapel Hill, NC.)*

TABLE **4-23** Mechanical Properties of Machinable Ceramic Materials in Clinical Use with CAD/CAM and Copy Milling Systems (Circa 1999)

	DICOR MGC	VITA MARK II	INCERAM ALUMINA
Manufacturer	Corning/Dentsply (USA)	Vita Zahnfabrik (Germany)	Vita Zahnfabrik (Germany)
Material type	Glass ceramic	Feldspathic porcelain	Glass-infiltrated alumina
Hardness (GPa)	3.72	6.94	9.82
Elastic modulus (GPa)	65	73	286
3-Pt. flexure strength (MPa)	229	122	446
Fracture toughness (MPa·m$^{1/2}$)	1.65	1.26	4.61

Adapted from Grossman DG: *Proceedings of the International Symposium on Computer Restorations*, Chicago, 1991, Quintessence; Seghi RR, Denri IL, Rosenstiel SF: *J Prosthet Dent* 74:145-150, 1995; Seghi RR, Sorensen JA: *Int J Prosthodont* 8:239-246, 1995; and Thompson JY, Bayne SC, Heymann HO: *J Prosthet Dent* 76:619-623, 1996.
CAD, Computer-aided design; *CAM,* computer-assisted manufacturing.

to adjacent tooth structure and light scattering from adjacent tooth structure into the restoration. Small restorations display color governed more by scattered light and are very esthetic. Larger restorations appear to be duller and less esthetic. Although this latter occurrence cannot be totally remedied, some color variation can be introduced by cutting troughs into the internal (tooth side) surface of CAD/CAM restorations. The troughs are then filled with varying shades of composite. This technique produces an optical effect of different dentin colors and enhances the overall esthetic appearance.

Composition, Structure, and Properties of Composite Cements. Although the dimensional accuracy and fit of machined restorations continues to improve, a weak link with CAD/CAM and copy milling systems is the *cement gap* along occlusal surfaces that may be wider than desired. Normal food abrasion produces cement loss and ditching. Wear of this type permits stain accumulation in marginal gaps and leaves exposed enamel and ceramic margins. Minimizing this gap depends on the computer digitization, design, and manufacturing steps being sufficiently accurate.

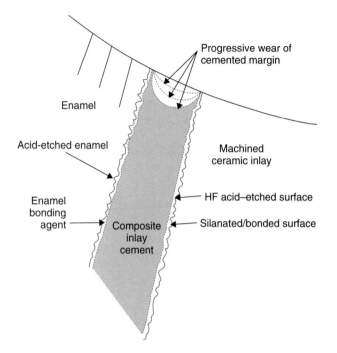

FIG. **4-91** Schematic summary of attaching ceramic CAD/CAM inlays to tooth structure. Enamel is etched for retention of bonding agents. Inlays are etched (with HF acid) and primed (silanated). The restoration is cemented with composite cement.

CAD/CAM restorations are routinely cemented with moderately filled composites (homogeneous microfills or hybrids). The composite cements are not as mechanically strong as composite restorative materials but do provide the best abrasion resistance because of the microprotection effect of closely spaced filler particles. Zinc phosphate and glass-ionomer cements are not recommended for use with milled ceramic restorations.[243]

Clinical Considerations. The clinical longevity of these restorations is difficult to project, because only relatively short-term clinical research information is available.[102,104,111,161] However, review of the earliest restorations of this type indicates that, although cement margins may degrade, the restorations themselves survive equally as well as amalgam or composite restorations of the same type. There is no evidence of postoperative sensitivity or secondary caries.

Major advantages of milled ceramics are excellent flexural strength and the ability to rigidly bond remaining tooth structure together. Occasional restoration fractures have been reported, but in most cases they are associated with restoration designs that are too thin and subject to stress concentration during flexure or fatigue fracture. It is still important to *use adequate thickness in the restoration design to resist flexure.*

Additionally, restorations from these systems are *repairable because* they are etchable, and defects can be restored using bonded composites. There should be no reason to completely replace the restoration unless it has undergone bulk fracture.

BOX **4-4** Acronyms for National and International Groups Interested in Dental Standards

NDA	National Dental Association
ADA	American Dental Association
CDMIE	Council on Dental Materials, Instruments, and Equipment
CDT	Council on Dental Therapeutics
ANSI	American National Standards Institute
ASC MD156	Accredited Standards Committee, Medical Devices
FDA	Food and Drug Administration
ASTM	American Society for Testing and Materials
FDI	Federation Dentaire Internationale
ISO	International Organizations for Standards
ISO TC106	ISO Technical Committee

SAFETY AND EFFICACY

The availability of dental materials of high quality and dependability is due in large part to the existence of standards for the safety and efficacy of such products. Yet, very few clinicians are aware of, or understand, the intricate system of voluntary and mandatory controls currently in place to accomplish this purpose.

STANDARDS PROGRAMS

The large number of organizations involved in standards programs and their acronyms are summarized in Box 4-4.

Standards programs can be broadly divided into dental *professional organizations,* larger *interest groups* that include all professional organizations, and *government agencies.* These hierarchies exist both within the United States and throughout the world as a whole. Fig. 4-92 attempts to interrelate these groups. In the discussion that follows, individual group activities are addressed. Most professional organizations attempt to coordinate their standards with other organizations so that a rational system of tests is involved in evaluating similar events.

Professional organizations develop *voluntary standards* that are often the basis for governmental *regulatory standards* whenever governments become involved. In many cases, the good faith standards and self-regulation of industry obviates the need for government involvement.

American Dental Association. For about 130 years, the ADA has been a reliable source of information on the safety and effectiveness of dental products. The *ADA Seal of Acceptance* program is designed to assist dental professionals and the public in making informed decisions about dental materials, instruments, equipment, and therapeutics.

The ADA's *Council on Scientific Affairs* (CSA) evaluates submitted products three times a year at its meetings.

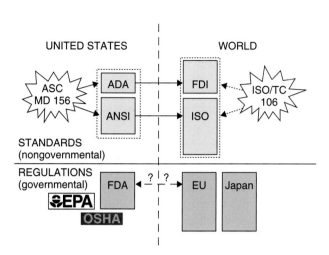

FIG. 4-92 Summary of key standards (voluntary) and regulations (mandatory). Dental professional standards communicate with standards organizations via liason groups (ADA with ANSI via ASC MD156; FDI with ISO via ISO/TC 106). A few countries have regulatory groups.

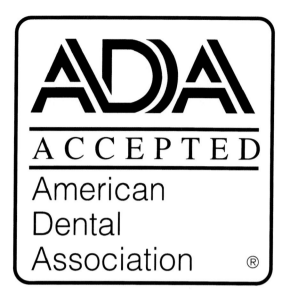

FIG. 4-93 ADA Seal of Acceptance. (Courtesy American Dental Association Council on Scientific Affairs, 211 East Avenue, Chicago, Ill.)

While following the *Provisions for Acceptance,* companies are encouraged to submit information on their products for review by the CSA. In many cases, the submission must also comply with product category guidelines and/or American National Standards Institute (ANSI)/ADA specifications. Criteria for acceptance of many products include data from clinical studies and/or ADA laboratory testing. For example, posterior composite and dentin bonding materials require submission of the results of two clinical studies that successfully meet the guidelines for the respective category. Dental amalgam and impression materials are examples of products that require company laboratory data and in-house testing by ADA laboratories. The CSA utilizes over 60 ANSI/ADA specifications and has developed over 50 product category guidelines to use to evaluate a submission.

Depending on the category, a product is *Accepted* for a period of 3 to 5 years, whereupon the product is then considered for reacceptance. Accepted products may use the ADA Seal (Fig. 4-93) in all advertising and promotional materials after demonstrating compliance with ADA advertising guidelines for claims of safety and efficacy.

American National Standards Institute. The ANSI is a clearinghouse for national standards. The Accredited Standards Committee (ASC) MD156 is a liaison group between the ADA and ANSI. It is an independent committee of both organizations sponsored by the ADA and accredited by ANSI for dentistry in the United States. ADA standards that are developed are submitted to ANSI for approval as national standards.

Food and Drug Administration. Since 1976, the Food and Drug Administration (FDA) has been charged with

regulating dental devices (including materials). In this role, they classify individual materials as Classes I, II, or III. Class I materials are simply required to be produced under conditions of good manufacturing practices to assure reproducibility and continuing safety. Class II materials are required to present evidence of meeting standards as well, such as the ADA standards for acceptance or certification. Class III materials are required, in addition, to submit evidence of safety and efficacy using biocompatibility and clinical data to show satisfactory performance in tissue culture tests, implantation tests, and/or usage tests. Tests for the relative safety of dental materials (biocompatibility) are described as part of ANSI/ADA document No. 41. These tests are in large part controversial because they are continually evolving and may be reinterpreted in light of new or more sophisticated understandings of biocompatibility.

American Society for Testing and Materials. The American Society for Testing and Materials (ASTM) is a nongovernmental group involved widely in the development of standards for test methods for use in industry. It has recently become interested in standards for dentistry (dental materials and devices) as well as the development of appropriate terminology, nomenclature, and test methods. ASTM's F-4 subcommittee has developed specifications for surgical implants. ASTM's F-8 subcommittee governs sports devices such as mouth guards. ASTM's D-2 committee is concerned with rubber products, such as rubber gloves.

Federation Dentaire Internationale. The worldwide voluntary federation of national dental organizations is known as the Federation Dentaire Internationale (FDI).

International Standards Organization. An International Standards Organization (ISO) or International

Organization for Standards exists for the purpose of developing international standards for all activities, not only dentistry. ISO is a nontreaty organization. ANSI is the United States member of ISO.

FDI maintains a permanent liaison with ISO through its ISO/TC106-Dentistry group. To the extent that each group coordinates its activities with each other, the ADA role has been a major one in initiating standards for a range of current standards organizations.

SAFETY FOR DENTAL PROFESSIONALS

Although numerous organizations and standards regulate the safety of dental materials with regard to the patient, quite different ones are concerned with the health of dental professionals. In many situations the scope and regulations of different groups are overlapping and inconsistent.

Occupational Safety and Health Administration. The *Occupational Safety and Health Administration (OSHA) is the U.S. federal agency charged with responsibility for maintaining safety in the workplace.* It differs from the organizations discussed previously, in that OSHA has the legal authority to enforce compliance. During 1970, the United States adopted a wide range of OSHA regulations, with the goal of reducing the potential for illness or injury to employees from chemical exposures. Many of these regulations were enforced only sparingly during the 1980s, and usually only for large businesses. *Since 1992, enforcement of these standards for dental offices and dental laboratories has been stricter.* OSHA has issued regulations involving a wide range of issues, including hazard communications, bloodborne pathogens, office water lines, and waste disposal.

Hazard communications include public posting of OSHA regulations, office record keeping, office emergency planning, office employee training, and office planning for workman's compensation. These processes involve *seven categories of responsibilities* described in the following paragraphs. The ADA provides dental professionals with detailed information in this regard.

First Category of Responsibility. To ensure that all employees are aware of the processes required to guarantee the safety and health of the employees, an *OSHA poster must be continuously displayed within the office (at one or more sites) so as to be seen by all personnel.* This location is most often a kitchen, apparel changing location, or employee lounge area. The poster is titled *Job Health and Safety Protection.*

Second Category of Responsibility. For many years, large businesses and laboratories have had to meet OSHA requirements involving hazardous chemicals to protect the health of their employees. The enforcement of these requirements has been extended recently to cover dental offices. Although modifications of office routines are required, dentistry can benefit from the prior experience of industry in refining the application of these safety principles. *Hazardous chemical materials are routinely managed by proper labeling and storage as well as by certifying that all office personnel are fully informed of possible risks and the necessary precautions in those regards.* The requirement for hazardous chemical labeling is waived for FDA-regulated items, such as most products in dental offices. However, the information about the nature of the chemical hazard and its management is still a responsibility of the office. This information is published on *material safety data sheets* (MSDSs) and is available from individual manufacturers. Manufacturers have the primary responsibility to determine whether an MSDS is required and to supply that information. Commercial chemicals generally are packaged with MSDSs. However, dental products often cannot conveniently include the MSDS, because the sheet is too big for the package in which materials are sold. Only some dental products include MSDSs, and therefore, absent MSDS information must be collected after the fact. The ADA maintains a list of available MSDSs by company (and code). Therefore it is relatively easy to check off required MSDSs. Some manufacturers have not supplied this information to the ADA and will not be listed. In that case, it is the responsibility of the dental office to contact the manufacturer directly and obtain the MSDSs if they are available. MSDS information is now available on the Internet both on manufacturer and OSHA home pages. However, permanent copies of MSDSs are still required within dental offices.

Most personnel in a dental office are not familiar with key information they need about materials to be able to make an informed judgment about relative risks or hazards. *Therefore the best approach is to inventory everything in the office (by company or supplier) and then check a published list for the presence or absence of an MSDS.*

These sheets must be available for review by all potentially exposed office personnel and should be stored in a central location with bold labeling or identification of the site. Most sheets are three-hole punched for convenient insertion into an *MSDS notebook.* A common recommendation is to label the notebook "MSDS" on the spine and on the front. *The notebook should be of a color that is distinct from any other notebooks or books* that might be in the same area. All *MSDSs should be organized within the notebook* in a logical fashion for locating easily.

MSDSs are typically a two- to four-page summary of the material's names, chemical reactivity, potential risks in storage or biologic contact, methods of managing emergencies, and summaries of key biologic information. A sample MSDS is shown in Fig. 4-94, with categoric sections indicated.

Third Category of Responsibility. The information, once collected, must be communicated to all employees on a regular basis. In the same notebook with the MSDSs, records should be kept on procedures and times for annual employee hazard communications training. This record should include information about nonroutine tasks such as clean-

3M General Offices
3M Center
St. Paul, Minnesota 55144-1000
612/733-1110
Duns No.: 00-617-3082   00-78
                                                          745

MATERIAL SAFETY
DATA SHEET   **3M**

DIVISION: DENTAL PRODUCTS
TRADE NAME:
  SCOTCHBOND MULTIPURPOSE ADHESIVE

3M I.D. NUMBER: 70-2010-0402-8

ISSUED: MAY 11, 1992
SUPERSEDES: APRIL 16, 1992
DOCUMENT: 05-4869-3

1. INGREDIENT

INGREDIENT	C.A.S. NO.	PERCENT	
BISPHENOL A DIGLYCIDYL ETHER DIMETHACRYLATE	1565-94-2	60.0 –	70.0
2-HYDROXYETHYL METHACRYLATE	868-77-9	30.0 –	40.0
DL-CAMPHORQUINONE	10373-78-1	<	1.0
N,N-DIMETHYLBENZOCAINE	10287-53-3	<	1.0
DIPHENYLIODONIUM HEXAFLUOROPHOSPHATE	58109-40-3	<	1.0

2. PHYSICAL DATA

```
BOILING POINT:............... > 95 F
VAPOR PRESSURE:.............. < 16 psi
VAPOR DENSITY:............... N/A
EVAPORATION RATE:........... N/A
SOLUBILITY IN WATER:........ N/A
SP. GRAVITY:................. 1.15 Water = 1
PERCENT VOLATILE:........... N/A
VOLATILE ORGANICS:.......... N/A
VOC LESS H2O & EXEMPT SOLVENT N/A
pH:......................... N/A
VISCOSITY:.................. 250 CPS Brkfld
MELTING POINT:.............. N/A
APPEARANCE AND ODOR:  Liquid, CLEAR, SLIGHTLY YELLOW, SLIGHT ACRYLATE ODOR
```

3. FIRE AND EXPLOSION HAZARD DATA

```
FLASH POINT:................ 214 F
FLAMMABLE LIMITS - LEL:..... N/A
FLAMMABLE LIMITS - UEL:..... N/A
AUTOIGNITION TEMPERATURE:... N/A
EXTINGUISHING MEDIA:
  Carbon dioxide, Dry chemical
SPECIAL FIRE FIGHTING PROCEDURES:
  Not applicable
UNUSUAL FIRE AND EXPLOSION HAZARDS:
  Not applicable.
NFPA-HAZARD-CODES: HEALTH 1  FIRE 1  REACTIVITY 0
                 UNUSUAL REACTION HAZARD: none
OSHA FIRE HAZARD CLASS: Not applicable
```

4. REACTIVITY DATA

```
STABILITY: Stable
INCOMPATIBILITY - MATERIALS TO AVOID:
  N/A

HAZARDOUS POLYMERIZATION: Will Not Occur
HAZARDOUS DECOMPOSITION PRODUCTS:
  N/A
```

5. ENVIRONMENTAL INFORMATION

```
SPILL RESPONSE:
  Observe precautions from other sections.  Ventilate area.  Cover with
  absorbent material.  Place in metal container.

USE PROTECTIVE GLOVES

RECOMMENDED DISPOSAL:
  Dispose of completely cured (or polymerized) material in a sanitary
  landfill.

  SINCE REGULATIONS VARY, CONSULT APPLICABLE REGULATIONS OR
  AUTHORITIES BEFORE DISPOSAL.

ENVIRONMENTAL DATA:
  Not applicable.

  NOT A MARINE POLLUTANT

REGULATORY INFORMATION:
  U.S. EPA Hazardous Waste Number = None (Not U.S. EPA Hazardous).
  Since regulations vary, consult applicable regulations or authorities
  before disposal.

SARA HAZARD CLASS:
  FIRE HAZARD: No  PRESSURE: No  REACTIVITY: No  ACUTE: Yes  CHRONIC: No
```

6. SUGGESTED FIRST AID

```
EYE CONTACT:
  Immediately flush eyes with large amounts of water for at least 15
  minutes. Get immediate medical attention.

SKIN CONTACT:
  Flush skin with large amounts of water. If irritation persists, call
  a physician. Wash contaminated clothing before reuse.

INHALATION:
  No need for first aid is anticipated.

IF SWALLOWED:
  Do not induce vomiting. Drink two glasses of water. Call a physician.

OTHER FIRST AID:
  MUCOSAL CONTACT: FLUSH WITH PLENTY OF WATER
```

7. PRECAUTIONARY INFORMATION

```
EYE PROTECTION:
  Avoid eye contact.

SKIN PROTECTION:
  Wear appropriate gloves when handling this material.  A pair of
  gloves made from the following material(s) are recommended: nitrile
  rubber.

VENTILATION PROTECTION:
  Not applicable.

RESPIRATORY PROTECTION:
  Not applicable..

PREVENTION OF ACCIDENTAL INGESTION:
  Do not ingest.

RECOMMENDED STORAGE:
  Store at room temperature.

FIRE AND EXPLOSION AVOIDANCE:
  Not applicable.

OTHER PRECAUTIONARY INFORMATION:
  N/A
```

EXPOSURE LIMITS

INGREDIENTS	VALUE	UNIT	TYPE	AUTH	SKIN*
BISPHENOL A DIGLYCIDYL ETHER DIMETHACRYLATE	NONE	NONE	NONE	NONE	
2-HYDROXYETHYL METHACRYLATE	NONE	NONE	NONE	NONE	
DL-CAMPHORQUINONE	NONE	NONE	NONE	NONE	
N,N-DIMETHYLBENZOCAINE	NONE	NONE	NONE	NONE	
DIPHENYLIODONIUM HEXAFLUOROPHOSPHATE	NONE	NONE	NONE	NONE	

```
* SKIN NOTATION: Listed substances indicated with "Y" under SKIN refer to
  the potential contribution to the overall exposure by the cutaneous route
  including mucous membrane and eye, either by airborne or, more particularly,
  by direct contact with the substance.  Vehicles can alter skin absorption.

  SOURCE OF EXPOSURE LIMIT DATA:
  - NONE: None Established
```

8. HEALTH HAZARD DATA

```
EYE CONTACT:
  Severe Eye Irritation: signs/symptoms can include redness, swelling,
  pain, tearing, cloudy appearance of the cornea, impaired vision and
  possible permanently impaired vision.

SKIN CONTACT:
  Allergic Skin Reaction: signs/symptoms can include redness, swelling,
  blistering, and itching.

  Mild Skin Irritation: signs/symptoms can include redness, swelling,
  and itching.

INHALATION:
  No adverse health effects are expected from inhalation exposure.

IF SWALLOWED:
  No adverse health effects are expected from swallowing.
```

SECTION CHANGE DATES

INGREDIENTS	SECTION CHANGED SINCE APRIL 16, 1992 ISSUE

Abbreviations: N/D - Not Determined N/A - Not Applicable

The information on this Data Sheet represents our current data and best
opinion as to the proper use in handling of this material under normal
conditions. Any use of the material which is not in conformance with this
Data Sheet or which involves using the material in combination with any
other material or any other process is the responsibility of the user.

FIG. 4-94 Example of a MSDS for a dentin bonding agent, containing information on the material's: (1) ingredients and identity, (2) physical (and chemical) characteristics, (3) fire and explosion hazard data, (4) reactivity data, (5) environmental precautions, (6) suggested first aid, (7) precautions for safe handling and use, and (8) health hazard data.

ing the dental unit suction reservoirs, training new employees, training service personnel for the office (e.g., janitorial personnel), and inventorying new materials, equipment, or devices that might require updating the MSDSs. This process is rigorously defined and the appropriate details can be obtained from OSHA and the ADA. Some of the details are emphasized in the following discussions.

Fourth Category of Responsibility. For safety in the general office environment and during servicing, sterilization, and maintenance of equipment and instruments, it is mandatory that precautionary measures (e.g., ventilation), personal protective equipment (e.g., protective gloves, apron, and goggles), and emergency equipment (e.g., eyewash fountain, fire extinguisher, and resuscita-

tor mask) be available and appropriately used. *These precautions should be reviewed at least annually.* Review of the *emergency equipment should be checked at least monthly.* A complete review of emergency preparedness for a small office for health and safety can generally be conducted in a matter of 10 to 15 minutes. This review requires only a small amount of time and minimizes employee and patient risks.

Fifth Category of Responsibility. Any incidents that require medical attention or involve loss of work should be documented. A range of forms is needed to: (1) maintain permanent records of incidents, follow-ups, and new preventive measures, (2) summarize incidents and dates for periodic review, and (3) file workman's compensation reports.

Sixth Category of Responsibility. In addition to OSHA's initial concern with hazard communications, relatively recent emphases have been placed on *universal precautions against exposure to bloodborne pathogens* and *waste disposal* for dental offices. Infection control practices for blood-borne pathogens have become much more sophisticated because of concern about the increase in hepatitis and human immunodeficiency virus (HIV) transmissions. These problems and related procedures for offices are discussed in detail in Chapter 8.

Waste disposal currently is not regulated by OSHA. It really involves collection, transport, and management operations. Within the dental office, the collection systems must necessarily be more sophisticated than in many businesses because of infection control regulations. *Trash must be separated on the basis of being: (1) biohazard waste (hazardous), (2) chemical waste (hazardous), or (3) regular (nonhazardous) waste. Nonhazardous waste can be placed in sanitary landfills. The other materials must be incinerated or buried in continuously managed waste disposal sites.*

Currently, most communities have focused only on medical waste. Containers, such as dentin bonding agent vials or precapsulated amalgam capsules, although considered chemical waste, can be disposed of in the nonhazardous waste. Waste transport may occur within a building and/or from the building to an approved disposal facility or site. *The owner of the office generating the waste is responsible for guaranteeing appropriate and safe transport for disposal.* However, there are numerous careless or unscrupulous transporters and managers of waste disposal, who are inadequately informed or unconvinced about the care needed. There is some responsibility for the dental office personnel to ensure the reliability of individuals providing these services.

Seventh Category of Responsibility. Finally there must be employee training and education programs at least annually with respect to hazards, management of blood-borne pathogens, and waste disposal. All new employees must be trained immediately. Records must be kept of the training procedures and training times. All individual records should be kept either in the MSDS notebook and/or in personnel records.

Environmental Protection Agency. All by-products of dental procedures end up as solid, liquid, or gaseous waste, and their disposal can be regulated by the *Environmental Protection Agency* (EPA). At the present time, most waste disposal is regulated by local authorities.

Hazardous gases or vapors, such as nitrous oxide, should be vented directly to the outside air or should be collected from the air using scrubbing devices, both to protect intraoffice individuals and to prevent inadvertent contamination of other local air systems.

Liquid wastes emptied into the sewer or drainage systems have some potential to contaminate the waste treatment plant or groundwater supplies. Therefore it is becoming increasingly important to separate hazardous liquids, such as waste solvents, for controlled disposal. Small amounts of water-based chemicals can be diluted and flushed into the sewer system. However, water-immiscible materials are best disposed of in alternative ways. Waste disposal of blood and body fluids into sanitary sewers is a commonly accepted practice.

Solid wastes include the trash from an office and the effluent disposed into the sewer system. Collected amalgam scrap should be recycled (see Mercury Management and Box 4-1). Amalgam scrap in wastewater is an important issue and separating devices are required in many regions to separate suspended solid (see Amalgam Waste Management, earlier in this chapter). Chairside and plumbing line filters are available for this purpose. The regulations across the United States are not yet uniform.

REFERENCES

1. Albers HA: *Tooth-colored restoratives: an introductory text for selecting, placing and finishing direct systems,* ed 8, Santa Rosa, 1986, Alto Books.
2. Allan DN: A longitudinal study of dental restorations, *Brit Dent J* 143:87-89, 1977.
3. Alster D et al: Polymerization contraction stress in thin resin composite layers as a function of layer thickness, *Dent Mater* 13:146-150, 1997.
4. Alster D et al: Tensile strength of thin resin composite layers as a function of layer thickness, *J Dent Res* 74:1745-1748, 1995.
5. American Dental Association: *Accepted dental therapeutics,* ed 40, Chicago, 1984, American Dental Association.
6. American Dental Association: *Dentist's desk reference: materials, instruments, and equipment,* ed 1, Chicago, 1981, American Dental Association.
7. American Dental Association Council on Scientific Affairs: Dental amalgam: update on safety concerns, *J Am Dent Assoc* 129:493-503, 1998.
8. American Dental Association Council on Scientific Affairs: Dental mercury hygiene recommendations, *J Am Dent Assoc* 130:1125-1126, 1999.
9. American Dental Association Council on Dental Materials, Instruments, and Equipment: Dental mercury hygiene: summary of recommendations in 1990, *J Am Dent Assoc* 122(9):112, 1991.
10. Ames BN, Gold LS: Too many rodent carcinogens: mitogenesis versus mutagenesis, *Science* 249:970-971, 1990.
11. Anderson JN: *Applied dental materials,* ed 6, London, 1976, Blackwell Scientific Publications.
12. Anusavice KJ: *Dental biomaterials III: dental materials for clinical practice,* ed 1, Gainesville, 1992, University of Florida.
13. Anusavice KJ: *Phillip's science of dental materials,* ed 10, Philadelphia, 1996, WB Saunders.
14. Arenholt-Bindslev D: Dental amalgam—environmental aspects, *Adv Dent Res* 6:125-130, 1992.
15. Arenholt-Bindslev D et al: Time-related bisphenol—A content and estrogenic activity in saliva samples collected in relation to placement of fissure sealants, *Clin Oral Investig* 99:120-125, 1999.
16. Avprox Incorporated: http://www.avprox.com.
17. Bader JD et al: Identifying children who will experience high caries increments, *Community Dent Oral Epidemiol* 14:198-201, 1986.

18. Bader JD, Shugars DA: Agreement among dentists' recommendations for restorative treatment, *J Dent Res* 72:891-896, 1993.

19. Baldissara P, Catapano S, Scotti R: Clinical and histological evaluation of thermal injury thresholds in human teeth: a preliminary study, *J Oral Rehabil* 24:791-801, 1997.

20. Bawden JW: Fluoride varnish: a useful new tool for public health dentistry, *J Public Health Dent* 58:266-269, 1998.

21. Bayne SC: CAD/CAM: science and technology, *Trans Acad Dent Mater* 2(1):3-7, 1989.

22. Bayne SC: Dental composites/glass ionomers: clinical reports. In effects and side effects of dental restorative materials proceedings, *Adv Dent Res* 6:65-77, 1992.

23. Bayne SC: The mercury controversy (editorial), *Quintessence Int* 22(4):247-248, 1991.

24. Bayne SC: What is the future of CAD/CAM materials and techniques? In *Symposium on esthetic restorative materials*, Chicago, 1993, American Dental Association Council on Dental Materials, Instruments, and Equipment.

25. Bayne SC, Barton RE: Dental materials for direct restorations. In Richardson RE, Barton RE, editors: *The dental assistant*, ed 6, Philadelphia, 1988, Lea & Febiger.

26. Bayne SC et al: A characterization of first-generation flowable composites, *J Am Dent Assoc* 129:567-577, 1998.

27. Bayne SC et al: Class V angulation, size, and depth effects on composite retention (abstract 1669), *J Dent Res* 71A:314, 1992.

28. Bayne SC et al: Clinical longevity of ten posterior composite materials based on wear (abstract 630), *J Dent Res* 70A:344, 1991.

29. Bayne SC et al: Long term clinical failures in posterior composites (abstract 32), *J Dent Res* 68A:185, 1989.

30. Bayne SC et al: 2-year clinical evaluation of Optibond stress-breaking DBA in Class-V's, *Trans Acad Dent Mater* 8:115, P-25, 1995.

31. Bayne SC, Fleming JE, Faison S: SEM-EDS analysis of macro and micro resin tags of laminates (abstract 1128), *J Dent Res* 61A:304, 1982.

32. Bayne SC, Swift Jr EJ: Solvent analysis of three reduced-component dentin bonding systems, *Trans Acad Dent Mater* 1:156, P-026, 1997.

33. Bayne SC, Taylor DF, Heymann HO: Protection hypothesis for composite wear, *Dent Mater* 8:305-309, 1992.

34. Bayne SC, Taylor DF, Zardiackas LD: *Biomaterials science*, ed 6, Chapel Hill, NC, 1992, Brightstar Publishing.

35. Beltran-Aguilar ED, Goldstein JW: Fluoride varnishes—a review of their clinical use, cariostatic mechanism, efficacy and safety, *J Am Dent Assoc* 131:589-596, 2000.

36. Bentley C, Drake CW: Longevity of restorations in a dental school clinic, *J Dent Educ* 50:594-600, 1986.

37. Bowen RL: Dental filling material comprising vinyl silane treated fused silica and a binder consisting of the reaction product of BIS phenol and glycidyl acrylate (US Patent 3,066,112), 1962.

38. Boyd ND et al: Mercury from dental "silver" tooth fillings impairs sheep kidney function, *Am J Physiol* 261(4 Pt 2): R1010-1014, 1991.

39. Braem M et al: In vivo evaluation of four posterior composites: quantitative wear measurements and clinical behavior, *Dent Mater* 2:106-113, 1986.

40. Bratel J, Haraldson T, Ottosson JO: Potential side effects of dental amalgam restorations. II: No relation between mercury levels in the body and mental disorder, *Eur J Oral Sci* 105:244-250, 1997.

41. Buonocore MG: Simple method of increasing the adhesion of acrylic filling materials to enamel surfaces, *J Dent Res* 34: 849-853, 1955.

42. Cagle CV: *Handbook of adhesive bonding*, ed 1, New York, 1973, McGraw-Hill.

43. Chai JY, Yeung T: Wettability of nonaqueous elastomeric impression materials, *Int J Prosthodont* 4:555-560, 1991.

44. Chang SB, Siew C, Gruninger SE: Factors affecting blood mercury concentrations in practicing dentists, *J Dent Res* 71: 66-74, 1992.

45. Charles AD: The story of dental amalgam, *Bull Hist Dent* 30: 2-6, 1982.

46. Choi KK, Condon JR, Ferracane JL: The effects of adhesive thickness on polymerization contraction stress of composite, *J Dent Res* 79:812-817, 2000.

47. Clemmensen S: Sensitizing potential of 2-hydroxyethyl-methacrylate, *Contact Dermatitis* 12:203-208, 1985.

48. Clinical Research Associates: Materials use survey, *CRA Newsletter* 19(10):3-4, 1995.

49. Clinical Research Associates: Use survey—1990, *CRA Newsletter* 14(12):1, 1990.

50. Collins CJ, Bryant RW: Finishing of amalgam restorations: a three-year clinical trial, *J Dent Res* 20:202-206, 1992.

51. Combe EC: *Notes on dental materials*, ed 4, Edinburgh, 1981, Churchill Livingstone.

52. Condon JR, Ferracane JL: Assessing the effect of composite formulation on polymerization stress, *J Am Dent Assoc* 131: 497-503, 2000.

53. Condon JR, Ferracane JL: Evaluation of composite wear with a new multi-mode oral wear simulator, *Dent Mater* 12: 218-226, 1996.

54. Cook WD: Factors affecting the depth of cure of UV-polymerized composites, *J Dent Res* 59:800-808, 1980.

55. Cooley RL, Stilley J, Lubow RM: Mercury vapor produced during sterilization of amalgam-contaminated instruments, *J Prosthet Dent* 53:304-308, 1985.

56. Crabb HSM: The survival of dental restorations in a teaching hospital, *Brit Dent J* 150:315-318, 1981.

57. Craig RG: *Dental materials—a problem oriented approach*, ed 1, St Louis, 1978, Mosby.

58. Craig RG: Overview of posterior composite resins for use in clinical practice. In Vanherle G, Smith DC, editors: *Posterior composite resin dental restorative materials*, Netherlands, 1985, Peter Szulc Publishing.

59. Craig RG: *Restorative dental materials*, ed 11, St Louis, 2001, Mosby.

60. Craig RG, Powers JM, Wataha JC: *Dental materials: properties and manipulation*, ed 7, St Louis, 2000, Mosby.

61. Cvar JF, Ryge G: Criteria for the clinical evaluation of dental restorative materials (US Dept HEW PHS, Publ No 7902244), Dental Health Center, San Francisco, 1973, US Government Printing Office.

62. Dauvillier BS et al: Visco-elastic parameters of dental restorative materials during setting, *J Dent Res* 79:818-823, 2000.

63. Davidson CL, Feilzer AJ: Polymerization shrinkage and polymerization shrinkage stress in polymer-based restoratives, *J Dent* 25:435-440, 1997.

64. Davidson CL, Van Zeghbroeck L, Feilzer AJ: Destructive stresses in adhesive luting cements, *J Dent Res* 70:880-882, 1991.

65. Davidson-Kaban SS et al: The effect of curing light variations on bulk curing and wall-to-wall quality of two types and various shades of resin composites, *Dent Mater* 13:344-352, 1997.

66. Dawson AS, Smales RJ: Restoration longevity in an Australian defense force population, *Aust Dent J* 37:196-200, 1992.

67. Demaree NC, Taylor DF: Properties of dental amalgams made from spherical alloy powders, *J Dent Res* 41:890-906, 1962.

68. Dental Recycling of North America: http://www.drna.com.

69. Disney JA et al: The University of North Carolina caries risk assessment study: further developments in caries risk assessment, *Community Dent Oral Epidemiol* 20:64-75, 1992.

70. Eames WB: Preparation and condensation of amalgam with low mercury-alloy ratio, *J Am Dent Assoc* 58(4):78-83, 1959.

71. Eames WB et al: Accuracy and dimensional stability of elastomeric impression materials, *J Prosthet Dent* 42:159-162, 1979.

72. Eastman J, Siegel RW: Nanophase synthesis assembles materials from atomic clusters, *Res Devel* 56-60, Jan 1989.

74. Elderton RJ: Longitudinal study of dental treatment in the general dental service in Scotland, *Brit Dent J* 155:91-96, 1983.

75. Ericson D, Derand T: Increase of in vitro curing depth of class II composite resin restorations, *J Prosthet Dent* 70:219-223, 1993.

76. Evans FG: *Mechanical properties of bone,* ed 1, Springfield, Ill, 1973, Charles C Thomas Publisher.

77. Fan PL, O'Brien WJ, Craig RG: Wetting properties of sealants and glazes, *Oper Dent* 4:100-103, 1979.

78. Feilzer AJ, De Gee AJ, Davidson CL: Relaxation of polymerization contraction shear stress by hygroscopic expansion, *J Dent Res* 69:36-39, 1990.

79. Feilzer AJ, De Gee AJ, Davidson CL: Quantitative determination of stress reduction by flow in composite restorations, *Dent Mater* 6:167-171, 1990.

80. Feilzer AJ, De Gee AJ, Davidson CL: Setting stresses in composites for two different curing modes, *Dent Mater* 9:2-5, 1993.

81. Feilzer AJ, De Gee AJ, Davidson CL: Setting stress in composite resin in relation to configuration of the restoration, *J Dent Res* 66:1636-1639, 1987.

82. Feilzer AJ et al: Influence of light intensity on polymerization shrinkage and integrity of restoration-cavity interface, *Eur J Oral Sci* 103:322-326, 1995.

83. Ferracane JL: *Materials in dentistry—principles and applications,* Philadelphia, 1995, JP Lippincott.

84. Freund M, Munksgaard EC: Enzymatic degradation of BisGMA/TEGDMA-polymers causing decreased microhardness and greater wear in vitro, *Scand J Dent Res* 98:351-355, 1990.

85. Fried K: Changes in innervation of dentine and pulp with age. In Ferguson DF, editor: *The aging mouth,* Basel, 1987, Karger.

86. Fung EY et al: Pharmacokinetics of bisphenol-A released from a dental sealant, *J Am Dent Assoc* 131:51-58, 2000.

87. Geurtsen W et al: Aqueous extracts from dentin adhesives contain cytotoxic chemicals, *J Biomed Mater Res* 48:772-777, 1999.

88. Geurtsen W et al: Cytotoxicity of 35 dental resin composite monomers/additives in permanent 3T3 and three human primary fibroblast cultures, *J Biomed Mater Res* 41:474-480, 1998.

89. Gold LS et al: Rodent carcinogens: setting priorities, *Science* 258:261-265, 1992.

90. Greener EH, Harcourt JK, Lautenschlager EP: *Materials science in dentistry,* Baltimore, 1972, Williams & Wilkins.

91. Grippo JO, Masi JV: Role of biodental engineering factors (BEF) in the etiology of root caries, *J Esthet Dent* 3:71-76, 1991.

92. Grossman DG: Structure and physical properties of Dicor/MGC glass-ceramic. *Proceedings of the International Symposium on Computer Restorations,* Chicago, 1991, Quintessence.

93. Guggenberger R, May R, Stefan KP: New trends in glass-ionomer chemistry, *Biomaterials* 19:479-483, 1998.

94. Hahn LJ et al: Dental "silver" tooth fillings: a source of mercury exposure revealed by whole-body image scan and tissue analysis, *FASEB J* 3:2641-2646, 1989.

95. Haines D, Berry DC, Poole DFG: Behavior of tooth enamel under load, *J Dent Res* 42:885-888, 1963.

96. Harada M: Minamata disease: methylmercury poisoning in Japan caused by environmental pollution, *Crit Rev Toxicol* 25:1-24, 1995.

97. Hasegawa J: Dental casting materials, *Trans Acad Dent Mater* 2(3):190-201, 1989.

98. Helkimo E, Carlsson GE, Helkimo M: Bite force and state of dentition, *Acta Odont Scand* 35:297-303, 1977.

99. Hench LL, Ethridge EC: *Biomaterials, an interfacial approach,* ed 1, New York, 1982, Academic Press.

100. Herø H, Okabe T, Wie H: Corrosion of gallium alloys in vivo, *J Mat Sci Mat Med* 8:357-360, 1997.

101. Herø H, Simensen CJ, Jorgensen RB: Structure of dental gallium alloys, *Biomaterials* 17:1321-1326, 1996.

102. Heymann HO et al: The clinical performance of CAD-CAM-generated ceramic inlays: a four-year study, *J Am Dent Assoc* 127:1171-1181, 1996.

103. Heymann HO et al: Tooth flexure effects on cervical restorations: a two-year study, *J Am Dent Assoc* 122:41-47, 1991.

104. Heymann HO et al: Two-year clinical performance of CEREC CAD/CAM-generated MGC inlays (abstract 814), *J Dent Res* 71A:207, 1992.

105. Heymann HO et al: Two-year clinical study of composite resins in posterior teeth, *Dent Mater* 2:37-41, 1986.

106. Hickel R et al: CAD/CAM—Fillings or the future? *Inter Dent J* 47:247-258, 1997.

107. Hörsted-Bindslev P et al: *Dental amalgam–a health hazard?,* Copenhagen, Denmark, 1991, Munksgaard.

108. Iler RK: *The chemistry of silica. Solubility, polymerization, colloid, and surface properties, and biochemistry,* New York, 1979, John Wiley & Sons.

109. Innes DBK, Youdelis WV: Dispersion strengthened amalgams, *J Can Dent Assoc* 29:587-593, 1963.

110. Inokoshi S et al: Dual-cure luting composites. I: Filler particle distribution, *J Oral Rehabil* 20:133-146, 1993.

111. Isenberg BP, Essig ME, Leinfelder KF: Three-year clinical evaluation of CAD/CAM restorations, *J Esthet Dent* 4:173-175, 1992.

112. Jaarda MJ et al: Measurement of composite resin filler particles by using scanning electron microscopy and digital imaging, *J Prosthet Dent* 69:416-424, 1993.

113. Johnson GH, Gordon GE, Bales DJ: Postoperative sensitivity associated with posterior composite and amalgam restorations, *Oper Dent* 13:66-73, 1988.

114. Jorgensen KD: The mechanism of marginal fracture of amalgam fillings, *Acta Odont Scand* 23:347-389, 1965.

115. Jorgensen KD: Occlusal abrasion of a composite resin with ultra-fine filler—an initial study, *Quintessence Int* 6:73-78, 1978.

116. Kaga M et al: Gallium alloy restorations in primary teeth: a 12-month study, *J Am Dent Assoc* 127:1195-1201, 1996.

117. Kinomoto Y et al: Comparison of polymerization contraction stresses between self and light-curing composites, *J Dent* 27:383-389, 1999.

118. Koch G, Petersson LG: Fluoride content of enamel surface treated with a varnish containing sodium fluoride, *Odontol Rev* 23:437-446, 1972.

119. Krejci I et al: Wear of ceramic inlays, their enamel antagonists, and luting cements, *J Prosthet Dent* 69:425-430, 1993.

120. Lammie GA: A comparison of the cutting efficiency and heat production of tungsten carbide and steel burs, *Brit Dent J* 90:251-259, 1951.

121. Lang BR, Jaarda M, Wang RF: Filler particle size and composite resin classification systems, *J Oral Rehabil* 19:569-684, 1992.

122. Larmas MA, Hayrynen H, Lajunen LHJ: Thermogravimetric studies on sound and carious human enamel and dentin as well as hydroxyapatite, *Scand J Dent Res* 101:185-191, 1993.

123. Lee WC, Eakle WS: Possible role of tensile stress in the etiology of cervical erosive lesions of teeth, *J Prosthet Dent* 52:374-380, 1984.

124. Leinfelder KF: Composites: current status and future developments. In *International state-of-the-art conference on restorative dental materials,* Bethesda, Md, 1986, National Institute of Dental Research.

125. Leinfelder KF: Wear patterns and rates of posterior composite resins, *Int Dent J* 37:152-157, 1987.

126. Leinfelder KF, Bayne SC, Swift EJ: Packable composites: overview and technical considerations, *J Esthet Dent* 11:234-249, 1999.

127. Leinfelder KF, Bayne SC, Swift Jr EJ: Packable composites: overview and technical considerations, *J Esthet Dent* 11:234-249, 1999.

128. Leinfelder KF et al: An in vitro device for determining wear of posterior composites (abstract 636), *J Dent Res* 70A:345, 1991.

129. Leinfelder KF et al: Burnished amalgam restorations: a two-year clinical evaluation, *Oper Dent* 3:2-8, 1978.

130. Leinfelder KF, Lemons JF: *Clinical restorative materials and techniques,* ed 1, Philadelphia, 1988, Lea & Febiger.

131. Letzel H: Four-year survival and failures of posterior composite restorations in a multicentre controlled clinical trial (abstract 197), *J Dent Res* 68A:206, 1989.

132. Letzel H et al: Materials influences on the survival of amalgam and composite restorations (abstract 1426), *J Dent Res* 69A:287, 1990.

133. Letzel H, Vrijhoef MMA: Survival rates of dental amalgam restorations (abstract 820), *J Dent Res* 61A:269, 1982.

134. Lutz F et al: In vivo and in vitro wear of potential posterior composites, *J Dent Res* 63:914-920, 1984.

135. Lutz F, Phillips RW: A classification and evaluation of composite resin systems, *J Prosthet Dent* 50:480-488, 1983.

136. 3M: Personal Air Monitoring Systems: 3600 mercury vapor monitor, http://www.mmm.com.US/safety/produts/ohes/.

137. Mackert JR: Dental amalgam and mercury, *J Am Dent Assoc* 122(8):54-61, 1991.

138. Mackert JR et al: Lymphocyte levels in subjects with and without amalgam restorations, *J Am Dent Assoc* 122(3):49-53, 1991.

139. Mahler DB: Standardizing amalgam marginal fracture evaluation (abstract 445), *J Dent Res* 65:219, 1986.

140. Mahler DB, Peyton FA: Photoelasticity as a research technique for analyzing stress in dental structures, *J Dent Res* 34:831-838, 1955.

141. Mahler DB, Terkla LC: Analysis of stress in dental structures. In *Dental Clinics of North America: symposium on dental materials,* Philadelphia, 1958, WB Saunders.

142. Mahler DB, Terkla LG, Eysden JV: Marginal fracture of amalgam restorations, *J Dent Res* 52:823-827, 1973.

143. Mandel ID: Amalgam hazards. an assessment of research, *J Am Dent Assoc* 122(8):62-65, 1991.

144. Mandikos MN: Polyvinyl siloxane impression materials: an update on clinical use, *Aust Dent J* 43:428-434, 1998.

145. Marshall GW, Sarkar NK, Greener EH: Detection of oxygen in corrosion products of dental amalgam, *J Dent Res* 54:904, 1975.

146. Marshall SJ, Marshall GW Jr: $Sn_4(OH)_6Cl_2$ and SnO corrosion products on amalgams, *J Dent Res* 59:820-823, 1980.

147. McCabe JF: *Applied dental materials,* ed 2, London, 1990, Blackwell Scientific.

148. McCabe JF: Resin-modified glass-ionomers, *Biomaterials* 19:521-527, 1998.

149. McCabe JF, Carrick TE: Output from visible-light activation units and depth of cure of light-activated composites, *J Dent Res* 68:1534-1539, 1989.

150. The mercury in your mouth: you can avoid amalgam fillings or even replace the ones you have, but should you? *Consumer Reports* 316-319, May 1991.

151. The mercury scare: if a dentist wants to remove your fillings because they contain mercury, watch your wallet, *Consumer Reports* 51(3):150-152, 1986.

152. Mertz-Fairhurst EJ et al: A comparative clinical study of two pit and fissure sealants: 7-year results in Augusta, Ga, *J Am Dent Assoc* 109:252-255, 1984.

153. Mertz-Fairhurst EJ et al: Ultraconservative and cariostatic sealed restorations: results at year 10, *J Am Dent Assoc* 129:55-66, 1998.

154. Meyer JM, Cattani-Lorente MA, Dupuis V: Compomers: between glass-ionomer cements and composites, *Biomaterials* 19:529-539, 1998.

155. Mitra SB, Li MY, Culler SR: Setting reaction of Vitrebond light cure glass ionomer liner/base. In Setting mechanisms of dental materials, *Trans Acad Dent Mater* 5(2):1-22, 1992.

156. Mjor IA: Frequency of secondary caries at various anatomical locations, *Oper Dent* 10:88-92, 1985.

157. Mjor IA: Placement and replacement of restorations, *Oper Dent* 6:49-54, 1981.

158. Molin C: Amalgam—fact and fiction, *Scand J Dent Res* 100:66-73, 1992.

159. Momoi Y et al: A suggested method for mixing direct filling restorative gallium alloy, *Oper Dent* 21:12-16, 1996.

160. Morin DL et al: Biophysical stress analysis of restored teeth: modeling and analysis, *Dent Mater* 4:77-84, 1988.

161. Mormann W, Krejci I: Computer-designed inlays after 5 years in situ: clinical performance and scanning electron microscope evaluation, *Quintessence Int* 23:109-115, 1992.

162. Morris HF: Veterans Administration Cooperative Studies Project No. 147. Part VIII: Plaque accumulation on metal ceramic restorations cast from noble and nickel-based alloys: a five-year report, *J Prosthet Dent* 61:543-549, 1989.

163. Mount GJ: Glass ionomer cements: clinical considerations, In *Clinical dentistry,* New York, 1984, Harper & Row.

164. Mount GJ: Restoration with glass-ionomer cement: requirements for clinical success, *Oper Dent* 6:59-65, 1981.

165. Munksgaard EC: Permeability of protective gloves to (di)methacrylates in resinous dental materials, *Scand J Dent Res* 100:189-192, 1992.

166. Munksgaard EC, Freund M: Enzymatic hydrolysis of (di)methacrylates and their polymers, *Scand J Dent Res* 98:261-267, 1990.

167. Nakabayashi N, Ashizawa M, Nakamura M: Identification of a resin-dentin hybrid layer in vital human dentin created in vivo: durable bonding to vital dentin, *Quintessence Int* 23:135-141, 1992.

168. Nash KD, Bentley JE: Is restorative dentistry on its way out? *J Am Dent Assoc* 122(9):79-80, 1991.

169. Nathanson D et al: In vitro elution of leachable components from dental sealants, *J Am Dent Assoc* 128:1517-1523, 1997.

170. National Institutes of Health: Consensus development conference statement on dental sealants in the prevention of tooth decay, *J Am Dent Assoc* 108:233-236, 1984.

171. National Institutes of Health: Effects and side effects of dental restorative materials—NIH Technology Assessment Conference Statement, *Natl Lib Med* 1-18, 1991.

172. Navarro MFL et al: Clinical evaluation of gallium alloy as a posterior restorative material, *Quintessence Int* 27:315-320, 1996.

173. Nicholson JW, Wasson EA: The setting of glass-polyalkenoate ("glass-ionomer") cements. In Setting mechanisms of dental materials, *Trans Acad Dent Mater* 5(2):1-14, 1992.

174. Noda M, Komatsu H, Sano H: HPLC analysis of dental resin composite components, *J Biomed Mater Res* 47:374-378, 1999.

175. Norman RD, Wilson NHF: Three-year findings of a multicentre trial for a posterior composite, *J Prosthet Dent* 59:577-583, 1986.

176. O'Brien WJ: *Dental materials and their selection*, ed 2, Chicago, 1997, Quintessence.

177. O'Brien WJ, Fan PL, Apostolides A: Penetrativity of sealants and glazes, *Oper Dent* 3:51-56, 1978.

178. O'Brien WJ, Ryge G: *An outline of dental materials and their selection*, ed 1, Philadelphia, 1990, WB Saunders.

179. Odom JG: Ethics and dental amalgam removal, *J Am Dent Assoc* 122(7):69-71, 1991.

180. Okamoto Y, Horibe T: Liquid gallium alloys for metallic plastic fillings, *Brit Dent J* 170:23-26, 1991.

181. Olea N et al: Estrogenicity of resin-based composites and sealants used in dentistry, *Environ Health Perspect* 104:298-305, 1996.

182. Opdam NJ et al: Marginal integrity and postoperative sensitivity in Class 2 resin composite restorations in vivo, *J Dent* 26:555-562, 1998.

183. Opdam NJ et al: A radiographic and scanning electron microscopic study of approximal margins of Class II resin composite restorations placed in vivo, *J Dent* 26:319-327, 1998.

184. Osborne JW, Berry TG: Zinc-containing high-copper amalgams: a 3-year clinical evaluation, *Am J Dent* 5:43-45, 1992.

185. Osborne JW et al: Clinical performance and physical properties of twelve amalgam alloys, *J Dent Res* 57:983-988, 1978.

186. Osborne JW, Summit JB: Direct-placement gallium restorative alloy: a 3-year clinical evaluation, *Quintessence Int* 30:49-53, 1999.

187. Osborne JW, Summitt JB: 2-year clinical evaluation of a gallium restorative alloy, *Am J Dent* 9:191-194, 1996.

188. Oysaed H, Ruyter IE, Sjovik-Kleven IJ: Release of formaldehyde from dental composites, *J Dent Res* 67:1289-1294, 1988.

189. Park JB: *Biomaterials: an introduction*, ed 1, New York, 1979, Plenum.

190. Patterson N: The longevity of restorations: a study of 200 regular attenders in a general dental practice, *Brit Dent J* 157:23-25, 1984.

191. Petersson LG: On topical application of fluorides and its inhibiting effect on caries, *Odontol Revy Suppl* 34:1-36, 1975.

192. Petersson LG et al: Effect of quarterly treatments with a chlorhexidine and a fluoride varnish on approximal caries in caries-susceptible teenagers: a 3-year clinical study, *Caries Res* 34:140-13, 2000.

193. Peyton FA: *Restorative dental materials*, ed 3, St Louis, 1968, Mosby.

194. Phillips RW: *Skinner's science of dental materials*, ed 9, Philadelphia, 1991, WB Saunders.

195. Phillips RW, Moore BK: *Elements of dental materials: for dental hygienists and dental assistants*, ed 5, Philadelphia, 1994, WB Saunders.

196. Port RM, Marshall GW: Characteristics of amalgam restorations with variable clinical appearance, *J Am Dent Assoc* 110:491-495, 1985.

197. Powers JM, Capp JA, Koran A: Color of gingival tissues of blacks and whites, *J Dent Res* 56:112-116, 1977.

198. Preston JD, Duret F: CAD/CAM in dentistry, *Oral Health* 87:17-27, 1997.

199. Pulgar R et al: Determination of bisphenol A and related aromatic compounds released from bis-GMA-based composites and sealants by high performance liquid chromatography, *Environ Health Perspect* 108:21-27, 2000.

200. Putnam JJ: Quicksilver and slow death, *National Geographic* 142(4):507-527, 1972.

201. Rakich DR et al: Effects of dentin bonding agents on macrophage mitochondrial activity, *J Endod* 24:528-533, 1998.

202. Reese JA, Valega TM: *Restorative dental materials: an overview*, vol 1, Guildford, Surrey, 1985, FDI, Biddles.

203. Rehfeld RL et al: Evolution of various forms of calcium hydroxide in the monitoring of microleakage, *Dent Mater* 7:202-205, 1991.

204. Reisbick MH: *Dental materials in clinical dentistry*, ed 1, Boston, 1982, John Wright PSG.

205. Retief DH, Mallory WP: Evaluation of two pit and fissure sealants: an in vitro study, *Pediatr Dent* 3:12-16, 1981.

206. Rinne VW: Aluminum foil pouch packaging in pre-measured amalgam capsules, *J Dent Res* 62:116-117, 1983.

207. Ripa LW: Occlusal sealing: rationale of the technique and historical review, *J Am Soc Prev Dent* 3:32-39, 1973.

208. Roberson TM et al: Five-year clinical wear analysis of 19 posterior composites (abstract 63), *J Dent Res* 67A:120, 1988.

209. Robinson AD: The life of a filling, *Br Dent J* 130:206-208, 1971.

210. Ross GK et al: Measurement of deformation of teeth in vivo (abstract 432), *J Dent Res* 71A:569, 1992.

211. Rothwell PS, Frame JW, Shimmin CV: Mercury vapor hazards from hot air sterilisers in dental practice, *Br Dent J* 142:359-365, 1977.

212. Roulet JF: *Degradation of dental polymers*, Basel, 1987, Karger.

213. Ruddell DE et al: Mechanical properties and wear behavior of condensable composites (abstract 407), *J Dent Res* 78:156, 1999.

214. Ruse ND: What is a "compomer"?, *J Can Dent Assoc* 65:500-504, 1999.

215. Ryge G: Clinical criteria, *Int Dent J* 30:347-358, 1980.

216. Santerre JP, Shajii L, Tsang H: Biodegradation of commercial dental composites by cholesterol esterase, *J Dent Res* 78:1459-1468, 1999.

217. Schafer TE et al: Estrogenicity of bisphenol A and bisphenol A dimethacrylate in vitro, *J Biomed Mater Res* 45:192-197, 1999.

218. Scheinin A et al: Multifactorial modeling for root caries predictions, *Community Dent Oral Epidemiol* 20:35-37, 1992.

219. Schmidt C: In vitro toothbrushing/dentifrice wear of resin-based materials used to seal or repair dental restorations

(Master's thesis), D.A.T.E., Division of Dental Hygiene, Department of Dental Ecology, School of Dentistry, Chapel Hill, NC, 1998, University of North Carolina.

220. Seghi RR, Denry IL, Rosenstiel SF: Relative fracture toughness and hardness of new dental ceramics, *J Prosthet Dent* 74:145-150, 1995.

221. Seghi RR, Sorensen JA: Relative flexural strength of six new ceramic materials, *Int J Prosthodont* 8:239-246, 1995.

222. Silverstone LM et al: Variation in the pattern of acid etching of human dental enamel examined by scanning electron microscopy, *Caries Res* 9:373-387, 1975.

223. Silvey RG, Myers GE: Clinical study of dental cements. VII. A study of bridge retainers luted with three different dental cements, *J Dent Res* 57:703-707, 1978.

224. Simmons JJ: The miracle mixture: glass ionomer and alloy powder, *Tex Dent J* 100:10-12, 1983.

225. Simonsen RJ: Retention and effectiveness of dental sealant after 15 years, *J Am Dent Assoc* 122(11):34-42, 1992.

226. Skinner EW, Phillips RW: Direct filling gold and its manipulation. In *Science of dental materials*, ed 6, Philadelphia, 1967, WB Saunders.

227. Smales RJ: Long-term deterioration of composite resin and amalgam restorations, *Oper Dent* 16:202-209, 1991.

228. Smales RJ et al: Prediction of amalgam restoration longevity, *J Dent* 19:18-23, 1991.

229. Smales RJ, Gao W: In vitro caries inhibition at the enamel margins of glass ionomer restoratives developed for the ART technique, *J Dent* 28:249-256, 2000.

230. Smales RJ, Webster DA, Leppard PI: Predictions of restoration deterioration, *J Dent* 20:215-220, 1992.

231. Smith DC: Development of glass-ionomer cement systems, *Biomaterials* 19:467-478, 1998.

232. Smith DL, Caul HJ: Alloys of gallium with powdered metals as possible replacement for dental amalgam, *J Am Dent Assoc* 53:315-324, 1956.

233. Soderholm KJ: Correlation of in vivo and in vitro performance of adhesive restorative materials: a report of the ASC MD156 task group for the adhesion of restorative materials, *Dent Mater* 7:74-83, 1991.

234. Soderholm KJ: Degradation of glass filler in experimental composites, *J Dent Res* 60:1867-1875, 1981.

235. Spencer P et al: Chemical characterization of the dentin/adhesive interface by Fourier transform photoacoustic spectroscopy, *Dent Mater* 8:8-10, 1992.

236. Stock A: Die gefahrlichkeit des quecksilberdampfes und der amalgame, *Med Klin* 22:1209-1212, 1250-1252, 1926.

237. Sturdevant JR et al: The 8-year clinical performance of 15 low-gold casting alloys, *Dent Mater* 3:347-352, 1987.

238. Sturdevant JR et al: Ten-year clinical analysis of 3 barium glass filled posterior composites (abstract 794), *J Dent Res* 71A:204, 1992.

239. Takahashi H, Finger WJ: Dentin surface reproduction with hydrophilic and hydrophobic impression materials, *Dent Mater* 7:197-201, 1991.

240. Taylor DF et al: Pooling of long term clinical wear data for posterior composites, *Am J Dentistry* 7(6):167-174.

241. Taylor NO, Paffenbarger GC, Sweeney WT: Inlay casting golds: physical properties and specification, *J Am Dent Assoc* 19:36-53, 1932.

242. Thompson JY, Bayne SC, Heymann HO: Mechanical properties of a new mica-based machinable glass ceramic for CAD/CAM restorations, *J Prosthet Dent* 76:619-623, 1996.

243. Thompson JY, Rapp MM, Parker AJ: Microscopic and energy dispersive x-ray analysis of surface adaptation of dental ce-

ments to dental ceramic surfaces, *J Prosthet Dent* 79:378-383, 1998.

244. Thompson VP, Williams EF, Bailey WJ: Dental resins with reduced shrinkage during hardening, *J Dent Res* 58:1522-1532, 1979.

245. Tomashov ND: *Theory of corrosion and protection of metals*, ed 1, New York, 1966, Macmillan.

246. Vanherle G, Lambrechts P, Braem M: Overview of the clinical requirements for posterior composites. In Vanherle G, Smith DC, editors: *Posterior composite resin dental restorative materials*, Netherlands, 1985, Peter Szulc.

247. Van Meerbeek B et al: Microscopy investigations: techniques, results, and limitations, *Am J Dent* 13:3D-18D, 2000.

248. Venugopalan R, Broome JC, Lucas LC: The effect of water contamination on dimensional change and corrosion properties of a gallium alloy, *Dent Mater* 14:173-178, 1998.

249. Vimy MF, Takahashi Y, Lorscheider FL: Maternal-fetal distribution of mercury (^{203}Hg) released from dental amalgam fillings, *Am J Physiol* 258(4-Pt2):R939-945, 1990.

250. Vimy MJ, Lorscheider FL: Intra-oral air mercury released from dental amalgam, *J Dent Res* 64:1069-1071, 1985.

251. Von Fraunhofer JA: *Scientific aspects of dental materials*, ed 1, London, 1975, Butterworth.

252. Vrijhoef MMA, Vermeersch AG, Spanauf AJ: *Dental amalgam*, Chicago, 1980, Quintessence.

253. Waterstrat RM: New alloys show extraordinary resistance to fracture and wear, *J Am Dent Assoc* 123(12):33-36, 1992.

254. Wilder AD et al: Five-year clinical study of UV polymerized posterior composites, *J Dent* 19:214-220, 1991.

255. Wilder AD et al: Long term clinical color-matching analysis for 30 dental composites (abstract 801), *J Dent Res* 71A:206, 1992.

256. Wilder AD Jr et al: Seventeen-year clinical study of ultraviolet-cured posterior composite Class I and II restorations, *J Esthet Dent* 11:135-142, 1999.

257. Wilkerson MD et al: Biaxial flexure strength and fracture toughness of flowable composites (abstract 779), *J Dent Res* 77:203, 1998.

258. Willems G et al: A classification of dental composites according to their morphological and mechanical characteristics. *Dent Mater* 8:310-319, 1992.

259. Willems G et al: Composite resins in the twenty-first century, *Quintessence Int* 24:641-658, 1993.

260. Willer J, Rossbach A, Weber H: Computer-assisted milling of dental restorations using a new CAD/CAM data acquisition system, *J Prosthet Dent* 80:346-353, 1998.

261. Wilson AD, Kent BE: A new translucent cement for dentistry—the glass ionomer cement, *Brit Dent J* 132:133-135, 1972.

262. Wilson HJ, McLean JW, Brown D: *Dental materials and their clinical applications*, ed 1, London, 1988, British Dental Association, William Clowes.

263. World Health Organization: *Environmental health criteria 118: inorganic mercury*, Geneva, Switzerland, 1991, World Health Organization.

264. Wu W, Cobb EN: A silver staining technique for investigating wear of restorative dental composites, *J Biomed Mater Res* 15:343-348, 1981.

265. Xu HHK: Dental composite resins containing silica-fused ceramic single-crystalline whiskers with various filler levels, *J Dent Res* 78:1304-1311, 1999.

266. Xu HHK et al: Ceramic whisker reinforcement of dental resin composites, *J Dent Res* 78:706-712, 1999.

267. Xu HHK et al: Cyclic contact fatigue of a silver alternative to amalgam, *Dent Mater* 14:11-20, 1998.

268. Xu HHK et al: Two-body sliding wear of a direct-filling silver alternative to amalgam, *Quintessence Int* 30:199-208, 1999.

269. Yamada H: *Strength of biological materials,* ed 1, Huntington NY, 1973, RE Krieger.

270. Yamauchi M, Woodley DT, Mechanic GT: Aging and cross-linking of skin collagen, *Biochem Biophys Res Commun* 158:898-903, 1988.

271. Yoshii E: Cytotoxic effects of acrylates and methacrylates: relationships of monomer structures and cytotoxicity, *J Biomed Mater Res* 37:517-524, 1997.

272. Zach L, Cohen G: Pulp response to externally applied heat, *Oral Surg Oral Med Oral Path* 19:515-530, 1965.

273. Zach L, Cohen G: Thermogenesis in operative techniques—comparison of four methods, *J Prosthet Dent* 12:977-984, 1962.

274. Zardiackas LD, Bayne SC: Fatigue characterization of nine dental amalgams, *Biomat* 6:49-54, 1985.

275. Zu JJK et al: Three-body wear of a hand-consolidated silver alternative to amalgam, *J Dent Res* 78:1560-1567, 1999.

5

Fundamental Concepts of Enamel and Dentin Adhesion

JORGE PERDIGÃO

EDWARD J. SWIFT, JR.

BASIC CONCEPTS OF ADHESION

The American Society for Testing and Materials (ASTM; specification D 907) defines adhesion as "the state in which two surfaces are held together by interfacial forces which may consist of valence forces or interlocking forces or both."[213] The word *adhesion* comes from the Latin *adhaerere* ("to stick to"). An adhesive is a material, frequently a viscous fluid, that joins two substrates together and solidifies, and therefore is able to transfer a load from one surface to the other. Adhesion or adhesive strength is the measure of the load-bearing capacity of an adhesive joint.[3] Four different mechanisms of adhesion have been described[6]:

1. Mechanical adhesion—interlocking of the adhesive with irregularities in the surface of the substrate, or adherend.
2. Adsorption adhesion—chemical bonding between the adhesive and the adherend. The forces involved may be primary (ionic and covalent) or secondary (hydrogen bonds, dipole interaction, or van der Waals) valence forces.
3. Diffusion adhesion—interlocking between mobile molecules, such as the adhesion of two polymers through diffusion of polymer chain ends across an interface.
4. Electrostatic adhesion—an electrical double layer at the interface of a metal with a polymer that is part of the total bonding mechanism.

Bonding of resins to tooth structure is a result of four possible mechanisms[286]:

1. Mechanical—penetration of resin and formation of resin tags within the tooth surface
2. Diffusion—precipitation of substances on the tooth surfaces to which resin monomers can bond mechanically or chemically
3. Adsorption—chemical bonding to the inorganic component (hydroxyapatite) or organic components (mainly Type I collagen) of tooth structure
4. A combination of the previous three mechanisms

For good adhesion, close contact must exist between the adhesive and the substrate (enamel or dentin). Furthermore, the surface tension of the adhesive must be lower than the surface energy of enamel and dentin. A major problem in bonding resins to tooth structure is that all methacrylate-based dental resins shrink during free-radical addition polymerization.[263] Therefore a dental adhesive should provide a strong initial bond to resist the stresses of resin shrinkage.[7]

Failures of adhesive joints occur in three locations, which are generally combined when an actual failure occurs: cohesive failure in the substrate; cohesive failure within the adhesive; and adhesive failure, or failure at the interface of substrate and adhesive.

RECENT TRENDS IN RESTORATIVE DENTISTRY

The introduction of enamel bonding,[56] the increasing demand for both restorative and nonrestorative esthetic treatments, and the ubiquity of fluoride have combined to transform the practice of operative dentistry.[328] The classic concepts of tooth preparation[38] advocated in the early 1900s have changed drastically over the last 20 years. This transformation in philosophy has resulted in a more conservative approach to tooth preparation, regarding not only the basic concepts of retention form, but also the resistance form of the remaining tooth structure. Bonding techniques allow more conservative tooth preparations, less reliance on macromechanical retention, and less removal of unsupported enamel.

The availability of new scientific information on the etiology, diagnosis, and treatment of carious lesions, as well as the introduction of reliable adhesive restorative materials, has substantially reduced the need for extensive tooth preparations. Adhesive composite restorations are used to replace carious dental tissues, to restore fractured teeth, and to replace missing enamel or dentin in the cervical areas of teeth. With improvements in materials, these indications have progressively shifted from the anterior segment only to posterior teeth as well. Adhesive restorative techniques are currently used to:

1. Change the shape and the color of anterior teeth.
2. Restore Classes I, II, III, IV, V, and VI carious or traumatic defects.
3. Restore teeth with amalgam using an adhesive technique.
4. Provide retention for metallic crowns or for porcelain-fused-to-metal crowns.
5. Bond all-ceramic restorations (Fig. 5-1).
6. Bond indirect resin-based restorations.

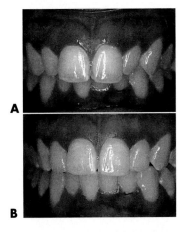

FIG. 5-1 **A**, Twenty-year-old patient with peg lateral incisors. Patient specifically requested ceramic restorations rather than direct composite resin. **B**, Porcelain veneers wrapping around the proximal surfaces were fabricated and bonded using a total-etch simplified dentin adhesive and a light-activated composite cement.

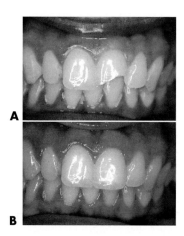

FIG. 5-2 **A,** Twenty-two-year-old patient fractured the maxillary left central incisor in an accident, but recovered the fractured fragment. **B,** Exposed dentin and peripheral enamel were etched with 35% phosphoric acid for 15 seconds. The fractured fragment was etched in the same manner. A dentin adhesive was applied to the etched surfaces and the fragment was adapted to the fractured area. After ensuring a tight and close adaptation, the area was light-cured for 40 seconds from the facial and 40 seconds from the lingual.

7. Seal pits and fissures of posterior teeth.
8. Bond orthodontic brackets.
9. Bond periodontal splints and conservative tooth-replacement restorations.
10. Repair existing restorations (composite, amalgam, or ceramic).
11. Provide foundations for crowns.
12. Desensitize exposed root surfaces.
13. Impregnate dentin that has been exposed to the oral fluids, making it less susceptible to caries.
14. Bond fractured fragments of anterior teeth (Fig. 5-2).
15. Bond prefabricated and cast posts.
16. Reinforce fragile roots internally.
17. Seal apical restorations placed during endodontic surgery.

ADVANTAGES OF ENAMEL ADHESION

As measured in the laboratory, bond strengths of composite to phosphoric acid-etched enamel usually exceed 20 MPa.[95,162,303] Such bond strengths provide adequate retention for a broad variety of procedures and prevent microleakage around enamel margins of restorations.[277] Adhesive restorations provide other benefits such as cusp reinforcement after tooth preparation.[302] Adhesive restorations substantially reinforce remaining enamel and dentin, making them less susceptible to fracture.[18,184,195]

ENAMEL ADHESION

Inspired by the industrial use of 85% phosphoric acid to facilitate adhesion of paints and resins to metallic surfaces, Buonocore envisioned the use of acids to etch enamel for sealing pits and fissures.[56] Since Buonocore's

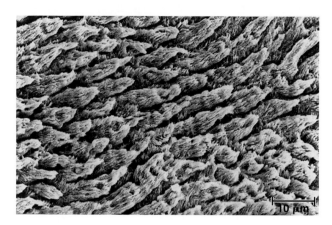

FIG. 5-3 Scanning electron micrograph of enamel etched with 36% phosphoric acid (Dentsply DeTrey, Konstanz, Germany) for 30 seconds.

introduction of the acid-etch technique, many dental researchers have attempted to achieve methods for reliable and durable adhesion between resins and tooth structure.

Acid-etching transforms the smooth enamel into a very irregular surface (Fig. 5-3), and also increases its surface free energy. When a fluid resin-based material is applied to the irregular etched surface, the resin penetrates into the surface, aided by capillary action. Monomers in the material polymerize, and the material becomes interlocked with the enamel surface (Fig. 5-4).[15,57] The formation of resin microtags within the enamel surface is the fundamental mechanism of adhesion of resin to enamel.[21,57,130] Fig. 5-5 shows a mold of an etched enamel surface visualized through the extensions of resin that penetrated the irregular enamel surface. The acid-etch technique has significantly changed the practice of restorative dentistry.

Enamel etching results in three different micromorphologic patterns.[123,281] Type I involves the dissolution of prism cores without dissolution of prism peripheries (Fig. 5-6). The Type II etching pattern is the opposite of Type I—the peripheral enamel is dissolved, but the cores are left intact (see Fig. 5-3). Type III etching is less distinct than the other two patterns. It includes areas that resemble the other patterns and areas whose topography is not related to enamel prism morphology.

Beginning with Buonocore's use of 85% phosphoric acid, various concentrations of phosphoric acid have been used to etch enamel. Gwinnett and Buonocore suggested the use of lower acid concentrations to prevent the formation of precipitates that could interfere with adhesion.[126] Application of 50% phosphoric acid for 60 seconds results in formation of a monocalcium phosphate monohydrate precipitate that can be rinsed off. However, concentrations below 27% may create a dicalcium phosphate monohydrate precipitate that cannot be easily removed and, consequently, may interfere with

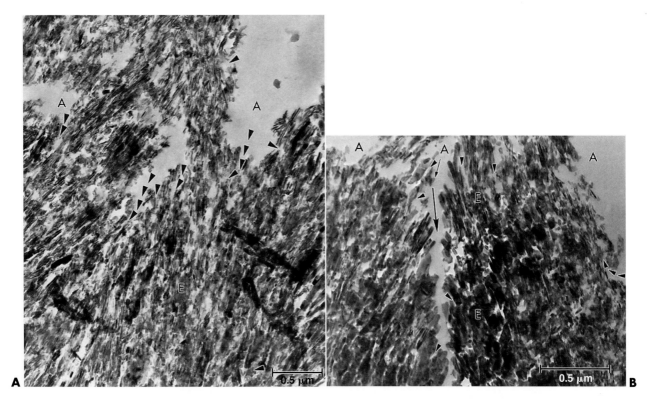

FIG. **5-4** **A** and **B,** Transmission electron micrographs of the enamel-adhesive interface following application of Single Bond (3M ESPE, St. Paul, Minnesota) per manufacturer's instructions. Acid etching with 35% phosphoric acid (3M ESPE, St. Paul, Minnesota) opened spaces between enamel prisms *(arrows),* allowing the permeation of resin monomers between the crystallites *(arrowheads). A,* Adhesive; *E,* enamel.

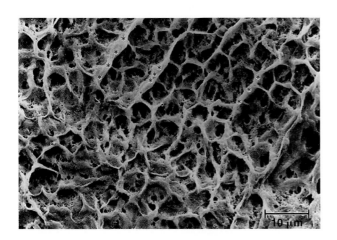

FIG. **5-5** Replica of enamel etched with 35% phosphoric acid (3M ESPE, St. Paul, Minnesota). Enamel was completely dissolved in 6N HCl for 24 hours. Note the resin extensions that correspond to the interprismatic spaces *(asterisks).*

adhesion.[66] Silverstone found that the application of 30% to 40% phosphoric acid resulted in very retentive enamel surfaces.[282] Concentrations above 40% seem to dissolve less calcium and result in etch patterns with poorer definition than when concentrations below 40% are used.[180] Consequently, most current phosphoric acid gels have concentrations of 30% to 40%, even though some studies using lower concentrations have reported similar adhesion values.[118,129,287]

An etching time of 60 seconds was originally recommended for permanent enamel using 30% to 40% phosphoric acid. While one study concluded that shorter etch times resulted in lower bond strengths,[182] other studies using scanning electron microscopy (SEM) showed that a 15-second etch resulted in a similar surface roughness as that provided by a 60-second etch.[18,21,206] Other in vitro studies have demonstrated similar bond strengths and microleakage for etching times of 15 and 60 seconds.[24,75,113,277] Clinically, reduced etching times do not appear to diminish the retention of pit-and-fissure sealants.[91,293]

DENTIN ADHESION

The classic concepts of operative dentistry have been challenged in the last two decades by the introduction of new adhesive techniques, first for enamel and then for dentin. Nevertheless, adhesion to dentin still remains difficult. Adhesive materials can interact with dentin in different ways—mechanically, chemically, or both.[14,15,41,201,330] The importance of micromechanical bonding, similar to what occurs in enamel bonding, has become accepted over the last decade.[14,96,329] Researchers now believe that dentin adhesion relies primarily on the penetration of adhesive monomers into the filigree of collagen fibers

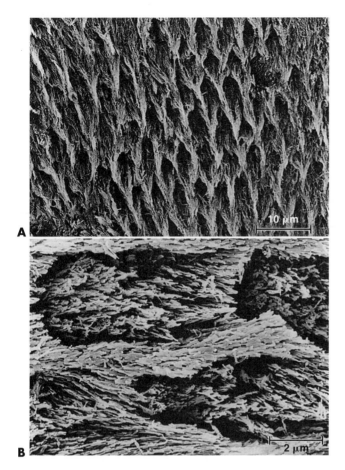

FIG. 5-6 Scanning electron micrograph of enamel etched with 35% phosphoric acid (Ultradent Products, South Jordan, Utah) for 2 minutes, denoting a Type I etching pattern.

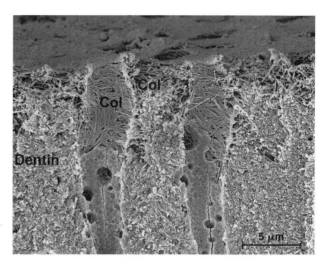

FIG. 5-7 Dentin etched with 32% phosphoric acid (Bisco, Inc., Schaumburg, Illinois). *Col,* Collagen exposed by the acid.

left exposed by acid etching (Fig. 5-7).[311,329] The various strategies currently used for bonding to dentin are summarized in Table 5-1.

CHALLENGES IN DENTIN BONDING

Substrate. Bonding to enamel is a relatively simple process, without major technical requirements or difficulties. Bonding to dentin, on the other hand, presents a much greater challenge. Several factors account for this difference between enamel and dentin bonding. Whereas enamel is a highly mineralized tissue composed of more than 90% (by volume) hydroxyapatite, dentin contains a substantial proportion of water and organic material, primarily Type I collagen (Fig. 5-8). Dentin also contains a dense network of tubules that connect the pulp with the dentin-enamel junction (Fig. 5-9). The tubules are lined by a cuff of hypermineralized dentin called peritubular dentin. The less-mineralized intertubular dentin contains collagen fibrils with the characteristic collagen banding (Fig. 5-10). The intertubular dentin is penetrated by submicron channels, which allow the passage of tubular liquid and fibers between neighboring tubules, forming intertubular anastomoses.

Dentin is an intrinsically hydrated tissue, penetrated by a maze of 1 to 2.5 μm diameter fluid-filled dentin tubules. Movement of fluid from the pulp to the dentin-enamel junction is a result of a slight but constant pulpal pressure.[50] Pulpal pressure has a magnitude of 25 to 30 mm Hg or 34 to 40 cm H_2O.[312,327]

Dentinal tubules enclose cellular extensions from the odontoblasts and therefore are in direct communication with the pulp (Fig. 5-11). Inside the tubule lumen, other fibrous organic structures (the *lamina limitans*) can be observed; these substantially decrease the functional radius of the tubule.

The relative area occupied by dentin tubules decreases with increasing distance from the pulp. The number of tubules decreases from about 45,000 per mm² close to the pulp, to about 20,000 per mm² near the dentin-enamel junction.[111] The tubules occupy an area of only 1% of the total surface near the dentin-enamel junction, whereas they comprise 22% of the surface close to the pulp.[218] The average tubule diameter ranges from 0.63 μm at the periphery to 2.37 μm near the pulp.[181]

Adhesion can be affected by the remaining dentin thickness after tooth preparation. Bond strengths are generally less in deep dentin than in superficial dentin.[192,296] Nonetheless, some dentin adhesives, such as those based on the 4-META monomer, do not seem to be affected by dentin depth.[306]

Whenever tooth structure is prepared with a bur or other instrument, residual organic and inorganic components form a "smear layer" of debris on the surface.[42,154] The smear layer fills the orifices of dentin tubules (forming smear plugs; see Fig. 5-12) and decreases dentin permeability by up to 86%.[226] The composition of the smear layer is basically hydroxyapatite and altered denatured collagen. This altered collagen may even acquire a gelatinized consistency as a result of the friction

TABLE 5-1   Adhesion Strategies

	ACID (A)	PRIMER (P)	FLUID RESIN (R)
Fourth-generation (multibottle total-etch adhesives) A + P + R	Removes the smear layer. Exposes both intertubular and peritubular collagen. Opens the tubules in a funnel configuration. Decreases surface-free energy.	Includes bifunctional molecules (simultaneously hydrophilic and hydrophobic). Envelops the external surface of collagen fibrils. Reestablishes the surface free energy to levels compatible with a more hydrophobic restorative material.	Includes monomers that are mostly hydrophobic, such as Bis-GMA; however, may contain a small percentage of hydrophilic monomers, such as HEMA. Copolymerizes with the primer molecules. Penetrates and polymerizes into the interfibrilar spaces to serve as a structural backbone to the hybrid layer. Penetrates into the dentin tubules to form resin tags.
SEPs (AP) + R		The SEP does not remove the smear layer, but fixes it and exposes about 0.5-1µm of intertubular collagen because of its acidity (pH=1.25-1.40). Smear plug impregnated with acidic monomers but is not removed. When it impregnates the smear plug, the SEP prepares the pathway for the penetration of the subsequently placed fluid resin into the microchannels that permeate the smear plug.	Utilizes the same type of fluid resin included in the fourth-generation adhesives. The resin tags form upon resin penetration into the microchannels of the primer-impregnated smear plug.
Fifth-generation (one-bottle total-etch adhesives) A + (PR)	Removes the smear layer. Exposes both intertubular and peritubular collagen. Opens the tubules in a funnel configuration. Decreases surface free energy.	The first coat applied on etched dentin works as a primer. The second coat (and the third, and fourth, and so on) acts as the fluid resin used in fourth-generation materials—it fills the spaces between the dense network of collagen fibers. When the manufacturer recommends only one coat, brushing it on for a few seconds may serve simultaneously as primer and adhesive layers.	
Self-etching adhesives (APR)	Etch enamel. Incorporate the smear layer into the interface. Being an aqueous solution of a phosphonated monomer, demineralizes and penetrates dentin simultaneously, leaving a precipitate on the hybrid layer. Forms a very thin adhesive layer of adhesive leading to low bond strengths; therefore a multicoat approach is recommended. More compatible with compomers than with composite.		

SEP, Self-etching primer.

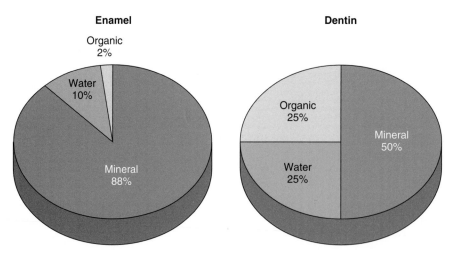

FIG. **5-8** Composition of enamel and dentin by volume percentage.

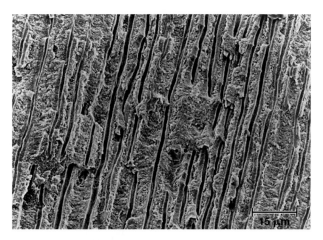

FIG. **5-9** Scanning electron micrograph of dentin that was fractured longitudinally.

and heat created by the preparation procedure.[88] Submicron porosity of the smear layer still allows for diffusion of dentinal fluid.[219]

The removal of the smear layer and smear plugs with acidic solutions may result in an increase of the fluid flow onto the exposed dentin surface. This fluid may interfere with adhesion,[42] because hydrophobic resins do not adhere to hydrophilic substrates even if resin tags are formed in the dentin tubules.[313]

Several additional factors affect dentin permeability. Besides the use of vasoconstrictors in local anesthetics, which decrease pulpal pressure and fluid flow in the tubules, other factors such as the radius and length of the tubules, the viscosity of dentin fluid, the pressure gradient, the molecular size of the substances dissolved in the tubular fluid, and the rate of removal of substances by

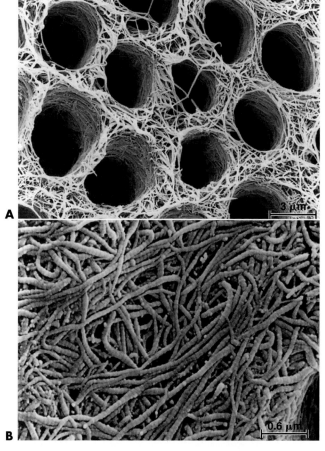

FIG. **5-10** **A,** Scanning electron micrograph of etched dentin showing exposed collagen fibers. **B,** A higher magnification shows the characteristic collagen banding in intertubular collagen. Superficial collagen was dissolved by collagenase to remove the most superficial collagen fibers that were damaged by tooth preparation.

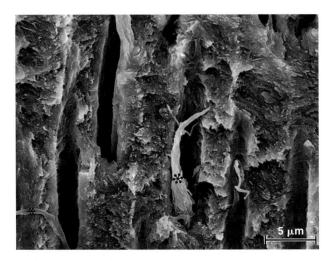

FIG. **5-11** Scanning electron micrograph of deep dentin displaying an odontoblastic process in a dentinal tubule *(asterisk).*

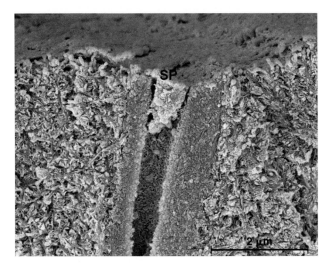

FIG. **5-12** Scanning electron micrograph of a smear plug blocking the entrance of a dentinal tubule. *SP,* Smear plug.

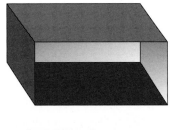

Occlusal class I preparation; C-factor = 5

Proximoocclusal class II preparation; C-factor = 2

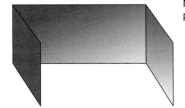

Mesioocclusodistal class II preparation; C-factor = 1

FIG. **5-13** Schematic representation of the C-factor.

the blood vessels in the pulp affect permeability.[220,251] All of these variables make dentin a dynamic substrate and consequently a very difficult substrate for bonding.[218,286]

Stresses at the Resin-Dentin Interface. Composites shrink as they polymerize, creating stresses of up to 7 MPa within the composite mass,[43,81,82,144] depending on the configuration of the preparation. When the composite is bonded to one surface only (such as in the case of a direct facial veneer), stresses within the composite are relieved by flow from the unbonded surface. However, stress relief within a three-dimensional bonded restoration is limited by its configuration factor, or C-factor.[98] For example, in an occlusal preparation, composite is bonded to five surfaces—mesial, distal, facial, lingual, and pulpal. The occlusal surface is the only "free" or unrestrained surface (Fig. 5-13). In such a clinical situation,

the ratio between the number of bonded surfaces and the number of unbonded surfaces is 5, giving the restoration a C-factor of 5. Stress relief is rather limited because flow can occur only from the single free surface.[80,98] Unrelieved stresses in the composite may cause internal bond disruption as well as marginal gaps around restorations that increase microleakage.[234]

Immediate bond strengths of approximately 17 MPa may be necessary to resist the contraction stresses that develop in the composite during polymerization to prevent marginal debonding.[81,199] Water sorption by the resin may compensate for the effect of the polymerization shrinkage because the resin may expand and seal off marginal gaps, but this occurs only over a relatively long period of time.[138] Water sorption is directly proportional to the resin content.[212]

Enamel bond strengths are usually sufficient to prevent the formation of marginal gaps by polymerization contraction stresses. These stresses may, however, be powerful enough to cause enamel defects at the margins.[167] Extension of the enamel cavosurface bevel may increase the enamel peripheral seal.[43,137]

Each time a restoration is exposed to wide temperature variations in the oral environment (such as drinking coffee and eating ice cream), the restoration undergoes volumetric changes of different magnitude than those of the tooth structure. This occurs because the linear coefficient of thermal expansion of the composite is about four times greater than that of the tooth structure.

Accordingly, microleakage around dentin margins is potentiated by this discrepancy in linear coefficient of thermal expansion between the restoration and the substrate.[12]

DEVELOPMENT OF DENTIN BONDING SYSTEMS

The Beginning. During the 1950s, it was reported that a resin containing glycerophosphoric acid dimethacrylate (GPDM) could bond to a hydrochloric acid–etched dentin surface.[55] (Table 5-2 provides a complete listing of the chemical names mentioned in this chapter.) The bond strengths of this primitive adhesion technique were severely reduced by immersion in water. A few years before that report, another researcher, Dr. Hagger, had used the same monomer chemically activated with sulfinic acid,[185,186] and that combination would later be commercially known as Sevriton Cavity Seal (Amalgamated Dental Company, London, England).

First-Generation Dentin Adhesives. The development of the surface-active comonomer NPG-GMA[41] was the basis for Cervident (S.S. White, Lakewood, New Jersey), which is considered a first-generation dentin bonding system.[17] Theoretically, this comonomer could chelate with calcium on the tooth surface to generate

TABLE 5-2	List of Chemical Abbreviations
BAC	Benzalkonium chloride
Bis-GMA	Bisphenol glycidyl methacrylate
BPDM	Biphenyl dimethacrylate
EDTA	Ethylene diamine tetra-acetic acid
GPDM	Glycerophosphoric acid dimethacrylate
HEMA	2-Hydroxyethyl methacrylate
10-MDP	10-Methacryloyloxy decyl dihydrogenphosphate
4-META	4-Methacryloxyethyl trimellitate anhydride
NPG-GMA	N-phenylglycine glycidyl methacrylate
PENTA	Dipentaerythritol penta-acrylate monophosphate
Phenyl-P	2-(Methacryloxy) ethyl phenyl hydrogen phosphate
PMGDM/ PMDM	Pyromellitic acid diethyl methacrylate
TGDMA/ TEGDMA	Triethylene glycol dimethacrylate
UDMA	Urethane dimethacrylate

water-resistant chemical bonds of resin to dentinal calcium.[4,5] However, the in vitro dentin bond strengths of this material were in the range of only 2 to 3 MPa.[256] Likewise, the in vivo results were discouraging; Cervident had very poor clinical results when used to restore cervical erosion lesions without mechanical retention.[156] Based on Carbon-13 NMR analysis, it appears that no ionic bonding actually develops between NPG-GMA and hydroxyapatite.[344]

Second-Generation Dentin Adhesives. In 1978, the Clearfil Bond System F (Kuraray, Osaka, Japan) was introduced in Japan.[256] Generally recognized as the first product of the second generation of dentin adhesives, it was a phosphate-ester material (phenyl-P and HEMA in ethanol). Its mechanism of action was based on the polar interaction between negatively charged phosphate groups in the resin and the positively charged calcium in the smear layer.[256] The smear layer was the weakest link in the system because of its relatively loose attachment to the dentin surface. Examination of both sides of failed bonds revealed the presence of smear layer debris.[87]

Several other phosphate-ester dentin bonding systems were introduced in the early 1980s, including Scotchbond (3M ESPE, St. Paul, Minnesota), Bondlite (Kerr Corporation, Orange, California), and Prisma Universal Bond (Dentsply Caulk, Milford, Delaware). These second-generation dentin bonding systems typically had in vitro bond strengths of only 1 to 5 MPa,[15,88] which was considerably below the 10 MPa value estimated as the threshold value for acceptable in vivo retention.[15] In addition to the problems caused by the loosely attached smear layer, these resins were devoid of hydrophilic groups, and therefore had large contact angles on intrinsically moist surfaces.[16] They did not wet dentin well nor penetrate the entire depth of the smear layer, and could not reach the superficial dentin to establish ionic bonding or resin extensions into the dentinal tubules.[88] Whatever bonding did occur was due to interaction with calcium ions.[62]

The in vitro performance of second-generation adhesives after 6 months was unacceptable.[148] The bonding material peeled off the dentin surface after water storage, indicating that the interface between dentin and some types of chlorophosphate-ester–based materials was unstable.[94,148] The in vivo performance of these materials was found to be clinically unacceptable 2 years after placement in cervical tooth preparations without additional retention such as beveling and acid etching.[321,329]

Third-Generation Dentin Adhesives. The concept of phosphoric acid-etching of dentin before application of a phosphate ester-type bonding agent was introduced by Fusayama and others in 1979.[109] However, because of the hydrophobic nature of the bonding resin, acid-etching did not produce a significant improvement in dentin bond strengths, despite the flow of the resin into the open dentinal tubules.[313,326] Furthermore, pulpal inflammatory responses were thought to be triggered by the application of acid on dentin surfaces, providing another reason for not using acid.[255,292] Nevertheless, continuing the etched dentin philosophy, Kuraray introduced Clearfil New Bond in 1984. This new phosphate-based material contained HEMA and a ten-carbon molecule known as 10-MDP, which includes a long hydrophobic and a short hydrophilic component.[4]

Most other third-generation materials were designed not to remove the entire smear layer, but rather to modify it and allow penetration of acidic monomers such as Phenyl-P or PENTA. Despite promising laboratory results,[238,239,335] some of the bonding mechanisms developed never resulted in satisfactory clinical results. For example, the impregnation of dentin with amino-group-containing substances was considered an important factor in the establishment of a chemical bond to collagen.[13,198] However, in vivo and in vitro reports using adhesives that supposedly impregnate dentin with such amino groups are contradictory.[158,239,335] It is possible that acidic conditioners/primers that create precipitates on dentin surfaces, such as the systems with oxalic acid, may block both dentin tubules and submicron porosities within the demineralized dentin, thus preventing resin penetration.[284]

Treatment of the smear layer with acidic primers was proposed using an aqueous solution of 2.5% maleic acid, 55% HEMA, and a trace of methacrylic acid (Scotchbond 2 [3M ESPE, St. Paul, Minnesota]).[4,6] Scotchbond 2 was the first dentin bonding system to receive "provisional" and "full acceptance" from the American Dental Association (ADA) in 1987.[329] With this type of smear layer treatment, manufacturers effectively combined the dentin etching philosophy advocated in Japan with the more cautious approach advocated in Europe and United States. The result was preservation of a modified smear layer with slight demineralization of the underlying intertubular dentin surface. Clinical results were mixed, with some reports of good performance[329] and some reports of poor performance.[320]

The removal of the smear layer with chelating agents, such as EDTA, was recommended in the original Gluma system (Bayer Dental, Leverkusen, Germany) before the application of a solution of 5% glutaraldehyde and 35% HEMA in water. However, the effectiveness of this system may have been impaired by the manufacturer's questionable recommendation of placing the composite over uncured unfilled resin.[329]

Fourth-Generation Dentin Adhesives. Although the smear layer acts as a "diffusion barrier" that decreases the permeability of dentin,[226] it can also be considered an obstacle that must be removed so that resin can be bonded to the underlying dentin substrate. Based on that consideration, fourth-generation dentin adhesives were introduced for use on acid-etched dentin.[92] Removal of the smear layer via acid-etching has led to significant improvements in the in vitro bond strengths of resins to dentin.[22,161,164,304]

Fourth-generation adhesives, such as All-Bond 2 (Bisco, Inc., Schaumburg, Illinois), OptiBond FL (Kerr Corporation, Orange, California), and Scotchbond Multi-Purpose (3M ESPE, St. Paul, Minnesota), are basically composed of (1) an acid etching gel that is rinsed off; (2) a solution of primers that are reactive hydrophilic monomers in ethanol, acetone, and/or water; and (3) an unfilled or filled fluid bonding agent. The latter generally contains hydrophobic monomers such as bisphenol glycidyl methacrylate (Bis-GMA), frequently combined with hydrophilic molecules such as HEMA.

Application of acid to dentin results in partial or total removal of the smear layer and demineralization of the underlying dentin.[88] Besides demineralizing intertubular and peritubular dentin, acids open the dentin tubules and expose a dense filigree of collagen fibers (see Figs. 5-7 and 5-14), thus increasing the microporosity of the intertubular dentin (Fig. 5-15).[235,329] Dentin is demineralized up to 7.5 μm, depending on the type of acid, application time, and concentration.[65,108,330]

Alterations in the mineral content of the substrate also change the surface free energy of dentin.[92,96] The adhesive system must have a low surface tension and the substrate must have a high surface free energy for adequate interfacial contact.[88,93,96] Substrates are characterized as having low or high surface energy. Of those materials used in dentistry, hydroxyapatite and glass-ionomer cement filler particles are high-energy substrates.[3] Collagen and composite have low energy surfaces.[3] Consequently, dentin consists of two distinct substrates, one of high-surface energy (hydroxyapatite) and one of low surface energy (collagen). Thus, after etching with acidic agents, the dense web of exposed collagen is a low-surface energy substrate.[93] In fact, there is a correlation between the ability of an adhesive to spread on the dentin surface and the concentration of calcium on that same surface.[216] An increase in the critical surface tension of dentin by surface-active components (such as primers) is highly desirable in this case, since a direct correlation between surface energy of dentin and shear bond strengths has been demonstrated.[30]

When primer and bonding resins are applied to etched dentin, they penetrate the intertubular dentin, forming a resin-dentin interdiffusion zone, or "hybrid layer." They also penetrate and polymerize in the open dentinal tubules, forming resin tags.

Fifth-Generation Dentin Adhesives. The development of dentin bonding systems is continuing at a rapid pace. In vitro dentin bond strengths have improved so

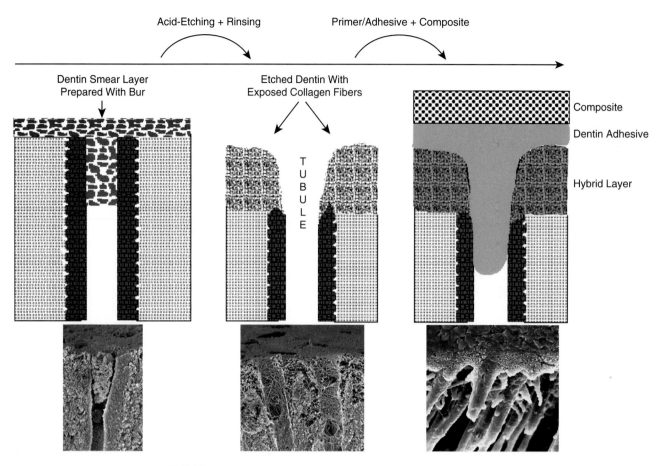

FIG. 5-14 Bonding of resin to dentin, using a "total-etch" technique.

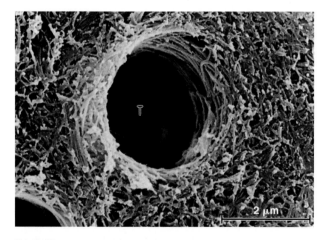

FIG. 5-15 Scanning electron micrograph of dentin that was kept moist after rinsing off the etchant. The abundant intertubular porosity will serve as a pathway for the penetration of the dentin adhesive. *T,* Dentinal tubule.

much that they approach the values of enamel bonding.[303,316] Therefore many current developments are directed at simplification of the bonding procedure. Nearly all dental materials manufacturers now have a "one-bottle" adhesive system available on the market. These combine the primer and bonding agent steps, but a separate etching step is still needed for the majority of adhesive systems.

When a commercially available adhesive proves to be satisfactory under in vitro conditions but takes several time-consuming steps to be applied in vivo, the clinician usually prefers a material that would be easier to apply. Manufacturers have been attempting to reduce the number of steps needed and the corresponding application time, making more user-friendly adhesive systems. Within the last several years, numerous simplified bonding systems have been released: One-Step (Bisco, Inc., Schaumburg, Illinois); Prime & Bond, Prime & Bond 2.1, and Prime & Bond NT (Dentsply Caulk, Milford, Delaware); Prime & Bond 2.0 (Dentsply DeTrey,

Konstanz, Germany); Single Bond (3M ESPE, St. Paul, Minnesota); OptiBond Solo and OptiBond Solo Plus (Kerr Corporation, Orange, California); PQ1 (Ultradent Products, South Jordan, Utah); Syntac Single Component, Syntac Sprint, and Excite (Ivoclar Vivadent, Schaan, Principality of Liechtenstein); Bond1 (Jeneric/Pentron, Wallingford, Connecticut), One Coat Bond (Coltène/ Whaledent Inc., Mahwah, New Jersey); Gluma One Bond (Heraeus Kulzer, South Bend, Indiana); and many others.

Another type of material with durable bonding to dentin has been marketed since the late 1970s, the glass-ionomer cements (GIC). These materials set via an acid-base reaction and also are called glass-polyalkenoate cements.[187] Although beyond the scope of this chapter, it should be noted that the recent developments in the area of GICs, namely their chemistry and in vitro bond strengths, have many characteristics in common with the development of the fifth-generation dentin adhesive systems.[187,316] In fact, some current adhesives (e.g., Single Bond and One Coat Bond) contain polyalkenoic acid derivatives.

Current Strategies. Table 5-3 shows the composition of some fifth-generation adhesive materials.

Total-Etch Dentin Adhesive Systems. Simultaneous application of an acid to enamel and dentin, known as the *total-etch* technique, is the most common strategy of dentin bonding (see Fig. 5-14). The total-etch technique was initiated in Japan by phosphoric acid etching of dentin before the application of a phosphate ester-type of bonding agent.[109] In spite of the obvious penetration of this early adhesive into the dentinal tubules, the application of phosphoric acid on dentin did not result in a significant improvement in bond strengths, possibly because of the hydrophobic nature of the phosphonated resin.[326] In addition, in the mid-1970s, some researchers had hypothesized that the application of acids to dentin might trigger inflammatory pulpal responses.[255,292] Based on these concerns, acids were believed to be contraindicated for direct application on dentin and the total-etch technique did not gain acceptance in Europe or the United States. However, newer adhesive systems (the fourth- and fifth-generation materials described in the previous section) based on the total-etch philosophy have proved successful both in vitro (Box 5-1) and in vivo.[302,329,333] Clinical retention rates have been reported to be very close to 100%, compared with a second-generation adhesive system having retention rates in the 50% range.[333] Laboratory bond strengths usually vary from 17 MPa to 30 MPa, which are very close to the values commonly obtained on enamel.[127,135,297]

| TABLE **5-3** | Composition of Several Fifth-Generation Adhesive Materials | | | |

ADHESIVE SYSTEM	ETCHANT	COATS RECOMMENDED	MANUFACTURER	COMPOSITION OF ADHESIVE
Dentastic Uno	38% H_3PO_4 for 15 seconds	2	Pulpdent	PMGDM, proprietary monomers, acetone
EasyBond	10% citric acid with 3% ferric chloride for 10 seconds on dentin and 30 seconds on enamel	2	Parkell	4-META, HEMA, dimethacrylate monomer, acetone
Excite	37% H_3PO_4 for 15 seconds	1	Ivoclar Vivadent	Phosphonate monomer, HEMA, cross-linking agents, fumed silica, 25% ethanol
Gluma Comfort Bond	20% H_3PO_4 for 20 seconds	3	Heraeus Kulzer	HEMA, 4-META, methacrylic polycarboxylic acid, glutaraldehyde, ethanol
One Coat Bond	15 % H_3PO_4 for 30 seconds	1	Coltène/ Whaledent	HEMA, UDMA, hydroxypropylmethacrylate, glycerol methacrylate, polyalkenoate methacrylized, amorphous silica, 5% water
One-Step	32% H_3PO_4 with BAC for 15 seconds	2	Bisco Inc.	Bis-GMA, BPDM, HEMA, acetone
OptiBond Solo	37.5% H_3PO_4 for 15 seconds	1	Kerr	Bis-GMA, GPDM, HEMA, silica, barium glass, sodium hexafluorosilicate, ethanol

Continued

TABLE 5-3 Composition of Several Fifth-Generation Adhesive Materials—cont'd

ADHESIVE SYSTEM	ETCHANT	COATS RECOMMENDED	MANUFACTURER	COMPOSITION OF ADHESIVE
Permaquick PQ1	35% H_3PO_4 for 15 seconds	1	Ultradent Products	TEGDMA, Canadian balsam (tree sap), 15% HEMA, 40% filler with fluoride, ethanol
Prime & Bond NT	34% H_3PO_4 (United States) for 15 seconds 36% H_3PO_4 (Europe) for 15 seconds	1	Dentsply	PENTA, UDMA + T-resin (cross-linking agent) + D-resin (small hydrophilic molecule), butylated hydroxitoluene, 4-ethyl dimethyl aminobenzoate, cetilamine hydrofluoride, acetone, silica nanofiller
Single Bond	35% H_3PO_4 for 15 seconds	2	3M ESPE	Bis-GMA, HEMA, dimethacrylates, polyalkenoic acid copolymer, initiator, water, ethanol
Tenure Quik with Fluoride	37% H_3PO_4 for 15 seconds	2	Den-Mat Corp.	Dimethacrylate resins, HEMA, PMDM, fluoride, initiator, acetone

BOX 5-1 Dentin Bond Strengths Associated with Several Generations of Adhesives

Second-generation adhesives—2 to 4 MPa
Third-generation adhesives—3 to 8 MPa
Fourth-generation adhesives—13 to 30 MPa
Fifth-generation adhesives—3 to 25 MPa

From Asmussen E, Munksgaard EC: *Int Dent J* 38:97-104, 1988; Barkmeier WW, Suh BI, Cooley RL: *J Esthet Dent* 3:148-153, 1991; Eick JD et al: *Quintessence Int* 22:967:977, 1991; Gwinnett AJ: *Am J Dent* 5:127-129, 1992; Gwinnett AJ, Kanca J: *Am J Dent* 5:315-317, 1992; Gwinnett AJ, Kanca J: *Am J Dent* 5:73-77, 1992; Perdigão J, Baratieri LN, Lopes M: *J Esthet Dent* 11:23-35, 1999; Perdigão J et al. *J Dent Res* 73:44-55, 1994; and Perdigão J, Ramos JC, Lambrechts P: *Dent Mater* 13:218-227, 1997.

Self-Etching Dentin Adhesive Systems. Simultaneous etching of enamel and dentin is the basis for most of the fourth- and fifth-generation dentin-enamel adhesives in use today (Fig. 5-16). These adhesive are therefore frequently called "total-etch" systems. The first systems based on this philosophy included acidic etchants with a lower concentration than the traditional 30% to 40% phosphoric acid. Some studies have indicated that low-concentration etchants (such as 2.5% nitric, 10% citric, 10% phosphoric, or 10% maleic) are as effective as 30% to 40% phosphoric acid when applied to enamel for 15 seconds.[1,35,39,120,127,129,135, 271] However, other studies have shown that such low-concentration acids have lower enamel bond strengths than conventional 30% to 40% phosphoric acid, when the manufac-

turers' recommended etching times were used.[252,298,317, 324] Clinically, the traditional frosted enamel surface often is not apparent after the application of weaker acids. Under SEM, enamel etched with 10% maleic acid or with 10% phosphoric acid for 15 seconds does not acquire the etching pattern characteristic of enamel etched with 30 % to 40% phosphoric acid for 15 to 30 seconds (Fig. 5-17).[236] The long-term clinical consequences of etching enamel with these low-concentration acids are not yet known. However, a clinical study in Class V restorations using maleic acid as the etchant demonstrated marginal staining in 10% of the restorations after 1 year and 30% after 3 years,[334] without jeopardizing the retention rate. The marginal staining was associated with minor defects on the enamel margins, which may have been a result of the enamel treatment with the maleic acid.

More recently, another type of acidic conditioner, the self-etching primers (SEPs), was introduced in Japan. These acidic primers include a phosphonated resin molecule that performs two functions simultaneously—etching and priming of dentin and enamel. Unlike conventional etchants, self-etching primers are not rinsed off. The bonding mechanism of SEPs is based on the simultaneous etching and priming of enamel and dentin without rinsing, forming a continuum in the substrate and incorporating smear plugs into the resin tags (Fig. 5-18).[232,338] In addition to simplifying the bonding technique, the elimination of rinsing and drying steps reduces the possibility of overwetting or overdrying, which can have a negative influence in adhesion.[161,164] However, the sealing of enamel margins in vivo may be com-

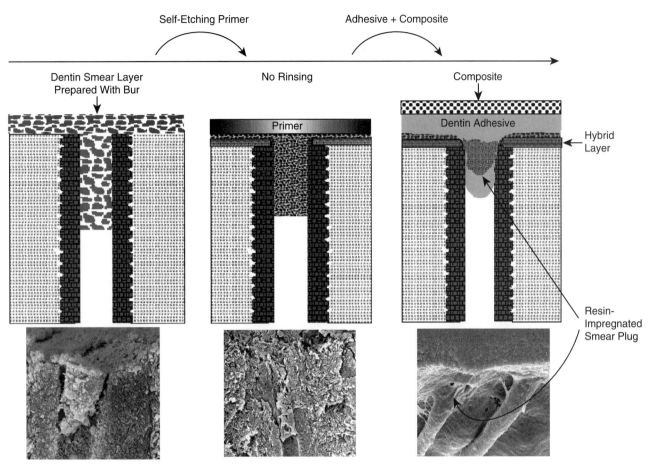

FIG. **5-16** Bonding to dentin using a self-etching primer.

promised because a perfect marginal integrity is not achieved.[102,210]

A clinical study using Clearfil Liner Bond 2 (Kuraray, Osaka, Japan), a self-etching primer, has demonstrated excellent retention in Class V restorations at three years, but 47% of the restorations had a score of "bravo" for marginal integrity.[175] An in vitro study involving the same adhesive material resulted in enamel bond strengths statistically similar to those obtained with the concomitant use of a separate acid etchant before the application of the primer.[232] However, when the fitting surface was observed under the SEM, the use of the self-etching primer resulted in a shallower etching pattern than when a conventional acid etchant was used.[232] Nevertheless, some in vitro studies using the same SEP reported bond strengths of 20 to 28 MPa, which are similar to those bond strengths obtained with phosphoric acid-etching of enamel.[19,117,232] These data raise questions about the

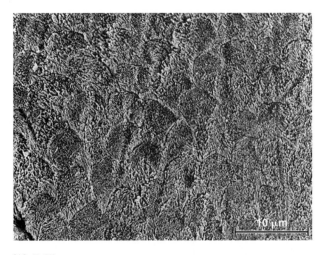

FIG. **5-17** Scanning electron micrograph of enamel etched with 10% phosphoric acid (Bisco, Inc., Schaumburg, Illinois) for 15 seconds. Note that the etching pattern is barely discernible, as opposed to the enamel shown in Figs. 5-3 and 5-6.

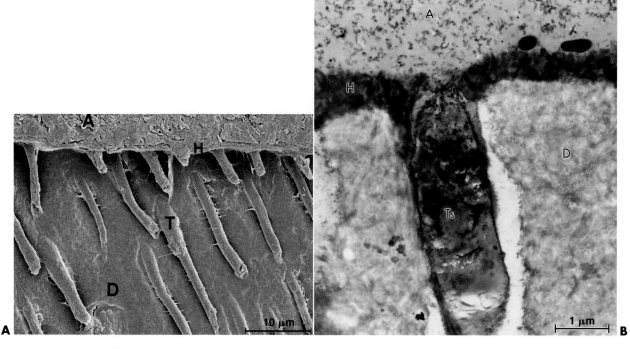

FIG. 5-18 **A,** Scanning electron micrograph of a resin-dentin interface formed with Clearfil SE Bond (Kuraray, Osaka, Japan) upon chemical dissolution of the superficial dentin. *A,* Adhesive; *D,* residual dentin; *H,* hybrid layer; *T,* resin tag. **B,** TEM micrograph of a resin-dentin interface formed with Clearfil SE Bond (Kuraray, Osaka, Japan) upon EDTA-decalcification and staining with uranyl acetate and lead citrate. *A,* Adhesive; *D,* residual dentin (appears gray because it was decalcified with EDTA); *H,* hybrid layer (appears dark because of decalcification followed by staining); *Ts,* resin tag that incorporates the smear plug.

definitive need for conventional acid-etching as a separate clinical procedure.

Following the trend toward simplification, two non-rinsing, self-etching materials have been introduced for use with polyacid-modified composites or compomers—Prompt L-Pop (3M ESPE, St. Paul, Minnesota) and NRC Non-Rinse Conditioner (Dentsply DeTrey, Konstanz, Germany). The former is a *self-etching adhesive,* while the latter is a *nonrinsing conditioner* combined with a one-bottle adhesive. Prompt L-Pop, according to its manufacturer, is an "all-in-one" adhesive system with etching, priming, and adhesive potentials all in one solution, whereas NRC requires the subsequent application of a separate adhesive, Prime & Bond NT (Dentsply DeTrey, Konstanz, Germany). The use of NRC instead of phosphoric acid does not seem to provide any advantage with either composites or compomers.[259] Although Prompt L-Pop results in enamel bond strengths similar to those obtained with a separate phosphoric acid etching step, some preliminary in vitro studies suggest that dentin bond strengths are significantly lower than those obtained with total-etch, one-bottle adhesives.

ROLE OF THE HYBRID LAYER

The role of the hybrid layer in dentin bonding is somewhat controversial. Data from one in vitro study indi-

cated that resin infiltration or "hybridization" of the dentinal tubules and intertubular dentin accounts for a substantial proportion of the bond of resin to dentin.[125] On the other hand, data from another study suggested that the collagen layer offers no quantitative contribution to the interfacial bond strength.[121] Studies of various adhesive systems report different results. A study with Prime & Bond 2.1 (Dentsply Caulk, Milford, Delaware) indicated that the removal of collagen fibers may actually increase bond strengths of resin to dentin.[152] Studies with One-Step (Bisco, Inc., Schaumburg, Illinois) indicated that the hybrid layer might not play any important role in the establishment of bond strengths.[152,166] For a multibottle adhesive system, All-Bond 2 (Bisco, Inc., Schaumburg, Illinois), one study reported that the presence or absence of the hybrid layer did not affect fracture toughness of resin-dentin interfaces.[11] In the case of All-Bond 2, a different mechanical behavior of the adhesive interface would be expected. The Young's modulus of the adhesive resin is 1.8 GPa, while the Young's modulus of the All-Bond 2-infiltrated hybrid layer was estimated to be 3.6 GPa.[268] Dentin has a Young's modulus in the range of 11 to 18 GPa.[11] Therefore the presence of the collagen layer would presumably allow for the establishment of a stress-relieving layer at the interface.

A study using a self-etching primer demonstrated that dentin bond strengths did not vary from 1 day to 6 months to 1 year in teeth subjected to occlusal function. It also showed that porosity in the hybrid layer increased significantly at 1 year, due to loss of resin between the collagen fibers.[264] Since these results were obtained with a hybrid layer being created by a self-etching primer, they cannot be generalized to total-etch adhesives. However, they do support the theory that collagen may play an important role in the strength of the resin-dentin interface.[264]

For most dentin adhesives, the ultramorphologic characterization of the transition between the hybrid layer and the unaffected dentin suggests that there is an abrupt shift from hybrid tissue to mineralized tissue, without any empty space or pathway that could result in leakage (Figs. 5-19 and 5-20). The demarcation line seems to consist of hydroxyapatite crystals embedded in the resin from the hybrid layer (see Fig. 5-20, B,C).

MOIST VERSUS DRY DENTIN SURFACES

Vital dentin is inherently wet; therefore, complete drying of dentin is difficult to achieve clinically.[164,165] Water has been considered an obstacle for attaining an effective adhesion of resins to dentin. With that in mind, research has shifted toward development of dentin adhesives compatible with humid environments. Most newer adhesives combine hydrophilic and hydrophobic monomers in the same bottle, dissolved in an organic solvent such as ethanol or acetone. The "wet-bonding" technique prevents the spatial alterations (i.e., collagen collapse) that occur upon drying demineralized dentin (Fig. 5-21; compare with Fig. 5-15). Such alterations may prevent the monomers from penetrating the labyrinth of nanochannels formed by dissolution of hydroxyapatite crystals between collagen fibers.[89,178] The use of adhesive systems on moist dentin is made possible by incorporation of the organic solvents acetone or ethanol in the primers or adhesives. Because the solvent can displace water from both the dentin surface and the moist collagen network, it promotes the infiltration of resin monomers throughout the nanospaces of the dense collagen web. The "wet bonding" technique has been shown repeatedly to enhance bond strengths because water preserves the porosity of collagen network available for monomer interdiffusion.[2,164,165,240] If the dentin surface is dried with air, the collagen undergoes immediate collapse and prevents resin monomers from penetrating (see Figs. 5-21 and 5-22).[61,231]

The clinician must be aware that pooled moisture should not remain on the tooth, because excess water can dilute the primer and render it less effective.[309,310] A glistening hydrated surface is preferred (Fig. 5-23).[302] Many clinicians, however, still dry the tooth preparation after rinsing away the etching gel to check for the classic etched enamel appearance. Because it is clinically

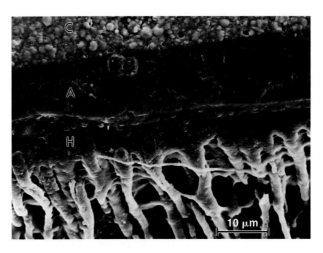

FIG. 5-19 Scanning electron micrograph of the transition between composite resin (C) adhesive (A), adhesive-hybrid layer (H), and hybrid layer-dentin.

impossible to dry enamel without simultaneously drying dentin, the dentin collagen collapses easily upon air-drying, resulting in the closing of the micropores in the exposed intertubular collagen.[310,311] For acetone-based, water-free dentin bonding systems, the etched dentin surface must be rewetted before applying the adhesive. Rewetting the dried etched dentin with water or with aqueous rewetting agents has been demonstrated to restore bond strength values and to raise the collapsed collagen network to a level similar to a "wet bonding" technique.[122,231,311] Some authors have suggested that the inclusion of water in the composition of some adhesives may result in rewetting the collagen fibers in areas that are not left fully moist, thus opening the interfibrillar spaces to the infiltration of the priming resin.[310,332] Therefore the simultaneous inclusion of both an organic solvent and water may be fundamental for the best infiltration of some adhesives into demineralized dentin. This could result in a less technique-sensitive procedure.[258]

When etched dentin is dried using an air syringe, bond strengths decrease substantially, especially for acetone- and ethanol-based dentin adhesive systems.[161,231,310] When water is removed, the elastic characteristics of collagen may be lost. The collapse of the collagen fibers upon drying may therefore be a result of the changes in the molecular arrangement. While in a wet state, wide gaps separate the collagen molecules from each other,[269] in a dry state, the molecules are arranged more compactly. This is because extrafibrillar spaces in hydrated Type I collagen are filled with water, while dried collagen has fewer extrafibrillar spaces (see Fig. 5-22) open for the penetration of the monomers included in the adhesive systems.[270] Water removal also may permit additional hydrogen bonds to form between collagen molecules that were previously bonded to water molecules, leaving no interfibrillar space.[260] During air-drying, water that occupies the interfibrillar

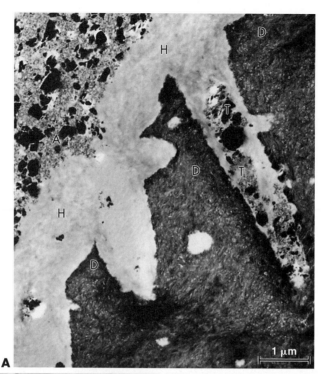

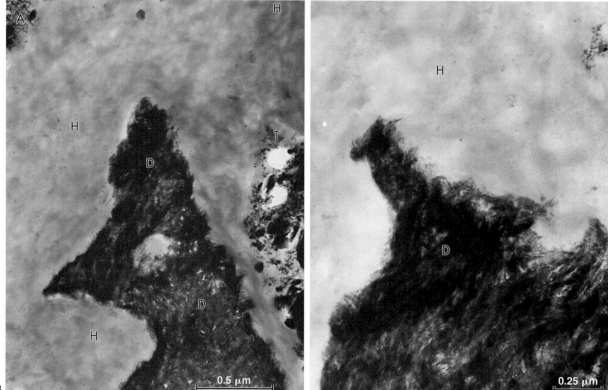

FIG. **5-20** Transmission electron micrograph of a resin-dentin interface formed with the adhesive PQ1 (Ultradent Products, South Jordan, Utah). This specimen was not decalcified or stained; therefore the unaltered dentin appears darker and the hybrid layer appears lighter. **A,** General view, showing the adhesive *(A),* the hybrid layer *(H),* a filled resin tag *(T),* and the unaffected dentin *(D).* **B,** Higher magnification of the transition between the hybrid layer and the unaffected dentin. Note the small amount of filler in the hybrid layer as small dark dots, which correspond with the fraction of the filler that fits the size of the space between individual collagen fibers in the etched dentin. **C,** Higher magnification of the same transition showing a gradual shift from demineralized dentin to unaffected dentin.

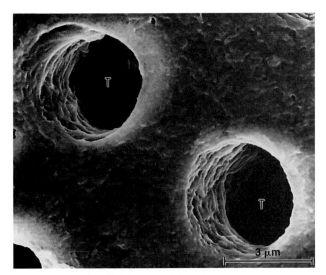

FIG. **5-21** Scanning electron micrograph of dentin collagen after acid etching with 35% phosphoric acid (Ultradent Products, South Jordan, Utah). Dentin was air-dried. The intertubular porosity disappeared as a consequence of the collapse of the collagen because of evaporation of water that served as a backbone to keep collagen fibers raised. *T*, Dentin tubule.

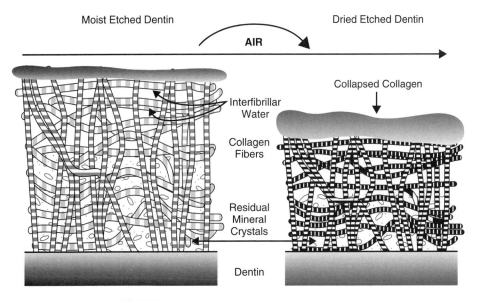

FIG. **5-22** Collapse of etched dentin by air-drying.

spaces previously filled with hydroxyapatite crystals is lost by evaporation, resulting in a decrease of the volume of the collagen network to approximately one third of its original volume.[61] When air-dried demineralized dentin is rewet with water, the collagen matrix may reexpand and recover its primary dimensions to the levels of the original hydrated state.[61,178,323] This spatial reexpansion occurs because the spaces between fibers are refilled with water and because Type I collagen itself is capable of undergoing expansion upon rehydration.[86] The stiffness of decalcified dentin increases when the tissue is dehydrated either chemically in water-miscible solvents, or physically in air.[178] The increase in stiffness is reversed when specimens are rehydrated in water. Therefore, rewetting dentin after air-drying to check for the enamel frosty aspect may be an acceptable clinical procedure.

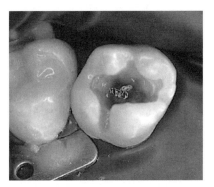

FIG. **5-23** Clinical aspect of moist dentin—a glistening appearance without accumulation of water.

In spite of numerous research papers focused on the low bond strengths associated with air-dried dentin,[161,162,178] the ultrastructural effects of drying dentin collagen during clinical procedures are not fully understood. Under the SEM, areas of detachment with incomplete peritubular hybridization have been observed, along with deficient penetration of the adhesive into the tubules.[231] The adhesive does not seem to penetrate etched dried intertubular dentin. Under the TEM, collagen fibers coalesce into a structure without individualized interfibrillar spaces. Rewetting reexpands this collapsed collagen.[178,231]

Clinically, it is very difficult to either assess or standardize the ideal amount of moisture that should be left on the dentin surface before the application of the adhesive system. Ideally, water should form a uniform layer without pooling (overwet) and without dry areas (overdried). Therefore air-drying with an air-water syringe after rinsing off the etching gel is not recommended because it cannot produce a uniform layer of water on the surface. A recent study demonstrated that the excess water after rinsing the etching gel can be removed with a damp cotton pellet, a disposable brush, or a tissue paper without adversely affecting bond strengths.[115]

ROLE OF PROTEINS IN DENTIN BONDING

Another important issue in dentin bonding is that drying demineralized dentin effectively increases the potential for the subsequent remineralization of that dentin.[151] It may, therefore, be debatable to state that air-drying has a deleterious effect on long-term stability and durability of dentin-resin bonded interfaces. In fact, no clinical study has ever supported this theory. By becoming insoluble upon air-drying, collagen may remain less susceptible to degradation. These exposed collagen fibers might be able to stretch upon tension and provide an elastic interface. Therefore this is one of numerous questions to be addressed in the area of dentin adhesion research. These questions pertain especially to extrapolations obtained from only empirical observations of bond strength studies.

The partial removal of phosphoproteins from root lesions may enhance the remineralization potential of those lesions.[67] This is important because acid-etching demineralizes dentin and may leave a layer of exposed collagen at the bottom of the hybrid layer.[168,265] If this collagen had the ideal environmental conditions for undergoing remineralization, nanoleakage at the bottom of the hybrid layer might be only an initial temporary phenomenon that could be arrested by the remineralization process. It has been reported that when demineralized dentin is restored with an adhesive system, the demineralized layer undergoes remineralization within 4 months.[308] Further studies are warranted to determine the effect of etching on the concentration of noncollagenous proteins and the role that these proteins

have for the stability and durability of the resin-dentin interfaces.

MICROLEAKAGE

Microleakage is the passage of bacteria and their toxins between restoration margins and tooth preparation walls.[25] Clinically, microleakage becomes important when one considers that pulpal irritation is more likely caused by bacteria than by chemical toxicity of restorative materials.[33,53,54] An adhesive restoration may not bond sufficiently to etched dentin to prevent gap formation at margins.[314] The smear layer alone may be a pathway for microleakage through the nanochannels within its core.[221]

Several studies have demonstrated that the pulpal response to restorative materials is related to the degree of marginal leakage.[51,52,189,190] Bacteria are able to survive and proliferate within the fluid-filled marginal gaps under composite restorations. If the restoration is hermetically sealed, bacteria will not survive.[33,189]

In some cases, pulpal inflammation may occur in the absence of bacteria. Some bacterial by-products, such as endotoxins, material from cell walls, and some elements derived from bacterial lipopolysaccharides, can cause damage to the pulpal tissue. This damage is initiated when leukocytes migrate into the pulp, sometimes as early as 72 hours after the pulp has been challenged.[31,34,48,51,336]

A useful property of dentin adhesives that remove the smear layer is that they may seal the resin-dentin interface and thus prevent exposure of the pulp-dentin complex to bacteria and their toxins. Several in vitro reports have demonstrated such sealing capacity for total-etch dentin adhesive systems,[128,132,280] but other studies have shown the occurrence of severe leakage associated with similar dentin adhesives.[104,266] Recent research also has demonstrated the presence of nanometer-sized pores underneath or within the resin-dentin interdiffusion area, despite the presence of gap-free restoration margins.[265,266] Therefore it is debatable whether the absence of marginal openings will result in a perfect seal between resin and dentin.[266] Bonding the resin to a preparation with cavosurface margins in enamel is still the best way to prevent microleakage.[302]

The occurrence of gaps at the resin-dentin interface may not cause immediate debonding of the restoration. For example, in spite of having demonstrated excellent marginal seal in vitro, OptiBond (Kerr Corporation, Orange, California) does not completely seal the interface in vivo.[234] Another report demonstrated 100% clinical retention in sclerotic dentin lesions at 1 year.[26] If a dentin adhesive system does not adhere intimately to the dentin substrate, an interfacial gap will eventually develop and bacteria will be able to penetrate through this gap.[263] In spite of the probability of incomplete seal of dentin margins, Class V clinical studies using total-etch dentin adhesive systems report no findings of pulpal inflammation and/or necrosis.[296,329] A plausible explanation for this apparent paradox is that a gap forms between the hybrid layer and the adhesive resin, leaving the tubules still plugged with resin tags (Fig. 5-24).[234]

In vitro microleakage studies generally involve Class V restorations. Specimens usually are thermocycled and sometimes mechanically loaded to simulate oral conditions.[79] To quantify microleakage, specimens are immersed in a disclosing solution, such as silver nitrate, basic fuchsin, or methylene blue. The dye penetrates the resin-dentin interface wherever gaps occur. After sectioning the teeth, the depth of dye penetration is usually measured and averaged for the sample size. However, the relationship between the laboratory testing and the oral cavity environment is ambiguous at best. Silver nitrate penetration may be a particularly demanding test of marginal seal because silver ions are smaller than the bacteria that usually live in the oral cavity.[246] Some authors have speculated that in vivo leakage is less than the corresponding dye penetration in vitro.[23]

BIOCOMPATIBILITY

Besides demineralizing the dentin surface, phosphoric acid removes the smear layer and opens the orifices of the tubules (see Fig. 5-14).[224,330] Despite past apprehension about potential acid penetration into the dentin tubules and pulp space, the interaction of etchants with dentin is limited to the superficial 1.9 to 5.8 µm.[229,235] Thus, it is unlikely that the acid is directly responsible for any injury to the pulp.[176,183] Acid penetration occurs primarily along the tubules,[275] with penetration of intertubular dentin occurring at a lower rate.[183] The effects of etchants on dentin are limited by the buffering effect of hydroxyapatite and other dentin components,[335] including the collagen, which may act as a barrier that reduces the rate of demineralization.[322] Marshall and others have elucidated the importance of pH regarding the effects of acids on dentin surfaces.[183] Etching rates increase dramatically with lower pH. Small differences in pH between acidic gels of similar phosphoric acid concentration may be responsible for distinct depths of dentin demineralization. Manufacturers add thickeners to facilitate handling and other modifiers (such as buffers, surfactants, and colorants) to their etching gels, and these may contribute to that phenomenon.

Another problem associated with etching dentin with acids is that current gel etchants are hypertonic.[225] Application of a hypertonic gel could osmotically draw fluid from the dentin toward the surface and alter the exposed collagen fibers. Ideally, one would use isotonic acids as dentin etchants, which have been reported to be well tolerated both by cell cultures and by monkey pulps.[194]

Several early studies suggested that acidic components included in restorative materials such as silicate cements would trigger adverse pulp reactions.[179,255] For

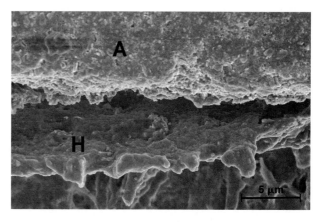

FIG. **5-24** Interfacial gap showing the top of the hybrid layer (H) with tag filling the tubular space. A, Adhesive.

several decades, the development of adhesive systems was limited by the belief that acids applied to dentin during restorative procedures caused pulpal inflammation. The use of bases and liners was considered essential to protect the pulp from the toxicity of restorative materials. This concept, however, has changed over the last 20 years.[33,53,73,74]

It has been demonstrated that dentin adhesive systems are well tolerated by the pulp-dentin complex in the absence of bacterial infection.[73] To prevent bacterial infection, restorations must be hermetically sealed. The pulp response to dentin adhesives, when teeth are restored in an ideal clinical environment, has been studied using histologic assessment of animal pulps, or in human premolars extracted for orthodontic reasons, and in third molars extracted for surgical reasons.[73,74,107,153,248,285,314,318,343] Some clinical studies also have reported normal pulp responses after the application of adhesive on the dentin-pulp complex when the pulp is macroscopically exposed,[145,163] although one report involved only one tooth. Another recent study showed that the newest dentin adhesive systems are not harmful when applied to exposed pulps.[72] However, several reports have shown that etching the pulp and applying a dentin adhesive directly on the exposed pulp tissue results in severe inflammation and eventual formation of pulpal abscesses.[131,143,215,288] The solution for this disparity would be long-term follow-up of patients in whom the pulp was treated with acid and adhesive. Ethical concerns, however, do not allow the routine use of pulpal etching in patients. It is known, however, that the thicker is the remaining dentin left between the pulpal aspect of the preparation and the pulp, the better is the prognosis for that specific pulp.[143] Certainly, the concept of pulp capping remains a controversial topic.

Adverse pulpal reactions after a restorative procedure may not be caused by the material used in that procedure, but by bacteria remaining in, or penetrating the preparation. In some cases, adverse reactions are caused by a combination of factors, such as the following:

1. Bacterial invasion of the pulp, either from the tooth preparation or from an existing carious lesion
2. Bacterial penetration into the pulp caused by a faulty restoration
3. Pressure gradient caused by excessive desiccation or by excessive pressure during cementation[32,47]
4. Traumatic injuries
5. Iatrogenic tooth preparation—excessive pressure, heat, or friction.[32]
6. Stress derived from polymerization contraction of composites and adhesives.

An important note on the biocompatibility issue is the importance of tooth preparations with enamel peripheries. When all margins are in enamel, polymerization shrinkage stresses at the interface are counteracted by strong enamel adhesion. Thus, marginal gaps are less likely to form, and the restoration is sealed against bacteria.

RELEVANCE OF IN VITRO STUDIES

The laboratory parameter most often measured in dentin adhesion is shear bond strength. Flat dentin surfaces are prepared in extracted human or bovine teeth, the adhesive system is applied, and a composite post is bonded over the adhesive. A shear force is then applied at the resin-dentin interface, most often using a knife-edge probe (Fig. 5-25). After testing, the specimens are usually evaluated to determine the nature of the fractures—adhesive, cohesive, or mixed.

The number of cohesive failures in the dentinal substrate increases with increasing bond strengths.[141] There may be, however, some misinterpretation of cohesive failures in dentin.[10] For example, a mean bond strength of 9.2 MPa has been reported to result in 82% of cohesive failures in dentin,[241] while the intrinsic strength of dentin has been reported to be in the range of 28.4 to 45.9 MPa.[132] Cohesive failures of dentin obtained during bond strength testing may result from anomalous stress distribution.[223]

A major disadvantage of shear bond strength testing is that it does not consider the three-dimensional geometry of tooth preparations and consequent variations in polymerization shrinkage vectors.[103,294] Additionally, it may not represent a true representation of a shear force. In vitro shear bond strength studies are therefore rather imprecise methods to evaluate the efficacy of dentin adhesive systems.[207,334]

Although these studies are only rough categorizing tools for evaluating the relative efficacy of bonding materials, they are, nevertheless, excellent tools for screening new materials and for comparing the same parameter among different adhesive systems.[106] The results of in vitro bond strength tests have been validated with clinical results because improvements seen in the laboratory environment from the second-generation to the fourth-generation adhesive systems have been confirmed in clinical trials.[329,333] Additionally, the combination of bond strength data with ultramorphologic analysis of adhesive interfaces supplies much useful information concerning the interaction of dentin bonding systems with dental substrates.[168]

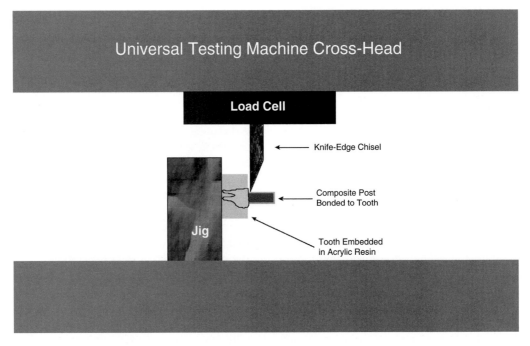

FIG. **5-25** Schematic representation of shear-bond strength testing.

One of the major concerns with laboratory bond strength testing is the wide range of results obtained for the same material in different testing sites. It is not uncommon for the same dentin adhesive system to have bond strengths of 20 MPa in one laboratory, while others report bond strengths below 10 MPa.[17,88] There is also some apprehension that no correlation can be established between bond strength and degree of resin penetration into the hybrid layer.[228,345] To illustrate this discrepancy, there have been reports of dentin adhesives that do not penetrate the whole depth of the demineralized dentin layer, but still result in bond strengths above 20 MPa.[90,305] In such cases, retention would be good, in spite of a deficient seal over time, which could be a triggering factor for nanoleakage phenomena.[265] Intuitively, one would expect an inverse relationship between bond strength and microleakage, but that relationship has not been confirmed.[105]

Clinical studies with dentin adhesive systems are expensive for manufacturers and take at least 18 months. Cost is a major concern, in part because of the constant developments in the area of adhesion, making new materials quickly obsolete. There is no financial incentive for the manufacturer to invest in a clinical study of a material that may not be on the market by the time the study is concluded. Consequently, in vitro studies are still used predominantly by manufacturers to anticipate the clinical behavior of their materials.

Several factors contribute to the questionable use of in vitro tests to predict clinical behavior. Among others, age and storage conditions of the teeth used, dentin depth, degree of sclerosis, tooth surface to be bonded, dentin roughness, and type of test used are variables that frequently are not controllable.[103,217,262,286] According to some authors, one of the major drawbacks of laboratory bond strength testing is the lack of simulated pulpal pressure to replicate the pulpal pressure that occurs in vivo.[217] However, other authors have reported that the pulpal pressure does not significantly interfere with bond strength results.[214]

Recently, a new bond strength testing methodology was introduced in dental research.[267] This new method, the microtensile test, allows for the assessment of bond strengths using bonded surfaces with a cross-sectional area in the range of only 0.5 to 1.5 mm^2 (Fig. 5-26). The new method carries several advantages over conventional shear and tensile bond strengths methods because it:

1. Permits the use of only one tooth to fabricate several bonded dentin/resin rods.
2. Allows for testing substrates of clinical significance, such as carious dentin, cervical sclerotic dentin, and enamel.[203]
3. Results in fewer defects occurring in the small-area specimens, as reflected in higher bond strengths.[243]

4. Allows for the testing of regional differences in bond strengths within the same tooth.[279]

CLINICAL FACTORS IN DENTIN ADHESION

Several clinical factors may influence the success of an adhesive restoration. First, the mineral content of dentin increases in different situations, including aged dentin, dentin in the vicinity of a carious lesion, and dentin exposed to the oral cavity in noncarious cervical lesions, in which the tubules become obliterated with tricalcium phosphate crystals.[203,347,348]

The dentin that undergoes these compositional changes is called "sclerotic dentin" and is much more resistant to acid-etching than "normal" dentin.[331] Consequently, the penetration of a dentin adhesive is limited.[84,139,331] Additionally, the clinical effectiveness of dentin adhesives is less in sclerotic cervical lesions than in normal dentin.[146,331] Nevertheless, some specific dentin adhesives may perform better in sclerotic dentin than in normal dentin.[325]

Some evidence indicates that masticatory forces may not only cause cervical noncarious lesions, but also may contribute to failure of Class V restorations.[46,146,147] Bruxism or any other eccentric movement may generate lateral forces that cause concentration of stresses around the cervical area of the teeth. Although this stress may be of very low magnitude, the fatigue caused by cyclic stresses may cause failure of bonds between resin and dentin.

The type of composite used may play an important role in clinical longevity of Class V restorations.[333] Composites shrink as they polymerize, but the amount of shrinkage depends on the inorganic load of each specific composite. Microfilled composites have a low elastic (or Young's) modulus, which means they are more able to relieve stresses caused by polymerization or by tooth flexure.[114,193,333] Materials that have a higher Young's modulus do not relieve stresses by flow; therefore they are unable to compensate for the stresses accumulated during polymerization. These stresses may be subsequently transferred to the adhesive interface and cause debonding.[333]

The low flow capacity of photoinitiated hybrid composites prevents them from flowing to compensate for the polymerization shrinkage. Polymerization is initiated on the surface of the restoration, close to the light source, eliminating this surface as a potential stress relief pathway.[170] Several methods have been advocated to

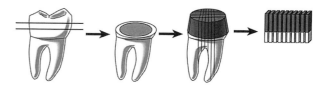

FIG. **5-26** Preparation of specimens for microtensile bond strength testing.

improve the flow capacity of composites used in Class II tooth preparations. One of those methods is the use of a flowable composite between the composite and the tooth wall. Conceptually, this flowable low-modulus composite would serve as a shock absorber[103,104] and simultaneously protect the interface against fatigue stresses.[169] Low-viscosity resins have been reported to decrease microleakage when used as part of dentin adhesive systems.[104,105,291] However, the use of flowable composites as the gingival increment of Class II preparations has not been proven effective clinically.

NEW CLINICAL INDICATIONS FOR DENTIN ADHESIVES

Desensitization. Dentin hypersensitivity is a common clinical condition that is difficult to treat because the treatment outcome is not consistently successful. Most authorities agree that the hydrodynamic theory[49] best explains dentin hypersensitivity. The equivalency of various hydrodynamic stimuli has been evaluated from measurements of the fluid movement induced in vitro and relating this to the hydraulic conductance of the same dentin specimen.[222]

Patients may complain of discomfort when teeth are subjected to temperature changes, osmotic gradients such as those caused by sweet or salty foods, or even tactile stimuli. It has been calculated that 40 million Americans may have some degree of dentin hypersensitivity at some point in their life,[272] while in other regions of the world the prevalence of dentin sensitivity may approach 50% of the population.[112,200] The cervical area of teeth is the most common site of hypersensitivity. Cervical hypersensitivity may be caused not only by chemical erosion, but also by mechanical abrasion or even occlusal stresses.[119,120]

Theories about the transmission of pain stimuli in dentin sensitivity suggest that pain is amplified when the dentinal tubules are open to the oral cavity.[76,254] Therefore dentin hypersensitivity can be a major problem for periodontal patients, who frequently have gingival recession and exposed root surfaces. The relationship between dentin hypersensitivity and the patency of dentin tubules in vivo has been established[76] and occlusion of the tubules seems to decrease that sensitivity.[172] It also has been suggested that the incorrect manipulation of some adhesive materials, namely those with acetone, may actually trigger postoperative sensitivity.[309,310]

Clinicians have used many materials and techniques to treat dentin hypersensitivity, including specific dentifrices, CO_2 laser irradiation, dentin adhesives, antibacterial agents, aldehydes, resin suspensions, fluoride rinses, fluoride varnishes, calcium phosphate, potassium nitrate, and oxalates, among others.[60,110,150,196,197,247,315,342,346,349]

More recently, dentin desensitizing solutions also have been used under amalgam restorations and crowns to prevent postoperative sensitivity.[274] The use of a dentin desensitizer before cementing full-coverage crowns is supported by studies that showed that dentin-desensitizing solutions do not interfere with crown retention, regardless of the type of luting cement used.[69,253,301]

The use of dentin adhesives to treat hypersensitive root surfaces has gained popularity over the last few years.[59,101] Reductions in sensitivity may result from formation of resin tags and a hybrid layer when a dentin adhesive is used.[202] The precipitation of proteins from the dentinal fluid in the tubules also may account for the efficacy of desensitizing solutions.[273] However, other factors may be involved in the action of dentin desensitizing solutions.[205,339] For example, the primers of the multibottle adhesive system All-Bond 2 (Bisco, Inc., Schaumburg, Illinois) have a desensitizing effect, even without consistent resin tag formation.[299] In a clinical study using the primer of the original Gluma adhesive system (an aqueous solution of 5% glutaraldehyde and 35% HEMA, currently marketed as Gluma Desensitizer [Heraeus Kulzer, South Bend, Indiana]), the desensitizing solution was applied to crown preparations.[99] The authors concluded that Gluma primer reduced dentin sensitivity through a protein denaturation process with concomitant changes in dentin permeability. This theory recently has been supported by studies using confocal microscopy,[273] which found the formation of transversal septa occluding the dentinal tubules following application of Gluma Desensitizer. However, another study found that Gluma Desensitizer did not have any effect on dentin permeability in vitro.[253]

Adhesive Amalgam Restorations. Marginal discoloration, recurrent caries lesions, and postoperative sensitivity are the most frequent consequences of the penetration of oral fluids and bacteria through gaps at the dentin-resin interface towards the pulp.[136]

Delayed interfacial marginal leakage occurs at the amalgam-preparation interface.[8] Corrosion products from amalgam seal the interface after a few months; however, this process may take more than 6 months for copper-rich amalgam alloys such as the spherical and blended amalgam alloys currently used in dentistry.[28,97] High-copper amalgam alloys undergo a much slower corrosion process than conventional amalgam alloys because of the elimination of the γ2 phase.[28] To overcome the inevitable marginal microleakage, dentin adhesive systems have been used both under mercury-based amalgam restorations and under gallium-based amalgam restorations.[85,211] It is now accepted that the use of adhesive systems beneath amalgam restorations reduces or prevents marginal leakage both in vivo and in vitro[27,29,261,276] and improves marginal integrity of the restoration[307] when compared to the use of a copal varnish. Additionally, dentin adhesives reinforce the amalgam restoration margins, making the cavosurface angle less susceptible to acidic demineralization in vitro.[245] However, despite anecdotal evidence to the contrary, postoperative sensitivity may be one clinical parameter that dentin adhesives do not improve over the use of copal varnishes.[116,171]

Several laboratory and clinical studies have shown that dentin adhesive systems such as All-Bond 2 (Bisco, Inc., Schaumburg, Illinois), Amalgambond Plus (Parkell, Farmingdale, New York), Panavia (Kuraray, Osaka, Japan), and Scotchbond Multi-Purpose Plus (3M ESPE, St. Paul, Minnesota) can be used to bond amalgam restorations.[27,68,249] The attachment mechanism between the adhesive and the amalgam is not fully understood, but it may be micromechanical entanglement of the uncured adhesive material with the setting amalgam mix during condensation of the amalgam (Fig. 5-27). This bonding mechanism actually may depend on the type of amalgam used; for example, spherical amalgam alloys typically have higher bond strengths than dispersed-phase or admixed amalgam alloys.[319]

Shear bond strengths between amalgam and dentin were in the range of 3 to 5 MPa in the late 1980s and early 1990s.[63,70,71,142,191,227] However, recent studies have demonstrated that some current adhesive systems provide bond strengths in the range of 10 to 14 MPa.[68,249] As a safety precaution, primary mechanical retention features are still recommended when an adhesive system is used with amalgam.

Some studies also suggest that the use of dual-cured filled liners may be beneficial for bonding amalgam to dentin.[68,188,249] The use of a self-cured filled adhesive liner has been shown to be as valuable under amalgam restorations as under composite restorations.[209] The additional adhesive liner may provide an increased retention to adhesive amalgam restorations, therefore allowing for preparations with lower demand for additional retention features such as dovetails, slots, holes, or even pins.[64,149,290] Moreover, marginal leakage has been shown to decrease when thick dual-cured or self-cured liners are used.[188]

Another advantage from the use of dentin adhesives under amalgam restorations is that the residual tooth structure becomes more resistant to fracture than when teeth are restored with a copal varnish and amalgam.[208,244] This reinforcing effect may not be as evident for wide tooth preparations as for narrow tooth preparations.[45]

Light-curing of the resin from the external tooth surface after condensing the amalgam into the preparation recently has been evaluated in vitro for three dual-cured adhesive systems.[250] The rationale behind the use of light-curing through the tooth walls was that some dual-cured adhesive systems might not be able to polymerize completely underneath the amalgam restoration. However, the mean bond strengths obtained for the groups in which the extra light-curing period was used were statistically similar to the mean bond strengths obtained when the dual-cured adhesive systems were used as per manufacturers' instructions (i.e., without additional light curing).[250]

Dentin adhesive systems also are used to bond fresh amalgam to existing amalgam restorations in repair procedures. The prognosis of this type of procedure is, however, unpredictable and can be unsuccessful.[133,134,174,257] The interfacial failure between fresh amalgam and old amalgam may be a result of the lack of micromechanical retention in the "old" amalgam restoration surface. Therefore dentin adhesive systems are not recommended for amalgam repair.

Indirect Adhesive Restorations. Current dentin adhesive systems are considered as universal adhesives because they bond to various substrates besides dentin.[20,22,159,328,337] Recent developments in adhesion technology have led to new indications for bonding to the tooth structure, such as indirect composite and ceramic restorations (crowns, inlays, onlays, and veneers). The use of a universal adhesive system in conjunction with a resin cement provides durable bonding of indirect restorations to tooth structure.[58]

Ceramic restorations (with the exception of aluminous-core porcelains such as In-Ceram High Strength Ceramic [Vita Zahnfabrik/Vident, Bäd Säckingen, Germany]) must be etched internally with 6% to 10% hydrofluoric acid (HF) for 1 to 2 minutes to create retentive microporosities (Fig. 5-28) analogous to those that occur in enamel upon etching with phosphoric acid. HF must be rinsed off carefully with running water for at least 2 minutes. Some clinicians use sandblasting with aluminum oxide particles in the internal surface of the restoration. However, mean bond strengths decrease when HF-etching is not used.[295] After rinsing off the HF and drying with an air syringe, a silane coupling agent is applied on the etched porcelain surface and air-dried. The coupling agent acts as a primer because it modifies the surface characteristics of etched porcelain. Because etched porcelain is an inorganic substrate, the coupling agent makes this surface more receptive to organic materials, the adhesive system, and composite

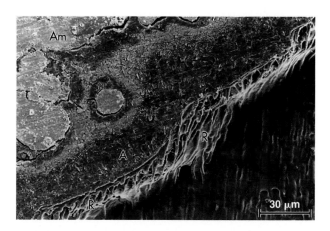

FIG. 5-27 Scanning electron micrograph of amalgam-resin-dentin interface showing the amalgam *(Am)*, the adhesive *(A)*, and resin tags *(R)*.

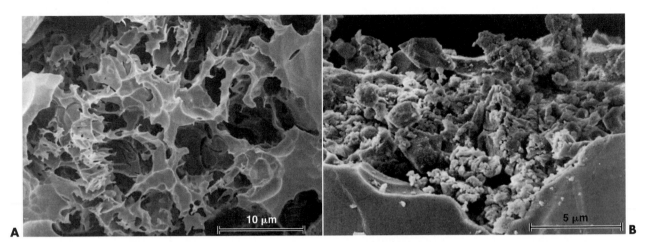

FIG. **5-28** Scanning electron micrograph of Vita (Vita Zahnfabrik/Vident, Bäd Säckingen, Germany) dental ceramic etched with 9.6% hydrofluoric acid for 2 minutes. **A,** Top view. **B,** Lateral view.

resin cement. Silane coupling agents were introduced in 1952 to bond organic with inorganic substances.[37] In 1962 this technology was transferred to dentistry to couple a Bis-GMA resin with inorganic particles to form a composite.[44] The use of silanes may actually increase the bond between composite and porcelain in the range of 25%.[83,204,278] Most luting resins are dual-cured (they polymerize both chemically and by light activation). However, some materials marketed as "dual-cure" do not polymerize efficiently in the absence of a curing light.[78,140,242]

Other circumstances exist in which porcelain bonding is of extreme importance. Fracture of all-ceramic or metal-ceramic restorations is not uncommon. It becomes very frustrating for the clinician who must decide whether to repair or to replace the fractured restoration.[157] Several methods for repairing porcelain restorations have been advocated. The creation of surface roughness (e.g., with a coarse diamond bur) on the porcelain surface allows its repair with a universal adhesive and composite.[100,157] Sandblasting with aluminum oxide particles is another method for roughening the porcelain surface for repair.[36] However, the use of HF on the roughened porcelain surface is still necessary to create deep microretentive porosities and facilitate mechanical retention.[174,278,295] If the internal surface of the porcelain restoration is treated adequately, the bond strengths between composite and porcelain surface often exceed 25 MPa, which has been considered a predictable value for clinical success.[9,173,283,289]

Indirect composite restorations also may be bonded to etched dental substrates using a universal adhesive system and a resin luting cement. One of the great advantages of indirect composite restorations is that polymerization shrinkage occurs outside the mouth. Additionally, the degree of monomer conversion is higher for indirect resin-based restorations.[155,160,177,340,341] However, this increased level of double bond conversion results in

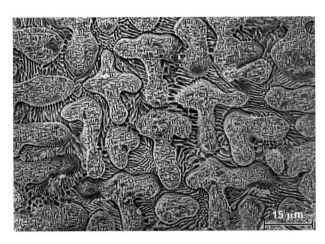

FIG. **5-29** Scanning electron micrograph of Rexillium III (Jeneric/Pentron, Wallingford, Connecticut) after electrochemical etching with 0.5N nitric acid for 5 minutes. *(Special thanks to Dr. Glen Imamura for preparing this specimen.)*

only a small amount of monomer double bonds on the internal surface of the indirect composite restoration, therefore decreasing the potential for bonding with the adhesive system and with the composite luting cement. To overcome this unsuitable bonding surface, the composite may be treated with surface activators to reestablish the surface energy (Composite Activator [Bisco, Inc., Schaumburg, Illinois], Activator-ArtGlass [Heraeus Kulzer, South Bend, Indiana]). Another alternative is sandblasting the bonding surface of the indirect restoration to expose an internal area where more double bonds may be present.[40] HF is contraindicated for treating indirect composites because it softens some composite materials.[300]

Cast metal restorations traditionally were cemented with zinc phosphate or polycarboxylate cements. With the advent of new adhesive techniques, the treatment of the internal surface of the metal restoration with acids (Fig. 5-29), sandblasting, or tin-plating (for gold) has resulted in high bond strengths between metal and tooth structure using resin cements.[36,77]

SUMMARY

Reliable bonding of resins to enamel and dentin has revolutionized the practice of operative dentistry. Improvements in dentin bonding materials and techniques are likely to continue. However, even as the materials themselves become better and easier to use, proper attention to technique and a good understanding of the bonding process remain essential for clinical success.

REFERENCES

1. Aasen SM, Ario PD: Bonding systems: a comparison of maleic and phosphoric acids (abstract 269), *J Dent Res* 72:137, 1993.
2. Abdalla AI, García-Godoy F: Bond strengths of resin-modified glass ionomers and polyacid-modified resin composites to dentin, *Am J Dent* 10:291-294, 1997.
3. Akinmade AO, Nicholson JW: Glass-ionomer cements as adhesives. I: Fundamental aspects and their clinical relevance, *J Mater Sci: Materials in Medicine* 4:95-101, 1993.
4. Albers HF: Dentin-resin bonding, *ADEPT Report* 1:33-42, 1990.
5. Alexieva C: Character of the hard tooth tissue-polymer bond. II: Study of the interaction of human tooth enamel and dentin with N-phenylglycine-glycidyl methacrylate adduct, *J Dent Res* 58:1884-1886, 1979.
6. Allen KW: Theories of adhesion. In Packham DE, editor: *Handbook of adhesion*, Essex, 1992, Longman Scientific & Technical.
7. al-Salehi SK, Burke FJ: Methods used in dentin bonding tests: an analysis of 50 investigations on bond strength, *Quintessence Int* 28:717-723, 1997.
8. Andrews JT, Hembree JH: Marginal leakage of amalgam alloys with high content of copper: a laboratory study, *Oper Dent* 5:7-10, 1980.
9. Appeldoorn RE, Wilwerding TM, Barkmeier WW: Bond strength of composite resin to porcelain with newer generation porcelain repair systems, *J Prosthet Dent* 70:6-11, 1993.
10. Armstrong SR, Boyer DB, Keller JC: Microtensile bond strength testing and failure analysis of two dentin adhesives, *Dent Mater* 14:44-50, 1998.
11. Armstrong SR et al: Effect of hybrid layer on fracture toughness of adhesively bonded dentin-resin composite joint, *Dent Mater* 14:91-98, 1998.
12. Asmussen E: Clinical relevance of physical, chemical, and bonding properties of composite resins, *Oper Dent* 10:61-73, 1985.
13. Asmussen E, Bowen RL: Adhesion to dentin mediated by Gluma: effect of pretreatment with various amino acids, *Scand J Dent Res* 95:521-525, 1987.
14. Asmussen E, Hansen EK, Peutzfeldt A: Influence of the solubility parameter of intermediary resin on the effectiveness of the Gluma bonding system, *J Dent Res* 70:1290-1293, 1991.
15. Asmussen E, Munksgaard EC: Bonding of restorative materials to dentine: status of dentine adhesives and impact on cavity design and filling techniques, *Int Dent J* 38:97-104, 1988.
16. Baier RE: Principles of adhesion, *Oper Dent* 5(suppl):1-9, 1992
17. Barkmeier WW, Cooley RL: Laboratory evaluation of adhesive systems, *Oper Dent* 5(suppl):50-61, 1992.

18. Barkmeier WW, Gwinnett AJ, Shaffer SE: Effects of enamel etching on bond strength and morphology, *J Clin Orthodont* 19:36-38, 1985.
19. Barkmeier WW, Los SA, Triolo PT Jr: Bond strengths and SEM evaluation of Clearfil Liner Bond 2, *Am J Dent* 8:289-293, 1995.
20. Barkmeier WW, Menis DL, Barnes DM: Bond strength of a veneering porcelain using newer generation adhesive systems, *Pract Periodont Aesthet Dent* 5:50-55, 1993.
21. Barkmeier WW, Shaffer SE, Gwinnett AJ: Effects of 15 vs 60 second enamel acid conditioning on adhesion and morphology, *Oper Dent* 11:111-116, 1986.
22. Barkmeier WW, Suh BI, Cooley RL: Shear bond strength to dentin and Ni-Cr-Be alloy with the All-Bond universal adhesive system, *J Esthet Dent* 3:148-153, 1991.
23. Barnes DM, Thompson VP, Blank LW, McDonald NJ: Microleakage of Class 5 composite resin restorations: a comparison between in vivo and in vitro, *Oper Dent* 18:237-245, 1993.
24. Bastos PAM et al: Effect of etch duration on the shear bond strength of a microfill composite resin to enamel, *Am J Dent* 1:151-157, 1988.
25. Bauer JG, Henson JL: Microleakage: a measure of the performance of direct filling materials, *Oper Dent* 9:2-9, 1984.
26. Bayne SC et al: One-year clinical evaluation of stress-breaking class V DBA design, *Trans Acad Dent Mater* 7:91, 1994.
27. Belcher MA, Stewart GP: Two-year clinical evaluation of an amalgam adhesive, *JADA* 128:309-314, 1997.
28. Ben-Amar A, Cardash HS, Judes H: The sealing of the tooth/amalgam interface by corrosion products, *J Oral Rehabil* 22:101-104, 1995.
29. Ben-Amar A et al: Long term sealing properties of Amalgambond under amalgam restorations, *Am J Dent* 7:141-143, 1994.
30. Benediktsson S et al: Critical surface tension of wetting of dentin (abstract 777), *J Dent Res* 70:362, 1987.
31. Bergenholtz G: Effect of bacterial products on inflammatory reactions in dental pulp, *Scand J Dent Res* 85:122-129, 1977.
32. Bergenholtz G: Iatrogenic injury to the pulp in dental procedures: aspects of pathogenesis, management and preventive measures, *Int Dent J* 41:99-110, 1991.
33. Bergenholtz G et al: Bacterial leakage around dental restorations its effect on the dental pulp, *J Oral Pathol* 11:439-450, 1982.
34. Bergenholtz G, Warfvinge J: Migration of leukocytes in dental pulp in response to plaque bacteria, *Scand J Dent Res* 90:354-362, 1982.
35. Berry TG et al: Effectiveness of nitric-NPG as a conditioning agent for enamel, *Am J Dent* 3:59-62, 1990.
36. Bertolotti RL, Lacy AM, Watanabe LG: Adhesive monomers for porcelain repair, *Int J Prosthodont* 2:483-489, 1989.
37. Bjorksten J, Yaeger LL: Vinyl silane size for glass fabric, *Mod Plast* 2(29):124, 128, 1952.
38. Black GV: *A work on operative dentistry in two volumes*, ed 3, Chicago, 1917, Medico-Dental Publishing.
39. Blosser RL: Time dependence of 2.5% nitric acid solution as an etchant for human dentin and enamel, *Dent Mater* 6:83-87, 1990.
40. Bouschlicher MR, Reinhardt JW, Vargas MA: Surface treatment for resin composite repair, *Am J Dent* 10:279-283, 1997.
41. Bowen RL: Adhesive bonding of various materials to hard tooth tissues. II: Bonding to dentin promoted by a surface-active comonomer, *J Dent Res* 44:895-902, 1965.
42. Bowen RL et al: Smear layer: removal and bonding considerations, *Oper Dent* 3(suppl):30-34, 1984

43. Bowen RL, Nemoto K, Rapson JE: Adhesive bonding of various materials to hard tooth tissue: forces developing in composite materials during hardening, *JADA* 106:475-477, 1983.

44. Bowen RL, Rodriguez MS: Tensile strength and modulus of elasticity of tooth structure and several restorative materials, *JADA* 64:378-387, 1962.

45. Boyer DB, Roth L: Fracture resistance of teeth with bonded amalgams, *Am J Dent* 7:91-94, 1994.

46. Braem M et al: Stiffness increase during the setting of dental composite resins, *J Dent Res* 66:1713-1716, 1987.

47. Brännström M: The effect of dentin desiccation and aspirated odontoblasts on the pulp, *J Prosthet Dent* 20:165-171, 1968.

48. Brännström M: Communication between the oral cavity and the dental pulp associated with restorative treatment, *Oper Dent* 9:57-68, 1984.

49. Brännström M, Linden LA, Astrom A: The hydrodynamics of the dental tubule and of pulp fluid: a discussion of its significance in relation to dentinal sensitivity, *Caries Res* 1:310-317, 1967.

50. Brännström M, Linden LA, Johnson G: Movement of dentinal and pulpal fluid caused by clinical procedures, *J Dent Res* 47:679-682, 1968.

51. Brännström M, Nordenvall J: Bacterial penetration, pulpal reaction and the inner surface of Concise Enamel Bond: composite fillings in etched and unetched cavities, *J Dent Res* 57:3-10, 1978.

52. Brännström M, Nyborg H: Cavity treatment with a microbicidal fluoride solution: growth of bacteria and effect on the pulp, *J Prosthet Dent* 30:303-310, 1973.

53. Brännström M, Nyborg H: Pulpal reaction to polycarboxylate and zinc phosphate cements used with inlays in deep cavity preparations, *J Am Dent Assoc* 94:308-310, 1977.

54. Brännström M, Vojinovic O, Nordenvall KJ: Bacteria and pulpal reactions under silicate cement restorations, *J Prosthet Dent* 41:290-295, 1979.

55. Buonocore M, Wileman W, Brudevold F: A report on a resin composition capable of bonding to human dentin surfaces, *J Dent Res* 35:846-851, 1956.

56. Buonocore MG: A simple method of increasing the adhesion of acrylic filling materials to enamel surfaces, *J Dent Res* 34:849-853, 1955.

57. Buonocore MG, Matsui A, Gwinnett AJ: Penetration of resin into enamel surfaces with reference to bonding, *Arch Oral Biol* 13:61-70, 1968.

58. Burke FJT, Watts DC: Fracture resistance of teeth restored with dentin-bonded crowns, *Quintessence Int* 25:335-340, 1994.

59. Calamia JR, Styner DL, Rattet AH: Effect of Amalgambond on cervical sensitivity, *Am J Dent* 8:283-284, 1996.

60. Camps J et al: Effects of desensitizing agents on human dentin permeability, *Am J Dent* 11:286-90, 1998.

61. Carvalho RM et al: In vitro study on the dimensional changes of dentine after demineralization, *Arch Oral Biol* 41:369-377, 1996.

62. Causton BE: Improved bonding of composite restorative to dentine: a study in vitro of the use of a commercial halogenated phosphate ester, *Br Dent J* 156:93-95, 1984.

63. Chang J et al: Shear bond strength of a 4-META adhesive system, *J Prosthet Dent* 67:42-45, 1992.

64. Charlton DG, Moore BK, Swartz, ML: In vitro evaluation of the use of resin liners to reduce microleakage and improve retention of amalgam restorations, *Oper Dent* 17:112-119, 1992.

65. Chiba M, Itoh K, Wakumoto S: Effect of dentin cleansers on the bonding efficacy of dentin adhesive, *Dent Mater J* 8:76-85, 1989.

66. Chow LC, Brown WE: Phosphoric acid conditioning of teeth for pit and fissure sealants, *J Dent Res* 52:1158, 1973.

67. Clarkson BH et al: Effects of phosphoprotein moieties on the remineralization of human root caries, *Caries Res* 25:166-173, 1991.

68. Cobb DS, Denehy GE, Vargas MA: Amalgam shear bond strength to dentin using single-bottle primer/adhesive systems, *Am J Dent* 12:222-226, 1999.

69. Cobb DS, Reinhardt JW, Vargas MA: Effect of HEMA-containing dentin desensitizers on shear bond strength of a resin cement, *Am J Dent* 10:62-65, 1997.

70. Cooley RL, Tseng EY, Barkmeier WW: Dentinal bond strengths and microleakage of a 4-META adhesive to amalgam and composite resin, *Quintessence Int* 22:979-983, 1991.

71. Covey DA, Moon PC: Shear bond strength of dental amalgam bonded to dentin, *Am J Dent* 4:19-22, 1991.

72. Cox CF et al: Biocompatibility of primer, adhesive and resin composite systems on non-exposed and exposed pulps of non-human primate teeth, *Am J Dent* 11:S55-S63, 1998.

73. Cox CF et al: Biocompatibility of surface-sealed dental materials against exposed pulps, *J Prosthet Dent* 57:1-8, 1987.

74. Cox CF, Suzuki S: Re-evaluating pulp protection: calcium hydroxide liners vs. cohesive hybridization, *JADA* 125:823-831, 1994.

75. Crim GA, Shay JS: Effect of etchant time on microleakage, *J Dent Child* 54:339-340, 1987.

76. Cuenin MF et al: An in vivo study of dentin sensitivity: the relation of dentin sensitivity and the patency of dentin tubules, *J Periodontol* 62:668-673, 1991.

77. Czerw RJ et al: Shear bond strength of composite resin to microetched metal with five newer generation bonding agents, *Oper Dent* 20:58-62, 1995.

78. Darr AH, Jacobson PH: Conversion of dual-cure luting cements, *J Oral Rehabil* 22:43-47, 1995.

79. Davidson CL, Abdalla AI: Effect of occlusal load cycling on the marginal integrity of adhesive Class V restorations, *Am J Dent* 7:111-114, 1994.

80. Davidson CL, de Gee AJ: Relaxation of polymerization contraction stresses by flow in dental composites, *J Dent Res* 63:146-148, 1984.

81. Davidson CL, de Gee AJ, Feilzer A: The competition between the composite-dentin bond strength and the polymerization contraction stress, *J Dent Res* 63:1396-1399, 1984.

82. Davidson CL, Feilzer AJ: Polymerization shrinkage and polymerization shrinkage stress in polymer-based restoratives, *J Dent* 25:435-440, 1997.

83. Diaz-Arnold AM, Schneider RL, Aquilino SA: Porcelain repairs: an evaluation of the shear strength of three porcelain repair systems (abstract 806), *J Dent Res* 66:207, 1987.

84. Duke ES, Lindemuth J: Polymeric adhesion to dentin: Contrasting substrates, *Am J Dent* 4:241-146, 1991.

85. Eakle WS et al: Mechanical retention versus bonding of amalgam and gallium alloy restorations, *J Prosthet Dent* 72:351-354, 1994.

86. Eanes ED, Lundy DR, Martin GN: X-ray diffraction study of the mineralization of turkey leg tendon, *Calcif Tissue Res* 6:239-248, 1970.

87. Eick JD: Smear layer: materials surface, *Proc Finn Dent Soc* 88:225-242, 1992.

88. Eick JD et al: The dentinal surface: its influence on dentinal adhesion. I. *Quintessence Int* 22:967:977, 1991.

89. Eick JD et al: Current concepts on adhesion to dentin, *Crit Rev Oral Biol Med* 8:306-335, 1997.

90. Eick JD et al: The dentinal surface: its influence on dentinal adhesion. III. *Quintessence Int* 24:571-582, 1993.

91. Eidelman E, Shapira J, Houpt M: The retention of fissure sealants using twenty-second etch time: a clinical trial. I. *J Dent Child* 51:422-424, 1984.

92. Eliades G: Clinical relevance of the formulation and testing of dentine bonding systems, *J Dent* 22:73-81, 1994.

93. Eliades GC: Dentine bonding systems. In Vanherle G, Degrange M, Willems G, editors: *State of the art on direct posterior filling materials and dentine bonding*, Leuven, 1993, Van der Poorten.

94. Eliades GC, Vougiouklakis GJ: ^{31}P-NMR study of P-based dental adhesives and electron probe microanalysis of simulated interfaces with dentin, *Dent Mater* 5:101-108, 1989.

95. el-Kalla IH, García-Godoy F: Saliva contamination and bond strength of single-bottle adhesives to enamel and dentin, *Am J Dent* 10:83-87, 1997.

96. Erickson RL: Surface interactions of dentin adhesive materials, *Oper Dent* 5(suppl):81-94, 1992.

97. Fayyad MA, Ball PC: Cavity sealing ability of lathe-cut, blend, and spherical amalgam alloys: a laboratory study, *Oper Dent* 9:86-93, 1984.

98. Feilzer A, de Gee AJ, Davidson CL: Setting stress in composite resin in relation to configuration of the restoration, *J Dent Res* 66:1636-1639, 1987.

99. Felton DA, Bergenholtz G, Kanoy BE: Evaluation of the desensitizing effect of Gluma dentin bond on teeth prepared for complete coverage restorations, *Int J Prosthodont* 4:292-298, 1991.

100. Ferrando JMP et al: Tensile strength and microleakage of porcelain repair materials, *J Prosthet Dent* 50:44-50, 1983.

101. Ferrari M et al: Clinical evaluation of a one-bottle bonding system for desensitizing exposed roots, *Am J Dent* 12:243-249, 1999.

102. Ferrari M et al: Effect of two etching times on the sealing ability of Clearfil Liner Bond 2 in Class V restorations, *Am J Dent* 10:66-70, 1997.

103. Finger WJ: Dentin bonding agents. Relevance of in vitro investigations, *Am J Dent* 184-188, 1988.

104. Fortin D, Perdigao J, Swift EJ: Microleakage of three new dentin adhesives, *Am J Dent* 7:315-318, 1994.

105. Fortin D et al: Bond strength and microleakage of current adhesive systems, *Dent Mater* 10:253-258, 1994.

106. Fritz UB, Finger WJ, Uno S: Resin-modified glass ionomer cements: bonding to enamel and dentin, *Dent Mater* 12:161-166, 1996.

107. Fuks AB, Funnel B, Cleaton-Jones P: Pulp response to a composite resin inserted in deep cavities with and without a surface seal, *J Prosthet Dent* 63:129-134, 1990.

108. Fukushima T, Horibe T: A scanning electron microscope investigation of bonding of methacryoyloxyalkyl hydrogen maleate to etched dentin, *J Dent Res* 69:46-50, 1990.

109. Fusayama T et al: Non-pressure adhesion of a new adhesive restorative resin, *J Dent Res* 58:1364-1370, 1979.

110. Gaffar A: Treating hypersensitivity with fluoride varnishes, *Compend Contin Educ Dent* 19:1088-1094, 1998.

111. Garberoglio R, Brännström M: Scanning electron microscopic investigation of human dentinal tubules, *Arch Oral Biol* 21:355-362, 1976.

112. Gillam DG et al: Perceptions of dentine hypersensitivity in a general practice population, *J Oral Rehabil* 26:710-714, 1999.

113. Gilpatrick RO, Ross JA, Simonsen RJ: Resin-to-enamel bond strengths with various etching times, *Quintessence Int* 22:47-49,1991.

114. Gladys S et al: Comparative physico-mechanical characterization of new hybrid restorative materials with conventional glass-ionomer and resin composite restorative materials, *J Dent Res* 76:883-894, 1997.

115. Goes MF, Pachane GCF, García-Godoy F: Resin bond strength with different methods to remove excess water from the dentin, *Am J Dent* 10:298-301, 1997.

116. Gordan VV et al: Effect of different liner treatments on postoperative sensitivity of amalgam restorations, *Quintessence Int* 30:55-59, 1999.

117. Gordan VV et al: Evaluation of adhesive systems using acidic primers, *Am J Dent* 10:219-223, 1997.

118. Gottlieb EW, Retief DH, Jamison HC: An optimal concentration of phosphoric acid as an etching agent: tensile bond strength studies. Part I. *J Prosthet Dent* 48:48-51, 1982.

119. Gray A, Ferguson MM, Wall JG: Wine tasting and dental erosion: case report, *Austr Dent J* 43:32-34, 1988.

120. Grippo JO: Abfractions: a new classification of hard tissue lesions of teeth, *J Esthet Dent* 3:14-19, 1991.

121. Gwinnett AJ: Altered tissue contribution to interfacial bond strength with acid conditioned dentin, *Am J Dent* 7:243-246, 1994.

122. Gwinnett AJ: Dentin bond strengths after air-drying and re-wetting, *Am J Dent* 7:144-148, 1994.

123. Gwinnett AJ: Histologic changes in human enamel following treatment with acidic adhesive conditioning agents, *Arch Oral Biol* 16:731-738, 1971.

124. Gwinnett AJ: Moist versus dry dentin: its effect on shear bond strength, *Am J Dent* 5:127-129, 1992.

125. Gwinnett AJ: Quantitative contribution of resin infiltration/hybridization to dentin bonding, *Am J Dent* 6:7-9, 1993.

126. Gwinnett AJ, Buonocore MG: Adhesion and caries prevention: a preliminary report, *Br Dent J* 119:77-80, 1965.

127. Gwinnett AJ, García-Godoy F: Effect of etching time and acid concentration on resin shear bond strength to primary tooth enamel, *Am J Dent* 5:237-239, 1992.

128. Gwinnett AJ, Kanca J: Interfacial morphology of resin composite and shiny erosion lesions, *Am J Dent* 5:315-317, 1992.

129. Gwinnett AJ, Kanca J: Micromorphology of the bonded dentin interface and its relationship to bond strength, *Am J Dent* 5:73-77, 1992.

130. Gwinnett AJ, Matsui A: A study of enamel adhesives: the physical relationship between enamel and adhesive, *Arch Oral Biol* 12:1615-1620, 1967.

131. Gwinnett AJ, Tay FR: Early and intermediate time response of the dental pulp to an acid etch technique in vivo, *Am J Dent* 11:S35-S44, 1998.

132. Gwinnett AJ, Yu S: Shear bond strength, microleakage and gap formation with fourth generation dentin bonding agents, *Am J Dent* 7:312-314, 1994.

133. Hadavi F et al: The influence of an adhesive system on shear bond strength of repaired high-copper amalgams, *Oper Dent* 16:175-180, 1991.

134. Hadavi F et al: Tensile bond strength of repaired amalgam, *J Prosthet Dent* 67:313-317, 1992.

135. Hallett KB, García-Godoy F, Trotter AR: Shear bond strength of a resin composite to enamel etched with maleic or phosphoric acid, *Austr Dent J* 39:292-297, 1994.

136. Hals E, Simonsen LT: Histopathology of experimental in vivo caries around silver amalgam fillings, *Caries Res* 6:16-33, 1972

137. Hansen EK: Effect of Scotchbond dependent on cavity cleaning, cavity diameter and cavosurface angle, *Scand J Dent Res* 92:141-147, 1984.

138. Hansen EK, Asmussen E: Comparative study of dentin adhesives, *Scand J Dent Res* 93:280-287, 1985.

139. Harnirattisai C et al: Adhesive interface between resin and etched dentin of cervical erosion/abrasion lesions, *Oper Dent* 18:138-143, 1993.

140. Hasegawa EA, Boyer DB, Chan DL: Hardening of dual-cured cements under composite resin inlays, *J Prosthet Dent* 66:187-192, 1991.

141. Hasegawa T, Retief DH: Laboratory evaluation of experimental restorative systems containing 4-META, *Am J Dent* 7:212-216, 1994.

142. Hasegawa T et al: A laboratory study of the Amalgambond Adhesive System, *Am J Dent* 5:181-186, 1992.

143. Hebling J, Giro EM, Costa CA: Biocompatibility of an adhesive system applied to exposed human dental pulp, *J Endod* 25:676-682, 1999.

144. Hegdahl T, Gjerdet NR: Contraction stresses of composite filling materials, *Acta Odontol Scand* 35:191-195, 1977.

145. Heitman T, Unterbrink G: Direct pulp capping with a dentinal adhesive resin system: a pilot study, *Quintessence Int* 11: 765-770, 1995.

146. Heymann HO et al: Examining tooth flexure effects on cervical restorations: a two-year clinical study, *JADA* 122:41-47, 1991.

147. Heymann HO et al: Twelve-month clinical study of dentinal adhesives in Class V cervical lesions, *JADA* 116:179-183, 1988.

148. Huang GT, Söderholm K-JM: In vitro investigation of shear bond strength of a phosphate based dentinal bonding agent, *Scand J Dent Res* 97:84-92, 1989.

149. Ianzano JA, Mastrodomenico J, Gwinnett AJ: Strength of amalgam restorations bonded with Amalgambond, *Am J Dent* 6:10-12, 1993.

150. Ide M et al: The role of a dentine-bonding agent in reducing cervical dentine sensitivity, *J Clin Periodontol* 25:286-290, 1998.

151. Inaba D et al: The influence of air-drying on hyper-remineralization of demineralized dentin: a study on bulk as well as on thin wet section of bovine dentin, *Caries Res* 29:231-236, 1995.

152. Inai N et al: Adhesion between collagen depleted dentin and dentin adhesive, *Am J Dent* 11:123-127, 1998.

153. Inokoshi S, Iwaku M, Fusayama T: Pulpal response to a new adhesive restorative resin, *J Dent Res* 61:1014-1019, 1982.

154. Ishioka S, Caputo AA: Interaction between the dentinal smear layer and composite bond strengths, *J Prosthet Dent* 61:180-185, 1989.

155. James DF, Yarovesky U: An esthetic inlay technique for posterior teeth, *Quintessence Int* 11:725-731, 1983.

156. Jendresen MD: Clinical performance of a new composite resin for Class V erosion (abstract 1057), *J Dent Res* 57:339, 1978.

157. Jochen DG, Caputo AA: Composite resin repair of porcelain denture teeth, *J Prosthet Dent* 38:673-679, 1997.

158. Jordan RE, Suzuki M, Davidson DF: Clinical evaluation of a universal dentin bonding resin: preserving dentition through new materials, *JADA* 124:71-76, 1993.

159. Kanca J: Dental adhesion and the All-Bond system, *J Esthet Dent* 3:129-132, 1991.

160. Kanca J: The effect of heat on the surface hardness of light-activated composite resins, *Quintessence Int* 20:899-901, 1989.

161. Kanca J: Effect of resin primer solvents and surface wetness on resin composite bond strength to dentin, *Am J Dent* 5: 213-221, 1992.

162. Kanca J: One Step bond strength to enamel and dentin, *Am J Dent* 10:5-8, 1997.

163. Kanca J: Replacement of a fractured incisor fragment over pulpal exposure: a case report, *Quintessence Int* 24:81-84, 1993.

164. Kanca J: Resin bonding to wet substrate: bonding to dentin. I. *Quintessence Int* 23:39-41, 1992.

165. Kanca J: Wet bonding: effect of drying time and distance, *Am J Dent* 9:273-276, 1996.

166. Kanca J, Sandrik J: Bonding to dentin: clues to the mechanism of adhesion, *Am J Dent* 11:154-159, 1998.

167. Kanca J, Suh BI: Pulse activation: reducing resin-based composite contraction stresses at the enamel cavosurface margins, *Am J Dent* 12:107-112, 1999.

168. Kato G, Nakabayashi N: Effect of phosphoric acid concentration on wet-bonding to etched dentin, *Dent Mater* 12: 250-255, 1996.

169. Kemp-Scholte CM, Davidson CL: Complete marginal seal of Class V resin composite restorations effected by increased flexibility, *J Dent Res* 69:1240-1243, 1990.

170. Kemp-Scholte CM, Davidson CL: Marginal integrity related to bond strength and strain capacity of composite resin restorative systems, *J Prosthet Dent* 64:658-664, 1990.

171. Kennington LB et al: Short-term clinical evaluation of postoperative sensitivity with bonded amalgams, *Am J Dent* 11: 177-180, 1998.

172. Kerns DG et al: Dentinal tubule occlusion and root hypersensitivity, *J Periodontol* 62:421-428, 1991.

173. Lacy AM et al: Effect of porcelain surface treatment on the bond to composite, *J Prosthet Dent* 60:288-291, 1988.

174. Lacy AM, Rupprecht R, Watanabe L: Use of self-curing composite resins to facilitate amalgam repair, *Quintessence Int* 23: 53-59, 1992.

175. Latta MA et al: Three-year clinical evaluation of the Clearfil Liner Bond 2 system (abstract 1030), *J Dent Res* 79:272, 2000.

176. Lee HL et al: Effects of acid etchants on dentin. *J Dent Res* 52:1228-1233, 1973.

177. Lopes LMP, Leitão JGM, Douglas WH: Effect of a new resin inlay/onlay restorative material on cuspal reinforcement, *Quintessence Int* 22:641-645, 1991.

178. Maciel KT et al: The effect of acetone, ethanol, HEMA, and air on the stiffness of human decalcified dentin matrix. *J Dent Res* 75:1851-1858, 1996.

179. Macko DJ, Rutberg M, Langeland K: Pulpal response to the application of phosphoric acid to dentin, *Oral Surg* 6:930-946, 1978.

180. Manson-Rahemtulla B, Retief DH, Jamison HC: Effect of concentrations of phosphoric acid on enamel dissolution, *J Prosthet Dent* 51:495-498, 1984.

181. Marchetti C, Piacentini C, Menghini P: Morphometric computerized analysis on the dentinal tubules and the collagen fibers in the dentine of human permanent teeth, *Bull Group Int Rech Sci Stomatol Odontol* 35:125-129, 1992.

182. Mardaga WJ, Shannon IL: Decreasing the depth of etch for direct bonding in orthodontics, *J Clin Orthodont* 16:130-132, 1982.

183. Marshall GW et al: Dentin demineralization: Effects of dentin depth, pH and different acids, *Dent Mater* 13: 338-343, 1997.

184. McCullock AJ, Smith BGN: In vitro studies of cuspal movement produced by adhesive restorative materials, *Br Dent J* 161:405-409, 1986.

185. McLean JW: Bonding to enamel and dentin (letter), *Quintessence Int* 26:334, 1995.

186. McLean JW, Kramer IRH: A clinical and pathological evaluation of a sulphinic acid activated resin for use in restorative dentistry, *Br Dent J* 93:255, 1952.

187. McLean JW, Nicholson JW, Wilson AD: Proposed nomenclature for glass-ionomer dental cements and related materials (guest editorial), *Quintessence Int* 25:587, 1994.

188. Meiers JC, Turner EW: Microleakage of dentin/amalgam alloy bonding agents: results after 1 year, *Oper Dent* 23:30-35, 1998.

189. Mejàre B, Mejàre I, Edwardsson S: Acid etching and composite resin restorations: a culturing and histologic study on bacterial penetration, *Acta Odontol Scand* 3:1-5, 1987.

190. Mejàre I, Mejàre B, Edwardsson S: Effect of a tight seal on survival of bacteria in saliva-contaminated cavities filled with composite resin, *Endod Dent Traumatol* 3:6-9, 1987.

191. Miller BH et al: Bond strengths of various materials to dentin using Amalgambond, *Am J Dent* 5:272-276, 1992.

192. Mitchem JC, Gronas DG: Effects of time after extraction and depth of dentin on resin dentin adhesives, *JADA* 113:285-287, 1986.

193. Miyazaki M et al: Effect of filler content of light-cured composites on bond strength to bovine dentine, *J Dent* 19:301-303, 1991.

194. Mjör IA, Hensten-Pettersen A, Bowen RL: Biological assessments of experimental cavity cleansers: correlation between in vitro and in vivo studies, *J Dent Res* 61:967-972, 1982.

195. Morin D, DeLong R, Douglas WH: Cusp reinforcement by the acid-etch technique, *J Dent Res* 63:1075-1078, 1984.

196. Moritz A et al: Long-term effects of CO₂ laser irradiation on treatment of hypersensitive dental necks: results of an in vivo study, *J Clin Laser Med Surg* 16:211-215, 1998.

197. Morris MF, Davis RD, Richardson BW: Clinical efficacy of two dentin desensitizing agents, *Am J Dent* 12:72-76, 1999.

198. Munksgaard EC: Amine-induced polymerization of aqueous HEMA/aldehyde during action as a dentin bonding agent, *J Dent Res* 69:1236-1239, 1990.

199. Munksgaard EC, Irie M, Asmussen E: Dentin-polymer bond promoted by Gluma and various resins, *J Dent Res* 64:1409-1411, 1985.

200. Murray L, Roberts AJ: The prevalence of self-reported hypersensitive teeth, *Arch Oral Biol* 39:129S-135S, 1994.

201. Nakabayashi N, Kojima K, Masuhara E: The promotion of adhesion by the infiltration of monomers into tooth substrates, *J Biomed Mater Res* 16:265-273, 1982.

202. Nakabayashi N, Nakamura M, Yasuda N: Hybrid layer as a dentin-bonding mechanism, *J Esthet Dent* 3:133-138, 1991.

203. Nakajima M et al: Tensile bond strength and SEM evaluation of caries-affected dentin using dentin adhesives, *J Dent Res* 74:1679-1688, 1995.

204. Newburg R, Pameijer CH: Composite resin bonded to porcelain with a silane solution, *JADA* 96:288-291, 1978.

205. Nikaido T et al: Effect of pulpal pressure on adhesion of resin composite to dentin: bovine serum versus saline, *Quintessence Int* 26:221-226, 1995.

206. Nordenvall K-J, Brännström M, Malmgren O: Etching of deciduous teeth and young and old permanent teeth: a comparison between 15 and 60 seconds of etching, *Am J Orthodont* 78:99-108, 1980.

207. Øilo G: Bond strength testing: what does it mean? *Int Dent J* 43:492-498, 1993.

208. Oliveira JP, Cochran MA, Moore BK: Influence of bonded amalgam restorations on the fracture strength of teeth, *Oper Dent* 21:110-115, 1996.

209. Olmez A, Cula S, Ulusu T: Clinical evaluation and marginal leakage of Amalgambond Plus: three-year results, *Quintessence Int* 28:651-656, 1997.

210. Opdam NJ et al: Marginal integrity and postoperative sensitivity in Class 2 resin composite restorations in vivo, *J Dent* 26:555-562, 1998.

211. Osborne JW, Summit JB: Mechanical properties and clinical performance of a gallium restorative material, *Oper Dent* 20:241-245, 1995.

212. Oysaed H, Ruyter IE: Water sorption and filler characteristics of composites for use in posterior teeth, *J Dent Res* 65:1315-1318, 1986.

213. Packham DE: *Adhesion*. In Packham DE, editor: *Handbook of adhesion*, Essex, 1992 Longman Scientific & Technical.

214. Pameijer CH, Louw NP: Significance of pulpal pressure during clinical bonding procedures, *Am J Dent* 10:214-218, 1997.

215. Pameijer CH, Stanley HR: The disastrous effects of the "total etch" technique in vital pulp capping in primates, *Am J Dent* 11:S45-S54, 1998.

216. Panighi M, G'Sell C: Influence of calcium concentration on the dentin wettability by an adhesive, *J Biomed Mater Res* 26:1081-1089, 1992.

217. Pashley DH: Dentin bonding: overview of the substrate with respect to adhesive material, *J Esthet Dent* 3:46-50, 1991.

218. Pashley DH: Dentin: a dynamic substrate—a review, *Scanning Microsc* 3:161-176, 1989.

219. Pashley DH: The effects of acid etching on the pulpodentin complex, *Oper Dent* 17:229-242, 1992.

220. Pashley DH: The influence of dentin permeability and pulpal blood flow on pulpal solute concentrations, *J Endod* 5:355-361, 1979.

221. Pashley DH, Depew DD, Galloway SE: Microleakage channels: scanning electron microscopic observation, *Oper Dent* 14:68-72, 1989.

222. Pashley DH et al: Fluid shifts across human dentine in vitro in response to hydrodynamic stimuli. *Arch Oral Biol* 41:1065-1072, 1996.

223. Pashley DH et al: The microtensile test: A review, *J Adhes Dent* 1:299-309, 1999.

224. Pashley DH et al: Permeability of dentin to adhesive agents, *Quintessence Int* 24:618-631, 1993.

225. Pashley DH, Horner JA, Brewer PD: Interactions of conditioners on the dentin surface, *Oper Dent* 5(suppl):137-150, 1992.

226. Pashley DH, Livingstone MJ, Greenhill JD: Regional resistances to fluid flow in human dentine in vitro, *Arch Oral Biol* 23:807-810, 1978.

227. Pashley EL et al: Amalgam buildups: Shear bond strength and dentin sealing properties, *Oper Dent* 16:82-89, 1991.

228. Paul SJ, Welter DA, Ghazi M, Pashley D: Nanoleakage at the dentin adhesive interface vs microtensile bond strength, *Oper Dent* 24:181-188, 1999.

229. Perdigão J: An ultra-morphological study of human dentine exposed to adhesive systems (doctoral thesis, ISBN 90-801303-4-6), Katholieke Universiteit te Leuven. Leuven, 1995, Van der Poorten.

230. Perdigão J, Baratieri LN, Lopes M: Laboratory evaluation and clinical application of a new one-bottle adhesive, *J Esthet Dent* 11:23-35, 1999.

231. Perdigão J et al: The effect of a re-wetting agent on dentin bonding, *Dent Mater* 15:282-295, 1999.

232. Perdigão J et al: Effects of a self-etching primer on enamel shear bond strengths and SEM morphology, *Am J Dent* 10:141-146, 1997.

233. Perdigão J et al: In vitro bond strengths and SEM evaluation of dentin bonding systems to different dentin substrates, *J Dent Res* 73:44-55, 1994.

234. Perdigão J et al: The interaction of adhesive systems with dentin, *Am J Dent* 9:167-173, 1996.

235. Perdigão J et al: A morphological field emission SEM study of the effect of six phosphoric acid etching agents on human dentin, *Dent Mater* 12:262-271, 1996.

236. Perdigão J, Lopes M: Dentin bonding: questions for the new millennium, *J Adhes Dent* 1:191-209, 1999.

237. Perdigão J, Ramos JC, Lambrechts P: In vitro interfacial relationship between human dentin and one-bottle dental adhesives, *Dent Mater* 13:218-227, 1997.

238. Perdigão J, Swift EJ: Adhesion of a total-etch phosphate ester bonding agent, *Am J Dent* 7:149-152, 1994.

239. Perdigão J, Swift EJ: Analysis of dental adhesive systems using scanning electron microscopy, *Int Dent J* 44:349-359, 1994.

240. Perdigão J, Swift EJ, Cloe BC: Effects of etchants, surface moisture, and resin composite on dentin bond strengths, *Am J Dent* 6:61-64, 1993.

241. Perinka L, Sano H, Hosoda H: Dentin thickness, hardness and Ca-concentration vs bond strength of dentin adhesives, *Dent Mater* 8:229-233, 1992.

242. Peutzfeldt A: Dual-cure resin cements: in vitro wear and effect of quantity of remaining double-bonds, filler volume and light-curing, *Acta Odontol Scand* 53:29-34, 1995.

243. Phrukkanon S, Burrow MF, Tyas MJ: The influence of cross-sectional shape and surface area on the microtensile bond test, *Dent Mater* 14:212-221, 1998.

244. Pilo R, Brosh T, Chweidan H: Cusp reinforcement by bonding of amalgam restorations, *J Dent* 26:467-472, 1998.

245. Pimenta LA et al: Inhibition of demineralization in vitro around amalgam restorations, *Quintessence Int* 29:363-367, 1998.

246. Pintado MR, Douglas WH: The comparison of microleakage between two different dentin bonding resin systems, *Quintessence Int* 19:905-907, 1988.

247. Quarnstrom F et al: A randomized clinical trial of agents to reduce sensitivity after crown cementation, *Gen Dent* 46:68-74, 1988.

248. Qvist V, Stoltze K, Qvist J: Human pulp reactions to resin restorations performed with different acid-etched restorative procedures, *Acta Odontol Scand* 47:253-263, 1989.

249. Ramos JC, Perdigão J: Shear bond strengths and SEM morphology of dentin-amalgam adhesives, *Am J Dent* 10:152-158, 1997.

250. Ramos JC et al: Effect of supplemental polymerization on the bond strengths of adhesive amalgam restorations (abstract 373), *J Dent Res* 77:678, 1998.

251. Reeder OW et al: Dentin permeability: determinants of hydraulic conductance, *J Dent Res* 57:187-193, 1978.

252. Reifeis PE, Cochran MA, Moore BK: An in vitro shear bond strength study of enamel/dentin bonding systems on enamel, *Oper Dent* 20:174-179, 1995.

253. Reinhardt JW, Krell KV: Effect of desensitizers and bonding agents on radicular dentin permeability (abstract 1332), *J Dent Res* 76:180, 1997.

254. Reinhardt JW, Stephens NH, Fortin D: Effect of Gluma desensitization on dentin bond strength, *Am J Dent* 8:170-172, 1995.

255. Retief DH, Austin JC, Fatti LP: Pulpal response to phosphoric acid, *J Oral Pathol* 3:114-122, 1974.

256. Retief DH, Denys FR: Adhesion to enamel and dentin, *Am J Dent* 2:133-144, 1989.

257. Roeder LB, DeSchepper EJ, Powers JM: In vitro bond strength of repaired amalgam with adhesive bonding systems, *J Esthet Dent* 3:126-128, 1991.

258. Romney RL, Dickens SH: Bonding to dry dentin with water-modified acetone-based primers (abstract 1948), *J Dent Res* 76:257, 1997.

259. Rosa BT, Perdigão J: Bond strengths of nonrinsing adhesives, *Quintessence Int* 31:353-358, 2000.

260. Rosenblatt J, Devereux B, Wallace DG: Injectable collagen as a pH-sensitive hydrogel, *Biomaterials* 15:985-995, 1994.

261. Royse MC, Ott NW, Mathieu G: Dentin adhesive superior to copal varnish in preventing microleakage in primary teeth, *Pediatr Dent* 18:440-443, 1996.

262. Rueggeberg FA: Substrate for adhesion testing to tooth structure: review of the literature, *Dent Mater* 7:2-10, 1991.

263. Ruyter IE: The chemistry of adhesive agents, *Oper Dent* 5(suppl):32-43, 1992.

264. Sano H et al: Long-term durability of dentin bonds made with a self-etching primer in vivo, *J Dent Res* 78:906-911, 1999.

265. Sano H et al: Microporous dentin zone beneath resin-impregnated layer, *Oper Dent* 19:59-64, 1994.

266. Sano H et al: Nanoleakage: Leakage within the hybrid layer, *Oper Dent* 20:18-25, 1995.

267. Sano H et al: Relationship between surface area for adhesion and tensile bond strength: evaluation of a micro-tensile bond test, *Dent Mater* 10:236-240, 1994.

268. Sano H et al: Tensile properties of resin-infiltrated demineralized human dentin, *J Dent Res* 74:1093-1102, 1995.

269. Sasaki N, Odajima S: Stress-strain curve and Young's modulus of a collagen molecule as determined by the x-ray diffraction technique, *J Biomechanics* 29:655-658, 1996.

270. Sasaki N et al: X-ray diffraction studies on the structure of hydrated collagen, *Biopolymers* 22:2539-2547, 1983.

271. Saunders WP, Strang R, Ahmad I: Shear bond strength of Mirage Bond to enamel and dentin, *Am J Dent* 4:265-267, 1991.

272. Scherman A, Jacobsen PL: Managing dentin hypersensitivity: what treatment to recommend to patients, *JADA* 123:57-61, 1992.

273. Schüpbach P, Lutz F, Finger WJ: Closing of dentinal tubules by Gluma desensitizer, *Eur J Oral Sci* 105:414-421, 1997.

274. Schwartz RS, Conn LJ Jr, Haveman CW: Clinical evaluation of two desensitizing agents for use under Class 5 silver amalgam restorations, *J Prosthet Dent* 80:269-273, 1998.

275. Selvig KA: Ultrastructural changes in human dentine exposed to a weak acid, *Arch Oral Biol* 13:719-734, 1968.

276. Sepetcioglu F, Ataman BA: Long-term monitoring of microleakage of cavity varnish and adhesive resin with amalgam, *J Prosthet Dent* 79:136-139, 1998.

277. Shaffer SE, Barkmeier WW, Kelsey WP: Effects of reduced acid conditioning time on enamel microleakage, *Gen Dent* 35:278-280, 1987.

278. Sheth J, Jensen M, Tolliver D: Effect of surface treatment on etched porcelain and bond strength to enamel, *Dent Mater* 4:328-337, 1998.

279. Shono Y et al: Regional measurement of resin-dentin bonding as an array, *J Dent Res* 78:699-705, 1998.

280. Sidhu SK: The effect of acid-etched dentin on marginal seal, *Quintessence Int* 25:797-800, 1994.

281. Silverstone LM: Fissure sealants: laboratory studies, *Caries Res* 8:2-26, 1974.

282. Silverstone LM et al: Variation in the pattern of acid etching of human dental enamel examined by scanning electron microscopy, *Caries Res* 9:373-387, 1975.

283. Simonsen RJ, Calamia JR: Tensile bond strength of etched porcelain (abstract 1154), *J Dent Res* 62:297, 1983.

284. Simpson MD et al: Effects of aluminum oxalate/glycine pretretament solutions on dentin permeability, *Am J Dent* 5: 324-328, 1992.

285. Snuggs HM et al: Pulpal healing and dentinal bridge formation in an acidic environment, *Quintessence Int* 24:501-509, 1993.

286. Söderholm K-JM: Correlation of in vivo and in vitro performance of adhesive restorative materials: a report of the ASC MD156 Task Group on test methods for the adhesion of restorative materials, *Dent Mater* 7:74-83, 1991.

287. Soetopo, Beech DR, Hardwick JL: Mechanism of adhesion of polymers to acid-etched enamel: effect of acid concentration and washing on bond strength, *J Oral Rehabil* 5:69-80, 1978.

288. Souza Costa CA, Hebling J, Hanks CT: Current status of pulp capping with dentin adhesive systems: a review, *Dent Mater* 16:188-197, 2000.

289. Stangel I, Nathanson D, Hsu CS: Shear bond strength of the composite bond to etched porcelain, *J Dent Res* 66:1460-1465, 1987.

290. Staninec M: Retention of amalgam restorations: undercuts versus bonding, *Quintessence Int* 20:347-351, 1989.

291. Staninec M, Kawakami M: Adhesion and microleakage tests of a new dentin bonding system, *Dent Mater* 9:204-208. 1993.

292. Stanley HR, Going RE, Chauncey HH: Human pulp response to acid pretreatment of dentin and to composite restoration, *JADA* 91:817-825, 1975.

293. Stephen KW et al: Retention of a filled fissure sealant using reduced etch time, *Br Dent J* 153:232-233, 1982.

294. Sudsangiam S, van Noort R: Do dentin bond strength tests serve a useful purpose? *J Adhes Dent* 1:57-67, 1999.

295. Suliman AA, Swift EJ, Perdigão J: Effects of surface treatment and bonding agents on bond strength of composite to porcelain, *J Prosthet Dent* 70:118-120, 1993.

296. Suzuki T, Finger WJ: Dentin adhesives: site of dentin vs. bonding of composite resins, *Dent Mater* 4:379-383, 1988.

297. Swift EJ, Bayne SC: Shear bond strength of a new one-bottle dentin adhesive, *Am J Dent* 10:184-188, 1997.

298. Swift EJ, Cloe BC: Shear bond strengths of new enamel etchants, *Am J Dent* 6:162-164, 1993.

299. Swift EJ et al: Prevention of root surface caries using a dental adhesive, *JADA* 125:571-576, 1994.

300. Swift EJ, LeValley BD, Boyer DB: Evaluation of new methods for composite repair, *Dent Mater* 8:362-365, 1992.

301. Swift EJ, Lloyd AH, Felton DA: The effect of resin desensitizing agents on crown retention, *J Am Dent Assoc* 128:195-200, 1997.

302. Swift EJ, Perdigão J, Heymann HO: Bonding to enamel and dentin: a brief history and state of the art, 1995, *Quintessence Int* 26:95-110, 1995.

303. Swift EJ, Perdigão J, Heymann HO: Enamel bond strengths of "one-bottle" adhesives, *Pediatr Dent* 20:259-262, 1998.

304. Swift EJ, Triolo PT: Bond strengths of Scotchbond Multi-Purpose to moist dentin and enamel, *Am J Dent* 5:318-320, 1992.

305. Tam LE, Pilliar RM: Fracture surface characterization of dentin-bonded interfacial fracture toughness specimens, *J Dent Res* 73:607-619, 1994.

306. Tao L, Tagami J, Pashley DH: Pulpal pressure and bond strengths of Superbond and Gluma, *Am J Dent* 4:73-76, 1991.

307. Tarim B et al: Marginal integrity of bonded amalgam restorations, *Am J Dent* 9:72-76, 1996.

308. Tatsumi T et al: Remineralization of etched dentin, *J Prosthet Dent* 67:617-620, 1992.

309. Tay FR et al: Resin permeation into acid-conditioned, moist, and dry dentin: a paradigm using water-free adhesive primers, *J Dent Res* 75:1034-1044, 1996.

310. Tay FR, Gwinnett AJ, Wei SHY: Micromorphological spectrum from overdrying to overwetting acid-conditioned dentin in water-free, acetone-based, single-bottle primer/adhesives, *Dent Mater* 12:236-244, 1996.

311. Tay FR, Gwinnett AJ, Wei SHY: Ultrastructure of the resin-dentin interface following reversible and irreversible rewetting, *Am J Dent* 10:77-82, 1997.

312. Terkla LG et al: Testing sealing properties of restorative materials against moist dentin, *J Dent Res* 66:1758-1764, 1987.

313. Torney D: The retentive ability of acid-etched dentin, *J Prosthet Dent* 39:169-172, 1978.

314. Torstenson B, Hordenvall KJ, Brännström M: Pulpal reaction and microorganisms under Clearfil Composite Resin in deep cavities with acid etched dentin, *Swed Dent J* 6:167-176, 1982.

315. Touyz LZ, Stern J: Hypersensitive dentinal pain attenuation with potassium nitrate, *Gen Dent* 47:42-45, 1999.

316. Triana R et al: Dentin bond strength of fluoride-releasing materials, *Am J Dent* 7:252-254, 1994.

317. Triolo PT et al: Effect of etching time on enamel bond strengths, *Am J Dent* 6:302-304, 1993.

318. Tsuneda Y et al: A histopathological study of direct pulp capping with adhesive resins, *Oper Dent* 20:223-229, 1995.

319. Turner EW, St Germain HA, Meiers JC: Microleakage of dentin-amalgam bonding agents, *Am J Dent* 8:191-196, 1995.

320. Tyas MJ, Chandler JE: One-year clinical evaluation of three dentine bonding agents, *Austr Dent J* 38:294-298, 1993.

321. Tyas MJ et al: Clinical evaluation of Scotchbond: three-year results, *Austr Dent J* 34:277-279, 1989.

322. Uno S, Finger WJ: Effects of acidic conditioners on dentine demineralization and dimension of hybrid layers, *J Dent* 24: 211-216, 1996.

323. van der Graaf ER, ten Bosch JJ: Changes in dimension and weight of human dentine after different drying procedures and during subsequent rehydration, *Arch Oral Biol* 38:97-99, 1993.

324. van der Vyver PJ, de Wet FA, Jansen van Rensburg JM: Bonding of composite resin using different enamel etchants, *J Dent Assoc South Africa* 52:169-172, 1997.

325. van Dijken JWV: Clinical evaluation of three adhesive systems in class V non-carious lesions, *Dent Mater* 16:285-291, 2000.

326. van Dijken JWV, Horstedt P: In vivo adaptation of restorative materials to dentin, *J Prosthet Dent* 56:677-681, 1986.

327. van Hassel HJ: Physiology of the human dental pulp, *Oral Surg Oral Med Oral Pathol* 32:126-134, 1971.

328. van Meerbeek B et al: The clinical performance of dentin adhesives, *J Dent* 26:1-20, 1998.

329. van Meerbeek B et al: Clinical status of ten adhesive systems, *J Dent Res* 73:1690-1702, 1994.

330. van Meerbeek B et al: Morphological aspects of the resin-dentin interdiffusion zone with different dentin adhesive systems, *J Dent Res* 71:1530-1540, 1992.

331. van Meerbeek B et al: Morphological characterization of the interface between resin and sclerotic dentine, *J Dent* 22:141-146, 1994.

332. van Meerbeek B et al: A TEM study of two water-based adhesive systems bonded to dry and wet dentin, *J Dent Res* 77: 50-59, 1998.

333. van Meerbeek B et al: Three-year clinical effectiveness of four total-etch dentinal adhesive systems in cervical lesions, *Quintessence Int* 27:775-784, 1996.

334. Versluis A, Tantbirojn D, Douglas WH: Why do shear bond tests pull out dentin? *J Dent Res* 76:1298-1307, 1997.

335. Wang J-D, Hume WR: Diffusion of hydrogen ion and hydroxyl ion from various sources through dentine, *Int Endod J* 21:17-26, 1988.

336. Warfvinge J, Dahlen G, Bergenholtz G: Dental pulp response to bacterial cell wall material, *J Dent Res* 64:1046-1050, 1985.

337. Watanabe F, Powers JM, Lorey RE: In vitro bonding of prosthodontic adhesives to dental alloys, *J Dent Res* 67:479-783, 1988.

338. Watanabe I, Nakabayashi N, Pashley DH: Bonding to ground dentin by a Phenyl-P self-etching primer, *J Dent Res* 73:1212-1220, 1994.

339. Watanabe T et al: The effects of primers on the sensitivity of dentin, *Dent Mater* 7:148-150, 1991.

340. Wendt SL: The effect of heat used as a secondary cure upon the physical properties of three composite resins: diametral tensile strength, compressive strength and marginal dimention stability. I. *Quintessence Int* 18:265-271, 1987.

341. Wendt SL: The effect of heat used as a secondary cure upon the physical properties of three composite resins: wear, hardness, and color stability. II. *Quintessence Int* 18:351-356, 1987.

342. West N, Addy M, Hughes J: Dentine hypersensitivity: the effects of brushing desensitizing toothpastes, their solid and liquid phases, and detergents on dentine and acrylic: studies in vitro, *J Oral Rehabil* 25:885-895, 1998.

343. White KS et al: Pulp response to adhesive resin systems applied to acid-etched vital dentin: damp versus dry primer application, *Quintessence Int* 25:259-268, 1994.

344. Wolinsky LE, Armstrong RW, Seghi RR: The determination of ionic bonding interactions of N-Phenyl Glycine and N-(2-hydroxy-3-methacryloxypropyl)-N-Phenyl Glycine as measured by Carbon-13 NMR analysis, *J Dent Res* 72:72-77, 1993.

345. Yanagawa T, Finger WJ: Relationship between degree of polymerization of resin composite and bond strength of Gluma-treated dentin, *Am J Dent* 7:157-160, 1994.

346. Yates R et al: The effects of a potassium citrate, cetylpyridinium chloride, sodium fluoride mouthrinse on dentine hypersensitivity, plaque and gingivitis: a placebo-controlled study, *J Clin Periodontol* 25:813-820, 1998.

347. Yoshiyama M et al: Regional bond strengths of resins to human root dentine, *J Dent* 24:435-442, 1996.

348. Yoshiyama M et al: Regional strengths of bonding agents to cervical sclerotic root dentin, *J Dent Res* 75:1404-1413, 1996.

349. Zhang C et al: Effects of CO_2 laser in treatment of cervical dentinal hypersensitivity, *J Endod* 24:595-597, 1998.

Fundamentals in Tooth Preparation

THEODORE M. ROBERSON

CLIFFORD M. STURDEVANT*

*This author is inactive this edition. See the Acknowledgments.

The discipline of operative dentistry harbors the essential knowledge of basic tooth restoration, which is of utmost importance to the dental student and dental practitioner. This basic knowledge must not be construed as simply treating a tooth, but rather in the context of treating a person. The physiologic and psychologic aspects of the patient must be given proper consideration. In the sense of local treatment, biologic and mechanical factors regarding care of tooth tissues and contiguous oral tissues are paramount. Procedural organization for tooth preparation is emphasized in this chapter. Nomenclature associated with tooth preparation, including the historical classification of carious lesions (*cavities*), also is presented.

In the past, most restorative treatment was due to caries (*decay*), and the term *cavity* was used to describe a carious lesion in a tooth that had progressed to the point that part of the tooth structure had been destroyed. Thus the tooth was cavitated (a breach in the surface integrity of the tooth) and was referred to as a *cavity*. Likewise, when the affected tooth was repaired, the cutting or preparation of the remaining tooth structure (to best receive a restorative material) was referred to as a *cavity preparation*.

Now many indications for treatment for teeth are not due to caries and, therefore, the preparation of the tooth is no longer referred to as *cavity preparation* but as *tooth preparation*, and the term *cavity* is used only as a historical reference.

DEFINITION OF TOOTH PREPARATION

Tooth preparation is defined as the mechanical alteration of a defective, injured, or diseased tooth to best receive a restorative material that will reestablish a healthy state for the tooth, including esthetic corrections where indicated, along with normal form and function. Included in the procedure of preparing the tooth is the removal of all defective or friable tooth structure because remaining infected or friable tooth structure may result in further caries progression, sensitivity or pain, or fracture of the tooth and/or restoration. This textbook covers such preparations, with the exception of preparation for either a three-quarter crown or full crown.

NEED FOR RESTORATIONS

Teeth need restorative intervention for various reasons. Foremost is the need to repair a tooth after destruction from a *carious lesion*. A large, extensive restoration may be required in treating a large carious lesion, or a smaller, more conservative restoration may restore the tooth to proper form and function when the lesion is small. Another common need is the *replacement or repair* of restorations with serious defects, such as improper proximal contact, gingival excess, defective open margins, or poor esthetics. Restorations also are indicated to restore proper form and function to *fractured teeth*. Such teeth present with minor to major tooth structure missing or with an incomplete fracture ("greenstick fracture"), resulting in a tooth that has compromised function and, many times, pain or sensitivity. A tooth may require a restoration to simply *restore form or function* absent as a result of congenital malformation. A careful assessment of other diagnostic factors must be undertaken before restoration of such teeth to avoid unnecessary restorative intervention. With an increasing number of older persons who are retaining their natural teeth, the prevalence of incomplete tooth fracture is expected to increase. The proper restoration of such fractured teeth requires early diagnosis and knowledgeable, skillful treatment.

As previously mentioned, an *esthetic* desire of a patient may be a reason for placing (and replacing) restorations. An increasing percentage of practitioners' operative treatments are solely as a result of patient desires to improve appearance (see Chapter 15). These may or may not involve complex tooth preparations. Restorations also are required for teeth simply as part of fulfilling *other restorative needs*. For example, when replacing a missing tooth with a fixed or removable partial denture, the teeth adjacent to the space usually require some type of restorative procedure to allow for adequate placement and/or function of the prosthesis. Lastly, a tooth may be restored in a preventive sense. Because caries is an infectious disease, the removal of the caries during the restoration of a tooth reduces the microorganisms involved in the disease and thereby may reduce the potential spread. However, it should be completely understood that *restorative intervention primarily repairs damage caused by caries and by itself does not rid the patient of the factors that caused the disease initially*. To accomplish an effective preventive program that places the patient into a low-risk status for developing future caries or periodontal disease, a complete assessment must be made of (1) the type and number of microorganisms present; (2) the patient's homecare ability, effectiveness, and motivation; (3) the need for antimicrobial therapy; and (4) dietary factors.

OBJECTIVES OF TOOTH PREPARATION

In general terms, the objectives of tooth preparation are to: (1) remove all defects and provide necessary protection to the pulp, (2) extend the restoration as conservatively as possible, (3) form the tooth preparation so that under the force of mastication the tooth or the restoration or both will not fracture and the restoration will not be displaced, and (4) allow for the esthetic and functional placement of a restorative material.

Much of the scientific foundation on which these objectives are executed was presented by Black.[4] For many years the Black tooth preparations, with few modifications, formed the basis for most operative preparation procedures. Modifications of Black's principles of tooth preparation have resulted from the influence of Bronner,[6] Ireland,[20] Markley,[25] R. Sturdevant,[43] Sockwell,[37] and

C. Sturdevant,[41] as well as from improvements in restorative materials, instruments, and techniques, and the increased knowledge and application of preventive measures for caries and periodontal disease.

In the past, most tooth preparations were very precise procedures, usually resulting in uniform depths, particular wall forms, and specific marginal configurations. Such precise preparations are still required for amalgam and cast metal restorations. However, because of the use of adhesive restorations, primarily composites, the degree of precision of tooth preparations has decreased. Many composite restorations may require only the removal of the defect (caries or defective restorative material) and friable tooth structure for tooth preparation, without specific uniform depths, wall designs, or marginal forms. This simplification of the tooth preparation process is due to the physical properties of the composite material and the strong bond obtained between the composite and tooth structure.

STAGES AND STEPS OF TOOTH PREPARATION

The preparation procedure is divided into two stages (initial and final), primarily to allow assessment of the beginning operator's knowledge and ability. While the separation into stages may facilitate better adherence to preparation principles and pulpal protection for all operators, it is particularly beneficial in an academic setting. Having student operators complete initial preparation before extensive caries excavation allows the attending faculty member to better assess the student's knowledge of, and ability to perform, proper preparation extensions. Each stage has several steps that are discussed comprehensively later in this chapter. It is important to realize that the stages do exist for specific reasons. The first stage of tooth preparation is referred to as the initial tooth preparation stage. In this stage, the mechanical alterations of the tooth are extended to sound tooth structure (sound dentin or enamel supported by noncarious dentin) in all directions (facially, lingually, gingivally, incisally or occlusally, mesially, and distally) while adhering to a specific, limited pulpal or axial depth (Fig. 6-1). In this way, the final dimensions of the restoration can be anticipated (minus any necessary bevels). The preparation walls are designed in the initial stage of tooth preparation to both retain the restorative material in the tooth and resist potential fracture of the tooth or restoration from masticatory forces delivered principally in the long axis of the tooth. Additional features for retaining the restorative material and protect-

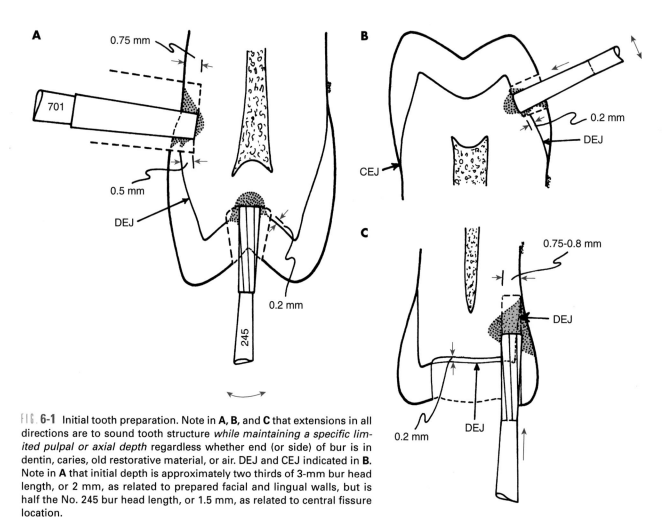

FIG. 6-1 Initial tooth preparation. Note in **A, B,** and **C** that extensions in all directions are to sound tooth structure *while maintaining a specific limited pulpal or axial depth* regardless whether end (or side) of bur is in dentin, caries, old restorative material, or air. DEJ and CEJ indicated in **B.** Note in **A** that initial depth is approximately two thirds of 3-mm bur head length, or 2 mm, as related to prepared facial and lingual walls, but is half the No. 245 bur head length, or 1.5 mm, as related to central fissure location.

ing against fracture may be deemed necessary as part of the final stage of tooth preparation. Guidelines for appropriate extensions during initial tooth preparation are discussed in detail later.

Final tooth preparation, the second stage of tooth preparation, is the completion of the tooth preparation. It includes excavating any remaining, infected carious dentin; removing old restorative material if indicated; protecting the pulp; incorporating additional preparation design features that both minimize the chance of tooth or restoration fracture against oblique forces and maximize the retention of the material in the tooth; finishing preparation walls, particularly regarding the margins; and performing the final procedures of cleaning, inspecting, and, sometimes, sealing the preparation before placement of the restorative material. (Bonded restorations seal the prepared tooth during the bonding process.) Specific final tooth preparation steps and features that relate to completing the preparation procedure are discussed in subsequent sections. (Treatment of the preparation walls for adhesive bonding of restorative materials is considered the first procedure in the insertion of the restoration.)

FACTORS AFFECTING TOOTH PREPARATION

Preparing a tooth to receive a restorative material is a comprehensive endeavor. As routine or mundane as it may seem, many factors affect the appropriate tooth preparation design for a given tooth. These factors must be considered for each restorative procedure contemplated, the end result being that no two preparations are the same. This section presents many of the factors that must be considered before any mechanical alteration of a tooth.

GENERAL FACTORS

Diagnosis. Before any restorative procedure, a complete and thorough diagnosis must be made. There must be a reason to place a restoration in the tooth. The reasons, as presented earlier, may include caries, fractured teeth, esthetic needs, or needs for improved form or function. A careful examination as described in Chapter 9 must be made to determine a diagnosis and subsequent treatment recommendation. An assessment of both pulpal and periodontal status will influence the potential treatment of the tooth, especially in terms of the choice of restorative material as well as the design of the tooth preparation.

Likewise, an assessment of the *occlusal relationships* must be made. Such knowledge often affects the design of the tooth preparation and the choice of material. The patient's concern for *esthetics* should be considered when planning the restorative procedure and will influence the restorative material selected. Esthetic considerations will also influence the tooth preparation by altering, in some situations, the extension or design.

The relationship of a specific restorative procedure with *other treatment* planned for the patient must be considered. For example, if the tooth is an abutment for a fixed or removable partial denture, the design of the restoration may need to be altered to accommodate maximum effectiveness of that prosthesis.

Lastly, the *risk potential* of the patient to further dental disease should be assessed. If appropriate, diagnostic tests should be performed to determine the risk the patient has for further dental caries. A high-risk patient may require altered treatment planning initially, until the risk factors are better controlled. This may mean that caries control procedures should be instituted, followed by more definitive treatment once the patient's homecare, dietary habits, and microbiologic assays are improved. Also, more conservative, less expensive restorative procedures may be planned initially until caries factors are controlled.

Knowledge of Dental Anatomy. Proper tooth preparation is accomplished through systematic procedures based on definite physical and mechanical principles. A prerequisite for understanding tooth preparation is knowledge of the anatomy of each tooth and its related parts. A gross picture, both internal and external, of the individual tooth being operated on must be visualized. The direction of the enamel rods, the thickness of the enamel and dentin, the size and position of the pulp, the relationship of the tooth to supporting tissues, and other factors must all be known to facilitate accurate judgment in tooth preparation.

Patient Factors. Patient factors must play an important role in determining the appropriate restorative treatment rendered. *The patient's knowledge and appreciation of good dental health* influence his or her desire for restorative care and may influence his or her choice of restorative materials. Certainly the patient's *economic status* is a factor in selecting the type of restorative care selected, and the patient's input in this regard must be obtained. Too often dentists predetermine what they believe is the patient's best economic alternatives and realize later that their assessment was incorrect and that other, more suitable, treatment alternatives should have been pursued.

The patient's *age* may be a factor in determining the restorative material and, consequently, the tooth preparation to be used. With increasing numbers of older adults in the population, their treatment may pose restorative considerations. Older adults who have physical or medical complications may require special positioning for restorative treatment as well as shorter, less stressful appointments. Such considerations may influence the type of procedure planned. Because many older adults will have new or replacement restorative needs that are completely or partially on the root surfaces, the treatment of many of these areas will be more complex. The prevalence of root-surface restorative needs is increasing significantly. Whether or not *adequate isolation of the operating site* can be obtained may affect the restorative material selection.

CONSERVATION OF TOOTH STRUCTURE

While one of the primary objectives of operative dentistry is to repair the damage from dental caries, the preservation of the vitality of the tooth is paramount. Although pulp tolerance to insult is usually favorable, the pulp should not be subjected to unnecessary abuse by the application of poor or careless operative procedures on the tooth. The less tooth structure removed, the less potential damage that may occur to the pulp.

Every effort should be made to make restorations as small as possible. The smaller the tooth preparation, the easier it is to retain the restorative material in the tooth. Small tooth preparations result in restorations that have less effect on both intraarch and interarch relationships, as well as esthetics. Naturally, the smaller the tooth preparation, the stronger is the remaining unprepared tooth structure.

Examples of conservative tooth preparation features are discussed later in this chapter as well as in the technique chapters of this textbook. Included in those features are concepts relating to: (1) *minimal extensions* of the tooth preparations, especially faciolingually and pulpally; (2) *supragingival margins;* and (3) *rounded internal line angles.*

RESTORATIVE MATERIAL FACTORS

The choice of restorative material affects the tooth preparation and is made by considering many factors. The patient's input into the decision is important. Economic and esthetic values are primary patient decisions. The ability to isolate the operating area and the extensiveness of the problem are factors that the operator must consider in recommending a material or material options to a patient.

An amalgam restoration requires a specific tooth preparation form that ensures: (1) retention of the material within the tooth and (2) strength of material in terms of thickness and marginal form. An indirect cast metal restoration also requires a specific tooth preparation form that provides: (1) draw or draft to provide seating of the rigid restoration, (2) a beveled cavosurface configuration to provide better fit, and (3) retention of the casting by virtue of prepared wall angles and heights.

As already stated, adhesive composite restorations do not typically require tooth preparations as precise as those for amalgam and cast metal restorations. Composite does not have low edge strength (as amalgam) and micromechanically "bonds" to the tooth structure. These features allow a reduction in the complexity of the tooth preparation. Other adhesive restorations may require more precise tooth preparations. Ceramic inlay restorations do require specific preparation depths and wall designs but do not require complex cavosurface marginal configurations. Adhesive amalgams still re-

quire the same tooth preparation as for nonadhesive amalgam restorations. Thus the type of tooth preparation is determined by the restorative material used.

NOMENCLATURE

Nomenclature refers to a set of terms used in communication by persons in the same profession that enables them to better understand one another. The prudent student will master these terms early in the study of dentistry, since their comprehension will aid in diagnosing and treating disease and defects of the teeth.

CARIES TERMINOLOGY

As stated in Chapter 3, dental caries is an infectious microbiologic disease that results in localized dissolution and destruction of the calcified tissues of the teeth. Moreover, caries is episodic with alternating phases of demineralization and remineralization, and these processes may be occurring simultaneously in the same lesion.

Location of Caries. Caries can be described according to location, extent, and rate.[16]

Primary Caries. Primary caries is the original carious lesion of the tooth. The etiology, morphology, control, and prevention of caries are presented in Chapter 3. Associated with certain areas of the teeth, variations of this pathologic condition fundamentally influence tooth preparation and therefore should be emphasized. Accordingly, three *morphologic types of primary caries* are evident in clinical observation, namely, carious lesions originating: (1) in enamel pits and fissures, (2) on enamel smooth surfaces, or (3) on root surfaces. Also described in the following sections are backward caries, forward caries, and residual caries. Of these, the terms *backward caries* and *forward caries* are rarely used.

Caries of Pit-and-Fissure Origin. Pit-and-fissure caries can form in the regions of pits and fissures usually resulting from the imperfect coalescence of the developmental enamel lobes. When such areas are exposed to those oral conditions conducive to caries formation, caries usually develops (Fig. 6-2, *A*). As caries progresses in these areas, sometimes very little evidence is clinically noticeable until the forces of mastication fracture the increasing amount of unsupported enamel. The caries forms a small area of penetration in the enamel at the bottom of a pit or fissure and does not spread laterally to a great extent until the *dentinoenamel junction (DEJ)* is reached. At that time, the disintegration spreads along the junction and begins to penetrate the dentin toward the pulp via the dentinal tubules. In diagrammatic terms, pit-and-fissure caries may be represented as two cones, base to base, with the apex of the enamel cone at the point of origin and the apex of the dentin cone directed toward the pulp.

Perfect coalescence of the enamel developmental lobes is indicated by faultless enamel areas termed *grooves and fossae.* Usually these areas are not susceptible to caries because they are cleansed by the rubbing of food during

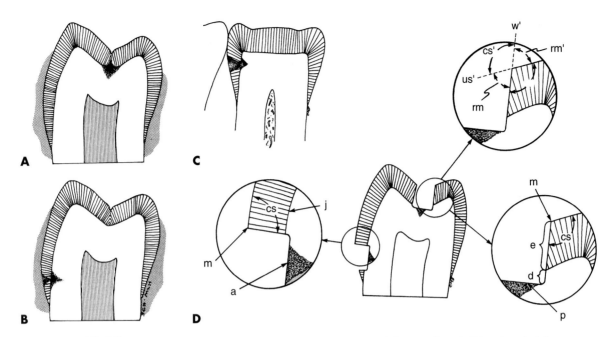

FIG. 6-2 Graphic example of cones of caries (decay) in pit and fissure of tooth **(A)** and on facial **(B)** and proximal **(C)** surfaces when caries has penetrated approximately same depth into dentin. Note differences in loss of enamel on external surfaces. **D,** Sectional view of initial stage of tooth preparations for lesions in **A** and **B** showing cavosurface angle *(cs);* axial wall *(a);* pulpal wall *(p);* enamel wall *(e);* dentinal wall *(d);* margin *(m);* and dentinoenamel junction *(j).* Note in upper exploded view that cavosurface angle *(cs)* can be visualized by imaginary projections *(w')* of the preparation wall and *(us`)* of the unprepared surface contiguous with margin, forming angle *cs'.* Angles *(cs)* and *(cs`)* are equal because opposite angles formed at the intersection of two straight lines are equal. Likewise, minimal restorative material angle *(rm)* is equal to angle *(rm')* .

mastication. However, in areas of no masticatory action in neglected mouths, caries may develop in a groove or fossa.

Caries of Enamel Smooth-Surface Origin. Smooth-surface caries does not begin in an enamel defect, but rather in a smooth area of the enamel surface that is habitually unclean, and is thereby continually, or usually, covered by plaque (see Fig. 6-2, *B* and *C*). It is emphasized in Chapter 3 that plaque is necessary for caries, and that additional oral conditions also must be present for caries to ensue. The disintegration in the enamel in smooth-surface caries also may be pictured as a cone, but with its base on the enamel surface and the apex at, or directed to, the DEJ. The caries again spreads at this junction in the same manner as in pit-and-fissure caries. Thus, the apex of the cone of caries in the enamel contacts the base of the cone of caries in the dentin.

Backward Caries. When the spread of caries along the DEJ exceeds the caries in the contiguous enamel, caries extends into this enamel from the junction and is termed *backward caries* (Fig. 6-3).

Forward Caries. Forward caries is wherever the caries cone in enamel is larger or at least the same size as that in dentin[26] (see Fig. 6-2, *A*).

Residual Caries. Residual caries is caries that remains in a completed tooth preparation, whether by operator intention or by accident. Such caries is not acceptable if at the DEJ or on the prepared enamel tooth

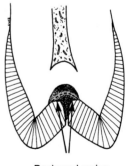

Backward caries

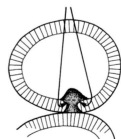

FIG. 6-3 Backward caries extends from DEJ into enamel.

wall (Fig. 6-4, *A* and *B*; see also Fig. 17-51). It may be acceptable, however, when it is *affected dentin,* especially near the pulp (see Affected and Infected Dentin).

Root-Surface Caries. Root-surface caries may occur on the tooth root that has been both exposed to the oral

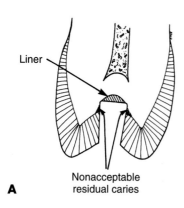

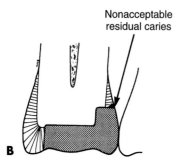

FIG. 6-4 Nonacceptable types of residual caries remaining after tooth preparation (A) at dentinoenamel junction and (B) on enamel wall of tooth preparation. In postoperative radiograph, B appears similar to secondary (recurrent) caries.

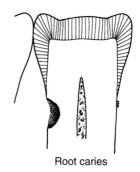

FIG. 6-5 Root-surface caries.

environment and habitually covered with plaque (Fig. 6-5; see also Fig. 9-5, *F*). Additional oral conditions (discussed in Chapter 3) conducive for caries also must be present and often are prevalent in the older population. *Root caries is usually more rapid than other forms of caries, and thus should be detected and treated early.* Root caries is becoming more prevalent because an increasing number of older persons are retaining more of their teeth and experiencing gingival recession, both of which increase the likelihood of root caries development.

Secondary (Recurrent) Caries. Secondary caries occurs at the junction of a restoration and the tooth and may progress under the restoration. It is often termed *recurrent caries.* This condition usually indicates that microleakage is present, along with other conditions conducive to caries (Fig. 6-6; see also Figs. 9-4, *D,* and 9-8, *C*).

Extent of Caries

Incipient Caries (Reversible). Incipient caries is the first evidence of caries activity in the enamel. On smooth surface enamel, the lesion appears opaque white when air-dried, and will seem to disappear (not be distinguishable from contiguous unaffected enamel) if wetted. (See *white spot [ws]* in Fig. 9-5, *D*.) This lesion of demineralized enamel has not extended to the DEJ, and the enamel surface is fairly hard and still intact (smooth to the touch). The lesion can be *remineralized* if immediate corrective measures alter the oral environment, including plaque removal and control. This le-

sion, then, may be characterized as *reversible.* A remineralized lesion usually is either opaque white, or a shade of brown-to-black from extrinsic coloration, has a hard surface, and appears the same whether wet or dry (see *brown spot [bs]* in Fig. 9-14, *C*).

Cavitated Caries (Nonreversible). In cavitated caries, the enamel surface is broken (not intact), and usually the lesion has advanced into dentin. Usually remineralization is not possible (see Fig. 9-5, *E*) and treatment by tooth preparation and restoration is often indicated.

Rate (Speed) of Caries

Acute (Rampant) Caries. Acute caries, often termed *rampant caries,* is when the disease is rapid in damaging the tooth. It is usually in the form of many, soft, light-colored lesions in a mouth and is infectious (see Fig. 9-5, *E*). Less time for extrinsic pigmentation explains the lighter coloration.

Chronic (Slow or Arrested) Caries. Chronic caries is *slow,* or it may be *arrested* following several active phases. The slow rate results from periods when demineralized tooth structure is almost remineralized (the disease is episodic over time because of changes in the oral environment). The condition may be in only a few locations in a mouth, and the lesion is discolored and fairly hard (see Fig. 9-19, *C*). The slow rate of caries allows time for extrinsic pigmentation. An arrested enamel lesion is brown-to-black, hard, and as a result of fluoride, may be more caries-resistant than contiguous, unaffected enamel (see Fig. 9-14, *C [bs]*). An arrested, dentinal lesion typically is "open" (allowing debridement from toothbrushing), dark and hard, and this dentin is termed *sclerotic* or *eburnated dentin* (see Fig. 9-19, *A [a]* and *B*).

Grooves and Fissures; Fossae and Pits.
On the enamel surface, grooves or fissures mark the location of the union of developmental enamel lobes (see Fig. 2-2). Where such union is complete, this "landmark" is only slightly involuted, smooth, hard, shallow, accessible to cleansing, and is termed a *groove.* (Note in Fig. 2-2 on the upper left illustration the good coalescence of the facial cusps to form an occlusofacial groove.) Where such union is incomplete, the landmark is sharply involuted to form a narrow, inaccessible canal of varying depths in

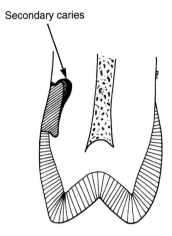

Secondary caries

FIG. 6-6 Secondary (recurrent) caries.

the enamel and is termed a *fissure* (note in Fig. 2-2 on the upper left illustration the mesial portion of the central fissure). A fissure may be a trap for plaque and other oral elements that together can produce caries, unless the surface enamel of the canal is fluoride rich (see Fig. 2-12). Caries-preventive treatment of fissured enamel is presented in Chapter 3; and corrective treatments are discussed in this chapter and subsequent technique chapters.

The distinction made between a groove and a fissure also applies to an enamel surface *fossa* that is nondefective and a *pit* that is defective.

Extension for Prevention, Enameloplasty, Sealant, and Preventive Resin or Conservative Composite Restoration. Black[4] noted that, in tooth preparations for smooth-surface caries, the restoration should be extended to areas that are normally self-cleansing to prevent recurrence of caries. This principle was known as *extension for prevention* and was broadened to include the extension necessary to remove remaining enamel defects, such as pits and fissures.

However, the practice of extension for prevention on smooth surfaces virtually has been eliminated because of the relative caries immunity provided by preventive measures, such as fluoride, improved oral hygiene, and proper diet. This has fostered a more conservative philosophy defining the factors that dictate extension on smooth surfaces to be the extent of caries or injury and the restorative material to be used.

Likewise, extension for prevention to include the full length of enamel fissures has been reduced by treatments that conserve tooth structure; therefore restored teeth are stronger and more resistant to fracture. Such treatments are enameloplasty (see Fig. 17-8), application of pit-and-fissure sealant (see Fig. 13-3), and the preventive resin[36] (see Fig. 13-5), or conservative composite restoration (see Fig. 13-17).

Enameloplasty is removal of a shallow, enamel developmental fissure or pit to create a smooth, saucer-shaped surface that is self-cleansing or easily cleaned. Not only

can this prophylactic procedure be applied to fissures and pits and deep supplemental grooves, but also to some shallow, smooth-surface enamel defects. More details regarding enameloplasty are presented later. Pit-and-fissure sealant application does not require any tooth preparation and is a preferred preventive method. For more advanced lesions, the preventive resin or conservative composite restoration may be used, whereby a small rotary cutting instrument or air abrasion is used to prepare fissures and pits, which are subsequently restored with composite and sealant (see Chapter 13).

Prophylactic Odontotomy. Prophylactic odontotomy[22] is presented only as a historical concept characterized by minimally preparing and filling with amalgam, developmental, structural imperfections of the enamel, such as pits and fissures, to prevent caries originating in these sites. *It is no longer advocated as a preventive measure.*

Affected and Infected Dentin. Fusayama has reported that carious dentin consists of two distinct layers, an *outer* and an *inner*.[14] This textbook refers to the outer layer as *infected dentin* (zones 4 and 5 discussed in Chapter 3) and the inner layer as *affected dentin* (zones 2 and 3 discussed in Chapter 3). *In tooth preparation, it is desirable that only infected dentin be removed, leaving the affected dentin, which then may be remineralized in a vital tooth following the completion of restorative treatment.* This principle for the removal of dentinal caries is supported by Fusayama's observation that the softening front of the lesion always precedes the discoloration front, which in turn always precedes the bacterial front[15] (Figs. 6-7 and 6-8).

Infected dentin has bacteria present and the collagen is irreversibly denatured. It is not remineralizable and must be removed. Affected dentin has no bacteria, is reversibly denatured, remineralizable, and should be preserved. To distinguish clinically between these two layers, the operator traditionally both observes the degree of discoloration (extrinsic staining) and tests the area for hardness by the feel of an explorer tine or a slowly revolving bur. Some difficulties occur with this approach because: (1) the discoloration may be very slight and gradually changeable in acute (rapid) caries, and (2) the hardness (softness) felt by the hand through an instrument may be an inexact guide. To differentiate between remineralizable and nonremineralizable dentin, staining carious dentin was proposed many years ago by Fusayama.[13] Use of these materials is more appropriate for very deep excavations. Many caries-staining products are available and are becoming more widely used.

In *chronic* (slow) *caries*, infected dentin usually is discolored and, because the bacterial front is close to the discoloration front, it is advisable in caries removal to remove all discolored dentin unless judged to be within 0.5 mm of the pulp (Fig. 6-9). Because in *acute* (rapid) *caries* the discoloration is very slight and the bacterial

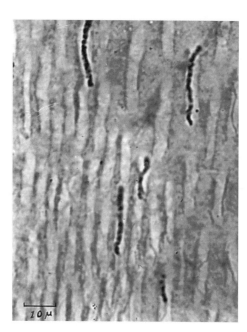

FIG. **6-7** Bacteria in dentinal tubules in the bacterial front of a carious lesion. *(Courtesy of Takao Fusayama and the* Journal of Dental Research.*)*

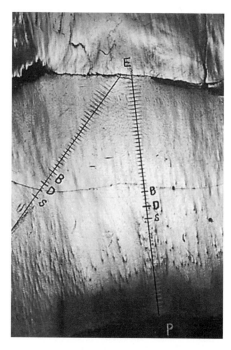

FIG. **6-8** Series of Knoop indentations parallel and oblique to dentinal tubules. *(E),* Dentinoenamel junction; *(B)* bacterial invasion front; *(D),* discoloration front; *(S),* softening front; *(P),* pulp chamber wall. *(Courtesy of Takao Fusayama and the* Journal of Dental Research.*)*

front is well behind the discoloration front, some discolored dentin may be left, although any "clinically remarkable" discoloration should be removed.[15]

NONCARIOUS TOOTH DEFECTS TERMINOLOGY

Abrasion. Abrasion is abnormal tooth surface loss resulting from direct friction forces between the teeth and external objects, or from frictional forces between contacting teeth components in the presence of an abrasive medium.[27] Abrasion may occur from (1) improper brushing techniques, (2) habits such as holding a pipe stem by the teeth, (3) tobacco chewing, or (4) vigorous use of toothpicks between adjacent teeth. Toothbrush abrasion is the most common example and is usually seen as a sharp, V-shaped notch in the gingival portion of the facial aspect of a tooth (see Fig. 9-11, *D*).

Erosion. Erosion is the wear or loss of tooth surface by chemicomechanical action (see Fig. 9-11, *A* and *B*). Regurgitation of stomach acid can cause this condition on the lingual surfaces of maxillary teeth (particularly anterior teeth). Other examples are the dissolution of the facial aspects of anterior teeth because of habitual sucking of lemons or the loss of tooth surface from ingestion of acidic medicines.

Abfraction. Recently, it has been proposed that the predominant causative factor of some of the cervical, wedge-shaped defects is a strong (heavy) eccentric occlusal force (shown as an associated wear facet) resulting in microfractures or abfractures. Such microfrac-

tures occur as the cervical area of the tooth flexes under such loads. This defect is termed *idiopathic erosion*[24] or *abfraction* (see Fig. 9-11, *C*).

Attrition. Attrition is mechanical wear of the incisal or occlusal surface as a result of functional or parafunctional movements of the mandible (tooth-to-tooth contacts) (see Fig. 9-11, *E*). Attrition also includes proximal surface wear at the contact area because of physiologic tooth movement.

Fractures. One of the more difficult and challenging defects of teeth, in both diagnosis and treatment, are fractures (see Figs. 9-12 and 9-18). The following types of fracture may occur.

Incomplete Fracture Not Directly Involving (Not Into) Vital Pulp. An incomplete fracture not directly involving a vital pulp is often termed a *greenstick fracture.* This condition is very sensitive, yet the patient can only specify which side of the mouth is affected rather than the specific tooth. It is most challenging to diagnose and treat (see Chapter 9 and Fig. 9-18).

Complete Fracture Not Involving (Not Into) Vital Pulp. Usually, pain is not associated with this condition (see Fig. 9-12), unless the gingival border of the fractured segment is still held by periodontal tissue. Restorative treatment (sometimes also periodontal) is indicated.

Fracture Involving (Into) Vital Pulp. This condition always results in pulpal infection and severe pain. If the tooth is restorable, immediate root canal therapy is indicated; otherwise the tooth must be extracted.

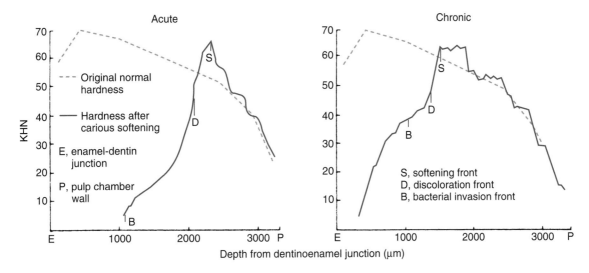

FIG. **6-9** Graphs comparing acute and chronic caries regarding closeness, hardness, and depth factors of the softening, discoloration, and bacterial invasion fronts. *(Courtesy of Takao Fusayama.)*

Nonhereditary Enamel Hypoplasia. Nonhereditary enamel hypoplasia occurs when the ameloblasts are injured during enamel formation, resulting in defective enamel (diminished form and/or calcification). It usually is seen on anterior teeth and first molars in the form of opaque white or light brown areas with smooth intact, hard surface (see Fig. 15-1, *B*), or of pitted or grooved enamel, which is usually hard and discolored and caused by fluorosis or high fever (see Fig. 15-34). The reader is referred to a textbook on oral pathology for additional information.

Amelogenesis Imperfecta. In amelogenesis imperfecta, the enamel is defective either in form or calcification as a result of heredity and has an appearance ranging from essentially normal to extremely unsightly.[34]

Dentinogenesis Imperfecta. Dentinogenesis imperfecta is a hereditary condition in which only the dentin is defective. Normal enamel is weakly attached and lost early. The reader is referred to a textbook on oral pathology.

TOOTH PREPARATION TERMINOLOGY

A prerequisite to the comprehension of terms in either tooth preparation or classification (following section) is a knowledge of all terms of tooth description as presented in dental anatomy, including the names and positions of tooth surfaces.

Simple, Compound, and Complex Tooth Preparations. A tooth preparation is termed *simple* if only one tooth surface is involved (see Fig. 6-12), *compound* if two surfaces are involved (see Fig. 6-15), and *complex* for a preparation involving three (or more) surfaces (see Fig. 19-1).

Abbreviated Descriptions of Tooth Preparations. For brevity in records and communication, the descrip-

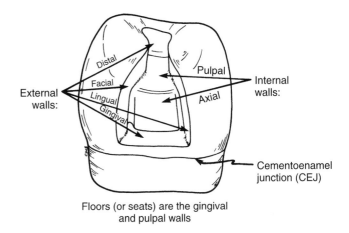

Floors (or seats) are the gingival and pulpal walls

FIG. **6-10** Illustration indicating external and internal walls.

tion of a tooth preparation is abbreviated by using the first letter, capitalized, of each tooth surface involved. Examples are: (1) an occlusal tooth preparation is an O (see Fig. 6-12); (2) a preparation involving the mesial and occlusal surfaces is an MO (see Fig. 6-15); and (3) a preparation involving the mesial, occlusal, and distal surfaces is an MOD (see Fig. 19-1).

Tooth Preparation Walls

Internal Wall. An internal wall is a prepared (cut) surface that does not extend to the external tooth surface (Fig. 6-10).

Axial wall. An axial wall is an internal wall parallel with the long axis of the tooth (see Fig. 6-10).

Pulpal wall. A pulpal wall is an internal wall that is both perpendicular to the long axis of the tooth and occlusal of the pulp (see Figs. 6-10 and 6-13 *[p]*).

External Wall. An external wall is a prepared (cut) surface that extends to the external tooth surface, and such a wall takes the name of the tooth surface (or aspect) that the wall is toward (see Fig. 6-10).

Floor (or Seat). A floor (or seat) is a prepared (cut) wall that is reasonably flat and perpendicular to those occlusal forces that are directed occlusogingivally (generally parallel to the long axis of the tooth). Examples are the pulpal and gingival walls (see Fig. 6-10). Such floors may be purposefully prepared to provide stabilizing seats for the restoration, thus distributing the stresses in the tooth structure, rather than concentrating them. This increases the *resistance form* of the restored tooth against postrestorative fracture. More regarding this type of resistance form is presented in a later section.

Enamel Wall. The enamel wall is that portion of a prepared external wall consisting of enamel (see Fig. 6-2, *D*).

Dentinal Wall. The dentinal wall is that portion of a prepared external wall consisting of dentin, in which mechanical retention features may be located (see Fig. 6-2, *D*).

Tooth Preparation Angles. Although the junction of two or more prepared (cut) surfaces is referred to as an angle, in fact, the junction is almost always "softened" so as to present a slightly rounded configuration (the exception being a tooth preparation for gold foil). In spite of this rounding, these junctions are still referred to as angles for descriptive and communicative purposes.

Line Angle. A line angle is the junction of two planal surfaces of different orientation along a line (see Fig. 6-14). An internal line angle is a line angle whose apex points into the tooth (see Fig. 6-14, *[fp]*). An external line angle is a line angle whose apex points away from the tooth (see Fig. 6-17, *[ap]*).

Point Angle. A point angle is the junction of three planal surfaces of different orientation (see Fig. 6-14, *[mfp]*).

Cavosurface Angle and Cavosurface Margin. The *cavosurface angle* is the angle of tooth structure formed by the junction of a prepared (cut) wall and the external surface of the tooth (see Fig. 6-2, *D*, *[cs]*). The actual junction is referred to as the *cavosurface margin* (see Fig. 6-2, *[m]*). The cavosurface angle may differ with the location on the tooth, the direction of the enamel rods on the prepared wall, or the type of restorative material to be used. This subject is discussed in greater detail later in this chapter and also in later chapters dealing with tooth preparations for different restorative materials. It should be noted in Fig. 6-2, *D*, that the cavosurface angle *(cs)* is determined by projecting the prepared (cut) wall in an imaginary line *(w')* and the unprepared enamel surface in an imaginary line *(us')* and noting the angle *(cs')* opposite to the cavosurface angle *(cs)*. (Recall that when two straight lines intersect, the opposite angles are equal). For better visualization, these imaginary projections can be formed by using two periodontal probes, one lying on the unprepared surface and the other on the prepared external tooth wall (Fig. 6-11).

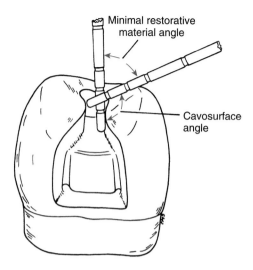

FIG. **6-11** Visualization of cavosurface angle and associated minimal restorative material angle.

Combination of terms. When discussing or writing a term denoting a combination of two or more surfaces, the *al* ending of the prefix word is changed to an *o*. Thus the angle formed by the lingual and incisal surfaces of an anterior tooth would be termed the *linguoincisal* line angle. A tooth preparation involving the mesial and occlusal surfaces is termed a *mesioocclusal* preparation, or an *MO* preparation (see Fig. 6-15); and a preparation involving mesial, occlusal, and distal surfaces is a *mesioocclusodistal* tooth preparation, or an *MOD* preparation (see Fig. 19-1). When referring to a combination of tooth preparation walls (i.e., stating line angles or point angles), the same nomenclature principle is used (see Figs. 6-13 and 6-14).

Dentinoenamel Junction. The DEJ is the junction of the enamel and dentin (see Fig. 6-2, *D*).

Cementoenamel Junction. The cementoenamel junction (CEJ) is the junction of the enamel and cementum (see Fig. 6-10). It also is referred to as the *cervical line*. Sometimes the enamel and cementum do not actually join, thereby leaving a narrow region of exposed dentin.

Enamel Margin Strength. One of the more important principles in tooth preparation is the concept of the *strongest enamel margin*. This margin has two significant features: (1) it is formed by full-length enamel rods whose inner ends are on sound dentin, and (2) these enamel rods are buttressed on the preparation side by progressively shorter rods whose outer ends have been cut off but whose inner ends are on sound dentin (see Figs. 6-1, *D*, and 17-6, *B*). Because enamel rods usually are perpendicular to the enamel surface, the strongest enamel margin results in a cavosurface angle greater than 90 degrees.

An enamel margin composed of full-length rods that are on sound dentin but are *not* buttressed tooth-side by shorter rods also on sound dentin is termed *strong* (but not the strongest). Generally, this margin will result in a 90-degree cavosurface angle (see Fig. 17-48, *C*).

An enamel margin composed of rods that do not run uninterrupted from the surface to sound dentin is termed unsupported, and this marginal enamel tends to split or fracture off, leaving a V-shaped ditch along the margin of a restoration (see Fig. 2-4, *A*). Usually, this weak enamel margin either has a cavosurface angle less than 90 degrees or no dentinal support.

Vertical (Longitudinal) and Horizontal (Transverse) Terminology. It is customary through habitual use to describe tooth preparation features or sections that are parallel (or nearly so) to the long axis of the tooth crown as *vertical,* such as vertical height of cusps, or vertical walls. However, sometimes the term *longitudinal* may be used in lieu of *vertical.* Tooth preparation features that are perpendicular (or nearly so) to the long axis of the tooth are termed *horizontal,* although sometimes referred to as *transverse.* When the terms *vertical (longitudinal)* and *horizontal (transverse)* are first used in a chapter, the parenthetical alternate may be included, but not thereafter.

Intracoronal and Extracoronal Tooth Preparations. An intracoronal tooth preparation is usually "boxlike," having both internal and external preparation walls (see Fig. 6-10). With a conservative tooth preparation for treatment of a small lesion, much of the tooth crown, as well as crown surface, is not involved. Nevertheless, the remaining tooth usually is weakened, and the restoration may or may not restore the tooth strength.

Conversely, the extracoronal preparation is usually "stumplike," having walls or surfaces that result from removal of most to all of the enamel. The extracoronal restoration, termed a *crown,* envelops the remaining tooth crown and thereby usually restores some of its strength. This textbook does not include extracoronal tooth preparation for crown restorations. However, included in Chapter 20 are *cast metal onlay restorations* that by design, encompass the transitional vertical tooth corners (line angles) and thereby strengthen the tooth against postrestorative fracture.

Anatomic Tooth Crown and Clinical Tooth Crown. The anatomic tooth crown is the portion of the tooth covered by enamel. The clinical tooth crown is the portion of the tooth exposed to the oral cavity.

CLASSIFICATION OF TOOTH PREPARATIONS

Classification of tooth preparations according to the anatomic areas involved as well as by the associated type of treatment was presented by Black and is designated as Class I, Class II, Class III, Class IV, and Class V.[4] Since Black's original classification, an additional class has been added, Class VI. Class I refers to pit-and-fissure lesions, whereas the remaining classes are smooth-surface lesions. Classification was originally based on the observed frequency of carious lesions on certain aspects of the tooth. Even though the relative frequency of caries

locations may have changed over the years, the original classification is still used, and the various *classes also are used to identify restorations* (i.e., a Class I amalgam restoration). This method of classification is used throughout this textbook.

Also used in this textbook is a classification of tooth preparations that primarily relates to a comparison between the more historical tooth preparation (conventional) and alterations from that type of preparation. The altered preparation designs are referred to as: (1) beveled conventional preparations and (2) modified preparations. Much of the detailed description of tooth preparation in this chapter focuses on conventional designs, although appropriate differences with the other two designs also are presented in this chapter and in the technique chapters. The conventional design preparation is typical for an amalgam restoration and includes the following characteristics: (1) uniform pulpal and/or axial wall depths, (2) cavosurface margin design that results in a 90-degree restoration margin, and (3) primary retention form derived from occlusally converging vertical walls. Beveled conventional designs are characterized as conventional preparations with beveling of some accessible enamel margins. Modified preparation designs may not have uniform axial or pulpal depths or occlusally converging vertical walls. Furthermore, thin cavosurface margins may result in more acute angles in the restoration. Amalgam tooth preparations only use conventional designs, whereas composite preparations may be any of the three designs.

Class I Restorations. All pit-and-fissure restorations are *Class I,* and they are assigned to three groups, as follows.

Restorations on Occlusal Surface of Premolars and Molars. The names of the walls, line angles, and point angles of an occlusal conventional tooth preparation are identified by the labels and legends in Figs. 6-12, 6-13, and 6-14, noting again that a preparation takes the name of the tooth surface (or aspect) that the wall is toward.

Restorations on Occlusal Two Thirds of the Facial and Lingual Surfaces of Molars. The names of the walls, line angles, and point angles of these tooth preparations are the same as those depicted for the preparations for Class V restorations (see later section).

Restorations on Lingual Surface of Maxillary Incisors. The names of the walls, line angles, and point angles of these tooth preparations also are the same as those depicted for the preparations for Class V restorations (see later section).

Class II Restorations. Restorations on the proximal surfaces of posterior teeth are *Class II.* A proximoocclusal (MO) conventional preparation illustrates and designates walls, line angles, and point angles (Figs. 6-15, 6-16, and 6-17). A distoocclusal preparation has the same walls, line angles, and point angles, except the distal wall (in the MO) is a mesial wall (in the DO);

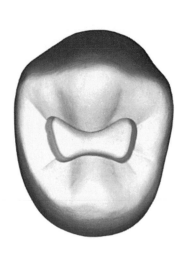

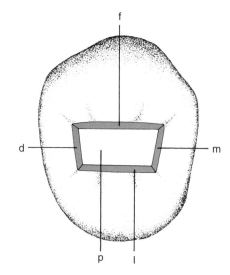

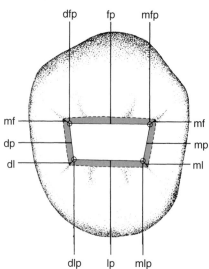

FIG. **6-12** Typical Class I tooth preparation for amalgam on maxillary premolar.

FIG. **6-13** Schematic representation (for descriptive purpose) of Fig. 6-12 illustrating tooth preparation *walls:* facial *(f)*, distal *(d)*, lingual *(l)*, mesial *(m)*, and pulpal *(p)*.

FIG. **6-14** Schematic representation (for descriptive purpose) of Fig. 6-12 illustrating tooth preparation line angles and point angles. *Line angles* are faciopulpal *(fp)*, distofacial *(df)*, distopulpal *(dp)*, distolingual *(dl)*, linguopulpal *(lp)*, mesiolingual *(ml)*, mesiopulpal *(mp)*, and mesiofacial *(mf)*. *Point angles* are distofaciopulpal *(dfp)*, distolinguopulpal *(dlp)*, mesiolinguopulpal *(mlp)*, and mesiofaciopulpal *(mfp)*.

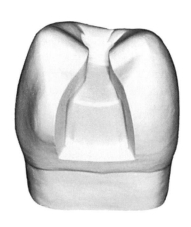

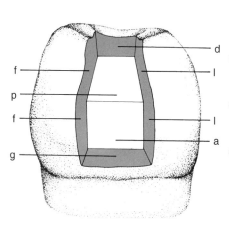

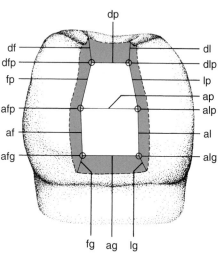

FIG. **6-15** Typical Class II mesioocclusal conventional tooth preparation for amalgam on maxillary premolar.

FIG. **6-16** Schematic representation (for descriptive purpose) of Fig. 6-15 illustrating tooth preparation *walls:* facial *(f)* of proximal and occlusal portions, gingival *(g)*, lingual *(l)* of proximal and occlusal portions, distal *(d)*, pulpal *(p)*, and axial *(a)*.

FIG. **6-17** Schematic representation (for descriptive purpose) of Fig. 6-15 illustrating tooth preparation line angles and point angles. *Line angles* are distofacial *(df)*, faciopulpal *(fp)*, axiofacial *(af)*, faciogingival *(fg)*, axiogingival *(ag)*, linguogingival *(lg)*, axiolingual *(al)*, axiopulpal *(ap)*, linguopulpal *(lp)*, distolingual *(dl)*, and distopulpal *(dp)*. Point angles are distofaciopulpal *(dfp)*, axiofaciopulpal *(afp)*, axiofaciogingival *(afg)*, axiolinguogingival *(alg)*, axiolinguopulpal *(alp)*, and distolinguopulpal *(dlp)*.

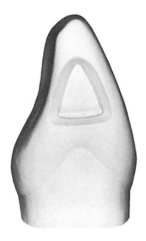

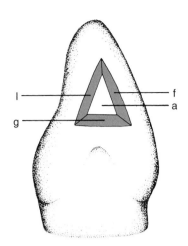

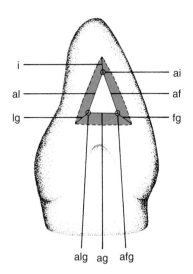

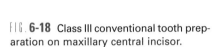

FIG. **6-18** Class III conventional tooth preparation on maxillary central incisor.

FIG. **6-19** Schematic representation (for descriptive purpose) of Fig. 6-18 illustrating tooth preparation *walls*: facial *(f)*, lingual *(l)*, gingival *(g)*, and axial *(a)*.

FIG. **6-20** Schematic representation (for descriptive purpose) of Fig. 6-18 illustrating tooth preparation line angles and point angles. *Line angles* are axiolingual *(al)*, linguogingival *(lg)*, axiogingival *(ag)*, faciogingival *(fg)*, axiofacial *(af)*, and incisal *(i)*. Point angles are axiolinguogingival *(alg)*, axiofaciogingival *(afg)*, and axioincisal *(ai)*. (Note that names for incisal line angle and point angle are exceptions to the general naming rule.)

and the line angles and point angles relating to a distal wall (in the MO) relate to a mesial wall (in the DO). An MOD preparation has similar walls, line angles, and point angles, but there is neither a mesial wall nor a distal wall, and therefore line angles and point angles associated with mesial and distal walls are not present.

Class III Restorations. Restorations on the proximal surfaces of anterior teeth that do *not* involve the incisal angle are *Class III*. Walls, line angles, and point angles of a representative conventional tooth preparation are identified in Figs. 6-18, 6-19, and 6-20. Note that the faciolingual line angle at the incisal is termed the *incisal line angle*; likewise, the faciolinguoincisal point angle is termed the *axioincisal point angle.*

Class IV Restorations. Restorations on the proximal surfaces of anterior teeth that *do* involve the incisal edge are *Class IV*. Walls, line angles, and point angles of a representative conventional tooth preparation are identified in Figs. 6-21, 6-22, and 6-23.

Class V Restorations. Restorations on the gingival third of the facial or lingual surfaces of all teeth (except pit-and-fissure lesions) are *Class V*. Walls, line angles, and point angles of a representative conventional tooth preparation on an anterior tooth are designated in Figs. 6-24, 6-25, and 6-26. For posterior teeth the incisal *(i)* becomes occlusal *(o).*

Class VI Restorations. Restorations on the incisal edge of anterior teeth or the occlusal cusp heights of posterior teeth are *Class VI*. Walls, line angles, and point angles of these tooth preparations are the same as those depicted for the preparations of occlusal pit-and-fissure lesions.

INITIAL AND FINAL STAGES OF TOOTH PREPARATION

Proper tooth preparation is accomplished through systematic procedures based on definite physical and mechanical principles. Also, the differences between clinically manifested physiologic and pathologic processes of teeth and supporting tissues must be recognized. Moreover, the physical properties and capabilities of the different restorative materials must be appreciated. All of these are determining factors in understanding proper tooth preparation. Without this background knowledge, plus additional information concerning the mechanics of cutting and patient management, the exercise of proper judgment for efficient and proper tooth preparation cannot be achieved.

As stated earlier, the tooth preparation procedure is divided into two stages, each with several steps. Each stage should be thoroughly understood, and each step should be accomplished as perfectly as possible. There are occasions, however, when the sequence is altered,

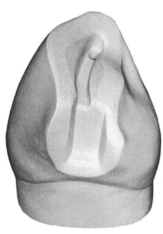

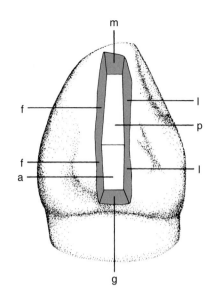

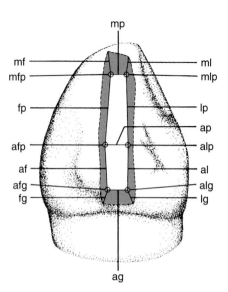

FIG. **6-21** Class IV conventional tooth preparation for inlay on maxillary canine.

FIG. **6-22** Schematic representation (for descriptive purpose) of Fig. 6-21 illustrating tooth preparation *walls:* facial *(f)* of proximal and incisal portions, gingival *(g)*, lingual *(l)* of proximal and incisal portions, axial *(a)*, and mesial *(m)*.

FIG. **6-23** Schematic representation (for descriptive purpose) of Fig. 6-21 illustrating tooth preparation line and point angles. *Line angles* are mesiofacial *(mf)*, faciopulpal *(fp)*, axiofacial *(af)*, faciogingival *(fg)*, axiogingival *(ag)*, linguogingival *(lg)*, axiolingual *(al)*, axiopulpal *(ap)*, linguopulpal *(lp)*, mesiolingual *(ml)*, and mesiopulpal *(mp)*. Point angles are mesiofaciopulpal *(mfp)*, axiofaciopulpal *(afp)*, axiofaciogingival *(afg)*, axiolinguogingival *(alg)*, axiolinguopulpal *(alp)*, and mesiolinguopulpal *(mlp)*.

but this is the exception and not the general rule (see Caries Control Restoration in Chapter 3). The stages are presented in the sequence in which they should be followed if consistent, ideal results are to be obtained. The division of the procedure into two stages also assists in assessing students' understanding and ability to properly execute the preparation. In an academic setting, the student should be instructed to accomplish the initial stage first. An evaluation of this stage should then occur before any steps in the final stage are initiated.

The stages and steps in tooth preparation are:

Initial Tooth Preparation Stage

Step 1: Outline form and initial depth
Step 2: Primary resistance form
Step 3: Primary retention form
Step 4: Convenience form

Final Tooth Preparation Stage

Step 5: Removal of any remaining infected dentin and/or old restorative material, if indicated
Step 6: Pulp protection, if indicated
Step 7: Secondary resistance and retention forms

Step 8: Procedures for finishing external walls
Step 9: Final procedures: cleaning, inspecting, sealing

As stated earlier, under certain circumstances this sequence is changed, such as extensive caries that may involve the pulp. Then it may be advisable to remove infected dentin earlier in the procedure. When this becomes necessary, it also is important to place the desired liner and/or base in the preparation at this time, especially if a pulp capping procedure is necessary (see Chapter 3). Normally, however, much of the caries is removed in completing the initial tooth preparation and any remaining infected dentin is removed later in the final stage.

Specific procedures and instrumentation are discussed in detail in later chapters that present the various classes of restorations in conjunction with the use of different restorative materials. *The discussion in this section is concerned with what should be accomplished and why,* and not specifically how it should be accomplished.

Before any restorative procedure can be undertaken, the environment in which the procedure will be done must be readied. *Most restorative materials require a moisture-free environment; otherwise, the physical properties of the material are compromised.* Chapter 10 of this textbook presents the methods of field isolation, ensuring maxi-

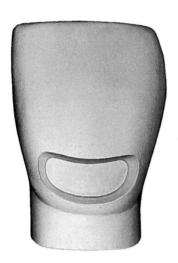

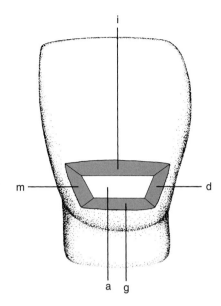

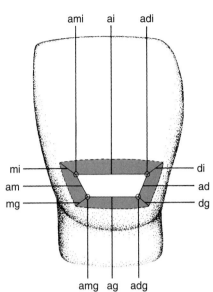

FIG. **6-24** Class V conventional tooth preparation.

FIG. **6-25** Schematic representation (for descriptive purpose) of Fig. 6-24 illustrating tooth preparation *walls*: mesial *(m)*, gingival *(g)*, distal *(d)*, incisal *(i)* (or occlusal *[o]* if preparation on posterior tooth), and axial *(a)*.

FIG. **6-26** Schematic representation (for descriptive purpose) of Fig. 6-24 illustrating tooth preparation line angles and point angles. *Line angles* are mesioincisal *(mi)* (or mesioocclusal *[mo]*), axiomesial *(am)*, mesiogingival *(mg)*, axiogingival *(ag)*, distogingival *(dg)*, axiodistal *(ad)*, distoincisal *(di)* (or distoocclusal *[do]*), and axioincisal *(ai)* (or axioocclusal *[ao]*). Point angles are axiomesioincisal *(ami)*, (or axiomesioocclusal *[amo]*), axiomesiogingival *(amg)*, axiodistogingival *(adg)*, and axiodistoincisal *(adi)* (or axiodistoocclusal *[ado]*).

mum effectiveness of the restorative material. In most cases, the use of the *rubber dam* best assures the correct isolation. Some operators prefer to place the rubber dam after the initial stage of tooth preparation but before excavating infected dentin and placing secondary retentive features.

Also, the treatment and management of the remainder of the oral environment must be considered. *Protecting the contiguous soft tissues in the operating site must be a primary objective.* Oral mucosa, lips, cheek, and tongue should be protected against deleterious effects from substances placed in the mouth during a restorative procedure as well as from possible mechanical injury caused by the procedure. Likewise, these tissues must be treated carefully so as not to cause any lasting harm. This requires specific actions that will provide appropriate soft tissue response. Proper manipulation of the gingiva requires appropriate use of retraction cord, protection by wedge placement, and development of restoration contours that engender postoperative gingival health. For years, it was recommended that restoration margins be extended into the gingival sulcus, a region thought to be immune to recurrent caries. It is now accepted that the gingival sulcus is not immune to recurrent caries. Moreover, soft tissue responds negatively to margins placed

in the crevice. *Therefore margins should be limited to supragingival locations whenever possible.* Obviously, the less the gingival tissue is affected by the restoration, the less likely future gingival harm will be caused by either the operative procedure or the restoration contour. Also, and just as important, less extension gingivally is more conservative of tooth structure, leaving the tooth stronger. Specific factors that best assure proper soft tissue health both during and after a restorative procedure are presented in the chapters describing the various operative restorative techniques.

INITIAL TOOTH PREPARATION STAGE

As stated earlier, *initial tooth preparation is the extension and initial design of the external walls of the preparation at a specified, limited depth so as to provide access to the caries or defect, reach sound tooth structure (except for later removal of infected dentin on the pulpal or axial walls), resist fracture of the tooth or restorative material from masticatory forces principally directed with the long axis of the tooth, and retain the restorative material in the tooth* (except for the Class V preparation). The preparation is extended internally no deeper than 0.2 mm (0.5 mm when restoring with direct gold) into dentin for pit-and-fissure lesions and 0.2 to 0.8 mm into dentin for smooth-surface lesions (the greater on root surfaces; see Fig. 6-1). This may necessitate additional deepening of the preparation in the excavation of any remaining faulty tooth structure, faulty old restorative material, or infected dentin during the final stage of tooth preparation. In this way, the operator can maximize the use of the preparation instrumentation before making changes and can perform the final preparation techniques with better access and visibility. However, when the carious lesion is very extensive, the sequence of these steps is altered to determine the pulpal involvement and protect the pulpal tissue as early in the procedure as possible. The steps in *initial tooth preparation* are: (1) developing the outline form and initial depth, (2) establishing primary resistance form, (3) establishing primary retention form, and (4) providing convenience form. These steps are discussed in detail in the following sections. Although these are listed as individual steps, in practice they often occur simultaneously.

Step 1: Outline Form and Initial Depth. The first step in initial tooth preparation is determining and developing the outline form while establishing the initial depth.

Definition. Establishing the *outline form* means: (1) placing the *preparation margins* in the positions they will occupy in the final preparation, except for finishing enamel walls and margins, and (2) preparing an *initial depth* of 0.2 to 0.8 mm pulpally of the DEJ position or normal root-surface position (*no deeper initially whether in tooth structure, air, old restorative material, or caries* unless the occlusal enamel thickness is minimal and greater dimension is necessary for strength of the restorative material). The greater depth is for extensions onto the root surface. Otherwise, the depth into dentin is not to exceed 0.2 to 0.5 mm, the deeper dimension necessary when placing secondary retention (see Fig. 6-1). The outline form must be visualized before any mechanical alteration to the tooth is begun. Occasionally, extensive caries, fractured enamel, and other conditions may prevent an accurate preoperative mental visualization at the onset of tooth preparation, although a dentist with sufficient clinical experience usually can do this. With the principles governing the outline form as a background, this preoperative visualization of the outline form acts as a deterrent to overcutting and overextension, which very often cause weak remaining tooth structure and an unesthetic restoration. Thus, it is very important to preoperatively assess the proposed tooth preparation extensions before mechanical removal of any tooth structure, chiefly enamel.

Principles. The three general principles, not without exception, on which outline form is established regardless of the type of tooth preparation being prepared are: (1) all friable and/or weakened enamel should be removed (recall previous Nomenclature section, Enamel Margin Strength), (2) all faults should be included, and (3) all margins should be placed in a position to afford good finishing of the margins of the restoration. The

third principle has ramifications that differ for pit-and-fissure preparations as compared with smooth-surface preparations.

Factors. In determining the outline form of a proposed tooth preparation, certain conditions or factors must first be assessed. These conditions affect the outline form and often dictate the extensions. Obviously the *extent of the carious lesion, defect, or faulty old restoration* affects the outline form of the proposed tooth preparation because *the objective is to extend to sound tooth structure, except in a pulpal direction.* There is one extension exception: occasionally, a tooth preparation outline for a new restoration will contact or extend slightly into a sound, existing restoration (e.g., a new MO abutting a sound DO; see Fig. 17-65, *A* and *B*). *This is sometimes an acceptable practice (i.e, to have a margin of a new restoration placed into an existing, sound restoration).*

In addition to these factors, esthetic and occlusal conditions affect the proposed preparation. *Esthetic considerations* not only affect the choice of restorative material, but also the design of the tooth preparation in an effort to maximize the esthetic result of the restoration. Correcting or improving *occlusal relationships* also may necessitate altering the tooth preparation to accommodate such changes, even when the involved tooth structure is not faulty (i.e., perhaps a cuspal form must be altered to effect better occlusal relationships). Likewise, the *adjacent tooth contour* may dictate specific preparation extensions that both secure appropriate proximal relationships and provide the restored tooth with optimal form and strength. Lastly, the desired *cavosurface marginal configuration* of the proposed restoration affects the outline form. Restorative materials that are more effective when having beveled margins require tooth preparation outline form extensions that must anticipate the final cavosurface position and form. All of these factors are discussed in subsequent chapters that present the clinical techniques for the various operative restorations.

Features. Generally the six specific, typical features of establishing proper outline form and initial depth are: (1) preserving cuspal strength, (2) preserving marginal ridge strength, (3) minimizing faciolingual extensions, (4) using enameloplasty, (5) connecting two close (less than 0.5 mm apart) faults or tooth preparations, and (6) restricting the depth of the preparation into dentin to a maximum of 0.2 mm for pit-and-fissure caries and 0.2 to 0.8 mm for the axial wall of smooth-surface caries (the greater depth indicated only for an extension gingivally onto the root surface). These features are discussed as they relate to both pit-and-fissure cavities and smooth surface cavities.

Outline form and initial depth for pit-and-fissure lesions. Outline form and initial depth in pit-and-fissure preparations are controlled by three factors: (1) the extent to which the enamel has been involved by the carious process, (2) the extensions that must be made along the fissures to achieve sound and smooth margins, and (3) the limited bur depth related to the tooth's original surface (real, or visualized if missing because of disease or defect) while extending the preparation to sound external walls that have a pulpal depth of approximately 1.5 to 2 mm and usually a maximum depth into dentin of 0.2 mm (see Fig. 6-1, *A* and *B*). It should be noted in Fig. 6-1, *A*, that this depth measured in relation to the location of the fissure itself is 1.5 mm.

Rules for establishing outline form for pit-and-fissure tooth preparation

1. Extend the preparation margin until sound tooth structure is obtained and no unsupported and/or weakened enamel remains.
2. Avoid terminating the margin on extreme eminences such as cusp heights or ridge crests.
3. If the extension from a primary groove includes one-half or more of the cusp incline, consideration should be given to *capping the cusp.* If the extension is two-thirds, the cusp-capping procedure is most often the proper procedure (Fig. 6-27), which removes the margin from the area of masticatory stresses.

4. Extend the preparation margin to include all of the fissure that cannot be eliminated by appropriate *enameloplasty* (Fig. 6-28; see also Figs. 17-8 and 20-5).
5. Restrict the pulpal depth of the preparation to a maximum of 0.2 mm into dentin (except when (1) preparing a tooth for a gold foil restoration, in which case the initial depth is 0.5 mm into dentin as described in Chapter 21) or (2) when the occlusal enamel has been worn thin. *To be as conservative as possible, the preparation for an occlusal surface pit-and-fissure lesion is first prepared to a depth of 1.5 mm, as measured at the central fissure.* Depending on the cuspal steepness angles, the facial and lingual prepared walls usually will be greater than 1.5 mm. As such an example, note in Fig. 6-1, *A*, that the initial depth is two thirds of a 3-mm long No. 245 bur blade, or 2 mm, as related to the prepared facial and lingual walls, but is only half the blade length, or 1.5 mm, as related to the preoperative central fissure location. However, once this depth is established, if remaining enamel pit or fissure is present on less than 50% of the pulpal floor, it is removed during the final stage of tooth preparation (see Step 5: Removal of Any Remaining Enamel

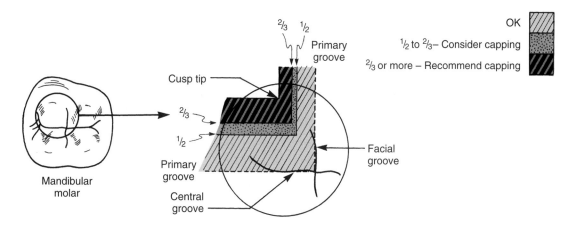

FIG. **6-27** Rule for cusp capping: If extension from a primary groove toward the cusp tip is no more than half the distance, then no cusp capping; if this extension is from one half to two thirds of the distance, then consider cusp capping; if the extension is more than two thirds of the distance, then usually cap the cusp.

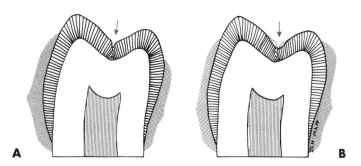

FIG. **6-28 A,** Enameloplasty on area of imperfect coalescence of enamel. **B,** No more than one-third of the enamel thickness should be removed.

Pit or Fissure, Infected Dentin, and/or Old Restorative Material, if Indicated). However, if the amount of pit or fissure remaining is greater than 50% of the pulpal floor, the entire pulpal floor is deepened (at this time of preparing outline form) to a maximum initial depth of 0.2 mm into dentin. This will mean 0.2 mm into dentin when extension is to sound tooth structure (i.e., a 0.2-mm dentinal wall, with the remainder of the wall formed in enamel). Thus, the actual depth of the preparation may vary from 1.5 mm, depending on the thickness of the enamel and the steepness of the cuspal inclines. *During this cutting procedure, the end of the bur may be in air (over a hole or caries depression), in old restorative material, or in caries.*

6. When two pit-and-fissure preparations have less than 0.5 mm of sound tooth structure between them, they should be joined to eliminate a weak enamel wall between them.

7. Extend the outline form to provide sufficient access for proper tooth preparation, restoration placement, and finishing procedures (see Step 4: Convenience Form).

In the application of these rules, adequate extension of the outline form cannot be overemphasized; however, the improvement of restorative materials and increased knowledge about caries have permitted a more conservative approach to preparation extension than was originally expressed by Black. Therefore conservative, minimal tooth preparation extension should be pursued while conforming to the sound principles of outline form.

Naturally the typical outline form varies with the anatomic form of the particular tooth being treated. In extending fissures or connecting pits and fissures on the occlusal surfaces of teeth, the margins usually do not assume a straight line from one point to another (see Fig. 6-32); rather, they follow smooth curves that preserve as much strong cusp structure as possible. Another example of this circumventing of cusps is the conventional Class I preparation on maxillary premolars in which tooth extension includes an occlusal fissure, mesial and distal pits, and facial and lingual radiating fissures (see Fig 13-5 for a conventional Class I composite preparation and Fig. 17-2 for a conventional Class I amalgam preparation). The outline form resulting from proper extension of this preparation somewhat resembles a butterfly in flight and is often referred to as *butterfly-type preparation*. The most narrow portion of the preparation, faciolingually, is between the cusp heights. *As much of the cusp incline as possible should be preserved in any preparation involving the occlusal surface,* provided that other principles are maintained at the same time. Outline form will vary from tooth to tooth and is dictated by these rules.

On the occlusal surfaces of molars, all developmental grooves should be included to the extent of their being fissured, with appropriate consideration first being given to use of enameloplasty, a sealant, or a preventive resin or conservative composite restoration (see Extension for Prevention: Enameloplasty, Sealant, Preventive Resin, or Conservative Composite Restoration). At times, this may necessitate extending onto the facial or lingual surfaces (particularly the facial surface of the mandibular molar and the lingual surface of the maxillary molar). The methods of including the facial or lingual fissures and pits are discussed under amalgam (Chapter 17), composite (Chapter 13), and gold restorations (Chapter 20).

For faulty pits on the lingual surfaces of maxillary anterior teeth and occlusal two-thirds of the lingual and facial surfaces of molars, the extent of caries or defect and provision of minimal manipulative access are the chief criteria for preparation extension.

Outline form and initial depth for smooth-surface lesions. Smooth-surface lesions occur in two very different locations: (1) proximal surfaces or (2) the gingival portion of the facial and lingual surfaces (see Fig. 6-2, *B* and *C*). For discussion of outline features and initial depth in initial tooth preparation, each location must be considered separately.

Proximal Surfaces (Classes II, III, and IV). The proximal surface presents another controlling factor in establishing outline form, namely, the location of the contact area in relation to the adjacent tooth.

Rules for establishing outline forms for proximal surface tooth preparations

1. Extend the preparation margins until sound tooth structure is obtained and no unsupported and/or weakened enamel remains. (Sometimes, unsupported but not friable enamel may remain in tooth preparations for bonded restorations.)

2. Avoid terminating the margin on extreme eminences such as cusp heights or ridge crests.

3. Extend the margins to allow sufficient access for proper manipulative procedures.

4. Restrict the axial wall pulpal depth of the proximal preparation to a maximum of 0.2 to 0.8 mm into dentin (the greater depth when the extension is onto the root surface; the lesser depth when no retention grooves will be placed). Typically, in this stage of tooth preparation for Class II amalgam restorations, which will have proximal retention locks, the cutting instrument (No. 245 bur) is positioned by being held parallel to the DEJ and thereby creating a cut approximately 0.3 mm into enamel with the remainder of the instrument diameter (approximately 0.5 mm) into dentin (see Fig. 6-1, *C*). During this initial cutting, portions of the instrument may be in air (from a void caused by

deeper caries) but it should not remove dentin caries that is deeper pulpally than 0.5 mm from the DEJ.

5. Usually, gingival margins of tooth preparations are extended apically of the proximal contact to provide a minimum clearance of 0.5 mm between the gingival margin and the adjacent tooth (see Fig. 17-44, *F*). Otherwise, this gingival extension is to sound tooth structure and no farther.

6. Likewise, the facial and lingual margins in proximal tooth preparations usually are extended into the respective embrasures to provide specified clearance between the prepared margins and the adjacent tooth. The purpose of this clearance is to place the margins away from close contact with the adjacent tooth so that the margins can be better visualized, instrumented, and restored (see Figs. 17-60, *A* and B; 17-63, *A* and B; 18-11; and 18-24). However, for a skilled operator it is permissible to leave the prepared facial or lingual margin in contact with the adjacent tooth, especially with Class II and Class III composite restorations. Obviously, proper margin preparation, matrix placement, and material insertion and finishing must be done.

In the Class II preparation involving two surfaces, the occlusal outline is governed by the factors that determine the placement of margins of pit-and-fissure lesions, and for inlays the preparation of a dovetail on the occlusal surface in the area of the occlusal pit opposite the involved proximal surface (see Chapter 20).

Note that when extending the proximal surface incisally *in Class III preparations, the incisal margin may be placed in the area of contact,* especially when an esthetic restorative material is used or when the incisal embrasure is not large enough to allow extension incisal of contact and still have a strong incisal angle of the tooth. An incisal margin of sound enamel in the contact area should not be extended incisally to clear the contact, unless necessary for instrumentation in tooth preparation or restoration, such as may be required in gold foil.

Gingival Portion of Facial and Lingual Surfaces (Class V). The outline form of Class V tooth preparations is governed ordinarily only by the extent of the lesion, except pulpally. Therefore extension mesially, gingivally, distally, and occlusally (incisally) is limited to reaching sound tooth structure; and during this initial tooth preparation, the bur depth is usually no deeper than 0.8 to 1.25 mm pulpally from the original (when unaffected) tooth surface. The lesser axial wall depth (0.8 mm) is at a gingival wall without an enamel portion (i.e., the margin is on the root surface; see Fig 6-1, A). The correct axial wall pulpal depth at the occlusal (incisal) wall is that which provides a 0.5 mm extension into dentin (the remainder being enamel). Infected caries deeper than these described depths should not be removed by the cutting instrument during this initial preparation stage.

Restricted and Increased Extensions. Conditions that may warrant consideration of restricted or reduced extensions for smooth-surface tooth preparations are: (1) proximal contours and root proximity, (2) esthetic requirements, and (3) the use of some tooth preparations for composite restorations.

Some conditions that may necessitate increased extensions for smooth-surface tooth preparations are: (1) mental or physical handicaps, (2) advanced age of the patient, (3) restoration of teeth as partial denture abutments or as units of a splint, (4) need for additional measures for retention and resistance form, and (5) need to adjust tooth contours.

Enameloplasty. Sometimes a pit or groove (fissured or not) does not penetrate to any great depth into the enamel and does not allow proper preparation of tooth margins, except by undesirable extension. This is always true of the end of a fissure. If such a shallow feature is removed and the convolution of the enamel is rounded or "saucered," the area becomes cleanable, finishable, and allows conservative placement of preparation margins. This procedure of reshaping the enamel surface with suitable rotary cutting instruments is termed enameloplasty (see Fig. 6-28). Specific applications of this procedure are covered and illustrated in detail in chapters pertaining to tooth preparations for inlay and amalgam restorations (see Figs. 17-8 and 20-5, *A* and B). *Enameloplasty does not extend the outline form.* The amalgam or gold restorative material is not placed into the recontoured area, and thus the only difference in the restoration is that the thickness of the restorative material at the enameloplastied margin (or pulpal depth of the external wall) is decreased. This differs from including adjacent faulty enamel areas in composite restorations because those areas are covered with the bonded composite material. Such inclusions may restore carious, decalcified, discolored, or poorly contoured areas.

The operator must be selective in the choice of areas on which enameloplasty is performed. Usually a fissure should be removed by normal preparation procedures if it penetrates to more than one-third the thickness of the enamel in the area. If one-third or less of the enamel depth is involved, the fissure may be removed by enameloplasty without preparing or extending the tooth preparation. This procedure is applicable also to supplemental grooves (fissured or not) extending up cusp inclines. If the ends of these grooves were included in the tooth preparation, the cusp could be weakened to the extent that it would need to be capped. Provided these areas are "saucered" by enameloplasty, the cusp strength can be retained and a smooth union effected between the restorative material and the enamel margin, because the grooved enamel is eliminated.

Another instance in which enameloplasty is indicated is on a shallow fissure that approaches or crosses a lingual or facial ridge (see Fig. 20-20). This fissure, if extended under tooth extension principles, would involve two surfaces of the tooth. Use of the enameloplasty procedure can often confine the tooth preparation to one surface and produce a smooth union of the tooth surface and restorative material. An example would be the lingual fissure of a mandibular first molar that terminates on the occlusolingual ridge. Conventional extension should terminate when approximately 2 mm of tooth structure remains between the bur and the lingual surface, and the remainder of the fissure then reshaped, provided the terminal portion of the fissure is no more than one-third of the enamel in depth. Otherwise, the tooth preparation must be extended onto the lingual surface (see Fig. 20-20).

As specific tooth preparations are detailed, several additional applications of enameloplasty will be cited. It also may be applied to teeth in which no preparation is anticipated. However, extreme prudence must be used in the selection of these areas and the depth of which the enamel is removed. This procedure should not be used unless the fissure can be made into a groove with a saucer base by a minimal reduction of enamel and unless centric contacts can be maintained. For composite preparations, it may be appropriate to seal shallow fissures with sealant or composite material, without any mechanical alteration to the fissure.

Step 2: Primary Resistance Form. While extending the external preparation walls to sound tooth structure, the shape and form of the preparation walls must be initiated. Depending on the restorative material to be used, and especially in Classes I, II, and IV restorations, the preparation wall design at this initial stage should provide for both protection against fracture from forces delivered in the tooth's long axis (primary resistance form) and retention of the material in the tooth against forces in reverse.

Definition. Primary resistance form may be defined as *that shape and placement of the preparation walls that best enable both the restoration and the tooth to withstand, without fracture, masticatory forces delivered principally in the* *long axis of the tooth.* (For protection principally against oblique forces, see Step 7—Secondary Resistance and Retention Forms, and Final Tooth Preparation Stage.) The relatively flat pulpal and gingival walls prepared perpendicular to the tooth's long axis help resist forces in the long axis of the tooth and prevent tooth fracture from wedging effects (Fig. 6-29).

Principles. The fundamental principles involved in obtaining primary resistance form are: (1) to use the box shape with a relatively *flat floor,* which helps the tooth resist occlusal loading by virtue of being at right angles to those forces of mastication that are directed in the long axis of the tooth; (2) to *restrict the extension* of the external walls (keep as small as possible) to allow strong cusp and ridge areas to remain with sufficient dentin support; (3) to have a *slight rounding* (coving) *of internal line angles* to reduce stress concentrations in tooth structure; (4) in extensive tooth preparations, to *cap weak cusps and envelope or include enough of a weakened tooth* within the restoration to prevent or resist fracture of the tooth by forces both in the long axis and obliquely (laterally) directed (most resistance to oblique or lateral forces is attained later in the final tooth preparation stage); (5) to provide enough *thickness of restorative material* to prevent its fracture under load; and (6) to bond the material to tooth structure when appropriate. Conventional and beveled conventional preparation designs provide these resistance form principles. Modified tooth preparation designs are for small-to-moderate size composite restorations and may not provide uniform pulpal or axial depths or minimal thickness for the material. However, any bonded restoration results in increased resistance form, as discussed later.

During extension of external walls to sound tooth in developing outline form in conventional Classes I and II preparations, the end of the cutting instrument prepares a relatively flat pulpal wall of uniform depth into the tooth (1.5 to 2 mm overall depth or 0.2 mm into dentin) (see Fig. 6-1, *A* and *C*). *The pulpal wall, therefore, is as flat as the original occlusal surface and the DEJ (these roughly paralleling each other).* This semblance of flatness (see

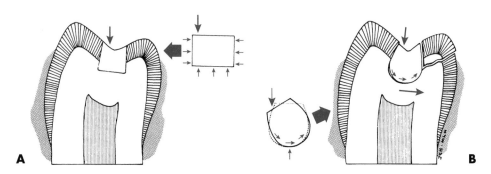

FIG. 6-29 Resistance forms must consider resistance of tooth to fracture from forces exerted on restoration. Flat floor **(A)** will help prevent restoration movement, whereas rounded pulpal floor **(B)** may allow a nonbonded restoration rocking action producing a wedging force, which may result in shearing of tooth structure.

Fig. 6-29) is perpendicular to those masticatory forces directed nearly in the long axis of the tooth, and thus is ideal for the stable seating of a restoration that can best *resist* such forces without fracture of the tooth (both wedging forces on the tooth or tilting forces on the restoration are unlikely). Following the same principle, in the proximal portion of conventional Class II preparations, the end of the cutting instrument prepares a *gingival wall (floor) that is flat* and relatively perpendicular to these forces. A modified preparation design for a composite restoration may resemble a scooped appearance, rather than having uniform depths or wall configurations. Such preparation form may not enhance resistance form, but the restoration is bonded and therefore adequate resistance to tooth or restoration fracture is obtained.

Minimally extended facial and lingual walls conserve dentin supporting the cusps as well as facial and lingual ridges, thereby maintaining as much strength of the remaining tooth structure as possible. This resistance is against obliquely delivered forces, as well as those in the tooth's long axis.

Internal and external angles within the tooth preparation are slightly rounded (coved) so that stresses in the tooth and restoration from masticatory forces will not be as concentrated at these line angles.[28] Rounding internal line angles (those with apices directed internally) reduces the stress on the tooth, thus *resistance* to fracture of the tooth is increased. Rounding external angles (those with apices directed externally [e.g., axiopulpal line angles]) reduces the stress on some restorative materials (amalgam and porcelain), thus increasing resistance to fracture of the restorative material. Details regarding these tooth preparation modifications are described in Chapters 14 and 17 to 20 (see Fig. 6-32).

A tooth weakened by extensive caries deserves consideration of the fourth principle (capping weakened cusp(s) and/or extending to include cusp[s] entirely) in obtaining primary resistance form during tooth preparation. In extensive caries, facial or lingual extension of the pulpal or gingival walls indicates: (1) reduction of weak cusps for capping by the restorative material (see rules for cusp reduction in the following Features section; see Figs. 6-27, 19-8, and 20-22), and/or (2) extension of gingival floors around axial tooth corners onto facial or lingual surfaces (see Figs. 17-71 and 20-25, *J* through *P*). Either of these features provides some *resistance* both to forces in the long axis and to those obliquely (laterally) directed.

Restorative material thickness affects the ability of a material to resist fracture. The minimal occlusal thickness for amalgam for appropriate resistance to fracture is 1.5 mm, cast metal 1 to 2 mm (depending on the region), and porcelain 2 mm. Composite restorative materials may have more acute marginal angles, and although no specific thickness dimension has been noted

for strength, most composite restorations are 1 to 2 mm thick.

Bonded restorations increase the strength of the weakened unprepared tooth structure.[5] Therefore enhanced resistance form results from bonding a material to the prepared tooth.

When considering the resistance form in anterior proximoincisal preparations (Class IV), one must recognize the narrowness faciolingually of the anterior teeth (and therefore the lesser dentinal support) in applying the principles of obtaining resistance form.

In pulpless teeth, special consideration is applied in obtaining resistance form because of the weakened nature of the remaining structure.[12] The weakened cusps may need to be reduced, enveloped, and covered with restorative material to prevent the cracking or splitting of the remaining tooth structure in accord with the fourth principle mentioned previously. Methods of cusp protection are discussed in Chapters 13, 17, 19, and 20. Placement of a bonded restoration into pulpless teeth may reduce the need for cusp reduction.

Factors. The need to develop resistance form in a preparation is a result of several factors. Certain conditions must be assessed to reduce the potential for fracture of either the restoration or the tooth. Foremost is the assessment of the occlusal contact on both the restoration and the remaining tooth structure. Obviously, the greater the occlusal force and contacts, the greater is the potential for future fracture (e.g., the further posterior the tooth, the greater is the effective masticatory force because the tooth is closer to the condyle head).

The amount of *remaining tooth structure* also affects the need and type of resistance form. Very large teeth, even though extensively involved with caries or defects, may require less resistance form consideration, especially in regard to capping cusps, because the remaining tooth structure is still bulky and strong enough to resist fracture. Weakened, friable tooth structure should always be removed in the preparation, but sometimes unsupported, but not friable, enamel may be left. This is usually for esthetic reasons in anterior teeth, especially on the facial surfaces of maxillary teeth where stresses are minimal and a bonded restoration typically is used.

The type of *restorative material* also dictates resistance form needs. Amalgam requires a minimum occlusal thickness of 1.5 mm for adequate strength and longevity in relation to wear. Cast metal requires less thickness to resist fracture but should still have a dimension of at least 1 mm in areas of occlusal contact, even though the marginal dimensions of cast metal restorations are thinner. Ceramics require a minimum dimension of 2 mm to resist bulk fracture. The dimensional needs of composite are more dependent on the occlusal wear potential of the restored area. In posterior teeth, the thickness requirement is greater than for anterior teeth. Composite can be used in thinner applications such as veneers or minor esthetic enhancements as long as the wear potential is considered.

The last factor relates to the enhancement of resistance form simply by bonding a restoration to the tooth. Bonding amalgam, composite, or ceramic to prepared tooth structure increases the strength of the remaining unprepared tooth, thereby reducing the potential for fracture.[5] In fact, the benefits of bonding procedures may permit the operator to leave a portion of the tooth in a more weakened state than usual or not to cap a cusp.

Features. The design features of tooth preparation that enhance primary resistance form are as follows and are discussed in more detail in the technique chapters:

1. Relatively flat floors
2. Box shape
3. Inclusion of weakened tooth structure
4. Preservation of cusps and marginal ridges
5. Rounded internal line angles
6. Adequate thickness of restorative material
7. Reduction of cusps for capping when indicated

Reduction of cusps, when indicated, occurs as early as possible in the preparation to improve access and visibility. Obviously the decision to reduce a cusp (for capping) is very important and should be approached judiciously. Although the cusp size and occlusal considerations may affect the decision, a basic rule guides the reduction of cusps during initial tooth preparation. This *rule* is: (1) cusp reduction should be *considered* when the outline form has extended *half the distance from a primary groove to a cusp tip,* and (2) cusp reduction usually is mandatory when the outline form has extended *two-thirds the distance from a primary groove to a cusp tip* (see Fig. 6-27). The exception to capping a cusp where extension has been two-thirds from a primary groove toward the cusp tip is when the cusp is unusually large and the operator judges that adequate cuspal strength remains, or when a bonded restoration is being used and the operator judges the bonding to provide for adequate remaining cuspal strength.

Although specific preparation form is necessarily associated with a bonded composite restoration, preparation walls left in a roughened state increase the surface area for bonding and therefore enhance both resistance and retention forms. More roughened preparation walls, enamel, and dentin may be prepared with coarse diamond instruments.

Step 3: Primary Retention Form. During initial tooth preparation, not only does the form and shape of the preparation need to provide resistance against fracture, but also the design of the preparation must provide for the retention of the restorative material in the tooth for nonbonded restorations (Fig. 6-30). Often, features that enhance the retention form of a preparation

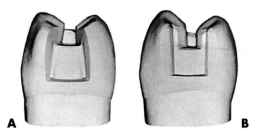

FIG. **6-30** Basic primary retention form in Class II tooth preparations for amalgam **(A)** with vertical external walls of proximal and occlusal portions converging occlusally and for inlay **(B)** with similar walls slightly diverging occlusally.

also enhance the resistance form (e.g., pins placed in a manner so that one portion of a tooth supports another portion of the tooth).

Definition. Primary retention form is that shape or form of the conventional preparation that resists displacement or removal of the restoration from tipping or lifting forces. In many respects, retention form and resistance form are accomplished in the same cutting procedure and are sometimes discussed together. Although they are separate entities, the same prepared form may contribute to both the resistance and retention qualities of the preparation.

The retention form developed during initial tooth preparation may be adequate to retain the restorative material in the tooth. Sometimes, however, additional retention features must be incorporated in the final stage of tooth preparation.

Principles. Because retention needs are related to the restorative material used, the principles of primary retention form vary depending on the material.

For *amalgam* restorations in most Class I and all Class II conventional preparations, the material is retained in the tooth by developing external tooth *walls that converge occlusally* (see Fig. 6-30, *A*). In this way, once the amalgam is placed in the preparation and hardens, it cannot dislodge without some type of fracture occurring. In these preparations, the facial and lingual walls of the occlusal portion of the preparation, as well as the proximal portion, converge toward the occlusal surface. This convergence should not be overdone for fear of leaving unsupported enamel rods on the cavosurface margin of the occlusal surface. The occlusal convergence of the proximal portion has several advantages in addition to producing retention. It allows slight facial and/or lingual extension of the proximal portion of the preparation in the gingival area while conserving the marginal ridge, thus reducing the forces of mastication on critical areas of the restoration. The cavosurface angle where the proximal facial and lingual walls meet the marginal ridge is a desirable 90 degrees because of the occlusal convergence of the preparation.

In other conventional preparations for amalgam (such as Classes III and V), the external walls diverge outwardly to provide strong enamel margins, and therefore *retention coves or grooves* are prepared in the dentinal walls to provide the retention form (see Step 7: Secondary Resistance and Retention Forms).

Adhesive systems provide some retention by micromechanically *bonding amalgam to tooth structure and also reducing or eliminating microleakage.*[2] However, until longevity studies demonstrate that bonding systems provide complete retention form, traditional retention features should be provided for amalgam restorations, especially for root-surface restorations.

Composite restorations primarily are retained in the tooth by a *micromechanical bond* that develops between the material and *etched and primed prepared tooth structure.* In such restorations, the enamel and dentin are etched by an acid and the dentin is primed with a dentin bonding agent. These procedures are discussed in a subsequent section, Final Tooth Preparation Stage, and in Chapters 11 to 15. Sometimes the tooth preparation for a composite restoration also requires the use of mechanical retention form, which is considered part of the final stage of preparation and is presented in Chapters 11 to 15. As an example, in a Class V composite tooth preparation on the root surface, groove retention may be recommended in addition to the use of a bonding system. Because of the strong and rapid bond that is developed between etched enamel and composite, the initial tooth preparation of many composite restorations should result in a beveled or flared (greater than 90 degrees) enamel marginal configuration that is ready to be etched. These would be considered the modified composite tooth preparations. Other conventional-type composite restorations may require a separate enamel beveling procedure that would be done in final tooth preparation. When bevels are placed on a conventional preparation, the design is then a beveled conventional preparation.

Cast metal (usually a gold alloy) *intracoronal restorations* rely primarily on almost parallel vertical (longitudinal) walls to provide retention of the casting in the tooth. During initial tooth preparation, the preparation walls must be designed not only to provide for draw or draft (in order for the casting to be placed into the tooth) but also to provide for an appropriate *small angle of divergence* (2 to 5 degrees per wall) from the line of draw that will enhance *retention form.* The degree of divergence needed primarily depends on the length of the prepared walls: the greater the vertical height of the walls, the more divergence is permitted and recommended, but within the range described.

In inlay and onlay preparations for cast metal restorations, the opposing vertical walls diverge outwardly by only a few degrees to each other and to a draw path that is usually perpendicular to the floor of the preparation (see Fig. 6-30, *B*). Having sufficient length of these almost parallel walls allows enough frictional resistance and mechanical locking of the luting agent into minute irregularities of both the casting and the preparation walls to counteract the pull of sticky foods. Close parallelism of prepared vertical walls is a principal retention form for cast metal restorations, another being the use of a luting agent that bonds to tooth structure.

In Class II preparations involving only one of the two proximal surfaces, an occlusal dovetail may aid in preventing the tipping of the restoration by occlusal forces. When an unusually large amount of retention form is required, the occlusal dovetail may be placed whether or not caries is on the occlusal surface. The dovetail simulates a Class I occlusal preparation in the area opposite the proximal involvement (see Fig. 20-6).

Another consideration in obtaining retention form, in addition to compensating for the forces of mastication, is the pull of sticky foods. In all cases, the preparation design must provide for the retention of the restorative material in the tooth. Although features of primary retention form are very important, sometimes additional, secondary retentive features are necessary in the final stage of tooth preparation, usually for nonbonded restorations.

Factors. The factors that affect primary retention form already have been presented.

Features. Likewise, the features of primary retention form already were presented.

Step 4: Convenience Form. *Convenience form is that shape or form of the preparation that provides for adequate observation, accessibility, and ease of operation in preparing and restoring the tooth.* On occasion, obtaining this form may necessitate extension of distal, mesial, facial, or lingual walls to gain adequate access to the deeper portion of the preparation. An example of this is the preparation and restoration of a mesial (or distal) root surface carious lesion (see Fig. 17-62). However, the arbitrary extension of facial margins on anterior teeth usually is contraindicated for esthetic reasons.

In preparations for gold foil, convenience form assumes an additional purpose other than accessibility for instrumentation (see Chapter 21). It includes establishing convenience points for the starting of foil condensation. These are prepared by deepening, or making more acute, one or more point angles of the preparation. Usually proper refinement of the line and point angles of Class I and Class V preparations is sufficient to produce the necessary convenience form, but additional accentuation may be practiced if desired. The most common application of convenience points is in the gingival area of proximal preparations and is for the convenience of the operator in starting the condensation of the foil. These angles or points are placed with small instruments and should not be "sunk" into the gingival floor.

The occlusal divergence of vertical (longitudinal) walls of tooth preparations for Class II cast restorations also may be considered as convenience form. Extending proximal preparations beyond proximal contacts is another convenience form procedure. Although exceptions may be made to such an extension, preparing the proximal walls to obtain clearance with an adjacent proximal surface affords better access to finish the preparation walls and the restorative material. For cast restorations, clearance with the adjacent proximal surface is mandatory to finish the preparation walls, make an accurate impression of the prepared tooth, and try in the casting.

FINAL TOOTH PREPARATION STAGE

Once the extensions and wall designs have fulfilled the objectives of initial tooth preparation, the preparation should be inspected carefully for other needs. With conservative amalgam or composite restorations, the preparation may be complete after initial tooth preparation except for: (1) sealing the prepared walls for amalgam or (2) etching and priming the prepared walls for the bonding agent(s) for amalgam or composite. Often, however, additional steps (steps 5 through 9) are needed in the final tooth preparation stage. These steps are discussed in the following sections.

Step 5: Removal of Any Remaining Enamel Pit or Fissure, Infected Dentin, and/or Old Restorative Material, if Indicated. In teeth in which the carious lesion is minimal, the carious enamel and dentin are probably removed in completing the initial tooth preparation. If, however, carious infected dentin remains after completion of the previous steps, it should be removed now.

Definition. Removal of any remaining enamel pit or fissure, infected dentin, and/or old restorative material is the elimination of any infected carious tooth structure or faulty restorative material left in the tooth after initial tooth preparation. The exception to the removal of infected carious tooth structure is when it is decided to perform an indirect pulp cap as described in Caries Control Restoration in Chapter 3. Removal of remaining enamel pit or fissure typically occurs as small, minimally extended excavations on isolated faulty areas of the pulpal floor. Removal of defective old restorative material is addressed later in this section. However, in dentin, as caries progresses, an area of decalcification precedes the penetration of microorganisms. This area of decalcification often appears discolored in comparison with undisturbed dentin, yet it does not exhibit the soft texture of caries. This dentin condition may be termed affected dentin and differs from infected dentin in that it has not been significantly invaded by microorganisms. It is accepted and appropriate practice to allow affected dentin to remain in a prepared tooth.

The use of color alone to determine how much dentin to remove is unreliable. One risks the commitment to overcut on the one hand and to leave infected dentin on the other hand. Often soft, acute (rapid) caries manifests itself entirely within the normal range of color for dentin; thus the eye may not differentiate among infected, affected, or unaffected, normal dentin. On the other hand, distinctly discolored dentin, certainly affected, is often sound and comparable in hardness to surrounding unaffected, normal dentin.

A clinical description of exactly where infected dentin stops and affected dentin begins is practically impossible. It is an empirical decision enhanced by practical knowledge and experience, although some chemical, "caries-disclosing" dyes may aid that decision. Fortunately the decision does not require exactness, for it is not necessary that all dentin invaded by microorganisms be removed. In shallow or moderately deep lesions, the removal of the masses of microorganisms and the subsequent sealing of the preparation by a restoration at best destroy those comparatively few remaining microorganisms and at worst reduce them to inactivity or dormancy.[32] Even in deep caries in which actual invasion of the pulp may have occurred, the recovery of the pulp requires only that, between virulence of the organisms and resistance of the host, a favorable balance be established for the pulp. This is often accomplished by removing all soft caries with its numerous organisms.[39] Leaving carious dentin at the DEJ area is not acceptable (see Fig. 6-4, *A*; see also Residual Caries).

After initial tooth preparation, the initial depths may result in old restorative material remaining on the pulpal or axial walls. *Any remaining old restorative material should be removed if any of the following conditions are present:* (1) the old material may affect negatively the esthetic result of the new restoration (i.e., old amalgam material left under a new composite restoration), (2) the old material may compromise the amount of anticipated needed retention (i.e., old glass-ionomer material having a weaker bond to the tooth than the new composite restoration using enamel and dentin bonding), (3) radiographic evidence indicates caries is under the old material, (4) the tooth pulp was symptomatic preoperatively, or (5) the periphery of the remaining old restorative material is not intact (i.e., there is some breach in the junction of the material with the adjacent tooth structure that may indicate caries under the old material). *If none of these conditions is present, the operator may elect to leave the remaining old restorative material to serve as a base, rather than risk unnecessary excavation nearer to the pulp, which may result in pulpal irritation or exposure.*

Techniques. When a pulpal or axial wall has been established at the proper initial tooth preparation position and a small amount of infected carious material remains, only this material should be removed, leaving a rounded, concave area in the wall. The level or position of the wall peripheral to the caries removal depression should not be altered.

In large preparations with extensive soft caries, the removal of infected dentin may be accomplished early in the initial tooth preparation. When the extensive caries is removed, the condition of both the pulp and the remaining tooth structure has a definite bearing on the type of restoration placed. For this reason, it is more expedient to remove extensive caries early in the tooth preparation before time and effort are spent in doing a tooth preparation for a certain restorative material that is then deemed inadequate for satisfactory restoration of the tooth.

Another instance in which the removal of caries is indicated early in tooth preparation is when a patient has numerous teeth with extensive caries. In one appointment, infected dentin is removed from several teeth and temporary restorations are placed. After all the teeth containing extensive caries are so treated, then individual teeth are restored definitively. This procedure stops the progress of caries and is often referred to as the *caries control technique* (see Chapter 3). It should be obvious that this practice allows many more teeth to remain serviceable than if a single, seriously involved tooth were treated to completion at the expense of others in the same condition in the same mouth.

Large areas of soft caries usually are best removed with spoon excavators by flaking up the caries around the periphery of the infected mass and peeling it off in layers. The bulk of this material is thus easily removed in a few large pieces.

Regarding the removal of the harder, heavily discolored dentin, opinions vary between the use of spoon excavators, round steel burs at very low speed, and round carbide burs rotating at high speeds. There are several considerations in the removal of this type of caries in deep-seated lesions, although basically the primary concern is for the pulp. Pulpal damage may result from the creation of frictional heat with the use of a bur. The pulp may become infected by forcing microorganisms into the dentinal tubules through excessive pressure with a spoon excavator, or it may be exposed when either instrument is used. The ideal method of removing this material would be one in which minimal pressure is exerted, frictional heat is minimized, and complete control of the instrument is available. *Consideration of these factors usually favors the use of a round carbide bur, in a high-speed handpiece, with air coolant and slow speed (just above stall-out).* This technique gives the operator complete control of the instrument, minimizes pressure and heat generation, and permits adequate vision of the area being operated on. *Examination of the area with an explorer following the removal of infected dentin is advisable, but should be done judiciously to avoid perforation into the pulp.* Caries that rapidly develops sometimes is relatively unstained, and unless the sense of touch is relied on to detect softness, the operator may unintentionally leave infected dentin. Ideally, removal of infected dentin should continue until the remaining dentin feels as hard as normal dentin. However, heavy pressure should not be applied with an explorer, or any other instrument, on what

is believed to be a thin layer of reasonably firm dentin next to a healthy pulp, for fear of creating an unnecessary pulpal exposure.

Removal of remaining old restorative material, when indicated, also is accomplished with use of a round carbide bur, at slow speed (just above stall-out) with air or air-water coolant. The water spray (along with high-volume evacuation) is used when removing old amalgam material to reduce the amount of *mercury vapor.*

Step 6: Pulp Protection, if Indicated. Although the placement of liners and bases is not a step in tooth preparation in the strict sense of the word, it is a step in adapting the preparation for receiving the final restorative material. Therefore a basic discussion of this subject follows.

The reason for using traditional liners or bases is to either protect the pulp or to aid pulpal recovery or both. However, often, neither liners nor bases are needed. When the thickness of the remaining dentin is minimal, *heat generated by injudicious cutting can result in a pulpal burn lesion, an abscess formation, or pulpal necrosis.* Thus a water or air-water spray coolant must be used with the high-speed rotary instrument. *Cutting the dentinal odontoblastic fibrils* that previously have not been exposed to any irritating episode such as caries or tooth wear will result in degeneration and death of the affected primary odontoblasts and their extensions. The involved tubules become open, dead tracts. Worse still, if the remaining dentin thickness is 1.5 mm or more and the cutting was done atraumatically using high speed with water or air-water spray, the pulp is not irritated enough to form replacement odontoblasts and therefore no reparative dentin is formed to seal the pulpal side of the dead tracts.

Other pulpal irritants that affect operative procedures are: (1) some ingredients of various materials; (2) thermal changes conducted through restorative materials; (3) forces transmitted through materials to the dentin; (4) galvanic shock; and, most importantly, (5) the ingress of noxious products and bacteria through microleakage.

Because the ingress of bacteria is most commonly associated with various pulpal responses, more emphasis should be given to the complete sealing of the prepared dentinal tubules. Effective tubular sealing will prevent penetration of bacteria or their toxins. Although one study[38] found calcium hydroxide to be more successful on vital pulp exposures on subhuman primates than bonding agents, other studies are reporting success using resin bonding agents on exposed pulps.[1,10,23] Although dentin bonding agents are being recognized as beneficial for dentinal sealing under any type of restorative material, another technique[46] also is being advocated. This technique results in the removal of the most coronal, potentially infected area of the pulpal tissue; placement of a calcium hydroxide liner over the excavated pulpal area; and then, placement of a resin-modified glass-ionomer liner over the calcium hydroxide. This technique is advocated when root canal therapy is not utilized on direct pulpal exposures. Currently, no scientific evidence supports this procedure. However, the pulpal tissue appears to be disinfected and necrosed by the calcium hydroxide and the area adequately sealed by the resin-modified glass ionomer, both of which may increase the success of a pulp-capping procedure.

As these technologies and techniques are developed further, more information will become available. If such technologies are scientifically substantiated, the presented use of liners, bases, and varnishes will be significantly altered if not eliminated. In spite of that likelihood, the following information is presented about traditional use of liners, bases, and varnishes/sealers.

Certain physical, chemical, and biologic factors should be considered in the selection of a traditional liner or base. The material used should be one that, under the circumstances, more nearly satisfies the needs of the individual tooth. The attainment of generic status by popularization is insufficient basis for selecting a particular material. Rather, selection should be based on an assessment of the anatomic, physiologic, and biologic response characteristics of the pulp, as well as the physical and chemical properties of the considered material.

In the following discussion of traditional liners and bases, the use of the term *liners is reserved for those volatile or aqueous suspensions or dispersions of zinc oxide or calcium hydroxide that can be applied to a tooth surface in a relatively thin film*[17] *and are used to affect a particular pulpal response.* Liners also may provide: (1) a barrier that protects the dentin from noxious agents from either the restorative material or oral fluids, (2) initial electrical insulation, and/or (3) some thermal protection. *Bases are considered those cements commonly used in thicker dimensions beneath permanent restorations to provide for mechanical, chemical, and thermal protection of the pulp.* Examples of bases include zinc phosphate; zinc oxide–eugenol; calcium hydroxide; polycarboxylate; and the most common, some type of glass ionomer.

A traditional liner is used to medicate the pulp when suspected trauma has occurred. The desired pulpal effects include both sedation and stimulation, the latter resulting in reparative dentin formation. The specific pulpal response desired dictates the choice of liner. If the removal of infected dentin does not extend deeper than 1 to 2 mm from the initially prepared pulpal or axial wall, usually no liner is indicated. *If the excavation extends into or very close to the pulpal tissue, a calcium hydroxide liner is usually selected to stimulate reparative dentin. In the past, if the excavation depth was between the above examples, a zinc oxide–eugenol liner may have been selected (except for composite restorations, for which it could impede the polymerization process) to provide a palliative, sedative pulpal response, thus decreasing the potential for postoperative sensitivity.* Now zinc oxide-eugenol liners

rarely are used and, instead, a glass-ionomer material would be used, but primarily as a base.

Both zinc oxide–eugenol and calcium hydroxide liners (chemosetting types that harden) in thicknesses of 0.5 mm or greater have adequate strength to resist condensation forces of amalgam[9] and provide protection against short-term thermal changes. However, when a very deep excavation occurs, it may be necessary to overlay the typical calcium hydroxide liner with a stronger base material. As a general rule, it is desirable to have approximately a 2-mm dimension of bulk between the pulp and a metallic restorative material. This bulk may include remaining dentin, liner, and/or base. The base materials offer greater pulpal protection from mechanical, thermal, and chemical irritants. However, *for composite restorative materials,* which are thermal insulators and passively inserted, *a liner of calcium hydroxide is indicated only when pulpal exposure or the excavation is judged to be within 0.5 mm of the pulp* and bases are not indicated.

The ability of calcium hydroxide to stimulate the formation of reparative dentin when it is in contact with pulpal tissue makes it the typical material of choice for application to very deep excavations and known pulpal exposures. As stated earlier, the use of resin bonding agents is also proposed for similar clinical situations. Very deep excavations may contain *microscopic pulpal exposures* that are not visible to the naked eye. Hemorrhage is the usual evidence of a vital pulp exposure, but with microscopic exposures, such evidence may be lacking. Nevertheless, these exposures are large enough to allow direct pulpal access for bacteria and fluids. *Liners and bases in exposure areas should be applied without pressure.* It is recommended to have approximately a 1-mm thickness of calcium hydroxide (chemoset) over near or actual exposures, which then may be overlaid with a base for amalgam or cast metal restorations.

When zinc phosphate, glass-ionomer, or polycarboxylate cement bases are used, tooth depth and the properties of prior liners determine the technique of placement. When there is known or suspected exposure to the pulp, care must be exercised against forcing material into the pulp chamber. Therefore it is essential to either first use a calcium hydroxide cement in adequate thickness or a nonpressure technique for placing an overlay base.

In instances when either an adequate thickness of calcium hydroxide liner has been placed over an exposure or the excavation is not deep enough to provide danger of forcing cement into the pulp chamber by pressure, a zinc-phosphate base material may be packed (condensed) into place. In these instances, the cement base is used in a puttylike consistency and may be conveyed to the preparation with a hand instrument. The cement base may then be shaped with appropriate hand instruments. A base of zinc phosphate placed in this manner has advantages of less free acid and often the elimination of the use of rotary instruments in forming the surface of the base.

Usually, however, a glass ionomer is used for most "base" needs. These materials effectively bond to tooth structure, contain fluoride, and have sufficient strength as a base. Furthermore, they are easily placed and contoured, when necessary. Because of their chemical and micromechanical bond to tooth structure, retentive preparation features are not required. These materials are excellent for bases under amalgam, gold, or ceramic restorations.

In tooth preparations for castings, deeply excavated areas must be covered with positively retained liner/base material that will withstand the subsequent procedural forces. Zinc phosphate, glass-ionomer, and polycarboxylate cements fulfill the requirements for such overlay base material. *Bases for cast restorations need to be positively retained against possible displacement in subsequent procedures.* Often undercuts resulting from removal of infected dentin provide retention for the cement base. However, for some tooth preparations, prepared undercuts must be provided to retain a nonbonding cement base. If this is the case, a small round bur is used to place small indentations in the excavation in dentin in areas away from the pulp. Usually two such undercuts opposing each other are sufficient to hold the cement base. The prepared undercuts need not be deeper than the diameter of the bur (see Figs. 20-10 and 20-11).

The protective qualities of zinc phosphate, polycarboxylate, and glass-ionomer cements are somewhat in proportion to the bulk of material used. Thus, a thin layer will not afford the protection of a thicker layer. However, *the level to which a base is built should never compromise the desired tooth preparation depth, resulting in inadequate restorative material thickness.*

No liner or base exhibits the crushing strength of amalgam. Therefore, in the placement of large amounts of these materials, *ideally there should be at least three seats, tripodally distributed, for the amalgam on sound dentin at the prescribed level of the pulpal wall in initial tooth preparation* (see Fig. 17-12, C). This will allow the restoration and the tooth structure, rather than the liner or base, to bear the load after the amalgam has set. However, when a bonded material is used, tripodal seats are less necessary.

Tooth varnish is a solution liner that was used in the past to seal dentinal tubules and was placed on all tooth preparation walls for amalgam and on dentinal walls of tooth preparations for cast gold, but was not used for composites. Tooth varnish usually was applied just before the insertion of an amalgam or cementation of a cast gold restoration. Two coats of tooth varnish were applied to the prepared surfaces for amalgams. Tooth varnish was the only material necessary for shallow excavations in such preparations. The varnish prevented penetration of materials into the dentin[18] and helped prevent microleakage.[44] Varnishes also helped reduce

postoperative sensitivity by reducing the infiltration of fluids and salivary components at the margins of newly placed restorations.[17]

Two coats of tooth varnish were applied to dentin surfaces (not on enamel walls) of tooth preparations for cast gold restorations. The varnish barrier helped reduce pulpal irritation from the luting cement.

Although varnishes were valuable in reducing postoperative sensitivity, their thin film thickness was insufficient to provide thermal insulation even when applied in two coats.[48] However, their presence significantly *reduced the diffusion of acid* from cements into dentin. Consequently, their use was recommended routinely, especially in deep preparations, with any restorative or cementing material containing acid.[17] *Tooth varnishes were not used under composites* because the solvent in the varnish could react with or soften the resin component in the composite, adversely affecting polymerization. Furthermore, the free monomer of the resin could dissolve the varnish film, rendering it ineffective.[17] Obviously, varnish was not to be applied to any prepared tooth walls that would be, or were, treated (etched and primed) for bonding. This textbook no longer recommends the use of tooth varnishes. Instead, sealers are recommended under nonbonded restorations and bonding systems are used for bonded restorations. The objective of both of these approaches is to seal the prepared dentin tubules. The nonbonded amalgam restoration should be sealed with Gluma Desensitizer[33] before amalgam placement. Similar materials may be used before cementing restorations with nonbonding luting agents. All bonded restorations (composites, amalgams, glass-ionomer–type materials and bonded indirect restorations) use various bonding systems that not only bond the material to the tooth but also seal the prepared tooth structure.

Darkening of tooth structure adjacent to an amalgam restoration is observed on occasion. This may be caused by the gradual diffusion of metallic ions into the dentin or by light passing through the translucent enamel that is reflected from the underlying amalgam.[28] Placement of a cement liner or base when replacing such a restoration decreases this unnatural appearance. This use of liner or base is for esthetic purposes rather than strictly for pulp protection. Completely sealing the prepared dentin before amalgam insertion prevents this diffusion.

Again, it should be mentioned that the historical use of traditional liners, bases, and varnishes has become obsolete as more focus is directed on the use of various agents to provide sealing of dentinal tubules. As evidence increases regarding the benefits of such materials, the use of traditional liners, bases, and varnishes may be limited only to clinical situations in which pulpal exposure has occurred; and yet, even that indication may eventually be eliminated in favor of the use of resin adhesives. Regardless of the materials used, protecting the pulp appropriately is mandatory for the successful restoration of teeth.

Step 7: Secondary Resistance and Retention Forms. After removal of any remaining enamel pit or fissure, infected dentin, and/or old restorative material (if indicated) and pulpal protection has been provided by appropriate liners and bases, additional resistance and retention features may be deemed necessary for the preparation. Many compound and complex preparations require these additional features. When a tooth preparation includes both occlusal and proximal surfaces, each of those areas should have independent retention and resistance features.

Because many preparation features that improve retention form also improve resistance form, and the reverse is true, they are presented together. *The secondary retention and resistance forms are of two types: (1) mechanical preparation features and (2) treatments of the preparation walls with etching, priming, and adhesive materials.* However, the second type is not really considered as a part of tooth preparation, but rather as the first step for the insertion of the restorative material. Regardless, some general comments are presented about such treatments.

Mechanical Features. A variety of mechanical alterations to the preparation enhance retention form, and these alterations require additional removal of tooth structure. They are discussed fully in the respective technique chapters but are briefly identified in the next five sections.

Retention locks, grooves, and coves. Vertically oriented retention locks and retention grooves are used to provide additional retention for proximal portions of some tooth preparations; the locks are for amalgams (see Fig. 17-54) and the grooves are for cast metal restorations (see Fig. 20-8). Horizontally oriented retention grooves are prepared in most Classes III and V preparations for amalgam (see Figs. 18-13 and 18-31) and in some root-surface tooth preparations for composite (see Fig. 12-41). Retention coves are appropriately placed undercuts for the incisal retention of Class III amalgams (see Fig. 18-14), occlusal portion of some amalgam restorations (see Fig. 17-38, *C* and *D*), some Class V amalgams (see Fig. 18-32), and occasionally for facilitating the start of insertion of certain gold foil restorations.

Retention locks in Class II preparations for amalgam restorations are generally thought to increase retention of the proximal portion against movement proximally due to creep. Also, they are believed to increase the resistance form of the restoration against fracture at the junction of the proximal and occlusal portions. In vivo studies do not substantiate the necessity of these locks in proximoocclusal preparations with occlusal dovetail outline forms or in MOD preparations.[42,47] However, they are recommended for extensive tooth preparations for amalgam involving, for example, wide faciolingual proximal boxes and/or cusp capping.

Groove extensions. Additional retention of the restorative material may be obtained by arbitrarily extending the preparation for molars onto the facial or lingual surface to include a facial or lingual groove. Such an extension when performed for cast metal restorations, results in additional vertical (longitudinal), almost-parallel walls for retention. This feature also enhances resistance for the remaining tooth due to envelopment (see Figs. 20-27, *I*, and 20-30, *I*).

Skirts. Skirts are preparation features used in cast gold restorations that extend the preparation around some, if not all, of the line angles of the tooth (see Figs. 20-29 and 20-30). When properly prepared, skirts provide additional, opposed vertical walls for added retention. The placement of skirts also significantly increases resistance form by enveloping the tooth, thereby resisting fracture of the remaining tooth from occlusal forces.

Beveled enamel margins. Both cast gold/metal and composite restorations include beveled marginal configurations. The bevels for cast metal may slightly improve retention form when there are opposing bevels, but are used primarily to afford a better junctional relationship between the metal and the tooth. Many enamel margins of composite restorations have a beveled or flared configuration to increase both the surface area of etchable enamel and to maximize the effectiveness of the bond by etching more enamel rod ends.

Pins, slots, steps, and amalgampins. When the need for increased retention form is unusually great, especially for amalgam restorations, several other features may be incorporated into the preparation. The use of pins and slots increases both retention and resistance forms (see Figs. 19-1 and 19-42). Amalgampins and properly positioned steps also improve retention form, but not to the extent of pins or slots. All of these procedures are described in Chapter 19.

Placement of Etchant, Primer, or Adhesive on Prepared Walls. In addition to mechanical alterations to the tooth preparation, certain alterations to the preparation walls by actions of various materials also afford increased retention, as well as resistance to fracture. Both enamel and dentin surfaces may be treated with etchants and/or primers for certain restorative procedures. Although such treatment is considered the first step in the insertion of the restorative material, some general comments are presented here.

Enamel wall etching. Enamel walls are etched for bonded restorations that use porcelain, composite, or amalgam materials. This procedure consists of etching the enamel by an appropriate acid, resulting in a microscopically roughened surface to which the bonding material is mechanically bound.

Dentin treatment. Dentinal surfaces may require etching and priming when using bonded porcelain, composite, or amalgam restorations. The actual treatment varies with the restorative material used, but for most composite restorations, a dentin bonding agent is recommended. Sometimes a glass-ionomer material is used as a base before the restoration of the tooth with another restorative material, usually amalgam. The advantages and disadvantages of this technique are presented in Chapters 11 through 19.

Lastly, it should be noted that retention of indirect restorations (fabricated extraorally) is enhanced by the luting agent used. Although not considered part of the tooth preparation, the cementation procedure does affect the retention of these restorations, and some cementing materials do require pretreatment of the dentin, resulting in varying degrees of micromechanical bonding.

Step 8: Procedures for Finishing the External Walls of the Tooth Preparation. Finishing the external walls of the preparation entails consideration of both degree of smoothness and cavosurface design, since each restorative material has its maximum effectiveness when the appropriate conditions are developed for that specific material. Not all preparations require special finishing of the external walls at this stage, because the walls may already have been finished during earlier steps in the preparation. This is particularly true for many composite preparations and most amalgam preparations.

Because most preparations have external walls in enamel, most of the following discussion relates to the appropriate finishing of enamel walls. Nevertheless, when a preparation has extended onto the root surface (no enamel present), the root-surface cavosurface angle should be either 90 degrees (for amalgam, composite, or porcelain restorations) or beveled (for intracoronal cast metal restorations). The 90-degree root-surface margin provides a butt joint relationship between the restorative material and the cementum/dentin preparation wall, a configuration that provides appropriate strength to both. The beveled root-surface margin for cast metal restorations provides the benefits addressed in later paragraphs of this section.

Definition. Finishing the preparation walls is the further development, when indicated, of a specific cavosurface design and degree of smoothness or roughness that produces the maximum effectiveness of the restorative material being used.

Objectives. The objectives of finishing the prepared walls are to: (1) create the best marginal seal possible between the restorative material and the tooth structure, (2) afford a smooth marginal junction, and (3) provide maximum strength of both the tooth and the restorative material at and near the margin. The following *factors* must be considered in the finishing of enamel walls and margins: (1) the direction of the enamel rods, (2) the support of the enamel rods both at the DEJ and laterally (preparation side), (3) the type of restorative material to be placed in the preparation, (4) the location of the margin, and (5) the degree of smoothness or roughness desired.

Theoretically, the enamel rods radiate from the DEJ to the external surface of the enamel and are perpendicular to the tooth surface. All rods extend full length from the dentin to the enamel surface. The rods converge from the DEJ toward concave enamel surfaces and diverge outwardly toward convex surfaces. In general, therefore, the rods converge toward the center of developmental grooves and diverge toward the height of cusps and ridges (see Fig. 6-2, *B* and *C*). In the gingival third of enamel of the smooth surfaces in the permanent dentition, the rods incline slightly apically (see Fig. 6-33).

In some instances, the rods of occlusal enamel appear to be harder than those of axial (mesial, facial, distal, lingual) enamel. This can be attributed to the amount of interlacing or twisting of the rods in the former as compared with the straight rods of the latter. Enamel with such interlacing of the rods is termed *gnarled enamel* (see Fig. 2-7).

Having a thorough knowledge of the direction of the enamel rods on various tooth surfaces, the operator should create all enamel walls so that all rods forming the prepared enamel wall have their inner ends resting on sound dentin. Enamel rods that do not run uninterrupted from the preparation margin to dentin tend to split off, leaving a V-shaped ditch along the cavosurface margin area of the restoration (see Fig. 17-48). This should not be interpreted that all enamel walls should consist of full-length rods. *The strongest enamel margin is one that is composed of full-length enamel rods supported on the preparation side by shorter enamel rods, all of which extend to sound dentin* (Fig. 6-31). The shorter enamel rods buttress the full-length enamel rods that form the margin, thus increasing the strength of the enamel margin (see Fig. 17-6, *B*).

An acute, abrupt change in an enamel wall outline form results in fracture potential, even though the enamel may have dentin support. This indicates that the preparation outline and walls should have smooth curves or straight lines. When two enamel walls join,

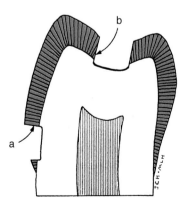

FIG. **6-31** All enamel walls must consist of either full-length enamel rods on sound dentin *(a)* or full-length enamel rods on sound dentin supported on preparation side by shortened rods also on sound dentin *(b)*.

the resulting line angle may be "sharp." If so, it should be slightly curved ("softened"). This slight rounding usually results in a similar curve at the margin. It is to be understood that this discussion is not about cavosurface (marginal) bevels. In other words, *line angles formed by the junction of enamel walls should be slightly rounded whether they are obtuse or acute* (Fig. 6-32).

Features. As already stated, finishing of external walls has two primary features: (1) the design of the cavosurface angle, and (2) the degree of smoothness or roughness of the wall.

The *design of the cavosurface angle* is dependent on the restorative material being used. Because of the low edge strength or friability of amalgam, a tooth preparation cavosurface angle of 90 degrees produces maximal strength for both the amalgam and the tooth. Thus, no bevels are placed at the cavosurface margin. On occlusal surfaces for Class I and Class II amalgam restorations, the incline planes of the cusp and the converging walls (for retentive purposes) of the preparation approximate the desirable 90-degree butt joint junction, even though the actual occlusal enamel margin may be greater than 90 degrees. However, as shown in Fig. 17-26, when extending the facial and lingual walls *to remove extensive occlusal caries, tilting the bur is often indicated to conservatively extend the margins and provide a 90- to 100-degree cavosurface angle. The extent of this alteration in bur orientation is dictated by the inclination of the contiguous unprepared enamel surfaces.*

Beveling the external walls is a preparation technique used for some materials such as intracoronal cast gold/metal and composite restorations. Occasionally, some margins in preparations for gold foil are beveled, but these bevels form a cavosurface angle much less obtuse than for gold/metal castings and composites.

Beveling can serve four useful purposes in the tooth preparation for a casting: (1) it produces a stronger enamel margin, (2) it permits a marginal seal in slightly undersized castings, (3) it provides marginal metal that is more easily burnished and adapted, and (4) it assists in adaptation of gingival margins of castings that fail to seat by a very slight amount. The bevel of the margin in a preparation for castings should produce a cavosurface angle that results in 30- to 40-degree marginal metal (see Figs. 20-12 to 20-14). The marginal gold alloy will be too thin and weak if the angle of the gold bevel is less than 30 degrees. If the angle is greater than 40 degrees, the marginal gold will be too thick and therefore too difficult to burnish satisfactorily. The steepness of cuspal inclines is a factor when beveling *occlusal margins,* even eliminating the need for a bevel when inclines are very steep. (See Fig. 20-14 for developing 140-degree occlusal cavosurface margins.) The *gingival margin* of a casting is a very critical one; an improper beveling of this area may lead to early failure of the restoration. Providing 30-degree beveled metal in this area results in a sliding, lap fit that definitely improves adaptation of metal to tooth at this margin (see Fig. 20-12).

Ceramic materials belong to that category of materials that contraindicated beveling the cavosurface margins. When amalgam is used, beveling also is contraindicated, except on the gingival floor of a Class II preparation when enamel is still present. In these instances, it is usually necessary to place a slight *bevel (approximately 15 to 20 degrees) only on the enamel portion of the wall to remove unsupported enamel rods.* This is necessary because of the gingival orientation of enamel rods in the cervical area of the tooth crown. This minimal bevel may be placed with an appropriate gingival margin trimmer hand instrument and, once placed, still results in a 90-degree amalgam marginal angle (Fig. 6-33). Sometimes the unsupported enamel rods are removed simply by an explorer tip pulled along the margin. If the angle of marginal amalgam is less than 80 to 90 degrees (90 degrees is best), it is likely to fracture because it has low edge strength. Such a fracture leaves a crevice at the interface. Thus, the external walls of amalgam preparations must be designed to result in an approximately 90-degree amalgam marginal angle.

Beveling enamel margins in composite preparations is primarily indicated for larger restorations that have increased retention needs. The use of a beveled marginal form with a composite tooth preparation may be advocated because the potential for retention is in-

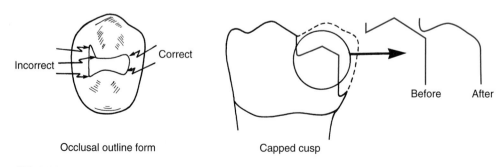

Incorrect   Correct

Occlusal outline form

Before   After

Capped cusp

F I G. **6-32** The junctions of enamel walls (and respective margins) should be slightly rounded, whether obtuse or acute.

creased by increasing the surface area of enamel available for etch and having a more effective area of etch obtained by etching the cut ends of the enamel rods. Other advantages of beveling composites are: (1) adjacent, minor defects can be included with a bevel, (2) esthetic quality may be enhanced by a bevel creating an area of gradual increase in composite thickness from the margin to the bulk of the restoration, and (3) the marginal seal may be enhanced.

The *degree of desired smoothness or roughness* is the second consideration in finishing external walls. Although both the selection of finishing instruments and the methods of finishing enamel walls are reserved for sections describing specific types of preparations, the reasoning for finishing procedures is reviewed in this section. The advent of high-speed cutting procedures has produced two pertinent factors related to finishing enamel walls: (1) the lessening of tactile sense and (2) the rapid removal of tooth structure. Performing enamel finishing with high speed can be, and is, accomplished by the highly skilled and experienced operator; however, in the hands of inexperienced operators, high speed can lead to overextension of margins, grooved walls, and/or rounded cavosurface angles, especially on proximal margins. If this method is used, *plain-cut fissure burs produce the finest surface.*[21] These burs produce a smoother surface than crosscut burs, diamonds, or carborundum stones.[7] In fact, at stall-out speeds with an air-turbine handpiece, an excellent finish is achieved with this type of bur.

In instances when proximal margins are left at minimal extension for esthetic reasons, rotating instruments (burs, stones, wheels, or discs) may not be usable because of lack of proper access. In such locations, *hand instruments* may need to be used. The planing action of a razor-sharp hand instrument can result in a smooth enamel wall, although it may not be as smooth as that achieved with other instruments.[40] Hand instruments such as enamel hatchets and margin trimmers may be used in planing enamel walls, cleaving enamel, and establishing enamel bevels. Their usefulness in this capacity should not be overlooked.

The restorative material used is the primary factor dictating the desired smoothness or roughness of an enamel wall. The prepared walls of inlay or onlay preparations require a very smooth surface to permit undistorted impressions and close adaptation of the casting to the enamel margins.[8] In areas of sufficient access, fine sandpaper discs can create a very smooth surface; however, proper use of hand instruments, plain fissure burs, or fine diamond stones also create satisfactory enamel margins for cast preparations. On the other hand, prepared walls and margins of composite restorations can be roughened, usually by a course diamond stone, to provide increased surface area for bonding.

Likewise, when using *gold foil or amalgam restorative materials, a very smooth preparation wall is not as desirable as for cast restorations.* When these materials are used, it has been demonstrated[29] that a more rough surface prepared wall markedly improves resistance to marginal leakage. This does not mean, however, that finishing of the enamel wall should be ignored, but it does indicate that no strict rule for the selection of the finishing instrument can be applied in all instances.

Step 9: Final Procedures: Cleaning, Inspecting, and Sealing. Final procedures in tooth preparation include the cleaning of the preparation, inspecting the preparation, and applying a sealer when indicated. Treatment of the preparation wall, when appropriate, with etchant, primer, or adhesive is reviewed but is considered the first step in material insertion. The first procedure includes removing all chips and loose debris that have accumulated, drying the preparation (do not desiccate), and making a final complete inspection of the preparation for any remaining infected dentin, unsound enamel margins, or any condition that renders the preparation unacceptable to receive the restorative material. Naturally, most of the gross debris has been removed during the preparation steps, but some fine debris usually remains on the prepared walls after all cutting is completed.

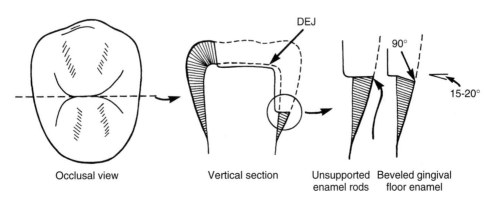

Occlusal view   Vertical section   Unsupported   Beveled gingival
                                                 enamel rods   floor enamel

F I G. **6-33** Vertical section of Class II cavity preparation. Gingival floor enamel (and margin) is unsupported on dentin and friable unless removed.

The usual procedure in cleaning is to free the preparation of visible debris with warm water from the syringe and then to remove the visible moisture with a few light surges of air from the air syringe. (Regarding moisture on the dentinal surface, be mindful that dentin bonding systems have specific requirements for etching, priming, and applying the bonding agent, which usually is hydrophilic). In some instances, debris will cling to the walls and angles despite the above efforts, and it may be necessary to loosen this material with an explorer or small cotton pellet. After all the visible debris has been removed, the preparation is dried free of visible moisture. It is important *not to dehydrate the tooth by overuse of air* or by the application of alcohol. Once the preparation has been cleaned adequately, it is *visually inspected* to confirm its appropriateness.

Composite restorations, which are bonded to the tooth, require some treatment of the preparation before insertion of the restorative material. This treatment usually includes etching the enamel and dentin and placing a dentin bonding agent. Some of these steps were presented earlier in this chapter (see Step 7—Secondary Resistance and Retention Forms) and are discussed in detail in Chapters 11 to 15. In all cases, the *smear layer* is either altered or removed and a hybrid layer is formed, which is characterized by an intermingling of the resin adhesive (bonding agent) with collagen fibrils of the intertubular dentin. This creates a strong mechanical bond between the composite and the dentin. Additional strong mechanical bonding occurs between the composite and the etched enamel, when enamel is present.

In accomplishing the final procedures before insertion of the restorative material, sterilization of the preparation may be considered. Although the term *sterilization* is used in the discussion of this topic, "disinfection" would be a more accurate term to describe the objective. However, because much of the literature uses the term "sterilization," it is used here as well. The act of sterilizing a preparation before inserting a restoration may be a logical procedure. Some operators do place medicaments in preparations for sterilization purposes, based on empirical factors. Others who have studied this procedure find the literature controversial on the subject of preparation sterilization.

The dentin tubule lumen, varying from 1 to 4 μm in diameter at varying distances between the DEJ and the pulp, certainly presents sufficient size for the entrance of microorganisms. Investigators have verified the presence of microorganisms in dentin tubules beneath preparation walls. However, this fact in no way indicates that caries is progressing or that failures will automatically result. As early as 1943, Besic[3] contended that caries in dentin stops or gradually ceases as soon as the carious lesion is closed to the oral environment, even if microorganisms remain in dentin. Investigators have noted that the number of bacteria in the dentin tubules is relatively small compared with the numerous microorganisms found in the superficial carious lesion. The question is whether these remaining organisms are capable of extending caries under the environmental circumstances of a restored tooth.[39]

Of course, the possible infection of the pulp is always a consideration when bacteria remain in a channel that terminates in the pulp chamber. In this respect, the resistance of vital tissue to the ingress of bacteria must be considered. In many instances, the presence of reparative dentin deposited as a result of pulpal insult constitutes a significant deterrent to bacterial progress. Another possible answer as to why all teeth with carious involvement do not eventually have pulpal infection is that bacteria may be in a dormant condition as the result of the more sealed environment of a restored tooth.

The basic considerations in preparation sterilization follow: (1) Is the agent used effective? (2) Is it capable of maintaining a sterile field? (3) Is it harmful to the pulp?

Early investigators[30] indicated that the common antiseptics once used routinely for preparation sterilization were effective only as a surface disinfectant when applied for a limited amount of time. Therefore, simply swabbing the preparation with such agents as silver nitrate, phenol, or ethyl alcohol only leads to a false sense of security. If some of these agents were allowed to remain for a longer period of time, to permit penetration of the tubules, irreparable pulpal damage would result.[11] In deep preparations microscopic pulp exposures are not always visible to the naked eye, and the placement of harmful sterilization agents in such preparations would likely produce pulpal damage.

Assuming that a surface disinfectant is successful, it is doubtful that the sterilization can exist for any appreciable length of time because of the difference between the thermal coefficients of expansion of the tooth and filling materials.[18,19] Although differing in amounts, marginal leakage has been demonstrated for most restorative materials.[31,44,45] However, a large percentage of unsterilized restorations exhibits no caries on the internal wall as a result of this oral fluid penetration; therefore it is possible that the natural defense mechanism of the tooth or the germicidal action of the restorative material destroys any invading bacteria. The germicidal or protective effect ranges from the fluoride content of some materials to the deposition of corrosive products at the interface of the preparation wall in an amalgam. Zinc oxide–eugenol cement has significant germicidal properties over an extended period of time. Therefore some protection from further carious action is afforded by some restorative materials.[35]

The objective of the previous discussion is not to determine whether preparation sterilization via medicaments is essential or nonessential in the practice of sound dentistry but to ascertain if it is justified in routine procedures. *The routine use of specific sterilization medicaments should no longer be a strong consideration.* However, as stated previously, the use of dentin bonding agents (for bonded restorations) and sealers (for nonbonded restorations) to effect a dentin tubular seal is recognized. *Eliminating bacterial penetration is so important that the use of dentin bonding agents or sealers will likely become universal (under all restorations).*

ADDITIONAL CONCEPTS IN TOOTH PREPARATION

A thorough understanding of the principles and concepts of tooth preparation must be obtained by an effective operative dentist. Applying those to a specific restorative procedure, combined with appropriate operating skills and proper handling of the restorative materials will result in successful treatment. Because many new techniques are being advocated for the restoration of teeth, the operator must assess each such proposed method of treatment on the basis of the fundamentals of tooth preparation presented in this chapter. Understanding these fundamental principles makes the assessment of new approaches easier and wiser.

Because amalgam and composite restorations are done more often than other operative procedures, most of the proposed new ways to restore teeth relate to these types of restorations.

AMALGAM RESTORATIONS

Several *new restorative techniques* have been advocated for use with amalgam restorations. In assessing these and future proposals, *the operator must remember the fundamental requirements for a successful amalgam preparation.* These prerequisites for success are: (1) 90-degree junctions of amalgam with tooth structure, (2) mechanical retention form, and (3) adequate thickness for the amalgam material.

Amalgam Box-Only Tooth Restorations. Box-only tooth preparations for amalgam may be advocated for some posterior teeth in which a proximal surface requires restoration, but the occlusal surface is not faulty (see Fig. 17-61). A proximal box is prepared and specific retention form is provided, but no occlusal step is included. Such restorations obviously are more conservative, in that less tooth structure is removed. That conservation of tooth structure must be weighed against possible loss of retention form provided by the occlusal step of a typical Class II amalgam preparation.

Amalgam Tunnel Tooth Restorations. In an effort to be conservative of tooth structure removal, others advocate a tunnel tooth preparation. This preparation joins an occlusal lesion with a proximal lesion by means of a prepared tunnel under the involved marginal ridge. In this way, the marginal ridge remains essentially intact.

In assessing this technique, the adequacy of preparation access may be controversial. Developing appropriately formed preparation walls and excavating caries may be compromised by lack of access and visibility. Whether or not the marginal ridge is preserved in a strong state also is controversial. This technique is controversial and not supported in this textbook.

Adhesive Amalgam Restorations. Other techniques advocated for amalgam restorations use adhesive systems. Some of these materials bond the amalgam material to tooth structure. Others seal the prepared tooth structure with an adhesive resin before amalgam placement. Although the proposed bonding techniques vary, the essential procedure is to prepare the tooth similar to typical amalgam preparations except that more weakened, remaining tooth structure may be retained. Next, the preparation walls are treated or covered with specific adhesive lining materials that mechanically bond to both the tooth and the amalgam. The amalgam is condensed onto or into this resin-lining material before polymerization and a bond develops between the amalgam and resin liner. The technique for the adhesive resin liner is different in that the adhesive resin is placed and polymerized before the amalgam placement.

COMPOSITE RESTORATIONS

Likewise, there are *new concepts* relating to the use of composite to restore teeth. Some of the newer concepts relating to preparations for composite restorations are presented in Chapters 11 to 15. In these chapters modified, more conservative, preparations are presented as well as preparations relating to expanded uses of composite such as for composite inlays, esthetic enhancements, the conservative composite restoration of posterior occlusal surfaces, the preventive resin restoration, veneers, and porcelain inlays cemented with composite materials. In addition to those concepts, several others should be addressed.

Again, it is *imperative that the operator understands the requirements of successful composite restorations* when assessing any proposed modifications. For a composite restoration to be successful, (1) most marginal enamel should have a beveled or flared form and all should be etched; (2) dentin bonding systems should be used; and (3) nonenamel (root surface) external walls should provide butt joint shapes, when necessary, and have appropriately placed mechanical retention form.

Composite Box-Only Tooth Restorations. The box-only preparations for composite restorations are similar to those for amalgam restorations, except the box form is less distinct, having "roughed out" marginal configurations rather than refined, 90-degree butt joints. The prepared tooth structure (both enamel and dentin) is etched and/or primed; which provides the retention form of the material in the tooth.

Composite Tunnel Tooth Restorations. The tunnel preparation, as described above, also has been advocated for composite restorations. Usually it also is advocated to use a glass-ionomer liner under the composite, and some suggest this preparation design be partially or completely restored with a glass-ionomer restorative material. The same disadvantages exist as with amalgam tunnel restorations and therefore this technique is not recommended in this textbook.

"Sandwich" Technique. Another proposed treatment is the use of a *glass-ionomer or flowable composite material as a liner* under some composite restorations. The advantages of this technique for glass-ionomer materials are purported to be: (1) the glass-ionomer material bonds both to the tooth structure and the composite, thereby increasing retention form; (2) fluoride contained in the glass-ionomer material reduces the potential for recurrent caries; and (3) the glass-ionomer material, because of its bond to tooth structure, provides a better seal when used at non-enamel margins. These suggested advantages are controversial. For the flowable composite as a liner under a composite, the purported advantages are: (1) it acts as a shock absorber, distributing stresses applied to the more rigid composite, and (2) it may reduce some of the negative effects of polymerization shrinkage.

Some considerations an operator must make about the "sandwich" technique are: (1) Is the retention increased or decreased? (2) Is the resistance form of the restoration compromised because the composite does not rest on tooth structure? (3) Does the preparation need to be deeper into the tooth to provide enough space for both materials? (4) Is the esthetic result sometimes compromised? (5) Do clinical research results support these claims?

BONDED RESTORATIONS STRENGTHEN WEAKENED TOOTH STRUCTURE

Another issue is that the placement of a bonded composite or bonded amalgam restoration will bind remaining portions of weakened tooth structure together. The bond created between etched enamel and composite is very strong and not only is adequate to hold the composite in the tooth, but also strengthens the remaining unprepared tooth structure. The use of a large composite restoration or a bonded amalgam may be a valid alternative to more complex and expensive cast restorations for badly broken-down posterior teeth. A consideration in using this concept must still be the occlusal relationship of the involved tooth. If some centric contact remains on a nonrestored portion of the occlusal surface, a large composite restoration may withstand any minor possible loss of surface integrity caused by wear. If, however, all the occlusal contact is on the restorative material, the wear rate of the composite may be greater even though the wear resistance of many composites is similar to amalgams. Wear of the bonded amalgam is not a problem.

Some of these new concepts in restoring teeth will become accepted methods of treatment. Because the adhesive amalgam and large bonded composite restorations are successful and can improve the strength of the tooth,

TABLE 6-1	Tooth Preparation: Amalgam Vs. Composite	
	AMALGAM	**COMPOSITE**
Outline form	Include fault	Same
	May extend to break proximal contact	Same
	Include adjacent suspicious area	No
		Seal these areas
Pulpal depth	Uniform 1.5 mm	Remove fault; not usually uniform
Axial depth	Uniform 0.2 to 0.5 mm inside DEJ	Remove fault; not usually uniform
Cavosurface margin	Create 90-degree amalgam margin	90 or greater degrees
Bevels	None (except gingival?)	Large preparation, esthetics, and seal
Texture of prepared walls	Smoother	Rough
Cutting instrument	Burs	Diamonds
Primary retention form	Convergence occlusally	None (roughness/bonding)
Secondary retention form	Grooves, slots, locks, pins, bonding	Bonding; grooves for very large or root-surface preparation
Resistance form	Flat floors, rounded angles, box-shaped, floors, perpendicular to occlusal forces?	Same for large preparations; No special form for small-to-moderate size preparations
Base indications	Provide ~2 mm between pulp and amalgam	Not needed
Liner indications	Ca(OH)$_2$ over direct or indirect pulp caps	Same
Sealer	Gluma Desensitizer when not bonding	Sealed by bonding system used

the need for their use is substantial. Because of the aging population, the need for the restoration of teeth having large existing, but failing restorations will be increased, and these treatment modalities may provide a technique that is relatively fast, inexpensive, stress free, and reliable.

SUMMARY

This chapter has addressed the principles of tooth preparation. Specific tooth preparation techniques are presented in various chapters later in the textbook. What should be apparent at this time is that a tooth preparation is determined by many factors, and each time a tooth is to be restored, each of these factors must be assessed. Tooth preparation for composite restorations is simpler and more conservative than for amalgam restorations because of the physical requirements necessary for amalgam (Table 6-1). If the principles of tooth preparation are followed, the success of any restoration is greatly increased. No two tooth preparations are the same.

To summarize, numerous factors should be considered before initiating a tooth preparation. Box 6-1 lists many of these factors, but it is not all inclusive.

The increasing bond strengths of enamel and dentin bonding are likely to result in significant emphasis on *adhesive restorations*. Likewise, *the improved ability to bond to tooth structure will likely continue to alter the entire tooth preparation procedure*. When materials can be effectively bonded to a tooth while restoring the inherent strength of the tooth, the need for refined tooth preparations is reduced or eliminated. The only factors necessary then for successful tooth restoration will be the ability and knowledge to: (1) completely remove infected dentin and friable enamel; (2) appropriately treat the enamel and dentin with etchant, primer, and adhesive; (3) properly manipulate the to-be-bonded restorative material;

and (4) contour the restoration to provide proper form and function. *Thus emphasis will shift away from traditional tooth preparation to knowledge of restorative materials and dental anatomy.*

REFERENCES

1. Akimoto N et al: Biocompatibility of Clearfil Liner Bond 2 and Clearfil AP-X systems on nonexposed and exposed primate teeth. *Quintessence Int* 29(3): 177-188, 1998.
2. Ben-Amar A: Reduction of microleakage around new amalgam restorations, *J Am Dent Assoc* 119:725, Dec 1989.
3. Besic FC: The fate of bacteria sealed in dental cavities, *J Dent Res* 22:349, 1943.
4. Black GV: *Operative dentistry*, ed 8, 2 vols, Woodstock, Ill, 1947-1948, Medico-Dental.
5. Boyer DB, Roth L. Fracture resistance of teeth with bonded amalgams. *Am J Dent* 7(2):91-94, 1994.
6. Bronner FJ: Mechanical, physiological, and pathological aspects of operative procedures, *Dent Cosmos* 73:577, 1931.
7. Cantwell KR, Aplin AW, Mahler DB: Cavity finish with high-speed handpieces, *Dent Progr* 1:42, Oct 1960.
8. Charbeneau GT, Peyton FA: Some effects of cavity instrumentation on the adaptation of gold castings and amalgam, *J Prosthet Dent* 8:514, 1958.
9. Chong WF, Swartz ML, Phillips RW: Displacement of cement bases by amalgam condensation, *J Am Dent Assoc* 74(1):97, 1967.
10. Cox CF, Suzuki S: Re-evaluating pulp protection: calcium hydroxide liners vs cohesive hybridization, *J Am Dent Assoc* 125: 823-831, 1994.
11. Englander HR, James VE, Massler M: Histologic effects of silver nitrate on human dentin and pulp, *J Am Dent Assoc* 57:621, 1958.
12. Frank AL: Protective coronal coverage of the pulpless tooth, *J Am Dent Assoc* 59:895, 1959.
13. Fusayama T: *A simple pain free adhesive restorative system by minimal reduction and total etching*, St Louis, 1993, Ishiyaku EuroAmerica.
14. Fusayama T: Two layers of carious dentin: diagnosis and treatment, *Oper Dent* 4:63-70, 1979.
15. Fusayama T, Okuse K, Hosoda H: Relationship between hardness, discoloration, and microbial invasion in carious dentin, *J Dent Res* 45(4):1033-1046, 1966.
16. Gilmore HW et al: *Operative dentistry*, ed 4, St Louis, 1982, Mosby.
17. Going RE: Status report on cement bases, cavity liners, varnishes, primers, and cleaners, *J Am Dent Assoc* 85:654, 1972.
18. Going RE, Massler M: Influence of cavity liners under amalgam restorations on penetration by radioactive isotopes, *J Prosthet Dent* 11:298, 1961.
19. Going RE, Massler M, Dute HL: Marginal penetration of dental restorations by different radioactive isotopes, *J Dent Res* 39:273, 1960.
20. Guard WF, Haack DC, Ireland RL: Photoelastic stress analysis of buccolingual sections of Class II cavity restorations, *J Am Dent Assoc* 57:631, 1958.
21. Hartley JL, Hudson DC: *Clinical evaluation of devices and techniques for the removal of tooth structure*, Randolph Air Force Base, Texas, 1959, Air University.
22. Hyatt TP: Prophylactic odontotomy: the ideal procedure in dentistry for children, *Dent Cosmos* 78:353, 1936.
23. Kanca J III: Replacement of a fractured incisor fragment over pulpal exposure: a long-term case report. *Quintessence Int* 27(12):829-832,1996.

░░░ **6-1**	Factors to Consider Before Tooth Preparation

Extent of caries	Extent of defect
Occlusion	Pulpal protection
Pulpal involvement	Contours
Esthetics	Economics
Patient's age	Patient's risk status
Patient's homecare	Bur design
Gingival status	Radiographic
Anesthesia	assessment
Bone support	Other treatment factors
Patient's desires	Patient cooperation
Material limitations	Fracture lines
Operator skill	Tooth anatomy
Enamel rod direction	Ability to isolate area
Extent of old restorative material	

24. Lee WC, Eakle WS: Possible role of tensile stress in the etiology of cervical erosive lesions of teeth, *J Prosthet Dent* 52(3): 374-380, 1984.

25. Markley MR: Restorations of silver amalgam, *J Am Dent Assoc* 43:133, Aug 1951.

26. Marzouk MA et al: *Operative dentistry*, ed 1, St Louis, 1985, Ishiyaku EuroAmerica.

27. Marzouk MA et al: *Operative dentistry*, ed 1, St Louis, 1985, Ishiyaku EuroAmerica.

28. Massler M, Barber TK: Action of amalgam on dentin, *J Am Dent Assoc* 47:415, 1953.

29. Menegale CM, Swartz ML, Phillips RW: Adaptation of restorative materials as influenced by the roughness of cavity walls, *J Dent Res* 39:825, 1960.

30. Muntz JA, Dorfman A, Stephan RM: In vitro studies on sterilization of carious dentin: evaluation of germicides, *J Am Dent Assoc* 30:1893, 1943.

31. Nelson RJ, Wolcott RB, Paffenbarger GC: Fluid exchange at the margins of dental restorations, *J Am Dent Assoc* 44:288, 1962.

32. Reeves R, Stanley HR: The relationship of bacterial penetration and pulpal pathosis in carious teeth, *Oral Surg* 22:59, July 1966.

33. Schupbach P, Lutz F, Finger WJ. Closing of dentinal tubules by Gluma Desensitizer. *Eur J Oral Sci*, 105:414-421, Oct 1997.

34. Shafer WG, Hines MK, Levy BM: *Textbook of oral pathology*, ed 4, Philadelphia: 1983, WB Saunders.

35. Shay DE, Allen TJ, Mantz RF: Antibacterial effects of some dental restorative materials, *J Dent Res* 35:25, Feb 1956.

36. Simonsen RJ: Preventive resin restoration, *Quintessence Int* 9(1):69-76, 1978.

37. Sockwell CL: Dental handpieces and rotary cutting instruments, *Dent Clin North Am* 15:219, Jan 1971.

38. Stanley HR: Criteria for standardizing and increasing credibility of direct pulp capping studies. *Amer J Dent* 11 (special issue): S17-S334, 1998.

39. Stanley HR: *Human pulp response to operative dental procedures*, Gainesville, Fla, 1976, Storter Printing.

40. Street EV: Effects of various instruments on enamel walls, *J Am Dent Assoc* 46:274, 1953.

41. Sturdevant CM et al: *The art and science of operative dentistry*, ed 1, New York, 1968, McGraw-Hill.

42. Sturdevant JR et al: Clinical study of conservative designs for Class II amalgams (abstract 1549), *J Dent Res* 67:306, 1988.

43. Sturdevant RE: A further study of inlay problems, *J Am Dent Assoc* and *Dent Cosmos* 25:611, 1938.

44. Swartz ML, Phillips RW: In vitro studies on the marginal leakage of restorative materials, *J Am Dent Assoc* 62:141, Feb 1961.

45. Swartz ML et al: Role of cavity varnishes and bases in the penetration of cement constituents through tooth structure, *J Prosthet Dent* 16:963, 1966.

46. Swift EJ, Trope M: Treatment options for the exposed vital pulp, *Pract Periodont Aesthet Dent* 11(6):735-739, 1999.

47. Terkla LG, Mahler DB, Eysden JV: Analysis of amalgam cavity design, *J Prosthet Dent* 29:204, Feb 1973.

48. Voth ED, Phillips RW, Swartz ML: Thermal diffusion through amalgam and various liners, *J Dent Res* 45:1184, 1966.

Instruments and Equipment for Tooth Preparation

STEPHEN C. BAYNE

JEFFREY Y. THOMPSON

CLIFFORD M. STURDEVANT*

DUANE F. TAYLOR*

*These authors are inactive this edition. See the Acknowledgments.

HAND INSTRUMENTS FOR CUTTING

The removal and shaping of tooth structure are essential aspects of restorative dentistry. Initially this was a difficult process accomplished entirely by the use of hand instruments. The introduction of rotary, powered cutting equipment was one of the truly major advances in dentistry. From the time of the first hand-powered dental drill to the present-day air-powered handpiece, tremendous strides have been made in the mechanical reduction of tooth structure, and thus in the ease with which teeth can be restored. Modern high-speed equipment has eliminated the need for many hand instruments for tooth preparation. Nevertheless, hand instruments remain an essential part of the armamentarium for quality restorative dentistry.

The early hand-operated instruments, with their large, heavy handles (Fig. 7-1) and inferior (by present standards) metal alloys in the blades, were cumbersome, awkward to use, and ineffective in many situations. Likewise, there was no uniformity of manufacture or nomenclature. Many dentists made their own hand instruments in an effort to find a suitable instrument for a specific need. As the commercial manufacture of hand instruments increased and dentists began to express ideas on tooth preparation, it became apparent that some scheme for identifying these instruments was necessary. G.V. Black,[6] among his many contributions to modern dentistry, is credited with the first acceptable *nomenclature for and classification of hand instruments.* His classification system enabled both dentists and manufacturers to communicate more clearly and effectively in regard to instrument design and function.

Modern hand instruments, when properly used, produce beneficial results for both the operator and the patient. It should be noted that some of these results can be satisfactorily achieved only with hand instruments, and not with rotary instruments. Preparation form dictates some circumstances in which hand instruments are to be used, whereas accessibility dictates others.

MATERIALS

Hand cutting instruments are manufactured from two main materials: *carbon steel* and *stainless steel.* In addition, some instruments are made with *carbide* inserts to provide more durable cutting edges. Carbon steel is harder than stainless steel, but when unprotected, it will corrode. Stainless steel remains bright under most conditions but loses a keen edge during use much more quickly than does carbon steel. Carbide, although hard and wear resistant, is brittle and cannot be used in all designs.

Other alloys of nickel, cobalt, or chromium are used in the manufacture of hand instruments, but they usually are restricted to instruments other than those used for the cutting of tooth structures.

Hardening and Tempering Heat Treatments. To gain maximal benefits from carbon steel or stainless steel, the manufacturer must submit them to two heat treatments: hardening and tempering. The hardening heat treatment hardens the alloy, but it also makes it brittle, especially when the carbon content is high. The tempering heat treatment relieves strains and increases toughness. These properties are optimized by the manufacturer. Subsequent heating of hand instruments during dental use can alter the original properties of the alloy and render it unserviceable. Flaming or improper sterilizing procedures can easily ruin a well-manufactured instrument.

Effects of Sterilization. Methods of sterilization are sporicidal cold disinfection, boiling water, steam under pressure (autoclave), chemical vapor, and hot air (dry heat). (See Chapter 8 for details regarding acceptable methods of sterilization.) Sterilizing carbon steel instruments by any of the first three methods causes *discoloration, rust, and corrosion.* However, several methods for protecting against or minimizing these problems are available. One method used by the manufacturer is to electroplate the instrument. This affords protection, except on the blade, where use and sharpening remove the plating. The plating also may pit or peel on the handle and shank under certain circumstances. A second method of protection is by use of rust inhibitors, which are soluble alkaline compounds. These are usually incorporated into commercial sporicidal cold disinfectant solutions, and special preparations are available for use in boiling water and autoclaves. The third method of minimizing the effect of moisture is to remove the instruments promptly at the end of the recommended

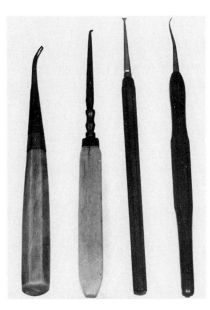

F I G. **7-1** Designs of some early hand instruments. These instruments were individually handmade, variable in design, and cumbersome to use. Because of nature of the handles, effective sterilization was a problem.

sterilizing period, dry them thoroughly, and place them in the instrument cabinet or on the tray setup. Leaving instruments exposed to moisture for extended periods or overnight is definitely contraindicated.

The boiling water or autoclave methods of sterilization do not produce discoloration, rust, or corrosion of stainless steel instruments. However, prolonged immersion in cold disinfectant solutions may cause rust. It is advisable to leave stainless steel instruments exposed to moisture only for the recommended time. Dry-heat sterilizers do not rust and corrode carbon steel instruments, but the high heat may reduce the hardness of the alloy, which would reduce the ability of the instruments to retain a sharp cutting edge.

The choice of alloy in the hand instrument is up to the operator, but whichever is selected to suit the immediate needs will soon prove unsatisfactory if proper manipulation and sterilization are not continually followed.

TERMINOLOGY AND CLASSIFICATION

Instrument Categories. The hand instruments used in the dental operatory may be categorized as: (1) cutting (excavators, chisels, and others) or (2) noncutting (amalgam condensers, mirrors, explorers, probes).[6] *Excavators* may be further subdivided into *ordinary hatchets, hoes, angle formers,* and *spoons. Chisels* are primarily used for cutting enamel and may be further subdivided into *straight chisels, curved chisels, bin-angle chisels, enamel hatchets,* and *gingival margin trimmers.* Other cutting instruments may be subdivided as *knives, files, scalers,* and *carvers.* In addition to the cutting instruments, there is also a very large group of noncutting instruments (see Fig. 17-21, *D* and *E*).

Instrument Design. Most hand instruments, regardless of use, are composed of three parts: *handle, shank,* and *blade* (Fig. 7-2). For many noncutting instruments, the part corresponding to the blade is termed the *nib.* The end of the nib, or working surface, is known as the *face.* The blade or nib is the working end of the instrument and is connected to the handle by the shank. Some instruments have a blade on both ends of the handle and are known as *double-ended instruments.* The blades are of many designs and sizes, depending on the function they are to perform.

Handles are available in various sizes and shapes. Early hand instruments had handles of quite large diameter and were grasped in the palm of the hand. A large, heavy handle is not always conducive to delicate manipulation. In North America, most instrument handles are small in diameter (5.5 mm) and light. They are commonly eight-sided and knurled to facilitate control. In Europe, the handles are often larger in diameter and tapered.

Shanks serve to connect the handles to the working ends of the instruments. They are normally smooth, round, and tapered. Shanks often have one or more bends to avoid the instrument having a tendency to twist in use when force is applied.

Enamel and dentin are difficult substances to cut and require the generation of substantial forces at the tip of the instrument. Hand instruments must be balanced and sharp. Balance allows for the concentration of force onto the blade without causing rotation of the instrument in the grasp. Sharpness concentrates the force onto a small area of the edge, producing a high stress (see Mechanical Properties in Chapter 4).

Balance is accomplished by designing the angles of the shank so that the cutting edge of the blade lies within the projected diameter of the handle and nearly coincides with the projected axis of the handle (Fig. 7-3; see also Fig. 7-2). For optimal antirotational design, the blade edge must not be off axis by more than 1 to 2 mm. All dental instruments and equipment need to satisfy this principle of balance.

Instrument Shank Angles. The functional orientation and length of the blade determines the number of angles necessary in the shank to balance the instrument. G.V. Black[5] classified instruments based on the number of shank angles, as *mon-angle* (one), *bin-angle* (two), or *triple-angle* (three).

Instruments with small, short blades may be easily designed in mon-angle form, while confining the cutting edge within the required limit. Instruments with longer blades or more complex orientations may require two or three angles in the shank to bring the cutting edge near to the long axis of the handle. Such shanks are termed *contra-angled.*

Instrument Names. Black classified all instruments by *name.* In addition, for hand cutting instruments, he developed a numeric *formula* to characterize the dimen-

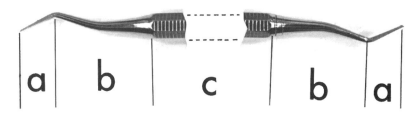

FIG. **7-2** Double-ended instrument illustrating three component parts of hand instruments: blade *(a)*, shank *(b)*, and handle *(c)*.

sions and angles of the working end (see the next section for details of the formula). Black's classification system[5] by instrument name categorized instruments by (1) function (e.g., scaler, excavator), (2) manner of use (e.g., hand condenser), (3) design of the working end (e.g., spoon excavator, sickle scaler), or (4) shape of the shank (e.g., mon-angle, bin-angle, contra-angle). These names were combined to form the complete description of the instrument (e.g., bin-angle spoon excavator).

Operative Cutting Instrument Formulas. Cutting instruments have *formulas* describing the dimensions and angles of the working end. These are placed on the handle using a code of three or four numbers separated by dashes or spaces (e.g., 10-8.5-8-14) (see Fig. 7-3). The first number indicates the *width of the blade* or primary cutting edge in tenths of a millimeter (0.1 mm) (e.g., 10 = 1 mm). The second number of a four-number code

indicates the *primary cutting edge angle,* measured from a line parallel to the long axis of the instrument handle in clockwise centigrades. The angle is expressed as a percent of 360 degrees (e.g., 85 = 85% × 360 degrees = 306 degrees). The instrument is positioned so that this number always exceeds 50. If the edge is locally perpendicular to the blade, then this number is normally omitted, resulting in a three-number code. The third number (second number of a three-number code) indicates the *blade length* in millimeters (e.g., 8 = 8 mm). The fourth number (third number of a three-number code) indicates the *blade angle,* relative to the long axis of the handle in clockwise centigrade (e.g., 14 = 50 degrees). For these measurements, the instrument is positioned so that this number is always 50 or less. The most commonly used hand instruments, including those specified in this text, are shown in Figs. 7-5 through 7-9 *with their formulas indicated.*

In some instances, an additional number on the handle is the manufacturer's identification number. It should not be confused with the formula number. It is simply to assist the specific manufacturer in cataloging and ordering.

Cutting Instrument Bevels. Most hand cutting instruments have on the end of the blade a *single bevel* that forms the *primary cutting edge.* Two additional edges, called *secondary cutting* edges, extend from the primary edge for the length of the blade (Fig. 7-4). *Bibeveled* instruments, such as ordinary hatchets, have two bevels that form the cutting edge (Fig. 7-5, *A*).

Certain single-beveled instruments, such as spoon excavators (Fig. 7-6) and gingival margin trimmers (Fig. 7-7, *B* and *C*), are used with a scraping or lateral cutting motion. Others, such as enamel hatchets (see Fig. 7-7, *A*), may be used with a planing or direct cutting motion, as well as a lateral cutting motion. For such single-beveled designs, the instruments must be made in pairs, having the bevels on opposite sides of the blade. Such instruments are designated as *right* or *left* beveled and are indicated by appending the letter R or L to the instrument formula. To determine whether the instrument has a *right* or *left bevel,* the primary cutting edge is held down and pointing away, and if the bevel appears on the right side of the blade, it is the right instrument of the pair. This instrument, when used in a scraping motion, is moved from right to left. The opposite holds true for the left instrument of the pair.

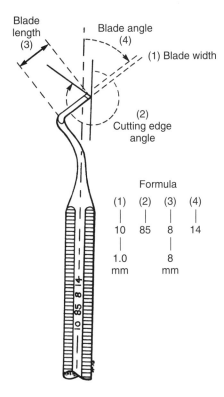

FIG. 7-3 Instrument shank and blade design (with primary cutting edge positioned close to handle axis to produce *balance*). The complete instrument formula (four numbers) is expressed as the *blade width* (1) in 0.1-mm increments, *cutting edge angle* (2) in centigrades, *blade length* (3) in millimeters, and *blade angle* (4) in centigrades.

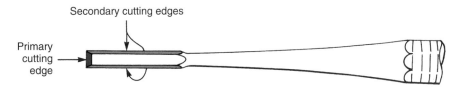

FIG. 7-4 Chisel blade design showing primary and secondary cutting edges.

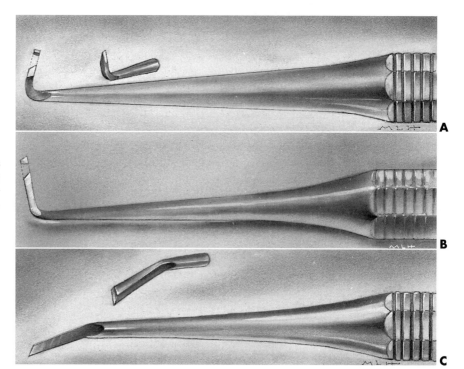

FIG. **7-5** Examples of hand instruments called *excavators* (with corresponding instrument formulas). **A,** Bibeveled ordinary hatchet (3-2-28). **B,** Hoe (4½-1½-22). **C,** Angle former (12-85-5-8).

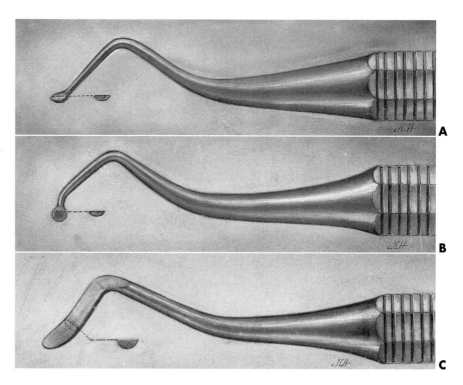

FIG. **7-6** Examples of hand instruments called *spoon excavators* (with corresponding instrument formulas). **A,** Bin-angle spoon (13-7-14). **B,** Triple-angle spoon (13-7-14). **C,** Spoon (15-7-14).

Thus one instrument is suited for work on one side of the preparation, and the other is suited for the opposite side of the preparation.

Most instruments are available with blades and shanks on both ends of the handle. Such instruments are termed *double-ended.* In many cases the right instrument of the pair is on one end of the handle, and the left instrument is on the other end. Sometimes similar blades of different widths are placed on double-ended instruments. Single-ended instruments may be safer to use, but double-ended instruments are more efficient because they reduce instrument exchange.

Instruments having the cutting edge perpendicular to the axis of the handle (Fig. 7-8), such as bin-angle chisels (see Fig. 7-8, *C*), those with a slight blade curvature (Wedelstaedt chisels) (see Fig. 7-8, *B*), and hoes (see Fig.

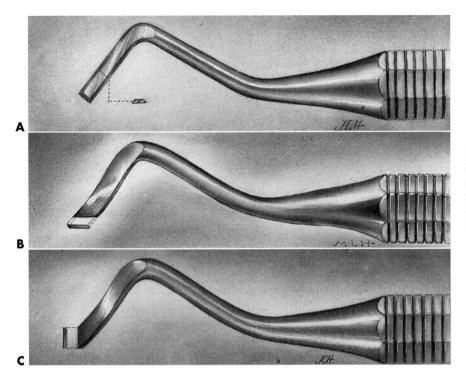

FIG. **7-7** Examples of hand instruments called *chisels* (with corresponding instrument formulas). **A,** Enamel hatchet (10-7-14). **B,** Gingival margin trimmer (12½-100-7-14). **C,** Gingival margin trimmer (12½-75-7-14).

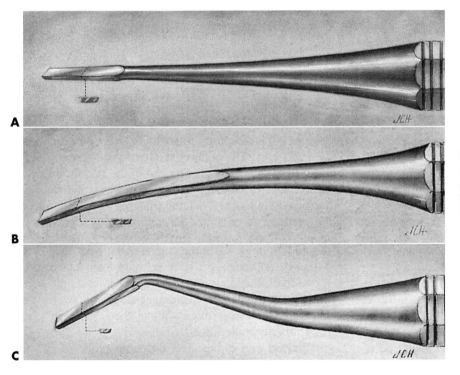

FIG. **7-8** Examples of hand instruments called *chisels* (with corresponding instrument formulas). **A,** Straight (12-7-0). **B,** Wedelstaedt (11½-15-3). **C,** Bin-angle (10-7-8).

7-5, *B),* are single-beveled and not designated as rights or lefts, but as having a *mesial bevel* or a *distal bevel.* If when one observes the inside of the blade curvature (or the inside of the angle at the junction of the blade and shank) the primary bevel is not visible, the instrument has a *distal bevel.* Conversely, if the primary bevel can be seen (from the same viewpoint) the instrument has a *mesial* or *reverse bevel* (see Fig. 7-8).

As previously described, instruments such as chisels and hatchets have three cutting edges, one primary and two secondary. These allow cutting in three directions, as the need presents. The secondary edges permit more effective cutting than the primary edge in several instances. They are particularly effective in work on the facial and lingual walls of the proximal portion of a proximoocclusal tooth preparation. The operator should not forget the usefulness of these secondary cutting edges because they enhance the use of the instrument.

CUTTING INSTRUMENT APPLICATIONS

The cutting instruments are used to cut hard or soft tissues of the mouth. Excavators are used for removal of caries and refinement of the internal parts of the preparation. Chisels are used primarily for cutting enamel.

Excavators. The four subdivisions of excavators are: (1) ordinary hatchets, (2) hoes, (3) angle formers, and (4) spoons.

An *ordinary hatchet excavator* has the cutting edge of the blade directed in the same plane as that of the long axis of the handle and is bibeveled (see Fig. 7-5, *A*). These instruments are used primarily on anterior teeth for preparing retentive areas and sharpening internal line angles, particularly in preparations for direct gold restorations.

The *hoe excavator* has the primary cutting edge of the blade perpendicular to the axis of the handle (see Fig. 7-5, *B*). This type of instrument is used for planing tooth preparation walls and forming line angles. It is commonly used in Classes III and V preparations for direct gold restorations. Some sets of cutting instruments contain hoes with longer and heavier blades, with the shanks contra-angled. These are intended for use on enamel or posterior teeth.

A special type of excavator is the *angle-former* (see Fig. 7-5, *C*). It is used primarily for sharpening line angles

and creating retentive features in dentin in preparation for gold restorations. It also may be used in placing a bevel on enamel margins. It is mon-angled and has the primary cutting edge at an angle (other than 90 degrees) to the blade. It may be described as a combination of a chisel and gingival margin trimmer. It is available in pairs (right and left).

Spoon excavators (see Fig. 7-6) are used for removing caries and carving amalgam or direct wax patterns. The blades are slightly curved and the cutting edges are either circular or clawlike. The circular edge is known as a *discoid*, whereas the clawlike blade is termed a *cleoid* (Fig. 7-9, *C* and *D*). The shanks may be bin-angled or triple-angled to facilitate accessibility.

Chisels. Chisels are intended primarily for cutting enamel and may be grouped as: (a) straight, slightly curved, or bin-angle; (b) enamel hatchets; and (c) gingival margin trimmers.

The *straight chisel* has a straight shank and blade, with the bevel on only one side. Its primary edge is perpendicular to the axis of the handle. It is similar in design to a carpenter's chisel (see Fig. 7-8, *A*). The shank and blade of the chisel also may be slightly curved (Wedelstaedt design) (see Fig. 7-8, *B*) or may be bin-angled (see Fig. 7-8, *C*). The force used with all these chisels is essentially a straight thrust. There is no need for a right and left type in a straight chisel, since a 180-degree turn of the instrument allows for its use on either side of the preparation. The *bin-angle* and *Wedelstaedt chisels* have

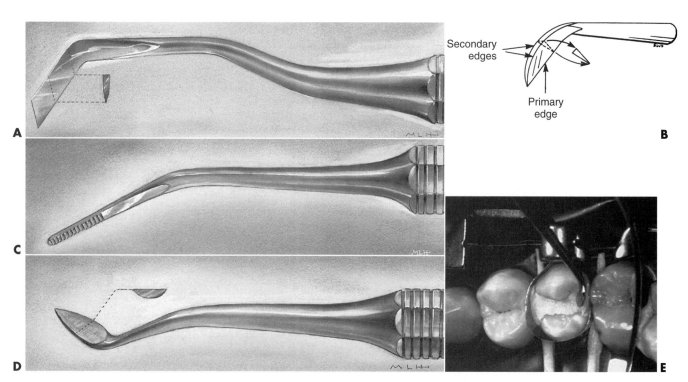

FIG. **7-9** Examples of other hand instruments for cutting. **A,** Finishing knife. **B,** Alternative finishing knife design emphasizing secondary cutting edges. **C,** Dental file. **D,** Cleoid blade. **E,** Discoid blade carving amalgam.

the primary cutting edges in a plane perpendicular to the axis of the handle and may have either a distal bevel or a mesial (reverse) bevel. The blade with a distal bevel is designed to plane a wall that faces the blade's inside surface (see Fig. 7-5, *A* and *B*). The blade with a mesial bevel is designed to plane a wall that faces the blade's outside surface (see Fig. 7-8, *B* and *C*).

The *enamel hatchet* is a chisel similar in design to the ordinary hatchet except that the blade is larger, heavier, and is beveled on only one side (see Fig. 7-7, *A*). It has its cutting edges in a plane that is parallel with the axis of the handle. It is used for cutting enamel and comes as right or left types for use on opposite sides of the preparation.

The *gingival margin trimmer* is designed to produce a proper bevel on gingival enamel margins of proximoocclusal preparations. It is similar in design to the enamel hatchet, except the blade is curved (similar to a spoon excavator), and the primary cutting edge is at an angle (other than perpendicular) to the axis of the blade (see Fig. 7-7, *B* and *C*). It is made as *right* and *left* types. It also is made so a right and left pair is either a mesial pair or a distal pair. When the second number in the formula is 90 to 100, the pair is used on the distal gingival margin. When this number is 85 to 75, the pair is used to bevel the mesial margin. *The 100 and 75 pairs are for inlay/onlay preparations with steep gingival bevels. The 90 and 85 pairs are for amalgam preparations with gingival enamel bevels that decline gingivally only slightly.* Among other uses for these instruments is the rounding or beveling of the axiopulpal line angle of two-surface preparations.

Other Cutting Instruments. Other hand cutting instruments, such as the knife, file, and discoid-cleoid instrument, are used for trimming restorative material rather than for cutting tooth structure.

Knives, known as finishing knives, amalgam knives, or gold knives, are designed with a thin, knifelike blade that is made in various sizes and shapes (see Fig. 7-9, *A* and *B*). Knives are used for trimming excess restorative material on the gingival, facial, or lingual margins of a proximal restoration or trimming and contouring the surface of a Class V restoration. Sharp secondary edges on the heel aspect of the blade are very useful in a scrape-pull mode.

Files (see Fig. 7-9, *C*) also can be used to trim excess restorative material. They are particularly useful at gingival margins. Blades of files are very thin, and teeth on the cutting surfaces are short. The teeth of the instrument are designed to make the file either a *push* or a *pull* instrument. Files are manufactured in various shapes and angles to allow access to restorations.

The *discoid-cleoid* (see Fig. 7-9, *D* and *E*) instrument is used principally for carving occlusal anatomy in unset amalgam restorations. It also may be used to trim or burnish inlay-onlay margins. The working ends of this instrument are larger than the discoid or cleoid end of an excavator.

HAND INSTRUMENT TECHNIQUES

There are four grasps used with hand instruments: (1) modified pen, (2) inverted pen, (3) palm-and-thumb, and (4) modified palm-and-thumb. *The pen grasp is not an acceptable instrument grasp* (Fig. 7-10, *A*).

Modified Pen Grasp. The grasp that permits the greatest delicacy of touch is the modified pen grasp (see Fig. 7-10, *B*). As the name implies, it is similar to that used in holding a pen, but not identical. Pads of the thumb, index, and middle fingers contact the instrument, while the tip of the ring finger (or tips of the ring and little fingers) is placed on a nearby tooth surface of the same arch as a *rest*. The palm of the hand generally is facing away from the operator. The pad of the middle finger is placed near the topside of the instrument; and by this finger working with wrist and forearm, cutting or cleaving pressure is generated on the blade. The instrument should not be allowed to rest on or near the first joint of the middle finger as in the conventional pen grasp (see Fig. 7-10, *A*). Although this latter position may appear to be more comfortable, it limits the application of pressure. Recall that a balanced instrument design allows the application of suitable force without the instrument tending to rotate in the fingers (see Fig. 7-3).

Inverted Pen Grasp. The finger positions of the inverted pen grasp are the same as for the modified pen grasp. However, the hand is rotated so that the palm faces more toward the operator (Fig. 7-11). This grasp is used mostly for tooth preparations utilizing the lingual approach on anterior teeth.

Palm-and-Thumb Grasp. The palm-and-thumb grasp is similar to that used for holding a knife while paring the skin from an apple. The handle is placed in the palm of the hand and grasped by all the fingers, while the thumb is free of the instrument and the *rest* is provided

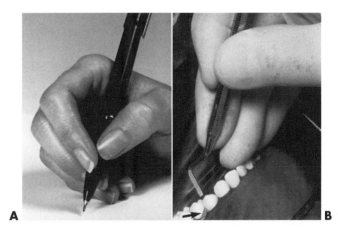

A **B**

FIG. **7-10** Pen grasps. **A,** Conventional pen grasp. Side of middle finger is on writing instrument. **B,** Modified pen grasp. Correct position of middle finger is near the "topside" of the instrument for good control and cutting pressure. The rest is tip(s) of ring finger (ring and little fingers) on tooth (teeth) of same arch. Note gingival wedge *(arrow)* serving as *guard.*

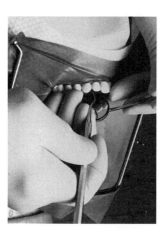

FIG. **7-11** Inverted pen grasp. Palm faces more toward operator. The rest is similar to that shown for modified pen grasp (see Fig. 7-10, *B*).

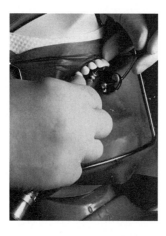

FIG. **7-12** Palm-and-thumb grasp. This grasp has limited use, such as preparing incisal retention in a Class III preparation on a maxillary incisor. The rest is tip of thumb on tooth in same arch.

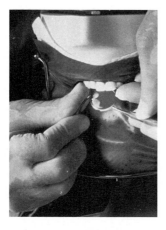

FIG. **7-13** Modified palm-and-thumb grasp. This modification allows greater ease of instrument movement and more control against slippage during thrust stroke compared to palm-and-thumb grasp. The rest is tip of thumb on tooth being prepared or adjacent tooth. Note how instrument is braced against pad and end joint of thumb.

by supporting the tip of the thumb on a nearby tooth of the same arch or on a firm, stable structure. For suitable control, this grasp requires careful utilization during cutting. An example of an appropriate use is holding a handpiece for cutting incisal retention for a Class III preparation on a maxillary incisor (Fig. 7-12).

Modified Palm-and-Thumb Grasp. The modified palm-and-thumb grasp may be used when it is feasible to rest the thumb on the tooth being prepared or the adjacent tooth (Fig. 7-13). The handle of the instrument is held by all four fingers whose pads press the handle against the distal area of the palm, as well as the pad and first joint of the thumb. Grasping the handle under the first joint of the ring and little fingers acts as a stabilizer. This grip fosters control against slippage.

The modified pen and inverted pen grasps are used practically universally. The modified palm-and-thumb grasp is usually used in the area of the maxillary arch and is best adopted when the dentist is operating from a rear-chair position.

Rests. A proper instrument grasp must include a firm rest to steady the hand during operating procedures. When the modified pen and inverted pen grasps are used, rests are established by placing the ring or ring and little fingers on a tooth (or teeth) of the same arch and as close to the operating site as possible (see Figs. 7-10 and 7-11). The closer the rest areas are to the operating area, the more reliable they are. When the palm-and-thumb grasps are used, rests are created by placing the tip of the thumb on the tooth being operated on, on an adjacent tooth, or on a convenient area of the same arch (see Figs. 7-12 and 7-13).

In some instances, it is impossible to establish a rest on tooth structure, and soft tissues must be used. Neither soft tissue rests nor distant hard tissue rests afford reliable control, and they reduce the force or power that can be used safely.

Occasionally, it is impossible to establish normal finger rests with the hand holding the instrument. Under these circumstances, instrument control may be gained using the forefinger of the opposite hand on the shank of the instrument or using an *indirect rest*, (i.e., the operating hand rests on the opposite hand, which rests on a stable oral structure).

Guards. Guards are hand instruments or other items, such as interproximal wedges, used to protect soft tissue from contact with sharp cutting or abrasive instruments (see Fig. 7-10, *B*).

SHARPENING HAND INSTRUMENTS

Selecting the proper hand cutting instrument and using the proper instrument grasp mean little if the instrument is not sharp. Instruments with dull cutting edges cause more pain, prolong operating time, are less controllable, and reduce quality and precision in tooth preparation. It is essential, therefore, that all cutting instruments be sharp. Resharpening requires little time and is very rewarding. The dentist or the assistant should habitually test for sharpness, and sharpen, when indicated, the hand instruments before they are placed in the tray setup, thus preventing delays in starting or completing an operation (see Sharpness Test).

Many types of sharpening equipment exist, including stationary sharpening stones, mechanical sharpeners, and stones that are used in the handpiece. One type or design usually does not accommodate the full variety of dental instruments with their various shapes of cutting edges. For efficient and effective sharpening, the dentist must seek out the most suitable equipment.

Stationary Sharpening Stones. The most frequently used sharpening equipment consists of a block or stick of abrasive material called a "stone." The stone is supported on a firm surface and the instrument is oriented and held by hand while being stroked against the stone surface. Stationary stones are often called *oilstones* because of the common practice of applying a coating of oil to them as an aid to the sharpening process. Sharpening stones are available in a variety of grits, shapes, and materials.

Stationary oilstones are available in coarse, medium, or fine grit. Only a fine grit stone is suitable for the final sharpening of dental instruments to be used for tooth preparation. Coarse and medium grits may be used for initial reshaping of a badly damaged instrument or for sharpening other dental equipment such as bench knives. Coarser stones cut more rapidly but produce a rougher surface. If the use of two or more grits is required, the coarser is used as little as needed for reshaping, and then the final sharpening is done with a fine stone.

Stationary stones can be obtained in various shapes including flat, grooved, cylindric, and tapered. The flat stones are preferred for sharpening all instruments with straight cutting edges; the other shapes are most useful for sharpening instruments with curved cutting edges. Cylindric stones are used for sharpening instruments with concave edges, and the tapered stones permit using a portion of the stone with a curvature matching that of the instrument.

Sharpening stones are made from any of several natural or synthetic materials. The normal manufacturing process for the synthetic materials involves pressing carefully sized particles of an abrasive into the desired shape and heating to form a solid. To retain sharp edges on the particles, the process must result in a porous material. The properties of the stone depend on the volume and size of the pores as well as on the composition and size of the abrasive. Four types of materials are in common use for sharpening stones: Arkansas stone, silicon carbide, aluminum oxide, and diamond.

Arkansas stone is a naturally occurring mineral containing microcrystalline quartz and traditionally has been the preferred material for fine sharpening stones. It is semitranslucent, white or gray in color, and hard enough to sharpen steel, but not carbide instruments. Arkansas stones are available in hard and soft varieties. The hard stone, although it may cut slower, is preferred because the soft stone scratches and grooves easily, rendering it useless. These stones should be lubricated with light machine oil before being used. This assists in the fineness of sharpening, prevents clogging of the stone pores, and avoids the creation of heat, which alters the temper of the steel blade. In fact, an Arkansas stone should be covered with a thin film of oil when stored. During the sharpening of an instrument, the fine steel cuttings remain on the stone and tend to fill up the pores of the stone; therefore, when the stone appears dirty, it should be wiped with a clean woolen cloth soaked in oil. If the stone is extremely dirty or difficult to clean, it may be wiped with a cloth soaked in alcohol.

Silicon carbide (SiC) is widely used as an industrial abrasive. It is the most commonly used material for grinding wheels and "sandpapers," as well as for sharpening stones. It is hard enough to cut steel effectively, but not hard enough to sharpen carbide instruments. SiC stones are available in many shapes in coarse and medium grits, but not in fine grits. As a result, they are not as suitable as other materials for final sharpening of dental instruments. SiC stones are normally of a dark color, often black or greenish black. These stones are moderately porous and require lubrication with a light oil to prevent clogging.

Aluminum oxide is increasingly used to manufacture sharpening stones. Aluminum oxide stones commonly are produced in various textures from different particle sizes of abrasive. Coarse and medium grit stones generally appear as speckled tan or brownish in color. Fine grit stones are usually white, have superior properties, and are less porous so that they require less lubrication during use. Either water or light oil is adequate as a lubricant.

Diamond is the hardest available abrasive and is most effective for cutting and shaping hard materials. It is the only material routinely capable of sharpening carbide as well as steel instruments. Diamond hones are small blocks of metal with fine diamond particles impregnated in the surface. The diamonds are held in place by an electroplated layer of corrosion-resistant metal. Most hones include grooved and rounded surfaces, as well as a straight surface, and are adaptable for sharpening instruments with curved blades. These hones are nonporous, but the use of a lubricant will extend the life of the hones. They may be cleaned with a mild detergent and a medium-bristle brush.

Mechanical Sharpeners. As high-speed rotary cutting instruments have been improved and their use has increased, the use of hand cutting instruments and the need for resharpening has decreased. As a result, some dental office personnel do not do enough hand sharpening to remain confident of their proficiency. Under such circumstances the use of a powered *mechanical sharpener* is of benefit.

The Rx Honing Machine is an example of a mechanical sharpener (Fig. 7-14). Basically this instrument moves a hone in a reciprocating motion at a slow speed, while the instrument is held at the appropriate angulation and supported by a rest. This is much easier than having to hold the instrument at the proper angulation while moving it relative to the hone. Interchangeable aluminum oxide hones of different shapes and coarseness are available to accommodate the various instrument sizes, shapes, and degrees of dullness. Restoration of the cutting edge is accomplished more easily and in less time than by other sharpening methods. This type of sharpener is also very versatile and, with available accessories, can fill almost all instrument sharpening needs.

Handpiece Sharpening Stones. Mounted SiC and aluminum oxide stones for use with both straight and angle handpieces are available in various sizes and shapes (see Other Abrasive Instruments). Those intended for use in straight handpieces, particularly the cylindric instruments with straight-sided silhouettes, are more useful for sharpening hand instruments than are the smaller points intended for intraoral use in the angle handpieces. Because of their curved periphery, it is difficult to produce a flat surface using any of these instruments. These stones also may produce somewhat inconsistent results because of the speed variables and the usual lack of a rest or guide for the instrument. However, satisfactory results can be obtained with minimal practice, especially on instruments with curved blades.

Principles of Sharpening. The majority of operative hand cutting instruments can be sharpened successfully on either a stationary stone or the mechanical sharpener. The secret to easy and successful sharpening is to sharpen the instrument at the first sign of dullness and not wait until the edge is completely lost. If this procedure is followed, a fine cutting edge is restored with a few strokes on a stationary stone or a light touch to the mechanical sharpener. At the same time, operating efficiency is not reduced by attempting to use an instrument that is getting progressively duller.

The choice of equipment used for sharpening is up to the dentist. In the use of any equipment, several *basic principles of sharpening* should be followed:

1. Sharpen instruments only after they have been cleaned and sterilized.
2. Establish the proper bevel angle (usually 45 degrees) and the desired angle of the cutting edge to the blade before placing the instrument against the stone, and maintain these angles while sharpening.

3. Use a light stroke or pressure against the stone to minimize frictional heat.
4. Use a rest or guide whenever possible.
5. Remove as little metal from the blade as possible.
6. Lightly hone the unbeveled side of the blade after sharpening, to remove the fine bur that may be created.
7. After sharpening, resterilize the instrument along with other items on the instrument tray setup.
8. Keep the sharpening stones clean and free of metal cuttings.

Mechanical Techniques. When chisels, hatchets, hoes, angle formers, or gingival margin trimmers are sharpened on a reciprocating honing sharpener, the blade is placed against the steady rest, and the proper angle of the cutting edge of the blade is established before starting the motor. Light pressure of the instrument against the reciprocating hone is maintained with a firm grasp on the instrument. A trace of metal debris on the face of a flat hone along the length of the cutting edge is an indication that the entire cutting edge is contacting the hone (see Fig. 7-14, *B*).

The mechanical sharpener is easily mastered with a little practice and is a quick method of sharpening hand instruments. Regardless of the type of mechanical sharpener used, the associated instructions for use should be thoroughly understood before an attempt is made to sharpen any type of instrument.

Handpiece stones are used chiefly for instruments with curved blades, especially for the inside curve of such blades. The handpiece should be run at a low speed. The instrument is held lightly against the stone with a modified pen grasp, and, whenever possible, the ring and little fingers of each hand should be touching each other to act as a rest or steadying force. When this method of sharpening is used, care must be exercised not to overheat the instrument being sharpened. The use of some form of lubricant or coolant is desirable. If oil is used, care should be exercised not to throw oil from the stone during sharpening, and the stone should be reserved for future sharpening use only.

An instrument such as an amalgam or gold knife has a wide blade with a very narrow edge bevel, unlike the wide bevel of a chisel or hatchet. It is difficult to maintain the narrow edge bevel by using a mechanical sharpener or a handpiece stone. This type of instrument should be sharpened on a stationary stone.

Stationary Stone Techniques. The stationary sharpening stone should be at least 2 inches wide and 5 inches long, since a smaller stone is impractical. It also should be of medium grit for hand cutting instruments. Before the stone is used, a thin film of light oil should be placed on the working surface. In addition to establishing the proper 45-degree angle of the bevel and the cutting edge

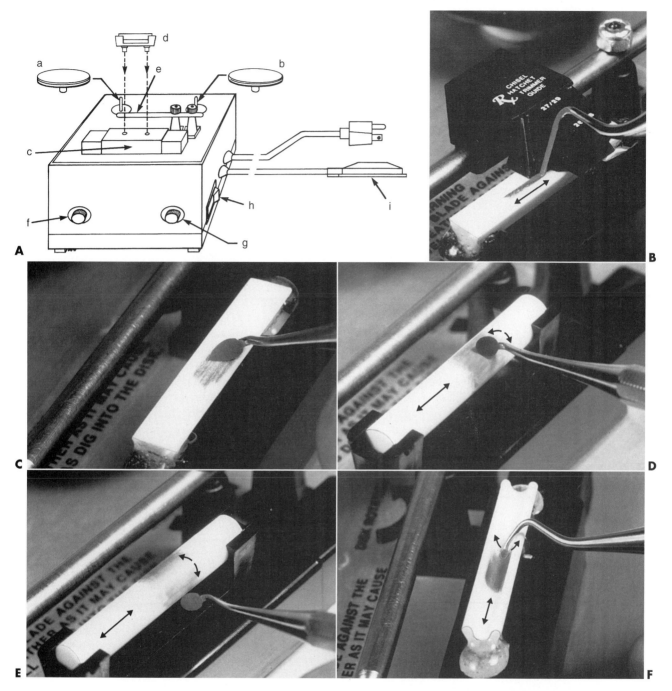

FIG. 7-14 Type of mechanical sharpener. **A,** R$_x$ Honing Machine System II has two spindle drives, one clockwise and the other counterclockwise, to which can be mounted diamond abrasive disk (a), RSC (rubberized SiC) disk (b), or leather polishing disk; hone (reciprocating) carriage (c) to which can be mounted vitreous alumina (coarse) or ceramic alumina (fine) abrasive hone (d); angle guide (see **B**) slides onto bar (e); knob for selecting disk or hone drive (f); speed control knob (g); on/off switch (h); and foot activating switch (i). **B,** Sharpening enamel hatchet. Note instrument guide on bar, and track of sharpening debris on reciprocating (two-headed arrow), ceramic hone. Track width should equal length of cutting edge. **C,** Sharpening cleoid carver on same hone. **D** and **E,** Sharpening discoid carver on snap-in round, reciprocating (two-headed arrow), ceramic hone. Note track of sharpening debris as instrument is moved in arc by operator around hone (arrows) to sharpen desired length of blade edge. **F,** Sharpening small discoid excavator on grooved, reciprocating (two-headed arrow), ceramic hone. Again note operator arcing movement of blade (arrows) in hone to sharpen desired length of cutting edge.

to the stone, several *fundamental rules* apply to using the stationary stone:

1. Lay the stone on a flat surface and do not tilt the stone while sharpening.
2. Grasp the instrument firmly, usually with a modified pen grasp, so it will not rotate or change angles while being sharpened.
3. To ensure stability during the sharpening strokes, use the ring and little fingers as a rest, and guide along a flat surface or along the stone. This prevents rolling or dipping of the instrument, which results in a distorted and uneven bevel.
4. Use a light stroke to prevent the creation of heat and the scratching of the stone.
5. Use different areas of the stone's surface while sharpening because this helps prevent the formation of grooves on the stone that impair efficiency and accuracy of the sharpening procedure.

When sharpening *chisels, hatchets,* or *hoes* on the stationary stone, grasp the instrument with a modified pen grasp, place the blade perpendicular to the stone, and then tilt the instrument to establish the correct bevel (Fig. 7-15). Establishing and maintaining this correct bevel is the most difficult part of sharpening on a stationary stone. One method that assists in establishing the proper bevel angle is to observe the oil on the stone while the instrument is tilted, in an effort to establish contact between the entire bevel and the stone. When oil is expressed evenly on all sides, then the entire bevel is touching the stone and the proper angle has been established to proceed with the sharpening strokes. If this alignment is altered during sharpening, discrepancies of the cutting edge and bevel will result. Using the finger rests and guides as illustrated in Fig. 7-15, the operator can slide the instrument back and forth along the stone. The motivating force should be from the shoulder so that the relationship of the hand to the plane of the stone is not changed during the stroke. Another technique is to move the stone back and forth while maintaining a constant position of the instrument.

The procedure for sharpening *angle formers* is essentially the same as that used for chisels, hatchets, or hoes, except that allowance must be made for the angle of the cutting edge to the blade.

Gingival margin trimmers require more orientation of the cutting edge to the stone before sharpening than a regular hatchet does. However, the same principle of establishing the proper bevel angle and cutting edge angle is the criterion for instrument position before sharpening. It may be expedient to use a palm-and-thumb grasp when sharpening a trimmer with a 95- or 100-centigrade cutting edge angle (Fig. 7-16).

When single-bevel instruments are sharpened, a thin, rough ridge of distorted metal, called a *burr* or *burr-edge,* collects on the unbeveled side of the blade. This burr is eliminated by a light stroke of the unbeveled side of the blade over the stone. This side of the blade is placed flat on the stone, and one short forward stroke is made. Burring can be kept to a minimum, however, if the direction of the sharpening stroke is only against the cutting edge of the blade, and the cutting edge does not contact the stone during the return stroke. Thus, the blade is touching the stone only on the forward sharpening stroke.

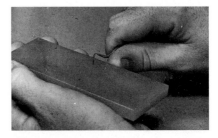

FIG. **7-16** Sharpening gingival margin trimmer. Palm-and-thumb grasp may be used while holding stone in opposite hand to establish proper cutting edge angle.

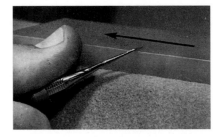

FIG. **7-17** Sharpening amalgam or gold knife. Place stone at edge of table so that blade may be tilted to form an acute angle with stone. Direction of sharpening movement of instrument along stone is indicated by arrow.

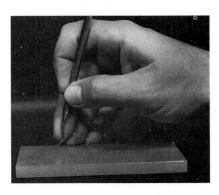

FIG. **7-15** Sharpening an instrument. Maintaining proper angle of bevel and angle of cutting edge to stone is aided by resting fingertips on stone.

The *amalgam* or *gold knife* has a very thin blade tapering to the sharpened edge. There is a narrow edge bevel on both sides of the blade. In sharpening this instrument, only the edge bevels should be honed. If the entire side of the blade is worked each time, the thin blade will soon disappear or become so thin that it will fracture under the slightest pressure. To sharpen the amalgam or gold knife, the blade is placed on the stone with the junction of the blade and shank immediately over the edge of the stone. The blade is then tilted to form a small acute angle with the surface of the stone, and the stroke is straight along the stone and toward the edge of the blade only (Fig. 7-17). The sharpening is accomplished on both sides of the blade, with the stroke always toward the blade edge. This method produces the finest edge and eliminates any burrs on the cutting edge.

The most difficult instruments to sharpen on a flat stone are the *spoon excavators* and *discoids.* Only the rounded outside surface of the spoon can be honed satisfactorily on a flat stone, and this involves a rotary movement accompanied by a pull stroke to maintain the curvature of the edge. The spoon is placed on the far end of the stone and held so that the handle is pointing toward the operator. As the instrument is pulled along the stone toward the operator, the handle is rotated gradually away from the operator, until it is pointing away from the operator at the end of the stroke. The instrument is picked up and placed at the far end of the stone, and the motion is repeated until the edge is honed. The stone either may be placed on a flat surface or held in the hand for this procedure (Fig. 7-18). To hone the flat inside surface of the blade, a small cylindric stone is passed back and forth over the surface (Fig. 7-19).

Other means of sharpening spoon excavators are achieved by using a grooved stone, mounted discs, or stones for use with a straight handpiece. However, there is a tendency to remove too much metal when handpiece stones are used.

Sharpness Test. Sharpness of an instrument can be tested by lightly resting the cutting edge on a hard plastic surface. If the cutting edge digs in during an attempt to slide the instrument forward over the surface, the instrument is sharp. If it slides, the instrument is dull. Only very light pressure is exerted in testing for sharpness.

The principles and techniques discussed provide sufficient background for the operator to use proper methods in sharpening other instruments not discussed. *It cannot be overemphasized that sharp instruments are necessary for optimal operating procedures.* It also has been

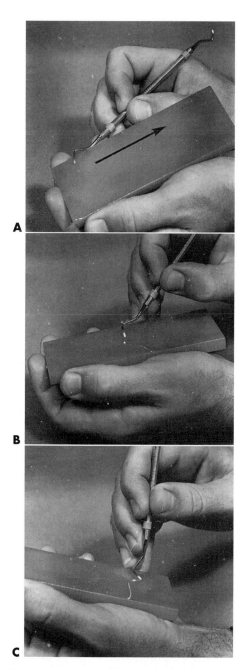

FIG. **7-18** Sharpening a spoon excavator. **A,** Beginning of stroke. **B,** Continuation of pull stroke while rotating handle in a direction opposite the stroke. **C,** Completion of stroke and handle rotation. Note that finger guides are used during entire stroke, which is in direction indicated by arrow.

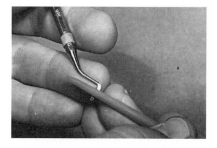

FIG. **7-19** Use of a small cylinder stone to hone inside surface of spoon excavators and discoid-cleoid instruments. **NOTE:** Gloving is not illustrated in Figs. 7-15 to 7-19 because sharpening is accomplished *after* sterilizing the washed instrument; after sharpening the instrument, it is sterilized again.

found prudent to have multiple tray setups so that a substitute instrument is available if necessary; or substitute sterile instruments should be available so that other sterile tray setups are not disrupted by the borrowing of instruments.

STERILIZATION AND STORAGE OF HAND CUTTING INSTRUMENTS

Because hepatitis A and B viruses have been found in the saliva of infected persons and evidence indicates that many dental personnel have hepatitis B infections, the importance of proper equipment and procedures for instrument sterilization must be emphasized. Sterilization in dental offices can be accomplished by autoclaving, dry-heat procedures, ethylene oxide equipment, and chemical vapor sterilizers. Boiling and chemical solutions (cold disinfection) do not sterilize instruments and should be considered as disinfection procedures only. The belief that only those instruments that puncture or cut soft tissue or are exposed to blood should be sterilized, and others only disinfected, is no longer valid as a precaution against cross-infections. Aseptic techniques are presented in other subject areas and are not be detailed here. Sterilization procedures for operative dentistry are presented in Chapter 8. Storage of any hand cutting instrument should be in a sterile, wrapped tray setup or in an individual sterile wrapping.

POWERED CUTTING EQUIPMENT
DEVELOPMENT OF ROTARY EQUIPMENT

The availability of some method of cutting and shaping of tooth structure is essential for the restoration of teeth. Although archeological evidence of dental treatment dates from as early as 5000 BC, little is known about the equipment and methods used then.[14] Early drills powered by hand are illustrated in Figs. 7-20 and 7-21. Much of the subsequent development leading to present powered cutting equipment can be seen as a search for improved sources of energy and means for holding and controlling the cutting instrument. This has culminated in the use of replaceable bladed or abrasive instruments held in a rotary handpiece, usually powered by compressed air.

A *handpiece* is a device for holding rotating instruments, transmitting power to them, and for positioning them intraorally. Handpieces and associated cutting and polishing instruments developed as two basic types, *straight* and *angle* (Fig. 7-22). Most of the development of methods for preparing teeth has occurred within the last 100 years.[34] Effective equipment for removal (or preparation) of enamel has been available only since 1947, when speeds of 10,000 rpm were first used, along with newly marketed carbide burs and diamond instruments. Since 1953, continued improvements in the design and materials of construction for both handpieces and instruments have resulted in equipment that is efficient and sterilizeable, much to the credit of manufacturers and the profes-

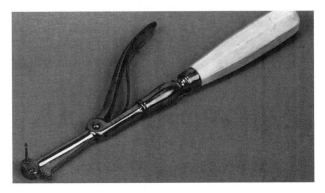

FIG. 7-21 Early angle hand drill for indirect access preparations (circa 1850). The bur is activated by squeezing the spring-loaded handle.

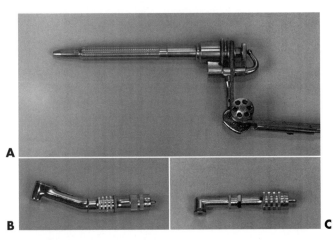

FIG. 7-22 Conventional designs of handpieces. **A,** Belt-driven straight handpiece. **B,** Gear-driven angle handpiece that attaches to front end of the straight handpiece. **C,** Gear-driven angle handpiece designed for cleaning and polishing procedures.

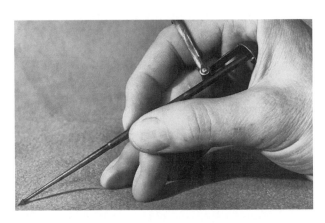

FIG. 7-20 Early straight hand drill for direct access preparations (circa 1800). Back end of bur shank fits into a finger ring while the front end is rotated with thumb and forefinger.

sion alike. Table 7-1 summarizes some of the more significant developments of rotary dental equipment.

One of the most significant advancements was the introduction of the *electric motor* as a power source in 1874. It was incorporated into a *dental unit* in 1914.[35] The initial handpiece equipment and operating speeds (maximum of 5000 rpm) remained virtually unchanged until

TABLE 7-1 | Evolution of Rotary Cutting Equipment in Dentistry

DATE	INSTRUMENT	SPEED (RPM)
1728	Hand-rotated instruments	300
1871	Foot engine	700
1874	Electric engine	1000
1914	Dental unit	5000
1942	Diamond cutting instruments	5000
1946	Old units converted to increase speed	10,000
1947	Tungsten carbide burs	12,000
1953	Ball bearings handpieces	25,000
1955	Water tubine angle handpiece	50,000
1955	Belt-driven angle handpiece (Page-Chayes)	150,000
1957	Air turbine angle handpiece	250,000
1961	Air turbine straight handpiece	25,000
1962	Experimental air bearing handpiece	(800,000)
2001	Air turbine handpiece	300,000

1946 (Fig. 7-23). The steel burs used at the time could not cut enamel effectively, even when applied with great force. With steel burs, increased speed and power resulted only in increased heat and instrument wear. Further progress was delayed until the development of instruments that could cut enamel. Diamond cutting instruments were developed in Germany around 1935, but were scarce in the United States until after World War II. In a 10-year period, starting in late 1946, cutting techniques were revolutionized. *Diamond instruments* and *tungsten carbide burs* capable of cutting enamel were produced commercially. Both instruments performed best at the highest speeds available and that prompted the development of higher speed handpieces. Obtaining speeds of 10,000 to 15,000 rpm was a relatively simple matter of modifying existing equipment by enlarging the drive pulleys on the dental engine. By 1950, speeds of 60,000 rpm and above had been attained by newly designed equipment employing speed-multiplying internal belt drives (Fig. 7-24).[34] They were found to be more effective for cutting tooth structure and for reducing perceived vibration.

The major breakthrough in the development of high-speed rotary equipment came with the introduction of *contra-angled handpieces with internal turbine drives* in the contra-angle head.[29] Early units were water driven but subsequent units were air driven (Figs. 7-25 and 7-26, *A*). Although most current *air-turbine handpieces* (Fig. 7-27) have free-running speeds of approximately 300,000 rpm, the small size of the turbine in the head limits their power output. The speed can drop to 200,000 rpm or less, with small lateral workloads during cutting, and the handpiece may stall at moderate loads.[36] This tendency to stall under high loads is an excellent safety feature for tooth preparation, since excessive pressure cannot be applied. Air-driven handpieces continue to be the most popular type of handpiece equipment because of the overall simplicity of design, ease of control, versatility, and patient acceptance. The external appearance of current handpieces is very similar to the earliest models.

The low torque and power output of the contra-angle turbines made them unsuitable for some finishing and

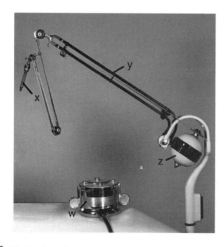

FIG. 7-23 Typical equipment when an electric motor is used as source of power: foot control with rheostat *(w)*, belt-driven straight handpiece *(x)*, three-piece adjustable extension arm *(y)*, and electric motor *(z)*.

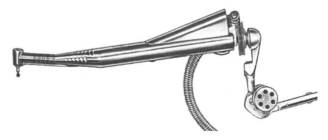

FIG. 7-24 Page-Chayes handpiece (circa 1955). The first belt-driven angle handpiece to operate successfully at speeds over 100,000 rpm.

polishing techniques, where large heavy instruments are needed. The application of the turbine principle to the *straight handpiece* eliminated the necessity of having an electric engine as part of a standard dental unit. The design of the straight handpiece turbine provided the desirable high torque for low-speed operation (see Fig. 7-26, *B*).

Increasing concern about patient-to-patient transfer of infectious agents has put emphasis on other aspects of handpiece performance. Recent advancements in both straight and angle handpieces allow repeated sterilization by several methods (see Chapter 8). However sterilization produces some damage to parts of the handpiece, thus necessitating more frequent service and repair. Other improvements of the angle handpiece include smaller head sizes, more torque, lower noise levels, and better chucking mechanisms. Since 1955, angle handpieces have had an air-water spray feature to provide cooling, cleansing, and improved visibility[32] (see Fig. 7-27). Most modern-angled handpieces also include fiber-optic lighting of the cutting site (see Fig. 7-27, *B*).

ROTARY SPEED RANGES

The rotational speed of an instrument is measured in revolutions per minute (rpm). Three speed ranges are generally recognized: low or slow speeds (below 12,000 rpm), medium or intermediate speeds (12,000 to 200,000 rpm), and high or ultrahigh speeds (above 200,000 rpm). The terms *low-speed, medium-speed,* and *high-speed* are used preferentially in this textbook. Most useful instruments are rotated at either low or high speed.

The crucial factor for some purposes is the surface speed of the instrument, the velocity at which the edges of the cutting instrument pass across the surface being cut. This is proportional to both the rotational speed and the diameter of the instrument, with large instruments having higher surface speeds at any given rate of rotation.

Although intact tooth structure can be removed by an instrument rotating at low speeds, it is a traumatic experience for both the patient and the dentist. Low-speed cutting is ineffective, time consuming, and requires a relatively heavy force application. This results in heat production at the operating site and produces vibrations of low frequency and high amplitude. Heat and vibration are the main sources of patient discomfort.[33] At low speeds, burs have a tendency to roll out of the tooth preparation and mar the proximal margin or tooth surface. In addition, carbide burs do not last long because their brittle blades are easily broken at low speeds. Many of these disadvantages of low-speed operation do not apply when the objective is some procedure other than cutting tooth structure. *The low-speed range is used for cleaning teeth, occasional caries excavation, and finishing and polishing procedures.* At low speeds, tactile sensation is better and there is generally less chance for overheating cut surfaces. The availability of a low-speed option is a valuable adjunct for many dental procedures.

At high speed, the surface speed needed for efficient cutting can be attained with smaller and more versatile cutting instruments. This speed is used for tooth prepa-

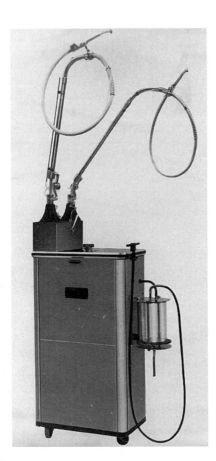

FIG. **7-25** Turbo-Jet portable unit (circa 1955). A small turbine in the head of the angle handpiece is driven by water circulated by a pump housed in the mobile base.

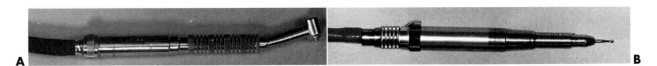

FIG. **7-26** Air-turbine handpiece. **A,** Borden Airotor handpiece (circa 1957) was first clinically successful air-turbine handpiece. Current air-driven handpieces are very similar in basic design. **B,** Air-turbine straight handpiece (circa 1980).

ration and removing old restorations. Other advantages are: (1) diamond and carbide cutting instruments remove tooth structure faster with less pressure, vibration, and heat generation; (2) the number of rotary cutting instruments needed is reduced because smaller sizes are more universal in application; (3) the operator has better control and greater ease of operation; (4) instruments last longer; (5) patients are generally less apprehensive because annoying vibrations and operating time are decreased; and (6) several teeth in the same arch can and should be treated at the same appointment.

Variable control to regulate the speed makes the handpiece more versatile. This allows the operator to easily obtain the optimal speed for the size and type of rotating instrument at any stage of a specific operation.

For infection control, all dental handpieces are now sterilized, but the process is accompanied with some challenges. Continual sterilization can produce degradation in clinical performance (longevity, power, turbine speed, fiber-optic transmission, eccentricity, noise, chuck performance, visibility angle, interocclusal clearance, water spray pattern).[23] Most handpieces require re-

oiling after sterilization, and excess oil may be sprayed during the start-up operation. It is therefore recommended to run the handpiece for a few seconds before initiating a dental procedure in which the deposition of oil spray onto tooth structure might interfere with processes, such as dental adhesion.

LASER EQUIPMENT

Lasers are devices that produce beams of coherent and very high intensity light. A large number of current and potential uses of lasers in dentistry have been identified that involve the treatment of soft tissues and the modification of hard tooth structures.[28,39] The word *laser* is an acronym for *"light amplification by stimulated emission of radiation."* A crystal or gas is excited to emit light photons of a characteristic wavelength that are amplified and filtered to make a coherent light beam. The effects of the laser depend on the power of the beam and the extent to which the beam is absorbed.

Several types are available (Table 7-2) based on wavelengths. The lasers range from long wavelengths (infrared), through visible wavelengths, to short wavelengths

TABLE 7-2 Laser Types by Source and Wavelength

TYPE	SOURCE	WAVELENGTH	MODE	OUTPUT
Infrared	CO_2	$10.60 \mu m$	Continuous	1000 W
	CO_2	$10.60 \mu m$	Pulsed	1000 mJ/p
	Ho:YAG	$2.06 \mu m$	Pulsed	800 mJ/p
	Nd:YAG	$1.06 \mu m$	Pulsed	1000 mJ/p
	Nd:YAG	$1.06 \mu m$	Continuous	100 W
Visible	HeNe	633 nm	Continuous	25 W
	Argon	514 nm, 488 nm	Continuous	20 W
Ultraviolet (Excimer)	XeF	351 nm	Pulsed	50 mJ/p
	XeCl	308 nm	Pulsed	300 mJ/p
	KrF	248 nm	Pulsed	1000 mJ/p
	ArF	193 nm	Pulsed	800 mJ/p

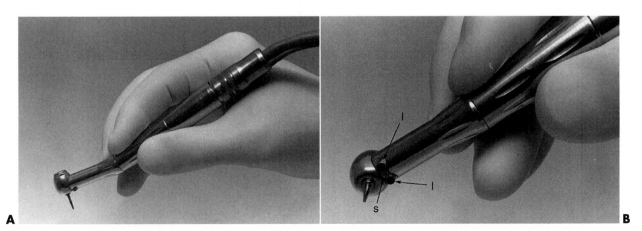

FIG. 7-27 Contemporary air-turbine handpiece (circa 1994). Most handpieces are being redesigned to withstand the rigors of routine sterilization. **A,** Contrangle air-turbine handpiece connected to air-water supply line. **B,** Ventral view of handpiece (Star 430SWL) showing port for air-water spray *(s)* onto bur at cutting site, and epoxied end of fiber-optic bundle *(l)* to shine light at cutting site.

(ultraviolet). Excimers are special ultraviolet lasers. At the present time, CO_2, Nd:YAG, and Er:YAG lasers have shown the most promise. For any application it is important to select the correct wavelength for absorption of the energy and prevention of side effects from heat generation.

Scientific and commercial lasers produce highly collimated beams, but such a beam is potentially dangerous in clinical situations. The collimated beam is directed via a flexible fiber-optic light pipe or mirror train to the point of application, where it is normally focused by a lens to a focal area near the tip.

Once the beam is focused, the total energy it delivers is a function of the intensity of the beam, the time of exposure, and the area affected. These are used to calculate the exposure dose (ED, Joules/cm^2). ED = (W)(t)/(A) where W is the power (watts) emitted from the light guide, t is the time (seconds) of the total exposure, and A is the area (cm^2) of the beam spot on the substrate.[26]

The effect of this energy depends on whether or not the wavelength of the energy is absorbed by the surface. The absorption wavelengths for various hard and soft tissues are different. The best results are obtained when the laser wavelength is matched to an absorption band of the substrate. In some cases, the substrate must be coated with an absorbing dye to facilitate beam interaction.

Interactions with the substrate can occur in photothermal, photochemical, or other ways. Generally, dental lasers produce photothermal effects, with soft or hard tissue being ablated by the action. At low temperatures, below 100° C, thermal effects denature proteins, produce hemolysis, and cause coagulation and shrinkage. Above 100° C, water in soft or hard tissues boils, producing explosive expansion. Above approximately 400° C, carbonization of organic materials is completed with the onset of some inorganic changes. As the temperature increases from 400° to 1400° C, inorganic constituents change in chemistry, may melt and/or recrystallize, and

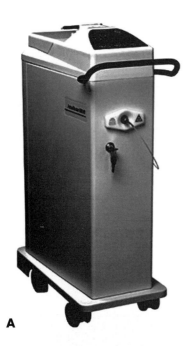

FIG. 7-28 Example of laser use. **A,** Nd:YAG laser unit with a power supply, control panel, fiber-optic wave guide, and probe. **B,** Laser probe and beam emanating from probe tip. **C,** Lased area on dentin (from Nd:YAG operated at 1.06 μm wavelength, 167 mJ/pulse, and 207 J/cm^2 power) showing physical modification produced by a single pulse. The hydroxyapatite crystals on the surface were melted and recrystallized with partial closure of the tubules. Surface roughness from tooth preparation was eliminated by the lasing. The area immediately adjacent to the lased site seemed to be unaffected. (**A,** Courtesy of American Dental Technologies, Inc., 5555 Bear Lane, Corpus Christi, Tex.; **B,** Courtesy of Dr. Art Vassiliadis, Sunrise Technologies, Freemont, Calif.; **C,** Courtesy of Dr. Joel White, Department of Restorative Dentistry, UCSF School of Dentistry, San Francisco, Calif.)

A

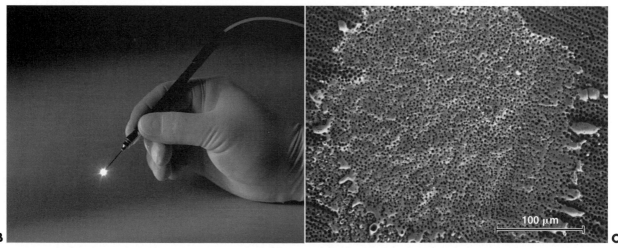

B

C

may vaporize. The actual temperatures depend on the initial composition of the tissue involved. When the laser and tissue are well matched, like the infrared lasers and enamel, energy can be absorbed very rapidly. Even low energy densities for short times can cause enamel to melt and recrystallize. High energy densities and/or longer times produce vaporization with drilling or cutting of the surface. For dentin, the same effects occur at lower energy densities. An example of lased dentin is shown in Fig. 7-28. Such surfaces can be produced to seal the dentin and assist bonding of restorative materials.

While infrared lasers produce their effects by heating at the focal point, ultraviolet laser beams involve photon energies coincident with bond energies of cellular constituents and are capable of directly disrupting the bonds that hold the molecules together.[11] For this reason, it is necessary to avoid those wavelengths that are absorbed by proteins such as DNA and RNA.

For dental applications, excessive heat must be avoided to protect the dental pulp.[20] High surface temperatures for short periods of time are acceptable, as long as there is sufficient time or path for heat dispersion. Lasers may be operated as continuous wave (cw) or pulsed (p) lasers. To control the beam energy, it is common to pulse the beam. Normally the operator can select the pulse rate (20 to 1000 Hertz or cycles per second) and pulse duration (1 to 50 microseconds). Pulsing occurs rapidly and is not the same as the operator turning the beam on or off. Local temperatures during lasing can reach many hundreds of degrees Celsius, but as long as the heat is dissipated effectively, pulpal temperatures will not be affected. Clinical studies indicate that lasers can be used correctly without causing pulpal damage.[38] Generally, pulpal temperature increases of more than 4.5° to 5.5° C are considered damaging.

Several lasers are of practical importance to medicine and dentistry (Table 7-3). The ones of most current interest to dentistry are Nd:YAG (Neodymium:yttrium-aluminum-garnet; wavelength = 1.064 μm; see Fig. 7-28, A), Er:YAG (Erbium:yttrium-aluminum-garnet; wavelength = 2.94 μm), or CO_2 (carbon dioxide; maximum

wavelength = 10.6 μm). Argon, helium-neon, Ho:YAG, and excimer lasers are being evaluated as well. A laser may produce more than one wavelength of photon energy. In the case of CO_2 lasers, the 9.6 μm peak is much more readily absorbed by hydroxyapatite than the standard 10.6 μm peak. This wavelength may be selected by filtration to eliminate longer wavelengths.

It is no longer a question of whether lasers will be used by dentistry but rather when they will become commonplace. Current units are relatively expensive and must be used frequently in a dental practice to justify the expense. At the moment, lasers are used primarily for either soft tissue applications (see Table 7-3) or hard tissue surface modification (see Fig 7-28, C). They generally are not used for tooth preparations because they are inefficient and awkward for removing large amounts of enamel or dentin, and that process with a laser can generate intolerable amounts of heat. Therefore lasers may never replace a high-speed dental handpiece. However, at least one commercial Ho:YAG laser instrument has been approved by the Food and Drug Administration (FDA) for use with hard tissues in primary teeth.[25]

Special safety precautions are prescribed when using a laser. A door is required to close off the room where lasers are being used, and appropriate signs are needed to indicate the presence of laser equipment. Eye protection is required for the operator, assistant, and patient to protect against any inadvertently reflected laser light. The FDA will most likely expand the number of sanctioned applications in the near future.

OTHER EQUIPMENT

Alternative methods of cutting enamel and/or dentin have been assessed periodically. In the mid-1950s, air-abrasive cutting was tested, but several clinical problems precluded general acceptance. Most importantly, no tactile sense was associated with air-abrasive cutting of tooth structure. This made it difficult for the operator to determine the cutting progress within the tooth preparation. Additionally, the abrasive dust interfered with visibility of the cutting site and tended to mechanically

TABLE 7-3 Suggested Dental Applications for Laser Types

	CO₂	Ho:YAG	Nd:YAG	HeNe	ARGON	EXCIMERS
Cutting and coagulation	X	X	X		X	
Stimulation of healing				X		
Analgesia (low power)			X	X		
Fissure sealing	X	X	X			X
Caries treatment	X	X	X			X
Composite curing					X	
Surface modification	X	X	X			X
Root canal	X	X	X			X
Apicoectomy	X	X	X			
Root sealing	X	X				X
Gingivectomy	X	X				

etch the surface of the dental mirror. Preventing the patient or office personnel from inhaling abrasive dust posed an additional difficulty.

Contemporary air-abrasion equipment (Fig. 7-29) is helpful for stain removal, debriding pit and fissures prior to sealing, and micro-mechanical roughening of surfaces to be bonded (enamel, cast metal alloys, or porcelain).[4] This approach works well when organic material is being removed and when only a limited amount of enamel or dentin is involved. Although promoted for caries excavation, air abrasion can not produce well-defined preparation wall and margin details that are possible with conventional rotary cutting techniques. Generally, the finest stream of abrading particles still generates an effective cutting width of at least 350 μm, far greater than the width of luted cement margins or the errors tolerable in most caries excavations. Roughening of surfaces to be bonded, luted, or repaired is an advantage, and can occur intraorally or extraorally, depending on the situation. However, roughening by air abrasion by itself is not a substitute for acid-etching techniques. While roughening improves bonding, acid-etching alone, or after roughening always produces a better bond than air abrasion roughening alone.[34]

Air abrasion techniques rely on the transfer of kinetic energy from a stream of powder particles on the surface of tooth structure or a restoration to produce a fractured Air abrasion techniques rely on the transfer of kinetic energy from a stream of powder particles on the surface of tooth structure or a restoration to produce a fractured surface layer, resulting in roughness for bonding or dis-

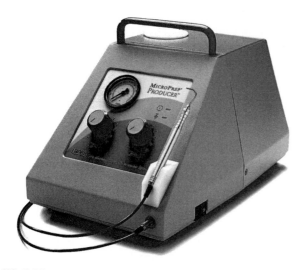

FIG. 7-29 Example of contemporary air-abrasion unit for removal of superficial enamel defects or stains, debriding pits and fissures for sealant application, or roughening surfaces to be bonded or luted. *(Courtesy of Lares Research, Chico, Calif.)*

FIG. 7-30 Schematic representation of range of variables associated with any type of air-abrasion equipment. The cleaning or cutting action is a function of kinetic energy imparted to the actual surface, and this is affected by variables concerning the particle size, air pressure, angulation with surface, type of substrate, and method of clearance. *(Courtesy of Barbara Kunselman [Master's thesis, 1999], School of Dentistry, University of North Carolina, Chapel Hill, NC.)*

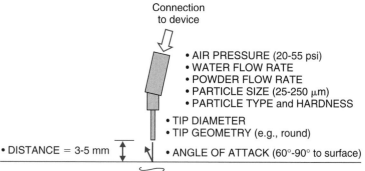

Connection to device

• AIR PRESSURE (20-55 psi)
• WATER FLOW RATE
• POWDER FLOW RATE
• PARTICLE SIZE (25-250 μm)
• PARTICLE TYPE and HARDNESS
• TIP DIAMETER
• TIP GEOMETRY (e.g., round)

• DISTANCE = 3-5 mm   • ANGLE OF ATTACK (60°-90° to surface)

• SUBSTRATE = Enamel, dentin, cementum, amalgam, composite, casting alloy, or ceramic

• MOTION (e.g., 12 mm/s scanning pattern)
• Duration (e.g., 2-20 seconds)

FIG. 7-31 Example of air-abrasion equipment used for tooth cleaning (Cavitron Jet, Dentsply Professional) showing the prophy tip and handle attached by a flexible cord to the control unit with the reservoir of powder and source of water. *(Courtesy of Dentsply Professional, 1301 Smile Way, York, PA, 17404-0807; phone: [800] 989-8826)*

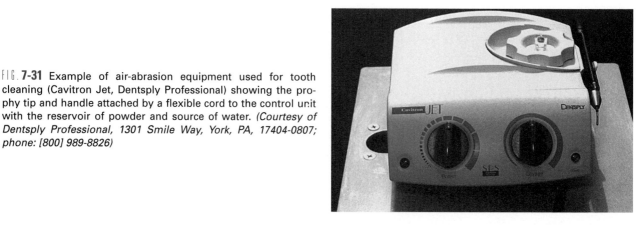

ruption for cutting. The energy transfer event is affected by many things, including powder particle, pressure, angulation, surface composition, and clearance angle variables (Fig. 7-30). The most common error for operators of air abrasion units is to hold the tip at the wrong distance from the surface, for the desired action. Greater distances significantly reduce the energy of the stream.[22] Short distances may produce unwanted cutting actions, such as when only surface stain removal is being attempted. The potential for unwanted cutting is a significant problem when employing an air-polishing device (e.g., Prophy Jet) to clean the surfaces of dentin and enamel.[3,7,12,31] However, when used properly, units designed for air-polishing tooth surfaces can be quite efficient and effective (Fig. 7-31).

ROTARY CUTTING INSTRUMENTS

The individual instruments intended for use with dental handpieces are manufactured in hundreds of sizes, shapes, and types. This variation is in part a result of the need for specialized designs for particular clinical applications or to fit particular handpieces, but much of the variation also results from individual preferences on the part of dentists. Since the introduction of high-speed techniques in clinical practice, a rapid evolution of technique and an accompanying proliferation of new instrument designs have occurred. Nevertheless, the number of instruments essential for use with any one type of handpiece is comparatively small, especially in the case of high-speed turbine handpieces.

COMMON DESIGN CHARACTERISTICS

In spite of the great variation among rotary cutting instruments, they have certain design features in common. Each instrument consists of three parts: (1) shank, (2) neck, and (3) head (Fig. 7-32). Each has its own function, influencing its design and the materials used for its construction. Note that there is a difference in the mean-

ing of the term "shank" as applied to rotary instruments and to hand instruments.

Shank Design. The *shank* is the part that fits into the handpiece, accepts the rotary motion from the handpiece, and provides a bearing surface to control the alignment and concentricity of the instrument. The shank design and dimensions vary with the handpiece for which it is intended. The American Dental Association Specification No. 23 for dental excavating burs[1] includes five classes of instrument shanks. Three of these (Fig. 7-33), the *straight handpiece shank,* the *latch-type angle handpiece shank,* and the *friction-grip angle handpiece shank,* are commonly encountered. The shank portion of the straight handpiece instrument is a simple cylinder. It is held in the handpiece by a metal chuck that accepts a range of shank diameters. Therefore precise control of the shank diameter is not as critical as for other shank designs. Straight handpiece instruments are now rarely used for preparing teeth, except for caries excavation. However, they are commonly used for finishing and polishing completed restorations.

The more complicated shape of the latch-type shank reflects the different mechanisms by which these instruments are held in the handpiece. Their shorter overall length permits substantially improved access to posterior regions of the mouth in comparison with straight handpiece instruments. Handpieces that use latch-type burs normally have a metal bur tube within which the instruments fit as closely as possible, while still permitting easy interchange. The posterior portion of the shank is flattened on one side so that the end of the instrument fits into a D-shaped socket at the bottom of the bur tube, causing the instrument to be rotated. Latch-type instruments are not retained in the handpiece by a chuck, but rather by a retaining latch that slides into the groove found at the shank end of the instrument. This type of instrument is used predominantly at low and medium speed ranges for finishing procedures. At these speeds,

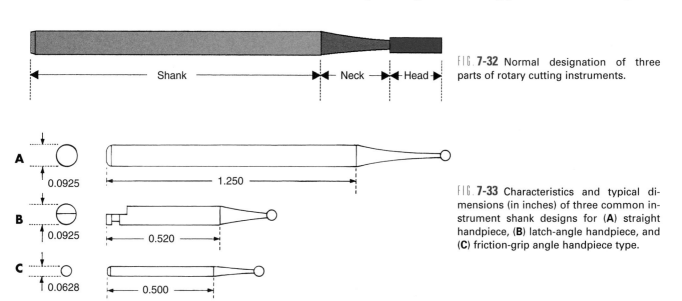

FIG. 7-32 Normal designation of three parts of rotary cutting instruments.

FIG. 7-33 Characteristics and typical dimensions (in inches) of three common instrument shank designs for (**A**) straight handpiece, (**B**) latch-angle handpiece, and (**C**) friction-grip angle handpiece type.

the small amount of potential wobble inherent in the clearance between the instrument and the handpiece bur tube is controlled by the lateral pressure exerted during cutting procedures. At higher speeds, the latch-type shank design is inadequate to provide a true-running instrument head, and as a result, an improved shank design is required for these speeds.

The friction-grip shank design was developed for use with high-speed handpieces. This design is smaller in overall length than the latch-type instruments, providing a further improvement in access to the posterior regions of the mouth. The shank is a simple cylinder manufactured to very close dimensional tolerances. As the name implies, friction-grip instruments originally were designed to be held in the handpiece by friction between the shank and a plastic or metal chuck. Newer handpiece designs have metal chucks that close to make a positive contact with the bur shank. Careful dimensional control on the shanks of these instruments is important, because for high-speed use, even minor variations in shank diameter can cause substantial variation in instrument performance and problems with insertion, retention, and removal.

Neck Design. As shown in Fig. 7-32, the *neck* is the intermediate portion of an instrument that connects the head to the shank. It corresponds to the part of a hand instrument called the shank. Except in the case of the larger, more massive instruments, the neck normally tapers from the shank diameter to a smaller size immediately adjacent to the head. The main function of the neck is to transmit rotational and translational forces to the head. At the same time, it is desirable for the operator to have the greatest possible visibility of the cutting head and the greatest manipulative freedom. For this reason the neck dimensions represent a compromise between the need for a large cross-section to provide strength and a small cross-section to improve access and visibility.

Head Design. The *head* is the working part of the instrument, the cutting edges or points that perform the desired shaping of tooth structure. The shape of the head and the material used to construct it are closely related to its intended application and technique of use. The heads of instruments show greater variation in design and construction than either of the other main portions. For this reason the characteristics of the head form the basis on which rotary instruments are usually classified.

Many characteristics of the heads of rotary instruments could be used for classification. Most important among these is the division into bladed instruments and abrasive instruments. Material of construction, head size, and head shape are additional characteristics that are useful for further subdivision. Bladed and abrasive instruments exhibit substantially different clinical performances, even when operated under nearly identical conditions. This appears to result from differences in the mechanism of cutting that are inherent in their design.

DENTAL BURS

The term *bur* is applied to *all rotary cutting instruments that have bladed cutting heads*. This includes instruments intended for such purposes as finishing metal restorations and surgical removal of bone, as well as those primarily intended for tooth preparation.

Historical Development of Dental Burs. The earliest burs, like those shown in Fig. 7-20, were handmade. Thus, they were both expensive and variable in dimension and performance. The shapes, dimensions, and nomenclature of modern burs are directly related to those of the first machine-made burs introduced in 1891.[35] Early burs were made of steel. *Steel burs* perform well, cutting human dentin at low speeds, but dull rapidly at higher speeds or when cutting enamel. Once dulled, the reduced cutting effectiveness creates increased heat and vibration.

Carbide burs, which were introduced in 1947, have largely replaced steel burs for tooth preparation. Steel burs now are used mainly for finishing procedures. Carbide burs perform better than steel burs at all speeds, and their superiority is greatest at high speeds.

All carbide burs have heads of cemented carbide in which microscopic carbide particles, usually tungsten carbide, are held together in a matrix of cobalt or nickel. Carbide is much harder than steel and less subject to dulling during cutting.

In most burs, the carbide head is attached to a steel shank and neck by welding or brazing. The substitution of steel for carbide in those portions of the bur where greater wear resistance is not required has several advantages. It permits the manufacturer more freedom of design in attaining the characteristics desired in the instrument and at the same time allows economy in the cost of materials of construction.

Although most carbide burs have the joint located in the posterior part of the head, others are sold that have the joint located within the shank and therefore have carbide necks as well as heads. Carbide is stiffer and stronger than steel, but it is also more brittle. A carbide neck subjected to a sudden blow or shock will fracture, whereas a steel neck will bend. A bur that is even slightly bent produces increased vibration and overcutting as a result of increased run-out. Thus, although steel necks reduce the risk of fracture during use, if bent they may cause severe problems. Either type can be satisfactory, and other design factors are varied to take maximal advantage of the properties of the material used.

Bur Classification Systems. To facilitate the description, selection, and manufacture of burs, it is highly desirable to have some agreed-upon shorthand designation, which represents all variables of a particular head design by some simple code. In the United States, dental burs traditionally have been described in terms of an arbitrary *numerical code* for head size and shape (e.g., 2 = 1-mm diameter round bur; 57 = 1-mm diameter straight fissure bur; 34 = 0.8-mm diameter inverted cone bur).[2] Despite the complexity of the system, it is still in common use. Other countries developed and used similarly arbitrary systems. Newer classification systems such as those developed by the International Dental Federation (Federation Dentaire Internationale [FDI]) and International Standards Organization (ISO) tend to use separate designations for shape (usually a shape name) and size (usually a number giving the head diameter in tenths of a millimeter [e.g., round 010; straight fissure plain 010; inverted cone 008]).[19,27]

Shapes. The term *bur shape* refers to the contour or silhouette of the head. The basic head shapes are round, inverted cone, pear, straight fissure, and tapered fissure (Fig. 7-34).

A *round bur* is spherical. This shape customarily has been used for such purposes as initial entry into the tooth, extension of the preparation, preparation of retention features, and caries removal.

An *inverted cone bur* is a portion of a rather rapidly tapered cone with the apex of the cone directed toward the bur shank. Head length is approximately the same as the diameter. This shape is particularly suitable for providing undercuts in tooth preparations.

A *pear-shaped bur* is a portion of a slightly tapered cone with the small end of the cone directed toward the bur shank. The end of the head either is continuously curved or is flat with rounded corners where the sides and flat end intersect. A normal-length pear bur (length slightly greater than the width) is advocated for use in Class I tooth preparations for gold foil. A long-length pear bur (length three times the width) is advocated for tooth preparations for amalgam.

A *straight fissure bur* is an elongated cylinder. Some advocate this shape for amalgam tooth preparation. Modified burs of this design with slightly curved tip angles are available.

A *tapered fissure bur* is a portion of a slightly tapered cone with the small end of the cone directed away from the bur shank. This shape is used for tooth preparations for indirect restorations, for which freedom from undercuts is essential for successful withdrawal of patterns and final seating of the restorations. Tapered fissure burs can have a flat end with the tip corners slightly rounded.

Among these basic shapes, variations are possible. Fissure and inverted cone burs may have half-round or domed ends. Taper and cone angles may be varied. The ratio of head length to diameter may be varied. In addition to shape, other features may be varied such as the number of blades, spiral versus axial patterns for blades, and continuous versus crosscut blade edges.

Sizes. In the United States, the number designating *bur size* also has traditionally served as a code for head design. This numbering system for burs was originated by the S.S. White Dental Manufacturing Company in 1891 for their first machine-made burs. It was both extensive and logical, so that other domestic manufacturers found it convenient to adopt it for their burs, as well. As a result, for over 60 years there was a general uniformity for bur numbers in the United States. Table 7-4 shows the correlation of bur head sizes with dimensions and shapes. It includes not only many bur sizes still in common use, but also others that have become obsolete.

The original numbering system grouped burs by 9 shapes and 11 sizes. The ½ and ¼ designations were added later when smaller instruments were included in the system. All original bur designs had continuous blade edges. Later, when crosscut burs were found to be more effective for cutting dentin at low speeds, crosscut versions of many bur sizes were introduced. This modification was indicated by adding 500 to the number of the equivalent noncrosscut size. Thus, a No. 57 with crosscut was designated No. 557. Similarly, a 900 prefix was used to indicate a head design intended for end-

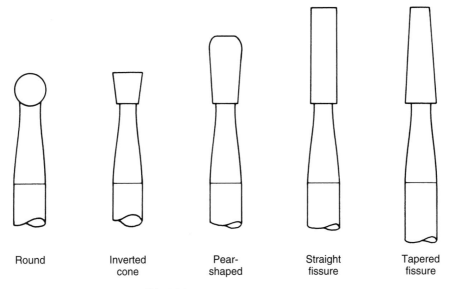

| Round | Inverted cone | Pear-shaped | Straight fissure | Tapered fissure |

FIG. 7-34 Basic bur head shapes.

cutting only. Except for differences in blade design, a No. 957, No. 557, and No. 57 bur all had the same head dimensions. These changes occurred gradually over time without disrupting the system. The sizes in common use in 1955 are shown in Table 7-5. The system changed rapidly thereafter, but where the numbers are still used, the designs and dimensions remain the same.

Modifications in Bur Design. As available handpiece speeds increased after 1950, particularly after the high-speed turbine handpieces were introduced, a new cycle of modification of bur sizes and shapes occurred. Numerous other categories have arisen as new variations in blade number or design have been created. Some of the numbers assigned to those burs were selected arbitrarily. With the introduction of new bur sizes and elimination of older sizes, much of the logic in the system has no longer been maintained, and many dentists and manufacturers no longer recognize the original significance of the numbers used for burs. The number of standard sizes that have continued in use has been reduced. This has been most obvious in the decreased popularity of large-diameter burs. The cutting effectiveness of carbide burs is greatly increased at high speeds.[9] This is particularly true of the small-diameter sizes, which did not have sufficient peripheral speed for efficient cutting when used at lower rates of rotation. As the *effectiveness of small burs has increased,* they have replaced larger burs in many procedures. *Three other major*

TABLE 7-4 | Original Bur Head Sizes (1891 to 1954)

HEAD SHAPES	HEAD DIAMETERS IN INCHES (mm*)												
	0.020 (0.5)	0.025 (0.6)	0.032 (0.8)	0.039 (1.0)	0.047 (1.2)	0.055 (1.4)	0.063 (1.6)	0.072 (1.8)	0.081 (2.1)	0.090 (2.3)	0.099 (2.5)	0.109 (2.8)	0.119 (3.0)
Round	1/4	1/2	1	2	3	4	5	6	7	8	9	10	11
Wheel		11 1/2	12	13	14	15	16	17	18	19	20	21	22
Cone		22 1/2	23	24	25	26	27	28	29	30	31	32	33
Inverted cone		33 1/2	34	35	36	37	38	39	40	41	42	43	44
Bud		44 1/2	45	46	47	48	49	50	51				
Straight fissure (flat end)	55 1/4	55 1/2	56	57	58	59	60	61	62				
Straight fissure (pointed end)		66 1/2	67	68	69	70	71	72	73				
Pear		77 1/2	78	79	80	81	82	83	84	85	86	87	88
Oval		88 1/2	89	90	91	92	93	94	95				

Courtesy of H.M. Moylan, S. S. White Dental Manufacturing Company.
*Millimeter values rounded to the nearest 0.1 mm.

TABLE 7-5 | Standard Bur Head Sizes—Carbide and Steel (1955 to Present)

HEAD SHAPES	HEAD DIAMETERS IN INCHES (mm*)												
	0.020 (0.5)	0.025 (0.6)	0.032 (0.8)	0.040 (1.0)	0.048 (1.2)	0.056 (1.4)	0.064 (1.6)	0.073 (1.9)	0.082 (2.1)	0.091 (2.3)	0.100 (2.5)	0.110 (2.8)	0.120 (3.0)	0.130 (3.3)
Round	1/4	1/2	1	2	3	4	5	6	7	8	9	10	11	
Wheel		11 1/2	12		14		16							
Inverted cone		33 1/2	34	35	36	37	38	39	40					
Plain fissure		55 1/2	56	57	58	59	60	61	62					
Round crosscut				502	503	504	505	506						
Straight fissure crosscut			556	557	558	559	560	561	562	563				
Tapered fissure crosscut				700	701		702		703					
End cutting fissure				957	958	959								
Round finishing				A	B	C	D		200		201		202	203
Oval finishing									218		219		220	221
Pear finishing									230		231		232	
Flame finishing				242	243	244	245	246						

Nonstandard excavating and finishing burs are not shown in this table.
*Millimeter values rounded to the nearest 0.1 mm.

trends in bur design are discernible: reduced use of crosscuts, extended heads on fissure burs, and rounding of sharp tip angles.

Crosscuts are needed on fissure burs to obtain adequate cutting effectiveness at low speeds, but at high speeds they are not needed. Because crosscut burs used at high speeds tend to produce unduly rough surfaces, many of the crosscut sizes originally developed for low-speed use have been replaced by noncrosscut instruments of the same dimension for high-speed use.[8] In many instances, the noncrosscut equivalents were available, thus a No. 57 bur might be used at high speed, whereas a No. 557 bur was preferred for low-speed use. Noncrosscut versions of the 700 series burs have become popular, but their introduction precipitated a crisis in the bur numbering system because no number had traditionally been assigned to burs of this type.

Carbide fissure burs with *extended head lengths* two to three times those of the normal tapered fissure burs of similar diameter have been introduced. Such a design would never have been practical using a brittle material such as carbide if the bur were to be used at low speed. The applied force required to make a bur cut at speeds of 5000 to 6000 rpm would normally be sufficient to fracture such an attenuated head. The extremely light applied pressures needed for cutting at high speed, however, permit many modifications of burs that would have been impractical at low speed.

The third major trend in bur design has been toward *rounding of the sharp tip corners.* Early contributions to this trend were made by Markley and Sockwell.[34] Because teeth are relatively brittle, the sharp angles produced by conventional burs can result in high stress concentrations and increase the tendency of the tooth to fracture. Bur heads with rounded corners result in lower stresses in restored teeth, enhance the strength of the tooth by preserving vital dentin, and facilitate the adaptation of restorative materials. Both carbide burs and diamond instruments of these designs last longer because there are no sharp corners to chip and wear. Such burs facilitate tooth preparation with desired features of a flat preparation floor and rounded internal line angles.

Many of these new and modified bur designs simplify the techniques and reduce the effort needed for optimal results. Although the development of new bur sizes and shapes has greatly increased the number of different types in current use, the number actually required for clinical effectiveness has been reduced. Most instruments recommended in this text for the preparation of teeth are illustrated in Fig. 7-35. The selection in-

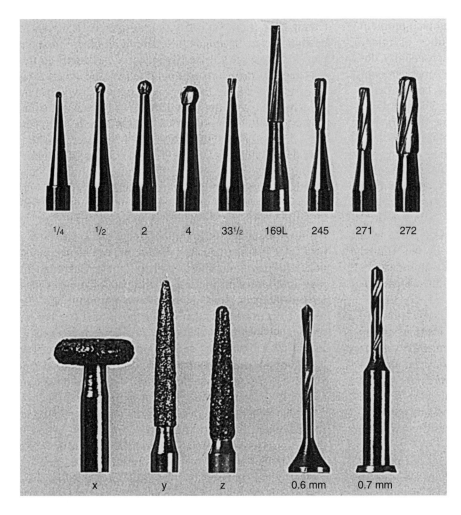

FIG. **7-35** Burs used in recommended procedures. Bur sizes ¼, ½, 2, 4, 33½, and 169L are standard carbide burs available from various sources. The 245, 271, and 272 burs are nonstandard carbide burs that do not conform to the current ADA standard numbering system. They are designed to combine rounded corners with flat ends and are available from several manufacturers. The diamond instruments shown are wheel (Star No. 110) *(x)*, flame (Star No. 265-8F) *(y)*, and tapered cylinder (R & R No. 770 x 7) *(z)*. Two sizes of twist drill are illustrated. Particular drills often are provided as specified by manufacturers of pin-retention systems.

| TABLE 7-6 | Names and Key Dimensions of Recommended Burs |

MANUFACTURER'S SIZE NUMBER	ADA SIZE NUMBER	ISO SIZE NUMBER	HEAD DIAMETER (mm)	HEAD LENGTH (mm)	TAPER ANGLE (DEGREES)	SHAPE
$1/_4$	$1/_4$	005	0.50	0.40	—	Round
$1/_2$	$1/_2$	006	0.60	0.48	—	Round
2	2	010	1.00	0.80	—	Round
4	4	014	1.40	1.10	—	Round
33S*	—	006	0.60	0.45	12	Inverted cone
$33^1/_2$	$33^1/_2$	006	0.60	0.45	12	Inverted cone
169	169	009	0.90	4.3	6	Tapered fissure
169L†	169L	009	0.90	5.6	4	Elongated tapered fissure
329	329	007	0.70	0.85	8	Pear, normal length
330	330	008	0.80	1.00	8	Pear, normal length
245‡§	330L	008	0.80	3.0	4	Pear, long length
271‡	171	012	1.20	4.0	6	Tapered fissure
272‡	172	016	1.60	5.0	6	Tapered fissure

*Similar to the No. $33^1/_2$ bur except that it is safe-sided end-cutting only.
†Similar to the No. 169 bur except for greater head length.
‡These burs differ from the equivalent ADA size by being flat ended with rounded corners. The manufacturer's number has been changed to indicate this difference.
§Similar to the No. 330 bur except for greater head length.

cludes standard head designs and modified designs of the types just discussed. Table 7-6 lists the significant head dimensions of these standard and modified burs.

A long-standing international problem related to the dimensions and designations of rotary dental instruments arose because each country developed its own system of classification. Dentists in the United States were not often aware of the problem because they predominantly used domestic products, and all U.S. manufacturers used the same system. The rapid rate at which new bur designs were introduced during the transition to high-speed techniques threatened to cause a complete breakdown in the numbering system. As different manufacturers developed and marketed new burs of similar design almost simultaneously, there was an increased risk of similar burs being given either different numbers or different burs the same number. Combined with an increased use of foreign products in the United States this has led to an increased interest in the establishment of international standards for dimensions, nomenclature, and other characteristics.

In recent years, progress toward the development of an international numbering system for basic bur shapes and sizes under the auspices of the International Standards Organization (ISO) has been slow. For other design features the trend instead appears to be toward the use of individual manufacturer's code numbers. Therefore, throughout the remaining text, the traditional U.S. numbers are used, where possible. The few exceptions are shown in Fig. 7-35 and Table 7-6.

Additional Features in Head Design. A large number of factors other than head size and shape are in-

volved in determining the clinical effectiveness of a bur design.[17,18] Fig. 7-36 shows a lateral view and a cross-sectional view of a No. 701 crosscut tapered fissure bur in which several of these factors are illustrated. The lateral view (see Fig. 7-36, A) demonstrates neck diameter, head diameter, head length, taper angle, blade spiral angle, and crosscut size and spacing as they apply to this bur size. Of these features *head length* and *taper angle* are primarily descriptive and may be varied within limits consistent with the intended use of the bur. This bur was originally designed for use at low speeds in preparing teeth for cast restorations. The taper angle therefore is intended to approximate the desired occlusal divergence of the lateral walls of the preparations, and the head length must be long enough to reach the full depth of the normal preparation. These factors do not otherwise affect the performance of the bur.

Neck diameter is important functionally because a neck that is too small will result in a weak instrument unable to resist lateral forces. Too large a neck diameter may interfere with visibility and the use of the part of the bur head next to the neck and may restrict access for coolants. As the head of a bur increases in length or diameter, the moment arm exerted by lateral forces increases, and the neck needs to be larger.

In comparison with these factors, two other design variables, the *spiral angle* and *crosscutting*, have considerably greater influence on bur performance. There is a tendency toward reduced spiral angles on burs intended exclusively for high-speed operation where a large spiral is not needed to produce a smoother preparation and a smaller angle, which produces more efficient cutting.

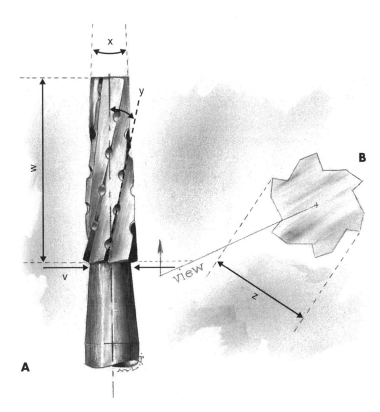

FIG. **7-36** Design features of bur heads (illustrated using No. 701 bur). **A,** Lateral view: neck diameter *(v),* head length *(w),* taper angle *(x),* and spiral angle *(y).* **B,** End view: head diameter *(z).*

As noted previously, crosscut bur designs have notches in the blade edges to increase cutting effectiveness at low and medium speeds. A certain amount of perpendicular force is required to make a blade grasp the surface and start cutting as it passes across the surface. The harder the surface, the duller is the blade, and the greater its length, the more force that is required to initiate cutting. By reducing the total length of bur blade that is actively cutting at any one time, the crosscuts effectively increase both the cutting pressure resulting from rotation of the bur and the perpendicular pressure holding the blade edge against the tooth.

As each crosscut blade cuts, it leaves small ridges of tooth structure standing behind the notches. Because the notches in two succeeding blades do not line up with each other, the ridges left by one blade are removed by the following one at low or medium speeds. However, at the high speed attained with air-turbine handpieces, the contact of the bur with the tooth is not continuous, and usually only one blade cuts effectively.[16] Under these circumstances, although the high cutting rate of crosscut burs is maintained, the ridges are not removed and a much rougher cut surface results.[8]

A cross-sectional view of the same No. 701 bur is shown in Fig. 7-36, *B.* This cross-section is made at the point of largest head diameter and is drawn as seen from the shank end. The bur has six blades uniformly spaced with depressed areas between them. These depressed areas are properly known as the *flutes.* The number of blades on a bur is always even because even num-

bers are easier to produce in the manufacturing process, and instruments with odd numbers of blades cut no better than those with even numbers. The number of blades on an excavating bur may vary from 6 to 8 to 10. Burs intended mainly for finishing procedures usually have 12 to 40 blades. The greater are the number of blades, the smoother is the cutting action at low speeds. Most burs are made with at least six blades because they may need to be used in this speed range. In the high-speed range, it appears that no more than one blade cuts effectively at any one time, and the remaining blades are, in effect, spares. The tendency for the bur to cut on a single blade is often a result of factors other than the bur itself. Nevertheless, it is important that the bur head be as symmetric as possible. Two terms are in common use to measure this characteristic of bur heads: *concentricity* and *runout.*

Concentricity is a direct measurement of the symmetry of the bur head itself. It measures how closely a single circle can be passed through the tips of all of the blades. Thus, concentricity is an indication of whether one blade is longer or shorter than the others. It is a static measurement not directly related to function. *Runout,* on the other hand, is a dynamic test measuring the accuracy with which all blade tips pass through a single point when the instrument is rotated. It measures not only the concentricity of the head, but also the accuracy with which the center of rotation passes through the center of the head. Even a perfectly concentric head will exhibit substantial runout if the head is off center on the axis of the bur, the bur neck is bent, the bur is not held straight in the handpiece chuck, or the chuck is eccentric relative to the handpiece bearings. The runout can never be less than the concentricity, and it is usually substantially greater. The runout is the more significant term clinically, because it is the primary cause of vibration during cutting and is the factor that determines the minimum diameter of the hole that can be prepared by a given bur. It is because of runout errors that burs normally cut holes measurably larger than the head diameter.

Bur Blade Design. The actual cutting action of a bur (or a diamond) takes place in a very small region at the edge of the blade (or at the point of a diamond chip). In the high-speed range, this effective portion of the individual blade is limited to no more than a few thousandths of a centimeter adjacent to the blade edge. Fig. 7-37 is an enlarged schematic view of this portion of a bur blade. Several terms used in the discussion of blade design are illustrated.

Each blade has two sides, the *rake face* (toward the direction of cutting) and *clearance face*, and three important angles, the *rake angle*, the *edge angle*, and the *clearance angle*. The optimal angles are dependent on such factors as the mechanical properties of the blade material, the mechanical properties of the material being cut, the rotational speed and diameter of the bur, and the lateral force applied by the operator to the handpiece, and thus to the bur.

The rake angle is the most important design characteristic of a bur blade. For cutting hard, brittle materials, a negative rake angle minimizes fractures of the cutting edge, thereby increasing the tool life. A rake angle is said to be negative when the rake face is ahead of the radius (from cutting edge to axis of bur) as is illustrated in Fig. 7-37. Increasing the edge angle reinforces the cutting edge and reduces the likelihood for the edge of the blade to fracture. Carbide bur blades have higher hardness and are more wear resistant, but they are more brittle than steel blades and require greater edge angles to minimize fractures. The three angles cannot be varied independently of each other. An increase in the clearance angle, for example, causes a decrease in the edge angle. The clearance angle eliminates rubbing friction of the clearance face, provides a stop to prevent the bur edge from digging into the tooth structure excessively, and reduces the radius of the blade back of the cutting edge to provide adequate flute space or clearance space for the chips formed ahead of the following blade.

Carbide burs normally have blades with slight negative rake angles and edge angles of approximately 90 degrees. Their clearance faces either are curved or have two surfaces to provide a low clearance angle near the edge and a greater clearance space ahead of the following blade.

DIAMOND ABRASIVE INSTRUMENTS

The second major category of rotary dental cutting instruments involves abrasive rather than blade cutting. *Abrasive instruments* are based on small, angular particles of a hard substance held in a matrix of softer material. Cutting occurs at a large number of points where individual hard particles protrude from the matrix, rather than along a continuous blade edge. This difference in design causes definite differences in the mechanisms by which the two types of instruments cut and in the applications for which they are best suited.

Abrasive instruments are generally grouped as diamond or other instruments. Diamond instruments have had great clinical impact because of their long life and great effectiveness in cutting enamel and dentin. Diamond instruments for dental use were introduced in the United States in 1942 at a time before carbide burs were available, and at a time when interest in increased rotational speeds was beginning to expose the limitations of

FIG. **7-37** Bur blade design. Schematic cross-section viewed from shank end of head to show rake angle, edge angle, and clearance angle.

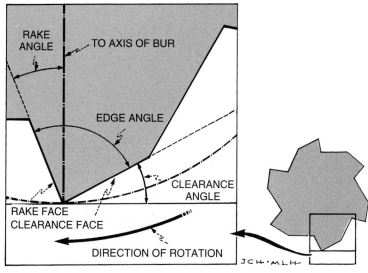
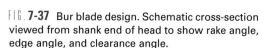

steel burs. The earliest diamond instruments were substitutes for previously used abrasive points of other types used for grinding and finishing. Their vastly superior performance in these applications led to their immediate acceptance. The shortage of burs as a result of wartime demands emphasized the relative durability of diamond instruments for cutting enamel and promoted the development of operative techniques employing them.

Terminology. Diamond instruments consist of three parts: a metal blank, the powdered diamond abrasive, and a metallic bonding material that holds the diamond powder onto the blank (Fig. 7-38).[30] The *blank* in many

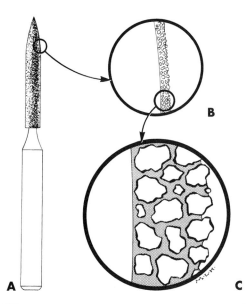

FIG. **7-38** Diamond instrument construction: **A,** overall view; **B,** detail of abrasive layer; and **C,** detail of particle bonding.

ways resembles a bur without blades. It has the same essential parts: head, neck, and shank.

The shank dimensions, like those for bur shanks, depend on the intended handpiece. The neck is normally a tapered section of reduced diameter that connects the shank to the head, but for large disc or wheel-shaped instruments it may not be reduced below the shank diameter. The head of the blank is undersized in comparison with the desired final dimensions of the instrument, but its size and shape determine the size and shape of the finished instrument. Dimensions of the head make allowance for a fairly uniform thickness of diamonds and bonding material on all sides. Some abrasive instruments are designed as a mandrel and a detachable head. This is much more practical for abrasive disks that have very short lifetimes.

The diamonds employed are industrial diamonds, either natural or synthetic, that have been crushed to powder and then carefully graded for size and quality. The shape of the individual particle is important because of its effect on the cutting efficiency and durability of the instrument, but the careful control of particle size is probably of greater importance. The diamonds generally are attached to the blank by electroplating a layer of metal on the blank while holding the diamonds in place against it. While the electroplating holds the diamonds in place, it also tends to cover much of the diamond surfaces. Some proprietary techniques do allow greater diamond exposure and more effective cutting.

Classification. Diamond instruments are currently marketed in a profusion of head shapes and sizes (Table 7-7), and in all of the standard shank designs. Most of the diamond shapes parallel those for burs (Fig. 7-39). This

TABLE **7-7**	Standard Categories of Shapes and Sizes for Diamond Cutting Instruments

HEAD SHAPES*	PROFILE VARIATIONS	SHANK VARIATIONS**
Round		With collar
Football	Pointed	
Barrel		
Cylinder	Flat-end, bevel-end, round-end, safe-end	
Inverted cone		With collar
Taper	Flat-end, round-end, safe-end	
Flame		
Curettage		
Pear		
Needle	Christmas tree	
Interproximal	Occlusal anatomy	
Pear		
Donut		
Wheel		

*See Fig. 7-39 for examples of head shapes.
**Most heads and shanks come in a range of dimensions.

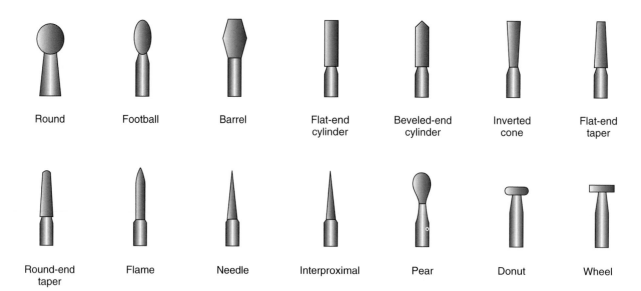

| Round | Football | Barrel | Flat-end cylinder | Beveled-end cylinder | Inverted cone | Flat-end taper |

| Round-end taper | Flame | Needle | Interproximal | Pear | Donut | Wheel |

FIG. **7-39** Characteristic shapes and designs for a range of diamond cutting instruments.

great diversity arose, in part, as a result of the relative simplicity of the manufacturing process. Because it is possible to make diamond instruments in almost any shape for which a blank can be manufactured, they are produced in many highly specialized shapes, on which it would be impractical to place cutting blades. This has been a major factor in establishing clinical uses for these points, which are not in direct competition with burs.

Head Shapes and Sizes. Diamond instruments are available in a wide variety of shapes and in sizes that correspond to all except the smallest diameter burs. The greatest difference lies in the diversity of other sizes and shapes in which diamond instruments are produced. Even with many subdivisions, the size range within each group is very large in comparison with that found among the burs. More than 200 shapes and sizes of diamonds are currently marketed.

Because of their design with an abrasive layer over an underlying blank, the smallest diamond instruments cannot be as small in diameter as the smallest burs, but a wide range of sizes is available for each shape. No one manufacturer produces all sizes, but each will usually offer an assortment of instruments, including the popular sizes and shapes. Because of the lack of uniform nomenclature for diamond instruments, it is often necessary to select them by inspection to obtain the desired size and shape. It is essential, therefore, to indicate the manufacturer when attempting to describe diamond instruments by catalogue number.

Diamond Particle Factors. The clinical performance of diamond abrasive instruments depends on the *size*, *spacing*, *uniformity*, *exposure*, and *bonding* of the diamond particles. Increased pressure causes the particles to dig into the surface more deeply, leaving deeper scratches and removing more tooth structure.

Diamond *particle size* is commonly categorized as coarse (125 to 150 μm), medium (88 to 125 μm), fine (60 to 74 μm), and very fine (38 to 44 μm) for diamond preparation instruments.[30] These ranges correspond to standard sieve sizes for separating particle sizes. When using large particle sizes, the number of abrasive particles that can be placed on a given area of the head is decreased. Thus, for any given force that the operator applies, the pressure on each particle tip is greater. The resulting pressure also is increased if diamond particles are more widely *spaced* so that fewer are in contact with the surface at any one time. The final clinical performance of diamond instruments is strongly affected by the technique used to take advantage of the design factors for each instrument.

Diamond finishing instruments use even finer diamonds (10 to 38 μm) to produce relatively smooth surfaces for final finishing with diamond polishing pastes. Surface finishes of less than 1 μm are considered clinically smooth (see Composites in Chapter 4) and can be routinely attained by using a series of finer and finer polishing steps.

Proper diamond instrument speed and pressure are the major factors in determining service life.[10] Properly used diamond instruments will last almost indefinitely. Almost the only cause of failure of diamond instruments is loss of the diamonds from critical areas. This results from the use of excess pressure in an attempt to increase the cutting rate at inadequate speeds.[15]

OTHER ABRASIVE INSTRUMENTS

Many types of abrasive instruments are used in dentistry in addition to diamond instruments. They were at one time extensively used for tooth preparation, but their use is now primarily restricted to shaping, finishing, and polishing restorations, both in the clinic and in the laboratory.

Classification. In these instruments, as in the diamond instruments, the cutting surfaces of the head are composed of abrasive particles held in a continuous matrix of softer material. Other than this and their use of standard shank designs, diamond instruments have little similarity in their construction. They may be divided into two distinct groups, molded instruments and coated instruments. Each uses various abrasives and matrix materials.

Molded abrasive instruments have heads that are manufactured by molding or pressing a uniform mixture of abrasive and matrix around the roughened end of the shank, or cementing a premolded head to the shank. In contrast to diamond instruments, molded instruments have a much softer matrix and wear during use. The abrasive is distributed throughout the matrix so new particles are exposed by the wear. These instruments are made in a full range of shapes and sizes. The mounted heads are often termed *points* as well as *stones*. Hard and rigid molded instrument heads use rigid polymer or ceramic materials for their matrix and commonly are used for grinding and shaping procedures. Other molded instrument heads use flexible matrix materials, such as rubber, to hold the abrasive particles. These are used predominantly for finishing and polishing procedures. Molded *unmounted discs* or *wheelstones* are made that attach by a screw to a mandrel of suitable size for a given handpiece that has a threaded hole in the end. This design permits the instruments to be changed easily and discarded economically.

The *coated abrasive instruments* are mostly discs that have a thin layer of abrasive cemented to a flexible backing. This construction allows the instrument to conform to the surface contour of a tooth or restoration. Most flexible discs are designed for reversible attachment to a mandrel. Coated abrasive instruments may be used in the finishing/smoothing procedures of certain enamel walls (and margins) of tooth preparations for indirect restorations, but most often in finishing procedures for restorations.

The abrasives are softer and less wear-resistant than diamond powder and, as a result, tend to lose their sharp edges and thus their cutting efficiency with use. When this happens to coated instruments, they are discarded. Molded instruments, in contrast, are intended to be partially regenerating by gradual loss of their worn outer layers, but may require that the operator reshape them to improve their concentricity. This is accomplished by applying a truing or shaping stone against the rotating instrument.

Materials. The *matrix materials* usually are phenolic resins or rubber. Some molded points may be sintered, but most are resin bonded. A *rubber matrix* is used primarily to obtain a flexible head on instruments to be

TABLE **7-8**	Hardness Values of Restorative Materials, Tooth Structure, and Abrasives		
	KNOOP HARDNESS (KHN)	BRINELL HARDNESS (BHN)	MOHS HARDNESS (VALUE)
Dentin	68	48	3-4
Enamel	343	300	5
Dental composite	41-80	60-80	5-7
Dental amalgam	110	—	4-5
Gold alloy (Type III)	—	110	—
MGC Dicor	330	—	—
Feldspathic porcelain	460	—	6-7
Pumice	—	—	6
Cuttlebone	—	—	7
Garnet	—	—	6.5-7
Quartz	800	600	7
Aluminum oxide	1500	1200	9
Silicon carbide	2500	—	9.5
Diamond	7000+	5000+	10

used for polishing. A harder, *nonflexible rubber matrix* is often used for molded SiC discs. The matrix of coated instruments is usually one of the phenolic resins.

Synthetic or natural abrasives may be used, including SiC, aluminum oxide, garnet, quartz, pumice, and cuttlebone. The hardness of the abrasive has a major effect on the cutting efficiency. Mohs hardnesses for important dental abrasives are shown in Table 7-8.

Silicon carbide (Carborundum) usually is used in molded rounds, tree or bud shapes, wheels, and cylinders of various sizes. These points are normally gray-green, available in various textures, usually fast cutting (except on enamel), and they produce a moderately smooth surface. Molded unmounted discs are black or a dark color, have a soft matrix, wear more rapidly than stones, and produce a moderately rough surface texture. These discs are termed *Carborundum discs* or separating discs.

Aluminum oxide is used for the same instrument designs as SiC. Points are usually white, rigid, fine textured, less porous, and produce a smoother surface than SiC.

Garnet (reddish) and *quartz* (white) are used for coated discs that are available in a series of particle sizes that ranges from coarse to medium-fine for use in initial finishing. These abrasives are hard enough to cut tooth structure and all restorative materials, with the exception of some porcelains.

Pumice is a powdered abrasive produced by crushing foamed volcanic glass into thin glass flakes. The flakes cut effectively, but break down rapidly. Pumice is used with rubber discs and wheels, usually for initial polishing procedures.

Cuttlebone is derived from the cuttlefish, a relative of squid and octopus. It is becoming scarce and is gradually being replaced by synthetic substitutes. It is a soft white abrasive, used only in coated discs for final finishing and polishing. It is soft enough that it reduces the risk of unintentional damage to tooth structure during the final stages of finishing.

CUTTING MECHANISMS

For cutting, it is necessary to apply sufficient pressure to make the cutting edge of a blade or abrasive particle dig into the surface. Local fracture occurs more easily if the strain rate is high (high rotary instrument surface speed) because the surface being cut responds in a brittle fashion.

The process by which rotary instruments cut tooth structure is complex and not fully understood. The following discussion of cutting addresses cutting evaluations, cutting instrument design, proposed cutting mechanisms, and clinical recommendations for cutting.

EVALUATION OF CUTTING

Cutting can be measured in terms of both effectiveness and efficiency. Certain factors may influence one, but not the other.[21] *Cutting effectiveness* is the rate of tooth structure removal (mm/min or mg/sec). Effectiveness does not consider potential side effects such as heat or noise. *Cutting efficiency* is the percentage of energy actually producing cutting. Cutting efficiency is reduced when energy is wasted as heat or noise. It is possible to increase effectiveness while decreasing efficiency. A dull bur, for example, may be made to cut faster than a sharp bur by applying a greater pressure, but experience indicates that this results in a great increase in heat production, and thus reduced efficiency.[37]

There is general agreement that increased rotational speed results in increased effectiveness and efficiency. Adverse effects associated with increased speeds are heat, vibration, and noise. *Heat has been identified as a primary cause of pulpal injury.* Air-water sprays do not prevent the production of heat, but do serve to remove it before it causes a damaging rise in temperature within the tooth.

BLADED CUTTING

The following discussion focuses on rotary bladed instruments, but is applicable to bladed hand instruments as well. Tooth structure, like other materials, undergoes both brittle and ductile fracture. *Brittle fracture* is associated with crack production, usually by tensile loading. *Ductile fracture* involves plastic deformation of material, usually proceeding by shear. Extensive plastic deformation also may produce local work hardening and encourage brittle fracture as well. Low-speed cutting tends to proceed by plastic deformation before tooth structure fracture. High-speed cutting, especially of enamel, proceeds by brittle fracture.

The rate of stress application (or strain rate) affects the resultant properties of materials. In general, the faster the rate of loading, the greater will be the strength, hardness, modulus of elasticity, and brittleness of a material. A cutting instrument with a large diameter and high rotational speed produces a high surface speed, and thus a high stress (or strain) rate.

Many factors interact to determine which cutting mechanism is active in a particular situation. The mechanical properties of tooth structure, the design of the cutting edge or point, the linear speed of the instrument's surface, the contact force applied, and the power output characteristics of the handpiece influence the cutting process in various ways.[9,24]

In order for the blade to initiate the cutting action, it must be sharp, must have a higher hardness and modulus of elasticity than the material being cut, and must be pressed against the surface with sufficient force. The high hardness and modulus of elasticity are essential to concentrate the applied force on a small enough area to exceed the shear strength of the material being cut.

As shown in Fig. 7-40, sheared segments accumulate in a distorted layer that slides up along the rake face of the blade until it breaks or until the blade disengages from the surface as it rotates. These chips will accumulate in the clearance space between blades until washed out or thrown out by centrifugal force.

Mechanical distortion of tooth structure ahead of the blade produces heat. Frictional heat is produced by both the rubbing action of the cut chips against the rake face of the blade and the blade tip against the cut surface of the tooth immediately behind the edge.

This can produce extreme temperature increases in both the tooth and the bur in the absence of adequate cooling. The transfer of heat is not instantaneous, and the reduced temperature rise observed in teeth cut at very high speeds may, in part, be caused by removal of the heated surface layer of tooth structure by a following blade before the heat can be conducted into the tooth.

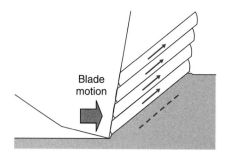

FIG. **7-40** Schematic representation of bur blade (end view) cutting a ductile material by shearing mechanism. Energy is required to deform the material removed and produce new surface.

ABRASIVE CUTTING

The following discussion is pertinent to all abrasive cutting situations, but diamond instruments are used as the primary example.[13] The cutting action of diamond abrasive instruments is similar in many ways to that of bladed instruments, but key differences result from the properties, size, and distribution of the abrasive. The very high hardness of diamonds provides superior resistance to wear. A diamond instrument that is not abused, has little or no tendency to dull with use. Individual diamond particles have very sharp edges, are randomly oriented on the surface, and tend to have large negative rake angles.

When diamond instruments are used to cut ductile materials, some material will be removed as chips, but much material will flow laterally around the cutting point and be left as a ridge of deformed material on the surface (Fig. 7-41). Repeated deformation work hardens the distorted material until irregular portions become brittle, break off, and are removed. This type of cutting is less efficient than that of a blade; therefore burs are generally preferred for cutting ductile materials such as dentin.

Diamonds cut brittle materials by a different mechanism. Most cutting results from tensile fractures that produce a series of subsurface cracks (Fig. 7-42). Diamonds are most efficient when used to cut brittle materials, and are superior to burs for the removal of dental enamel. Because a diamond prepares a rougher tooth surface, diamonds may be preferred for use in tooth preparation for bonded restorations. The roughened prepared surface increases the surface area, and therefore, the bonding potential.

Diamond abrasives are commonly used for milling in CAD/CAM or copy-milling applications (see Machined Restorations in Chapter 4).

CUTTING RECOMMENDATIONS

Overall, the requirements for effective and efficient cutting include using a contra-angle handpiece, air-water spray for cooling, high operating speed (above 200,000 rpm), light pressure, and a carbide bur or diamond instrument. *Carbide burs are better for end-cutting, produce lower heat, and have more blade edges per diameter for cutting.* They are effectively used for punch cuts to enter tooth structure, intracoronal tooth

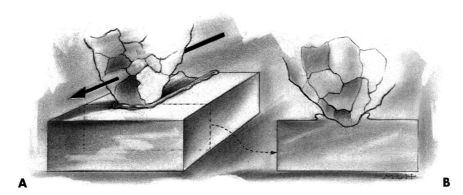

FIG. **7-41** Schematic representation of an abrasive particle cutting ductile material. **A,** Lateral view. **B,** Cross-sectional view. Material is displaced laterally by passage of an abrasive particle, work hardened, and subsequently removed by other particles.

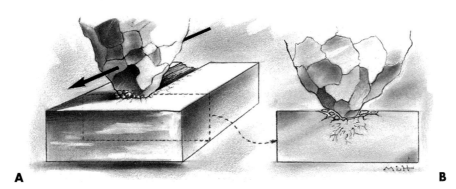

FIG. **7-42** Schematic representation of abrasive particle cutting brittle material. **A,** Lateral view. **B,** Cross-sectional view. Subsurface cracks caused by the passage of abrasive particles intersect, undermining small pieces of material, which are then easily removed by following abrasive particles.

preparation, amalgam removal, small preparations, and secondary retention features. Diamond instruments have higher hardness, and coarse diamonds have very high cutting effectiveness. *Diamonds are more effective than burs for both intracoronal and extracoronal tooth preparations, beveling enamel margins on tooth preparations, and enameloplasty.*

HAZARDS WITH CUTTING INSTRUMENTS

Almost everything done in a dental office involves some risk to the patient, dentist, and/or auxiliaries. For the patient, there are *pulpal dangers* from the tooth preparation and restoration procedures. There are also *soft tissue dangers.* Everyone is potentially susceptible to *eye, ear,* and *inhalation dangers.* However, careful adherence to normal precautions can eliminate or minimize most risks associated with cutting instrument use.

PULPAL PRECAUTIONS

The use of cutting instruments can harm the pulp by exposure to mechanical vibration, heat generation, desiccation and loss of dentinal tubule fluid, and/or transection of odontoblastic processes. As the thickness of remaining dentin decreases, the pulpal insult (and response) from heat or desiccation increases. Slight to moderate injury produces a localized, protective pulpal response in the region of the cut tubules. In severe injury, destruction extends beyond the cut tubules, often resulting in pulpal abscess and death of the pulp. These pulpal sequelae (recovery or necrosis) take from 2 weeks to 6 months or longer, depending on the extent and degree of the trauma. Although a young pulp is more prone to injury, it also recovers more effectively when compared with an older pulp, in which the recuperative powers are slower and less effective.

Enamel and dentin are good thermal insulators and will protect the pulp if the quantity of heat is not too great and the remaining thickness of tissue is adequate. The longer the time of cutting and the higher the local temperature produced, the greater is the threat of thermal trauma. *The remaining tissue is effective in protecting the pulp in proportion to the square of its thickness.* Steel burs produce more heat than carbide burs because of inefficient cutting. Burs and diamond instruments that are dull or plugged with debris do not cut efficiently, resulting in heat production. When used without coolants, diamond instruments generate more damaging heat than carbide burs.

The most common *instrument coolants* are *air or air-water spray.* Air alone as a coolant is not effective in preventing pulpal damage because it needlessly desiccates the dentin and damages the odontoblasts (see Chapter 2). Air has a much lower heat capacity than water and is much less efficient in absorbing unwanted heat. An air coolant alone should be used only when visibil-

ity is a problem, such as during the finishing procedures of tooth preparations. At such times, air coolant combined with both lower speed and light intermittent application, should be used to enhance vision and minimize trauma. Air-water spray is universally used to cool, moisten, and clear the operating site during normal cutting procedures. In addition, the spray lubricates, cleans, and cools the cutting instrument, thereby increasing its efficiency and service life. A well-designed and properly directed air-water spray also helps keep the gingival crevice open for better vision when gingival extension is necessary. The use of a water spray and its removal by an effective high-volume evacuator are especially important when old amalgam restorations are removed because they decrease mercury vapor release and increase visibility.

During normal cutting procedures a layer of debris, described as a *smear layer,* is created that covers the cut surfaces of the enamel and dentin (see Chapters 2 and 6). The smear layer on dentin is moderately protective because it occludes dentinal tubules and inhibits the outward flow of tubular fluid and the inward penetration of microleakage contaminants. However, the smear layer is still porous. When air alone is applied to dentin, local desiccation may produce fluid flow and affect the physiologic status of the odontoblastic processes in the underlying dentin (review Chapter 2 for hydrodynamic sequelae). *Air is applied only to the extent of removing excess moisture, leaving a glistening surface.*

SOFT TISSUE PRECAUTIONS

The lips, tongue, and cheeks of the patient are the most frequent areas of soft tissue injury. The handpiece should never be operated unless there is good access and vision to the cutting site. A rubber dam is very helpful in isolating the operating site. When the dam is not used, the dental assistant can retract the soft tissue on one side with a mouth mirror, cotton roll, and/or evacuator tip. The dentist can usually manage the other side with a mirror and/or cotton roll. If the dentist must work alone, the patient can help by holding a retraction-type saliva ejector evacuator tip, after it is positioned in the mouth.

With air-turbine handpieces, the rotating instrument does not stop immediately when the foot control is released. The operator must either wait for the instrument to stop or be extremely careful when removing the handpiece from the mouth so as not to lacerate soft tissues. The large disc is one of the most dangerous instruments used in the mouth. Fortunately such discs are seldom indicated intraorally. They should be used with light, intermittent application and with extreme caution.

The dentist and the assistant must always be aware of the patient's response during the cutting procedures. A sudden reflex movement by the patient, such as gagging, swallowing, or coughing could result in serious injury. If an accident does occur in which soft tissue is damaged, the operator should remain calm and control any hemorrhage with a pressure pack. The patient should be told what has happened, and medical assistance should be obtained if needed.

The chance of mechanical pulpal involvement may be greater if a hand excavator is used to remove the last portions of soft caries in a deep preparation. When the remaining dentinal wall is thin, the pressure exerted on the excavator may be sufficient to break into the pulp chamber. Therefore a round bur may be used at a low speed with light, intermittent pressure for caries removal. Air-turbine handpieces should be operated just above stalling speed to improve tactile sense for caries removal. Proceed with caution and inspect the area frequently.

EYE PRECAUTIONS

The operator, assistant, and patient should wear glasses with side shields to prevent eye damage from airborne particles during operative procedures utilizing rotary instrumentation. When using high speeds, particles of old restorations, tooth structure, bacteria, and other debris are discharged at high speeds from the patient's mouth. Sufficiently strong high-volume evacuation applied by the dental assistant near the operating site helps alleviate this problem. However, *protective glasses are always indicated when rotary instrumentation is being used.* The dentist is more likely to receive injury than is the assistant or the patient, because of being in a more direct path of such particles. If an eye is injured, it should be covered by a clean gauze pad until medical attention can be obtained.

In addition to routine air-borne debris, occasionally *airborne particles may be produced by matrix failure of molded abrasive cutting instruments.* Hard matrix wheels may crack or shatter into relatively large pieces. Soft abrasive wheels or points may increase in temperature during use, causing the rubber matrix to explosively debond from the abrasive into fine particles.

Furthermore, precautions must be taken for prevention of eye injury from unusual light sources, such as visible light-curing units and laser equipment. Dental personnel and patients should be protected from high-intensity visible light using colored plastic shields (attached to the fiber-optic tip). Laser light can be inadvertently reflected from many surfaces in the dental operatory; therefore the operatory should be closed, and everyone should wear protective goggles (see Laser Equipment).

EAR PRECAUTIONS

Various sounds are known to affect people in different ways. Soft music or random sounds like rainfall usually have a relaxing or sedative effect. Loud noises are generally annoying and may contribute to mental and physical distress. A noisy environment decreases the ability to concentrate, increases accident proneness, and reduces overall efficiency. Extremely loud noises such as explosions, or continuous exposure to high noise levels can cause permanent damage to the hearing mechanism.

An objectionable high-pitched whine is produced by some air-turbine handpieces at high speeds. Aside from the annoying aspect of this noise, there is some possibility that hearing loss can result from continued exposure.

Potential damage to hearing from noise depends on: (1) the intensity or loudness (decibels [db]), (2) frequency (cps), and (3) duration (time) of the noise, as well as (4) the susceptibility of the individual. Increased age, existing ear damage, disease, and medications are other factors that can accelerate hearing loss.

Normal ears require that the intensity of sound reach a certain minimum level before the ear can detect it. This is known as the *auditory threshold.* It can vary with frequency and exposure to other sounds. When subjected to a loud noise of short duration, a protective mechanism of the ear causes it to lose some sensitivity temporarily. This is described as a *temporary threshold shift.* If sufficient time is allowed between exposures, recovery will be complete. Extended or continuous exposure is much more likely to result in a *permanent threshold shift* with persistent hearing loss. The loss may occur for all frequencies, but often affects high frequency sounds more severely.

A certain amount of unnoticed noise (ambient noise level) is present even in a quiet room (20 to 40 db). An ordinary conversation averages 50 to 70 db in a frequency range of 500 to 2500 cps.

Turbine handpieces with ball bearings, free running at 30 pounds air pressure, may have noise levels as high as 70 to 94 db at high frequencies. Noise levels in excess of 75 db in frequency ranges of 1000 to 8000 cps may cause hearing damage. There is considerable variation in noise levels among handpieces by the same manufacturer. Handpiece wear and eccentric rotating instruments can cause increased noise. Protective measures are recommended when the noise level reaches 85 db with frequency ranges from 300 to 4800 cps. Protection is mandatory in areas where the level transiently reaches 95 db. The effect of excessive noise levels depends on exposure times. Normal use of a dental handpiece is one of intermittent application that generally is less than 30 minutes per day. Earplugs can be used to reduce the level of exposure but have several drawbacks. Room soundproofing helps and can be accomplished with absorbing materials used on walls and floors. Antinoise devices can be used to cancel unwanted sounds as well.

INHALATION PRECAUTIONS

Aerosols and vapors are created by cutting tooth structure and restorative materials. Both aerosols and vapors are a health hazard to all present. The aerosols are fine dispersions in air of water, tooth debris, microorganisms, and/or restorative materials. Cutting amalgams or composites produce both submicron particles and vapor. The particles that may be inadvertently inhaled have the potential to produce alveolar irritation and tissue reactions. Vapor from cutting amalgams is predominantly mercury and should be eliminated, as much as possible, by careful evacuation near the tooth being operated on. The vapors generated during cutting or polishing by thermal decomposition of polymeric restorative materials (sealants, acrylic resin, composites) are predominantly monomers. They may be efficiently eliminated by careful intraoral evacuation during the cutting or polishing procedures.

A rubber dam protects the patient against oral inhalation of aerosols or vapors, but nasal inhalation of vapor and finer aerosol may still occur. Disposable masks worn by dental office personnel filter out bacteria and all but the finest particulate matter. However, they do not filter out either mercury or monomer vapors. The biologic effects of mercury hazards, as well as appropriate office hygiene measures, were discussed in Chapter 4.

REFERENCES

1. American Dental Association: Council on Dental Research adopts standards for shapes and dimensions of excavating burs and diamond instruments, *J Am Dent Assoc* 67:943, 1963.
2. American National Standards Institute: American Dental Association Specification No. 23 for dental excavating burs, *J Am Dent Assoc* 104:887, 1982.
3. Atkinson DR, Cobb CM, Killoy WJ: The effect of an air-powder abrasive system on in vitro root surfaces, *J Periodontol* 55: 13-18, 1984.
4. Berry EA III, Eakle WS, Summitt JB: Air abrasion: an old technology reborn, *Compend Contin Educ Dent* 20(8):751-759, 1999.
5. Black GV: *Operative dentistry*, ed 8, Woodstock, Ill, 1947, Medico-Dental.
6. Black GV: *The technical procedures in filling teeth*, 1899, Henry O. Shepard.
7. Boyde A: Airpolishing effects on enamel, dentin and cement, *Brit Dent J* 156:287-291, 1984.
8. Cantwell KR, Aplin AW, Mahler DB: Surface characteristics of tooth structure after cutting with rotary instruments, *Dent Progr* 1(1):42-46, 1960.
9. Eames WB, Nale JL: A comparison of cutting efficiency of air-driven fissure burs, *J Am Dent Assoc* 86:412-415, 1973.
10. Eames WB, Reder BS, Smith GA: Cutting efficiency of diamond stones: effect of technique variables, *Oper Dent* 2(4): 156-164, 1977.
11. Frentzen M, Koort HJ, Thiensiri I: Excimer lasers in dentistry: future possibilities with advanced technology, *Quintessence Int* 23:117-133, 1992.
12. Galloway SE, Pashley DH: Rate of removal of root structure by use of the Prophy-Jet device, *J Periodontol* 58:464-469, 1987.
13. Grajower R, Zeitchick A, Rajstein J: The grinding efficiency of diamond burs, *J Prosthet Dent* 42:422-428, 1979.
14. Guerini V: *A history of dentistry*, Philadelphia, 1909, Lea & Febiger.
15. Hartley JL et al: Cutting characteristics of dental burs as shown by high speed photomicrography, *Armed Forces Med J* 8(2):209, 1957.
16. Hartley JL, Hudson DC: Modern rotating instruments: burs and diamond points, *Dent Clin North Am* 737, Nov 1958.
17. Henry EE: Influences of design factors on performance of the inverted cone bur, *J Dent Res* 35:704-713, 1956.
18. Henry EE, Peyton FA: The relationship between design and cutting efficiency of dental burs, *J Dent Res* 33:281-292, 1954.
19. International Standards Organization: *Standard ISO 2157: head and neck dimensions of designated shapes of burs*, Geneva, Switzerland, 1972, International Standards Organization.
20. Jeffrey IWM et al: CO_2 laser application to the mineralized dental tissues—the possibility of iatrogenic sequelae, *J Dent* 18:24-30, 1990.
21. Koblitz FF et al: *An overview of cutting and wear related phenomena in dentistry*. In Pearlman S, editor: *The cutting edge* (DHEW Publication No. [NIH] 76-670), Washington, DC, 1976, US Government Printing Office.
22. Kunselman B: *Effect of air-polishing shield on the abrasion of PMMA and dentin* (thesis). D.A.T.E., Division of Dental Hygiene, Department of Dental Ecology, School of Dentistry, Chapel Hill, NC, 1999, University of North Carolina.
23. Leonard DL, Charlton DG: Performance of high-speed dental handpieces, *J Am Dent Assoc* 130:1301-1311, 1999.
24. Lindhe J: Orthogonal cutting of dentine, *Odontol Revy* (Malma) 15(suppl 8):11-100, 1964.
25. McCann D: FDA OKs lasers for children, hard tissues, *ADA News*, Oct 29, 1998.
26. Merritt R: Low-energy lasers in dentistry, *Brit Dent J* 172:90, 1992.
27. Morrant GA: Burs and rotary instruments: introduction of a new standard numbering system, *Brit Dent J* 147(4):97-98, 1979.
28. Myers TD: Lasers in dentistry, *J Am Dent Assoc* 122:46-50, 1991.
29. Nelson RJ, Pelander CE, Kumpula JW: Hydraulic turbine contra-angle handpiece, *J Am Dent Assoc* 47:324-329, 1953.
30. Nuckles DB: Status report on rotary diamond instruments, Council on deutal materials and devices, *J Am Dent Assoc* 97(2):233-235, 1978.
31. Peterson LG et al: The effect of a jet abrasive instrument (Prophy Jet) on root surfaces, *Swed Dent J* 9:193-199, 1985.
32. Peyton FA: Effectiveness of water coolants with rotary cutting instruments, *J Am Dent Assoc* 56:664-675, 1958.
33. Peyton FA: Temperature rise in teeth developed by rotating instruments, *J Am Dent Assoc* 50:629-630, 1955.
34. Sockwell CL: Dental handpieces and rotary cutting instruments, *Dent Clin North Am* 15(1):219-244, 1971.
35. SS White Dental Manufacturing Company: *A century of service to dentistry*. Philadelphia, 1944, SS White Dental Manufacturing.
36. Taylor DF, Perkins RR, Kumpula JW: Characteristics of some air turbine handpieces, *J Am Dent Assoc* 64:794-805, 1962.
37. Westland IN: The energy requirement of the dental cutting process, *J Oral Rehab* 7(1):51, 1980.
38. White JM et al: Effects of pulsed Nd:YAG laser energy on human teeth: a three-year follow-up study, *J Am Dent Assoc* 124:45-51, 1993.
39. Zakariasen KL, MacDonald R, Boran T: Spotlight on lasers—a look at potential benefits, *J Am Dent Assoc* 122:58-62, 1991.

8

Infection Control

JAMES J. CRAWFORD

RALPH H. LEONARD, JR.

CHAPTER OUTLINE

EXPOSURE RISKS AND EFFECT OF INFECTIONS ON DENTISTRY

Pervasive increases in serious transmissible diseases over the last few decades have created global concern and impacted the treatment mode of all American health care practitioners. Every health care specialty that involves contact with mucosa, blood, or blood-contaminated body fluids is now regulated. The goal is to ensure compliance with universal barriers and other methods to minimize infection risks.

While the objective of operative dentistry has been to provide the highest standard of care, a prevailing concern has been to minimize the patient's anxiety of treatment. Providing a supportive, informal, relaxed, and nonthreatening operatory environment has been one emphasis. Although that concern has not waned, emphasis has now expanded to assuring and demonstrating to patients that they are well protected from risks of infectious disease. Universal use of treatment gloves, masks, protective eyewear, overgarments, plastic barriers to protect equipment, proper use of disinfectants, and instrument sterilization now work together to provide a professional health care atmosphere that conveys conscientious protection and treatment according to sound principles of infection control in keeping with current regulation (Fig. 8-1). Information on regulations, diseases, and infection control presented here is based on a manual developed by the authors.[48]

ENVIRONMENT OF THE DENTAL OPERATORY

To comprehend the problem of microbial contamination that confronts dentistry, it is necessary to examine the dental treatment environment. Because it was poorly understood in the past, personnel went unprotected from unseen exposures.

For most of the twentieth century, general dentistry was routinely practiced without barriers to protect eyes, nose, mouth, and hands as shown in Fig. 8-2. Not until 1991 were dental personnel required to wear gloves, masks, gowns, and protective eyewear while treating patients.

Microbial exposures in the dental operatory involve both airborne contamination (see Fig. 8-2) (an exposure concern for personnel) and digital contamination of surfaces (i.e., hands soiled with saliva that repeatedly contact operatory equipment and surfaces and return to the patient's mouth during treatments). Digital contamination is an exposure concern for both patients and personnel.

Airborne Contamination. A high-speed handpiece is capable of creating airborne contaminants from both bacterial residents in the dental unit water spray system and from microbial contaminants from saliva, tissues, blood, plaque, and fine debris cut from carious teeth (see Fig. 8-2). With respect to size, these airborne contaminants exist in the form of spatter, mists, and aerosols. *Aerosols* consist of invisible particles ranging from 50 μm to approximately 5 μm that can remain suspended in the air and breathed for hours.[88] Aerosols and larger particles may carry agents of any respiratory infection borne

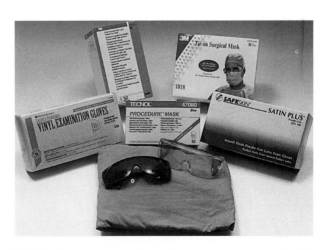

FIG. **8-1** Personal protective equipment worn to comply with OSHA's Bloodborne Disease Standard.

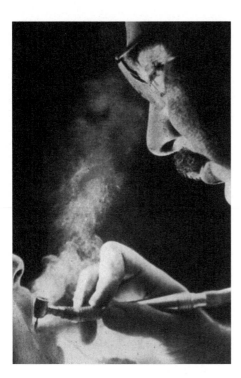

FIG. **8-2** Dentistry as it may have been practiced in the past. Rotary instrumentation can expose personnel to heavy spatter of more than 50-μm particles and mists. Aerosol particles of less than 5 μm remain suspended and can reach the alveoli if not stopped by a barrier. Air purification is a growing concern. *(Courtesy of Laminaire Corporation, Palm Beach Gardens, Fla.)*

by the patient. However, no scientific evidence indicates that fine aerosols have transmitted the bloodborne infection caused by hepatitis B virus (HBV).[61,101] There is even less likelihood that aerosols have transmitted human immunodeficiency virus (HIV), as evidenced by the extremely low transmissibility of HIV in both dental procedures and homes of infected persons.[18,28,29,31] *Mists* that become visible in a beam of light, consist of droplets estimated to approach or exceed 50 μm. Heavy mists tend to gradually settle from the air after 5 to 15 minutes.[12] Both aerosols and mists produced by the cough of a patient with unrecognized active pulmonary or pharyngeal tuberculosis (TB) are very likely to transmit the infection.[26] However, it has not been shown that oral fluids of tubercular patients aerosolized during a dental treatment can transmit TB.[12] *Spatter* consists of particles generally larger than 50 μm and are even visible splashes. Spatter has a distinct trajectory, usually falling within 3 feet of the patient's mouth, thus having the potential for coating the face and outer garments of the attending personnel.[12] Spatter or splashing of mucosa is considered a potential route of infection for dental personnel by bloodborne pathogens.[28,38]

Barrier protection of personnel using masks, protective eyewear, gloves, and gowns is now a standard requirement for dental procedures. A pretreatment mouthrinse, rubber dam, and high velocity air evacuation also

can reduce exposure risks.[12,38] To help reduce exposure to airborne particles capable of transmitting respiratory infections, adequate air circulation should be maintained and masks should be kept in place until air exchange in the room has occurred or until personnel leave the operatory.[26]

Hand-to-Surface Contamination. With saliva-contaminated hands, the hygienist, dentist, and assistant could repeatedly contact or handle unprotected operatory surfaces during treatments if not careful. The invisible trail of saliva left on such contaminated surfaces often defies either awareness or effective cleanup. Poorly cleaned soiled surfaces provide another source of gross environmental contamination to potentially contaminate both personnel and patients. In fact, *cross-contamination* of patients by such contaminated surfaces was documented in a clinical office radiology setting.[9,126]

Another study used water-soluble red-fluorescent poster paint (plain water-soluble fluorescent-red tempera in water) as a visible substitute for saliva to elevate awareness and facilitate problem solving in infection control. In this study, a hygienist was photographed treating a manikin fitted with dentures wetted with the red paint[71,125] (Fig. 8-3). The results demonstrated how extensively surfaces were smeared, how time-consuming, expensive, and difficult the contaminated surfaces were to clean, and how difficult it was to identify, clean, and disinfect objects covered with actual films of invisible saliva. Red poster paint is still used for dramatic training exercises, workshops, and poster displays to demonstrate or evaluate contamination control in dental operatories.

Another study used an invisible fluorescent dye added to the water delivered to the handpiece to evaluate airborne contamination of personnel during dental treatments.[12] Data were gathered after cutting natural teeth that had been placed into a teaching manikin. After only 5-minute treatments, fluids from the artificial mouth coated and contaminated personnel, equipment, and other environmental surfaces. This contamination was more pervasive and greater than that illustrated in the red dye studies.

Bacteriologic contamination of dental operatory surfaces also was investigated in 10 private dental offices after the surfaces were cleaned and disinfected.[71] Sampling confirmed widespread residual contamination with oral bacteria. Thus contamination was not controlled by conscientious use of cleaning and disinfecting procedures. Items or areas still contaminated after cleaning included handpieces; unprotected lamp handles; air-water syringe handles; control switches on the patient's chair; tubes, jars, and canisters of treatment materials; seat edges and rests of the dentist's and assistant's chairs; faucet knobs; cabinet, drawer, and operatory tray handles; room light switches, and operatory telephones. It is not difficult to understand how telephone handles at the receptionists' desks also became heavily contaminated with saliva bacteria. Before handpiece sterilization requirements, handpieces and other equipment found contaminated were cleaned only by wiping with disinfectant before reuse. (When nondental offices that were never disinfected were sampled as controls, phone handles and other similar surfaces were comparatively devoid of saliva bacteria.) Amalgam mixing equipment, light-curing units, and camera equipment are also subject to heavy contamination by soiled hands. *Maintaining no contamination of these items and areas is a priority objective today.*

From these studies, it is apparent that controlling contamination of equipment and personnel is essential to protect both patients and personnel in this operatory zone of potential heavy contamination. Barrier protection of personnel and equipment, instrument sterilization, and methods of avoiding direct contact with various surfaces are required.[12,38,71]

Cross-Infections. Most information on cross-infection and infection control concepts has been derived from data collected in hospitals. Among hospital patients and personnel, cross-infection and the routes of transmission come directly under the scrutiny of physicians, nurses, and surveillance of infection control personnel. However, in dental and other outpatient treatment settings, evidence of oral or systemic cross-infections is much more difficult to obtain. Such patients may have contracted infections elsewhere, before or after having a dental treatment. Patients infected usually are not aware of the source of their infection and go elsewhere for diagnosis and treatment of nonoral infections. Infection outbreaks are usually detected in patients or personnel only when they occur in clusters recognized by other health providers or are detected by epidemiologic studies and investigative surveys of personnel.

Patient Vulnerability. Although infection risks for dental patients have not been as well investigated as those of hospital patients, they appear to be low. Nine cluster cases of dentist-to-patient transmission of HB and one cluster case of HIV have been documented since 1971. Since 1986, when infection control practices became widespread, no cluster cases of HB transmission to patients have been reported that were related to dentistry.[18,20,21,55]

Personnel Vulnerability. When dental personnel experience exposure to saliva, blood, and possible injury from sharp instrumentation while treating patients, they are more vulnerable to infections if they have not had the proper immunizations or used the proper protective barriers. It is unfortunate that the need for proper control of exposures and infections was not realized before the occurrence of the bloodborne infection hepatitis B (HB), which poses a serious threat to all dental personnel[49] (see Impact of Hepatitis B). Fear that HIV would take a similar or worse toll did not materialize, pri-

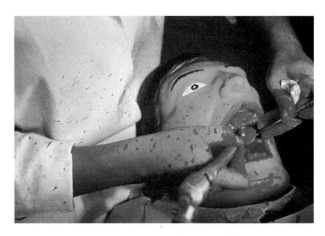

FIG. **8-3** Distribution of saliva spatter during a dental hygiene procedure. There is a need to wear a long-sleeved overgarment, mask, protective eyewear, and gloves.

marily because of the implementation of adequate infection control principles and surveillance. Patient-to-dental health care worker transmission of occupational disease is low.[20] Dental personnel who have treated infectious patients on a daily basis for years in hospital dental services have found infection control methods to be highly effective.[53] Infection control (IC) has helped dramatically allay risks and concerns of personnel in the private dental office, as well as instilling confidence in a safe environment for both patients and personnel. Private dentists continue to use IC as a way to build their practice.

Epidemiologic information about HB, hepatitis C, HIV, and other relevant infections is important. Examining the impact of these serious diseases provides the impetus to both use and improve effective methods of IC. It also may resist complacency about the risks from current and emerging diseases. Vulnerability of dental personnel before the institution of IC standards provides the best barometer of the potential for infection transmission in dentistry. Findings related to HBV and HIV illustrate this point.

IMPACT OF HEPATITIS B

HB was the first infectious disease to gain attention as a risk for health care personnel who have blood and body-fluid contact. General physicians and surgeons experienced HB infection rates of 19% and 28%, respectively. From 1982 to 1986, various blood sample studies in the United States showed that 14% to 28% of general dentists, 13% of dental assistants, and 17% of dental hygienists had evidence of past infection with HB.[2,44,49,93] If only 20% of the approximately 120,000 dentists in the United States had been infected by 1982, 24,000 dentists would have had HB. HB is transmitted sexually as well as parenterally. Transmission has been shown to occur in 23% to 42% of heterosexual partners of infected persons.[61,62] From these data, 5000 to 10,000 sexual partners, spouses, or families of the dentists with hepatitis may have been infected. If we apply the 2% mortality rate that characterizes HB, within 20 to 30 years after initial infection, 480 of the dentists who were infected with HB by 1982 will have died.

Fortunately a vaccine has dramatically curtailed HB infection among dental personnel who have been effectively immunized. However, IC procedures remain a major concern to prevent cross-infection among patients.[38]

IMPACT OF HIV AND AIDS

In view of the high HB infection rate among dental personnel, epidemiologists anticipated that acquired immune deficiency syndrome (AIDS) would decimate the workforce population in dentistry. By the mid-1980s HIV had infected approximately 1 million persons in the United States, most of whom were high-risk persons in metropolitan areas. By 1988, of over 1,000 dentists surveyed in high-risk areas who practiced with bare hands, only one was found infected who claimed no other exposure risks. Infections have since been suspected in five more dentists without other apparent risks. However, no dentists for whom negative HIV blood tests were established at the time of job-related exposure have acquired job-related HIV infection.[37,76]

Public alarm was intense when a Florida dentist with clinical AIDS transmitted his unique strain of HIV to six patients in his large dental practice.[25,87] No other instance of clinician-to-patient transmission of HIV has been established in dentistry. That isolated Florida instance of HIV transmission contrasts dramatically with the transmissibility of HB. Twenty reports have documented that over 300 patients treated by HB-infected health care workers acquired HB. Nine of the reports in the United States listed over 140 patients infected with HB by dental practitioners that caused several deaths.[43,55] Evidence indicates that the Florida cluster of HIV infections and most treatment-related HB infections from infected clinicians to patients could have been prevented by conscientious use of IC procedures.[20,37] The unfortunate Florida outbreak was nonetheless tragic for the individuals and families involved. The ensuing public demand for required testing of all health care personnel was reduced to voluntary testing, and states were required to enforce Public Health Service guidelines for IC in all health care facilities.[58] However, public *concern still focuses unprecedented attention on the standards of IC used in all health care professions, particularly in dentistry.*[23,24,29,30,58]

Despite the deficit in patient infection data and despite the misplaced concern regarding the transmissibility of HIV infection in dentistry, the Florida cluster of HIV infections and Occupational Safety and Health Administration (OSHA) regulations have provided an intense impetus to strengthen and control aseptic standards in all health care disciplines in a brief time span.[95] Dental students and auxiliary personnel, as well as patients, are all the final beneficiaries of the dramatic

changes that have occurred. *IC is now accepted as a standard of care by dentists.*[7,8]

In 1991, the American Association of Dental Schools (AADS) published curriculum guidelines to be used in dental schools for teaching the dental care of patients with bloodborne infectious diseases.[8] The guidelines specify a comprehensive array of basic and clinical topics including a description of transmissible infections, their epidemiology and mechanisms of transmission, principles and methods of IC, use of barriers, instrument sterilization, and disinfection. The topics must be taught with the prevailing concept of universal precautions (i.e., treating all patients as infectious). The content was not intended to be presented in a separate course, but to be integrated into existing courses as appropriate. *This chapter integrates applicable topics on transmissible diseases, epidemiology, and IC specified by the AADS curriculum guidelines into the teaching and practice of operative dentistry.* Content also includes information regarding federal and other requirements related to IC.

To meet clinical AADS guidelines and state and other requirements, dental schools must prepare and maintain a written manual of IC policies and procedures.[7] The manual standardizes and documents policies and procedures to protect patients and personnel as well as training students, faculty, and personnel in those regards. It is convenient to include required OSHA, state, and other regulations in sections of the same manual. Private dental offices develop an office IC manual for the same reasons. Much of the content in this chapter can be adapted to such a manual.

FEDERAL AND STATE REGULATIONS TO REDUCE EXPOSURE RISKS FROM PATHOGENS IN BLOOD AND OTHER SOURCES OF INFECTION

The term *infection control program* (IC program) has a long tradition in hospital usage. *IC programs,* such as those recommended by the Centers for Disease Control and Prevention (CDC) and the American Dental Association (ADA), *are designed to protect both patients and personnel.*[5,38]

The federal OSHA uses a different term, *exposure control plan,* for required office programs designed to protect personnel against risks of exposure to infection. Guidelines and requirements of other agencies that pertain to areas of IC not covered by OSHA are discussed in the next section. State occupational safety and health agencies are now enforcing regulations finalized by the federal OSHA, whose *Final Rule* (or *The Standard*) on occupational exposure to bloodborne pathogens was published in December, 1991.[95]

The OSHA rule derives from the original *Occupational Safety and Health Act* passed by the U.S. Congress in 1970.[121] This Act identified employers' obligations to protect employees from occupational risks. That Act has been the basis for all subsequent federal safety and health regulations. According to the Act, each employer must furnish employees with a place and conditions of employment free from recognized hazards that presently cause, or are likely to cause, death or serious harm to employees. The Act created the Occupational Safety and Health Agency (OSHA) in the U.S. Department of Labor. In the late 1980s labor unions petitioned OSHA in federal courts to extend chemical hazards protection standards to employees in the health care professions. Shortly thereafter, concern about transmitting HIV to health care workers stimulated the unions to take similar action to obtain the OSHA regulation of blood and body-fluid exposure among health care personnel.

Thus the Act covers two regulated programs of compliance: (1) an OSHA Hazard Communications program concerning risks from environmental and chemical hazards in the workplace (see Safety and Efficacy in Chapter 4), and (2) an OSHA Bloodborne Pathogens program that addresses control of "occupational exposure to blood and other potentially infectious materials.[95,96] The OSHA hazard communications program, which also must be implemented in every dental office, applies mainly to chemicals.[96]

Other dental office requirements, relating to environmental safety features also should be recorded in the same office manual and include maintenance of a complete first aid kit, full oxygen tank, pocket resuscitation masks, a fire evacuation plan, fire extinguishers with annual inspection and actual personnel training updated, and general environmental safety provisions such as clear passageways without mechanical obstructions, clearly marked exits, electrical safety (e.g., ground fault outlets near sinks), and adherence to radiation and nitrous oxide safety standards. An Occupational Safety and Health poster, stating the obligations of employers and employees to follow health and safety regulations, and workers rights and recourses, must be displayed in a convenient place for employees to see. State OSHA offices may be consulted to obtain specific information, manuals, documents, posters, and so on. County and state Environmental Protection Agency (EPA) offices should be consulted regarding requirements for storage and disposal of infectious waste.

All aspects of the OSHA bloodborne pathogens program to protect employees were required in every dental office by July 6, 1992.[95] Federal Law 42, passed by Congress in 1991, required state public health departments to apply similar standards or follow the CDC guidelines of IC to all dental care personnel to ensure protection of patients.[58] Thus, under Federal and State laws, "employers (including dentists operating nonincorporated offices) must comply with IC regulations.

Copies of the *OSHA Bloodborne Pathogens Standard of 1991* are available from the U.S. Government Printing Office, Superintendent of Documents, Washington, DC 20402 (specify GPO order no. 069-001-0040-8). A federal translation of the standard (but not a substitute) for dentistry can be requested free of charge by sending a return address label to the OSHA Publications Office, Room N-3101, 200 Constitution Ave. NW, Washington DC 20210, or it can be downloaded from OSHA's website. Required copies of regulations, posters, reporting forms, and other materials for training purposes are available from local state offices of the Division of Labor or of the Occupational Safety and Health Agency. Helpful brochures and manuals that provide copies of regulations, forms, and more detailed instructions also are available from some state health department divisions of dental health or from state and national dental associations.

PREPARING A WRITTEN OSHA OFFICE EXPOSURE CONTROL PLAN (SUMMARY)

Exposure Control Plan. A written exposure control plan must be accessible to employees with exposure risks. The plan must be reviewed and updated at least annually and when alterations in procedures create new occupational exposures.

The office exposure control plan applies to all operatory and laboratory personnel at risk for an exposure (i.e., dentist, hygienist, dental assistant, and dental laboratory technicians, as well as dental equipment repair personnel and laundry and custodial personnel who handle waste or laundry from operatories). These are persons who have regular, potential contact with blood and body fluids. This exposure determination shall be made without regard to use of personal protective equipment. All such persons must be listed in the exposure control plan by name, job, and kind of exposure potential (e.g., intraoral treatments, exposure to spatter of blood-contaminated oral fluids, cleaning and sterilizing of sharp instruments). Dentists who are employed by an office, corporation, or institution also are listed as personnel to whom all rules apply. Receptionists who never assist or work in the operatory and who do not have contact with blood or body fluid–contaminated charts would be exempt. If personnel do encounter blood and/or body fluid-contamination on charts or other items, then they must be listed. Appropriate training, immunization, protective equipment, and materials must be provided for all at-risk personnel. Clerical hospital personnel who handle blood-contaminated forms have shown elevated HB infection rates. Paper cuts were a likely mechanism of transfer.[99]

Dental students do not come directly under OSHA regulations unless they are employees of the school with duties that involve bloodborne pathogen exposure. However, in compliance with Federal and State policies, school accreditation requirements, and university policies, all dental schools have an IC manual of standard operating procedures that applies to students. These policies usually are based on the school's OSHA exposure control plan for faculty and staff. As future employers or employees, dental students will have to become acquainted with OSHA's exposure control plan.

A simple implementation schedule must be prepared to document how and when various aspects of compliance with the exposure control plan are provided for new and old employees. This can be done by notating a copy of the OSHA regulation.[95,122]

The OSHA exposure control plan uses terms that require definition. *Exposure* is defined in the OSHA regulation as, "specific eye, mouth, other mucous membrane, nonintact skin, or parenteral contact with blood or other potentially infectious materials (OPIM) that results from performance of an employee's duties."[79] *Only in dentistry is saliva considered a potentially infectious material, since oral manipulations and dental treatments routinely cause saliva to become contaminated with the patient's blood.* *Universal precautions* means that all patients and blood-contaminated body fluids are treated as infectious.

Means of compliance are expressed in the OSHA terminology of environmental safety engineers. *Work practice controls and engineering controls* are terms that describe precautions (e.g., careful handling of sharp instruments, and not putting hands into sharps containers) and use of devices to reduce contamination risks (e.g., using high-volume suction, rubber dam, and protective sharps containers). *Personal protective equipment* (PPE) is the term used for barriers, such as gloves, gowns, or masks. *Housekeeping* is a term that relates to cleanup of treatment-soiled operatory equipment, instruments, counters, and floors, as well as to management of used gowns and waste. Housekeeping also relates to cautions for servicing contaminated equipment and using only mechanical means to clean contaminated broken glass.

Standard operating procedures (SOPs) is a term used in former OSHA regulations for step-by-step descriptions of tasks. Such task descriptions are preferred for training new personnel and comprise part of the training manual.

Obtain and read a copy of the *Final OSHA Rule on Bloodborne Pathogens* to be apprised of complete and exact regulatory details.[95] Following is a summary of the current OSHA regulations specifying what employers must furnish, directions employers must provide, and compliance required of employees:

1. Employers must provide HB immunization to employees without charge within 10 days of employment. The employer also must provide a copy of the OSHA regulations on bloodborne pathogens from which this information is taken to the health care professional responsible for providing the HB vaccine.

2. Employers must require that universal precautions be observed to prevent contact with blood and other potentially infectious materials. Saliva is considered a blood-contaminated body fluid in relation to dental treatments.[28-30,38]

3. Employers must implement engineering controls to reduce production of contaminated spatter, mists, and aerosols. Examples are use of a rubber dam, high-volume suction, rubber prophy cup instead of brushes, scaling instruments for patients with respiratory infections instead of cavitron, and hard-wall containers to avoid contact with disposable and reusable sharps.[42,50,90]

4. Employers must implement work practice control precautions to minimize splashing, spatter, or contact of bare hands with contaminated surfaces. Never contact telephones, switches, door handles, or faucet handles with soiled gloves. The subsequent items (5 to 18) also are work practice control regulations.

5. Employers must provide facilities and instruction for washing hands after removing gloves, and for washing other skin immediately or as soon as feasible after contact with blood or potentially infectious materials (Figs. 8-4, 8-5, and 8-6). Flush eye or mucosa immediately or as soon as feasible after any contact with blood or potentially infectious materials.

6. Employers must prescribe safe handling of needles and other sharp items. Needles must not be bent or cut. When it can be shown necessary, needles may be resheathed with mechanical aids or other one-handed techniques (see Chapter 10).

7. Employers must prescribe disposal of single-use needles, wires, carpules, and sharps as close to the place of use as possible, as soon as feasible, in hard-walled, leakproof containers that are closable, from which needles cannot be easily spilled. Containers must be red or bear a biohazard label and must be kept upright and closed when moved (see Chapter

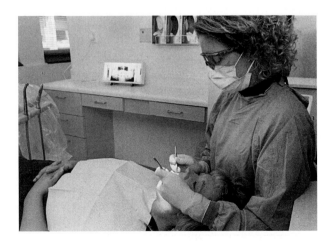

FIG. **8-4** In current dental practice PPE provides barriers against spatter and aerosols during patient treatments.

10). Teeth must not be discarded into trash but can be given to the patient or discarded into sharps containers.

8. Contaminated reusable sharp instruments must not be stored or processed in a manner that requires employees to reach hands into containers to retrieve them. Use a basket or cassette to place instruments into and retrieve them from soaking pans and ultrasonic cleaners. Use biohazard-labeled or red pans that are leakproof and puncture resistant.

9. Employers must prohibit eating, drinking, handling contact lenses, and application (but not wearing) of facial cosmetics in contaminated environments such as operatories and cleanup areas. Ban storage of food and drinks in refrigerators or other spaces where blood or infectious materials are stored.

10. Place blood and contaminated specimens (e.g., impressions that have not been well-cleaned and well-disinfected, teeth, biopsy specimens, blood specimens, and culture specimens) to be shipped, transported, or stored into suitable closed containers that prevent leakage. An adequately strong plastic bag can be used for impressions. The surface of all containers must be clean or enclosed in another clean, red, or biohazard-labeled container.

11. At no cost to employees, employers must provide them with necessary PPE and clear directions for use of appropriate universal barrier protection in treating all patients and for all other contact with blood or other infectious materials (see Figs. 8-1 and 8-4). PPE must not allow blood or other potentially infectious material to pass through to contaminate personal clothing, skin, or mucous membranes.

Namely, employers must provide protective gloves, or hypoallergenic gloves as needed; appropriate protective body clothing such as gowns, "the type and characteristics will depend upon the task and degree of exposure anticipated"[95]; protective eyewear, chin-length face shields, goggles, or glasses with solid protective side shields; masks; pocket resuscitation masks for cardiopulmonary resuscitation (CPR); and surgical caps or shoe covers to be worn when required for surgery or whenever heavy contamination can be reasonably anticipated.

12. Ensure that employees correctly use and discard PPE or properly prepare it for reuse. Provide adequate facilities to discard gowns or laundry in the location where they are used. Note: A face shield does not substitute for a mask.

13. As soon as feasible after treatments, attend to housekeeping requirements including floors, countertops, sinks, and other environmental equipment that are subject to contamination. Also included are the use of protective covers that are changed after each appointment, or thoroughly clean and disinfect contaminated surfaces and operatory equipment items that cannot be covered, discarded, or removed and sterilized. (See Operatory Asepsis, and Procedures, Materials, and Devices for Cleaning Instruments Before Sterilization for details.)

14. Employers must provide a written schedule for cleaning and decontaminating equipment, work surfaces, and contaminated floors. For contaminated spills, prescribe an appropriate method of cleaning and then applying disinfecting methods. Broken glassware that may be contaminated must

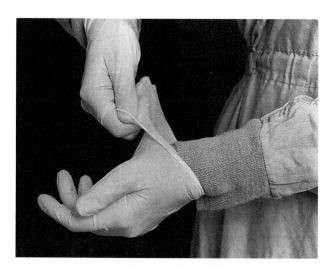

FIG. 8-5 To remove a contaminated glove, pinch the palm side of the outer cuff surface with the gloved fingers of the other hand. Pull off the glove, inverting it. Both gloves can be removed simultaneously in this manner. Alternately, after removing one, insert bare fingers under the cuff to grasp and pull off the remaining glove. Discard gloves safely.

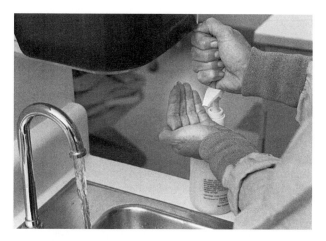

FIG. 8-6 To wash hands after removing treatment gloves, operate the pump as shown with the clean underside of a wrist. Also, operate faucet handles the same way to avoid contamination or use foot controls. Never touch the handles with contaminated gloves.

be cleaned with mechanical means, and never with gloved hands.

15. Contaminated equipment that requires service must first be decontaminated, or a biohazard label must be used to indicate contaminated parts.

16. Contaminated sharps are regulated waste; discard in hard-walled containers. For OSHA purposes in dentistry, regulated waste also means: (1) liquid or semiliquid blood or other potentially infectious materials, (2) contaminated items that would release blood or other potentially infectious materials in a liquid or semiliquid state if compressed, and (3) items that are caked with blood or other potentially infectious materials and are capable of releasing these materials during handling. Properly dispose of such regulated waste in biohazard-labeled or red closable bags or other labeled containers that prevent leakage. Containers contaminated on the outside must be placed in a secondary container. The secondary container also must be closable, prevent leakage, and be red or biohazard-labeled. Containers or bags must be closed when moved. If outsides of reusable containers are likely to become contaminated, they must be inspected, decontaminated, and cleaned on a regularly scheduled basis, and as soon as feasible if they become visibly contaminated. Cabinets or other storage areas on the premises in which blood-contaminated waste is stored must be identified by a biohazard label.

17. Place reusable contaminated sharp instruments into a basket in a hard-walled container for transportation to the clean-up area. Personnel must not reach hands into containers of contaminated sharps.

18. Employers must provide laundering of protective garments used for universal precautions at no cost to employees. Handle contaminated laundry as little as possible without sorting or rinsing. Bag all soiled linens where they are used in a color-coded bag recognized as requiring universal precautions.

Emergency and Exposure Incident Plan. An emergency and exposure incident plan must be developed for employees. A separate plan is needed for students if they use different medical care resources or methods for reporting exposure incidents.

A person must be identified who is the program coordinator and contact person when emergencies arise. That person also may become the trainer for office personnel. OSHA dictates an exposure incident plan that emphasizes documentation of incidents and their follow-up. During training sessions, personnel must be told what to do in an emergency, but documenting a plan of medical emergency care is an equally important aspect of employee protection. Five *requirements of an incident plan* should be addressed:

1. Exposures to mucosa may not be associated with an injury, or an exposure incident may involve minor or severe injury (e.g., from a cutting instrument). Rapid and thorough cleaning of a wound or washing a splashed eye or mouth as quickly as possible is the most important first step to minimize infection risks. Blood tends to collect on the surface of puncture wounds created by solid pointed instruments, so washing puncture wounds is just as important. Persons must be identified in the office to provide any help, direction, or transportation needed to obtain medical care. A brief written plan should be formulated of how to rapidly access medical attention. This content should comprise the first part of the exposure incident plan. Sufficient time will still be available for a designated responsible person to contact the patient and transmit medical records as well as other information to the attending physician, as presented next.

2. The exposure source patient's written permission must be obtained to copy and convey his or her medical history to the attending physician or to obtain other medical records regarding the patient. However, knowledge of risk behavior, blood test results, or other pertinent information usually can be conveyed verbally in confidence without permission in case of exposure. Consult local laws. Some states only prescribe transmission of the name, address, and phone number of the patient and the name and phone number of the patient's physician to the physician attending the exposed person. The patient's physician is then contacted by the examining physician who deals with testing the patient.

3. As directed by OSHA regulations, employers must provide a copy of the exposure incident plan and explain it to employees. Employers must document the route and circumstances of the exposure, identifying the source patient when possible. Employers must provide and pay for exposure incident evaluation and follow-up evaluations for an exposed employee unless paid for by workman's compensation.

4. If other local regulations do not prevail, employers must also: (1) identify and contact the source patient if possible; (2) obtain the source person's permission to be tested, unless he or she is already known to be infected; (3) have the source person's blood tested, as soon as feasible, for evidence of current HIV and HBV infection by a health care professional (e.g., if blood is available, some states permit testing without permission in exposure instances); (4) provide results to the exposed employee in confidence (state laws often require counseling of the source patient for HIV testing as well as the exposed person); (5) test the employee's blood, with his or her permission, as soon as feasible; (6) hold any available sample of the employee's blood for 90 days if consent is not given

for HIV testing to provide for a change of mind; and (7) provide postexposure prophylaxis to the employee when medically indicated according to recommendations of the U.S. Public Health Service.

5. The attending physician must be provided with a copy of OSHA regulations from which this information is taken, documentation collected regarding the incident, results of the source person's tests, and employee's immunization records and any other relevant medical records. A written report from the attending physician must be obtained by the employer and provided to the employee within 15 days of the evaluation completion stating that the employee has been informed of results, possible infection consequences, and any further evaluation or treatment needed that relates to the exposure incident. Unrelated diagnoses or findings remain confidential.

Training of Personnel Required by OSHA. Occupational safety guidelines require that new office personnel who will have contact with blood and blood-contaminated body fluids receive initial training in IC. Moreover, retraining is required annually and whenever the exposure control protocol changes.[95]

During inspections, OSHA representatives interview employees rather than supervisors to evaluate their understanding of universal precautions, exposures, and how to protect themselves. *Training of personnel* must contain the following elements as listed in the OSHA standard:

1. An accessible copy of the regulatory text of this standard and an explanation of its contents
2. A general explanation of the epidemiology and symptoms of bloodborne diseases
3. An explanation of the modes of transmission of bloodborne pathogens
4. An explanation of the employer's exposure control plan and the means by which employees can obtain a copy of the written plan
5. An explanation of the appropriate methods for recognizing tasks and other activities that may involve exposure to blood and other potentially infectious materials
6. An explanation of the use and limitations of methods that will prevent or reduce exposure, including appropriate engineering controls, work practices, and PPE
7. Information on the types, proper use, location, removal, handling, decontamination, and disposal of personal protective equipment
8. An explanation of the basis for selection of personal protective equipment
9. Information on the HB vaccine, including information on its efficacy, safety, method of administration,

benefits of being vaccinated, and that the vaccine and vaccination will be offered free of charge
10. Information on the appropriate actions to take and persons to contact in an emergency involving blood or other potentially infectious materials
11. An explanation of the procedure to follow if an exposure incident occurs, including the method of reporting the incident and the medical follow-up that will be made available
12. Information on the postexposure evaluation and follow-up that the employer is required to provide for the employee following an exposure incident
13. An explanation of the signs and labels and/or color-coding required by the OSHA standard
14. An opportunity for interactive questions and answers with the person conducting the training session[95]
15. Additional specific information must be provided regarding the details and cleanup schedules specific for employees' operatory and facilities.

OSHA-Required Records. Job classification and immunization and medical records of personnel must be kept for 30 years by the office or a designated physician for OSHA inspection, or disposed of according to requirements. Training records must be kept for 3 years from the date of training. Exposure incidents must be tabulated and posted according to OSHA requirements. Details are provided in the regulations.[95] An interpretation of these regulations for dentistry has since been published.[122] Some variations from these and other OSHA regulations may later be specified for dentistry as a result of petitions made by the ADA. Consult current information.

REGULATIONS OF OTHER AGENCIES

State public health services and dental licensing boards complete the spectrum of IC regulatory agencies. Most specify the IC guidelines of the ADA and the U.S. Public Health Service CDC, but focus more upon tasks and procedures necessary for patient protection in dentistry.[5,31,38,46,47]

REGULATION OF INFECTED HEALTH CARE PERSONNEL

Concerns about the possible transmission of AIDS from infected health care personnel to patients has led the U.S. Public Health Service to recommend additional precautions. *All health care personnel who perform invasive, exposure-prone treatments are urged to voluntarily obtain testing for HBV and HIV infections.*[23]

Exposure-prone procedures include simultaneous use of the operator's fingers and sharp instrumentation in a highly confined or poorly visualized anatomic site, such as the mouth, where tissues are cut or bleeding can occur. Clinical persons are considered infected when they test positive for antibody against HIV or for surface antigen and e antigen of HB. *Infected health care personnel are advised not to perform exposure-prone procedures unless they have sought counsel from an expert review panel and been advised under what circumstances they may continue to perform these procedures according to the experience and skill of the clinical person involved.*

As defined by the CDC, a review panel may consist of the worker's physician, an infectious disease specialist with expertise in epidemiology of HIV and HBV transmission, another health care professional with expertise in the type of procedures performed, and a local public health official.[23]

OSHA-REQUIRED TRAINING ON BLOODBORNE PATHOGENS

AIDS/HIV INFECTION

AIDS is the last stage of a debilitating, eventually fatal human disease. AIDS may develop in 1.5 to 11 or more years after an initial infection with *HIV*.[6,54] (HIV-1 is the predominant type; HIV-2 is a type found in some West African emigrants.) HIV is a relatively fragile ribonucleic acid (RNA) retrovirus that is easily destroyed in the dry state in 1 to 2 minutes by most disinfectants.[5,28,29,109]

HIV EPIDEMIOLOGY AND TRANSMISSION

Since its recognition in 1981, HIV has infected several million people in the United States and, by 1998, produced AIDS in over 688,000 persons.[18,24] HIV is transmitted mainly by blood, blood-contaminated body fluids, semen, and vaginal fluids. High-risk behaviors or situations that define high-risk groups include having multiple sex partners of the same or opposite sex; having a sexual partner that is high-risk or infected; intravenous drug abuse; hemophiliac treatment; blood transfusion before spring, 1985; and infants born to an infected parent.[3,24,63,65] *Casual, nonsexual contact, including social kissing and sharing towels or food among family members in a household with an AIDS victim, has not transmitted the infection.*

In 1990, AIDS was predominately distributed among males with promiscuous homosexual and bisexual behavior (54%), intravenous drug users (23%), and heterosexuals with multiple sexual partners (5%). Women comprised 12% of those with AIDS; most were intravenous drug abusers, and others were sexually infected.[24] A wide incidence of HIV infection was found in studies of prostitutes reported in 1987 (none in Las Vegas, 19% in Miami, and 69% in Newark).[66] Persons transfused with infected blood or blood products, such as hemophiliacs, comprised approximately 2% or more of AIDS cases. According to a 1990 U.S. Public Health Service study of students at 19 colleges, 1 per 200 male and 1 per 5000 female college students were found infected with HIV.[65] Infection rates were less than 1 per 1000 at 10 colleges, and ranged from 0.1% to 1% at the remaining nine sur-

veyed. By 1990, children infected with HIV by infected parents were seen in growing numbers, from birth to 9 years of age. They comprised 0.3% to 1.4% of AIDS cases reported.[24]

PROGRESSION OF HIV INFECTION INTO AIDS

In simple terms, after a prolonged quiet state of 1.5 to possibly 11 years after infection, the AIDS virus begins to destroy cells that control the normal immunity of the body against infections and tumors. At that time, the body becomes more and more vulnerable to many common viruses and microbes found in our normal environment. Commonly harmless parasites and fungi are then able to cause severe and often fatal pneumonia or cerebral infections.[6,54]

Upon entering the blood or tissues, HIV can only attach to certain docking sites that it finds projecting from the surfaces of certain white blood cells. Helper lymphocytes critical to the normal functioning of the immune system are covered with these sites. Immunologists have labeled these cells T-helper lymphocytes because the thymus has an important function in preparing them to function. The surface attachment sites are termed *category designation four* (CD4) glycoprotein antigens. Once attached, virus RNA can enter and infect the lymphocyte.[68]

The important point is that the cells commonly infected, termed *T4 (CD4) helper lymphocytes*, are critical to normal cellular and antibody functions that protect us against many bacteria, fungi, virus-infected cells, and tumors or cancers. Other cells, such as macrophages, neurologic glial cells, colon/rectal cells, and possibly some connective tissue cells, also have the CD4 glycoprotein surface sites to which HIV can attach. Colon cells, for example in male homosexual interactions, may serve as infection sites. It is not known whether mucosal cells of other body cavities may serve as initial infection sites as well. Various susceptible cells and perhaps cells in the bone marrow may serve as reservoirs of the virus in a prolonged latent or quiet incubation stage when HIV sometimes cannot be detected in the blood.[68]

HIV is termed an *RNA retrovirus,* one that needs complementary deoxyribonucleic acid (DNA) formed within the nucleus of a host cell (termed a provirus form) to reproduce the HIV. As HIV gains entry into the lymphocytes, reverse transcription of viral RNA begins, resulting in formation of double-stranded viral DNA in the infected cells. Once inserted into the cell's genetic structure (genome), this DNA becomes HIV provirus. HIV DNA may then divide and reproduce along with the cell's nuclear DNA for years. Antibody tests are now available to detect HIV provirus DNA fragments that regulate production of various parts of HIV structure (i.e., core proteins, gag; viral envelope, env; reverse transcriptase, pol).[3,68]

One drug found helpful in prolonging the health of HIV-infected persons is zidovudine (formerly azidothymidine [AZT]). This drug is one of a group of the dide-oxy nucleoside drugs that interferes with reverse transcriptase action necessary to complete HIV infection of human cells.[68] Other drugs and combinations of drugs ("cocktails") are currently on the market or being researched that show promise in battling the AIDS virus.

After remaining latent during the prolonged incubation period in infected helper lymphocyte cells, the HIV commences to replicate. The lymphocytes die, releasing virus into the blood, and thus the numbers of essential helper lymphocytes are drastically reduced. When helper cell counts fall below 200 per mm^3 in the blood, many different opportunistic infections and tumors appear. Conditions are such that it becomes increasingly difficult to treat until *Pneumocystis* infection of the lungs is fatal, or until HIV or other infection of the brain causes death.[54] Levels of virus in the blood usually increase at this time but are still very low compared with huge viral concentrations of HBV reached in the blood of patients with HB.[3] At the authors' institution, patients with T4 helper cell counts of 200 per mm^3 or less may benefit from the protective facilities, nursing care, and treatment expertise offered by the hospital dental service clinicians.

SYMPTOMS AND ORAL MANIFESTATIONS

Within 3 months of infection, temporary flulike symptoms of pharyngitis, myalgia, fatigue, fever, or diarrhea may occur when antibody to HIV becomes detectable. After prolonged incubation of approximately 1.5 to 11 years, the dentist may detect any of several early signs of AIDS, signaling gradual failure of the immune system.[6,69] (Refer to Chapter 9 for color illustrations of orofacial manifestations of AIDS.) Easily detected during examination are one or two cervical lymph nodes, especially below the mandible, that persist for more than 3 months. Nodes may be attached and painless, or movable, painful, and infected. Undifferentiated non-Hodgkins lymphoma cancers may arise in lymph nodes, or may appear in the mandible as well as in the central nervous system, eyes, bone marrow, and other vital organs.[6]

Persistent oral candidiasis is often seen with easily dislodged white curdlike patches scattered over the tongue. In AIDS, such infection may not easily respond to treatment, and often recurs, developing into atrophic candidiasis, or cheilitis at the angles of the lips. Painful herpes stomatitis is also somewhat common. Untreated herpes or candidiasis may extend into esophagitis or laryngitis, impairing speech.[6]

Red, brownish-to-purple blotches that persist on the oral mucosa and skin of the individual typify a sarcoma of the capillaries, termed *Kaposi's sarcoma*. Oral lesions often develop into tumors that may require surgery and radiation therapy. Kaposi's sarcoma is often found on oral tissues of male homosexuals. Human papilloma virus can cause flat to cauliflower-like oral warts to develop.[6]

A persistent, severe, recurrent gingivitis and periodontitis typical of AIDS is a common finding that brings patients for dental care. The gingivitis may persist despite good plaque control.[69]

Early systemic signs of illness progressing toward AIDS are marked by weight loss of up to 50 pounds within a few months, and chronic fever or night sweats that persist for 3 months or more.[6,54] Early detection, and medical treatment of HIV infection is beneficial to the majority of patients. Current treatments are summarized in the annual *Journal of the American Dental Association* supplement update, *Facts about AIDS for the Dentist.*[6]

SEROLOGY OF HIV INFECTION

HIV infection is detected by blood tests (enzyme-linked immunoassay [EIA], Western Blot, and fluorescent antibody tests) that detect antibodies formed against the virus. Tests for anti-HIV antibody are often positive within 3 months after infection; most are positive by 6 months; 1% take up to 12 months to become positive. A second positive test is necessary to confirm positive serologies.

Serologic tests for the virus and provirus DNA also have been developed. Tests for T4/T8 (or CD4/CD8) lymphocyte ratios are used to indicate progress of the HIV infection. One criterion for starting zidovudine therapy is a T4 helper cell count below 500 per mm^3 of blood.[6]

HIV RISKS FOR CLINICAL PERSONNEL

Of all American health care workers injured by needles and sharp instruments used to treat HIV-infected persons, only 0.3% or less have become infected with HIV. This contrasts with 30% of workers who become infected with HB following parenteral exposure to infected blood.[29] Among all U.S. health care personnel, *documented* occupationally related HIV infections now total 54. (None were established among dental personnel).[18,20,21] An additional 134 HIV infections are considered possible occupational transmissions (including six in dental personnel).

As was pointed out in the introduction, dental personnel have almost miraculously been spared infection with HIV. Thousands of unprotected dentists who unknowingly treated HIV-infected patients must have been exposed to HIV infection as the epidemic mounted during the 1980s before gloves and other barriers came into common use. Only six dentists who claim no other exposure risks appear to have acquired HIV infection by occupational exposure.[18,20,21,29] Testing for evidence of prior HIV infection at the time of exposure was not commonly performed in dentistry until the 1990s. Because none of the infected dentists had such baseline blood tests, their HIV infections cannot be firmly linked to time and circumstance of clinical exposure.

HIV infection has developed in a nurse and a technician spattered with HIV-infected blood. Five other medical personnel have acquired HIV infection related to spatter of infected blood to their nonintact skin. The serologic status for HIV in these persons was apparently not known when they were exposed.[18,20,21,29] *Therefore personnel are required to protect eyes, mucosa, skin, and hands from spatter and direct contact with blood and blood-contaminated body fluids during dental treatments of all patients.*[122] *Precautions also must be made to minimize risks of injuries with sharp instrumentation.*

Patients seriously ill enough with AIDS to be seen in a hospital setting also may harbor transmissible respiratory infections, such as TB and cytomegalovirus (CMV) infection.[22,60] As indicated in the section Epidemiology of Other Infection Risks, transmission of drug-resistant TB from immunocompromised patients is a growing concern. Personnel without adequate barrier protection should avoid exposure to coughing, saliva-spatter, and heavy aerosols from HIV-infected persons with signs of respiratory infection. This applies especially to pregnant women, since CMV can be detrimental to the newborn infant of a mother recently infected with CMV. CMV is also bloodborne.

HIV RISKS FOR DENTAL PATIENTS

With proper use of IC measures in dental practice, the risk for a dental patient of contracting HIV from office personnel or from other patients is extremely low. HIV has not been transmitted to dental patients from infected clinical personnel anywhere in the United States, with the exception of one unique outbreak.[20,25,37] In a circumstance that has been unique through 1999, a group of six patients was found to be infected with the same strain of HIV that infected the Florida dentist who treated them.[20,25,37] The patients had no other apparent source of exposure other than the dentist who persisted in treating patients while having symptoms of well-developed AIDS. Use of adequate IC measures was questionable. Therefore some kind of doctor-to-patient transmission seems likely. At this time, no other instances of patients being infected with HIV by infected dentists or physicians have been reported. One or more alleged HIV cross-infections between patients attributed to contaminated dental equipment have come under investigation.[21]

HIV DATA RELATED TO INFECTION CONTROL

Data that provide a better understanding of disease agents, their survival qualities, and clinical transmission potentials help us institute effective IC. The following HIV data are somewhat reassuring and help explain the amazingly low occupational risk of HIV infection for dental personnel.[6,76]

1. Unlike HB virus, HIV usually has been found in very low levels in blood of infected persons. This is especially true of asymptomatic persons who are the most

difficult to recognize and would be most likely to be treated in private offices.[30,77]

2. HIV was detected in only 28 of 50 samples of blood from infected persons. In saliva from infected persons, HIV was detectable in only 1 of 83 samples.[63] Counts of virus per milliliter of blood fluctuate, but may increase as antibody to HIV core protein declines.[3,77]

3. In dried infected blood, 99% of HIV has been found by CDC investigators to be inactive in approximately 90 minutes.[30] Longer survival data on larger numbers of HIV grown in laboratory cell cultures have created false impressions about HIV survival in dried infected blood. However, when kept wet, the virus may survive for 2 or more days.[112] Caution is required with containers of used needles in which the virus may remain wet.

4. HIV is killed by all methods of sterilization. When used properly, all disinfectants except some quaternary ammonium compounds are said to inactivate HIV in less than 2 minutes.[6,30,119]

5. HIV has been transmitted by blood-contaminated fluids that have been heavily spattered or splashed.[25] However, aerosols, such as those produced during dental treatments, have not been found to transmit HB or HIV infection.[30,100]

6. Barriers have proven successful in protecting dental personnel in hospital dentistry and in all other dental clinics against HIV and even more transmissible viral infections at the authors' institution for over 10 years.

A recent concern for the immunocompromised person, as well as for dental personnel, is airborne transmission of multidrug-resistant *Mycobacterium tuberculosis*.[5,22,26]

VIRAL HEPATITIS: AGENTS, EPIDEMIOLOGY, AND INFECTION

In the 8 years after AIDS was recognized, 38,000 persons developed the disease. During that same period, an estimated 38,400 persons died from HB, related cirrhosis, or liver carcinoma.[24,33,36]

Infective inflammation of the liver, termed *hepatitis,* can be caused by infection with five varieties of hepatitis viruses labeled A to E. The type of infection is specifically diagnosed by serologic testing. A, B, and C types of hepatitis are roughly equally divided among viral hepatitis cases detected in population surveys, with type A being the most prevalent. Types B, C, and D are bloodborne infections. Types A and E are fecal-borne infections.[33,78] A new bloodborne virus, hepatitis G, has been detected in a group of high-risk hospitalized dental patients who had liver disease that was associated with other viral agents or conditions.[117] Its importance and contribution to liver disease is not clear.

HB is found in 1 of 100 to 1 of 500 persons in the general population, including dental patients. Incidence has peaked in areas in association with high rates of intravenous (IV) drug abuse and closely follows the incidence of HIV infection.[28,43,44]

According to a 1998 CDC report, 1 in 55 persons (1.8%) in the U.S. population may carry type C hepatitis.[19,78,97] Type C accounts for one third of liver transplants and over 8000 deaths per year.[19]

VIRAL HEPATITIS INFECTION, SYMPTOMS, AND CLINICAL FINDINGS

HBV must enter the circulating blood to reach the liver where the viral DNA causes infected hepatic cells to reproduce the virus. Symptoms usually appear after 2 to 4 months of incubation. Extensive liver damage and illness occur rapidly in approximately 2 of 10 infected persons. Symptoms and signs include nausea, vomiting, chronic fatigue, mental depression, fever, joint aches, darkened urine, jaundice, elevated liver enzymes, and possibly diarrhea or rash. Mortality is 2% or less, but tends to be 2% or higher in persons over 30 years of age.[35,43] (CMV and Epstein-Barr virus [EBV] infections also may produce jaundice and elevated liver enzymes.)

Only 2 of 10 persons infected with HB show symptoms. The remaining eight persons are usually unaware of their infection. For this reason, it is impossible to detect most HB-infected persons by medical history. Whether infected persons are symptomatic or not, they can transmit HB. Usually within 1 year, 9 of the 10 persons develop immunity to HB and are no longer infectious. Unfortunately, 1 of 10 infected persons remains infected and infectious, often for the remainder of life. Acute cirrhosis may be fatal within a number of months. If illness was not severe and chronic infection persists, in 20 to 30 years increased risks of cirrhosis or hepatocellular carcinoma may prove fatal. The possibility of such an outcome produces an overall hepatitis mortality rate of 2%. There is no specific treatment against the virus after infection occurs.

Other types of hepatitis produce symptoms somewhat similar to those of HB.[33,43,44,78] Type A has a shorter incubation of approximately 1 month, with lower mortality. Persons infected with type A do not remain infected or infectious beyond 8 weeks after symptoms subside. Type C hepatitis is often (75%) anicteric (without jaundice), being detected by an elevation of liver enzymes and serologic tests. Type C hepatitis becomes chronic in 75% to 85% of persons infected, causing them to remain infectious.[19]

Type D, or delta hepatitis virus, has a curious makeup. It has no outer coating and relies upon cells infected with HBV to provide the required outer layer. Once types B and D infect a person together, usually by the same route and source, the infection becomes much more severe and many times more fatal than infection with HB alone. Protection against HB also protects against type D, but not types A, C, or E.[33,36,78]

TRANSMISSION OF VIRAL HEPATITIS

The transmission of viral hepatitis types B, C, and D is mainly by blood, IV drug abuse, and sexual contact. Up to billions of HBV may occur per milliliter of infectious blood.[29] HBV is also found in saliva at lower concentrations. HB can be transmitted by contamination of broken skin, the mouth, or eyes with blood-contaminated saliva. One in three exposed persons may be infected with HB. In studies performed during dental treatments of HBV-infected persons, aerosolization of HBV could not be detected by tests for HB surface antigen.[100]

HB is transmitted in the population by the same routes as HIV infection. Unlike HIV, however, HBV has been transmitted to family members by prolonged associations that may involve repeated saliva or blood contamination (e.g., by shared shaving utensils, traces of blood left on bathroom towels, or perhaps extensive sharing of unwashed tooth brushes, or by drinking after one another). *In public, however, neither HIV nor HBV are transmitted by casual contact.*[33,54] Persons with risks for HIV infection are also more likely to be carriers of HBV. Up to 90% of HIV-infected persons have been infected with HBV. Mothers infected with HBV have nearly a 50% chance of infecting their infants at birth. If a mother's infection is recognized, infants can be easily and safely protected with antiserum at birth. If not, up to 90% of infected infants remain carriers for life and have the same increased risk of fatal liver cancer or cirrhosis in 20 to 30 years as adult carriers.

Hepatitis A is excreted from the infected liver into the bile. Both hepatitis A and E are transmitted by the fecal-oral route. Poor hygiene and contaminated food and water are common routes of infection. These types are not a major concern in dentistry.

Blood transfusions were a major source of type B hepatitis until 1985 and of type C hepatitis until 1991. A test for type C hepatitis was developed in 1990. Testing instituted in hospitals since 1986 for type B and since 1991 for hepatitis C has virtually eliminated transfusions as a source of infections. A remaining problem is to detect infectious donors during incubation.[19,78]

INFECTION RISKS FOR PERSONNEL FROM HEPATITIS B AND C VIRUSES

Personnel can be infected by parenteral exposure; mucosal exposure to infected blood or blood-contaminated saliva; and by spatter of blood contamination to eyes, mouth, or broken skin.[29] Paper cuts from blood contaminated request forms appear to have transmitted HB.[99] Plain saliva also can be weakly infectious. Aerosolized, blood-contaminated saliva and respiratory secretions that can transmit many respiratory infection viruses and tuberculosis have not been shown to transmit HB.[12,26,33,42,82]

One in three parenteral exposures of nonvaccinated personnel to HB-infected blood has resulted in HB infection.[43] In contrast to the 1 of 300 nonvaccinated persons who develop HIV following parenteral exposure to HIV infected blood, 100 of 300 persons parenterally exposed to HBV will develop HB.

With a 2% mortality rate for HB, 2 of 100 HBV-exposed persons may die, compared with 1 of 300 HIV-exposed persons. Thus a parenteral blood exposure of a nonimmune person to HBV carries at least twice the mortality risk of a similar HIV exposure. This mortality risk from HB infection could be 6.6 times that of HIV exposure when studies are compared that showed only 1 of 1000 HIV infections per HIV exposure. This latter figure may more closely relate to HIV exposures in dentistry.

Fortunately, a vaccine is readily available against HBV. Mortality rates for personnel from HB exposure could approach zero.[33] Patient protection still depends on effective use of IC procedures.

Hepatitis C virus (HCV) exposure risks for personnel have been documented and appear to be low.[75] IC should minimize risks. Data indicate infection rates from parenteral exposure with HCV-infected blood to be between the rates for HB and HIV infection—approximately 6 of 300 persons parenterally exposed to HCV infected blood, or 1 of 50.[19,75,97]

SEROLOGIC TESTS RELATED TO HEPATITIS A, B, AND C

Serologic tests are available for several antigens of HBV and for the serum antibodies individuals produce against them.[33,43] Testing a blood sample for hepatitis B surface antigen (HbsAg) is used to determine the presence of infection by detecting the protein associated with the surface of the HB virus in the blood. The test is used to detect persons who are infected, whether they are symptomatic or not. Testing for HB e antigen (HBeAg) determines presence of an HB antigen found in blood when HB virus concentrations are high and relate to the person's ability to infect others.

Testing for anti-HBc (antibody against HB core antigen) can detect antibody against a virus core protein that becomes positive in virtually all persons a few months after infection and remains positive for years thereafter. The antibody is used as a marker for previous HB infection, but this antibody is not protective.

A test for anti-HBs (anti-HB surface antigen) is performed to determine the presence of antibodies that can protect against future HB infection. Detection of anti-HBs means that the person has been infected and has recovered or has been immunized with a vaccine.

Hepatitis A virus (HAV) is detected by a test for anti-HAV antibody. Recent infection is indicated by an immunoglobulin M class of anti-HAV antibody.[78] An anti-HCV test and a polymerase chain reaction (PCR) test for HCV-RNA are available for testing patients and clinical personnel.[19] Blood for transfusion and other blood products are now screened for type C hepatitis.

A test for anti-hepatitis D virus can detect superinfection with hepatitis D in persons infected with HB infection.[43] Testing would be especially indicated when the infection appears to be severe and progressing rapidly.

DATA RELATED TO CONTROL OF HEPATITIS B

HBV is a relatively stable DNA hydrophilic virus that can withstand drying on surfaces, and presumably upon equipment and clothing, for over 7 days.[16] Up to 1 billion virus particles of HBV can be found per milliliter of infected blood. Disinfectants selected for their ability to inactivate TB and hydrophilic viruses appear able to inactivate HBV.[15,57] All forms of sterilization destroy the virus.[31,57]

IMMUNIZATION AGAINST HEPATITIS A, B, AND C

A vaccine against type A hepatitis has been developed and found effective and is recommended for the dentist, dental student, and auxiliary personnel clinical trials.[91,103] HAVRIX vaccine (Smith Kline Beecham Biologicals) and VAOTA vaccine (Merck & Co., Inc.) are available. Type B hepatitis is effectively prevented by either of two genetically engineered vaccines now derived from bread yeast, Engerix-B (Smith Kline and French Laboratories) and Recombivax B (Merck Sharp and Dohme).[38] The antigenic protein of these genetically engineered vaccines is identical to the purified viral surface protein antigen used in the original "killed" vaccine derived from the serum of HB-infected persons.

Vaccination against HBV requires one dose followed with another, 1 month later, and a third dose 6 months after the first. Hepatitis vaccines must be given in the arm, not the hip. Both vaccines (yeast and human derived) have as few or fewer side effects compared to other injected vaccines. Protection of those who form antibodies is virtually 100%. One in 30 persons vaccinated may not respond to the vaccine. Follow-up testing is recommended to confirm immunity 1 month after immunization is completed because dental personnel are considered at high risk for HB infection.[28,33] Protective immunoglobulin is available for HBV-exposed persons who have no immunity.

No vaccine is available against hepatitis C. Because the virus mutates rapidly in infected persons, a vaccine may be difficult or impossible to develop. Nor is a protective immunoglobulin available for exposed persons.[19]

TESTS FOR HEPATITIS B ANTIBODY AND BOOSTERS

Persons with a history of exposure to HB and those who have worked in dentistry for several years may prefer to be tested for anti-HBs before being immunized to see if they need the vaccine. A test for antigen (HBsAg) is useful to detect an asymptomatic carrier (chronically infected) state. Persons who are carriers (HBsAg positive) cannot produce antibody, and they would want to test family contacts and immunize those not already exposed.

After a period of 1 to 6 months after vaccination against HB is completed, it is important that dental personnel (as high-risk persons) obtain a test to determine if protective anti-HB surface antigen antibodies (anti-HBs) were formed.[28,33] One or more in 30 vaccinated adults under 40 years of age may not respond to three vaccine injections. Still higher percentages of persons over 40 years do not respond because the immune response gradually lessens with age.[33]

Three or more years after vaccination, many dental personnel realize that they have never had a follow-up antibody test. Usually their antibody level is often undetectable by then, and their ability to respond cannot be evaluated without a booster. Many prefer to save the cost of an initial test by getting a booster dose and a test a month later.

Routine boosters are not recommended for the general health care profession during the first 6 to 9 years after immunization.[23,33,72,81,123] A booster effect is usually experienced upon infection in a person who has produced antibodies. Because of the crisis situation that can surround an exposure, the time it takes to obtain test results after an exposure, and the problem in dentistry of often never knowing when a small exposure has occurred, dental personnel often prefer to have their blood tested with a radioimmunoassay test for anti-HBs to check immunity. If test results are below 10 serum ratio units, they should take a booster dose of HB antigen. This is in keeping with the recommendation for having a booster dose when a known exposure occurs and antibody in a previously immunized person is deficient.[33]

EPIDEMIOLOGY OF OTHER INFECTION RISKS

Agencies are concerned that dental personnel and patients are protected against risks of all infections borne by blood, saliva, and respiratory secretions. Routine medical histories are important, but cannot be relied upon to detect infected patients or for selective use of "universal precautions" for individual patients. *All patients must be considered infectious.* In addition to HIV and hepatitis B, C, and D (discussed previously), other transmissible infections of concern include infectious mononucleosis (EBV infection), CMV, herpes simplex I and II, and tuberculosis.[27,38,60,71] Without barrier protection, hands and mucosa of eyes and mouth of treatment personnel are especially vulnerable to infection with herpes viruses.[12,49,89,90,129] Agents of measles, mumps, other childhood infections, and some other respiratory infections also are transmissible, especially in indistinguishable early stages of infection.[27,70] Measles and mumps can be severe in adults. (See Chapter 9, Patient Assess-

ment, Plate 9-1, showing oral manifestations associated with communicable diseases.)

In 1990, 23% of measles infections occurred in persons over 19 years of age. The mortality rate was 0.3%; one third of fatal cases involved nonimmunized adults.[27] Measles outbreaks among college students have been severe.[32]

Multidrug-resistant tuberculosis (MDR-TB) bacteria are an increasing concern.[22] They are resistant to two or more of the more common therapeutic drugs and are highly transmissible by aerosols produced by coughing. Infections seldom become active in healthy adults, but an active infection can remove a clinical person from practice for months until the infection is controlled and is no longer transmissible. Infection with MDR-TB can be rapidly fatal for immunocompromised persons.[22]

The least familiar disease is CMV infection, a sexually and blood-transmitted disease that often resembles infectious mononucleosis. Especially during pregnancy, a newly infected woman is faced with possible intrauterine or perinatal infection of her infant. Developmental defects can occur in 5% to 10% of infected infants resulting in neuromuscular, auditory, and visual impairments.[60] This is just another infection to which operatory personnel are vulnerable, but it can be prevented by universal use of barrier protection.

Personnel should avail themselves to immunizations against measles, polio, and tetanus. Annual or semiannual skin tests for tuberculosis (PPD) are urged and may soon be required for dental personnel. HB immunization is a federal OSHA requirement unless an employee documents his or her understanding of the risks and his or her refusal. Current regulations require employers to pay for HB immunization, but not for confirmatory testing a month after immunization is complete. Employers or workmen's compensation must pay for serologic testing of employees following exposure incidents related to HIV and HBV. Measles vaccination is required for persons born after 1956, or they must show proof of immunity for admission to most colleges.[34] This is also an excellent requirement for dental personnel.

Immunization against viral influenza and pneumococcal pneumonia may be elected and are advisable. Mumps immunization is highly desirable for male and female personnel who lack a history of immunization or childhood infection. Diphtheria and pertussis immunizations usually are obtained during infancy. Vaccines to prevent HIV, HCV, and other common infections may still be developed in years to come.[19]

EXPOSURE ASSESSMENT PROTOCOL

OSHA does not regulate students. However, dental students are required to follow the same exposure protocol incident plan as dental employees, but with any appropriate differences for students such as source of medical care.[7,58] This plan requires that if blood-contaminated body fluid from a patient is spattered to mucous membranes or comes into contact with the broken or punctured skin of a clinical person, or if exposure is produced by cut or puncture with a contaminated sharp instrument, the protocol must be followed immediately before the patient leaves. If possible, the patient's potential to transmit hepatitis B, C, and HIV infection is determined and the student's susceptibility to HB is determined. The attending physician who helps with these determinations then provides, if indicated, HB immunoglobulin, hepatitis booster, anti-HIV testing, and counseling (see OSHA Regulation).[95]

MEDICAL HISTORY

The medical history serves the following purposes: (1) to detect any unrecognized illness that requires medical diagnosis and care; (2) to identify any infection or high risk that may be important to a clinical person exposed during examination, treatment, or cleanup procedures; (3) to assist in managing and caring for infected patients; and (4) to reinforce use of adequate IC procedures, bearing in mind that general history taking is not capable of detecting all infectious persons. Only conscientious use of universal precautions provides safety. Symptoms of persistent respiratory illness, night sweats, chronic fatigue, and weight loss can be symptomatic of either tuberculosis or HIV infection. With increasing occurrence of MDR-TB bacteria, a dentist's medical history of HIV-infected dental patients and others at high risk should be kept abreast of any current medical care and surveillance from the patient's physician. Be aware of the relationship of all infections (and their characteristics) when taking a medical history and performing an initial general examination at each appointment. (Refer to Chapter 9 for more detail.)

PERSONAL BARRIER PROTECTION

Gloves. OSHA regulations specify that all clinical personnel must wear treatment gloves during all treatment procedures. After each appointment, or if a leak is detected, remove gloves, wash hands, and put on fresh gloves (see Figs. 8-5 and 8-6). Gloves must not be washed or used for more than one patient. Inexpensive disposable well-fitting treatment gloves are available for chairside use. They should be dispensed carefully to avoid contaminating others in the box. The value of gloves was emphasized by finding that without gloves, occult blood persisted under dentists' fingernails for several days after patient contact.[4] Gloves also help prevent very painful and transmissible herpetic infections to fingers (Whitlow) and hands.[82,86]

Treatment gloves cannot protect against punctures. Gloves that become penetrated or torn can imbibe patient fluids and therefore should be removed and the hands washed. Instead of acting as a barrier, gloves worn for more than one patient or for prolonged periods can harbor blood and saliva-borne microorganisms. Gloves must not be washed with hand soaps. Washing reduces glove integrity, leaving personnel more vulnerable. Instead of attempting to wash gloved hands before opening drawers or handling items adjacent to the operatory, use tongs, a paper towel, or a food handler's overglove to prevent contamination.

Dental personnel with chronic HBV or HIV infection should curtail any treatment activities that would jeopardize the patient. *All personnel with weeping or draining lesions that could infect patients should abstain from patient contact.*[23] Dry, nondraining lesions should be kept well protected from clinical contamination.

Increased marketing competition has reduced glove prices and improved quality of latex treatment gloves appreciably. Viruses have been found to penetrate no more than one intact latex glove out of 100.[74] Gloves must meet new Food and Drug Administration (FDA) regulations: less than 4% can have a leak detectable by a water test.[59] Some companies set their standards at less than 2% to 3%. Store boxes of gloves out of sunlight and store multiple boxes in tightly closed, heavy plastic bags to minimize oxidation. If in doubt about a supplier's gloves, contact the distributor about FDA regulations and manufacturing standards of the product. Products that do not meet FDA standards and advertising claims are subject to removal from the market if consumers report lack of compliance.

While cleaning and sorting used sharp instruments, wear puncture-resistant utility gloves. Nitrile latex gloves are preferred; they can be washed inside and out, disinfected, or steam autoclaved, as needed. Wear treatment gloves inside the heavy gloves if they must be shared. With the advent of wearing latex gloves for several hours each day, dental personnel should be aware that the possibility of latex allergy or hypersensitivity is a growing concern for all dental health care workers as well as for patients. In July 1991, the U.S. FDA requested that all cases of allergic reactions to latex be reported. The concern among dental health care workers is due to the frequent changes of gloves, which exposes them to the latex protein allergens. The symptoms associated with latex allergy or hypersensitivity should not be confused with the physical irritation caused by handwashing. Currently, there is no cure for latex allergy. Avoidance of latex products is the best treatment.

Instructions for Handwashing. At the beginning of a routine treatment period, remove watches, jewelry, and rings, or at least those with enlarged projections or stones that can penetrate gloves; then wash hands with a suitable cleanser. Lather hands for at least 10 seconds, rubbing all surfaces, and rinse. Use a clean brush to scrub under and around nails. Repeat at least once to remove all soil. Washing hands well when changing gloves is required.[64,95] Even good quality surgical gloves develop minor pinholes or leaks during vigorous use. Washing minimizes infection risks due to leakage. Before surgery use a prescribed surgical scrub, washing and rinsing from hands toward elbows. (Reserve a separate brush to clean instruments.)

Hand cleansers containing a mild antiseptic like 3% PCMX (p-chloro, meta-xylenole) or chlorhexidine are preferred to control transient pathogens and to suppress overgrowth of skin bacteria.[56] Hand cleansers with 4% chlorhexidine may have broader activity for special cleansing (e.g., for surgery, when a glove leaks, or when a clinical person experiences an injury), but they can be hazardous to eyes.[73,113] PCMX cleansers have been found equally effective, nonirritating, and preferable for routine use.[113] Newer nonopaque chlorhexidine products used especially for surgical scrubs may be less irritating to the hands of some individuals upon prolonged use.[48]

Protective Eyewear, Masks, and Hair Protection. Protective eyewear may consist of goggles, or glasses with solid side-shields. Wear a mask to protect against aerosols. Face shields are appropriate for heavy spatter, but a mask is still required to protect against aerosols that drift behind the shield.[12,95] Spatter also can pass under the edge of a short shield and strike the mouth. Antifog solution for eyewear can be obtained from opticians or product distributors.

Put on eyewear with clean hands before gloving, and remove it with clean hands after gloves are removed. Grasp eyewear by the temple pieces. Grasp the mask only by the string or band at the sides or back of the head to remove it (Fig. 8-7). *Change the mask between every patient or whenever it becomes moist or visibly soiled.* Discard the mask when the patient is dismissed after treatment instead of wearing it around the neck where contaminated edges can rub against the neck. Avoid touching facewear during treatments to avoid cross-contamination.

When eyewear or shields are removed they should be cleaned and disinfected. (To save time, have clean replacement eyewear available while disinfecting used eyewear.) Remove eyewear by grasping the temple pieces with clean fingers; place eyewear on a paper towel and spray with a water-based disinfectant that is allowed to stand for at least 5 minutes. Next, while wearing gloves (for protection against any contamination on lenses), wash eyewear well, and reapply disinfectant for 10 minutes, or preferably allow it to soak in a 1:50 to 1:100 solution of 5% hypochlorite bleach, or other disinfectant solution that does not damage eyewear. (One-half ounce of bleach in a quart of water provides an acceptable 1:65 dilution.) Rinse well and dry. If preferred, goggles that can be autoclaved are available from dental distributors.

Masks with the highest filtration are rectangular, folded types used for surgeries.[40] Dome-shaped masks are adequate barriers against spatter and are considered to prevent HB and HIV infection.[28,100] They are not adequate to hold back measles, influenza, and other aerosolborne respiratory viruses or tuberculosis bacteria. To best protect against aerosols, press edges of the rectangular mask close around the bridge of the nose and face. Masks have been rated according to porosity and effectiveness.[40] Consult claims and test data of mask manufacturers and compare before choosing a mask.

Hair should be kept back out of the treatment field. Hair can trap heavy contamination that, if not washed away, can be rubbed back from a pillow onto the face at night. Personnel must protect their hair with a surgical cap when encountering heavy spatter (e.g., from an ultrasonic scaling device).

Protective Overgarments. An overgarment must be protective of clothing and skin (see Fig. 8-4). Used overgarments should require a minimum of handling and should be easily laundered. *Overgarments must be changed whenever becoming moist or visibly soiled.* Operatory clothing becomes highly spattered with invisible saliva and traces of blood throughout the day. HB and many other microbes can live on dry materials for 1 or more days.[16,61,71,120] Spatter is heavy to the upper surface of the wrists and forearms.[12] Spatter remains on uncovered arms most of the day if not protected by long sleeves. Large cuffs of clinic coat sleeves drag across patient napkins and mouths, become grossly contaminated, and cross-contaminate patients.[128] Therefore sleeves with knit cuffs that tuck under gloves are preferred. If not covered, arms must be washed after each patient if spatter was created. Most office sinks are not deep or wide enough for effective, routine arm washing.

A simple, lightweight garment that covers the arms and chest up to the neck as well as the lap when seated appears to provide adequate protection. Cloth made of cotton or cotton/synthetic fiber like an isolation garment material appears to be thick enough to protect skin

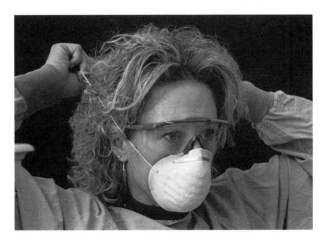

FIG. **8-7** Remove the mask as shown. Grasp the mask ties or elastic band behind the head instead of grasping the contaminated mask. Before treatment, put on mask and eyewear before washing and gloving hands. After treatment, remove gloves, then eyewear and mask, and wash hands.

and street clothing from the spatter of most dental treatments. If surgeries or other treatments produce splashing that wets or penetrates a garment, change it as soon as possible, and clean the skin.

Wearing contaminated garments home or out of the clinical area should not occur. Such garments can contaminate family members who sort, handle, and launder soiled clothing, or may infect young children who cling to adults' clothing. Contamination with HBV, TB, and respiratory viruses (e.g., respiratory syncytial virus) are of most concern.

Used overgarments are removed and placed directly into a laundry bag with a minimum of handling or sorting before leaving the clinical area. Guidelines call for managing used clinic garments to avoid handling or sorting (e.g., searching pockets, removing name tags). Persons handling soiled clinical garments must wear protective gloves. Laundering must be provided by the employer.

Laundering with a regular cycle with regular laundry detergent is considered acceptable, following manufacturer's directions.[28] Hot water up to 70° C or cool water containing 50 to 150 ppm of chlorine provided by liquid laundry bleach would provide more antimicrobial action. Use of a hot air dryer and/or ironing is also beneficial.[28,64]

DISPOSAL OF CLINICAL WASTE

Infected blood and other liquid clinical waste generally can be poured down a sanitary sewer or drain designated for that purpose, but not mercury, silver, or other heavy metal chemicals. Aseptic precautions, cleaning, and disinfection must be applied to the basin around the drain. Adding 3 ounces of 5% hypochlorite in water (household bleach) to each 30 ounces of fluid collected in surgical aspiration bottles is recommended before disposing the fluid down the drain.

Contaminated materials such as used masks, gloves, blood/saliva-soaked sponges, cotton rolls, and so on, must be discarded safely. OSHA regulations presented previously describe rules and required labels regarding regulated sharps and soft waste disposal. OSHA labeling requirements may differ from local protection agency requirements. As pathologic waste, excised tissues require separate disposal and may not be discarded into the trash.

Federal EPA and local environmental protection or control agencies regulate the management and disposal of blood-contaminated waste. This usually applies to waste when it leaves the dental office or clinic. Local county and state regulations must be consulted.

Judgment is essential in bagging medical waste so injury or direct contact with liquids does not take place because HIV and HBV can survive beyond a few days while wet. Separating needles and sharps into hard-walled, leak-proof, and sealable containers and out of

soft trash has provided adequate safety. Nevertheless, local laws governing waste disposal range from the adequate recommendations of the CDC to regulations requiring more strict management and tracking of waste disposal, usually at an added expense.[28,30] Consult local city, county, and state regulations.

NEEDLE DISPOSAL

Goals for needle disposal are to: (1) dispose of needles in a hard-walled, leakproof, and sealable container, which has the OSHA biohazard label; (2) locate the needle-disposal container in the operatory close to where the needle will be used; and (3) avoid carrying unsheathed contaminated needles or containers in a manner that could endanger others or would allow the needles to be accidentally spilled (see Chapter 10).[95] If numbers of approved disposal containers are limited, move the well-closed container to where it is needed during cleanup. Follow local regulations for disposal of the container.

PRECAUTIONS TO AVOID INJURY EXPOSURE

Pointed instruments without a hollow lumen have minimal capacity to transmit infected blood into a puncture site. However, the same principles that apply to needles should be reasonably translated and applied to used burs, wires, and sharp instruments from the operatory. Use great care in passing instruments and syringes with unsheathed needles to another person. Turn sharp and curved ends away from the recipient's hand.

Two-handed resheathing of needles is not permitted. A needle sheath holder or other safety device or technique should be used for the operator to resheath the needle with only one hand (see Chapter 10).[95]

Remove burs from handpieces when finished, or if left in the handpiece in a hanger, point the bur away from your hands and body. Hanging handpieces upside down in some types of hangers can angle the bur away from the operator. *Carefully and deliberately rehang a handpiece when a cutting instrument must be left in it.*

OVERVIEW OF ASEPTIC TECHNIQUES

The concept of asepsis is to prevent cross-contamination—all items that are touched with saliva-coated hands must be rendered free of contamination before treating the next patient. These contaminated items can be discarded; protected by disposable covers; or removed, cleaned, and sterilized. Do not directly touch what you do not want to contaminate. A few simple rules help avoid wasting costly time and effort between patient appointments.

During each appointment:
1. Remember, whatever is touched is contaminated.
2. Directly touch only what has to be touched (*anticipate your needs*).

3. Use one of the following to control contamination:
   A. Clean and sterilize it.
   B. Protect surfaces and equipment that are not sterilized with disposable, single-use covers (barriers). Discard them after every appointment. Use disposable covers on portable items (e.g., curing lamp handles, amalgam mixers, and plastic air-water syringe tips).
   C. Use a paper towel, tongs, or plastic baggie over gloves to briefly handle equipment or to open cabinets and drawers to get things not anticipated during setup.
   D. Scrub and disinfect noncritical surfaces as well as possible. These include any countertops that cannot be covered (and may collect aerosols or spatter) or things that may be accidentally touched, such as room door handles and light switches. With practice, these areas should not become contaminated.

When consistently practiced, these concepts of asepsis can reduce exposure risks, reduce cross-infection risks, and reduce cleaning and disinfecting numerous items in the operatory between appointments. Good asepsis practice also will reduce or eliminate the need to clean or disinfect nonoperatory areas of the dental office because office personnel will avoid contaminating these areas. Examples of items found contaminated in studies of dental offices include telephones, faucet handles, switches, cabinet and drawer handles, radiography controls, lamp handles, door handles, charts, and pens.[71] Evidence of potential cross-contamination and cross-infection risks for patients and personnel related to contact with contaminated surfaces was presented in the chapter introduction.[9,71]

With treatment-soiled gloves, avoid unnecessary contact with all switches, drawers, dispensers, or surfaces on the unit that need not be touched. Use the wrist, arm, or paper towel to operate faucet handles and soap dispenser handles. Use a paper towel to handle the phone, drawer pulls, and charts, and a tongue blade to operate uncovered switches. Rest your gloved writing hand on a paper towel when it is necessary to record findings while charting a patient. Pull a slender clear bag over a pen, tip first, then pop the tip through the plastic end, and tie the bag snugly in a knot at the other end; discard the bag between patients (Fig. 8-8).

Use single-use plastic bags on control unit and chair back, foil or plastic "baggies" on lamp handles, and adherent plastic sheets or a plastic bag on the radiography cone (Fig. 8-9). Use a thin plastic overglove, or a gauze or paper towel to avoid contaminating other objects. Use foot controls for faucets, dental chair, and radiography button. *In addition, cover light-curing units and amalgamators with custom-fitting plastic barriers to avoid contamination.*

Once a day, or as needed, use any water-based tuberculocidal disinfectant licensed by the EPA to clean and disinfect other environmental surfaces in the operatory and laboratory.

OPERATORY ASEPSIS

Protection of Operatory Surfaces: Rationale, Materials, and Methods. Operatory surfaces that will be repeatedly touched or soiled are best protected with disposable covers (barriers) that can be discarded after each treatment (see Fig. 8-9).[38,48,125] Changing covers eliminates cleaning and disinfecting the surface; saves time, effort, and expense; and can be more protective. White paper sheets ("white newsprint") are useful for workbenches and operatory surfaces on which dry contaminated materials are placed. For dental unit trays,

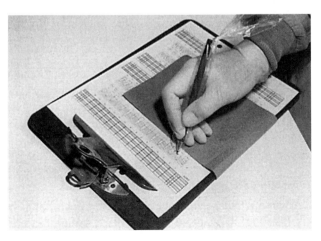

FIG. **8-8** Protect charts from contamination. When charting must be performed without help, rest your writing hand on a paper towel and cover the pen. Note that cuff of the glove should overlap cloth overgarment. Surfaces of both glove and plastic bag must not contaminate the chart and its contents.

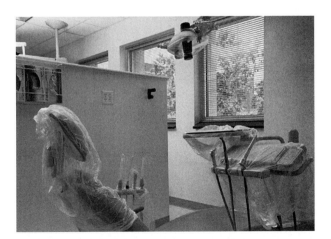

FIG. **8-9** Specially designed or generic plastic bags are used to cover the chair and unit as shown. Changing bags after each patient is more effective and more rapid than disinfection. Damage to equipment from disinfectants also is avoided. Do not routinely disinfect surfaces that have been covered.

paper, or plastic film, or surgical pack wraps (paper or towels) should cover the entire tray, including edges.

Special-sized commercial plastic bags and covers designed for dentistry are available and offer both a good fit and ease of dispensing. They are worthwhile investments for a dental practice. Materials from commercial plastics supply companies or restaurant supply companies are cheaper and are used in many clinics and offices. Plastic film, sandwich bags, or a small sheet of foil wrap have proven serviceable for covering operatory light handles. Removable lamp handles that can be sterilized also can be used. (Plastic or foil wrap is less expensive and covers far better than gauze sponges.) Use plastic film to cover dental control units that cannot be covered with bags. Inexpensive large clear plastic bags are used in numerous offices to cover chair back, control unit, and hose supports. Bags used by dry cleaning establishments also can be used to cover chairs and arms. Clear plastic 15-gallon waste container bags fit many chair backs, control units, and x-ray equipment. Plastic, restaurant, silverware bags fit suction handles, and air/water syringe handles (see Fig. 8-9).

After each appointment, discard and replace bags and covers without cleaning and disinfecting covered equipment items. If covers come off, become torn, or otherwise allow equipment to become contaminated, thoroughly clean and disinfect the item before recovering it for the next appointment.

Preparation of Semicritical Items (Attached to the Dental Unit for Reuse) and Noncritical Items (Supporting or Environmental). Instruments that contact cut tissues or penetrate tissues are considered to be critical items that require thorough cleaning and sterilization for reuse.[14,38,48,57] A number of items attached to the dental unit are used intraorally. They are either handled by gloved hands coated with blood and saliva or may touch mucosa. CDC guidelines consider these semicritical items.[38,57] Items that are not ordinarily touched during treatments are termed noncritical items.

Semicritical Items. Semicritical items that touch mucosa are the air/water syringe tip, suction tips, prophy angle, and handpieces. Others (air/water syringe handle, suction hose ends, lamp handle, and switches) are handled or touched interchangeably with treatment instruments that become contaminated with blood and saliva. Semicritical items must be removed for cleaning and sterilization unless they are either disposable or can be protected from contamination with disposable plastic covers. This applies especially to air-water syringe tips.

Semicritical items should not be disinfected only. As stated before, they should be covered, cleaned and sterilized, or discarded. Some bacteria often remain after use of the best disinfectant.[71,77,85] However, when a cover comes off, or when disinfection is the only recourse, semicritical items must be scrubbed clean, preferably at the sink; disinfected; and then wiped again using a fresh,

alcohol sponge. Surface disinfection is not adequate for items with a lumen such as air-water syringe tips.

Noncritical Items. Noncritical items are environmental surfaces such as chairs, benches, floors, walls, and supporting equipment of the dental unit that are not ordinarily touched during treatments. Lengths of hoses that connect equipment to the control unit become spattered but need not be touched. Contaminated noncritical items require cleaning and disinfection.

Disinfection is always at least a two-step procedure: the initial step involves vigorous scrubbing of the surfaces to be disinfected and wiping them clean; the second step involves wetting the surface with a disinfectant and leaving it wet for the time prescribed by the manufacturer. Many water-based disinfectants contain detergents that make them effective cleaners. So, some products can be used for both steps. However, there is no such thing as a "one-step disinfectant." The disinfectant step must always be preceded by cleaning.

Wear protective utility gloves to clean equipment that cannot be covered. For cleaning and disinfecting environmental surfaces, nitrile latex utility gloves are preferred. Disinfectants can penetrate treatment gloves to irritate covered skin, and these less sturdy gloves are prone to small tears. Use a water-based disinfectant cleaner (e.g., a synthetic phenolic complex disinfectant), a chlorhexidine antiseptic scrub, or other suitable cleaner to scrub equipment. Next, wipe items dry with a paper towel. Then, wet them with an EPA-registered disinfectant or one with an FDA premarket review, and leave them wet for the time specified by the disinfectant manufacturer.

Although uncovered chair arms may become spattered and need to be covered or disinfected, the chair itself is considered a noncritical item. Areas of the chair not contaminated by spatter need not be disinfected, except for housekeeping purposes. Chair backs and control units are covered to protect control buttons from operator gloved finger contamination and spatter, as well as from the damaging effects of disinfectants, and time for disinfecting is saved. A total chair cover can provide the same or more advantages.

Disinfectants. Preferred disinfectants are those that can inactivate polio or coxsackieviruses (because they are nonlipid viruses similar to HB in resistance).[5,14,15,57] Disinfectants must be active against *Mycobacterium* species, common respiratory viruses, and common bacterial hospital pathogens (e.g., *Staphylococcus and Pseudomonas* species). All such disinfectants readily inactivate HIV in 1 to 2 minutes.

Glutaraldehydes at concentrations used for instrument disinfection are far too toxic to be used on operatory surfaces and take at least 20 minutes to kill *Mycobacterium* species.

Unfortunately, the reliability of testing disinfectants against mycobacteria and HB is controversial and criteria for evaluating disinfectants are being revised.[107] Preferred disinfectants registered by the EPA include: 1:10 to 1:100 dilutions of 5% hypochlorite in water (household bleach); plain dilute iodine solutions; iodophor disinfectants containing phosphoric acid; water-based synthetic complex phenolic derivatives containing 9% o-phenyl-phenol and 1% o-benzyl-p-chlorophenol diluted 1 ounce to 1 quart of water to give 0.3% final concentration of synthetic complex phenols; 79% ethyl alcohol sprays containing 0.1% phenylphenol, or other ethyl alcohol disinfectants containing 60% or more alcohol.[41] (Isopropyl alcohol may be used, but ethyl alcohol is preferred.) Activity of disinfectants is reduced by organic debris or blood. Iodines are especially sensitive to the presence of blood.[41,116] Whereas most disinfectants can be applied with paper towels or gauze pads, some types of cellulose paper or fiber react with iodine to produce a greenish, black, or blue color reaction, which usually indicates inactivation. Most water-based disinfectants are effective for removing dried blood. Alcohols tend to harden whole blood that is dried on surfaces, making the surfaces difficult to clean.[92] (Alcohols were used to harden and fix blood films on glass slides in hematology laboratories). Disinfectants containing 70% to 79% ethyl alcohol are considered the most effective disinfectants on cleaned surfaces.[41,44,116]

Regarding disinfection, remember these two principles: (1) *Disinfection cannot occur until fresh disinfectant is reapplied to a thoroughly cleaned surface*,[46,57] and (2) *disinfection does not sterilize*.[71, 102,116]

Chlorine and iodine found in some disinfectants can react with or be absorbed by the plastic in some types of dispensing bottles, which must be refilled with fresh solution daily. Consult and follow manufacturer's directions in this regard.

Manufacturers specify a time to leave items wet with disinfectant for disinfection. This is usually 10 minutes. Most disinfectants, except plain phenol, appear to be active in approximately 5 minutes according to manufacturer data. Equipment left wet until the next patient is seated has usually been wet for at least 5 minutes. But this should be taken into careful consideration. Data on kill times should be obtained from the manufacturer. After sufficient time, wet items can be dried with a paper towel.

Step-by-Step Preparation of the Dental Chair, Dental Unit, and Instruments. As well as not being acceptable for semicritical items, the disinfectants generally considered most active against microorganisms are, unfortunately, the most drying or destructive to plastic chair covers and equipment. This again validates the use of covers wherever possible. When covers are used, the effectiveness of the disinfectants becomes less critical and protecting equipment is easier.

Following is an example of step-by-step SOPs for preparation of the dental chair, dental unit, and instru-

ments between appointments. (Remember, do not disinfect surfaces and items covered with plastic drape after each treatment unless the plastic cover was torn or came off during treatment.)

1. With hands still gloved after the last treatment, remove and invert chair back cover, discard cotton rolls and other disposable materials into the cover, and discard cover into the operatory trash bin. Remove and discard gloves aseptically.

2. Wash hands with antiseptic hand soap, rinse, and dry. Place three paper towels on the seat of the dental chair for later placement of air/water syringe and ends of suction hoses. Put on nitrile latex utility gloves.

3. With the used suction tip, clean saliva and debris from the cuspidor trap if present. Discard disposable suction tip into the operatory trash bin.

4. Remove (unscrew) from the anesthetic syringe the resheathed needle, and discard it with all other sharp disposable items in a sharps container. Using a Stick-shield is advised (see Chapter 10). *Remove the anesthetic cartridge before removing the needle to decrease the risk of an occupational needlestick. Handling needles without using a protective one-handed capping device and gathering instruments without heavy protective gloves account for most injury exposure incidents.*

5. Place any loose sharp instruments and instrument cassettes into a perforated metal basket, and then lower the basket into disinfectant solution in a covered hard-walled pan. Return the air/water syringe tip, handpieces, and pan of instruments to the cleanup area. Using handles provided, remove the basket of instruments, rinse, and then place into the ultrasonic cleaner.

6. Before handling disinfectant-dispensing bottles, wash utility gloves (on hands) with antiseptic scrub, rinse, and dry.

7. Spray any used bottles, containers, tubes, and unused burs with disinfectant, and wipe with a paper towel. Spray again, and leave damp with disinfectant as they are put away. Spraying in this manner has been found effective.[116] However, if there is a concern about breathing any irritating or possibly harmful aerosols that are produced, apply the disinfectant with any disposable material that will not inactivate the disinfectant.

8. Remove the air/water syringe (now minus its removable tip) and suction hoses from the hangers on the control unit. Remove the plastic covers from hose ends and discard. Lay the air/water syringe and suction hose ends on the paper towels previously placed on the dental chair.

9. Invert, remove, and discard plastic drapes from the control unit (Fig. 8-10); remove and discard protective covers from lamp handles, and surface covering

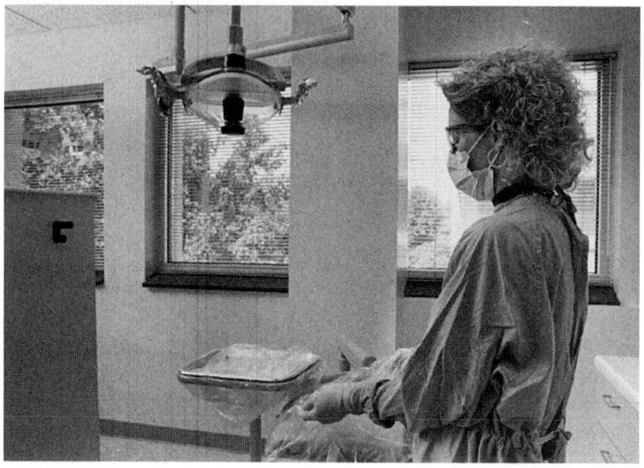

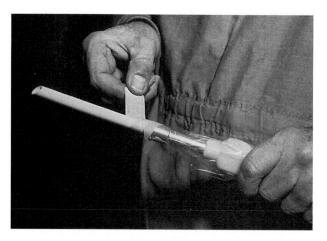

FIG. **8-10** Wear suitable protective gloves to undrape the unit. Remove hoses from their hangers and lay them on paper towels on the chair. Pull the draping bag off of the control unit so it will invert. Pull a clean bag over the unit from the front with clean hands and tuck it around the back and bottom. Cover equipment support arms as well.

FIG. **8-11** Install the suction tip and cover it with a slender plastic bag. Push the tip through the end of the bag and continue sliding the bag to cover the handle area of the hose. Wrap a piece of suitable tape at the bag/tip junction, as shown, to secure the bag against creeping and prevent exposing the handle to contamination. After use, the bag comes off with the plastic tip for easy removal and disposal.

from the side table. These disposables may be placed into the large bag removed from the control unit.

10. For any controls and switches that were not covered, wet a paper towel with disinfectant spray and wipe lamp switch and controls that were contaminated. (Do not spray control switches.) Wipe any contaminated surfaces not previously covered: side table, arms of dental chair, contaminated drawer handles, radiographic viewbox switch, and paper towel dispenser. Discard wet paper towels.

11. Use a second towel wet with disinfectant to rewet these items and leave them wet. (Paper towels neutralize iodine disinfectants and should not be used to apply them.)

12. Spray the outside and inside of the cuspidor, if present, with disinfectant. Use two paper towels to prevent gloves from contacting the cuspidor while first wiping the outside and then the inside of the cuspidor. Discard towels. Wipe any overspray of disinfectant from the operatory floor. Discard towels into the trash bin.

13. Spray any contaminated faucet handles, sink countertop, and trash disposal openings with disinfectant and wipe dry with paper towel. Discard towel and respray areas with disinfectant and leave damp.

14. Wash utility gloves (still on hands) with strong antiseptic hand scrub or disinfectant cleaner, rinse thoroughly, and dry them with paper towels. Discard towels into trash bin. Remove utility gloves and rehang them in the operatory. Wash hands. Contaminated utility gloves can be cleaned and disinfected. Nitrile latex gloves can be autoclaved.

To prepare the unit for the next patient, gloves need not be worn if only clean surfaces that have been pro-

tected with covers are touched. Use a paper towel or treatment glove to handle questionable surfaces such as hoses. The unit is prepared as follows:

1. Pull a large clear plastic bag-cover over the dental control unit from the front and tuck excess up under the unit (see Fig. 8-10). Split the bag up one side to cover mobile delivery system units with large surfaces.

2. Pull another bag down over the chair back; also cover chair arms.

3. Install suction and air/water syringe tips. Place a slender bag over each tip, pushing the tip through the end of the bag and then sliding the bag down to cover all of the handle. For the suction tip, wrap autoclave tape at the tip/bag junction to secure the bag against creeping and to prevent contamination of the handle area of the hose (Fig. 8-11). It usually is not necessary to tape the bag onto the air-water syringe. Press handles into the forked hangers on the unit that are covered by the plastic bag (Fig. 8-12).

4. Install sterilized handpieces. A plastic sleeve may be used to cover the motor-end of the low-speed handpiece that is not sterilized (see Fig. 8-9). Rehang handpieces. If the plastic film obstructs the electric eye in the hanger, use a small finger to pull out the film when the handle is removed.

5. Set out materials and instrument packs; open packs, being careful not to touch sterilized instruments with bare hands.

6. Seat the patient and put on a clean mask, eyewear, and gloves.

Protection of Complex Devices Against Contamination. Cameras, light-curing units, lasers, intraoral cameras, air abrasion units, and so on, are examples of com-

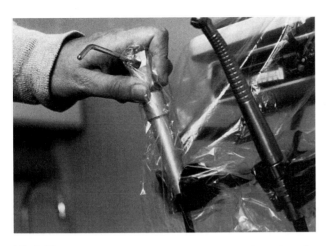

FIG. **8-12** Replace equipment attached to hoses by using the device to simply press the loose plastic film into the forked holder.

plex devices that must be protected against contamination. They are used in the operatory and cannot be sterilized or even readily disinfected. Clear plastic bags of suitable size obtained from plastics or dental supply companies are effective single-use protective barriers.

PROCEDURES, MATERIALS, AND DEVICES FOR CLEANING INSTRUMENTS BEFORE STERILIZATION

According to ADA guidelines and CDC specifications, instruments that touch mucosa or penetrate tissues must be cleaned and then sterilized before reuse (Box 8-1).[5,38]

Principles and Procedures for Handling and Cleaning Instruments After Treatment. Instrument cleaning procedures should be designed to be effective while avoiding risks such as grasping and scrubbing groups of single- and double-ended sharp instruments. Instrument grasping and scrubbing are the most exposure-prone tasks encountered after treatments, even when protective utility gloves are worn.

The safest and most efficient instrument cleaning procedures involve ultrasonic cleaning of used instruments kept in a perforated basket or cassette throughout the cleaning procedure.[17,44,50,115] Wear protective utility gloves at all times to handle contaminated containers and instruments.

Some dentists require all instruments to be placed directly into the sterilizer and steam sterilized before cleaning. They believe the increased safety of handling heat-processed instruments outweighs any disadvantages. Depending on the sterilizer, contaminated instruments may be placed directly into the sterilizer in an empty pan or cassette, or they may be submerged in a detergent solution containing a rust inhibitor. Contact the manufacturer of your sterilizer for guidance in this regard.

Procedures for Instrument Processing. Transport to the cleanup area instrument cassettes and any loose instruments in a perforated metal basket lowered by han-

BOX **8-1**   *Dos* and *Don'ts* of Instrument Recycling

DO THE FOLLOWING:
- Wear protective puncture-resistant gloves to handle used instruments.
- Keep instruments wet in an antibacterial solution before cleaning.
- Use an ultrasonic cleaning device.
- Test and maintain the ultrasonic device periodically.
- Use good quality sterilizer equipment.
- Read the operator's manual and follow operation instructions for the sterilizer.
- Have sterilizers annually inspected regarding gaskets, timer, valves, temperature and pressure gauges.
- Use proper water or chemicals to operate, clean and maintain sterilizer.
- Place only dry instruments in the sterilizer.
- Use a wrap that will be penetrated by the steam or gas used.
- Load the sterilizer loosely; leave air space between large packs.
- Read sterilizer temperature and pressure gauges daily.
- Use the complete sterilizer monitoring system outlined; use indicators daily and spore tests weekly.
- Keep a record of daily indicators and spore tests.

DON'T DO THE FOLLOWING:
- Place wet instruments into any type of sterilizer unless so instructed.
- Overwrap cloth packs or use impermeable wraps for steam or chemical vapor pressure sterilization.
- Use closed, nonperforated trays, foil, canisters, or other sealed containers in gas or steam sterilizers.
- Overload or cram packs together in the sterilizer.
- Decrease the required time for sterilization.
- Add instruments to a sterilizer without restarting the cycle.
- Sterilize viability control strips supplied with spore tests.

dles into a disinfectant detergent solution contained in a covered hard-walled pan.

Note that organic debris on instruments is likely to reduce activity of the disinfectant. Soaking used instruments before cleaning primarily keeps fresh debris from drying but also helps soften and loosen any dried debris. Leave instruments in their basket or cassette while rinsing them well. Next, move the cassettes or basket of instruments into an ultrasonic cleaning device for cleaning (Fig. 8-13), rinse them again, and then carefully inspect the instruments for debris.[17,115] Use tongs to remove any instruments left uncleaned. Remove the debris from these instruments individually, keeping hands well protected with utility gloves. Dip instruments likely to rust into a rust inhibitor such as fresh rust-retarding cleaning solution (e.g., solution from Health Sonics Corp., Pleasanton, California). Drain and air-dry instruments

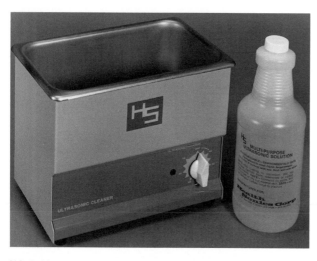

FIG. **8-13** An example of a commercial ultrasonic cleaner with a rust-inhibiting soaking and cleaning solution is shown. *(Courtesy of Health Sonics Corp., Pleasanton, Calif.)*

in cassettes or carefully spill the basket of instruments onto an absorbent towel on a tray. Wet instruments can be patted with a thickly folded towel. Treat both the towels and tray as contaminated items. Still wearing protective gloves, properly package the instruments together with internal and external sterilization indicators suited to the sterilization process used.[17]

Protective utility gloves made of nitrile latex are the most puncture resistant and are obtainable from dental suppliers. These gloves can be washed and wiped with disinfectant or autoclaved after use as needed. Household utility gloves are not suitable for handling and cleaning sharp instruments.

Instrument containers are used as specified by the following OSHA regulations:

1. Immediately, or as soon as possible after use, place contaminated reusable sharps into appropriate containers until they are properly reprocessed. Containers must be puncture resistant, properly labeled or color coded, and leakproof on sides and bottom. Cover the container to transport the instruments to the cleanup area.
2. Reusable contaminated sharps shall not be stored or processed in a manner that requires employees (with or without protective gloves) to reach by hand into containers where these sharps have been placed.[95,122]

If instruments can be securely enclosed in a cassette (Fig. 8-14), rewrapping the cassette in its sturdy sterilization wrapping paper may be considered by OSHA authorities to provide sufficient protection against injury or contamination while transporting the instruments. This option should be verified with local OSHA authorities. Otherwise, the OSHA criteria are met by placing instruments into a basket or cassette with attachable handles,

or by using other methods that avoid hand-reaching into the hard-walled containers to place, process, and remove used instruments.

Some OSHA consultants have prescribed that used instruments be placed in a hard-walled container of disinfectant soaking or holding solution before removing the instruments from the operatory. Although soaking is desirable to prevent debris from hardening on instruments, the OSHA regulation does not appear to address such holding solutions.

A disinfectant holding solution for transporting and/or soaking used instruments should contain a detergent, be economical so it can be discarded frequently, not corrode instruments in a reasonable time, be one of the least inactivated by organic debris, not give off toxic aldehyde vapors, and have 10-minute well-verified antimicrobial claims against TB and preferably against polio or coxsackievirus. Some concentrated phenolic-derivative products that must be diluted for use and a product recommended by an ultrasonic device manufacturer (Health Sonics Corp., Pleasanton, California) meet most of these criteria reasonably well. However, no product is currently considered able to completely disinfect soiled instruments, so protective gloves must still be worn until the instruments have been fully wrapped for sterilization.

When it is necessary to clean instruments by hand, use a suitable brush along with a disinfectant cleaner. Severe irritation, infection of unprotected eyes, or both can result from spatter of the disinfectant, detergents, or chlorhexidine gluconate hand cleansers often used to scrub instruments. Hand injury from double-ended instruments is the other main risk as indicated before.

Wear heavy gloves, eye protection, a mask or a face shield, and a protective garment or apron to protect against spatter. Use a long-handled pan-scrubbing brush. Grasp the mid-handle portion of only a few instruments at a time with fingers and thumb to protect the palm and to rotate the instruments. Brush away from yourself, down into the sink, using at least 5 strokes per end while rotating them. Pay attention to removing visible soil and debris. Rinse with an aerated stream of water to avoid spatter.

Scrape or use an appropriate solvent cleaner to remove coatings such as plaster, wax, cement, and impression material. When finished cleaning, use heavy gloves, disinfectant, and paper towels to clean up spattered or contaminated surfaces around the sink.

Ultrasonic Cleaners and Solutions. Ultrasonic cleaning is the safest and most efficient way to clean sharp instruments (see Fig. 8-13). Burs should be ultrasonically cleaned as well. To contain burs, place them in a fine screen basket, metal tea ball, or bur caddy. Some hinged instruments (e.g., some brands of orthodontics pliers) should not be submerged in ultrasonic or disinfectant cleaning solutions if hinges will corrode or rust. Consult the manufacturer.

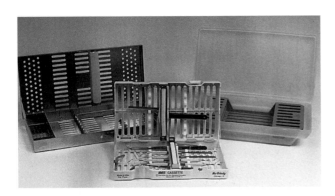

FIG. 8-14 Examples of three cassettes designed to hold instruments while they are cleaned and sterilized, supplied by Health Science Products, Birmingham, Ala. (*left*), Hu-Friedy, Chicago, Ill. (*center*), and Zirc Dental Products, Inc., Minneapolis, Minn. (*right*).

Ultrasonic cleaning can be one to nine times more effective than hand cleaning if the ultrasonic device functions properly and is used as directed by the manufacturer.[115] An ultrasonic cleaning device should provide fast and thorough cleaning without damage to instruments; have a lid, well-designed basket, and audible timer; and be engineered to prevent electronic interference with other electronic equipment and office communication systems.

1. Observe operating precautions.
2. Operate the tank at one-half to three-fourths full of cleaning solution at all times. Use only cleaning solutions recommended by ultrasonic device manufacturers. Change solutions as directed. An antimicrobial cleaning solution is preferred. Studies sponsored by one company indicated that their antibacterial solution remained free of contamination for approximately 3 days of continued reuse (Health Sonics Corp., Pleasanton, California).
3. Operate the ultrasonic cleaner for 5 minutes or longer as directed by the manufacturer to give optimal cleaning, possibly up to 1 minute per instrument.
4. Coatings such as plaster, wax, cement, and impression material can be removed with an appropriate solvent cleaner and then placed in a beaker in the ultrasonic device. Consult ultrasonic device manufacturers or dental product distributors.
5. Verify ultrasonic performance monthly or when poor performance is suspected by using a foil test as described below. Devices that have less than two transducers do not pass the foil test and are not suitable for instrument cleaning. Performance of ultrasonic devices used without periodic testing and maintenance is often poor.[39]

To perform an ultrasonic cleaner foil test, remove the basket from the device. Add solution to the tank, and operate the device for 5 minutes to expel dissolved gases as directed by the manufacturer. Measure the depth of the solution and the length (longest dimension) of the tank. From a roll of aluminum foil, cut a sheet approximately 1 inch more than the depth of the solution in the metal tank. Cut the length 1 inch less than the length of the tank. Hold the foil like a curtain vertically submerged in the solution in the center of the tank approximately one-half inch above the bottom. (Caution: do not immerse fingers.) Without allowing the edges of the curtain to touch the tank, operate the device for exactly 20 seconds. Upon close inspection, every square one-half inch of the foil should show small visible indentations or perforations if the ultrasonic device functions properly. The foil test can be performed in the midline, front, and rear areas of the tank to determine uniformity. Labeled foil sheets can be filed to document test results. (This method was adapted from directions of Health Sonics Corp., Pleasanton, California.)

Instrument Containment. Cloth packs, wraps, tubes of nylon film, or commercial paper/plastic bags are suitable for instrument containment if they are compatible with the method and temperature of sterilization. Various kinds of instrument trays and cassettes (see Fig. 8-14) are manufactured to contain instruments at chairside, and they can be placed in an ultrasonic cleaner, rinsed, and packaged ready for sterilization. Cassettes provide convenience, safety in handling and cleaning batches of instruments, and maintenance of instrument organization for efficient use.

STERILIZATION

Infectious dental patients are often undetected. Sterilization provides a method of instrument recycling that can be monitored and documented to show that conditions for control of disease transmission were indeed established. Because most instruments contact mucosa and/or penetrate oral tissues, it is essential that reused instruments be thoroughly cleaned and sterilized by accepted methods that can be routinely tested and monitored.[5,38,46] Heat sterilization takes less time than high-level sporicidal disinfection, which is required when heat or gas sterilization cannot be used. It is important to recognize that sterilization practices were found unreliable in 15% to 31% of dental offices surveyed where routine monitoring was not used to evaluate and maintain correct sterilization performance.[98]

The four accepted methods of sterilization are:

1. Steam pressure sterilization (autoclave)
2. Chemical vapor pressure sterilization (chemiclave)
3. Dry heat sterilization (dryclave)
4. Ethylene oxide sterilization

Each method and each commercial modification has very specific requirements regarding timing, temperature, suitable packaging of materials, and kinds of items and materials that can be safely and effectively sterilized.[43,45,46] Ignoring any of these specifications can prevent sterilization or damage materials or instruments.

It is best to evaluate office needs and examine various sterilizer capabilities and then carefully select one or two methods of sterilization. Kinds and sizes of sterilization equipment depend on the treatment instrumentation used in the practice. Stainless steel instruments and mirrors used for operative, endodontic, periodontics, or dental hygiene procedures can be sterilized by any accepted method. Both high- and low-speed handpieces are best autoclaved. Burs, discussed later, can be safely sterilized by dry heat or chemical vapor in a chemiclave or in a gas sterilizer, but they may rust or corrode if not protected from steam in the autoclave. Metal impression trays can be sterilized by any method, but dry heat above 345° F may remove soldered handles. Orthodontic pliers of high quality stainless steel will resist corrosion in an autoclave; lower quality stainless steel found in some pliers must be sterilized by dry heat or chemical vapor. Towels and towelpacks of instruments needed for surgery are best sterilized by autoclaving; chemical vapor pressure sterilization does not penetrate cloth well. Perhaps the widest variety of instruments would be found in pediatric dentistry and thus may require more than one sterilization method.

A sterilizer will be used every day of practice. Choose reliable sterilization equipment of proper size and cycle time compatible with needs of the practice. Patient load, turnaround time for instrument reuse, size of instrument inventory and instrument variety, and instrument quality must all be balanced against the type and size of sterilizer selected and the number of auxiliary personnel employed. Some offices have personnel come in at night to clean and sterilize instruments. Careful planning toward a central goal is more practical, effective, and economical than adapting several sterilization methods. Sterilizer modification and development is changing more rapidly now than ever before. Choosing equipment that is well established still is the safest and most reliable approach.

STEAM PRESSURE STERILIZATION (AUTOCLAVING)

Sterilization with steam under pressure is performed in a steam autoclave (Fig. 8-15). For a light load of instruments, the time required at 250° F (121° C) is a minimum of 15 minutes at 15 lbs of pressure. Time for wrapped instruments can be reduced to 7 minutes if the temperature is raised to approximately 273° F (134° C) to give 30 pounds of pressure. Time required for the sterilizer to reach the correct temperature is not included. Bench models may be automatic or manually operated. Manual sterilizers should have both a temperature and pressure gauge so temperatures can be related to corre-

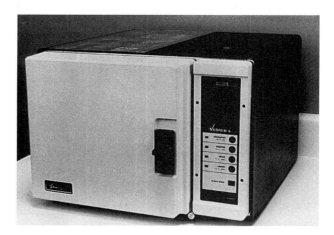

FIG. 8-15 An example of a steam pressure sterilizer (autoclave). *(Courtesy of Pelton and Crane, Charlotte, NC.)*

sponding temperatures required for sterilization. Unlike hospital autoclaves, bench models depend on gravity flow to distribute steam throughout the load rather than first evacuating air from the sterilizer and then refilling it with steam. Therefore bench models require more caution against the use of large or tightly packed loads. Steam must enter and circulate around packs easily. Instrument pans or other impermeable instrument containers must be left open so steam can enter. Except for containers of solutions, all metal items must be dry. Moisture evaporating from instruments can slow the heating process. Sterilization must be tested routinely (see Monitors of Sterilization).[5,38]

Advantages of Autoclaves. Autoclaving is the most rapid and effective method for sterilizing cloth surgical packs and towel packs. Other methods are not suitable for processing cloth packs. Automated models are available, although they still can be misused or fail almost as often as nonautomated ones; they must be evaluated with a biologic spore test monitoring system.

Disadvantages of Autoclaves. Items sensitive to the elevated temperature cannot be autoclaved. Autoclaving tends to rust carbon steel instruments and burs. Steam appears to corrode the steel neck and shank portions of some diamond instruments and carbide burs.

Sterilization of Burs in Autoclaves. For autoclave sterilization, burs can be protected by keeping them submerged in a small amount of 2% sodium nitrite solution.[49,50] Sodium nitrite crystals (not nitrate) can be obtained from distributors of scientific products and chemicals, or a pharmacy. Add 20 g (⅔ oz) of nitrite to 1 L of pure water. Store tightly sealed. After ultrasonic cleaning, burs can be rinsed and placed into any small metal or glass beaker with a perforated lid (e.g., a metal salt shaker). Fill the beaker with sufficient fresh nitrite solution to have it above the burs, approximately 1 cm. Leave the container uncovered or use a perforated cover. Place the container of burs and fluid into the sterilizer, and

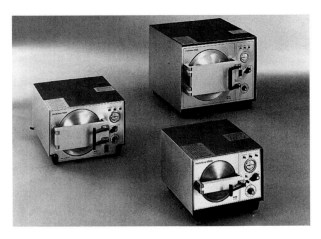

FIG. 8-16 Chemical vapor pressure sterilizer (Chemiclave). *(Courtesy of MDT Biologic Co., Rancho Dominguez, Calif.)*

operate a normal sterilization cycle. Discard the fluid from the container through the perforated lid. Use sterile forceps to place the burs into a sterilized bur holder or tray. Store the burs dry. Before use, any nitrite residue can be wiped away, or rinsed off with clean or sterile water, if desired.

CHEMICAL VAPOR PRESSURE STERILIZATION (CHEMICLAVING)

Sterilization by chemical vapor under pressure is performed in a Chemiclave (MDT Biologic Co., Rancho Dominguez, California) (Fig. 8-16). Chemical vapor pressure sterilizers operate at 270° F (131° C) and 20 pounds of pressure. They are similar to steam sterilizers and have a cycle time of approximately half an hour. Like ethylene oxide sterilizers, they must be used with a prescribed chemical and should be properly labeled to satisfy OSHA's Chemical Hazard Communication Standard. Newer models appear to handle aldehyde vapors well; vapors from older models must be safely vented. Loading cautions similar to those for autoclaving must be used. Water left on instruments loaded into the chamber can defeat sterilization.

Advantages of Chemiclaves. Carbon steel and other corrosion-sensitive burs, instruments, and pliers are said to be sterilized without rust or corrosion.

Disadvantages of Chemiclaves. Items sensitive to the elevated temperature will be damaged. Instruments must be lightly packaged in bags obtained from the sterilizer manufacturer. Towels and heavy cloth wrappings of surgical instruments may not be penetrated to provide sterilization. Routinely use biologic spore test monitoring strips to confirm heat penetration of heavy packs before using them (see Monitors of Sterilization). Only fluid purchased from the sterilizer manufacturer can be used. Load only dry instruments, and check the door gasket for leaks to avoid frequent sterilization monitoring failures.

DRY HEAT STERILIZATION

Conventional Dry Heat Ovens. Dry heat sterilization is readily achieved at temperatures above 320° F (160° C).[47] Conventional professional dry heat ovens that have been sold for instrument sterilization have heated chambers that allow air to circulate by gravity flow (gravity convection). Packs of instruments must be placed at least 1 cm apart to allow heated air to circulate. Individual instruments must actually be heated at 320° F for 30 minutes to achieve sterilization.[50] Increasing the total time by 50% as a safety factor is recommended. Total time required also depends on the efficiency of the oven for its size, the size of the load, and how instruments are packaged. Foil wrap or special nylon bags are used. Approximately 60 to 90 minutes may be required to sterilize a medium load of lightly wrapped instruments in an oven set at a range of 335° to 345° F. Temperatures vary at least 5° above and below the setting, so a range rather than a specific temperature must be set.

Use of a sterilizer not reviewed by the FDA for instrument sterilization or using one inappropriately may result in the dentist being liable for any adverse consequences.

Without careful calibration, more sterilization failures are obtained with gravity convection dry heat ovens than any other type of sterilizer. The only accurate way to calibrate a sterilization cycle in most relatively inexpensive industrial and professional dry heat ovens is by using an external temperature gauge (pyrometer) attached to a thermocouple wire. The other end of the wire is extended inside the oven and tied to an instrument in a centrally located pack to measure its exact temperature. Battery-operated pyrometers are available from scientific supply companies.

Short-Cycle, High-Temperature Dry Heat Ovens. A rapid high-temperature process that uses a forced-draft oven (a mechanical convection oven that circulates air with a fan or blower) is available. It reduces total sterilization time to 6 minutes for unwrapped and 12 minutes for wrapped instruments (Fig. 8-17) (Cox Manufacturing Corp. and Dentronics Corp.). These short-cycle high-temperature dry heat ovens operate at approximately 370° to 375° F. Chamber size of one brand is limited to processing about one set of instruments at a time, but is more effective for wrapped instruments and also may be adapted for a shorter heat disinfection cycle (consult the Cox Manufacturing Corp.).

Confirm that a sterilizer manufacturer has obtained premarket review by the FDA for their instrument sterilization device before purchasing a rapid dry heat sterilizer. Unfortunately, this requirement has not prevented some clinicians from adapting nonprofessional equipment for office use. Legal professionals have begun to anticipate how a jury may view use of home roasting ovens to sterilize professional treatment instruments. Moderately priced small ovens manufactured

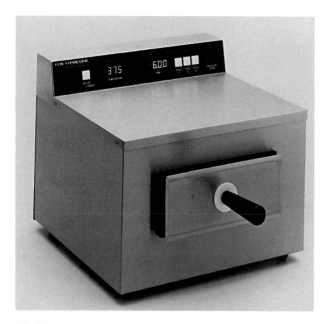

F I G. **8-17** Cox rapid heat transfer dry heat sterilizer. *(Courtesy of E.T.M. Corporation, Monrovia, Calif.)*

for industrial and scientific use by industrial manufacturers (e.g., Blue M Co., Blue Island, Illinois) are usually more accurate and reliable than ovens designed for home use. Careful calibration with a pyrometer to ensure that instruments reach and maintain sterilization temperatures is imperative. Once again, obtain evidence of FDA review of the equipment for instrument sterilization, or obtain legal advice before purchasing and using this type of oven for instrument sterilization.

Proper, weekly monitoring of all sterilizers, including dry heat ovens, is imperative. Some sterilization monitoring services now refuse to monitor sterilizers that do not have premarket review by the FDA.

Advantages of Dry Heat Sterilization. Carbon steel instruments and burs do not rust, corrode, or lose their temper or cutting edges if they are well dried before processing. Industrial forced-draft hot air ovens usually provide a larger capacity at a reasonable price. Rapid cycles are possible at high temperatures.

Disadvantages of Dry Heat Sterilization. High temperatures may damage more heat-sensitive items, such as rubber or plastic goods. Sterilization cycles are prolonged at the lower temperatures. Heavy loads of instruments, crowding of packs, and heavy wrapping easily defeat sterilization. Cycles are not automatically timed on some models. Inaccurate calibration, lack of attention to proper settings, and adding instruments without restarting the timing are other common sources of error.

ETHYLENE OXIDE STERILIZATION

Ethylene oxide sterilization is the best method for sterilizing complex instruments and delicate materials. However, you must verify that the sterilizer you plan to use

has a premarket review by the FDA in order to sterilize handpieces. Automatic devices sterilize items in several hours and operate at elevated temperatures well below 100° C. Less expensive devices operate overnight to produce sterilization at room temperature (Fig. 8-18). Both types meet OSHA requirements. Porous and plastic materials absorb the gas and require aeration for 24 hours or more before it is safe for them to contact skin or tissues. Units with large chamber sizes hold more instruments or packs per cycle; however, they are very expensive. Some chamber designs or sizes are better suited to accept stacks of instrument trays. Manufacturers should be consulted to obtain detailed information about these sterilizers. Consult IC texts or dental product distributors (e.g., Anderson Products Co., Haw River, North Carolina; 3M Co., Minneapolis, Minnesota).

BOILING WATER

Boiling water does not kill spores and cannot sterilize instruments. However, heat can reach and kill bloodborne pathogens in places that liquid sterilants and disinfectants used at room temperature cannot reach. Boiling is a method of high-level disinfection that has been used when actual sterilization cannot be achieved (e.g., in case of a sterilizer breakdown).[14] Well-cleaned items must be completely submerged and allowed to boil at 98° to 100° C (at sea level) for 10 minutes. *Great care must be exercised that instruments remain covered with boiling water the entire time.* Simple steaming is not reliable. Pressure cooking, similar to steam autoclaving, is preferred and would be required at high altitudes.

NEW METHODS OF STERILIZATION

Various new methods of sterilization are under investigation and development. The microwave oven has major limitations for sterilizing metal items, by either damaging the machine or not reaching all sides of the instruments. Research efforts to overcome such limitations are ongoing in industry. Ultraviolet light is not highly effective against RNA viruses such as HIV and is not very effective against bacterial spores.[109,114] Incomplete exposures of all surfaces and poor penetration of oil and debris are other limitations. Ultraviolet irradiation may be useful for sanitizing room air to help control tuberculosis bacteria.[26]

One valuable guide to whether a commercial device is an effective sterilizer rests upon whether the FDA can find it equivalent to other effective and proven devices now in common use. Before purchasing any medical device in question, require the manufacturer to provide documentation of FDA premarketing review.

MONITORS OF STERILIZATION

Sterilization assurance not only protects patients from cross-infections, but also protects personnel from the infections of previous patients as well. Effective instrument sterilization is assured by routine monitoring of instrument sterilization and has become a standard of care. Monitoring services are provided by most major schools.

In microbiology literature, *sterilization is defined as killing all forms of life, including the most heat-resistant forms, bacterial spores.* For instruments that can penetrate tissues, this provides control of spore-forming tetanus and gas gangrene species, as well as all pathogens borne by blood and secretions. For instrumentation used in body cavities that routinely touch mucosa, sterilization provides a margin of safety for assuring destruction of HB, mycobacteria, and other pathogenic bacteria and viruses that can become involved in cross-infections.

Weekly sterilization monitoring of highly efficient automated sterilizers in hospitals has been mandated for many years by the Joint Commission of Accreditation of Hospitals (Chicago, Illinois), an organization formed by the profession to monitor and accredit its own performance. Many state examining or disciplinary boards have now provided that type of regulation. Defense against litigation also has become a concern of professional liability insurers. Despite the high quality of large automated hospital sterilizers, most are monitored more frequently than those in dental offices.

In dental offices, sterilization must be monitored weekly with biologic spore tests using heat-resistant spores and tested daily with color-change process-indicator strips.[5,38] Documentation of routine monitoring in a daily-entry sterilization notebook allows confirmation of sterilizer operator performance, as well as the proper functioning of the equipment. Problems are identified and corrected. Evidence of sterilization assurance is also available when unavoidable localized or systemic posttreatment infections occur and instrument sterilization may be questioned. Sterilization monitoring has four components: (1) a sterilization indicator on the instrument bag, stamped with the date it is sterilized, (2) daily color-change process-indicator strips, (3) weekly biologic spore test, and (4) documentation notebook.

Sterilization Indicators and Date. Sterilization indicators, both tapes and bags, are marked with heat-sensitive dyes that change color easily upon exposure to heat or sterilization chemicals. Such heat-sensitive markers are important to identify and differentiate those packs that have been in the sterilizer from those that have not. Used alone, these indicators are not an adequate measure of sterilization conditions. Sterilization is task-dependent as much as time- and temperature-dependent. Always date the packs and rotate. If not used, packs need to be sterilized again in 1, 6, or 12 months, depending on the type of wrap and manufacturer's claims. Ask manufacturers of indicators and instrument packaging materials for data on their products.

Process Indicator Strips. Process indicator strips provide an inexpensive, qualitative, daily monitor of steril-

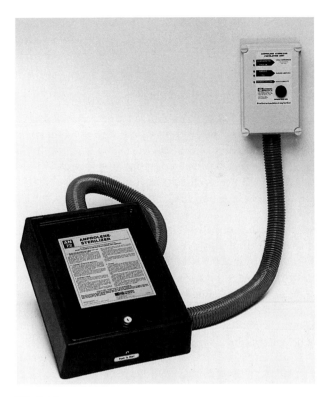

FIG. **8-18** Room temperature ethylene oxide sterilizer. *(Courtesy of Anderson Products Company, Burlington, NC.)*

izer function, operation, and heat penetration into packs. Place one of the inexpensive color-change process indicator strips into every surgical pack and in at least one operative instrument pack in the center of each load. Chemicals on the strip change color slowly, somewhat relative to the temperature reached in the pack. As soon as the pack is opened, the strip can immediately identify breakdowns and gross overloading. The strip is not an accurate measure of sterilization time and temperature exposure.

Biologic Monitoring Strips. A biologic monitoring spore test strip is the accepted weekly monitor of adequate time and temperature exposure. Spores dried on absorbent paper strips are calibrated to be killed when sterilization conditions are reached and maintained for the necessary time to kill all pathogenic microorganisms. An assistant processes a spore strip in a pack of instruments in an office sterilizer each week. Tests can be evaluated in the office. However, by sending the strip to a licensed reference laboratory for testing, the dentist obtains independent documentation of monitoring frequency and sterilization effectiveness. In the event of failure, such laboratory personnel provide immediate expert consultation to help resolve the problem.

Documentation Notebook. In a notebook, affix a single dated, initialed, indicator strip to a sheet or calendar for each workday, followed by a weekly spore strip report. The notebook provides valuable sterilization documentation. Dated sterilized instrument packs, bags, and trays provide the final evidence of the sterilization program.

LIQUID STERILANTS AND HIGH-LEVEL DISINFECTANTS

Liquid sterilants are those that can kill bacterial spores in 6 to 10 hours. These sterilants are high-level disinfectants and are EPA registered. Sterilants used for high-level disinfection of items for reuse are glutaraldehydes at 2% to 3% concentrations. Greater dilutions are not encouraged for repeated use.

Organic matter and oxidation reduce activity of reused disinfectant baths. Placing wet items into disinfectant trays dilutes the solution. The level does not change because solution is carried out when the instruments are removed. Despite reuse claims of several weeks' duration, studies have shown that disinfectants in heavy use often lost activity during the second week.[105] Therefore it is wise to place fresh disinfectant into trays on Monday, and discard it at the end of Friday.

Glutaraldehydes are irritating, sensitizing to skin and respiratory passages, and can be toxic as indicated in manufacturers' safety data sheets.[57] Keep trays tightly covered in a well-vented area. Do not use 2% or greater glutaraldehyde solutions to wipe counters or equipment (e.g., dental unit and chair). Most glutaraldehydes require 20 minutes to kill tuberculosis bacteria in contrast with some synthetic phenol complexes and alcohols that act in 10 minutes or less and are much less toxic.

Uses of High-Level Disinfection. According to the CDC, instruments that penetrate tissues or contact mucosa are termed *critical* or *semicritical* and require cleaning and heat or gas sterilization before reuse.[31,38,57] Few, if any, instruments now exist that cannot be heat sterilized. High-level disinfection is used mainly for plastic items that enter the mouth and that cannot withstand heat sterilization. Plastic cheek retractors, photographic mirrors, and similar heat-sensitive devices should be replaced with metal types that can be heat sterilized. Disinfection for 20 to 90 minutes in glutaraldehyde germicides is not appropriate for instruments used in the mouth. Most require 6 or more hours for sterilization. Liquid sterilants cannot process prepackaged instruments or be completely monitored with biologic indicators.

Prophy cups should be discarded and never disinfected for reuse. Used anesthesia carpules and anesthesia needles must be discarded after a patient appointment and never be disinfected or heat sterilized for reuse.

TYPES OF INSTRUMENTS AND STERILIZATION METHODS

Periodontal, restorative, and endodontic instruments are readily processed by autoclave or chemical vapor pressure sterilization. Carbon steel instruments and burs, if dried well before sterilizing, are best sterilized by dry heat and chemical vapor pressure sterilizers because these methods reduce the risk of rust.

DENTAL CONTROL UNIT WATER SYSTEMS AND HANDPIECE ASEPSIS

The high-speed handpiece is one component of a complex system of instrumentation operated by the dental operatory master control unit. Within the head of the handpiece and supported by delicate bearings, a turbine assembly holds and rotates the cutting instrument at the speeds preferred for tooth preparation. The handpiece is attached by flexible plastic lines to the dental unit that controls air and water supplied to the handpiece. A small orifice located below the neck of the handpiece near the bur supplies either a jet of air to blow away cutting debris or an air-water spray emitted from the same orifice to lubricate and clean the cutting site; this spray cools the cutting bur as well.

These components comprise a complex system that is vulnerable to several unique kinds of contamination by and through the handpiece. Oral fluid contamination problems of rotary equipment and especially the high-speed handpiece involve: (1) contamination of handpiece external surfaces and crevices, (2) turbine chamber contamination that enters the mouth, (3) water spray retraction and aspiration of oral fluids into the water lines of older dental units, (4) growth of environmental aquatic bacteria in water lines, and (5) exposure of personnel to spatter and aerosols generated by intraoral use of rotary equipment.[1,12,50,52,70]

If not controlled, external and internal contamination of this equipment by oral fluids holds infection potentials for dental patients. Even sterilization of handpieces cannot control contamination related to water spray retraction and bacterial colonization of water lines that holds infection potentials for immunocompromised patients.

HANDPIECE SURFACE CONTAMINATION CONTROL

Blood and saliva contaminate the surfaces of handpieces during various dental treatments. Irregular surfaces and especially crevices around the bur chuck are difficult to clean and disinfect, especially by a brief wipe with a disinfectant-soaked sponge.

Submersion of a high-speed handpiece in a high-level disinfectant has not been an option accepted by manufacturers. In tests, thorough scrubbing and applying the best disinfectants to inoculated smooth handpiece surfaces reduced numbers of simple test bacteria but did not completely eliminate them.[102] *Only sterilization can approach complete IC of handpiece surfaces.*

TURBINE CONTAMINATION CONTROL

Contaminated oral fluids may be drawn back into the turbine chamber by negative pressure created either by a

Venturi effect during operation or when the turbine continues to spin whenever the drive air is stopped. Oral fluids also may enter around worn bearing seals, or be aspirated into the vent holes in the top of older hand-chuck operated handpieces or possibly into the air-water spray orifice that communicates with the turbine chamber in some handpieces. The question is whether debris that contains viable microbes in the turbine chamber may then be vented from holes in the top of the turbine chamber during the next treatment, as indicated by some investigators.[51,79,80]

Although turbine contamination can be demonstrated experimentally under extreme conditions on a laboratory bench, it is not clear under what conditions this may occur during clinical treatments, nor have air-driven high-speed handpieces been clearly implicated in this manner of cross-infection. Cross-contamination potentials of water-driven handpieces that have been used in a hospital have been demonstrated more easily.[53]

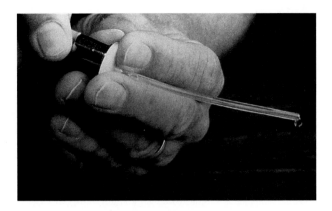

FIG. **8-19** This device is used to detect retraction of water supplied to the high-speed handpiece by older units when the foot control is released. If water moves back into the plastic tube, a new check valve is needed in the handpiece waterline to prevent retraction of oral fluids during treatments. *(Courtesy of A-DEC, Inc. Newberg, Ore.)*

WATER RETRACTION SYSTEM CORRECTION

Dental unit water control systems made before the mid- to late 1980s used water lines that easily expanded when air-water spray was used and gradually contracted when water pressure was relieved. Handpieces had an annoying tendency to continue to drip immediately after having been used. To overcome the problem in those units, a device was installed that retracted water in the line whenever the spray was stopped. Unfortunately, more than just water could be retracted. Following use, oral bacteria have been readily recovered from water samples obtained from the handpieces and water lines of those older dental units.[10,51]

Agencies recommend correcting water retraction by placing a one-way check valve in the water line.[31,45,47] Unfortunately check valves clog and fail. Systems should be tested monthly if not weekly to verify lack of water retraction.[52] A simple, inexpensive water retraction testing device is available from major dental supply companies that takes only approximately 1 minute to use (Fig. 8-19).[51]

The industry also has responded to correct the retraction problem. Since 1988, nearly all manufacturers have manufactured dental control units that simply cut off the water spray without retraction. The best solution for older dental control units, unless the units can be overhauled, is to replace them with newer units that do not retract.[38,51,52]

INHERENT WATER SYSTEM CONTAMINATION

Microbes exist in the dental unit waterline as free-floating bacteria and as a sessile form known as *biofilm*. The microorganisms in the biofilm produce a protective polysaccharide matrix that provides them a mechanism for surface attachment and retention to the waterline.[11,127] This matrix, which can be 30 to 50 μm thick, af-fords the biofilm flora resistance to antimicrobial agents on the order of 1500 times greater than normal free-floating bacteria. Because of this resistance to antimicrobial agents, once the biofilm is established, it is very difficult to remove.

Bacterial growth in biofilms on the inner walls of dental unit water lines is a universal occurrence unless steps are taken to control it.[11] Counts of bacteria that are shed from the biofilms into water of the dental unit may range from thousands to hundreds of thousands of bacteria per milliliter.[1,13,84,110] This bioload could be compared with bacterial counts of some foods (e.g., juices, milk, yogurt) except that the bacterial types present are not carefully controlled. The main inhabitants are opportunistic, gram-negative, aquaphilic bacteria. Similar species are found in biofilms that form in swimming pools or wherever nonsterile water remains in prolonged contact with habitable surfaces. The bacteria may include atypical *Mycobacteria*, *Pseudomonas*, and possibly *Legionella* bacteria, which can present an infection risk to immunocompromised persons.[67,83,101,104] Flushing or sterilizing high-speed handpieces cannot be expected to overcome this potential source of contamination of patients and personnel that extends throughout the dental unit water system.

The public health threat of biofilm in dental unit waterlines has not been established. However, as the characteristics of the population changes, the link between biofilm bacteria and infection may be verified. The ADA recommended that IC measures be established and followed such that dental unit treatments would contain less than 200 colony-forming units (cfu) per milliliter of bacteria by the year 2000.[111] Suggested mechanisms to accomplish this goal of 200 cfu/ml include use of microbial point-of-use filters and independent water systems. The uses of biocide solutions to treat the waterlines

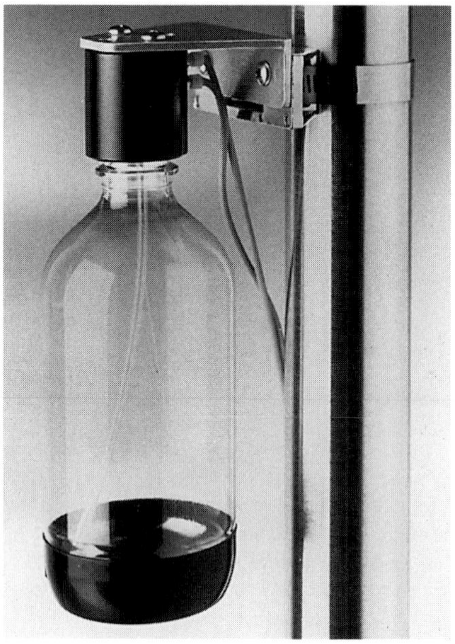

FIG. 8-20 A water reservoir can provide uncontaminated water to the syringe and to cool the high-speed bur if the reservoir and waterlines downstream are disinfected regularly. *(Courtesy of A-DEC, Inc., Newberg, Ore.)*

overnight and as a continuous addition to the treatment water also have been investigated.[127]

Although much work is currently being done in the area of the biofilm and dental unit water line contamination, one has to be careful in selecting which system to use to control the biofilm. Clean water reservoir systems combined with disinfection or sterilization of equipment downstream have been developed by several companies (Fig. 8-20).[77,84]

Disinfectants, such as an iodophore or diluted sodium hypochlorite, used to clean the system must then be flushed out of the system with clean, boiled, or sterile water before use. Always remove the handpiece before disinfecting the system because 0.5% sodium hypochlorite solution and other strong chemicals will damage the high-speed handpiece and other metal products. Very dilute biocides that are used continuously in the treatment water must be thoroughly researched because some of them can decrease composite bond strengths to enamel and dentin.[106,118] As stated earlier, once the biofilm is generated, it can be difficult to remove. Therefore, educating dental personnel and periodically monitoring compliance with procedures is paramount for the success in preventing dental unit waterline contamination.[11]

CONTROL OF CONTAMINATION FROM SPATTER AND AEROSOL

Concerns regarding contamination from spatter and aerosol created by rotary equipment are valid. Operating this equipment in the mouths of patients spatters oral fluids and microorganisms onto the attending clinical personnel, and aerosols can readily be inhaled. Aero-

solization of mycobacteria that cause pulmonary tuberculosis (*Mycobacterium tuberculosis*) has always been a concern, although an infectious patient coughing in the waiting room or operatory is clearly much more likely to infect others.[26] *Annual tuberculin testing of personnel has been a standard IC recommendation in dentistry.* There is also concern about nosocomial airborne transmission of multidrug-resistant strains of mycobacteria that have exhibited an 85% infection rate and have been lethal for 75% of infected immunocompromised persons in 16 weeks.[22,26] This poses a concern for health of dental personnel as well.

The rubber dam and high-volume evacuation (HVE) are very important and helpful methods for reducing exposure to contamination[42,90] (see Chapter 10). HVE can be up to 80% effective in reducing aerosol contamination. However, there is no way to completely eliminate airborne contamination, unless some method of continuous air purification can be used. Without the universal use of personal barriers, drapes, and/or effective cleanup procedures, personnel, and subsequent patients can be subjected to oral fluid-borne contamination.

STERILIZATION OF HANDPIECES AND RELATED ROTARY EQUIPMENT

Prophy angles, latch angles, burs, and rotary stones used in the mouth must be cleaned and sterilized for reuse. All such items are readily sterilized by three or more methods of sterilization. Carbon steel burs require special protection in the autoclave (see Sterilization of Burs in Autoclave). Handpieces are semicritical instrumentation requiring sterilization.[5,38] Few brands now exist on the market that cannot be routinely autoclaved. *Sterilization of handpieces must be monitored and documented.* The motor end of the attached low-speed handpiece can be covered by pulling a disposable, single use, slender plastic bag up over it and pushing (popping) the handpiece through the sealed end of the bag so the bag covers the motor end and part of the hose (see Fig. 8-9). Otherwise scrub and disinfect the motor-end for each reuse if it cannot be sterilized.

STEAM STERILIZATION OF HANDPIECES

Autoclave sterilization of handpieces is one of the most rapid methods. If proper cleaning and lubricating is performed as prescribed by the manufacturer, good utility is obtainable with regular autoclaving. Fiber optics dim with repeated heat sterilization in a number of months to a year, apparently due to oil residue and debris baked on the ends of the optical fibers. Cleaning with detergent solution and wiping ends of optics with alcohol or other suitable organic solvents may prolong use before factory servicing. Manufacturers are improving methods of preparing handpieces for sterilization. Consult the manufacturer's for current advice and warnings.

Procedures for Handpieces With a Metal-Bearing Turbine. Scrub metal-bearing high-speed handpieces and the sheath or cone of the low-speed straight handpiece at the sink with running water and detergent. See manufacturer's directions for further cleaning and lubrication before and after sterilization. Bag the handpiece and sheath and autoclave them. *Note: when first operating a freshly lubricated handpiece, keep it in a plastic bag or the sterilization bag to avoid breathing the vaporized lubricant.*

Procedure for Handpieces With a "Lube-Free" Ceramic-Bearing Turbine. Follow manufacturer's directions for cleaning high-speed handpieces with lubrication-free ceramic-bearing turbine (Den-Tal-Ez, Inc., Lancaster, Pennsylvania). For this type of handpiece, avoid using chemicals that will damage internal parts. Consult manufacturer's most current directions supplied with each handpiece for preparation of handpieces for sterilization. Attention to directions on cleaning fiber optics at both ends of the handpiece (e.g., with isopropyl alcohol) will prolong service life. Bag and autoclave the handpiece.

OTHER METHODS OF HANDPIECE STERILIZATION

Chemical vapor pressure sterilization recommended for some types of handpieces apparently works well with ceramic-bearing handpieces, yet may impair others. Always obtain the handpiece manufacturer's recommendations.

Ethylene oxide (ETOX) gas is the gentlest method of sterilization used for handpieces. Internal and external cleaning are important. Otherwise, preparation of handpieces before sterilization is not as critical because no heat is involved. In some types of ETOX sterilizers, gas appears to penetrate high-speed handpieces. However, oil left in handpieces can impair sterilization. Be sure to confirm with the manufacturer that the sterilizer has premarket review and approval from the FDA for sterilizing handpieces.

ETOX processing takes the handpiece out of circulation for several hours or overnight. Some practitioners have purchased enough low-cost handpieces to treat their maximum number of patients seen per day, and use overnight ETOX sterilization. This approach may be effective with adequate handpiece cleaning and disassembly. However, the FDA may not agree with use of certain types of ETOX sterilizers for sterilizing handpieces. Further research on the effectiveness and any limitations of ETOX handpiece sterilization still may be needed. (Consult the manufacturer or Anderson Products, Haw River, North Carolina.)

Dry heat sterilization of handpieces is generally not recommended. A rapid, high-temperature, dry heat disinfection process was under evaluation for handpieces. Check with the handpiece manufacturer and the sterilizer manufacturer (Cox Sterilizer Co.) regarding use of this process and obtain information regarding FDA review from the manufacturer.

INFECTION CONTROL FOR IMPRESSIONS AND RELATED REGISTRATIONS

FACTORS IN MAKING IMPRESSIONS AND ASSOCIATED REGISTRATIONS THAT WILL BE SENT TO A REMOTE LABORATORY

Precautions are required for IC in making impressions and associated bite registrations, just as for other operative procedures. Universally apply barrier protection for personnel against contamination from mucosa, saliva, and blood by use of adequate PPE, such as gloves, mask, and appropriate overgarment.

To eliminate any chance of cross-contamination when sizing impression trays, place the tray in a plastic baggy before it is tried in the mouth. After the appropriate size has been determined, remove the baggy and proceed with impression making. Indicate the tray size on the patient's chart to eliminate further try-ins.

For IC, custom resin trays for impressions made with nonaqueous rubber impression materials are used once and then discarded. Likewise, stock trays are used only once and discarded.

Before making the impression and associated bite registrations, use clean, gloved hands to dispense as many materials and disposable items as possible. This avoids contaminating their containers. Whenever possible, use unit dose packaged materials, or use a paper towel or plastic film to handle tubes and other reused containers. Least satisfactory, but adequate, is wiping material containers with a disinfectant after the procedures. A satisfactory disinfectant should be an EPA-approved tuberculocidal disinfectant.

CONCEPTS FOR TRANSPORTING IMPRESSIONS AND ASSOCIATED REGISTRATIONS TO A REMOTE LABORATORY

For transport to a remote laboratory, impressions and associated bite registrations are regulated by OSHA's specifications for handling and transporting specimens of blood or other potentially infectious materials (OPIM) such as blood-contaminated saliva: "Potentially infectious materials shall be placed in a container which prevents leakage during collection, handling, processing, storage, transport, or shipping (to the laboratory). Labeling or color coding is required when such specimens/containers leave the facility."[95]

Controversy exists over two choices that may be used for preparing a potentially infectious item for transport: (1) send it well cleaned (rinsed) and undisinfected in a biohazard-labeled, heat-sealed, plastic bag; or (2) débride, clean (rinse), and adequately disinfect it, place it in a sealed transport bag labeled with the precautions taken, and assume responsibility for the aseptic condition of the item. In either case, most laboratories will disinfect the item (a second time in the second choice) to ensure protection of laboratory personnel. Disinfecting twice is time wasted, and multiple exposures to disinfectant should be avoided.[85] The simplest and best approach may be the first. It avoids confusion over whether the item (e.g., an impression) is properly disinfected in the office, saves office time and materials for disinfection, and removes office liability. Special labeling of the item regarding potential contamination is not necessary (except for always having the OSHA biohazard label) if no item is disinfected and every item is assumed infected (thus satisfying the concept of universal precautions). This was the choice adopted in 1992 by the Washington State Department of Health Dental Disciplinary Board.[124] Satisfactory labeling requires that the prescription include the type of impression material. The National Association of Dental Laboratories recommends disinfecting all items received from the dental office and disinfecting all appliances before shipping them from the laboratory.[94]

Inexpensive, biohazard-labeled, heat-sealable bags are commercially available in various sizes made of sturdy clear plastic, and they are stamped with warnings to transporters and personnel (e.g., Seal-A-Case, Infection Control Services, Inc., P. O. Box 1389, Kent, WA 98035) (Fig. 8-21). The U.S. Postal Service also has specifications for double, leak-proof packaging and external labeling of such packaging if contaminated items must be sent by the U.S. Postal Service. Similar bags also are available for returning finished items to the office. They have no biohazard labels, but provide stamped instructions in green lettering advising office personnel that the contents are precleaned and disinfected, and to handle the enclosed items appropriately for delivery to the patient (Fig. 8-22). Generic, heat-sealable bags are available but must be appropriately labeled.

Procedures for Handling and Transporting Silicone (Vinyl Polysiloxane) or Rubber-Based Impression Material and Any Associated Registrations to a Remote Laboratory.

IC procedures regarding the nonaqueous rubber impression and any associated registration are as follows:

1. Before the patient appointment, prepare one or more industrially clean, strong, clear, heat-sealable, biohazard-labeled plastic bag(s) of appropriate size, one for containing the scheduled impression and a separate one for any associated interocclusal registration. (Do not place any other item along with an impression in a bag to prevent the possibility of pressure-deformation of the impression caused by the additional item). Place each bag into an open canister of suitable size so that the bag's open end extends above

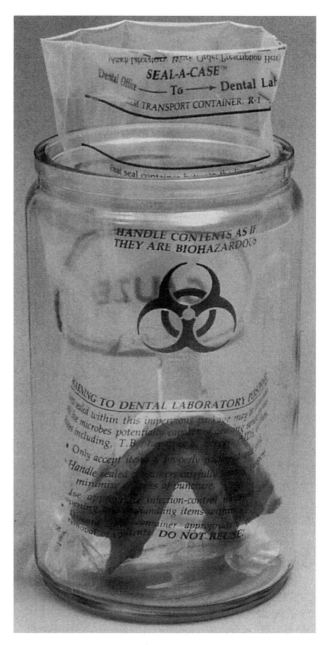

FIG. 8-21 The dentist or dental assistant prepares a potentially infectious impression for transport (to remote laboratory or to on-site laboratory) by rinsing the impression and then placing it in a biohazard-labeled plastic bag without contaminating the bag's outer surface.

the rim of the supporting canister, allowing a slight folding downward and outward of the bag's open edge. This helps keep it open and also prevents contamination of the bag's outer surface during insertion of the item.

2. Remove the impression, interocclusal registration, or device from the mouth, and while still wearing barriers (gowns, gloves, and so on) remove any attached debris and rinse the item well with running tap water for 15 seconds to remove saliva and blood.

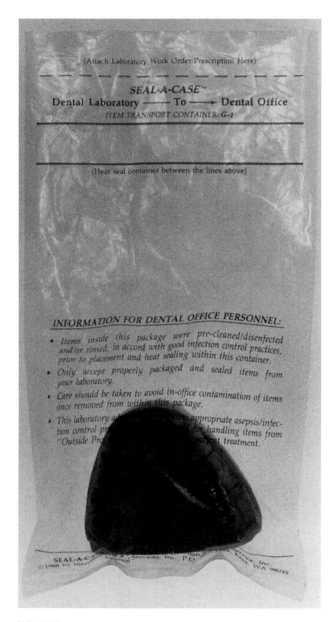

(Attach Laboratory Work Order/Prescription Here)

SEAL-A-CASE™
Dental Laboratory —— To —→ Dental Office
ITEM TRANSPORT CONTAINER: G-1

(Heat seal container between the lines above)

INFORMATION FOR DENTAL OFFICE PERSONNEL:

- *Items inside this package were pre-cleaned/disinfected and/or rinsed, in accord with good infection control practices, prior to placement and heat sealing within this container.*
- *Only accept properly packaged and sealed items from your laboratory.*
- *Care should be taken to avoid in-office contamination of items once removed from within this package.*
- *This laboratory o_____ _____ appropriate asepsis/infection control pr_____ _____ handling items from "Outside Pr_____ _____ __t treatment.*

SEAL-A-C___ ____ Services, Inc., P.O. ____on, ____ce, Inc.
©1988 by Tolo_____ _____, WA 98035

FIG. 8-22 The laboratory disinfects appliance and then transports it in a heat-sealed bag to the dentist.

3. After rinsing, and while still wearing barriers, place the impression (or other item) into the designated, prepared bag without touching the bag's outer surface.
4. Now, remove the gloves because they are contaminated. With clean hands, close the bag while touching only the bag's clean outer surface, and heat-seal it.
5. Tape the prescription to the bag.
6. Attach a note or use a bag appropriately lettered to alert the laboratory that the item(s) in the bag was (were) débrided and rinsed, but not disinfected. Communication with laboratory personnel also can state that this is how any item will be sent unless the labo-

ratory has different requirements. Place the bag(s) into a suitable box and send it to the remote laboratory. Laboratory personnel will proceed with disinfecting the items sent. Treat all potentially infectious items alike. Laboratory precautions and disinfection should be the same whether a patient has an infection or not. Only if a laboratory person has an exposure incident should the patient's history become important.

If the nonaqueous rubber impression is to be poured in the dental office, the impression must be disinfected before the cast is formed.

Procedures for Handling and Transporting Items From an Aqueous Impression Material Technique (Using Alginate [Irreversible Hydrocolloid], Reversible Hydrocolloid, or Polyether Impressions) and Any Associated Registrations to a Remote Laboratory. If the aqueous impression is to be poured in-office and the resultant cast and associated items transported to a remote laboratory, IC procedures are as follows:

1. Thoroughly rinse the impression under tap water (15 seconds recommended) to remove any saliva or blood. Handle the impression carefully to prevent distortion.
2. Disinfect the impression by spraying until thoroughly soaked with a hospital level disinfectant. The product with the shortest contact time allows less distortion. An acceptable alternative is to follow the manufacturer's recommendation for a particular disinfectant.
3. With clean hands, thoroughly rinse the disinfected impression under tap water to avoid prolonged exposure to the disinfectant and because any residual disinfectant can adversely affect surface hardness of the stone cast.
4. Shake excess water from the impression and pour the cast immediately. One reversible hydrocolloid manufacturer (Van R, 600 E. Hueneme Rd., Oxnard, CA 93033) offers two alternatives to immediate pouring of the impression after disinfection: (1) submerge the impression into a 2% potassium sulfate solution for (up to) 20 minutes, and then remove, shake off excess, and pour the impression; (2) place the impression into a humidor (for up to 4 hours with no temperature change), remove, submerge into the 2% potassium sulfate solution for 20 minutes, remove, shake-off excess, and pour the impression. (To make the potassium sulfate solution, Van R supplies the crystals and instructs the user to dissolve one capful of crystals to 1 pint of water.)
5. The cast from a disinfected impression does not need disinfecting.
6. Carefully package the cast for shipment to the remote laboratory; associated items (such as an interocclusal registration) that are from the mouth, must be rinsed, disinfected, and then rinsed again. These may then

be shipped along with the cast, but packaged to avoid harming it. Include also a written note stating that the impression and associated registration were disinfected and that the cast should not be subjected to a disinfection procedure that might compromise accuracy.

If the dentist desires to utilize a nearby commercial laboratory (having expeditious courier service) for pickup of the aqueous impression and associated items, and for the disinfection and subsequent handling of these items, the IC procedures described in the previous section should be followed.

PROCEDURES FOR HANDLING IMPRESSIONS AND ASSOCIATED REGISTRATIONS FOR AN ON-SITE LABORATORY

Laboratory personnel are required to wear a clean uniform or laboratory jacket, coat, or gown, and the dentist supplies these. Disposable mask, protective eyewear, and protective gloves also are supplied, and their use is required when there is potential for exposure to dust or spatter.

Convey impressions and associated items removed from the mouth to the on-site laboratory technician using the same procedures described in the previous section (for transport to a remote laboratory). These procedures should maintain the outside surfaces of the bag in an uncontaminated condition, as well as protect the contents from accidental spillage.

Additional IC measures for handling these items in the on-site laboratory are as follows:

1. A designated area must be available to receive the items. Personnel receiving them must wear disposable treatment gloves.
2. All incoming items to the dental laboratory must be properly labeled. With gloved hands, disinfect impressions (and associated registrations) by submerging (for 10 minutes) in 1:10 dilution (0.5%) of household liquid chlorine bleach (5.25% sodium hypochlorite) prepared fresh daily, or other accepted tuberculocidal disinfectant. As long as blood is not visible, containers can then be discarded in regular trash.
3. With gloved hands, spray articulators and any related equipment that have been contaminated, and which cannot be sterilized, with an alcohol disinfectant (see Operatory Asepsis) because chlorine in the hypochlorite-type disinfectant may damage the metal.
4. With clean hands, thoroughly rinse the impression under tap water (15 seconds) to remove any residual disinfectant, and follow manufacturer's directions for any additional procedures for treating the impression and forming the cast.
5. All outgoing items must be properly cleaned and placed in a leakproof bag or appropriate container before leaving the laboratory.
6. Contaminated countertops and work surfaces must be cleaned of debris and disinfected daily. After cleaning, spray surfaces with disinfectant, wipe dry with paper towels, and respray with disinfectant. Leave surfaces wet.

When repairing or polishing intraoral appliances, do not use the same pumice for new work and repair work. For repairs, wear protective gloves. Premeasure pumice in small amounts (e.g., on small disposable paper or plastic trays); discard after use. Wet pumice with a mixture of green soap and a disinfectant. *Do not use water only.* After using pumice in a repair, disinfect the appliance again for 10 minutes. Disinfect model trimmers and pumice pans at the end of the day.[108] Maintain an adequate supply of wheels for repairs so they can be sterilized with steam in an autoclave before reuse. Disinfectants cannot be expected to adequately prepare them for safe reuse.[38,57,86,94]

SUMMARY AND OTHER INFORMATION SOURCES

It is not possible in one chapter, even as comprehensive as this, to provide all the detail on disease updates, tests, vaccines, barriers, SOPs, sterilization methods, and equipment. IC and auxiliary persons are referred to other more detailed literature and texts in the reference list, and are advised to attend continuing education programs to expand and update their IC information.[5,38,39,48,89,129]

REFERENCES

1. Abel LC et al: Studies on dental aerobiology. IV: Bacterial contamination of water delivered by dental units, *J Dent Res* 50:1567-1569, 1971.
2. Ahtone J, Goodman RA: Hepatitis B and dental personnel: transmission to patients and prevention issues, *J Am Dent Assoc* 106(2):219-222, 1983.
3. Allain J-P et al: Long-term evaluation of HIV antigen and antibodies to p 24 and p 41 in patients with hemophilia, *N Engl J Med* 317:1114-1121, 1987.
4. Allen A, Bryan R: Occult blood accumulation under fingernails, *J Am Dent Assoc* 105:358-362, Sept 1982.
5. American Dental Association: Infection control for the dental office and dental laboratory, *J Am Dent Assoc* 123(suppl): 1-8, Aug 1992.
6. American Dental Association: Facts about AIDS for the dental team, ed 3, *J Am Dent Assoc* 119(suppl):1-9, July 1991.
7. Association of Dental Schools: Recommended clinical guidelines for infection control in dental education institutions, *J Dent Educ* 55:621-630, 1991.
8. Association of Dental Schools: Curriculum guidelines for the dental care management of patients with bloodborne infectious diseases, *J Dent Educ* 55:609-619, 1991.
9. Autio KK et al: Studies on cross-contamination in the dental office, *J Am Dent Assoc* 100 (3):358-361, 1980.

10. Bagga BSR et al: Contamination of dental unit cooling water with oral microorganisms and its prevention, *J Am Dent Assoc* 109:712-716, 1984.

11. Bednarsh HS, Eklunk KJ, Mills S: Check your dental unit water IQ, *Dent Assist* 5-8, Jan-Feb 1997.

12. Bentley CD, Burkhart NW, Crawford JJ: Evaluating spatter and aerosol contamination during dental procedures, *J Am Dent Assoc* 125:579-584, May 1994.

13. Blake GC: The incidence and control of bacterial infection in dental spray reservoirs, *Br Dent J* 115:413-416, 1963.

14. Bond WW et al: Effective use of liquid chemical germicides on medical instruments: instrument design problems. In Block SS, editor: *Disinfection, sterilization, and preservation,* ed 4, Philadelphia, 1991, Lea & Febiger.

15. Bond WW et al: Inactivation of hepatitis B by intermediate to high-level disinfectant chemicals, *J Clin Microbiol* 18: 535-538, 1983.

16. Bond WW et al: Survival of hepatitis B virus after drying and storage for one week, *Lancet* 7:550-551, March 1981.

17. Burkhart NW, Crawford JJ: Critical steps after cleaning: removing debris after sonication, *J Am Dent Assoc* 128: 456-463, 1997.

18. Centers for Disease Control: *HIV/AIDS Surveillance Report* 10(2):26, 1998.

19. Centers For Disease Control: Recommendations for prevention and control of hepatitis C virus (HCV) Infection and HCV-related chronic disease, *MMWR Morbid Mortal Wkly Rep* 47(No. RR-19):1-39, 1998.

20. Centers for Disease Control: Public health service guidelines for the management of health-care worker exposures to HIV and recommendations for postexposure prophylaxis, *MMWR Morbid Mortal Wkly Rep* 47(No. RR-7):1-34, 1998.

21. Centers for Disease Control: Surveillance for occupationally acquired HIV infection—United States, 1981-1982, *MMWR Morbid Mortal Wkly Rep* 41(No. 43):823-825, 1992.

22. Centers for Disease Control: Nosocomial transmission of multidrug-resistant tuberculosis among HIV-infected persons—Florida and New York, 1988-1991. *MMWR Morbid Mortal Wkly Rep* 40:585-591, 1991.

23. Centers for Disease Control: Recommendations for preventing transmission of human immunodeficiency virus and hepatitis B virus to patients during exposure prone invasive procedures, *MMWR Morbid Mortal Wkly Rep* 40(RR-8):1-9, 1991.

24. Centers for Disease Control: Update: acquired immunodeficiency syndrome, United States, 1981-1991, *MMWR Morbid Mortal Wkly Rep* 40(No. 22):358-368, 1991.

25. Centers for Disease Control: Update: transmission of HIV infection during invasive dental procedure—Florida, *MMWR Morbid Mortal Wkly Rep* 40(No.2):21-28, 1991.

26. Centers for Disease Control: Guidelines for preventing transmission of tuberculosis in health-care settings, with special focus on HIV-related issues, *MMWR Morbid Mortal Wkly Rep* 39(RR17):1-29, 1990.

27. Centers for Disease Control: Measles—United States, 1990, *MMWR Morbid Mortal Wkly Rep* 40(No. 22):369-372, 1990.

28. Centers for Disease Control: Guidelines for prevention of transmission of HIV and HBV to health care and public safety workers, *MMWR Morbid Mortal Wkly Rep* 38(No. S-6), 1989.

29. Centers for Disease Control: Update: Universal precautions for prevention of transmission of human immunodeficiency virus, hepatitis B virus, and other bloodborne pathogens in health-care settings, *MMWR Morbid Mortal Wkly Rep* 37: 377-387, 1988.

30. Centers for Disease Control: Recommendations for prevention of HIV transmission in health-care settings, *MMWR Morbid Mortal Wkly Rep* 36(suppl 2S):1S-18S, 1987.

31. Centers for Disease Control: Recommended infection-control practices for dentistry, *MMWR Morbid Mortal Wkly Rep* 35(No. 15):237-242, 1986.

32. Centers for Disease Control: Measles on a college campus—Ohio, *MMWR Morbid Mortal Wkly Rep* 34(7):89-90, 1985.

33. Centers for Disease Control, Immunization Practices Advisory Committee: Recommendation of the Immunization Practices Advisory Committee: Protection against viral hepatitis, *MMWR Morbid Mortal Wkly Rep* 39(No. S-2):1-26, 1990.

34. Centers for Disease Control, Immunization Practices Advisory Committee: Measles prevention: recommendations of the Immunologic Practices Committee, *MMWR Morbid Mortal Wkly Rep* 38:(S-9), 1989.

35. Centers for Disease Control, Immunization Practices Advisory Committee: Recommendations for protection against viral hepatitis, *MMWR Morbid Mortal Wkly Rep* 34 (22):314, 1985.

36. Centers for Disease Control, Immunization Practices Advisory Committee: Inactivated hepatitis B virus vaccine, *MMWR Morbid Mortal Wkly Rep* 31:317-328, 1982.

37. Centers for Disease Control and Prevention: Update: investigations of persons treated by HIV-infected health-care workers—United States, *MMWR Morbid Mortal Wkly Rep* 42(No. 17):329-337, 1993.

38. Centers for Disease Control and Prevention: Update: recommended infection-control practices for dentistry, *MMWR Morbid Mortal Wkly Rep* 142(No. RR-8):1-12, 1993.

39. Christensen RP: Ultrasonic cleaning equipment, *Clin Res Assoc Newsletter* 13(No. 8):1-3, Aug 1989.

40. Christensen RP et al: Efficiency of 42 brands of face masks and two face shields in preventing inhalation of airborne debris, *Gen Dent* 39:414-421, 1991.

41. Christensen RP et al: Antimicrobial activity of environmental surface disinfectants in the absence and presence of bioburden, *J Am Dent Assoc* 119:493-504, 1989.

42. Cochran MA, Miller CH, Sheldrake MA: The efficiency of the rubber dam as a barrier to the spread of microorganisms during dental treatment, *J Am Dent Assoc* 119:141-144, 1989.

43. Cottone JA: Recent developments in hepatitis: new virus, vaccine and dosage recommendations, *J Am Dent Assoc* 120: 501-508, 1990.

44. Cottone JA, Terezhalmy GT, Molinari JA, editors: *Practical infection control in dentistry*. Philadelphia, 1991, Lea & Febiger.

45. Council on Dental Materials, Instruments and Devices, American Dental Association: Dental units and water retraction, *J Am Dent Assoc* 116:417-420, 1988.

46. Council on Dental Therapeutics, Council on Dental Materials Instruments and Equipment, American Dental Association: *Monograph series on dental materials and therapeutics: safety and infection control in the dental office,* Chicago, 1990, American Dental Association.

47. Council on Dental Therapeutics, Council on Dental Practice, Council on Dental Materials Instruments and Equipment, American Dental Association: Infection control recommendations for the dental office and dental laboratory, *J Am Dent Assoc* 116:241-248, 1988.

48. Crawford JJ: *Clinical asepsis in dentistry: regulations, infection control*, Chapel Hill, NC, 1992, CIC Publishing Co.

49. Crawford JJ: State of the art: practical infection control in dentistry. In Mitchell E, Cottone J, editors: Proceedings of the National Symposium on hepatitis B and the dental profession, *J Am Dent Assoc* 110:629-633, 1985.

50. Crawford JJ: Sterilization, disinfection, and asepsis in dentistry. In Block SS, editor: *Disinfection, sterilization, and preservation*, Philadelphia, 1983, Lea & Febiger.

51. Crawford JJ, Broderius C: Evaluation of a dental unit designed to prevent retraction of oral fluids. *Quintessence Int* 21:47-51, 1989.

52. Crawford JJ, Broderius C: Control of cross infection risks in the dental operatory: prevention of water retraction by bur cooling spray systems. *J Am Dent Assoc* 116:695-687, 1988.

53. Crawford JJ, Fine J: Infection control in hospital dentistry. In Zambito R: *Hospital dentistry*, St Louis, 1997, Mosby.

54. DeVita VT Jr, Hellman S, Rosenberg SA, editors: *AIDS etiology, diagnosis, treatment, and prevention*, Philadelphia, 1985, JB Lippincott Co.

55. DiMaggio SL: State regulation and the HIV-positive health care professional: a response to a problem that does not exist, *Am J Law Med* 19:497-521, 1995

56. Ehrenkranz NJ, Alfanso BC: Failure of bland soap handwash to prevent hand transfer of patient bacteria to urethral catheters, *Inf Cont Hosp Epid* 12:654-662, 1991.

57. Favero MS, Bond WW: Chemical disinfection of medical materials. In Block SS, editor: *Disinfectiuon, sterilization, and preservation*, ed 4, Philadelphia 1991, Lea & Febiger.

58. Federal law 42 U.S. Code Section #300, ee-2 (Oct. 28, 1991).

59. Food and Drug Administration: Medical devices: patient examination and surgeons' gloves; adulteration. Final Rule, 21CFR Part 800. *Federal Register* 55 (No. 239):51254-52158, Dec 12, 1990.

60. Forbes B: Acquisition of cytomegalovirus infection: an update, *Clin Microbiol Rev* 2:204-216, 1989.

61. Francis D, Favero MS, Maynard JE: Transmission of hepatitis B virus, *Semin Liver Dis* 1(1):27-32, 1981.

62. Francis D et al.: Occurrence of hepatitis A, B, non-A/non-B in the United States, *Am J Med* 76:69, Jan 1984.

63. Friedland GH, Klein RS: Transmission of the human immunodeficiency virus, *N Engl J Med* 317:1125-1135, 1987.

64. Garner JS, Favero MS: *Guideline for handwashing and hospital environmental control* (HHS Pub. No.99-1117), Atlanta, 1985, Public Health Service, Centers for Disease Control.

65. Gayle HD et al: Prevalence of the human immunodeficiency virus among university students, *N Engl J Med* 323:1538-1541, 1990.

66. Glasel M: High-risk sexual practices in the transmission of AIDS. In DeVita VT Jr, Hellman S, Rosenberg SA, editors: *AIDS etiology, diagnosis, treatment, and prevention*, Philadelphia, 1985, JB Lippincott.

67. Gold J: Mycobacterial infections in immunosuppressed patients, *Semin Resp Inf* 13:160-165, 1986.

68. Greene WC: The molecular biology of human immunodeficiency virus type 1, *N Engl J Med* 324:308-317, 1991.

69. Greenspan D, Greenspan CA, Winkler JR: Diagnosis and management of oral manifestations of HIV infection and AIDS, *Infect Dis Clin North Am* 2:373-385, 1988.

70. Gwaltney JM Jr, Hendley JO: Transmission of experimental rhinovirus infection by contaminated surfaces, *Am J Epidemiol* 116:828-833, 1989.

71. Hackney RW: Using a biological indicator to detect potential sources of cross-contamination in the dental operatory, *J Am Dent Assoc* 129:1567-1577, Nov 1998.

72. Hadler SC et al: Long-term immunogenicity and efficacy of hepatitis B vaccine in homosexual men, *N Engl J Med* 315:209-214, 1986.

73. Hamed LM et al: Hibiclens keratitis, *Am J Ophthalmol* 104:50-56, 1987.

74. Klein RS, Freeman K, Taylor PE, Stevens CE: Occupational risk for hepatitis C virus infection among New York City dentists, *Lancet* 338(8782-8783):1539-1542, 1991.

75. Klein RS et al: Low occupational risk of human immunodeficiency virus infection among dental professionals, *N Engl J Med* 318:86-90, 1988.

76. Klein RC, Party E, Gershey EL: Virus penetration of examination gloves, *Biotechniques* 9:196-199, 1990.

77. Lange J, Goudsmit J: Decline of antibody reactivity to HIV core protein secondary to increased production of HIV antigen, *Lancet* 19, Feb 19, 1987.

78. Lettau LA: The A,B,C,D, and E of viral hepatitis: Spelling out the risks for health care workers, *Inf Cont Hosp Epidemiol* 13:77-81, 1992.

79. Lewis DL, Arens M, Appleton SS, et al: Cross-contamination potential with dental equipment, *Lancet* 340:1252-1254, Nov 21, 1992.

80. Lewis DL, Boe RK: Cross-infection risks associated with current procedures for using high-speed dental handpieces. *J Clin Microbiol* 30:401-406, 1992.

81. Lo K-J et al: Long-term immunogenicity and efficacy of hepatitis B vaccine in infants born to HBeAg-positive HBsAg-carrier mothers, *Hepatology* 8:1647-1650, 1988.

82. Manzella JP: An outbreak of herpes simplex virus type 1 gingivostomatitis in a dental hygiene practice, *JAMA* 252:2019-2022, 1984.

83. Martin MV: The significance of the bacterial contamination of dental unit water systems, *Br Dent J* 163:152-154, 1987.

84. McEntegart MG, Clark A: Colonization of dental units with water bacteria, *Br Dent J* 134:140-142, 1973.

85. Merchant VA: Infection control in the dental laboratory: concerns for the dentist, *Compend Contin Educ Dent* 14:(3)382-391, 1993.

86. Merchant VA, Molinari JA, Sabes WR: Herpetic whitlow: report of a case with multiple recurrences, *Oral Surg* 55:568-571, 1983.

87. Meskin LH: HIV update: misinformation persists, *J Am Dent Assoc* 130(soft):1260-1261, 1999.

88. Micik RE et al: Studies on aerobiology. I: Bacterial aerosols generated during dental procedures, *J Dent Res* 48:49-56, 1969.

89. Miller CH, Palenik CJ: *Infection control and management of hazardous materials for the dental team*, ed 2, St Louis, 1998, Mosby.

90. Miller RL, Micik RE: Air pollution and its control in the dental office, *Dent Clin North Am* 22:453, 1978.

91. Mitchell E: ADA Council recommends hepatitis vaccine for dentists, students, and auxiliary personnel, *ADA News* 13:1, Aug 8, 1982.

92. Molinari JA: How to choose and use environmental surface disinfectants. In Cottone JA, Terezhalmy GT, Molinari JA, editors: *Practical infection control in dentistry*, Baltimore, 1996, Williams & Wilkins.

93. Moriarty JD, Crawford JJ: Evaluation of an independent sterile water reservoir system for highspeed instrumentation (abstract No. 855), *J Dent Res* 55, 1976.

94. National Association of Dental Laboratories: *A complete program of infection control for dental laboratories*, Alexandria, VA, 1989, National Association of Dental Laboratories.

95. Occupational Safety and Health Administration: Bloodborne pathogens (Section 1910, 1030 [26 U.S.C. 635]), *Federal Register* 56(235):64175-64181, 1991.

96. Occupational Safety and Health Administration: Hazard Communications Standard, *Federal Register,* Aug 24, 1987.

97. Organization for Safety & Asepsis Procedures: Disease update: hepatitis C, *Focus* 8:1-4, 1998.

98. Palenik CJ et al: A survey of sterilization practices in selected endodontic offices, *J Endodont* 12:206-209, 1986.

99. Pattison CP et al: Epidemic hepatitis B in a clinical laboratory: possible association with computer card handling, *J Am Dent Assoc* 230:854-857, 1974.

100. Peterson NJ, Bond WW, Favero MS: Air sampling for hepatitis B surface antigen in a dental operatory, *J Am Dent Assoc* 99:465-467, 1979.

101. Polinsky B: Clean dental unit water reservoir to control mycobacteria and aquaphilic bacteria, *Control* 5:5, 1990.

102. Poole P, Summers T, Crawford JJ: Comparison of ultrasonic versus swabbing methods to evaluate handpiece disinfection, *Control* 6:4, 1991.

103. Raloff J: Successful hepatitis A vaccine debuts, *Science News* 142:103, 1992.

104. Reinthaler FF, Ascher FM, Stunzer D: Serologic examination for antibodies against Legionella species in dental personnel, *J Dent Res* 67:942-943, 1988.

105. Robinson RAN et al: A suspension method to determine reuse life of chemical disinfectants during clinical use, *Appl Microbiol* 54:158-164, 1988.

106. Roberts HW et al: Dental waterline antimicrobials' effect on dentin shear bond strength (abstract no. 1011), *J Dent Res* 78:232, 1999.

107. Rutala WA, Cole EC: Ineffectiveness of hospital disinfectants against bacteria, a collaborative study, *Infect Control* 8:501-506, 1987.

108. Sabatini B: Keeping the laboratory clean and safe; how to prevent cross-contamination, *Dental Teamwork* 4(No. 6):23-24, 1991.

109. Satter SA, Springthorpe VS: Survival and disinfectant inactivation of the human immunodeficiency virus: a critical review, *Rev Infect Dis* 1(13):430-447, 1991.

110. Sawyer DR et al: Bacterial contamination of the highspeed dental handpiece and the water it delivers, *Virginia Dent J* 53:14-23, 1976.

111. Shearer B: ADA statement on dental unit waterlines, *J Am Dent Assoc* 127:185-189, 1996.

112. Slade JS et al: The survival of human immunodeficiency virus in water, sewage, and sea water, *Water Science and Technology* 21:55-59, 1989.

113. Soulsby ME, Barnett JB, Maddox S: Brief report: the antiseptic efficiency of chlorxylenol-containing vs. chlorhexidine gluconate-containing surgical scrub preparations, *Infect Control* 7:223-226, 1986.

114. Spire B et al: Inactivation of lymphadenopathy-associated virus by heat, gamma rays, and ultraviolet light, *Lancet* 188-189, Jan 26, 1985.

115. Stubbs B et al: A quantitative biological assay to evaluate presterilization cleaning methods, *Transmissions: Society for Inf Cont in Dent* 7:4, 1992.

116. Summers T, Poole P, Crawford J: Statistical evaluation of cleaning methods and chemicals for disinfecting handpieces, *Transmissions: Society for Infect Control in Dent* 6:2, 1991.

117. Takata Y et al: Hepatitis G virus in a high-risk subgroup of hospitalized dental patients, *Oral Surg Oral Med Oral Path Oral Radiol Endod* 4:442-445, 1999.

118. Taylor TL, Leonard RH, Mauriello SM, et al: Effect of DUWL biocides on enamel bond strengths (abstract no. 237), *J Dent Res* 77:135, 1998.

119. Thomas DL et al: Occupational risk of hepatitis C infections among general dentists and oral surgeons in North America, *Am J Med* 100:41-45, 1996.

120. Thomas LE et al: Survival of herpes simplex and other selected microorganisms on patient charts: potential source of infection, *J Am Dent Assoc* 111:462-464, 1985.

121. U.S. Congress: *Occupational Safety and Health Act of 1970,* Sections 6 and 8, (29 U. S. C. 655, 657), CFR Part 1911 and Sec. of Labor's Orders Nos. 9-83 (48 FR 35736) and 29 CFR Part 1910, 1970.

122. U.S. Department of Labor, OSHA, *Controlling occupational exposure to bloodborne pathogens in dentistry,* Washington DC, 1992, US Government Printing Office.

123. Wainwright RB et al: Duration of immunogenicity and efficacy of hepatitis B vaccine in Yupik Eskimo population, *JAMA* 261:2362-2366, 1989.

124. Washington State Department of Health, Dental Disciplinary Board: Small business economic impact statement, *Infect Control* 246-816-720, March 3, 1992.

125. Whitacre RJ, Robins SK, Crawford JJ: *Dental Asepsis,* Seattle, Wash, 1979, Stoma.

126. White SC, Glaze S: Interpatient microbial cross-contamination after dental radiographic exam, *J Am Dent Assoc* 96:801-804, 1978.

127. Williams JF, Andrews N, Santiago JI: Microbial contamination of dental unit waterlines: Current preventive measures and emerging options, *Compend Contin Edu Dent* 17(7):691-708, 1996

128. Williams N, Shay DE, Hasler JF: Indications of the sanitation level in a dental clinic, *J Balt Coll Dent Surg* 31:18-34, 1976.

129. Wood PR, editor: *Cross infection control in dentistry,* Aylesbury, England, 1992, Wolf Publishing.

9

Patient Assessment, Examination and Diagnosis, and Treatment Planning

DANIEL A. SHUGARS

DIANE C. SHUGARS

CHAPTER OUTLINE

Pretreatment considerations consisting of patient assessment, examination and diagnosis, and treatment planning are the foundation of sound dental care. These considerations follow a stepwise progression as the diagnosis and treatment plan depend on thorough assessment and examination of the patient.

Planning of dental treatment is a challenging and rewarding undertaking for the dentist. This endeavor is no longer the sole province of the treating dentist, however. Heightened consumer awareness and interest in personal health has resulted in increased participation by the patient in decisions about treatment. The financing of nearly one half of dental care in the United States by private dental insurance[30] also has prompted third-party payers' interest in treatment decisions.

Growing attention to using only the most effective and appropriate treatment has spawned interest in numerous activities. For example, research, providing knowledge of what treatments work best in certain situations, is expanding the knowledge base of dentistry.[6] This has led to an interest in translating results of research into practice activities and hopefully enhanced care for patients. This movement has been termed *evidence-based dentistry,* which is defined as the "conscientious, explicit, and judicious use of current best evidence in making decisions about the care of individual patients."[54] It is anticipated that the systematic reviews that emerge from the focus on evidence-based dentistry will provide practitioners with a distillation of the available knowledge about various conditions and treatments. As evidence-based dentistry continues to expand, professional associations will become more active in the development of guidelines and parameters that will assist dentists and their patients in making informed and appropriate decisions. Currently, the American Dental Association and other specialty associations have begun promulgating practice parameters that can be used for this purpose.[55]

The first section of this chapter describes several aspects of patient assessment that includes a review of the patient's chief complaint, medical condition and history, sociologic and psychologic conditions, dental history, and an evaluation of the patient's risk for dental disease. The second section, devoted to examination and diagnosis, reviews the clinical examination of orofacial soft tissues, clinical and radiographic examinations of teeth and periodontium, and clinical examination of the occlusion. The second section also reviews special considerations for the examination of a patient in pain. A brief discussion of the need for and characteristics of informed consent also is included in the second section. The final section discusses types of treatment plans, indications for operative treatment, and sequencing of dental procedures with an emphasis on interdisciplinary aspects of treatment planning.

Three pretreatment considerations—medical review, examination, and diagnosis—are necessary during each of the initial, emergency, reevaluation, and recall visits. The *routine initial visit* involves obtaining detailed information for treatment planning. An *emergency visit* requires collecting basic information and then focusing on the patient's chief complaint. A *reevaluation appointment* requires updating patient information and evaluating previous treatment. In contrast, a *recall appointment* demands reviewing the patient assessment information and comparing the patient's current status with previous conditions. Regardless of the type of visit, however, the dentist must routinely evaluate the patient's systemic condition, along with the status of the teeth, periodontium, occlusion, and facial structures.

Pretreatment assessment must be thorough and systematic. The results of this assessment must be recorded accurately in the *patient record.* Accurate records are maintained for proper patient care and for medical, legal, and forensic purposes.

PATIENT ASSESSMENT

INFECTION CONTROL

Before the examination and diagnosis of teeth, periodontium, and orofacial soft tissues, attention is given to infection control (IC), the patient's chief complaint, medical review, sociologic and psychologic review, dental history, and risk assessment.

Before, during, and after any patient visit, appropriate IC measures must be instituted. For this information the reader is referred to Chapter 8.

CHIEF COMPLAINT

Before initiating any treatment, it is important to determine the patient's chief complaint, or the problem that initiated the patient's visit. Record the complaint verbatim in the dental record. The patient should be encouraged and guided to discuss all aspects of the current problem, including onset, duration, symptoms, and related factors. This information is vital to establish the need for specific diagnostic tests and to determine the cause and treatment of the complaint.

MEDICAL REVIEW

The patient or legal guardian completes a standard, comprehensive *medical history form* (Fig. 9-1). This form is the focus of the preexamination *patient interview,* which helps identify conditions that could alter, complicate, or contraindicate proposed dental procedures. For instance, the practitioner may identify: (1) *communicable diseases* that require special precautions, procedures, or referral; (2) *allergies or medications* that may contraindicate the use of certain drugs; (3) *systemic diseases and cardiac abnormalities* that demand less strenuous procedures or prophylactic antibiotic coverage; and (4) *physiologic changes associated with aging* that may alter clinical presentation and influence treatment. The practitioner also

ADA. Health History Form

Medical Alert	Condition	Premedication	Allergies	Anaest.		Date

Name_____   Home Phone (_____)_____   Business Phone (_____)_____
          Last   First   Middle

Address _____   City_____   State _____ Zip Code_____
          P.O. Box or Mailing address

Occupation_____   Height_____ Weight_____ Date of Birth ___/___/___ Sex ☐ M ☐ F

SS# _____ Emergency Contact _____ Relationship _____ Phone (_____)_____

If you are completing this form for another person, what is your relationship to that person? _____
                                                                                                    Name   Relationship

For the following questions, please (X) whichever applies, your answers are for our records only and will be kept confidential in accordance with applicable laws. Please note that during your initial visit you will be asked some questions about your responses to this questionnaire and there may be additional questions concerning your health. This information is vital to allow us to provide appropriate care for you. This office does not use this information to discriminate.

Dental Information

Yes	No	Don't Know		Yes	No	Don't Know	
☐	☐	☐	Do your gums bleed when you brush?	☐	☐	☐	Have you ever had orthodontic (braces) treatment?
☐	☐	☐	Are your teeth sensitive to cold, hot, sweets or pressure?	☐	☐	☐	Do you have headaches, earaches or neck pains?
☐	☐	☐	Have you had any periodontal (gum) treatments?	☐	☐	☐	Do you wear removable dental appliances?
☐	☐	☐	Have you had a serious/difficult problem associated with any previous dental treatment? If so, explain _____				

How would you describe your current dental problem?_____

Date of your last dental exam _____ Date of last dental x-rays _____

What was done at that time?_____

How do you feel about the appearance of your teeth? _____

Medical Information

Yes	No	Don't Know	
☐	☐	☐	Are you in good health?
☐	☐	☐	Has there been any change in your general health within the past year?

Do you have any of the following diseases or problems: **If you answer yes to any of the 3 items below, please stop and return this form to the receptionist.**

Yes	No	Don't Know	
☐	☐	☐	Active Tuberculosis
☐	☐	☐	Persistent cough greater than a 3 week duration
☐	☐	☐	Cough that produces blood
☐	☐	☐	Are you now under the care of a physician? If so, what is/are the condition(s) being treated? _____

Date of last physical examination _____

Physician(s) NAME _____ PHONE _____ ADDRESS _____ CITY/STATE/ZIP
             NAME _____ PHONE _____ ADDRESS _____ CITY/STATE/ZIP

Yes	No	Don't Know	
☐	☐	☐	Have you had any serious illness, operation, or been hospitalized in the past 5 years? If so, what was the illness or problem? _____
☐	☐	☐	Are you taking or have you recently taken any medicine(s) including non-prescription medicine? If so, what medicine(s) are you taking?

Prescribed _____

Over the counter _____

Natural or herbal preparations _____

Yes	No	Don't Know	
☐	☐	☐	Have you taken any diet drugs such as Pondimin (fenfluramine), Redux (dexphenfluramine) or phen-fen (fenfluramine-phentermine combination)?
☐	☐	☐	Do you drink alcoholic beverages? If yes, how much alcohol did you drink in the last 24 hours? _____ In the past month? _____
			If yes, _____# of drinks per day for _____# of years
☐	☐	☐	Are you alcohol and/or drug dependent? If so, have you received treatment? (Check one) ☐ Yes ☐ No
☐	☐	☐	Do you use drugs or other substances for recreational purposes? If yes, please list_____
			Frequency of use (daily, weekly, etc.) _____ Number of years of recreational drug use _____
☐	☐	☐	Do you use tobacco (smoking, snuff, chew)? If so, how interested are you in stopping? (Check one) ☐ Very ☐ Somewhat ☐ Not interested
☐	☐	☐	Do you wear contact lenses?

Allergies Are you allergic to or have you had a reaction to: (Please fill out both columns)

Yes	No	Don't Know		Yes	No	Don't Know	
☐	☐	☐	Local anesthetics	☐	☐	☐	Latex
☐	☐	☐	Aspirin	☐	☐	☐	Iodine
☐	☐	☐	Penicillin or other antibiotics	☐	☐	☐	Hay fever/seasonal
☐	☐	☐	Barbiturates, sedatives, or sleeping pills	☐	☐	☐	Animals
☐	☐	☐	Sulfa drugs	☐	☐	☐	Food (Specify)_____
☐	☐	☐	Codeine or other narcotics	☐	☐	☐	Other (Specify)_____

To yes responses, specify type of reaction _____

Please complete both sides

FIG. **9-1** A comprehensive medical review form is the focus of the patient interview. This form helps the practitioner identify conditions that may affect dental treatment or require referral to a physician. *(From The American Dental Association.)*

Yes No Don't Know

(Women Only)

☐ ☐ ☐ Are you pregnant?
☐ ☐ ☐ Nursing?
☐ ☐ ☐ Taking birth control pills?

☐ ☐ ☐ Have you had an orthopedic total joint (hip, knee, elbow, finger) replacement? If so when was this operation done? _____
☐ ☐ ☐ Have you had any complications or difficulties with your prosthetic joint?
☐ ☐ ☐ Has a physician or previous dentist recommended that you take antibiotics prior to your dental treatment? If so, what antibiotic and dose?
  Name of physician or dentist* _____ Phone _____

NOTE TO PATIENT: A new report (July 1997) prepared and endorsed by the American Dental Association and the American Academy of Orthopaedic Surgeons has recommended that antibiotic prophylaxis before dental treatment is not indicated for most dental patients with artificial orthopedic prosthetic joints. This office will be glad to discuss this report with you and provide a copy of it to you and your orthopedic surgeon/physician.

Please (X) if you have or had any of the following diseases or problems.

Yes	No	Don't Know		Yes	No	Don't Know		Yes	No	Don't Know	
☐	☐	☐	Abnormal bleeding	☐	☐	☐	Disease, drug, or radiation-induced immunosurpression	☐	☐	☐	Neurological disorders.
☐	☐	☐	AIDS or HIV infection								If yes, specify _____
☐	☐	☐	Anemia	☐	☐	☐	Diabetes. If yes, specify below:	☐	☐	☐	Osteoporosis
☐	☐	☐	Arthritis				○ Type I (Insulin dependent)	☐	☐	☐	Persistent swollen glands in neck
☐	☐	☐	Rheumatoid arthritis				○ Type II	☐	☐	☐	Respiratory problems.
☐	☐	☐	Asthma	☐	☐	☐	Dry mouth				If yes, specify below:
☐	☐	☐	Blood transfusion	☐	☐	☐	Eating disorder.				○ Emphysema,
			If yes, date _____				If yes, specify _____				○ Bronchitis, etc.
☐	☐	☐	Cancer/chemotherapy/radiation treatment	☐	☐	☐	Epilepsy	☐	☐	☐	Severe headaches
				☐	☐	☐	Fainting spells or seizures	☐	☐	☐	Severe or rapid weight loss
☐	☐	☐	Cardiovascular disease.	☐	☐	☐	G.E. reflux	☐	☐	☐	Sexually transmitted disease
			If yes, specify below:	☐	☐	☐	Glaucoma	☐	☐	☐	Sinus trouble
			○ Angina	☐	☐	☐	Hemophilia	☐	☐	☐	Sleep disorder
			○ Arteriosclerosis	☐	☐	☐	Hepatitis, jaundice or liver disease	☐	☐	☐	Sores or ulcers in the mouth
			○ Artificial heart valves	☐	☐	☐	Recurrent infections	☐	☐	☐	Stroke
			○ Coronary insufficiency				Indicate type of infection	☐	☐	☐	Systemic lupus erythematosus
			○ Coronary occlusion				_____	☐	☐	☐	Thyroid problems
			○ Damaged heart valves	☐	☐	☐	Kidney problems	☐	☐	☐	Tuberculosis
			○ Heart attack	☐	☐	☐	Low blood pressure	☐	☐	☐	Ulcers
			○ Heart murmur	☐	☐	☐	Mental health disorders.	☐	☐	☐	Excessive urination
			○ High blood pressure				If yes, specify below:	☐	☐	☐	Do you have any disease, condition, or problem not listed above that you think I should know about? Please explain:
			○ Inborn heart defects				_____				
			○ Mitral valve prolapse				_____				
			○ Pacemaker								_____
			○ Rheumatic heart disease	☐	☐	☐	Malnutrition				_____
☐	☐	☐	Chest pain upon exertion	☐	☐	☐	Migraines				_____
☐	☐	☐	Chronic pain	☐	☐	☐	Night sweats				_____
☐	☐	☐	Persistent diarrhea								

NOTE: Both doctor and patient are encouraged to discuss any and all relevant patient health issues prior to treatment.
I certify that I have read and understand the above. I acknowledge that my questions, if any, about inquiries set forth above have been answered to my satisfaction. I will not hold my dentist, or any other member of his/her staff, responsible for any action they take or do not take because of errors or omissions that I may have made in the completion of this form.

_____
Signature of Patient/Legal Guardian   Date

For completion by dentist

Comments on patient interview concerning health history _____
_____

Significant findings from questionnaire or oral interview _____
_____

Dental management considerations _____

_____
Signature of Dentist   Date

Health History Update: On a regular basis the patient should be questioned about any medical history changes, date and comments notated, along with signature.

Date	Comments	Signature of patient and dentist
_____	_____	_____
_____	_____	_____
_____	_____	_____

FIG. 9-1, cont'd

may identify a need for medical consultation or referral before initiating dental care. All of this information is carefully detailed in the patient's permanent record and is used as needed to shape subsequent treatment.

Communicable Diseases. During the medical interview, the dentist must recognize the clinical manifestations of common infectious diseases because their presence can affect patient management and may constitute potential transmission hazards within the dental practice. *The dentist is sometimes the first health professional to identify a patient with a contagious disease.* Moreover, many communicable diseases are transmissible through the dental setting unless appropriate IC measures are taken (see Chapter 8).

Of particular concern is the detection and prompt treatment of oral infections in *immunocompromised patients*. These individuals are at high risk of developing life-threatening illnesses due to the suppression of appropriate immune responses to infectious agents. This immunosuppression may be caused directly by diseases of the immune cells (e.g., leukemia, lymphomas, infection with the human immunodeficiency virus [HIV]) or indirectly by the use of immunosuppressive drugs and therapies (e.g., drug administration to prevent rejection of transplanted tissues and irradiation therapy for some cancers). The oral manifestations of bacterial, fungal, and viral infections in these immunocompromised individuals can develop into extensive, aggressive, and painful lesions that occur in characteristic or uncharacteristic locations and too often result in lethal dissemination to vital organs. Therefore, careful examination, detection, and aggressive treatment of oral and perioral lesions in this population are critical steps in maintaining the health of immunocompromised patients.

A comprehensive treatise of the numerous oral and perioral manifestations associated with communicable diseases is beyond the scope of this book. The reader is referred to texts on oral medicine, oral microbiology, and oral pathology for additional information. A list of recommended readings is included at the end of this chapter. The more common infectious diseases and associated orofacial lesions are reviewed in this section. Some of the clinical symptoms associated with contagious diseases that should be familiar to the dentist are listed in Table 9-1, and the intraoral and extraoral manifestations are shown in Plate 9-1. The dentist must be capable of detecting and identifying these manifestations either during the medical interview or during the clinical examination of soft tissues of the head (intraoral and extraoral) and neck (see Examination of Orofacial Soft Tissues).

Herpes Simplex Virus. This infectious disease is one of the most common nonrespiratory viral diseases affecting humans. Transmitted primarily through saliva, the herpes simplex virus (HSV) preferentially infects the skin, mucous membranes, eyes, and nervous tissues.[44]

The two HSV types tend to affect different regions of the body; type 1 involves the oral and perioral tissues ("above the waist"), whereas type 2 involves the genital and surrounding areas ("below the waist"). However, oral infections with HSV type 2 and genital infections with HSV type 1 are becoming more common, and their disease manifestations are clinically indistinguishable. In relatively healthy patients, infections are localized to the skin and mucous membranes. However, virus dissemination within the immunosuppressed individual or newborn may lead to serious sequelae such as esophagitis, pneumonitis, hepatitis, meningitis, or viral encephalitis.[43]

Primary infection with HSV type 1 usually occurs in children and is typically subclinical, but may be preceded by malaise, headache, irritability, fever, lymphadenopathy, and pharyngitis. Oral manifestations of primary HSV infection present as *primary herpetic gingivostomatitis,* an intraoral condition characterized by intensely red gingiva and small, painful vesicles (fluid-filled lesions) on the lips, facial mucosa, palate, pharynx, tonsils, or gingiva (see Plate 9-1, *A*). After the lesions rupture, they appear as shallow ulcers with irregular red borders ("halo") and may be covered by a gray pseudomembranous covering (see Plate 9-1, *B*). Symptoms may last from 10 to 14 days before resolving. It is important to note that infectious virus is present during this period and can be easily transmitted to others via contact with lesions and infected saliva.

During *primary infection,* the virus gains access to the nerve endings adjacent to the point of entry. HSV then retreats along the nerve to the sensory ganglia (trigeminal ganglion for oral lesions) where it lies dormant until reactivated by one of several factors (e.g., stress, sunlight, trauma, fatigue, or allergy). Upon reactivation, the virus travels down the nerve to the epithelium, where it produces secondary herpetic lesions on the lips (*herpes labialis,* commonly known as *fever blisters* or *cold sores*) (see Plate 9-1, *C*) or, less frequently, within the oral cavity. These *secondary herpetic lesions,* usually seen in adults, are frequently preceded by a burning or tingling sensation at the site where a single vesicle or cluster of vesicles subsequently develops. Intraoral, herpetic lesions occur in clusters, have well-defined borders, and are confined to the attached tissues of the palate, gingiva, and alveolar ridges (see Plate 9-1, *B*). Topical or systemic administration of the antiviral drug acyclovir or its derivatives valacyclovir and famciclovir reduces the duration and severity of HSV-related symptoms if given before the onset of skin lesions.[10] However, the extensive lesions seen in immunosuppressed patients infected with HSV require lengthy systemic therapy for complete resolution.

HSV infections also are of particular concern to those delivering patient care. *Herpetic whitlow,* HSV infection of the finger, has been documented among dental professionals (see Plate 9-1, *D*). This painful lesion arises from contact of infected oral secretions with broken skin of the finger. In addition, ocular infection with HSV may occur following autoinoculation from an oral infection, with potentially serious consequences of scarring and blindness. *The routine use of gloves and protective eyewear during patient treatment significantly reduces the occupational exposure to HSV.*

Chickenpox (Varicella) and Shingles (Zoster). Infection with the varicella-zoster virus (VZV) presents as chickenpox (varicella) during initial exposure and as shingles (zoster) in reactivated (or recurrent) disease. Chickenpox, a common and relatively mild childhood disease, is easily transmitted by airborne droplets and direct contact. Following an incubation period of 2 to 3 weeks, infected individuals frequently complain of malaise and fever. A rash typically appears on the trunk and spreads centrifugally to the head and extremities (see Plate 9-1, *E*). The rash is later replaced by crops of vesicles, which rupture and crust. Lesions frequently appear on the oral mucosa as nonpainful, blisterlike ulcers that resemble aphthous ulcers (see Plate 9-1, *F*).

After acute infection, the virus remains dormant indefinitely in the dorsal root ganglia of the affected sensory nerves. Reactivation in the form of shingles or zoster may occur decades later in the immunocompetent adult over the age of 50 or at any age in the immunosuppressed individual. Reactivation of virus replication occurs along the sensory distribution of the affected nerve (dermatome) and is frequently accompanied by itching and neuralgia. Skin lesions also occur characteristically along the unilateral dermatome distribution and appear as vesicles that erupt and ulcerate (see Plate 9-1, *G*). In the relatively healthy adult, the active disease is brought under control within a few days. However, in older persons or the severely immunocompromised, the lesions may resolve slowly and neural pain may persist for several months. Treatment includes palliative agents to decrease itching and pain and the antiherpetic drugs acyclovir, famciclovir or valacyclovir to limit the duration and intensity of symptoms.[10] A newly approved varicella vaccine is recommended for healthy children, patients with chronic diseases or immunosuppressive conditions such as leukemia, and susceptible health care workers.

An infected patient with chickenpox can transmit the virus via the respiratory route for 1 to 5 days following the appearance of the rash. Treating an infected patient in the dental office during that period may disseminate the infection to other susceptible patients and to dental personnel. *Routine dental care should be postponed in patients with chickenpox until all lesions have crusted.*

Condyloma Acuminatum (Venereal Warts). Condyloma acuminatum, more commonly referred to as *venereal warts,* is caused by the human papillomavirus. This transmissible and autoinoculable disease affects the anogenital skin and mucosa. Oral lesions initially present as soft pink nodules on the gingiva or other mucosal surface. These nodules may remain flat with well-defined margins or may coalesce to form raised, papillomatous ("cauliflower-like") clusters (see Plate 9-1, *H*). Typically asymptomatic, lesions may be localized or scattered throughout the mouth and frequently recur. Because some lesions have premalignant potential, removal by surgical excision, cryosurgery, or laser therapy and histologic evaluation are recommended.

Respiratory Viruses. Arguably the most frequently transmitted diseases within the dental environment are those caused by respiratory viruses. This group of viruses includes both viruses whose primary disease manifestations directly affect the respiratory tract (e.g., rhinoviruses, respiratory syncytial viruses, and influenza viruses) and viruses that are transmitted via respiratory secretions but manifest themselves through other organ systems (e.g., rubeola, rubella). Transmission occurs through inhalation of or direct contact with droplets and aerosols. Depending on the etiologic agent, symptoms may include sneezing, cough, low-grade fever, headache, malaise, conjunctivitis, and rash. In the immunocompetent individual, these respiratory infections are usually self-limiting and have few serious sequelae. Newly developed antiviral medications such as inhaled zamamivir for influenza virus infection reduced the duration and severity of symptoms in clinical trials and are awaiting approval by the Federal Drug Administration (FDA). However, in the immunocompromised or medically compromised patient, serious morbidity and mortality may result. The antiviral agent amantadine may provide relief in these severe situations. Annual vaccination for influenza viruses is recommended, especially in older persons and other highly susceptible populations. Vaccines are not currently available for the other respiratory viruses.

Rubeola (Measles). Rubeola, also known as *measles,* is a highly contagious viral childhood disease that spreads via respiratory secretions. Following an incubation period of 10 to 12 days, virus multiplication in the upper respiratory tract and conjunctivae causes prodromal symptoms of dry cough, sore throat, headache, low-grade fever, and conjunctivitis. During this prodromal stage, characteristic intraoral lesions known as *Koplik spots* may appear on the facial mucosa opposite the first and second maxillary molars. These lesions resemble white grains of sand set within red, inflamed patches. Following the prodromal period, a red maculopapular rash appears on the head and face and quickly extends to the extremities. Pharyngitis is commonly present. Because virus shedding occurs during the prodromal period and for about 2 days after the appearance of the rash (before the disease can be recognized), measles is spread rapidly throughout populated regions and can quickly escalate to epidemic proportions. However, since widespread vaccination began in 1973, the number and

TABLE 9-1 | Communicable Diseases of Concern in Dentistry

INFECTIOUS AGENT	ROUTE OF TRANSMISSION	DISEASE
Herpes simplex virus (HSV) types 1 and 2	Congenital; oral (saliva); sexual; direct contact with lesions	Oral/genital herpes Primary herpetic gingivostomatitis Herpes labialis Herpetic whitlow (finger) Keratoconjunctivitis (eye)
Varicella-zoster virus (VZV)	Aerosols; respiratory droplets; direct contact with lesions	Chickenpox, or varicella (primary infection) Shingles, or zoster (reactivated infection)
Human papilloma virus	Direct oral or sexual contacts with lesions	Venereal warts, or *condylomata acuminatum*
Respiratory viruses (e.g., rhinoviruses, respiratory syncytial virus, influenza viruses)	Direct contact with respiratory droplets; aerosols	Respiratory infections (e.g., cold, flu)
Paramyxoviruses	Direct contact with respiratory droplets; aerosols	Rubeola or measles Mumps
Togavirus	Direct contact with respiratory droplets; aerosols	Rubella, or German measles
Epstein-Barr virus (EBV)	Direct contact with saliva	Infectious mononucleosis
Hepatitis B virus (HBV)	Blood; sexual; perinatal; present in all body fluids, including saliva	Hepatitis, cirrhosis of the liver, hepatocellular carcinoma
Human immunodeficiency virus (HIV)	Blood; sexual; perinatal	Opportunistic infections Neoplastic lesions (e.g., Kaposi's sarcoma) Wasting syndrome Acquired immune deficiency syndrome (AIDS)
Mycobacterium tuberculosis	Respiratory droplets; aerosols; saliva; ingestion; direct contact	Pulmonary tuberculosis (TB) dissemination to the intestines, kidney, bones, meninges, lymph nodes, and oral structures
Neisseria gonorrhoeae	Sexual contact	Gonorrhea (i.e., oral lesions; gonococcal arthritis; infections of the skin, eye, heart, and meninges)
Treponema pallidum	Sexual contact, congenital	Syphilis (i.e., oral lesions; disseminated infections to other organs, including the central nervous system [CNS] and heart)

INFECTIOUS AGENT	ROUTE OF TRANSMISSION	DISEASE
Vesicles that rupture to form multiple shallow ulcers; inflamed gingiva may be present; lesions frequently recur when reactivated by various stimuli (e.g., stress)	Acyclovir, penciclovir, or valacyclovir Topical ointment Systemic use in severe cases	Lesions of HSV type 1 are usually found above the waist, while those of HSV type 2 usually occur below the waist; herpetic infections may be severe and potentially life threatening in newborns and immunosuppressed individuals
Vesicular lesions associated with chickenpox appear initially on the trunk and scalp; shingles follow a unilateral dermatome distribution	Acyclovir, penciclovir, valacyclovir, vidarabine, or famciclovir Topical and systemic use	VZV infections may have serious, fatal consequences in neonates and immunocompromised individuals
Flat or raised nodules that may coalesce into cauliflower-like clusters; typically asymptomatic; lesions frequently recur	Surgical or chemical removal	Certain lesions may progress to precancerous and cancerous growths
Sneezing, sore throat, fever, headache, and malaise	Prophylactic prevention for flu by vaccination or treatment with amantadine or rimantadine Palliative treatment for colds	Probably the most frequently transmitted diseases within dental practices
Rubeola—cough, conjunctivitis, fever, maculopapular rash, and Koplik's spots Mumps—salivary gland enlargement, headache, fever, and malaise	Childhood vaccination and palliative treatment	Serious infections may lead to life-threatening pneumonia
Low-grade fever, sore throat, and mild exanthematous rash of short duration	Childhood vaccination and palliative treatment	May cause congenital defects in neonates, including mental retardation, heart defect, deafness, and retarded growth
Lymphadenopathy, fever, and petechiae	None	Infection is rarely serious
Fever, malaise, anorexia, gastrointestinal distress, chills, and icteric symptoms of liver damage (e.g., jaundice, dark urine, pale stool)	Vaccination and palliative care Treatment of chronic hepatitis with α-interferon may be beneficial	HBV infection is a serious occupational hazard to unprotected dentists and dental personnel
Acute—flu-like symptoms (early in the illness), fever, weight-loss, chills, and lymphadenopathy Chronic—lymphadenopathy, intraoral lesions (e.g., herpes labialis), hairy leukoplakia, candidiasis, extreme weight loss, and HIV-associated periodontal diseases	No curative treatment is available Therapy with reverse transcriptase inhibitors, protease inhibitors, and similar medications may slow disease progression	HIV infection is a progressively debilitating and ultimately fatal illness that spans the clinical spectrum of no symptoms (asymptomatic period) to frank AIDS
Persistent cough, night sweats, and loss of energy and appetite	Multidrug chemotherapy (e.g., isoniazid and rifampin), rest, and proper nutrition	The incidence of TB is rising, largely because of poor sanitary and living conditions, growing numbers of persons with AIDS, and reactivated diseases
Urethral or vaginal discharge, pharyngitis, and oral lesions (rarely)	Penicillin	One of the most prevalent sexually transmitted diseases
Primary—lymphadenopathy and chancre Secondary—generalized rash, bone lesions, and red patches on mucosal membranes Tertiary syphilis—gummas, involvement of the CNS and circulatory system	Penicillin	Syphilis has been nicknamed "the great imitator" because of the varied clinical manifestations accompanying the infection

geographic extent of measles outbreaks have been limited. Although this infection is usually self-limiting, secondary infection of the lesions with staphylococci or other bacteria may result.

Rubella (German Measles). Rubella, commonly called *German measles,* results from infection with a togavirus, a virus distinct from the causative agent of rubeola. Rubella is an usually mild disease characterized by fever, transient rash, and vesicular eruption, features that closely resemble rubeola but are of shorter duration. Like rubeola, rubella is transmitted by droplets from the mouth, nose, and throat, and is communicable before symptoms appear. Although rare, oral lesions appear as rose-colored lesions of the palatal mucosa and the posterior region of the oral cavity. The disease is usually benign and self-limiting; however, secondary staphylococcal infections may develop, and infection during the first trimester of pregnancy can cause serious congenital defects in the fetus. *Female dental professionals and the spouses of male dental professionals should be protected by vaccination and by adherence to proper IC measures.*

Mumps. Bilateral or unilateral enlargement of the parotid, submandibular, and/or sublingual glands is the hallmark of mumps, a childhood disease. The paramyxovirus, the etiologic agent of mumps, is transmitted via respiratory droplets and saliva. Following an incubation period of 2 to 5 weeks, symptoms include headache, malaise, weight loss, fever, and swollen, tender salivary glands. Infected individuals are considered infectious approximately 2 days before swelling is noted, and remain infectious until approximately 9 days after swelling subsides. Although mumps can be an uncomfortable illness, it has few serious sequelae and an effective vaccine is available. Because this viral infection is spread by saliva via droplet dissemination and direct contact, care must be taken to limit transmission in the dental practice.

Infectious Mononucleosis. Primary infection with the *Epstein-Barr virus* (EBV) results in infectious mononucleosis (IM), an acute illness characterized by generalized lymphadenopathy, mild fever, and petechiae (pin-point subsurface hemorrhages) typically at the border of the hard and soft palates. Although the virus is present in saliva and exudates, IM is not very contagious and is transmitted mainly by direct contact with infected saliva (hence the nickname, "kissing disease"). IM typically lasts from 1 to 4 weeks but may linger for several months or longer. No specific treatment is available for IM and serious complications rarely develop.

Hepatitis B Virus. The hepatitis B virus (HBV) is readily transmitted through body fluids such as blood and saliva, and represents a *significant occupational hazard for the dental professional.* Fortunately, an effective vaccine is readily available for protection against HBV. Follow-up evaluation of immunization also is important to ensure that an appropriate immune response is generated. However, up to two thirds of acutely infected individuals report no symptoms and are unaware that they harbor the virus.[32] *Because both symptomatic and asymptomatic infected patients can transmit the virus, universal precautions must be taken with all patients to prevent disease transmission.*[25] During the acute stage of infection, individuals may exhibit vague symptoms of nausea, gastrointestinal distress, muscular aches, low-grade fever, chronic fatigue, or jaundice (yellowing of the skin and sclera). No distinct oral changes are associated with HBV infection. Other aspects of HBV infection are detailed in Chapter 8.

Hepatitis C Virus. Another contagious virus that causes chronic liver disease is hepatitis C virus (HCV) (see Chapter 8). Formerly referred to as *non-A, non-B hepatitis,* HCV infection leads to hepatitic disease in 60% to 85% of cases, is strongly associated with liver cirrhosis, portal hypertension, and hepatocellular carcinoma and is a leading cause of non–alcohol-associated liver transplantation in this country.[14] Most infected individuals are unaware of their infection and diagnosis is oftentimes delayed for several years until end-stage disease has developed.[25] HCV transmission occurs primarily through blood. Although present in saliva and other body fluids, no report has described viral transmission through blood-free saliva. No vaccine is available and immune globulin is not an effective postexposure prophylaxis. In clinical trials, experimental therapies using α-interferon, ribavirin, and viral protease inhibitors have shown modest short-term improvements in reducing viral titer, stabilizing or restoring liver function, and slowing tissue destruction in the liver. The long-term effects of these therapies and their usefulness in postexposure prophylaxis and acute disease are not known. Although the risk of HCV occupational transmission in the dental setting is low, strict adherence to universal precautions is recommended to reduce exposure to blood and blood-contaminated saliva.

Human Immunodeficiency Virus. The majority of individuals infected with the human immunodeficiency virus (HIV) present with some type of intraoral manifestation, many of which may be detected early in the disease course.[27,51] Lesions associated with HIV may arise from either newly acquired infections or from reactivation of opportunistic infections, asymptomatic infections that usually are held in check by a competent immune system. However, during the course of HIV disease, the immune response slowly deteriorates, allowing these opportunistic infections to reappear and cause significant morbidity and mortality. Aggressive management of HIV disease through potent antiretroviral medication use and therapies to reconstitute the immune response may resolve or reduce the severity of oral manifestations. However, lesions may reappear when drug-resistant viral strains arise in infected patients. HIV-associated lesions arise from various sources:

fungal infections (candidiasis), *viral infections* (herpetic lesions, hairy leukoplakia, warts), *bacterial infections* (HIV-associated periodontal diseases) and *neoplastic origin* (Kaposi's sarcoma), in addition to those of *generalized or undetermined origin* (lymphadenopathy, aphthouslike ulcers, or HIV-associated salivary gland disease). Clinical manifestations not previously discussed in this section are briefly addressed.

Oral Candidiasis. The most prevalent oral infection in HIV-infected individuals, oral candidiasis, a fungal infection, often presents as the initial manifestation and frequently predicts the likelihood of other opportunistic infections.[27,51] Although occasionally observed in older patients, the detection of these lesions is strongly suggestive of HIV infection in a young person without a known cause such as xerostomia ("dry mouth") or therapy with antibiotics, corticosteroids, or other immunosuppressive drugs.

Candidiasis appears on oral mucosa as one of four distinct forms: (1) pseudomembranous, (2) hyperplastic, (3) atrophic or erythematous, or (4) angular cheilitis. *Pseudomembranous candidiasis,* or *thrush,* is characterized by white or yellow plaques that can be easily wiped off to reveal erythematous surfaces that easily bleed (see Plate 9-1, *I*). The *hyperplastic form* also appears as light-colored plaques, but cannot be removed by scraping. The *atrophic form* occurs as smooth, red patches, more commonly on palatal tissues, facial mucosa, or the dorsal surface of the tongue. *Angular cheilitis* appears as fissures or ulcers radiating from the corners of the mouth and are frequently associated with white plaques. Candidiasis is generally diagnosed by its clinical appearance and confirmed by staining with potassium hydroxide. If left untreated, oral candidiasis can extend into the esophagus and develop into a potentially life-threatening illness. In most cases, oral candidiasis can be treated effectively with topical antifungal agents such as nystatin, clotrimazole, or ketoconazole; however, refractory cases may require systemic antifungal chemotherapy (e.g., fluconazole).

Hairy Leukoplakia. First reported by Greenspan and others[28] in 1984, oral hairy leukoplakia (HL) describes an adherent, filamentous white plaque that exhibits a characteristic corrugated or "hairy" appearance (see Plate 9-1, *J*). The lesion is typically observed on parakeratinized mucosa on the lateral border of the tongue, and may occur unilaterally or bilaterally. However, HL may extend to cover the dorsal surface of the tongue and also can appear on facial mucosa. This lesion is caused by the EBV, is usually asymptomatic, and has no known premalignant potential. Removal of the lesion may be indicated for esthetic reasons.

Kaposi's Sarcoma. HIV-infected patients may present with Kaposi's sarcoma (KS), a malignancy involving the endothelial covering of blood vessel walls. This lesion is often an initial manifestation of the severe stage of HIV disease known as *acquired immune deficiency syndrome (AIDS).* Over half of patients with mucocutaneous KS exhibit oral and perioral lesions.[51] The clinical appearance of oral KS is variable, but typically presents as blue, purple, or brown raised areas on the palate (see Plate 9-1, *K*), and also may be present on the tongue, gingiva, or other oral structures. Nearly two thirds of patients with oral KS have associated symptoms of pain or difficulty in swallowing.[22]

HIV-Associated Periodontal Diseases. Unusual clinical forms of periodontal diseases have been described in persons infected with HIV.[18,51] These lesions include linear gingival erythema (LGE), necrotizing ulcerative gingivitis (NUG), necrotizing ulcerative periodontitis (NUP) and necrotizing ulcerative stomatitis (NUS).

LGE (formerly called *HIV-associated gingivitis,* or *HIV-G*) is characterized by a distinct linear erythema limited to the marginal gingiva and the absence of mucosal ulceration (see Plate 9-1, *L*). Petechiae are frequently an associated finding. Spontaneous bleeding or bleeding upon probing of the involved gingiva may be present even in patients with meticulous home care. Unlike conventional gingivitis, this atypical gingivitis is not associated with plaque accumulation and poor oral hygiene, but rather can appear in areas with little or no plaque. Although the etiology has not been clearly defined, studies demonstrating an association between oral candidiasis and LGE suggest that the lesion may arise from a local fungal infection or candidal-induced altered immune response that makes the individual particularly susceptible to subgingival bacteria.[39] Treatment consists of removal of dental plaque if present and daily use of an antimicrobial oral rinse containing 0.12% chlorhexidine. The use of antifungal medications is not indicated because LGE does not progress to more serious forms of periodontal disease and typically resolves with the use of chlorhexidine alone.

Necrotizing and ulcerative forms of periodontal diseases also have been described in immunosuppressed HIV-infected persons. NUG, NUP (formerly called *HIV-associated periodontitis*) and NUS are periodontal lesions considered to represent different points on a spectrum of severity and extent of tissue destruction.[50] NUG involves isolated areas of soft tissue ulceration and necrosis limited to interdental gingival papillae. NUP presents all the features of NUG, but also includes rapid destruction of the periodontal attachment and alveolar bone, deep seated pain, and tooth mobility. NUS appears when tissue destruction and necrosis extend beyond periodontal tissues to affect adjacent areas such as the palate. The intense pain, spontaneous bleeding, and fetid odor associated with all of these lesions often drive patients to seek dental care. Patients may respond to an aggressive course of débridement involving scaling and root planing, irrigation of affected tissues with a 10% povidone-iodine solution (which also has a topical anesthetic effect), systemic antibiotics effective against both aerobic and anaerobic bacteria (e.g., metronidazole, clindamycin), twice daily rinses with chlorhexidine, and reinforcement of oral hygiene practices. However, recurrence is common and refractory lesions may require further treatment by a specialist.

Lymphadenopathy. Lymphadenopathy, or swollen lymph glands, is an almost invariant feature of HIV infection. Lymphadenopathy may be present at any time throughout the course of infection. Manual palpation of the superficial lymph nodes of the neck will reveal the presence of cervical lymphadenopathy during the extraoral clinical examination.

Aphthous Ulcers. Aphthouslike ulcerations may develop during the course of HIV infection. These recurrent ulcers usually appear as solitary lesions that persist and may be associated with ulcers of the esophagus and pharynx. Unlike HSV lesions, aphthous ulcers are confined to movable mucosa (e.g., buccal mucosa, floor of mouth). The application of topical corticosteroids can hasten healing in many instances; however, systemic corticosteroid therapy may be required for lesions resistant to topical treatment.

Salivary-Gland Disease. Some HIV-infected individuals complain of xerostomia, with or without enlargement of parotid and minor salivary glands, during the early stage of infection. Although the cause of this salivary-gland disease is unclear, the xerostomia and glandular swelling both may be managed by conventional means and antiretroviral therapy.

Tuberculosis. Tuberculosis (TB) is a highly contagious granulomatous disease caused by the slow-growing, rod-shaped, acid-fast bacillus *Mycobacterium tuberculosis*. This bacillus is transmitted via inhalation of respiratory droplets and aerosols (e.g., sputum and saliva), ingestion, or direct inoculation. Initial infection usually occurs in the lungs or intestines, depending on the route of transmission. However, dissemination to other regions such as the bones, meninges, kidneys, skin, lymph nodes, and oral structures may occur. Unless aggressively treated with multidrug chemotherapy, the unhealed bacterial lesions *(tubercles)* persist indefinitely within walled-off regions of the lungs and body tissues. *Caseation* (cheeselike) *necrosis* results as dead cells accumulate in the center of the tubercles. These caseous lesions may eventually heal by fibrosis and calcification to form radiodense *Ghon complexes* detectable upon radiographic evaluation of the lungs. However, in a small percentage of infected individuals, the lesions do not heal, and they release infectious particles that disseminate throughout the body to seed other organs *(miliary tuberculosis).*

Accurate diagnosis of TB is a common and serious problem because the infection may not be suspected or recognized. Furthermore, symptoms (e.g., fatigue, cough, excessive weight loss, low-grade fever, recurrent night sweats) resemble those of other infectious diseases, such as HIV. Oral lesions, which occur rarely and are usually secondary to pulmonary involvement, include tuberculosis gingivitis, tuberculosis of the lips, and persistent exudative ulcers of the tongue. Because these oral lesions may mimic squamous cell carcinoma, differential diagnosis should include one of several tests for TB: the skin test (PPD), sputum culture, and chest radiograph.

TB remains one of the most widespread and persistent human transmissible infections worldwide. Historically, the incidence of TB in developed countries has decreased because of effective chemotherapeutic agents and isolation procedures; however, TB remains a major cause of disease and death in underdeveloped and developing third-world countries. Unfortunately, the recent emergence of drug-resistant strains of *Mycobacterium tuberculosis* coupled with increasing poverty, homelessness, crowding, and rising numbers of persons with AIDS has led to the *resurgence of TB as a significant public health problem in this country.* Older persons who were infected in the 1920s and 1930s and continued to harbor persistent bacillus represent an important and growing source of TB. These individuals may experience a reactivation of their disease with deterioration of their immune response with aging.

The TB-infected patient represents a significant occupational hazard for dental personnel. Open lesions and infected sputum and saliva are highly contagious. Moreover, the outer lipid coating ("spore") of the bacillus allows the organism to survive in dried fluids for extended periods of time and renders it resistant to many germicidal agents. Therefore, *dental personnel must adhere to proper IC measures, which include personal protective barriers (e.g., eyewear, mask, and gloves) during patient treatment and the appropriate use of tuberculocidal disinfectants and sterilants* (see Chapter 8).

Gonorrhea. The bacterium *Neisseria gonorrhoeae*, a gram-negative diplococci, is the etiologic agent for gonorrhea, one of the most prevalent sexually transmitted diseases today. This organism is spread by direct contact with infected mucosal lesions of the urogenital tract, eyes, and oral cavity. Following an incubation period of 2 to 21 days, infected individuals may experience purulent urethral or vaginal discharge and pharyngitis. Rare oral lesions appear as patchy edema and erythema of the tonsillar regions and uvula, and as vesicles at the site of primary contact. Diagnosis is made by culture of the organism or microscopic examination of the discharge. Although this infection is effectively treated with penicillin, the emergence of penicillin-resistant strains of gonorrhea has heightened the awareness of gonorrhea as a serious public health threat.

Syphilis. Caused by the bacteria *Treponema pallidum*, syphilis may be acquired congenitally or through direct contact with infected mucous membranes of the oral, genital, and anorectal regions. Syphilis is characterized by three stages. Primary syphilis of the oral cavity appears as a hard ulcer (chancre) of the lip, tongue, gingiva, or palate. Unless treated with an antibiotic such as penicillin, primary syphilis may progress to secondary syphilis. A red maculopapular rash on the body, highly infectious erythematous patches on mucous membranes, bone defects, and recurrences characterize the secondary form. Continued progression can lead to tertiary syphilis with neurologic or cardiovascular involvement. Lesions may present intraorally as *gummas,* granulomatous lesions on the palate or tongue, which may erode and/or affect the central nervous system (CNS). Although individuals in the tertiary stage are not infectious, untreated individuals in the primary and secondary stages are highly contagious.

In summary, dental professionals must be aware of the signs and symptoms of infectious diseases and their routes of transmission for the proper evaluation, diagnosis, and management of patients. *Because these contagious diseases may be spread from the infected patient to the dental team and to other patients, meticulous attention to IC practices is essential.*

Allergies or Medications. The patient interview should include a discussion of any allergies or medications noted on the medical history form. Sometimes patients report that they are "sensitive" or allergic to local anesthetic. They often refer to having had a reaction after the injection of "Novocaine." These alleged reactions are often attributable to excessive anesthetic deposited over too short a time, or, more likely, to an intravascular deposition. However, patients may be allergic to preservatives in topical and injectable local anesthetics. Therefore *when any patient relays a history of "sensitivity" from injected dental anesthetic, the dentist must believe the patient until further investigation* (be it verbal questions and answers, or allergic testing in a sophisticated life-support environment) *disproves the patient's belief of an allergy.* These precautions are necessary because *anaphylactic shock following an allergic reaction can be immediate and life threatening.*

Medications used by the patient also can affect diagnosis and treatment. Certain medications can modify normal salivary flow and composition, alter normal appearance of oral soft tissues, or affect the metabolism and/or therapeutic effect of other pharmacologic agents. For example, *tricyclic antidepressants* may render patients extremely sensitive to epinephrine, antiepileptic agents may cause gingival enlargement, and antibiotics may reduce the efficacy of oral contraceptives.

Systemic Diseases and Cardiac Abnormalities. The presence of systemic diseases or cardiac abnormalities may require that treatment be altered (see Chapter 10). Of special note are patients with certain heart disorders. The manipulation of mucosal surfaces during dental procedures or even the patient's home care procedures may release bloodborne bacteria that lodge on abnormal or damaged heart valves or in the filial tissues, possibly resulting in increased risk of bacterial endocarditis. Patients with cardiac conditions such as valvular defects or heart murmurs may be at an increased risk of acquiring bacterial endocarditis following surgical and dental procedures. Patients who have used the "fen-phen" combination of appetite suppressants fenfluramine and phentermine for weight loss also are susceptible to valvular heart disease. Patients at risk for bacterial endocarditis should be treated prophylactically with an appropriate antibiotic before dental treatment. The reader is referred to the latest recommendations by the American Heart Association for information regarding antibiotic-dosing regimens, specific cardiac conditions for which endocarditis prophylaxis is recommended, and the dental procedures requiring coverage.[17] As a screening test for underlying diseases such as hypertension, the patient's pulse and blood pressure should be taken and recorded. This information provides a baseline for monitoring changes in the patient's health over time and for managing medical emergencies. High blood pressure, a sign of hypertension, is defined as having systolic blood pressure of at least 140 mm Hg or diastolic blood pressure of at least 90 mm Hg. Two or more blood pressure readings should be taken during the initial patient visit to determine the average blood pressure for that patient. A blood pressure reading is recommended at each subsequent visit before initiating an invasive dental procedure, including restorative treatment and prophylaxis. If any patient presents with a systolic blood pressure exceeding 180 mm Hg and/or diastolic blood pressure exceeding 110 mm Hg, *routine dental treatment should be deferred until acceptable levels are achieved, and the patient should be referred for medical evaluation.*[26]

Physiologic Changes Associated With Aging. With the lengthening life span and increased retention of teeth by older patients, dentists are treating more *geriatric patients* in their practices. Americans 65 years of age or older represented 13 percent of the total population in the United States in 1995.[2] By 2013, this number is expected to increase to 30 percent, largely because of the "graying" of the baby boom generation.[2] In general, patients (especially women) are living longer, are more highly educated, enjoy greater financial independence, and are expected to spend a greater proportion of their income on health care compared to their younger counterparts.[2]

It is important to thoroughly understand the medical and dental background of older patients. The geriatric population can experience significant age-related changes in behavior and diet, as well as in oral and systemic health. Older persons generally have more medical, physical, and mental problems than their younger counterparts. The majority of older persons have at least one chronic disease (e.g., heart disease, renal dysfunction), and many suffer from two or more serious, oftentimes interrelated diseases.[8] Many older persons have some impairment that limits their ability to perform daily activities such as tooth brushing due to mental disorders (e.g., depression, Alzheimer's disease) and physical ailments (e.g., arthritis).

Prescription medication use is rampant among the older adult population, with nearly 50% of persons aged 75 years or older taking at least two medications each day.[8] Several medications and illnesses can alter oral physiology, oral hygiene, and dental health, necessitating changes in treatment. For example, *xerostomia*, or reduced salivary flow, is a significant potential side effect of over 200 prescription medications, including anticholinergic, adrenergic-blocking, antipsychotic, antihistamine, diuretic, and antihypertensive medications.[3] Xerostomic medications may result in increased caries incidence, mucosal alterations, and plaque retention. The use of salivary stimulants such as sugar-free candy drops, artificial saliva, or pilocarpine in more serious cases, along with lowering drug dosage, may lessen or relieve this symptom. Additional considerations include the limited use of vasoconstrictors in patients with advanced cardiovascular disease, reduced dosages of diazepam to prevent oversedation due to poor renal/hepatic clearance with aging, and interactions between drugs prescribed for dental purposes and the patient's other medications (e.g., epinephrine, antidepressants).

Several normal physiologic changes may occur in older patients[7] and should not be mistaken for pathologic conditions. For example, the skin and blood vessels lose their elasticity because of degeneration of the elastic connective tissue and delayed healing following surgical procedures may result. Bones become more brittle and easily broken with advancing age. Sensory impairment may lead to hearing loss, visual changes, and alterations in taste and smell. Dental and mucosal changes also may be associated with the aging process. A tooth can change shape because of many years of attrition, abrasion, and wear of proximal surfaces. Variations in pulpal anatomy, physiology, and color changes due to extrinsic staining can occur with age and may lead to increased brittleness of the teeth. A continuous thickening of the cementum is frequently noted and is most pronounced in the apical regions. The gingivae can become edematous and friable, with a loss of stippling, and recede. Salivary flow rate may decrease with advanced age as a result of deposition of fatty and fibrous tissues within salivary glands.[57] The diminished salivary flow results in loss of elasticity of the oral mucosa and increased caries rate. An understanding that these physiologic or metabolic changes are not pathologic is essential for proper operative treatment planning for the geriatric patient.

Of primary importance in planning dental therapy is the biologic or physiologic age of the older patient, not the chronologic age. Factors such as genetic predisposition, physical or mental capabilities, and the presence of chronic disease may make an individual's biologic age older or younger than his or her chronologic age. Consideration of these factors in the treatment plan is crucial for the long-term success of any dental treatment of the older patient.

SOCIOLOGIC AND PSYCHOLOGIC REVIEW

During initial visits the clinician should ascertain the patient's attitudes, priorities, expectations, and motivations toward dental care. Attitudinal information combined with assessment of the patient's dental appreciation, educability, habits, parental history, occupation, and financial situation can indicate the patient's commitment to dental care. This commitment contributes to the overall success of dental treatment. As with every facet of patient assessment and examination, it is essential to maintain and update records of discussions and clinical findings.

During this portion of the pretreatment assessment, the dentist must begin to explore patient's preferences for dental care. The results of this exploration will affect the dentist's treatment recommendations.

DENTAL HISTORY

The dental history consists of reviewing previous dental experiences and current dental problems. Review of the dental history reveals information about past dental problems and treatment. Frequency of dental care and perceptions of that care may be indications of the patient's future behavior. Obviously, if a patient has difficulty tolerating certain types of procedures or has encountered problems with previous dental care, an alteration of the treatment or environment may help avoid future complications. Also, this discussion may lead to identification of other problems such as areas of food impaction, inability to floss, areas of pain, and broken restorations and/or tooth structure. It is critical to understand past experiences to provide optimal care in the future.

Finally, it is important to know the date and type of available radiographs to ascertain the need for additional radiographs and minimize the patient's exposure to unnecessary ionizing radiation. The FDA guidelines[42] help direct the type and frequency of radiographs needed according to patient condition and risk factors (Table 9-2).

RISK ASSESSMENT

Few diseases known to man are caused by a single factor. Instead most diseases have been shown to be associated with numerous behavioral/sociodemographic, physical/environmental, microbiologic, or host factors. In addition, every patient possesses a different set of *risk factors* and as such presents a challenge to determine the likelihood that disease is present or will occur in the future. For example, patients who possess several of the

TABLE 9-2 | Guidelines for Prescribing Dental Radiographs for Dentate Adults

NEW PATIENTS	RECALL PATIENTS		
ALL NEW PATIENTS TO ASSESS DENTAL DISEASES	CLINICAL CARIES OR HIGH-RISK FACTORS FOR CARIES*	NO CLINICAL CARIES AND NO HIGH-RISK FACTORS FOR CARIES*	PERIODONTAL DISEASE OR A HISTORY OF PERIODONTAL TREATMENT
Individualized radiographic examination consisting of posterior bitewings and selected periapicals; a full-mouth intraoral radiographic examination is appropriate when the patient has clinical evidence of generalized dental disease or a history of extensive dental treatment	Posterior bitewing examination at 12- to 18-month intervals	Posterior bitewing examination at 24- to 36-month intervals	Individualized radiographic examination consisting of selected periapical and/or bitewing radiographs for areas where periodontal disease (other than nonspecific gingivitis) can be demonstrated clinically

*See Table 9-3 for caries risk factors.

TABLE 9-3 | Risk Factors for Caries

FACTORS	HIGH-RISK CHARACTERISTICS
NON-ORAL	
Age	Less than 18 or more than 65 years old
Socioeconomic status	Lower status
Medical condition	Reduced salivation
Medications	Reduced salivation
Fluoride history	Lack of fluoride during tooth development
Dietary habits	High intake of refined carbohydrates; tobacco and alcohol use
Genetic predisposition	Family history of disease
General health	Debilitation and decreased ability to give self-care
ORAL	
Tooth anatomy and composition	Development fissures and low fluoride content
Oral flora/plaque	High levels of *mutans streptococci* (see Chapter 3)
Previous infections and restorations	History of extensive restoration
Restorations	Defective restorations
Oral hygiene (e.g., skills, knowledge, motivation)	Poor oral hygiene

risk factors shown in Table 9-3 should be considered at high risk for dental caries. This assessment will then be used to guide treatment. A patient at high risk for dental caries should receive aggressive intervention to remove or alter as many risk factors as possible. Alternatively, regular monitoring and reassessment of the condition may be appropriate for a patient at low risk for dental caries.

Risk assessment is a relatively young science in the health care professions. Unfortunately no valid standardized means of determining caries risk are available. Historically dentists have relied on their knowledge of the disease process in combination with their experiences and intuition to estimate the risk levels for their patients. To properly prescribe and determine appropriate preventive and therapeutic strategies, the dentist must consider the patient's overall risk status in the context of the current level of understanding of both disease progression and management options. Though such understanding is not yet perfected, certain conditions place patients at a higher risk for dental disease. Knowing this, dentists should try to identify and assess risk factors for dental disease during the initial oral examination and subsequent patient appointments.

EXAMINATION AND DIAGNOSIS

This section describes the examination and diagnosis of problems with orofacial soft tissues, teeth, restorations, periodontium, and occlusion. Special considerations for evaluating the patient presenting with pain also are reviewed. In practice, each tooth is evaluated individually by using a combination of clinical and radiographic examinations and appropriate adjunctive tests. However, for the purpose of presentation, the clinical examination, radiographic survey, and use of adjunctive diagnostic aids are discussed separately.

GENERAL CONSIDERATIONS

Clinical *examination* is the "hands-on" process of observing both normal and abnormal conditions. *Diagnosis* is a determination and judgment of variations from normal. During the clinical examination the dentist must be keenly sensitive to subtle signs, symptoms, and variations from normal to detect pathologic conditions and etiologic factors. Meticulous attention to detail generates a base of information for diagnosing the patient's general physical health and specific dental problems.

As alluded to in the previous section on IC, *universal IC measures* should be adhered to throughout the examination procedure. Certainly before any "hands-on" examination, standard precautions must be taken to avoid the transmission of disease. These precautions include the sterilization/disinfection of all instruments, supplies, and operatory surfaces and the use of barrier techniques such as gloves, masks, protective eyewear, and gowns, consistent with prevailing standards (see Chapter 8).

While following accepted barrier techniques, the initial step in the clinical examination includes an observation of the patient's general physical health and oral condition to determine the presence of potentially harmful *communicable diseases* (see Plate 9-1 and Table 9-1). However, as emphasized in Chapter 8, some individual disease carriers such as those infected with HIV or HBV may not be identified during medical review and clinical examination. This underscores the necessity for routine and universal IC for all dental patients.

An additional preliminary consideration is a cursory examination of the general tooth alignment and occlusal relationship because this information is helpful in the subsequent detailed examination.

Charting and Records. The oral health record should include the following categories of information: identification data, which includes all of the patient personal information such as telephone number, whom to contact in case of emergency, and other relevant data; medical history, which includes the medical history form and the dentist's interpretation and discussion of that information; dental history; clinical examination; diagnosis; treatment planning; documentation of informed consent; progress notes; and completion notes.[15]

Although various formats are available for recording a patient's dental condition, an acceptable *charting system* should conform to certain standards.[1] The chart should be: (1) *uncomplicated* (easily understood by the dentist and staff and be an effective and accurate means of recording dental conditions); (2) *comprehensive* (noting all dental conditions, both normal and abnormal, and a detailed representation of location, nature, and size of all restorations); (3) *accessible* (part of the permanent patient record and easily accessible for referencing during treatment or recall appointments); and (4) *current* (allowing for continual updating as treatment is rendered and as dental or medical conditions change). If these guidelines are followed, the findings of a thorough and systematic examination can be maintained for each patient.

Normal and abnormal clinical and radiographic findings are noted on a detailed chart as a permanent part of the patient's record. For example, Fig. 9-2 displays the clinical and radiographic findings as recorded in an electronic patient record. The growing use of computers in the dental office is providing a range of new and comprehensive technologies. Among these is the electronic patient record. Although issues related to patient confidentiality are a continuing concern, it is expected that the majority of practices in the United States will soon employ electronic patient records instead of the traditional paper form. Early versions of the electronic records have developed the means by which digital radiography and intraoral photographs can be incorporated into the chart as well. A growing number of practitioners are using intraoral photographs to both supplement routine dental charting and provide an educational tool for patients.

The exact location and condition of all teeth, restorations, defects and caries, and soft and hard tissues are necessary for many reasons, including:

- *Proper care*—Thorough charting of existing conditions provides basic information for an accurate, comprehensive treatment plan.
- *Third-party communication*—Accurate records of the patient's conditions are useful in communicating with third-party payment agencies.
- *Practice audits and quality assessment*—Dental charts and records are the foundation of many quality assurance programs because the content, completeness, and accuracy of records are used as measures of the care provided.
- *Legal proceedings*—The dental record is considered legal, admissible evidence in arbitration of contended negligence or malpractice.
- *Forensic uses*—In many instances, the dental record is the only means of identifying a deceased person.

Tooth Denotation System. To expedite the designation of teeth during examination and charting, a denotation system is used. Several denotation systems are in use, but the one used in this text is the *universal system.* In this system, the teeth are numbered from 1 to 32 starting with the maxillary right third molar and continuing around the arch to the left third molar, then continuing with the mandibular left third molar as No. 17 and ending with the right third molar as No. 32.

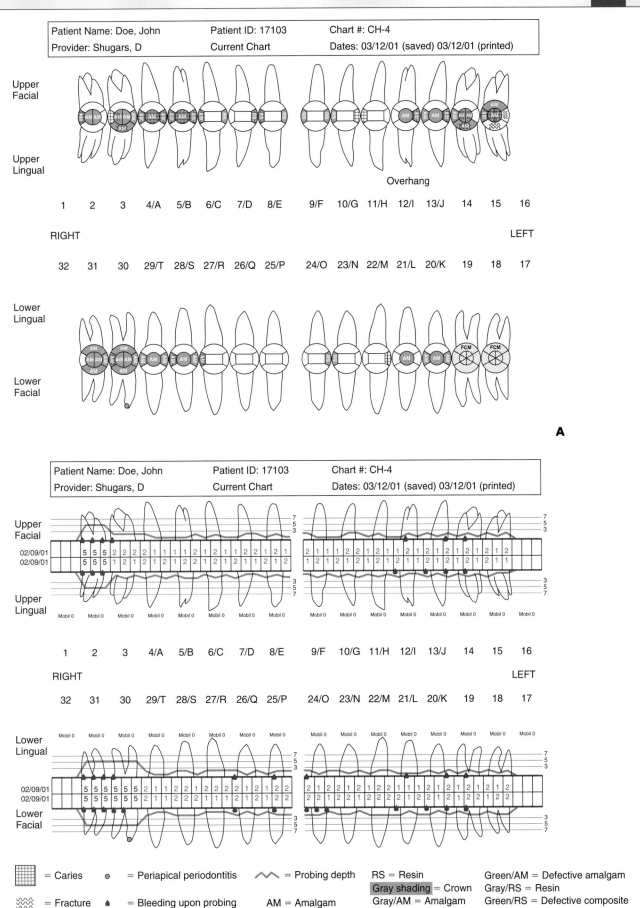

FIG. 9-2 A, An appropriate restorative charting system designates location, type, and extent of existing restorations and presence of disease and defects, all of which become part of the permanent patient record. The results of the periodontal examination are also included in the record.

Continued

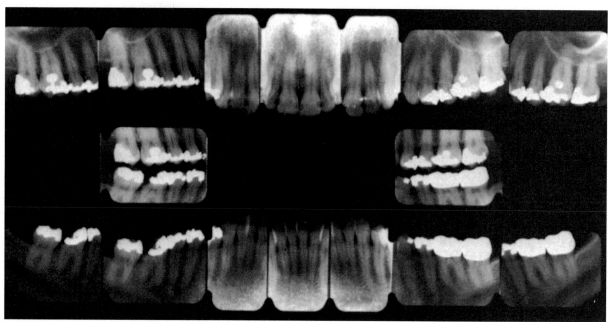

B

TREATMENT PLAN

Group	Planned	Code	Tooth	Surface	Description	Fees	Accepted
1	02/09/01	0150			Comprehensive Oral Evaluation	63.00	Yes
1	02/09/01	0210			Full Series	75.00	Yes
1	02/09/01	4341		LR	Perio Root Planing per Quad	168.00	Yes
1	02/09/01	4341		UR	Perio Root Planning per Quad	168.00	Yes
1	02/09/01	4249		LR	Crown Lengthening	630.00	Yes
1	02/09/01	7286			Biopsy of Oral Tissue	133.00	Yes
1	02/09/01	1110			Cleaning Adult	43.00	Yes
1	02/09/01	1204			Topical Application of Fluoride	19.00	Yes
1	02/09/01	3330			Root Canal (3 canals)	675.00	Yes
2	02/09/01	2950	30		Crown Build-up	139.00	Yes
2	02/09/01	2330	27	D	Tooth Colored Resin	75.00	Yes
2	02/09/01	2160	28	MOD	Amalgam	109.00	Yes
2	02/09/01	2330	6	D	Tooth Colored Resin	75.00	Yes
2	02/09/01	2330	7	M	Tooth Colored Resin	75.00	Yes
2	02/09/01	2330	8	D	Tooth Colored Resin	75.00	Yes
2	02/09/01	2330	10	D	Tooth Colored Resin	75.00	Yes
2	02/09/01	2330	11	M	Tooth Colored Resin	75.00	Yes
2	02/09/01	2330	22	D	Tooth Colored Resin	75.00	Yes
3	02/09/01	2790	2		Cast Crown High Noble Metal	664.00	Yes
3	02/09/01	2643	3	MOL	Porcelain Onlay 3 Surfaces	580.00	Yes
3	02/09/01	2630	4	MOD	Porcelain Inlay 3 Surfaces	520.00	Yes
3	02/09/01	2630	5	MOD	Porcelain Inlay 3 Surfaces	520.00	Yes
3	02/09/01	2620	12	DO	Porcelain Inlay 2 Surfaces	433.00	Yes
3	02/09/01	2630	13	MOD	Porcelain Inlay 3 Surfaces	520.00	Yes
3	02/09/01	2160	14	MOL	Amalgam	109.00	Yes
3	02/09/01	2790	15		Cast Crown High Noble Metal	664.00	Yes
3	02/09/01	2750	30		Crown Porcelain Fused to Metal	721.00	Yes
					TOTALS:	**7,478.00**	

C

FIG. **9-2, cont'd** **B,** Radiographic findings obtained from this full-mouth series are correlated with the findings of the clinical examination and noted in the patient's record. Most electronic patient records provide a system for coding various clinical conditions. **C,** The results of the medical history, interview, and clinical examination, along with an assessment of the patient's treatment preferences, are used to generate a properly sequenced treatment plan.

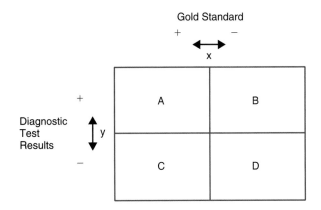

FIG. 9-4 Contingency table for interpretation of diagnostic tests.

Cell A = true positives
Cell B = false positives
Cell C = false negatives
Cell D = true negatives
Sensitivity = A/A + C
Specificity = D/B + D
Positive predictive value = A/A + B
Prevalence = A/A + B + C + D

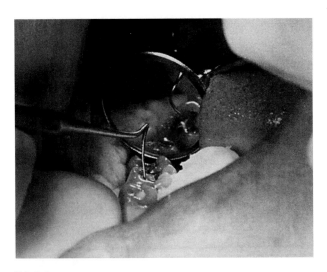

FIG. 9-3 An accurate clinical examination requires a clean, dry, well-illuminated mouth. Cotton rolls are placed in the vestibular space and under the tongue to maintain dryness and enhance visibility.

Preparation for Clinical Examination. A chairside assistant familiar with the terminology, denotation system, and charting procedure can survey and record the teeth and existing restorations to save chair time for the dentist. Subsequently, the dentist will perform the examination, confirm the charting, make a diagnosis, and develop the treatment plan. The clinical examination is performed systematically in a clean, dry, well-illuminated mouth. Proper instruments including a mirror, explorer, and periodontal probe are required. A routine for charting should be established such as starting in the upper right quadrant with the most posterior tooth and progressing around the maxillary and mandibular arches. An accurate examination can occur only when the teeth are clean and dry. This may require initial scaling, flossing, and a toothbrushing prophylaxis before final clinical examination of the teeth. A cotton roll in the vestibular space and another under the tongue will maintain dryness and improve vision (Fig. 9-3). Dental floss is useful in determining overhanging restorations, improper contours, and open contacts.

Interpretation and Use of Diagnostic Tests. The diagnostic effort of health professionals has been enhanced by the use of principles adopted from the discipline of *clinical epidemiology.* This analytic approach is a means of improving the interpretation of diagnostic tests. It relies on a "2 × 2" contingency table (Fig. 9-4). These tables are created from data derived from clinical studies. Such studies compare the results of a diagnostic test with those obtained from a "gold standard" (knowledge of the actual condition) to determine how well the test diagnoses the "true" condition. The results

of the diagnostic tests, positive or negative, are shown across the rows of the table, and the results of a gold standard or the "truth" are displayed in the columns. Thus, cell A of the table contains those cases that the test identifies as being positive (or diseased) and confirmed by the gold standard. These cases are termed *true positives.* Cell B contains all cases for which there is a positive finding from the diagnostic test but a negative finding with the gold standard. This cell denotes *false positives.* Cell C includes those cases identified by the diagnostic test as not being diseased but found by the gold standard to be diseased. Findings in this cell are termed *false negatives.* The final cell, cell D, includes *true negatives.* In cell D the diagnostic test accurately identifies the nondiseased cases that are truly negative as confirmed by the gold standard. Thus, an ideal diagnostic test would result in most cases being assigned to cells A or D with few or no false positives (cell B) and false negatives (cell C).

Once the basics of this table are understood, several additional features can be put to good use by the diagnostician. The first concept is *test sensitivity.* The sensitivity of a test is calculated as the number of true positives (A) divided by the number of total positive cases (A + C). This term indicates the proportion of those with disease in a population that are identified positively by the test. In contrast, *test specificity* is the proportion of those without disease properly classified by the diagnostic test and is the ratio of true negatives (D) to all negatives (B + D). Therefore, sensitivity and specificity relate to the proportion of cases in a population, diseased or not, that are predicted accurately by the diagnostic test. In contrast, the *positive predictive value* of a test is calculated by dividing the true positives (A) by all cases tested as positive by the diagnostic test (A + B). The positive predictive value denotes the proportion of cases that test positive and are in fact diseased.

Using these concepts, a clinician knows that if a diagnostic test has a high positive predictive value, there is a greater likelihood that a patient with a positive test does have the disease. Thus, if there is a positive result using a test with a high positive predictive value, the clinician has greater assurance that the diagnosed condition does actually exist. A test with low sensitivity indicates that there is a high probability that many of the cases with negative results will possess the disease and go undiagnosed (C). Finally, tests with high specificity suggest that patients without the disease are highly likely to test negative.

These concepts are widely used in medical practice. Although many of the necessary studies have not been conducted to develop these probabilities for dental conditions, interest in the use of clinical epidemiology in the dental profession has been growing. In the future, more studies will be conducted to provide this information for clinicians, and one should be prepared to take advantage of their use.

EXAMINATION OF OROFACIAL SOFT TISSUES

The reader is again referred to Plate 9-1 for a review of oral manifestations of contagious diseases and to Table 9-1 for clinical symptoms.

As with the other aspects of the clinical examination, soft tissue evaluation requires a systematic approach. Begin by examining the submandibular glands and cervical nodes for abnormalities in size, texture, mobility, and sensitivity to palpation. Then, palpate the masticatory muscles for pain or tenderness. Next, start in one area of the mouth and follow a routine pattern of visual examination and palpation of the cheeks, vestibules, mucosa, lips, lingual and facial alveolar mucosa, palate, tonsillar areas, tongue, and floor of the mouth. A thorough evaluation of all these structures is necessary before operative care is initiated. It is ill advised to plan restorative procedures for a patient while a life-threatening disease process goes undiagnosed because a thorough examination was not conducted.

EXAMINATION OF TEETH AND RESTORATIONS

Clinical Examination for Caries. *Dental caries* is diagnosed by one or all of the following: (1) visual changes in tooth surface texture or color, (2) tactile sensation when an explorer is used judiciously, (3) radiographs, and (4) transillumination.[31] Several technologies have emerged that show promising results for the clinical diagnosis of caries. These include electrical conductance[5] and laser fluorescence.[21] Chapter 3 has a further discussion of available tests for caries detection. The examination is aided by knowledge of the likelihood of overall caries risk (see Table 9-3), and patterns of susceptibility. For example, the patient's dental history, oral hygiene,

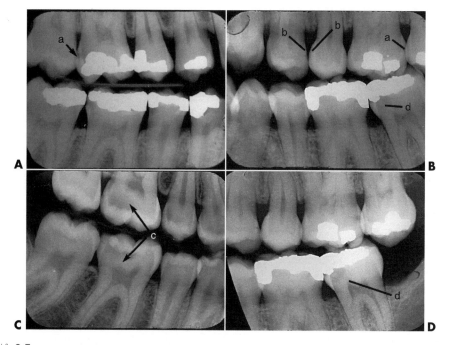

FIG. 9-5 Caries can be diagnosed radiographically as translucencies in the enamel or dentin. **A** and **B,** Proximal caries tends to occur bilaterally *(a)* and on adjacent surfaces *(b).* **C,** Occlusal caries *(c).* **D,** Recurrent caries gingival to an existing restoration *(d).* This same recurrent caries *(d)* is also shown in **B.**

diet, and age may suggest a certain pattern of caries activity. Caries also tends to occur bilaterally and on adjacent proximal surfaces (Fig. 9-5, *A* and *B*). If caries is found on the occlusal surface and a proximal surface in one tooth on one side of the arch, then the chances are increased that it will occur in the same locations on the opposite side. If caries is found on the proximal surface of one tooth, then the adjacent tooth's proximal surface also is suspect. In the clinical examination for caries, every accessible surface of each tooth must be inspected for localized changes in color, texture, and translucency.

Caries is most prevalent in the *faulty pits and fissures of the occlusal surfaces* where the developmental lobes of the posterior teeth failed to coalesce, partially or completely (Fig. 9-6, *B*). It is important to remember the distinction between primary occlusal grooves/fossae and occlusal fissures/pits. *Primary occlusal grooves/fossae* are smooth "valley/saucer" landmarks indicating the region of complete coalescence of developmental lobes. Normally, such *grooves/fossae are not susceptible to caries* because they are not niches for plaque (and bacteria), and furthermore are frequently cleansed by the rubbing action of food during mastication. Conversely, occlusal fis-

sure and pits are deep, tight, crevices/holes in enamel where the lobes failed to coalesce, partially or completely (see Fig. 2-12). Fissures and pits are detected visually.

Historically, sharp explorers have been used to diagnose fissure caries. However, numerous studies have found that use of an explorer for this purpose did not increase diagnostic validity compared to visual inspection alone.[38,40,51] Moreover, use of the dental explorer for this purpose was found to fracture enamel and serve as a source for transferring pathogenetic bacteria among various teeth.[19,58] Use of an explorer in diagnosing fissure caries is strongly discouraged.

An occlusal surface is examined visually and radiographically.[5,36] The visual examination is conducted in a dry, well-illuminated field. Through direct vision and reflecting light through the occlusal surface of the tooth, the occlusal surface is diagnosed as diseased if there is chalkiness or apparent softening/cavitation of tooth structure forming the fissure/pit or brown gray discoloration radiating peripherally from the fissure/pit. Radiographic diagnosis should be made from a bitewing radiograph when radiolucency is apparent beneath the occlusal enamel surface emanating from the

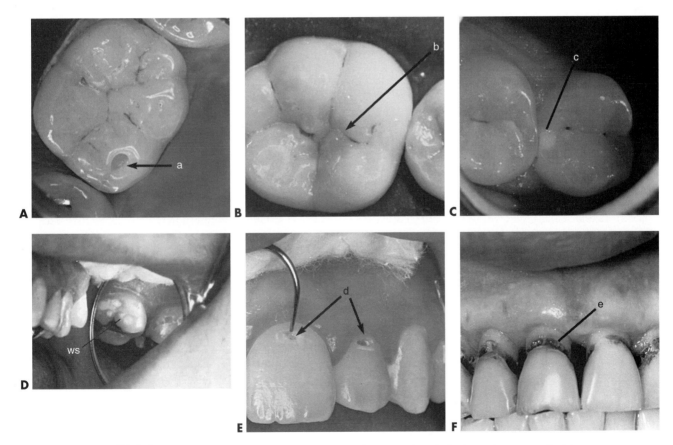

FIG. **9-6** Caries can be diagnosed clinically by careful inspection. **A,** Carious pit on cusp tip *(a)*. **B,** Loss of translucency and change in color of occlusal enamel *(b)* due to a carious fissure. **C,** White chalky appearance or shadow under marginal ridge *(c)*. **D,** Incipient smooth-surface carious lesion, or a white spot *(ws)*, has intact surface. **E,** Smooth-surface caries can appear white or dark, depending on the degree of extrinsic staining *(d)*. **F,** Root-surface caries *(e)*.

dental enamel junction. In contrast, a nondiseased occlusal surface will have either grooves or fossae that have shallow tight fissures, which exhibit superficial staining with no radiographic evidence of caries. The superficial staining is extrinsic and occurs over several years of oral exposure in a person with low caries risk. The radiographic detection of occlusal carious lesions in otherwise clinically sound teeth has been reported.[34] Thus careful inspection of high quality bitewing radiographs is critically important.

Precarious or carious pits are occasionally present on *cusp tips* (see Figs. 9-6, *A*, and 17-110). Typically these are the result of developmental enamel defects. *Carious pits and fissures* also occur on the *occlusal two thirds of the facial or lingual surface of the posterior teeth* and on the *lingual surface of maxillary incisors* (see Caries Diagnosis in Chapter 3 for the criteria for the diagnosis of caries in pits and fissures). Occlusal enamel can be evaluated for loss of translucency and change in color, which are characteristic of caries (see Fig. 9-6, *B*). This change in color can be dark gray and should not be confused with the noncarious fissures/pits that often become merely stained over time.

Proximal surface caries, one form of *smooth-surface caries,* is usually diagnosed radiographically (see Fig. 9-5, *A*). However, it also may be detected by careful visual examination either following tooth separation or through fiber-optic transillumination (FOTI).[31] When caries have invaded the proximal surface enamel and have demineralized the dentin, a white chalky appearance or a shadow under the marginal ridge may become evident (see Fig. 9-6, *C*). Careful probing with an explorer on the proximal surface may detect cavitation, which is defined as a break in the surface contour of enamel. The use of all examination methods is helpful in arriving at a final diagnosis.

Brown spots on intact, hard proximal surface enamel adjacent to and usually gingival to the contact area are often seen in older patients whose caries activity is low (see Fig. 9-15, *C*). These discolored areas are a result of extrinsic staining during earlier caries demineralizing episodes, each followed by a remineralization episode. Such a spot is no longer carious and is, in fact, usually more resistant to caries as a result of fluorhydroxyapatite formation. *Restorative treatment is not indicated.* These arrested lesions sometimes challenge the diagnosis because of faint radiographic evidence of the remineralized lesion.

Proximal-surface caries in anterior teeth may be identified by radiographic examination, visual inspection (transillumination optional), and/or probing with an explorer. *Transillumination* is accomplished by placing the mirror or light source on the lingual side of the anterior teeth and directing light through the teeth. Proximal surface caries, if other than incipient, appears as a dark area along the marginal ridge when light is directed through the tooth. In addition to transillumination, tactile exploration of the anterior teeth is appropriate to detect cavitation because the proximal surfaces generally are more visible and accessible than in the posterior regions. Small *incipient lesions* may be detectable only on the radiograph.

Another form of *smooth-surface caries* often occurs on the *facial and lingual surfaces* of the teeth, particularly in gingival areas that are less accessible for cleaning. The earliest clinical evidence of *incipient caries* on these surfaces is a *white spot* that is visually different from the adjacent translucent enamel and will partially or totally disappear from vision by wetting. Drying again will cause it to reappear (Fig. 9-6, *D*). This disappearing-reappearing phenomenon distinguishes the smooth-surface incipient carious lesion from the white spot resulting from nonhereditary enamel hypocalcification (see Clinical Examination for Additional Defects). Both types of white spots are undetectable tactilely because the surface is intact, smooth, and hard. For the carious white spot, preventive treatment discussed in Chapter 3 should be instituted to promote *remineralization* of the lesion.

The presence of several facial (or lingual) smooth-surface carious lesions within a patient's dentition suggests a high caries rate. In a caries-susceptible patient, the gingival third of the facial surfaces of maxillary posterior teeth and the gingival third of the facial and lingual surfaces of the mandibular posterior teeth should be evaluated carefully because these teeth are at a greater risk for caries. Advanced smooth-surface caries will exhibit discoloration and demineralization and will feel soft to penetration by the explorer. The discoloration can range from white to dark brown, with rapidly progressing caries usually being light in color (Fig. 9-6, *E*). With slowly progressing caries in a patient with low caries activity, darkening occurs over time because of extrinsic staining, and remineralization of decalcified tooth structure occasionally may harden the lesion. Such an *arrested lesion* may at times be rough, although cleanable (see Fig. 9-20), and a restoration is not indicated except for esthetics. The dentin in an arrested remineralized lesion is termed *eburnated* or *sclerotic*.

In patients with attachment loss, extra care must be taken to inspect for *root-surface caries*, carious lesions that occur on the cemental surfaces of teeth. A combination of cemental exposure, dietary changes, systemic diseases, and medications that affect the amount and character of saliva can predispose a patient, especially an older individual, to root-surface caries. It is not unusual to find caries at the cementoenamel junction (CEJ) or more apically on the cementum in older patients or in patients who have undergone periodontal surgery (Fig. 9-6, *F*). Early in its development, root caries appears as a well-defined discolored area adjacent to the gingival margin, typically near the CEJ. Root caries is found to be softer than the adjacent tissue and typically lesions spread laterally around the CEJ. Although no clinical criteria are universally accepted for the diagnosis of root caries, there is general agreement that softened cemental/dental tooth structure compared to the surrounding surface is characteristic.[24] Active root caries is detected by the presence of softening and cavitation.[33,49] Although root-surface caries may be detected on radiographic examination, a careful, thorough clinical examination is critical. One of the more difficult diagnostic challenges is a patient who has attachment loss with no gingival recession, thereby limiting accessibility for clinical inspection. These rapidly progressing lesions are best diagnosed using vertical bitewings. However, differentiation of a carious lesion from cervical burnout radiolucency is essential.[48]

Regardless of the location or type of carious lesions, a careful, thorough clinical examination is critical in the diagnosis of caries and for confirmation of radiographic evidence of the disease.

Clinical Examination of Amalgam Restorations. Evaluation of all restorations must be done systematically in a clean, dry, well-lighted field. Clinical evaluation of *amalgam restorations* requires visual observation, application of tactile sense with the explorer, use of dental floss, interpretation of radiographs, and knowledge of the probabilities that a given condition is sound or at risk for further breakdown.

At least 10 distinct conditions may be encountered when amalgam restorations are evaluated: (1) amalgam "blues," (2) proximal overhangs, (3) marginal ditching, (4) voids, (5) fracture lines, (6) lines indicating the interface between abutted restorations, (7) improper anatomic contours, (8) marginal ridge incompatibility, (9) improper proximal contacts, (10) recurrent caries, and (11) improper occlusal contacts.

Discolored areas or *amalgam blues* are often seen through the enamel in teeth that have amalgam restorations (Fig. 9-7). This bluish hue results either from the leaching of corrosion products of amalgam into the dentinal tubules or from the color of underlying amalgam as seen through translucent enamel. The latter occurs when the enamel has no dentin support, such as in undermined cusps, marginal ridges, and regions adjacent to proximal margins. When other aspects of the restoration are sound, amalgam blues are not indicative of caries, do not warrant classifying the restoration as defective, and require no further treatment. However, replacement of the restoration may be considered for elective improvement of esthetics or for areas under heavy functional stress that may require a cusp capping restoration to prevent possible tooth fracture.

Proximal overhangs are diagnosed visually, tactilely, and radiographically (Fig. 9-8). The amalgam-tooth junction is evaluated by moving the explorer back and forth across it. If the explorer stops at the junction and then moves outwardly onto the amalgam, an overhang is present. Overhangs also can be confirmed by the catching or tearing of dental floss. Such an overhang can be a plaque trap, provide an obstacle to good oral hygiene, and result in inflammation of the adjacent soft tissue. If causing problems, an overhang should be corrected, and this often indicates replacement of the defective restoration.

Marginal gap or *ditching* is the deterioration of the amalgam-tooth interface as a result of wear, fracture, or improper tooth preparation (Fig. 9-9, *A*). It can be diagnosed visually or by the explorer dropping into an opening as it crosses the margin. Shallow ditching less than 0.5 mm deep usually is not a reason for restoration replacement[37] because such a restoration usually looks worse than it really is. The eventual self-sealing property of amalgam allows the restoration to continue serving adequately if it can be satisfactorily cleaned and maintained. However, if the ditch is too deep to be cleaned or jeopardizes the integrity of the remaining restoration or tooth structure, the restoration should be replaced.[36] In addition, secondary caries is frequently found around

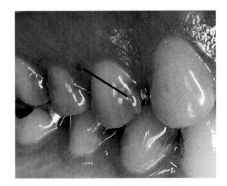

FIG. **9-7** Discoloration *(a)* by amalgam is a bluish hue (amalgam blues) seen through a thin shell of enamel of a tooth. In the absence of any other problems this condition does not indicate replacement.

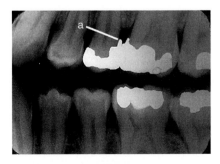

FIG. **9-8** Proximal overhang *(a)* can be diagnosed radiographically.

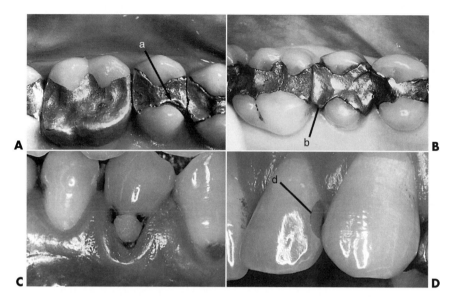

FIG. **9-9** Restorations can be diagnosed clinically as being defective by observing the following: **A**, Significant marginal ditching *(a)*. **B**, Improper contour *(b)*. **C**, Recurrent caries. **D**, Esthetically displeasing dark staining *(d)*.

marginal gaps near the gingival wall and thus warrants replacement.[46]

Voids other than ditching also occur at the margins of amalgam restorations. If the void is at least 0.3 mm deep and is located in the gingival third of the tooth crown, then the restoration is judged as defective and should be repaired or replaced. Accessible small voids in other marginal areas where the enamel is thicker may be corrected by recontouring or repairing with a small restoration.

A careful clinical examination will detect any *fracture line* across the occlusal portion of an amalgam restoration. A line that occurs in the isthmus region generally indicates fractured amalgam and thus a defective restoration that needs replacing (Fig. 9-10, *A*). However, care must be taken to evaluate correctly any such line, especially if it is in the midocclusal area because this may be an *interface line,* a manifestation of two abutted restorations, each accomplished at a separate appointment (see Fig. 9-10, *B*). If other aspects of the abutted restorations are satisfactory, replacement is not necessary.

Amalgam restorations should duplicate the *normal anatomic contours* of the teeth. Restorations that impinge on the soft tissue, have inadequate embrasure form or proximal contact, or prevent the use of dental floss should be classified as defective, indicating recontouring or replacement (see Fig. 9-9, *B*).

The marginal ridge portion of the amalgam restoration should be *compatible with the adjacent marginal ridge.* Both ridges should be at approximately the same level and display correct occlusal embrasure form for passage of food to the facial and lingual surfaces and for proper proximal contact area. If the marginal ridges are not compatible and are associated with poor tissue health, food impaction, or the inability of the patient to floss, the restoration is defective and should be recontoured or replaced.

The *proximal contact area* of an amalgam restoration should touch (a "closed" contact) the adjacent tooth at the proper contact level and with correct embrasure form. If the proximal contact of any restoration is suspected to be inadequate, it should be evaluated with dental floss and/or visually by trial angulations of a mouth mirror (held lingually when viewing from the facial aspect) to reflect light and actually see if there is a space at the contact ("open" contact). For this viewing, the contact must be free of saliva. If the contact is "open" and is associated with poor interproximal tissue health and/or food impaction, the restoration should be classified as defective and replaced. An "open" contact typically is annoying and even distressing to the patient; thus correcting the problem usually is a very appreciated service.

Recurrent caries at the marginal area of the restoration is detected visually, tactilely, or radiographically and is an indication for repair or replacement (see Figs. 9-5, *D*, and 9-9, *C*).

Inadequate occlusal contacts on an amalgam restoration may cause improper, deleterious occlusal functioning and/or undesirable tooth movement. Such a condition warrants correction or replacement.

Clinical Examination of Cast Restorations. Cast restorations should be evaluated clinically in the same manner as amalgam restorations. If any aspect of the restoration is not satisfactory or is causing tissue harm, it should be classified as defective and considered for recontouring, repair, or replacement.

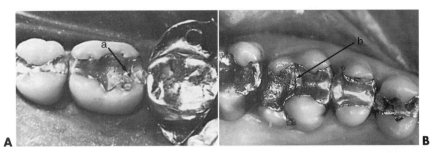

FIG. **9-10** Lines across the occlusal surface of an amalgam restoration may be: **A,** a fracture line *(a)* that indicates replacement, or **B,** an interface line *(b)* that indicates two restorations placed at separate appointments, which by itself is not sufficient indication for replacement.

Clinical Examination of Composite and Other Tooth-Colored Restorations. Tooth-colored restorations should be evaluated clinically in the same manner as amalgam and cast restorations. If there is an improper contour or proximal contact, an overhanging proximal margin, recurrent caries, or other condition that impairs cleaning, the restoration is considered defective. Corrective procedures include recontouring, polishing, repairing, or replacing.

One of the main concerns with anterior teeth is esthetics. If a tooth-colored restoration has dark marginal staining or is discolored to the extent that it is esthetically displeasing and the patient is unhappy with the appearance, the restoration should be judged defective (see Fig. 9-9, *D*). Marginal staining that is judged noncarious may be corrected by a small repair restoration along the margin. Occasionally the staining is superficial and can be removed by resurfacing.

Clinical Examination for Additional Defects. A thorough clinical examination occasionally discloses localized intact, hard white areas on the facial (Fig. 9-11) or lingual surfaces, or on cusp tips of the teeth. Generally these are *nonhereditary hypocalcified areas of enamel* that may have resulted from factors such as childhood fever, trauma, or fluorosis that occurred during the developmental stages of tooth formation. Another cause of hypocalcification is arrested and remineralized incipient caries, which leaves an opaque, discolored, and hard surface (see Fig. 9-15, *C*). When smooth and cleanable, such areas do not warrant restorative intervention unless they are esthetically offensive to the patient. These areas remain visible regardless if the tooth is wet or dry. Recall that in contrast, the smooth surface incipient carious lesion also is opaque white when dried. Therefore care must be exercised to distinguish the incipient carious lesion from nonhereditary developmental enamel hypocalcification.

Chemical erosion is the loss of surface tooth structure by chemical action in the continued presence of demineralizing agents (acids). The resulting defective surface is smooth. Although these agents are predominant causative factors, it is generally recognized that tooth-

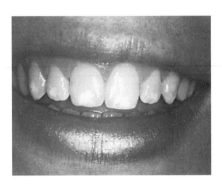

FIG. **9-11** Nonhereditary hypocalcified areas on facial surfaces. These areas may result from numerous factors but do not warrant restorative intervention unless they are esthetically offensive or cavitation is present.

brushing is a contributing factor. Exogenous acidic agents, such as lemon juice (by lemon sucking), cause crescent or dished defects (rounded as opposed to angular) on the surfaces of exposed teeth (Fig. 9-12, *A*), while endogenous acidic agents, such as gastric fluids, cause generalized erosion on the lingual, incisal, and occlusal surfaces (see Fig. 9-12, *B*). The latter defective surfaces are associated with the binge-purge syndrome in *bulimia,* or with *gastroesophageal reflux.*

In contrast to chemical erosion, *idiopathic erosion* is thought by some to explain the cervical, wedge-shaped defect (angular as opposed to rounded) that is similar to the defect customarily associated with toothbrush abrasion (subsequently presented), but where the predominant causative factor (as proposed) is heavy force in eccentric occlusion shown in an associated wear facet, resulting in flexuring (elastic bending) of the tooth (see Fig. 9-12, *C*). It is further hypothesized that the bending force produces tension stress in the affected wedge-shaped region on the tooth side away from the tooth bending direction, resulting in loss of surface tooth structure by microfractures and is termed an "abfracture."[29] Proponents of this hypothesis also add that the microfractures can foster loss of tooth structure from toothbrush abrasion and from acids in the diet and/or plaque. The resulting defect has smooth surfaces.

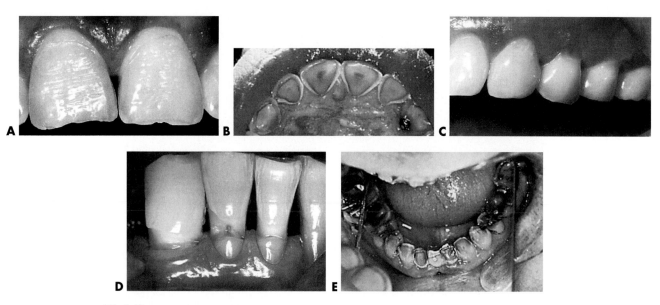

FIG. **9-12** Erosion. **A,** Crescent-shaped defects on enamel facial surfaces caused by exogenous demineralizing agent (from sucking lemons several years previous to the time of the photograph). **B,** Generalized erosion caused by endogenous fluids. **C,** Idiopathic erosion lesion at the DEJ is hypothesized to be associated with abnormal occlusal force. **D,** Wedge-shaped lesions caused by abrasion from toothbrush. **E,** Generalized attrition caused by excessive functional or parafunctional mandibular movements.

Abrasion is abnormal tooth surface loss resulting from direct frictional forces between the teeth and external objects, or from frictional forces between contacting teeth in the presence of an abrasive medium. Such wear is caused by improper brushing techniques or other habits such as holding a pipe stem between the teeth, tobacco chewing, and chewing on hard objects such as pens or pencils. Toothbrush abrasion is the most common example and is usually seen as a sharp wedge-shaped notch in the gingival portion of the facial aspects of the teeth (see Fig. 9-12, *D*). The surface of the defect is smooth. The presence of such defects does not automatically warrant intervention. Rather, it is important to determine and eliminate the cause.

Attrition is mechanical wear of the incisal or occlusal tooth structure as a result of functional or parafunctional movements of the mandible. Although a certain degree of attrition is expected with age, it is important to note abnormally advanced attrition (see Fig. 9-12, *E*). If significant abnormal attrition is present, the patient's functional movements must be evaluated and inquiry made about any habits creating this problem such as tooth grinding, or *bruxism,* usually due to stress. In some older patients, the enamel of the cusp tips (or incisal edges) is worn off resulting in cupped-out areas because the exposed, softer dentin wears faster than the surrounding enamel. Sometimes these areas are an annoyance because of food retention or the presence of peripheral, ragged, sharp enamel edges. Slowing such wear by appropriate restorative treatment is indicated. The sharp edges can result in tongue or cheek biting, and rounding

these edges does not resolve the problem but does improve comfort.

Fracture or *craze lines* in a tooth are often visible, especially with advancing age, and should be considered as potential cleavage planes for possible future fractures. Appropriate dye materials or light reflected from a dental mirror aid in detecting fracture lines. Any tooth that has an extensive restoration and weakened cusps should be identified as being susceptible to future fracture (Fig. 9-13) and should be considered for a cusp-protecting restoration. Deep developmental fissures across marginal or cusp ridges are cleavage planes, especially in the tooth weakened by caries or previous restoration. A minor fracture of a tooth can often be treated by recontouring and polishing. If the fracture is more extensive, the tooth should be restored. The examination and diagnosis of the incomplete fracture of a posterior tooth is presented in a subsequent section, Examination of the Patient in Pain.

The dental examination also may reveal *dental anomalies* that include variations in size, shape, structure, or number of teeth such as *dens in dente, macrodontia, microdontia, gemination, concrescence, dilaceration, amelogenesis imperfecta,* and *dentinogenesis imperfecta.* Thorough discussion of these anomalies is beyond the scope of this text; the reader should refer to an oral pathology textbook for additional information.

Radiographic Examination of Teeth and Restorations. Dental radiographs are an indispensable part of the contemporary dentist's diagnostic armamentarium. As with most things in life, however, the use of diagnos-

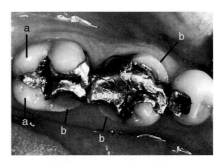

FIG. 9-13 Extensively restored teeth with weakened *(a)* and fractured *(b)* cusps. Note the distal developmental fissure in the second molar, which further predisposes the distal cusps to fracture.

BOX 9-1 Clinical Situations for Which Radiographs May Be Indicated

Previous periodontal or root canal therapy
History of pain or trauma
Familial history of dental anomalies
Clinical evidence of periodontal disease
Large or deep restorations
Deep carious lesions
Malposed or clinically impacted teeth
Swelling
Mobility of teeth
Fistula or sinus tract infection
Growth abnormalities
Oral involvement in known or suspected systemic disease
Evidence of foreign objects
Abutment teeth for fixed or removable partial prosthesis
Unexplained bleeding
Unexplained sensitivity of teeth
Unusual tooth morphology, calcification, or color
Missing teeth with unknown reason

tic ionizing radiation is not without risks. Exposure to any amount of ionizing radiation can potentially result in a range of adverse affects. Therefore the diagnostic yield or potential benefit that could be gained from a radiograph must be weighed carefully against the financial costs and the potential adverse affects of exposure to radiation. Several technologies including digital radiography are now available and are designed to enhance diagnostic yield and reduce radiation exposure.

To assist the clinician with assessing the risks and benefits, the FDA sponsored a panel of dental experts to develop radiograph selection criteria for dental patients. Their report specifies guidelines based on patient age and risk of dental disease for prescribing dental radiographs.[42] As a general rule, patients at higher risk for caries or periodontal disease should receive more frequent and more extensive radiographic surveys. Table 9-2, adapted from the FDA guidelines, lists the preferred types of radiographs and the intervals at which they should be used for the dentulous adult patient. Specific clinical situations for which radiographs may be indicated are also shown in Box 9-1.

For diagnosis of proximal-surface caries, restoration overhangs, or poorly contoured restorations, posterior bitewing and anterior periapical radiographs are most helpful. When interpreting the radiographic presentation of proximal tooth surfaces, it is necessary to know the normal anatomic picture presented in a radiograph before any abnormalities can be diagnosed. In a radiograph, proximal caries appears as a dark area or a radiolucency in the proximal enamel at or gingival to the contact of the teeth (see Fig. 9-5, *A*). This radiolucency typically is triangular and has its apex toward the den-

toenamel junction (DEJ). Moderate-to-deep occlusal caries can be seen as a radiolucency extending into dentin (see Fig. 9-5, *C*). Some defective aspects of restorations also may be identified radiographically. These include improper contour, overhangs (see Fig. 9-8), and recurrent caries gingival to restorations (see Fig. 9-5, *D*). Pulpal abnormalities such as *pulp stones* and *internal resorption* may be identified in the anterior periapical radiographs (Fig. 9-14, *A* and *B*). The height and integrity of the marginal periodontium may be evaluated from the bitewing radiographs. Periapical radiographs are helpful in diagnosing changes in the periapical periodontium such as *periapical abscesses, dental granulomas,* or *cysts* (see Fig. 9-14, *C*). Impacted third molars, supernumerary teeth, and other congenital or acquired abnormalities also may be discovered upon periapical radiographic examination. However, it should be kept in mind that the sensitivity and specificity of dental radiographs will vary according to the diagnostic task.

Always interpret dental radiographs cautiously. Remember the limitation imposed by interpreting a dental film is that the film is a two-dimensional representation of a three-dimensional mass. In addition, the dentist should realize that the interpretation of dental radiographs would produce a certain number of false-positive and false-negative diagnoses. For instance, misdiagnosis can occur when *cervical burnout* (the radiographic picture of the normal structure and contour of the cervical third of the crown) mimics caries (Fig. 9-15, *A* through *C*). Furthermore, a Class V lesion or a radiolucent tooth-colored restoration may be radiographically superimposed on the proximal area, mimicking proximal caries (Fig. 9-15, *D* and *E*). Finally, although caries may be more extensive clinically than it appears radiographically, approximately 60% of teeth with radiographic proximal lesions in the outer half of dentin are likely to be noncavitated[53] and therefore treatable with remineralization measures. Although radiographs are excellent diagnostic media, they do have limitations. The only way to guard against these limitations is to continually correlate clinical and radiographic findings.

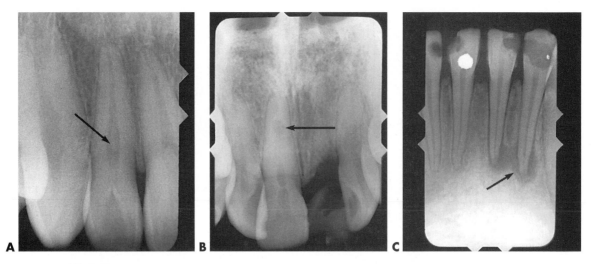

FIG. **9-14** Pulpal abnormalities. **A,** Pulp stone. **B,** Internal resorption. **C,** Periapical abscess, granuloma, or cyst.

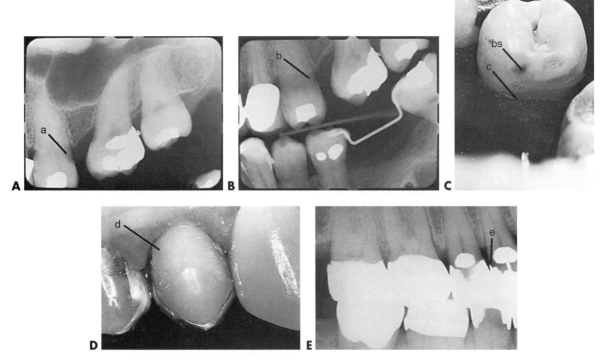

FIG. **9-15** **A,** A misleading radiographic appearance can be caused by cervical burnout, which mimics caries *(a)*. **B,** Caries is not visible on a radiograph from a different angle *(b)*. **C,** Caries also not detectable clinically *(c)*. Brown spot *(bs)* is a remineralized, arrested, incipient carious lesion. **D,** A Class V lesion or tooth-colored restoration *(d)* can mimic proximal caries **(E)** by superimposing a radiolucent area on proximal aspect of tooth *(e)*.

Adjunctive Aids for Examining Teeth and Restorations. Adjunctive aids or tests, such as the *percussion test, palpation, thermal tests, electric pulp test,* and *test preparation,* are useful when further information is needed to discern the health of the teeth and supporting structures. Remember, however, that these are only aids in arriving at a diagnosis. Positive results on only one test should not be considered conclusive because a test is seldom 100% accurate. Rather, all available information, including history, examination, radiographs, and other test results, and comparable findings on adjacent and contralateral teeth should be used in concert to confirm the diagnosis.

A *percussion test* is performed by gently tapping the occlusal or incisal surfaces of the suspected tooth and adjacent teeth with the end of the handle of a mouth mirror

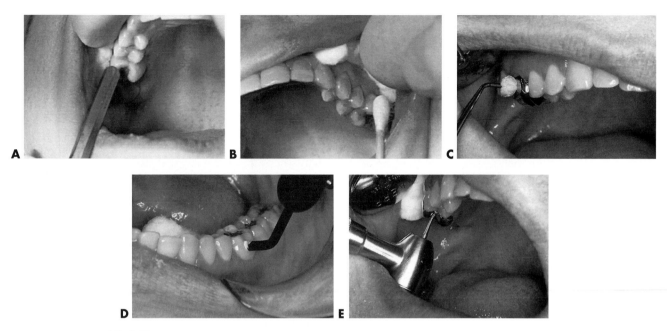

FIG. **9-16** Diagnostic aids for examining teeth. **A,** Percussion. **B,** Cold test. **C,** Heat test with hot gutta-percha. **D,** Electric pulp test. **E,** Test preparation.

to determine the presence of tenderness (Fig. 9-16, *A*). Pain on percussion suggests possible injury to the periodontal membrane from pulpal or periodontal inflammation. Care must be taken when interpreting a positive response on maxillary teeth because teeth in close proximity to the maxillary sinuses also may exhibit pain on percussion when the patient is suffering from maxillary sinusitis.

Palpation is performed by rubbing the index finger along the facial and lingual mucosa overlying the apical region of the tooth. An alveolar abscess in an advanced stage or other periapical pathosis may cause tenderness to palpation. Palpation also can reveal nontender swellings that may be overlooked otherwise.

An indication of pulp vitality can be obtained through the results of thermal tests, an electric pulp test, and a test cavity. In addition, before any tooth is restored with a casting, pulpal evaluation should be performed. To conduct a *thermal test,* a cotton applicator tip sprayed with a freezing agent (HistoFreeze, Fisher Brand, Fisher Scientific, Pittsburgh, PA 15219) or hot gutta-percha is applied directly to the tooth (see Fig. 9-16, *B* and *C*). Hot and cold testing should elicit from the healthy pulp a response that will subside within a few seconds following removal of the stimulus. Pain lasting 10 to 15 seconds or less after stimulation by heat or cold suggests a *hyperemia,* an inflammation that may be reversed by timely removal of the irritant. Intense pain of longer duration from hot or cold usually suggests *irreversible pulpitis,* which can only be treated by endodontic therapy or extraction. Pain that results from heat but is quickly relieved by cold also suggests irreversible pulpitis. Lack of response to thermal tests may indicate that the pulp is necrotic. Adjacent and/or contralateral unaffected

teeth should be tested for baseline comparisons because the duration of pain may differ among individuals.

The *electric pulp tester* also has value in determining the vitality of the dental pulp (see Fig. 9-16, *D*). The electric pulp tester is placed on the tooth and not on a restoration. A small electric current delivered to the tooth causes a tingling sensation when the pulp is vital and no response when the pulp is nonvital. It is important to obtain readings on adjacent and contralateral teeth so the tooth in question can be evaluated relative to the responses of the other teeth. Results of an electric pulp test should not be the sole basis for a pulpal diagnosis because false positives or false negatives can occur. Instead, electric pulp test results provide additional information that, when combined with other findings, may lead to a diagnosis. Electric pulp testing is sometimes not possible in teeth with large or full-coverage restorations.

A *test preparation* can be performed to help in the evaluation of pulpal vitality when a large restoration in the tooth may be resulting in false-negative responses with other evaluation methods. This test in particular is an option for diagnosing questionable pulpal vitality of a tooth contemplated for a replacement casting restoration. By using a round bur and no anesthetic, a test preparation is made through the existing restoration into the dentin (see Fig. 9-16, *E*). Lack of sensitivity (response) when the dentin is cut may indicate a nonvital pulp. However, sclerosed dentin can result in a false-negative response. Moreover, on a multiple-rooted tooth, one region of the dentin may respond, whereas there may be no response at another site, possibly indicating a degeneration of a portion of the pulp. Furthermore, heat generated by the bur might cause a response, but the pulp may not be healthy. Although there are indications for the test preparation, its use and the diagnostic information attained are limited.

When extensive restorative therapy is contemplated, *study casts* are helpful in providing an understanding of occlusal relationships, developing the treatment plan, and educating the patient. Accurately mounted study casts provide an opportunity for a thorough evaluation of the tooth interdigitation, the functional occlusion, and any occlusal abnormalities that may need treatment. For example, study casts provide for further evaluation of the plane of occlusion; tilted, rotated, or extruded teeth; cross-bites; plunger cusps; wear facets and defective restorations; coronal contours; proximal contacts; and embrasure spaces between the teeth. Combined with clinical and radiographic findings, study casts allow the practitioner to develop a treatment plan without the patient present, thus saving valuable chair time. When a proposed plan of treatment is discussed with the patient, study casts can be valuable educational media in helping the patient understand and visualize existing conditions and the need for proposed treatment.

Additional aids for diagnosis of additional problems are discussed in later sections of this chapter, and these include transillumination, the biting test, mobility testing, the anesthetic test, and occlusal analysis.

REVIEW OF PERIODONTIUM

Determination of operative treatment should occur only after the status of the *periodontium* has been evaluated. Because the periodontium and the teeth must exist in a mutually beneficial physiologic environment, an accurate diagnosis of the periodontal condition is critical to the planning of operative treatment.

Clinical Examination. The periodontium is evaluated clinically through a series of steps. The gingival color and texture are important indices of periodontal health. Healthy gingiva is light pink in color, firm, knife-edged, and stippled, whereas unhealthy gingiva is often red; soft; edematous; and has a glazed, smooth surface. The depth of the gingival sulcus around each tooth is determined by systematic probing using a specialized instrument (periodontal probe) having a round-ended, thin

shaft with millimeter indications (Fig. 9-17, *A*). A patient may be screened for periodontal disease using the periodontal screening and recording (PSR) technique.[35,47] In using the PSR, the examiner measures the sulcus depth around selected teeth and records the worse affected site in each sextant using a 1 to 4 system. If certain thresholds are met, a complete periodontal examination is conducted. In a complete examination, the sulcus depth is assessed at six locations around each tooth, three facially (mesiofacial, midfacial, distofacial), and three lingually (mesiolingual, midlingual, and distolingual). A sulcus depth greater than 3 mm and sites that bleed upon probing should be recorded in the patient's chart (see Fig. 9-2, *C*). The presence of a pocket (a sulcus depth greater than 3 mm) or the presence of hemorrhage or exudate may indicate periodontal disease.

The next step in probing is to evaluate the presence of bifurcation or trifurcation involvement. These regions should be explored with a furcation probe and classified according to the amount of penetration. The presence of furcation involvement reduces the long-term prognosis of the tooth and affects the restorative treatment plan.

After probing is completed, it is imperative to note areas of *gingival recession* and areas with a minimum or lack of attached gingiva, especially if these areas are near a tooth surface that requires a subgingival restorative margin (see Fig. 9-17, *B*). With a lack of attached gingiva in these areas, restorative manipulations such as margination, temporization, and impressions are more difficult and can further aggravate the gingival problem (see Fig. 9-17, *C*).

Teeth should be evaluated for *mobility* and noted with appropriate classification (1, 2, or 3). Class 1 mobility is barely distinguishable mobility (physiologic) in a faciolingual direction of only a few tenths of a millimeter (total); class 2 is mobility (nonphysiologic) in any transverse direction greater than a few tenths up to 1 mm; and class 3 mobility (nonphysiologic) is greater than 1 mm in any transverse direction. Teeth that can be depressed or rotated also are scored as class 3. Mobility signifies loss of bone support or the result of improper occlusal forces, either of which could affect subsequent operative treatment. The occlusal relationship of the

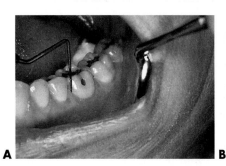
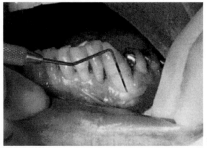
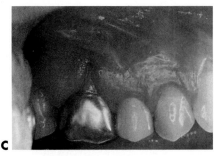

A **B** **C**

FIG. **9-17** Periodontal examination. **A,** Probing to measure sulcus depth. **B,** Lack of attached gingiva next to a tooth requiring restoration with a subgingival margin. **C,** Gingival recession.

teeth should be closely evaluated. Well-positioned occlusal contacts are necessary to prevent occlusal trauma to the periodontium. Nonphysiologic mobility observed during functional contacts should be recorded because this information is useful in treatment planning.

The presence of *plaque,* debris, and inflammation, and the general level of home care must be noted for two reasons. First, the teeth cannot be properly restored when they are covered by debris and surrounded by unhealthy tissues that bleed easily. The gingiva should be firm and healthy so that restorative procedures can be performed in a clean, dry field. Second, the long-term prognosis of any operative treatment is highly dependent on the long-term periodontal health and the patient's ability to keep the restoration and tooth surfaces clean.

Restorations should be *correctly contoured* to maintain proper periodontal health. Proximal, facial, and lingual surfaces should not be overcontoured because such contouring can impinge on the soft tissue or act as a plaque trap. Physiologic proximal contacts should be achieved to prevent interproximal food impaction and tooth movement and to foster during mastication proper movement of food facially and lingually as a result of correct lingual, occlusal, and facial embrasures.

Radiographic Examination. *Radiographs* are another valuable aid in assessing periodontal health. Bitewing radiographs, exposed at the proper angulation, are the best means of radiographically assessing bone levels. Vertical bitewing radiographs are recommended for patients with periodontitis involving substantial bone loss. Localized or generalized bone loss, vertical or horizontal, should be noted.

Radiographs aid in determining the relationship between the margins of existing or proposed restorations and the bone. A *biologic width* of at least 2 mm is required for the junctional epithelium and connective tissue attachments located between the base of the sulcus and the alveolar bone crest (Fig. 9-18, *A*). In addition to this physiologic dimension, the restoration margin should be placed occlusally as far away as possible from the base of the sulcus to foster gingival health. Encroachment on this biologic width may cause breakdown and apical migration of the attachment apparatus. The attachment breakdown and apical migration are in response to the inflammatory process caused by bacterial plaque that accumulates at the inaccessible restoration margins. The final position of a proposed gingival margin, which is dictated by the existing restoration, caries, or retention features, must be estimated to determine if *crown-lengthening* procedures are indicated before restoration (see Fig. 9-18, *B*). These procedures involve the surgical removal of the gingiva and/or bone to create a longer clinical crown, and thus provide more tooth structure for placing the restoration margin and for increasing retention form.

Because of the obvious importance of the periodontium, operative procedures must continually be performed with respect, understanding, and concern for the periodontium. Therefore the relationship of the periodontium and operative procedures always must be considered.

EXAMINATION OF OCCLUSION

Several reasons exist for completing a thorough occlusal examination for developing an analysis and understanding of the patient's occlusion before initiating restorative care. First, the operator can establish the patient's presenting condition before any alterations. This documentation includes the identification of signs of occlusal trauma, such as enamel cracks or tooth mobility, and notation of occlusal abnormalities that contribute to pathologic conditions, such as bone loss. Second, the potential effect of proposed restorative treatment on the occlusion can be assessed. For example, the potential of proposed restorations to provide a beneficial and harmonious occlusion must be determined. Third, the effect of the current occlusal scheme on proposed restorative treatment

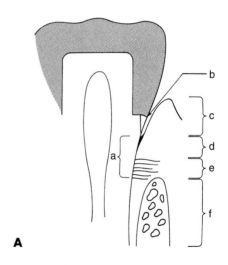

A

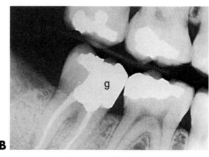

B

FIG. **9-18 A,** Biologic width *(a)* is the physiologic dimension needed for the junctional epithelium *(d)* and the connective tissue attachment *(e),* which is measured from the base of the sulcus *(c)* to the level of the bone crest *(f).* The margin of the restoration *(b)* must not violate this dimension. **B,** Tooth with an existing restoration *(g)* that encroaches on the biologic width requires crown-lengthening procedures before placement of a new restoration.

can be identified, and the existing occlusion altered if needed before placement of restorations.

The static and dynamic occlusion must be carefully examined (see Chapter 2). Although not all occlusal abnormalities require treatment, the clinician always must be able to identify deviations from normal and be prepared to treat, refer, or make allowances for these problems in any planned therapy. A description of the patient's static anatomic occlusion in maximum intercuspation (MI), including the relationship of the molars and canines (Angle's Classes I, II, or III), and the amount of *vertical overlap* (overbite) and *horizontal overlap* (overjet) of the anterior teeth should be recorded. The presence of missing teeth and the relationship of the maxillary and mandibular midlines should be evaluated. The appropriateness of the occlusal plane and the positions of malposed teeth should be identified. Supererupted teeth, spacing, fractured teeth, and marginal ridge discrepancies should be noted. The dynamic functional occlusion in all movements of the mandible (right, left, forward, and all excursions in between) should be evaluated. This evaluation also includes assessing the relationship of the teeth in centric relation, which is when the condyle head is in its most retruded (unforced) contact position. Functional movements of the mandible are evaluated to determine if *canine guidance* or *group function* exists. The presence and amount of *anterior guidance* is evaluated to note the degree of potential posterior disclusion. *Non–working side contacts* are recorded so that they may be eliminated and any planned restorative care for involved teeth will not perpetuate these contacts. Any mobility of teeth during function is identified. Movement of the mandible from maximum intercuspation to maximum opening is observed; any clicking of the joint(s) during such movement may be an indication of a pathologic condition.

Teeth are examined for abnormal wear patterns. If signs of abnormal wear are present, the patient is queried as to the presence of any contributing habits such as nocturnal bruxism or parafunctional habits. The examination also should disclose possible unfavorable occlusal relationships, such as a *plunger cusp,* which is a pointed cusp "plunging" deep into the occlusal plane of the opposing arch. A plunger cusp may be contacting the lower of two adjacent marginal ridges of different levels, or contacting directly between two adjacent marginal ridges in maximum intercuspation, or positioned in a deep fossa. These may result in food impaction or tooth/restoration fracture.

The results of the occlusal analysis should be included in the dental record and considered in the restorative treatment plan. Acceptable aspects of the occlusion must be preserved and not altered during treatment. When possible, improvement of the occlusal relationship is desirable; assuredly, abnormalities must not be perpetuated in the restorative treatment.

EXAMINATION OF THE PATIENT IN PAIN

One of the most perplexing yet challenging problems a dentist encounters is the treatment of patients who have pain in the jaws or teeth. Such problems often can test the dentist's diagnostic skills. The cause of discomfort must be determined before relief can be provided. The problem can be identified and treated by carefully piecing together subjective information from the patient and objective information from the clinical examination supplemented with appropriate diagnostic tests.

Regardless of whether the patient is new to the practice or is a patient of record, the medical history must be reviewed to identify potential health-related problems. The patient is then asked to describe various characteristics of the pain, particularly: (1) the onset and duration, (2) stimuli, (3) spontaneity, (4) intensity, and (5) factors that relieve it (Box 9-2). After carefully listening to the patient's thorough description of the nature of the problem, the practitioner guides the discussion to obtain more information. During this discussion the dentist begins to formulate an idea about the potential cause of the pain and a means for verifying it. Care should be taken, however, not to focus too quickly; instead, all possible sources of pain must be considered: systemic, pulpal, periapical, periodontal, restorative, degenerative, and neoplastic.

After assessing the subjective symptoms described by the patient and developing a preliminary diagnosis, the dentist should apply *objective tests* to confirm the diagnosis. These include a *percussion test* to determine possible inflammation in the periodontal ligament (PDL), *palpation* to examine for any tenderness in the apical region, and *transillumination* to check for cracks or caries in the tooth as well as for tooth color changes that may indicate loss of vitality. If a tooth is suspected of having a pulpal problem, *electric pulp testing* combined with *thermal testing* may assist in the diagnosis. *Periodontal probing* helps rule out periodontal abscess. The *integrity of restorations* is evaluated by examining them for fractures, recurrent caries, wear marks, shiny spots, or mobility (looseness).

One of the more challenging diagnostic problems is to locate the offending, posterior tooth that has an *incomplete fracture* not directly involving the pulp chamber/canal(s) of a vital pulp. If the chief complaint is, "When I chew on this side it hurts," the examiner must be especially alert for an *incomplete fracture of a vital posterior tooth.* Frequently the patient gives a history of seeking relief from the dentist over an extended period. Sensitivity to cold usually is an additional complaint. All fracture lines in the enamel of the teeth on the affected side of the arches, maxillary and mandibular, should be noted. Such lines usually are found in the remaining enamel of teeth weakened by extensive caries or restorations. Particularly suspect are those fracture lines emanating from enamel developmental fissures (natural

BOX 9-2 Patient Inventory for Diagnosing Dental Pain

For the diagnosis of dental pain, an inventory of information should be obtained from the patient interview and clinical and radiographic examinations:

QUESTIONS ASKED OF THE PATIENT

1. Can you point to the tooth or area that bothers you? _____
   Top right   Top left   Top front
   Bottom right   Bottom left   Bottom front
2. When did you first notice the pain or discomfort? _____
3. How long has it hurt? _____
4. Circle any of the following that describe(s) the character of your pain.
   Pulsating   Dull   Sudden   Constant
   Nagging   Sharp   Off and on
5. Is the pain spontaneous?   Yes   No
6. Does the pain wake you up at night?   Yes   No
7. What makes it hurt?

Heat	Yes	No	Don't know
Cold	Yes	No	Don't know
Sweets	Yes	No	Don't know
Chewing/biting	Yes	No	Don't know
Air	Yes	No	Don't know
Other			

8. How long does the pain last? _____
9. What relieves the pain? _____

CLINICAL EXAMINATION

1. Caries	Yes	No	
2. Extensive restoration	Yes	No	
3. Sensitive to percussion	Yes	No	
4. Sensitive to palpation	Yes	No	
5. Response to cold test	Normal	No response	Pain lingers
6. Response to heat test	Normal	No response	Pain lingers

7. Periodontal pocket depths   ML ____   L ____   DL ____   MF ____   F ____   DF ____

8. Mobility	Yes	No
9. Wear facets or signs of occlusal trauma	Yes	No
10. Tooth Slooth* test	Yes	No
11. Craze lines emanating from developmental fissures	Yes	No
12. Exposed root surface	Yes	No
13. Presence of sinus tract	Yes	No
14. Tooth discoloration	Yes	No
15. Other		_____

RADIOGRAPHIC EXAMINATION

1. Caries	Yes	No
2. Extensive restoration	Yes	No
3. Periapical pathology		
Widened periodontal ligament	Yes	No
Radiolucent lesion	Yes	No
4. Root fracture	Yes	No
5. Bone levels		
Furcation		_____
Interproximally		_____

*Tooth Slooth and Tooth Slooth II, Professional Results, Inc., Laguna Niguel, California.

cleavage planes), extending through marginal or cusp ridges, and then extending gingivally in axial surface enamel, thus leaving the included cusps liable to this incomplete fracture under occlusal load (Fig. 9-19). The incompletely fractured cusp causes *sharp pain when masticatory pressure is released* resulting in the fractured dentinal surfaces rubbing together creating hydrodynamic pressures in the dentinal tubules to thus elicit pulpal pain; also, the fractured dentinal surfaces become hypersensitive because of salivary contamination. Often it is difficult to determine which tooth is affected; however, a differential diagnosis frequently can be made with a biting *test*. This is accomplished by placing the Tooth Slooth (Tooth Slooth and Tooth Slooth II, Profes-

sional Results, Inc., Laguna Niguel, California) over each suspect cusp and asking the patient to bite and then release (see Fig. 9-19, *A* and *B*). Sharp pain on release of pressure helps to identify the offending tooth and its partially fractured component. Typically, if the fracture does not enter the dental pulp or is not in the root, a properly designed cast restoration (with extracoronal resistance features) often provides relief, because the fractured part is either removed during preparation or is encompassed by the restoration.

An *incomplete fracture that exposes the vital pulp of a posterior tooth* is characterized by symptoms different from those given for an incomplete fracture without pulpal exposure; in a short time the former will result in severe,

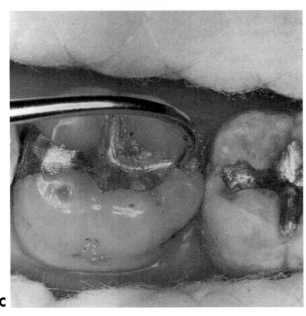

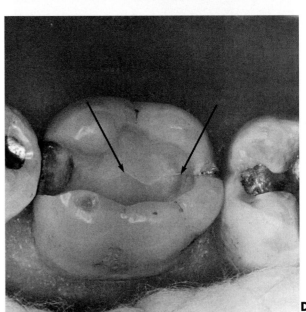

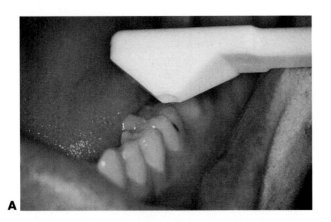

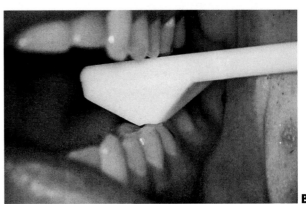

FIG. **9-19 A,** The Tooth Slooth is used to detect an incomplete fracture of a posterior tooth. The end with the small divot or depression is placed on the suspected cusp. The patient is instructed to close so that the opposite tooth engages the grooved, flat side of the Tooth Slooth. **B,** The patient is instructed to apply biting pressure on the plastic instrument and to move the mandible slowly side to side and then release quickly. **C,** Tooth that yielded a positive response to the rubber wheel test, indicating a possible incomplete fracture. **D,** Removal of existing restoration confirms diagnosis of an incomplete fracture.

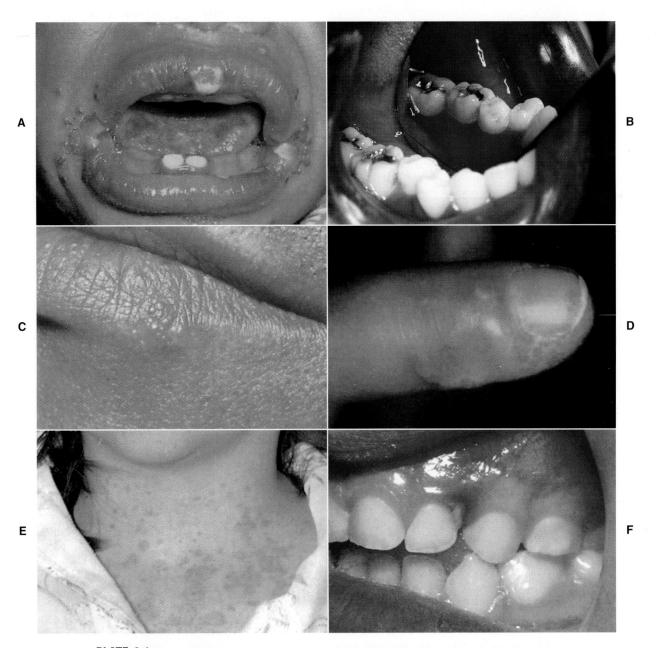

PLATE 9-1 Intraoral and extraoral manifestations associated with communicable diseases. **A,** Primary herpetic gingivostomatitis. **B,** Herpes simplex lesions (gingival mucosa). **C,** Herpes labialis. **D,** Herpetic whitlow (index finger). **E,** Chickenpox (rash on the trunk). **F,** Chickenpox (gingival lesion).   *Plate continued next page.*

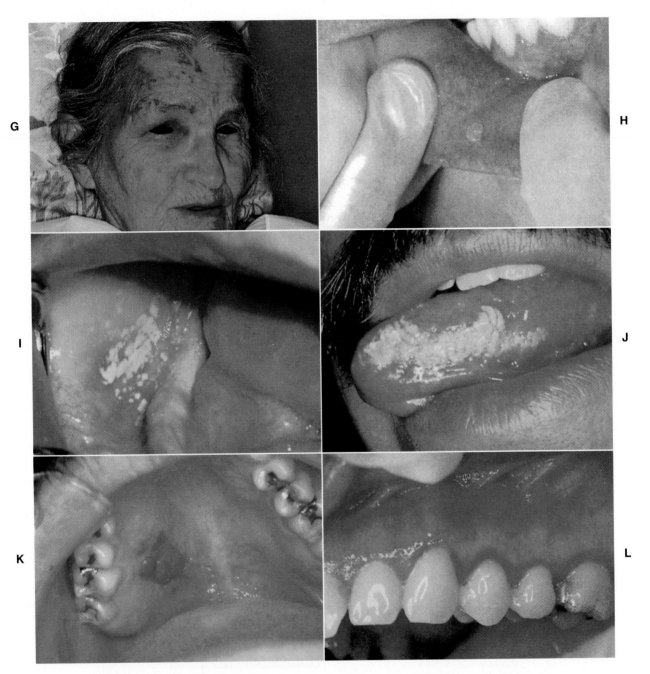

PLATE 9-1, continued from previous page. G, Herpes zoster (shingles), supraorbital dermatome distribution. **H,** *Condylomata acuminatum* (also called *venereal warts*). **I,** Pseudomembranous candidiasis (facial mucosa). **J,** Hairy leukoplakia (lateral border of the tongue). **K,** Kaposi's sarcoma (maxillary palate). **L,** Linear gingival erythema. *(A, E, and F, Courtesy of Dr. William F. Vann; B and C, Courtesy of Dr. Lauren Patton; D, Courtesy of Dr. James Crawford; G, Courtesy of Dr. Diane C. Shugars; H to K, Courtesy of Centers for Disease Control and Prevention, Atlanta; L, Courtesy of Dr. James R. Winkler.)*

almost constant, throbbing pain from irreversible pulpitis. Sometimes temporary relief follows pulpal death, but intervention therapies of root canal treatment or tooth extraction are indicated for long-term success. The choice of these therapies depends on several factors, including restorability, usefulness, supporting tissue, and patient preferences.

If the patient is unable to localize the arch in which the offending tooth is located, an *anesthetic test* may be used. The suspected tooth is anesthetized to determine if the patient gains any relief. If the symptoms subside, the offending tooth likely has been identified.

Exposed root surfaces can result in sharp, annoying pain. For treatment refer to the later section Treatment of Root Surface Sensitivity.

Along with a discussion of the patient's symptoms and a thorough clinical examination and the use of adjunctive tests, a radiograph of the involved region may provide additional information. Radiographs are useful in identifying significant interdental or periradicular bone loss associated with pulpal pathosis. Also, deep restorations and pulpal abnormalities can be detected through radiographic evaluation.

After diagnosis of the probable cause of pain, appropriate treatment should be instituted. Occasionally, examination findings may be so inconclusive that the patient may need to be advised that no definitive treatment is indicated at the moment and that it is best to wait for the symptoms to change or localize. Finally, treatment should be as conservative as possible. This means that unless otherwise indicated, the most palliative form of treatment should be initiated first.

A thorough and exacting examination of the orofacial soft tissue, teeth, periodontium, and occlusion provides adequate information on which to base a diagnosis. Only after abnormalities of these structures are diagnosed and recorded should the treatment planning process begin. A treatment plan and subsequent treatment are only as effective as the quality of information obtained during the examination.

TREATMENT PLANNING
GENERAL CONSIDERATIONS

A *treatment plan* is a carefully sequenced series of services designed to eliminate or control etiologic factors, repair existing damage, and create a functional, maintainable environment (see Fig. 9-2, *C*). A sound treatment plan depends on thorough patient evaluation, dentist expertise, understanding of indications and contraindications, and a prediction of the patient's response to treatment. An accurate *prognosis* for each tooth and for the patient's overall dental health is central to a successful treatment plan. To establish a prognosis, the practitioner must be able to forecast possible results given

the patient's current condition and knowledge of the possible outcomes of contemplated treatment.

The development of a dental treatment plan for a patient consists of four steps: (1) examination and problem identification, (2) decision to recommend intervention, (3) identification of treatment alternatives, and (4) selection of the treatment with the patient's involvement. *Step one*, examination and diagnosis, discussed in detail in the second part of this chapter, results in a list of dental problems. *Step two*, deciding to intervene, is dependent upon a determination that a tooth is diseased, restoration is defective, or that either tooth or restoration is at some increased risk of further deterioration if intervention does not occur. If any of these conditions exist, then intervention is recommended to the patient. *Step three*, identification of treatment alternatives, involves establishing the list of one or more reasonable interventions from the set of possible alternatives. Treatment alternatives for a specific condition can include periodic reevaluation to monitor the condition, chemotherapeutics (e.g., applications of fluoride to promote remineralization or antimicrobials to reduce bacteria), recontouring defective restorations or irregular tooth surfaces, repair (patching a defective restoration), and restoration. This list of reasonable treatment alternatives is based on the current knowledge of the effectiveness of the treatment, the prevailing standards of care, and both clinical and nonclinical patient factors. *Step four*, selection of the treatment, is conducted in consultation with the patient. The patient is advised of the reasonable treatment alternatives and their related risks and benefits. After the patient is fully informed, the doctor and patient can select a course of action that is most appropriate for that patient.

Treatment plans are influenced by patient preferences, motivation, systemic health, emotional status, and financial capabilities. The dentist's knowledge, experience, and training; laboratory support; dentist-patient compatibility; the availability of specialists; and functional, esthetic, and technical demands also can modify a treatment plan. Even when modification is necessary, the practitioner is ethically and professionally responsible for providing the best level of care possible. For instance, if a tooth ideally should be treated with a cast restoration but the patient is unable to afford this care, then optimal treatment would consist of a large, multisurface, amalgam or composite restoration. Although this is optimal rather than ideal treatment, it does not give the dentist license to perform an inadequate restoration. The best restoration possible should be done under the circumstances.

Finally, a treatment plan is not a static list of services. Rather, it is a multiphase and dynamic series of events. Its success is determined by its suitableness to meet the patient's initial and long-term needs. A treatment plan should allow for reevaluation and be adaptable to meet the changing needs, preferences, and health conditions of the patient. Therefore the patient must realize that the plan may have to be altered as conditions change.

TREATMENT PLAN SEQUENCING

Treatment plan sequencing is the process of scheduling the needed procedures into a time frame. Proper sequencing is a critical component of a successful treatment plan. Certain treatments must naturally follow others in a logical order, while other treatments can or must occur concurrently and thus require coordination. Complex treatment plans often should be sequenced in phases, including an urgent phase, a *control phase*, a *reevaluation phase*, a *definitive phase*, and a *maintenance phase*.[20] However, for most patients, the first three phases are accomplished as a single phase.

Generally, the concept of "greatest need" guides the order in which treatment is sequenced. *This concept dictates that what the patient needs most is performed first.*

Urgent Phase. The urgent phase of care begins with a thorough review of the patient's medical condition and history. As described earlier in the chapter, a patient presenting with swelling, pain, bleeding, or infection should have these problems managed as soon as possible and certainly before initiation of subsequent phases.

Control Phase. The control phase of treatment is meant to: (1) eliminate active disease such as caries and inflammation, (2) remove conditions preventing maintenance, (3) eliminate potential causes of disease, and (4) begin preventive dentistry activities. The goals of this phase are to remove etiologic factors and stabilize the patient's dental health. Examples of control phase treatment include extractions; endodontics; periodontal debridement and scaling; occlusal adjustment as needed; caries removal; replacement or repair of defective restorations, such as those with gingival overhangs; and use of caries control measures (as described in Chapter 3).

As part of the control phase, the dentist should develop a plan for the management and prevention of dental caries. After the patient's caries status and caries risk have been determined, chemical, surgical, behavioral, mechanical, and dietary techniques (Box 9-3) can be used to improve host resistance and alter the oral flora. Chapter 3 presents a detailed discussion of caries diagnosis, prevention, treatment, and control.

Reevaluation Phase. The holding phase is a time between the control and definitive phases that allows for resolution of inflammation and time for healing. Home care habits are reinforced, motivation for further treatment is assessed, and initial treatment and pulpal responses are reevaluated before definitive care is begun.

Definitive Phase. After the dentist reassesses initial treatment and determines the need for further care, the patient enters the corrective or definitive phase of treatment. This may include endodontic, periodontic, ortho-

dontic, oral surgical, and operative procedures before fixed or removable prosthodontic treatment. This phase is discussed in detail in a following section, Interdisciplinary Considerations in Operative Treatment Planning.

Maintenance Phase. This phase includes regular recall examinations that (1) may reveal the need for adjustments to prevent future breakdown and (2) provide an opportunity to reinforce home care. The frequency of reevaluation examinations during the maintenance phase depends in large part on the patient's risk for dental disease. A patient who has stable periodontal health and a recent history of no caries should have longer intervals (e.g., 9 to 12 months or longer) between recall visits. In contrast, those at high risk for dental caries and/or periodontal breakdown should be examined much more frequently (e.g., 3 to 4 months).

INTERDISCIPLINARY CONSIDERATIONS IN OPERATIVE TREATMENT PLANNING

When an operative procedure is performed during the control or definitive phases, there are general guidelines for when operative treatment should occur relative to other forms of care. Following is a discussion of how to sequence operative care with endodontic, periodontal, orthodontic, oral surgical, and prosthodontic treatments.

Endodontics. All teeth to be restored with large or cast restorations should have a pulpal/periapical evaluation. If indicated, they should have endodontic treatment before restoration is completed. Also, a tooth previously endodontically treated that shows no evidence of healing, or has an inadequate fill, or a fill exposed to oral fluids should be evaluated for retreatment before restorative therapy is initiated.[41]

Periodontics. Generally, periodontal treatment should precede operative care, especially when improved oral

---

BOX 9-3 Prevention and Management of Caries

Chemical—Use of antimicrobial agents to alter the oral flora and administration of topical fluoride to stimulate remineralization
Surgical—Removal of diseased tooth structure and replacement of missing tooth structure with restorative material
Behavioral—Application of appropriate techniques to help the patient develop the skills, knowledge, and attitudes to alter deleterious dietary intake and improve oral hygiene
Mechanical—Mechanical alteration of tooth surfaces at high risk (e.g., sealants), removal of overhangs, reestablishment of proximal contacts, and restoration of defective contours
Dietary—Alteration of the character of the diet
Other—Stimulation of salivary flow through increased chewing, alteration of medications, and use of artificial saliva

hygiene, initial scaling, and root planing procedures can create a more desirable environment for performing operative treatment. Obviously a tooth with a questionable periodontal prognosis should not receive an extensive restoration until periodontal treatment provides a more favorable prognosis. However, if a tooth has a good periodontal prognosis, operative treatment can occur before or after periodontal treatment as long as the operative treatment is not compromised by the existing tissue condition. Treatment of deep carious lesions often requires caries control, amalgam or composite foundations, temporization and/or root canal therapy before periodontal treatment. The correction of gross restorative defects in restoration contours (such as open contacts, gingival overhangs, and poor embrasure form) is considered a part of initial periodontal therapy, and such corrections enhance a favorable tissue response. If periodontal surgical procedures are required, permanent restorations such as inlays/onlays, crowns, and prostheses should be delayed until the surgical phase is completed. However, teeth planned for cast restorations can be prepared and temporized before periodontal surgery. This approach permits confirmation of the restoration prognosis before surgery and allows improved access for the surgical procedure.

Patients with gingivitis and early periodontitis generally respond favorably to improved oral hygiene and scaling/root planing procedures. More advanced periodontitis patients may require surgical pocket elimination/reduction procedures or various regenerative procedures. An increase in the zones of attached gingiva and the elimination of abnormal frenal tension should be provided by corrective periodontal surgical procedures around teeth receiving restorations with subgingival margins. In addition, any teeth requiring restorations that may encroach on the biologic width of periodontium should have appropriate crown-lengthening surgical procedures performed before the final restoration is placed. Usually a minimum of 6 weeks is required following the surgery before final restorative procedures.

Orthodontics. Orthodontic therapy may include extrusion or realignment of teeth to provide favorable interdental spacing, stress distribution, function, and esthetics. All teeth should be free of caries before orthodontic banding. Treatment of caries may include the placement of amalgam and composite restorations. There are few indications for cast restorations before orthodontic treatment is completed.

Oral Surgery. In most instances impacted, unerupted, and hopelessly involved teeth should be removed before operative treatment. This is especially true when second molars that are to receive cast restorations may be damaged or dislodged during removal of third molars. In addition, soft tissue lesions, complicating exostoses, and improperly contoured ridge areas should be eliminated or corrected before final restorative care.

Occlusion. The occlusion should be evaluated and, if indicated, adjusted to establish a static anatomic occlusion with stable maximum intercuspation that is nearly coincident with retruded contact position. This includes eliminating nonfunctional interferences and establishing appropriate guidance patterns before extensive restorative therapy is undertaken. Occlusal adjustment should occur before the definitive restoration phase but may occur at any time (see Occlusion in Chapter 2).

Fixed and Removable Prosthodontics. Preferably, restorations should be completed before placing cast restorations. Occasionally, a large amalgam or composite restoration is placed as a foundation (see Chapters 13 and 19) to provide improved retention for a full crown. For use as a foundation, retention features must be placed well inside the restoration so the material will remain after preparation for a crown. In removable prosthodontic dentistry, *tooth preparations and restorations should allow for the design of the removable partial denture.* This includes allowance for rests, guide planes, and clasps. Moreover, the design of the operative restoration and the selection of appropriate restorative materials must correlate with design of the contemplated removable prosthesis.

INDICATIONS FOR OPERATIVE TREATMENT

In the development of an *operative treatment plan,* all information must be assessed before making tooth-specific decisions. The following sections provide general guidelines for operative treatment planning. Specific indications for restorations will be reviewed in the chapters in which those restorations are discussed. It should be noted that the benefits of bonding materials to tooth structure have resulted in increased emphasis to at least seal all prepared tooth structures, and, in most cases to actually bond the restorative material. This approach includes not only composite restorations, but also many amalgam and indirect restorations.

Operative Preventive Treatment. Before discussing restorative care, it is important to emphasize that the *primary goal of dentistry is to prevent disease,* and thus operative preventive treatment is emphasized. As described in detail in Chapter 3, a caries-preventive program should be instituted for the caries-active or high-risk patient (see Box 9-3). This program should include *altering the oral environment* to encourage remineralization of incipient smooth-surface lesions and treating caries-prone pits and fissures and incipient pit-and-fissure caries with sealants. (Recall from Chapter 3 that incipient lesions are entirely within enamel.) Therefore, occurrence of new lesions decreases along with remineralization of incipient lesions as bacterial habitats are disrupted daily, diet is improved, and fluoride is incorporated into the enamel. The rationale for these treatments is described in Chapter 3, and the technique for sealant application is presented in Chapter 13. Also, extensive acute caries must be immediately eradicated by the caries control restoration (described in Chapter 3) to help suppress the infectious disease.

Restoration of Incipient Lesions. Although nonsurgical measures are the treatment of choice for managing incipient carious lesions, several criteria may indicate that tooth preparation and restoration are indicated. These criteria are used to assess present and future carious activity of the lesion. An experienced clinician is able to judge patient factors and make a decision as to whether sufficient indication exists to treat the lesion by a restoration. *Poor oral hygiene* and a *low frequency of routine dental care in unmotivated patients* would suggest restoration of some incipient lesions to prevent continued deterioration. A *history of caries or numerous restorations* on the contralateral surfaces or throughout the mouth may suggest that the incipient lesion should be restored. If there is a distinct variation in color when the area is transilluminated and *cavitation or a defect is present,* the lesion no longer is incipient and should be restored. Also, if radiographic evidence indicates that the *lesion extends to the DEJ,* the lesion should be assessed carefully and if appropriate, restored as early and as conservatively as possible to preserve the strength and esthetics of the remaining tooth. Finally, the *degree of caries susceptibility* and the *age of the patient* also must be considered. If caries susceptibility is low or if the patient is free of caries, the lesion is judged to be at lower risk and should not be restored, but appropriate recording, initiation of remineralization strategies, and regular periodic monitoring are indicated.

Esthetic Treatment. Among many segments of the U.S. population, interest in improved esthetics is growing. As a result, a range of treatments has been developed to manage a wide array of esthetic concerns. Chapter 15 describes these conservative esthetic treatments. They include esthetic recontouring of the anterior teeth, vital bleaching, and microabrasion. These conservative approaches have well-documented outcomes. In addition to these conservative techniques, advances in direct composite restorations have permitted the closure of diastemas, recontouring of teeth, and other tooth additions by means other than extensive full-coverage restorations.

Treatment of Abrasion, Erosion, and Attrition. Abraded or eroded areas should be considered for restoration only if one or more of the following exists: (1) the area is cariously involved, (2) the defect is sufficiently deep to compromise the structural integrity of the tooth, (3) intolerable sensitivity exists and is unresponsive to conservative desensitizing measures, (4) the defect contributes to a periodontal problem, (5) the area is to be involved in the design of a removable partial denture, (6) the depth of the defect is judged to be close to the pulp, or (7) the patient desires esthetic improvements.

Areas of significant attrition that are worn into dentin and are sensitive or annoying should be considered for restoration. However, before cast restorations are used, a complete occlusal analysis and an in-depth interview with the patient regarding the etiology should be conducted to reduce contributing factors. Also, biteguard therapy should be considered.

Treatment of Root-Surface Caries. Root caries is not uncommon in geriatric and postperiodontal treatment patients. Increases in the number of geriatric patients in the patient population and tooth retention have emphasized this growing problem. Areas with root-surface caries usually should be restored when there is clinical or radiographic evidence of cavitation. However, care must be exercised to distinguish the *active* root-surface carious lesion from the root-surface lesion that once was active but has become *inactive* (arrested) (Fig. 9-20, *A* and *B*). The latter lesion shows *eburnated dentin (sclerotic dentin)* that has darkened from extrinsic staining, is firm to the touch of an explorer, may be rough but is cleanable, and is seen in patients (usually older) whose oral hygiene and diet in recent years are good. Generally these lesions should not be restored except when the patient elects.

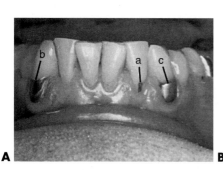
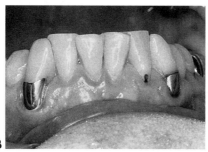
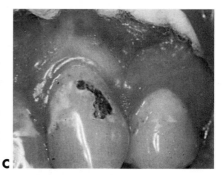

A　　　　　**B**　　　　　**C**

FIG. **9-20** **A,** Arrested, root surface carious lesion (40 years old) *(a)* showing darkened, eburnated (sclerotic) dentin. Lesion should not be restored unless esthetically objectionable. Also a gold inlay restoration (20 years old) *(b)* and amalgam restoration (36 years old) *(c).* **B,** Same patient as shown in **A,** but 12 years later (lesion 52 years old, gold inlay 32 years old, amalgam restoration 48 years old). **C,** Arrested carious lesions on facial surface of canine. Both lesions feel hard to explorer, are cleanable, and should not be restored except to improve esthetics.

If it is determined that the lesion needs restoration, it can be restored with amalgam or tooth-colored materials. Dentin adhesive restorative materials have enhanced the restorative treatment of root-surface caries.

Obviously prevention is preferred over restoration. It is recommended that appropriate preventive steps, such as improvements in diet and oral hygiene and fluoride treatment with or without cementoplasty,[46] be taken in hopes of avoiding carious breakdown and the need for restoration.

Treatment of Root-Surface Sensitivity. It is not unusual for patients to complain of root-surface sensitivity, which is annoying sharp pain usually associated with gingival recession and exposed root surfaces. Several theories have been advanced to explain the unusual sensitivity and response of such exposed dentin to a stimulus or irritation. The most accepted theory is the *hydrodynamic theory,* which postulates that the pain results from indirect innervation caused by dentinal fluid movement in the tubules that stimulates mechanoreceptors near the predentin (see the Pulp-Dentin Complex in Chapter 2). Some of the causes of such fluid shifts are temperature change, air-drying, and osmotic pressure. *Any treatment that can reduce these fluid shifts by partially or totally occluding the tubules may help reduce the sensitivity.*

Dentinal hypersensitivity is a particular problem in patients immediately after periodontal surgery that results in the clinical exposure of root surfaces. Numerous forms of treatment have been used to provide relief, such as topical fluoride, fluoride rinses, oxalate solutions, dentin bonding agents, sealants, iontophoresis, and desensitizing toothpastes. Although all of these methods have met with varying degrees of success, dentin-bonding agents provide the best rate of success. When these conservative methods fail to provide relief, restorative treatment is indicated.

Repairing and Resurfacing Existing Restorations. Many times amalgam, composite, or cast restorations can be repaired or recontoured as opposed to complete removal and replacement. There is growing evidence to suggest that the removal and replacement results in the "cycle of rerestoration" that leads to larger and larger tooth preparations and the resultant trauma to the tooth and supporting structures.[9] In addition, resurfacing or repair of composites,[16] as well as repair of cast restorations, have been shown to be effective.[23] In addition, amalgam restorations with localized defects can be repaired[13] with amalgam or with unfilled sealant resins.[44] Thus if a restoration has an isolated defect, which when explored operatively can be confirmed that all carious tooth structure has been removed, it is acceptable and many times preferable to repair or recontour. Further reshaping of overcontoured restorations is an acceptable form of treatment.

Replacement of Existing Restorations. Generally, a restoration should not be replaced unless: (1) it has significant discrepancies, (2) the tooth is at risk for caries or fracture, or (3) the restoration is an etiologic factor to adjacent teeth or tissue.[4] In many instances, recontouring or resurfacing the existing restoration can delay replacement.

Some indications for replacing restorations are as follows: (1) marginal void, especially in the gingival one third, that cannot be repaired; (2) poor proximal contour or a gingival overhang that contributes to periodontal breakdown; (3) a marginal ridge discrepancy that contributes to food impaction; (4) overcontour of a facial or lingual surface resulting in plaque gingival to the height of contour and resultant inflammation of gingiva overprotected from rubbing-cleansing action of food bolus or toothbrush; (5) poor proximal contact that is either open, resulting in interproximal food impaction and inflammation of impacted gingival papilla, or improper in location or size; (6) recurrent caries that cannot be adequately treated by a repair restoration; and (7) ditching deeper than 0.5 mm of the occlusal amalgam margin that is judged carious or caries-prone. By itself, the presence of shallow ditching around an amalgam restoration is not an indication for replacement.

Indications for replacing tooth-colored restorations include: (1) improper contours that cannot be repaired, (2) large voids, (3) deep marginal staining, (4) recurrent caries, and (5) unacceptable esthetics. Restorations that have only light marginal staining and are judged noncarious can be corrected by a shallow, narrow, marginal repair restoration.

Indications for Amalgam Restorations. Dental amalgam has proven to be a very good restorative material. Although its indications for use have decreased, it is still recognized as a successful restorative material. The use of amalgam in dentistry has been the source of controversy. Although the use of amalgam is considered safe, there are the perceived adverse effects on the environment by mercury and amalgam waste resulting as amalgam is removed from the teeth. Chapter 4 presents a more complete discussion of the issue, and Chapters 16 through 19 present the current indications for amalgam restorations.

Indications for Direct Composite and Other Tooth-Colored Restorations. The direct application of composite is indicated for the treatment of many lesions or faults in both anterior and posterior teeth. Detailed indications for composite and other tooth-colored restorations are presented in Chapters 11 through 15. The use of composite as a restorative material for posterior teeth has increased significantly. The American Dental Association has both supported the use of composite for many Class I and Class II restorations and indicated that such restorations should have a clinical longevity similar to amalgam restorations. Thus, direct composite restorations are appropriately indicated for most clinical applications, anteriorly and posteriorly.

Indications for Indirect Tooth-Colored Restorations.
Tooth-colored restorations that are indirectly fabricated out of the mouth may be indicated for Classes I and II due to esthetics, strength, and other bonding benefits (see Chapter 14). Moreover, because of the potential of bonded restorations to strengthen remaining tooth structure, indirect tooth-colored restorations also may be selected for the conservative restoration of weakened posterior teeth in esthetically critical areas.

Indirect tooth-colored restorations include: (1) processed composite, (2) feldspathic porcelain, (3) cast ceramic, and (4) computer-generated (computer-aided design [CAD]/computer-assisted machining [CAM]) inlays and onlays. Although all types offer superior physical characteristics when compared to direct composite restorations, they also are more costly because of the indirect process required for fabrication or the expense of CAD/CAM equipment.

Although *processed composite* restorations possess improved wear resistance over direct composites, they are indicated primarily for conservative Class I and Class II preparations in low-to-moderate stress areas. *Feldspathic porcelain* inlays and onlays for Class I and II restorations are highly esthetic but suffer from a relatively high incidence of fracture, especially if subjected to heavy occlusal forces. Porcelain restorations also have the potential to wear opposing tooth structure.

Cast ceramic inlays and onlays for Class I and Class II preparations offer excellent marginal fit, low abrasion to opposing tooth structure, and superior strength compared to processed composite or feldspathic porcelain. They offer an excellent esthetic alternative to cast metal restorations.

Computer-generated ceramic restorations for Class I and Class II preparations possess high strength and low abrasiveness and are highly esthetic because of the intrinsic coloration and highly polishable nature of the material. Onlays and inlays can be generated with this system. Because these restorations are fabricated chairside (CEREC System), only one appointment is required for placement as compared to the two appointments required for the other types of indirectly fabricated tooth-colored restorations.

Indications for Cast Metal Restorations. Although indications for intracoronal castings are few, a gold onlay that caps all of the cusps and includes some of the axial tooth line angles (see Chapter 20) is an excellent restoration. Cast metal restorations may be the treatment of choice for patients undergoing occlusal rehabilitation. Also, teeth with deep subgingival margins are well treated with cast restorations because, compared to amalgam and composite restorations, they provide a better opportunity for control of proximal contours and for restoration of the difficult subgingival margin. Specific indications for cast metal restorations are presented in Chapter 20.

TREATMENT PLAN APPROVAL

As noted earlier in this chapter, informed consent has become an integral part of modern day dental practice.[56] One aspect of informed consent is to provide the patient with the necessary information about the alternative therapies available to manage their oral conditions. For nearly all conditions, there is usually more than one alternative. These alternatives need to be presented to the patient and the advantages and disadvantages of each discussed. In addition, the patient needs to be informed of the risks associated with each alternative therapy. Many times a reasonable alternative is not to intervene but instead monitor the condition. Finally, the cost of treatment alternatives needs to be discussed with the patient. Once the dentist is sure that the patient has a full and complete understanding of the alternative treatments, their associated risks and benefits, and the results of possible nontreatment, then treatment can proceed.[11,12]

SUMMARY

Proper diagnosis and treatment planning play a critical role in the quality of dental care. Each patient must be evaluated individually in a thorough and systematic fashion. After the patient's condition is understood and recorded, a treatment plan can be developed and rendered.

A successful treatment plan carefully integrates and sequences all necessary procedures indicated for the patient. There are few absolutes in treatment planning; the available information must be considered carefully and incorporated into a plan to fit the needs of the individual. Patients should have an active role in the process; they should be made aware of the findings, be advised of the risks and benefits of the proposed treatment, and be given the opportunity to help decide the course of treatment.

Examination, diagnosis, and treatment planning are extremely challenging and rewarding for both the patient and the dentist if done thoroughly and properly with the patient's best interest in mind.

REFERENCES

1. American Dental Association: *The dental patient record: structure and function guidelines,* Chicago, 1987, American Dental Association.
2. American Dental Association Council on Access, Prevention and Interpersonal Relations: Providing dental care in long-term dental care facilities: a resource manual, Chicago, 1997, American Dental Association.
3. American Hospital Formulary Service: *AHFS drug information.* GK McEvoy, editor. Bethesda, 1999, Board of the American Society of Health-System Pharmacists, Inc.
4. Anusavice K: Criteria for placement and replacement of dental restorations: an international consensus report, *Int Dent J* 38(3):193-194, 1988.
5. Ashley PF et al: Occlusal caries diagnosis: an in vitro histological validation of the Electronic Caries Monitor (ECM) and other methods, *J Dent* 26(2):83-88, 1998.

6. Bader JD, Shugars DA: Variation, treatment outcomes, and practice guidelines in dental practice, *J Dent Educ* 59(1):61-95, 1995.

7. Berg R, Morgenstern NE: Physiological changes in the elderly, *Dental Clin North Am* 41(4):651-668, 1997.

8. Berkey DB et al: The old-old dental patient: The challenge of clinical decision-making, *J Am Dent Assoc* 127(3):321-332, 1996.

9. Brantley CF et al: Does the cycle of rerestoration lead to larger restorations? *J Am Dent Assoc* 126(10):1407-1413, 1995.

10. Cassady KA, Whitley RJ: New therapeutic approaches to the alphaherpesvirus infections, *J Antimicrob Chemother* 39(2): 119-128, 1997.

11. Christensen GJ: Educating patients about dental procedures, *J Am Dent Assoc* 126(3):371-372, 1995.

12. Christensen GJ: Educating patients: a new necessity, *J Am Dent Assoc* 124(8):86-87, 1993.

13. Ciprano TM, Santos JF: Clinical behavior of repaired amalgam restorations: a two-year study, *J Prosthet Dent* 73(1):8-11, 1995.

14. Cleveland J et al: Risk and prevention of hepatitis C virus infection: implications for dentistry, *J Am Dent Assoc* 130(5): 641-647, 1999.

15. Collins D: What a dentist should know about the oral health record, *Northwest Dent* 75(1):35-37, 1996.

16. Crumpler DC et al: Bonding to re-surfaced posterior composites, *Dent Mater* 5(6):417-423, 1989.

17. Dajani AS et al: Prevention of bacterial endocarditis: recommendations by the American Heart Association, *J Am Dent Assoc* 128(8):1142-1151, 1997.

18. EC-Clearinghouse on Oral Problems Related to HIV Infection and WHO Collaborating Centre on Oral Manifestations of the Human Immunodeficiency Virus: Classification and diagnostic criteria for oral lesions in HIV infection, *J Oral Pathol Med* 22:289-291, 1993.

19. Ekstrand K et al: Light microscope study of the effect of probing occlusal surfaces, *Caries Res* 21(4):368-374, 1987.

20. Fasbinder DJ: Treatment planner's toolkit, *Gen Dent* 47(1): 35-39, 1999.

21. Ferreira-Zandona AG et al: An in vitro comparison between laser fluorescence and visual examination for detection of demineralization in occlusal pits and fissures, *Caries Res* 32(3): 210-218, 1998.

22. Ficarra G et al: Kaposi's sarcoma of the oral cavity: a study of 134 patients with a review of the pathogenesis, epidemiology, clinical aspects, and treatment, *Oral Surg Oral Med Oral Pathol* 66(5):543-550, 1988.

23. Fitch DR et al: Amalgam repair of cast gold crown margins: a microleakage assessment, *Gen Dent* 30(4):328-333, 1982.

24. Galan D, Lynch E. Epidemiology of root caries, *Gerodontology* 10(2):59-71, 1993.

25. Gillcrist JA: Hepatitis viruses A, B, C, D, E and G: implications for dental personnel, *J Am Dent Assoc* 130(4):509-520, 1999.

26. Glick M: New guidelines for prevention, detection, evaluation and treatment of high blood pressure, *J Am Dent Assoc* 129(11):1588-1594, 1998.

27. Greenspan D, Greenspan JS: HIV-related oral disease, *Lancet* 348(9029):729-733, 1996.

28. Greenspan D et al: Oral "hairy" leukoplakia in male homosexuals: evidence of association with both papillomavirus and a herpes-group virus, *Lancet* 2(8407):831-834, 1984.

29. Grippo JO: Abfractions: a new classification of hard tissue lesions of teeth, *J Esthet Dent* 3(1):14-19, 1991.

30. Health Care Financing Agency. Personal health care expenditures, by type of expenditure and source of funds: selected calendar years 1990-1997. Available online at *http://www. hcfa.gov./stats//NHE-Proj/proj1998/tables/table8b.htm*. Accessed Dec 1999.

31. Hintze H et al: Reliability of visual examination, fiber-optic transillumination, and bite-wing radiography, and reproducibility of direct visual examination following tooth separation for the identification of cavitated carious lesions in contacting approximal surfaces, *Caries Res* 32(3):204-209,1998.

32. Hoofnagle JH: Type B hepatitis: virology, serology and clinical course, *Semin Liver Dis* 1(1):7-14, 1981.

33. Katz RV: The clinical identification of root caries, *Gerodontology* 5(1):21-24, 1986.

34. Kaugers GE et al: Radiographically detected class I carious lesions in clinically sound teeth, *Gen Dent* 268-270, May-June 1994.

35. Khocht A et al: Assessment of periodontal status with PSR and traditional clinical periodontal examination, *J Am Dent Assoc* 126:1658-1665, 1995.

36. Kidd EA et al: Diagnosis of secondary caries: a laboratory study, *Br Dent J* 176(4):135-139, 1994.

37. Kidd EAM et al: Marginal ditching and staining as a predictor of secondary caries around amalgam restorations: a clinical and microbiological study, *J Dent Res* 74(5):1206-1211, 1995.

38. Kidd EAM et al: Occlusal caries diagnosis: a changing challenge for clinicians and epidemiologists, *J Dent* 21(6):323-331, 1993.

39. Lamster IB et al: Epidemiology and diagnosis of HIV-associated periodontal diseases, *Oral Dis* 3:S141-S148, 1997.

40. Lussi A: Validity of diagnostic and treatment decisions of fissure caries, *Caries Res* 25(4):296-303, 1991.

41. Madison M, Wilcox LR: An evaluation of coronal microleakage in endodontically-treated teeth. Part III: in vivo study, *J Endod* 14(9):455-458, 1998.

42. Matteson SR et al: The report of the panel to develop radiographic selection criteria for dental patients, *Gen Dent* 39(4): 264-270, 1991.

43. Merchant VA: Herpes viruses and other microorganisms of concern in dentistry, *Dent Clin North Am* 35(2):283-298, 1991.

44. Mertz-Fairhurst EJ et al: Clinical performance of sealed composite restorations placed over caries compared with sealed and unsealed amalgam restorations, *J Am Dent Assoc* 115(5): 689-694, 1987.

45. Miller CS: Viral infections in the immunocompetent patient, *Dermatol Clin* 14(2):225-241, 1996.

46. Mjor IA: Frequency of secondary caries at various anatomical locations, *Oper Dent* 10(3):88-92, 1985.

47. Nasi JH: Background to, and implementation of, the Periodontal Screening and Recording (PSR) procedure in the USA, *Inter Dent J* 44(5 suppl 1):585-588, 1994.

48. Newbrun E: Problems in caries diagnosis, *Int Dent J* 43(2): 133-142, 1993.

49. Newwitter DS et al: Detection of root caries: sensitivity and specificity of a modified explorer, *Gerodontics* 1(2):65-67, 1985.

50. Patton LL, McKaig R: Rapid progression of bone loss in HIV-associated necrotizing ulcerative stomatitis, *J Periodont* 69(6): 710-716, 1998.

51. Patton LL, van der Horst C: Oral infections and other manifestations of HIV disease, *Infect Dis Clin North Am* 13:879-900, 1999.

52. Penning C et al: Validity of probing for fissure caries diagnosis, *Caries Res* 26(6):445-449,1992.

53. Pitts NB, Rimmer PA: An in vivo comparison of radiographic and directly assessed clinical caries status of posterior

approximal surfaces in primary and permanent teeth, *Caries Res* 26(2):146-152, 1992.

54. Sackett DL et al: Evidence-based medicine: What it is and what it isn't, *Br Med J* 312(7023):71-72, 1996.

55. Shugars DA, Bader JD: Practice parameters in dentistry: where do we stand? *J Am Dent Assoc* 126(8):1134-1143, 1995.

56. Sfikas PM: Informed consent and the law, *J Am Dent Assoc* 129(11):1471-1473, 1998.

57. Vissink A et al: Aging and saliva: a review of the literature, *Spec Care Dentist* 16(3):95-103, 1996.

58. Yassin OM: In vitro studies of the effect of a dental explorer on the formation of an artificial carious lesion, *J Dent Child* 62(2):111-117, 1995.

SUGGESTED READINGS

Gillchrist JA: Hepatitis viruses A, B, C, D, E and G: implications for dental personnel, *J Am Dent Assoc* 130:509-520, 1999.

Glick, M: *Dental management of patients with HIV,* Chicago, 1994, Quintessence.

Miller CS: Viral infections in the immunocompetent patient, *Dermatol Clin* 14:225-241, 1996.

Richman DD, Whitley RJ, Hayden FG, editors: *Clinical virology,* New York, 1997, Churchill Livingstone.

Samaranayake LP: *Essential microbiology for dentistry,* New York, 1996, Churchill Livingstone.

Slots J, Taubman MA, editors: *Contemporary oral microbiology and immunology,* St Louis, 1992, Mosby.

Preliminary Considerations for Operative Dentistry

ALDRIDGE D. WILDER, JR.

KENNETH N. MAY, JR.*

CLIFFORD M. STURDEVANT*

*These authors are inactive this edition. See the Acknowledgments.

In this chapter the routine chair-side preoperative procedures (before actual tooth preparation) are addressed. Primarily, these include patient and operator positions, pain control, and isolation of the operating field. The preliminary procedures of occlusal considerations and infection control are discussed in Chapters 2 and 8, respectively.

PREOPERATIVE PATIENT AND DENTAL TEAM CONSIDERATIONS

In preparation for a clinical procedure it is important to ensure that patient and operator positions are properly selected, that instrument exchange between the dentist and assistant are efficient, and that magnification is used if needed.

PATIENT AND OPERATOR POSITIONS

An appreciation of efficient patient and operator positions is beneficial for the welfare of both persons. The patient who is in a comfortable position is more relaxed, has less muscular tension, and is more capable of cooperating with the dentist. By using proper operating positions and good posture, the operator experiences less physical strain and fatigue and reduces the possibility of developing musculoskeletal disorders.

The practice of dentistry is demanding and stressful. Physical problems may arise if appropriate operating positions are neglected. Most restorative dental procedures can be accomplished while seated. Positions that create unnecessary curvature of the spine or slumping of the shoulders should be avoided. When the back and chest are held in an upright position with the shoulders squared, proper breathing and circulation are promoted. At times, circumstances prevent maintaining this position while operating, but it should be the basic body position. Proper balance and weight distribution on both feet is essential when operating from a standing position. Generally, any uncomfortable or unnatural position that places undue strain on the body should be used only rarely. The health and fitness of the dentist are significant factors contributing to physical endurance and productivity.

Chair and Patient Positions. Chair and patient positions are important considerations. Modern dental chairs are designed to provide total body support in any chair position. An available chair accessory is an adjustable headrest cushion or an articulating headrest attached to the chair back. A contoured or lounge-type chair provides complete patient support and comfort. Chair design and adjustment permit maximal operator access to the work area. The adjustment control switches should be conveniently located. Some chairs are also equipped with programmable operating positions. To improve infection control, chairs with a foot switch for patient positioning are recommended.

The patient should have direct access to the chair. The chair height should be low, the backrest upright, and the armrest adjusted to allow the patient to get into the chair. After the patient is seated, the armrest is returned to its normal position. The headrest cushion is positioned to support the head and elevate the chin slightly away from the chest. In this position neck muscle strain is minimal and swallowing is facilitated. The chair is then adjusted to place the patient in a reclining position.

The most common patient positions for operative dentistry are almost supine or reclined 45 degrees (Fig. 10-1). The choice of patient position varies with the operator, the type of procedure, and the area of the mouth involved in the operation. In the almost supine position, the patient's head, knees, and feet are approximately the same level. The patient's head should not be lower than the feet; the head should be positioned lower than the feet only in an emergency, as when the patient is in syncope. When the operation is completed, the chair should be placed in the upright position so the patient can leave the chair easily and gracefully, preventing undue strain or loss of balance.

Operating Positions. Operating positions may be described by the location of the operator or by the location of the operator's arms in relation to patient position. For a right-handed operator, there are essentially three positions—right front, right, and right rear. These are sometimes referred to as the 7-, 9-, and 11-o'clock positions, respectively (Fig. 10-2, *A*). For the left-handed

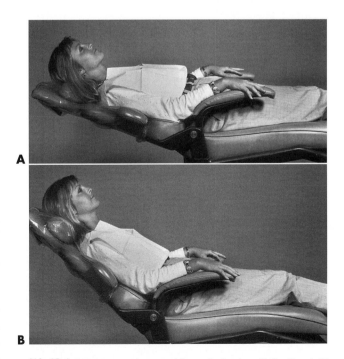

A

B

FIG. **10-1** Common patient positions. **A,** Supine. **B,** Reclined 45 degrees. Both are recommended for sit-down dentistry. Use depends on the arch being operated upon.

operator, the three positions are left front, left, and left rear, or the 5-, 3-, and 1-o'clock positions, respectively. A fourth position, direct rear or 12-o'clock position, has application for certain areas of the mouth. All of the positions discussed may be used from the standing or seated operating position, though to relieve stress on the operator's legs and support the operator's back, most dental treatment is delivered from a seated position. As a rule, the teeth being treated should be at the same level as the operator's elbow. The operating positions described here are for the right-handed operator; the left-handed operator should substitute *left* for *right*.

Right Front Position. This right front position facilitates examination and work on mandibular anterior teeth (see Fig. 10-2, *B*), mandibular posterior teeth (especially on the right side), and maxillary anterior teeth. It is often advantageous to have the patient's head rotated slightly toward the operator.

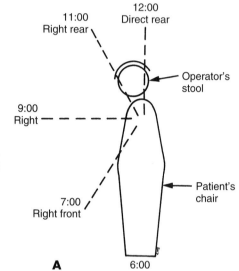

FIG. **10-2** Operating positions indicated by arm approach to the patient. **A,** Diagrammatic operator positions; **B,** right front; **C,** right; **D,** right rear; and **E,** direct rear.

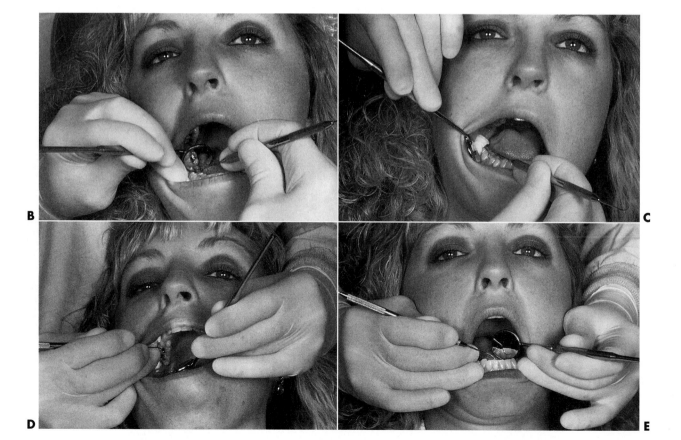

Right Position. In the right position, the operator is directly to the right of the patient (see Fig. 10-2, *C*). This position is convenient for operating on the facial surfaces of the maxillary and mandibular right posterior teeth and the occlusal surfaces of the mandibular right posterior teeth.

Right Rear Position. The right rear position is the position of choice for most operations. Most areas of the mouth are accessible and can be viewed directly or indirectly using a mouth mirror. The operator is behind and slightly to the right of the patient. The left arm is positioned around the patient's head (see Fig. 10-2, *D*). When operating from this position, the lingual and incisal (occlusal) surfaces of the maxillary teeth are viewed in the mouth mirror. Direct vision may be used on mandibular teeth, particularly on the left side, but the use of a mouth mirror is advocated for light reflection, retraction, and visibility.

Direct Rear Position. The direct rear position has somewhat limited application and is primarily used for operating on the lingual surfaces of mandibular anterior teeth. The operator is located directly behind the patient and looks down over the patient's head (see Fig. 10-2, *E*).

General Considerations. Several general considerations regarding chair and patient positions are also important. The operator should not hesitate to rotate the patient's head backward or forward or from side-to-side to accommodate the demands of access and visibility of the operating field. Minor rotation of the patient's head is not uncomfortable to the patient and allows the operator to maintain his or her basic body position. As a rule, when operating in the maxillary arch, the maxillary occlusal surfaces should be oriented approximately perpendicular to the floor. When operating in the mandibular arch, the mandibular occlusal surfaces should be oriented approximately 45 degrees to the floor. Patients are usually very cooperative in allowing the operator to position the head where it is most advantageous to the operator. Sacrificing good operating posture in most instances is unnecessary (Fig. 10-3).

The face of the operator should not come in close proximity to that of the patient. The ideal distance, similar to that for reading a book, should be maintained. However, small, detailed, or inaccessible tooth preparations may require closer proximity for adequate visibility. Maintaining an appropriate working distance from the patient is important for the operator to master in the early stages of learning. Another important aspect of proper operating position is to minimize body contact with the patient. A proper operator does not rest forearms on the patient's shoulders or hands on the patient's face or forehead. The patient's chest should not be used as an instrument tray. Unnecessary contact is unpleasant to many patients and should not be practiced.

From most positions the left hand should be free to hold the mouth mirror to reflect light onto the operating field to view the tooth preparation indirectly or to retract the cheek or tongue. In certain instances it is more appropriate to retract the cheek with one or two fingers of the left hand than to use a mouth mirror. However, it is often possible to retract the cheek and reflect light with the mouth mirror at the same time.

When operating for an extended period, the operator will find a certain amount of rest and muscle relaxation can be obtained by changing operating positions. Operating from a single position for an entire day, especially if standing, produces unnecessary fatigue. Changing positions, if only for a short time, reduces muscle strain and lessens fatigue.[36]

Operating Stools. A variety of operating stools are available for the dentist and dental assistant. The design of the stool is important. The stool should be on casters for mobility. It should be sturdy and well balanced to prevent tipping or gliding away from the dental chair. The seat should be well padded with smooth cushion edges and should be adjustable up and down. The backrest should be adjustable forward and backward as well as up and down. The assistant's stool should have a foot ring to permit proper leg position. Operator stools do not have a footrest. Comfortable, well-designed stools help reduce tension and fatigue.

Some of the advantages of a seated work position are lost if the operator uses the stool improperly. The operator should not be balanced on the stool, using it as a third leg of a tripod. The operator should sit back on the cushion, using the entire seat and not just the front edge. The upper body should be positioned so that the spinal column is straight or bent slightly forward and supported by the back rest of the stool. Some operator and assistant stools have backrests with curved extensions that offer additional body support. The thighs should be parallel to the floor, and the lower legs should be perpendicular to the floor. If the seat is too high, its

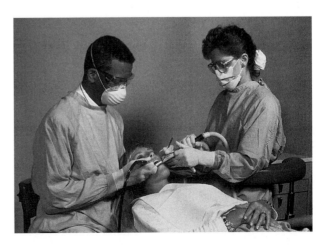

FIG. **10-3** Recommended seating positions for operator and chairside assistant, with the height of the operating field approximately at elbow level of the operator.

front edge will cut off circulation to the user's legs. Feet should be flat on the floor. Of course, this ideal position cannot be maintained at all times, but it should be used as much as possible.

The seated work position for the assistant is essentially the same as for the operator, except that the stool is 4 to 6 inches higher for maximal visual access. It is important, therefore, that the stool for the assistant have an adequate footrest so that a parallel thigh position can be maintained with good foot support. When properly seated, both the operator and assistant are capable of providing dental service throughout the day without an unnecessary decline in efficiency and productivity because of muscle tension and fatigue.

INSTRUMENT EXCHANGE

All instrument exchange between the operator and assistant should occur in the exchange zone below the patient's chin and several inches above the patient's chest. Instruments should not be exchanged over the patient's face. During the procedure the operator should anticipate and inform the assistant of the next instrument required; this allows the instrument to be brought into the exchange zone for a timely exchange. An experienced assistant will anticipate the operator's instrument needs before they are verbalized.

During proper instrument exchange it should not be necessary for the operator to remove his or her eyes from the operating field. The operator should rotate the instrument handle forward to cue the assistant to exchange instruments. Any sharp instrument should be exchanged with appropriate deliberation. The assistant should take the instrument from the operator, rather than the operator dropping it into the assistant's hand, and vice versa. The exchange need not be forceful, nor should it be conducted as if the instrument were a feather. Each person should be sure that the other has a firm grasp on the instrument before it is released. To maximize operating efficiency, whether treating one tooth or several, each instrument should be used completely before proceeding to the next instrument. This will minimize the number of instrument exchanges necessary for each procedure.

MAGNIFICATION

Another key to the success of clinical operative dentistry is visual acuity. The operator must be able to see clearly to attend to the details of each procedure. Normal accommodation of the operator's eyes is necessary to maintain proper working distance. The aging process causes a loss of accommodation. After the age of 40, operators may require magnifying lenses to compensate for this loss. The use of magnification before loss of accommodation facilitates attention to detail, acclimates the operator to magnifying lenses early, and does not adversely affect vision. Magnifying lenses have a fixed focal length that often requires the operator to maintain

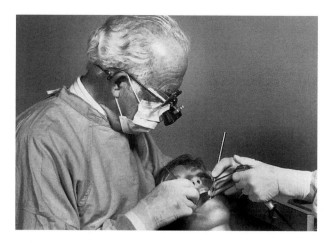

FIG. **10-4** Use of magnification with surgical telescopes.

a proper working distance, which ensures good posture. Several types of magnification devices are available, including bifocal eyeglasses, loupes, and surgical telescopes (Fig. 10-4). The use of eyeglasses also provides some protection from eye injury.

PAIN CONTROL

Historically, the public has associated dental treatment with pain. This is no longer valid, because techniques for the elimination of pain, including atraumatic needle injection, have been available for years and are essential to a successful dental practice. Local anesthesia for operative dentistry must be profound, often to depths required for pulpal anesthesia. The following information, if understood and practiced, should eliminate pain associated with dental procedures. For additional information the reader is referred to Malamed's *Handbook of Local Anesthesia*.[22]

LOCAL ANESTHESIA

Injection is used to achieve local anesthesia in restorative dentistry. The administration of local anesthesia to all tissues in the operating site is recommended for most patients to eliminate pain and reduce salivation associated with tooth preparation and restoration. To administer effective anesthesia the dentist must have a thorough knowledge of the patient's physical and emotional status and an understanding of the effects of the drug to be injected and the advantages and disadvantages of adding vasoconstrictors.

A *therapeutic dose* of a drug is the smallest amount that is effective when properly administered and does not cause adverse reactions. An *overdose* of a drug is an excessive amount that results in an overly elevated local accumulation or blood level of the drug, which causes adverse reactions. The normal healthy patient can safely receive as many as five to eight cartridges of anesthetic per appointment. Each 1.8-ml cartridge contains anesthetic, either with or without a vasoconstrictor (e.g., lidocaine 2% [anesthetic] with epinephrine 1:100,000

TABLE 10-1 Maximum Recommended Doses of 2% Lidocaine with Epinephrine 1:100,000 (Based on 36 mg per Cartridge)

PATIENT WEIGHT		MAXIMUM DOSE	MAXIMUM NUMBER OF CARTRIDGES
45 kg	100 lbs	200 mg	5.5 cartridges
68 kg	150 lbs	300 mg*	8 cartridges*
90 kg	200 lbs	300 mg*	8 cartridges*

From Malamed SF: *Handbook of local anesthesia,* ed 4, St Louis, 1997, Mosby.
*Absolute maximum of 300 mg.

TABLE 10-2 Maximum Recommended Doses of Other Commonly Used Local Anesthetics

LOCAL ANESTHETIC	MG/CARTRIDGE	MG/KG	MG/LB	MAXIMUM MG
Articaine 4% with epinephrine 1:200,000	72	7	3.2	500
Articaine 4% with epinephrine 1:100,000	72	7	3.2	500
Bupivacaine 0.5% with epinephrine 1:200,000	9	1.3	0.6	90
Etidocaine 1.5% + epinephrine 1:200,000	27	8	3.6	400
Lidocaine 2% with epinephrine 1:100,000	36	4.4	2.0	300
Lidocaine 2% with epinephrine 1:50,000	36	4.4	2.0	300
Mepivacaine 3% plain	54	4.4	2.0	300
Mepivacaine 2% with levonordefrin 1:20,000	36	4.4	2.0	300
Prilocaine 4% plain	72	6	2.7	400
Prilocaine 4% with epinephrine 1:200,000	72	6	2.7	400

From Malamed SF: *Handbook of local anesthesia,* ed 4, St Louis, 1997, Mosby.

[vasoconstrictor], lidocaine 2% plain [no vasoconstrictor]). The number of permissible cartridges increases as body weight increases. According to Malamed, the maximum recommended dose (MRD) of 2% lidocaine with epinephrine 1:100,000 is 4.4 mg/kg, or 2.0 mg/lb, to an absolute maximum of 300 mg (Table 10-1). (The maximum recommended dosages of other commonly used local anesthetics are listed in Table 10-2.) Tables 10-1 and 10-2 allow the operator to calculate the maximum dose for a specific agent depending on the weight of the patient. However, these dosages are averages, and the dentist must be alert to adverse systemic effects when injected dosages approach the recommended limits.[22]

Local anesthetics have different durations of action for both pulpal and soft tissue anesthesia. Pulpal (deep) anesthesia varies from 30 to 90 or more minutes. Soft tissue anesthesia varies from 1 to 9 hours depending on the specific agent and whether a vasoconstrictor is included. Local anesthetics are selected based on the estimated length of the clinical procedure and the degree of anesthesia required (Box 10-1). Two (or more) anesthetic agents can be administered when needed. However, the total dose of both anesthetics should not exceed the lower of the two maximum doses for the individual agents. Anesthetics are also available in amide and ester types. Hypersensitivity and allergic reactions in affected patients are much less frequent with the amide type of local anesthetic.[22]

BOX 10-1 Approximate Duration of Action of Local Anesthetics*

SHORT DURATION (PULPAL ABOUT 30 MINUTES)
Lidocaine 2%
Prilocaine 4% (infiltration)
Mepivacaine 3%

INTERMEDIATE DURATION (PULPAL 60 MINUTES)
Articaine 4% + epinephrine 1:100,000
Articaine 4% + epinephrine 1:200,000
Lidocaine 2% + epinephrine 1:50,000
Lidocaine 2% + epinephrine 1:100,000
Mepivacaine 2% + levonordefrin 1:20,000
Prilocaine 4% (nerve block)
Prilocaine 4% + epinephrine 1:200,000

LONG DURATION (PULPAL 90 OR MORE MINUTES)
Bupivacaine 0.5% + epinephrine 1:200,000
Etidocaine 1.5% + epinephrine 1:200,000 (nerve block)

From Malamed SF: *Handbook of local anesthesia,* ed 4, St Louis, 1997, Mosby.
*Note that these anesthetics are all from the amide category.

Patient Factors

Cardiovascular System. Before administering any drug, the condition of the cardiovascular system (CVS) (heart and blood vessels) must be assessed. At minimum, blood pressure, heart rate, and rhythm should be evaluated and recorded for all patients. For example, a patient with a systolic pressure greater than 200 and a diastolic pressure greater than 115 should not receive invasive, elective dental treatment until the blood pressure is reduced.[22]

Malamed[22] has suggested that any resting patient with a pulse rate below 60 or above 110 be questioned further. Athletes in good physical condition may have a lower heart rate, but without this information, the lower heart rate may indicate a heart block. Additionally, five or more "missed beats" (premature ventricular contractions) per minute with no obvious cause is an indication for medical consultation. Patients with valvular heart disease or a predisposition to bacterial endocarditis should have prophylactic antibiotics prescribed before dental treatment; the American Heart Association defines the recommended regimen for these antibiotics.[12]

Overdose of any vasoconstrictor causes a rise in blood pressure, elevated heart rate, and possible dysrhythmias. These symptoms may also occur if retraction cord treated with epinephrine is applied to abraded gingiva, resulting in a rapid uptake of the drug into the circulatory system. With careful operative dentistry, gingiva should be minimally abraded, even in subgingival tooth preparations.

Central Nervous and Respiratory Systems. The central nervous system (CNS) is more easily affected by an overdose of injected anesthetic drugs than the CVS. Anesthetics do depress the CNS, but when administered properly for local anesthesia, they cause very little or no clinical evidence of depression. However, at minimum to moderate overdose levels, depression is manifested in excitation (e.g., talkativeness, apprehension, sweating, elevated blood pressure and heart rate, elevated respiratory rate) or drowsiness. At moderate to high overdose levels there could be tonic-clonic seizure activity, followed by generalized CNS depression, depressed blood pressure, reduced heart rate (less than 60 beats/second), depressed respiratory rate, and respiratory arrest. With lidocaine and procaine, the usual progression of excitatory signs and symptoms described previously may not be seen, and the first clinical evidence of overdose may be mild sedation or drowsiness.[22]

The respiratory system is not affected by properly administered therapeutic doses of anesthetic drug. However, the system may be depressed and arrested by CNS depression due to overdose.

Allergy. Malamed[22] states that documented, reproducible allergy is an absolute contraindication for administration of local anesthetic. When a patient reports a history of "sensitivity" or "reaction" to an injected dental anesthetic, the dentist must believe the patient until further investigation disproves the patient's claim. Anaphylactic shock from an allergic reaction can be immediate and life threatening. Fast or intramuscular injection of anesthetic are both reasons for allergy-like reactions reported by patients. Some patients have a bona fide allergy to bisulfite, an antioxidant used in anesthetic cartridges as a preservative for the vasoconstrictor.[22]

Any special condition of the patient should be recorded in the chart. For example, health status of the CVS, CNS, respiratory system, liver, kidneys, and thyroid gland should be noted, as should the patient's age, allergies, and pregnancy status. A medical history form must be completed and signed by the patient (see Chapter 9).

Benefits

Cooperative Patient. When a local anesthetic appropriate for the procedure is properly administered, patient anxiety and tension should be minimal. The appreciation and trust of the patient for the dentist (and dental assistant) is expressed in a more relaxed and cooperative attitude. Physically and emotionally, both patient and dentist benefit from a relatively calm environment.

Salivation Control. Saliva control is a primary reason for desiring profound anesthesia for most patients. For years, it has been observed that complete anesthesia of all tissues (teeth and gingival tissues) in the dental operating site results in a near cessation of salivation.[39] Sometimes a tooth is not sensitive and does not require anesthesia. However, if all other sensations from the operating site are eliminated, salivation is controlled.

Hemostasis. The term *hemostasis*, as used in operative dentistry, is the temporary reduction in blood flow and volume in tissue (ischemia) where a vasoconstrictor is used. The alpha effect of the vasoconstrictor causes constriction of the small blood vessels; thus the affected tissue bleeds less if cut or abraded. The principle function of a vasoconstrictor in operative dentistry is the prolongation of anesthesia because of reduced blood flow to and from the anesthetized site. Without epinephrine, anesthesia from 1 ml of lidocaine 2% will last only 5 to 10 minutes; with epinephrine, the anesthesia will last 40 to 60 minutes. Reduced blood flow helps keep the patient's blood level of anesthetic and vasoconstrictor at a low level by reducing the rate of absorption into the circulatory system.

Operator Efficiency. Local anesthesia greatly benefits both dentist and patient and is very beneficial for successful tooth preparation and restoration. It improves operator efficiency, and usually the patient is calmer and more cooperative. This may reinforce the dentist's confidence and calmness, which, in turn, may promote more efficient treatment. Without distractions or management problems from the patient, the dentist can focus on the treatment and its completion in a reasonable time frame.

Administration

Psychology. Patients have varying degrees of concern about receiving an intraoral injection. A concentrated effort by the dentist and dental assistant is required to make the procedure more acceptable, and a positive approach is desirable with all patients during this phase of treatment. Probably the greatest positive effect is achieved by a caring manner, rather than by what is said. Words such as *pain, sting, hurt,* and *inject* should not be used, because no matter what else is said, the patient will only remember these potentially fear-invoking words. The operator must use a kind, considerate, and understanding approach. Every assurance should be made that comfort of the patient is paramount and that the teeth and soft tissues will be treated with care. Such assurances, confidently and softly spoken, are welcomed during the administration of local anesthesia. One example is, "I may be taking longer than you expected, but we are giving the solution slowly to be kind to your tissues." Patients who feel secure (safe from pain and in caring hands) will gratefully accept local anesthesia. The art of tactfully keeping the syringe and needle from view of the patient should be practiced. Here the chairside assistant can be a tremendous help.

Technique Steps and Principles. Since profound, painless anesthesia of both the teeth and contiguous soft tissues is so important in operative dentistry, salient features of a recommended technique for infiltration anesthesia of a maxillary canine are presented. Technique instructions for both injection and infection control (particularly avoiding accidental needlestick) are described, and the following principles for injection of local anesthetic and epinephrine are applicable for infiltration and conduction anesthesia. *Infiltration anesthesia* involves a supraperiosteal or field block where deposition is near the nerve ends in the operating site. *Conduction anesthesia* involves a nerve block where deposition is near a nerve trunk at a distance from the operating site.

In this example of infiltration anesthesia, the needle entry spot and direction are different from that presented in some local anesthesia textbooks. Aspiration as well as slow deposition of solution is emphasized. For other local anesthesia injections (inferior alveolar, Gow-Gates mandibular, posterior superior alveolar, infraorbital, mental, and periodontal ligament), the reader is referred to a textbook in local anesthesia.

The routine supine position of the patient helps prevent vasodepressor syncope because it maintains blood supply and blood pressure to the brain. As a precaution, the upper torso should never be more than 10 degrees below the horizontal plane, as this may cause respiratory distress due to the force of viscera against the diaphragm. Occasionally, patients may complain of difficulty in breathing except when sitting upright or standing (orthopnea), in which case a compromise in patient position is necessary. Another exception to the supine position is when symptoms suggest an epinephrine overdose; in this case, a semierect or sitting position is best since it minimizes any further elevation in cerebral blood pressure. Symptoms of overdose include fear, perspiration, weakness, pallor, palpitations, anxiety, and restlessness.[22]

The syringe must have an aspirating feature. When anesthetic is administered, aspiration is second in importance only to slow deposition of solution. For this purpose, the rod (piston) has a harpoon on its cartridge end and a thumb ring on the other end (see Fig. 10-5, *H*). The harpoon engages the cartridge plunger, resulting in its potential reverse movement to create negative pressure when the operator's thumb (in the ring) pulls back gently.

Injection into infected tissue should be avoided because of the risk of spreading the infection. Also, the anesthetic becomes less effective because the tissue is acidic rather than basic. Alternative approaches, such as nerve block, should be used.

Disposable needle. The sheath covers the needle and the cap covers the reverse end (cartridge end) of the disposable needle (see *s* and *c* in Fig. 10-5, *B*). For each patient (appointment) the dental assistant selects a sheathed, capped, new disposable needle of the desired length and gauge. The sheathed needle comes sterile from the manufacturer. The needle remains sheathed, except for setting the harpoon and testing the syringe preparedness (see later principles), until the moment of entry at the injection site. This helps prevent accidental needlestick, which among other things indicates needle replacement. For each patient appointment, using a new, sterile needle contaminated only by that patient's oral tissue eliminates crossinfection via the needle. Keeping the sheath in place ensures that the needle is sharp. When the needle contacts the firm periosteal tissue or bone, a minute barb can be formed that will cause pain on withdrawal or during subsequent reinjection.

The needle must be sufficiently long that its full length is never out of sight (never completely within tissue). This means that in the unlikely event a needle breaks at the hub junction there will be some of the needle exposed for grasping and withdrawal.

Needles of 27-gauge are generally recommended, although some operators prefer the 30-gauge, short needle for infiltration anesthesia of the maxillary teeth. The 30-gauge needle may not allow aspiration, and some authorities believe that it does not pierce or move in tissue easier than the 27-gauge needle. Also, the 30-gauge, long needle may deviate during injection for conduction anesthesia of the inferior alveolar nerve.

Prop/guard card. The dental assistant inserts the sheathed needle end into the prop/guard card (Stik-Shield, Tacoma, Washington) (see Fig. 10-5, *A* to *D*) and removes the cap on the reverse end of the needle (see Fig. 10-5, *E*). The dental assistant then inserts the reverse end of the needle into the hole at the threaded end of the syringe and screws the sheathed needle to a full seating position against the nose of the syringe (see Fig. 10-5, *F* and *G*). The guard card protects both hands. The card will hit the nose of the syringe before the needle could stick the hand holding the syringe.

The dental assistant inserts the cartridge and sets the harpoon or lays the propped (by card) syringe on a tray or countertop (see Fig. 10-5, *H*) behind the patient for the operator to insert the cartridge, set the harpoon, remove the sheath, and test for preparedness.

Anesthetic cartridge. Using a new cartridge for each patient is imperative. Because some ingredients do not have an extended shelf life, the anesthetic cartridge should not be over 18 months past the date of manufacture. The expiration date is printed on the packing container. Some manufacturers place an expiration date on the cartridge. The diaphragm end of the cartridge should not be contaminated by contact with potentially infected surfaces. The cartridge should not be immersed in a sterilizing solution (cold sterilizing solution or alcohol) because this can diffuse through the diaphragm and cause tissue damage. Cartridges should not be exposed to sunlight and should be stored at room temperature.[22]

Anesthetic solution. The weakest solution of anesthetic that will be effective should be used. Lidocaine 2% with 1:100,000 epinephrine is commonly used in operative dentistry and is generally recommended. One milliliter (half a cartridge) provides infiltration anesthesia for 40 to 60 minutes for anterior teeth.

The addition of a vasoconstrictor to the anesthetic solution is necessary to prolong anesthesia by decreasing the rate of absorption of the anesthetic into the blood. Moreover, the vasoconstrictor may reduce the potential of anesthetic toxicity. As previously described, the vasoconstrictor in the anesthetic solution administered by infiltration is useful in reducing occasional hemorrhage by producing slight, transient ischemia of cut or abraded soft tissue.

Before its use, the anesthetic solution should be warmed to approximately body temperature. Otherwise, the relatively cold solution will contribute to the pain of injection. There is approximately a 30° difference between room temperature and body temperature. The anesthetic cartridge can be warmed in an anesthetic warmer, usually heated by a low-watt light bulb, or the cartridge can be held tightly in the palm of the hand for 10 to 15 seconds.

Anesthetic syringe. The anesthetic syringe includes a rod (or piston) that has a harpoon (or barb) on the cartridge end and a thumb ring on the other end. The harpoon and thumb ring are features that allow the operator to aspirate during the injection. The harpoon engages the cartridge plunger. During injection, and using the thumb ring, the operator should periodically reverse the movement of the rod to create negative pressure causing aspiration. Periodic aspiration during injection is important to ensure that the solution is not being injected into a blood vessel. If the tip of the needle is in the vessel, blood will be aspirated into the cartridge, thus indicating the need to reposition the needle. For patient safety and comfort, periodic aspiration is as important as slow deposition of the anesthetic solution.

FIG. **10-5** **A,** Prop/guard (Stik-Shield) card. The periphery of the hole *(h)* is indexed *(i)* (four pairs of short cuts) to accept four external ridges *(r)* of the sheath *(s)* shown in **B. B,** Sheath (s) covers the injection portion of the needle, and the cap *(c)* covers the reverse end (cartridge needle). Sheath and cap are joined by spot plastic weld *(w)*. Note external ridge *(r)*. **C,** With fingers of one hand holding prop/guard card printed-side up (as well as supporting it), the dental assistant *(DA)* uses the ends of the thumb, index, and middle fingers of other hand to press the last one third of the sheath through the hole while lining up external ridges to coincide with card indices. (Do not at this time jar cap [on reverse end] loose with hand.) **D,** Dental assistant applies thumb pressure *(arrow)* on the end of the cap to fully insert sheath to its collar. (Do not at this time loosen cap by any twisting motion.) **E,** Dental assistant's left hand holds sheath (card on sheath) and presses down on countertop in a stationary position *(left arrow)* while fingers of right hand "twist-break" plastic weld at cap/sheath union and then deliberately move the cap off of the reverse-end needle. Note horizontal right arrow depicting movement of hand (away from needle), which discards the cap. **F,** Dental assistant's left hand, still holding carded sheathed needle, now inserts the reverse-end needle into the hole in the threaded end of the syringe held by other hand (kept at last 3 inches away from card), and, **G,** then screws the sheathed needle clockwise onto syringe threads to a full-seating position against syringe nose. Note protection of both hands by guard card during such threading. Harpoon *(h)* is utilized later. **H,** Dental assistant lays prepared syringe (minus anesthetic cartridge) on the countertop or tray behind the patient, propped up because of the guard card and ready for the operator. Note harpoon *(h)* on piston end.

Assembly of the syringe. To assemble the syringe the assistant or operator picks up the syringe, and while holding the piston fully retracted, inserts the cartridge (see Fig. 10-5, *I* and *J*). The cartridge needle should be diaphragm-centered. If it is not, the assistant or operator guides the axial alignment of the cartridge so that the needle pierces the center of the diaphragm as the spring-loaded, retracted piston is slowly released. If the cartridge needle is malpositioned or bent as the cartridge is loaded, leaking can occur as the injection is initiated. The distasteful solution may drip freely into the patient's mouth. If so, the injection must be aborted, and another cartridge must be placed properly in the syringe.

The harpoon is set into the cartridge plunger by a light, quick thrust from the palm of the hand on the thumb ring (see Fig. 10-5, *N*). Too strong a blow may crack or break the cartridge.

The sheath should be removed out of the patient's view, carefully moving it away from the needle and syringe-holding hand, which is stationary on the tray or countertop (see Fig. 10-5, *K* and *L*). The prop/guard card protects the hand during sheath removal (see Fig. 10-5, *L*). It also props the sheath, preventing contamination (Fig. 10-5, *M*).

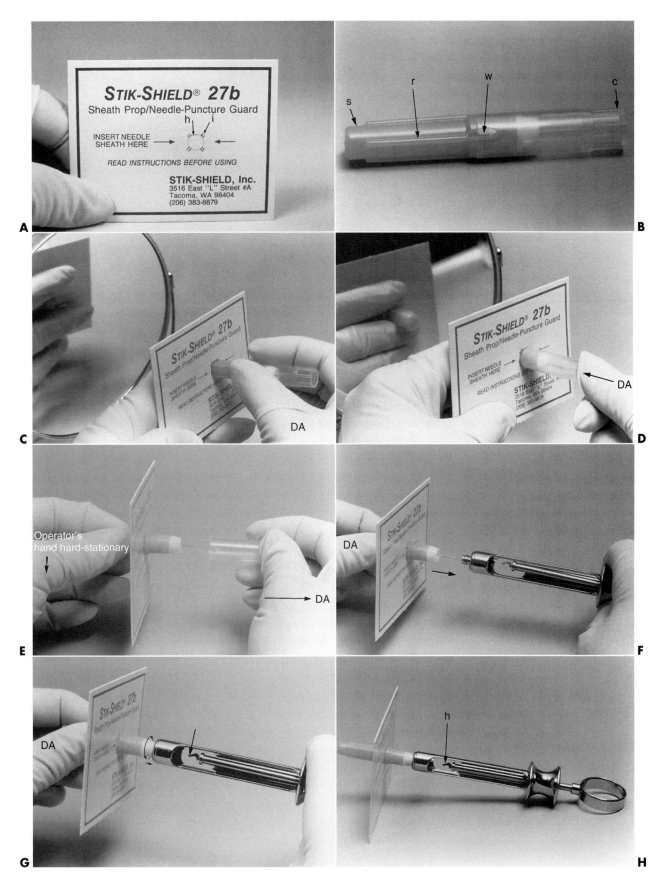

F I G. 10-5 For legend, see opposite page.

Continued

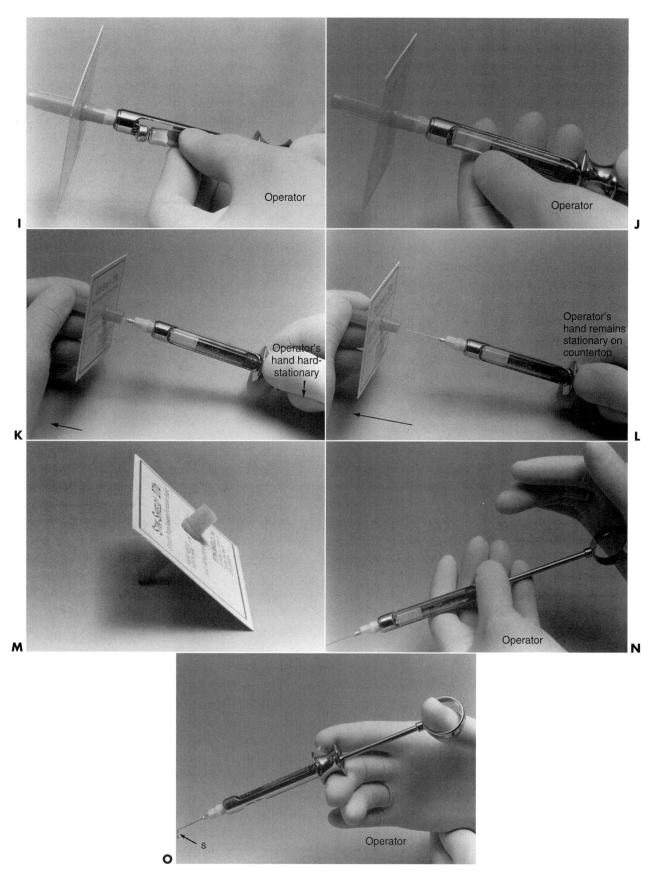

Operator

Operator

Operator's hand hard-stationary

Operator's hand remains stationary on countertop

Operator

Operator

S

FIG. 10-5, cont'd For legend, see opposite page.

FIG. **10-5, cont'd I** and **J,** While fully retracting the spring-loaded, moveable, rear cartridge seat of syringe by hand retraction of piston, the operator or assistant (behind the patient), inserts the cartridge, rearward end first **(I)** and then "drops" the forward end (diaphragm end) of the cartridge into position **(J)** without dragging across or bending the reverse-end needle. Then the operator or assistant slowly releases piston retraction, moving the rear cartridge seat and cartridge forward, allowing the reverse-end needle to pierce diaphragm. (Leakage of cartridge during later attempted deposition is usually caused by a bent, reverse-end needle poorly centered on the diaphragm.) **K** and **L,** With the syringe propped by the card on countertop (or tray) behind the patient, the operator or assistant holds the sheath by the fingers of one hand (card protected) and the syringe by the other hand, which is kept stationary **(K)** as sheath is loosened and removed away from needle **(L). M,** Guard card now props sheath. **N,** Operator or assistant sets the harpoon by gentle palm-thump of thumb ring, and then **(O)** tests the syringe for preparedness by thumb pressure moving plunger forward 1 to 2 mm while verifying emission of solution *(s)* from needle without leakage at the forward end of the syringe body.

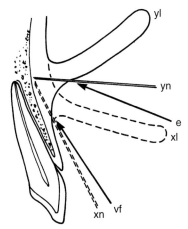

Lip position *yl* and needle direction *yn* recommended

FIG. **10-6** Recommended entry spot *(e),* direction of needle *(yn),* and lip position *(yl)* for infiltration anesthesia of maxillary canine. Direction of needle *xn* and lip position *xl* are not recommended. Vestibular fornix *vf* is the junction of the loose and fixed mucosa.

The assembled syringe is tested by pressing the plunger forward 1 to 2 mm to verify that it slides easily and ensure that the solution is emitted from the needle tip without leakage (see Fig. 10-5, *O*).

If preparation of the injection site has previously been accomplished by gauze-wiping of the entry site and the 1- to 2-minute placement of topical anesthetic (see the next principles), the injection procedure follows.

Topical anesthetic. Before needle entry, the mucosa at the injection site should be wiped free of debris and saliva by a sterile gauze. After wiping, apply a lidocaine topical anesthetic ointment for a minimum of 1 to 2 minutes to the proposed entry spot (using a cotton-tipped swab, limiting the area of application to the swab dimension). This procedure is often started immediately after positioning the patient in the chair and following the gauze wiping. The chairside assistant may perform the gauze wipe and application of topical anesthetic.

The use of topical anesthetic is generally recommended. However, good injection technique including a slow deposition rate (approximately 60 seconds per cartridge), a warmed cartridge, and the use of sharp needles are more important factors in a painless injection than the use of topical anesthetic.

Injection site. If in place, remove the needle sheath in a one-person procedure with the hand protected by the shield (see Fig. 10-5, *K* and *L*). With the left hand (right-handed operator) gently raise the lip outward and upward to identify the vestibular fornix, or mucogingival junction, where the attached gingiva joins the alveolar mucosa (Fig. 10-6). Holding the lip high enough, vi-

sualize the location of the root end and predict the injection site in the alveolar mucosa: (1) as it is stretched perpendicular, or nearly so, to the long axis of the tooth, and (2) toward the periosteal target area, which is very near the root end of the tooth to be operated on (see Fig. 10-6). The injection site should be 5 to 10 mm lateral of the mucogingival line, thereby allowing some freedom of needle movement without causing tissue tension. If the needle is held parallel to the tooth long axis, rather than at an angle as recommended, the tendency is to enter too close to the attached mucosa. This results in the needle being inserted too close to the very sensitive periosteal lining, inviting pain from touching or stripping the periosteum from the bone. The needle tip should not be close to the periosteum until it has reached its target area.

Injection. Knowing the injection site and with the needle directed properly, do two things simultaneously in preparation for the injection: (1) apply a slight, gentle tug to the lip (outward and upward) to have the entry spot tissue slightly taut, and (2) insert the needle about 3 mm into the mucosa (all the bevel under the epithelium). The slight, gentle tug while tensing the tissue, coupled with topical anesthesia, masks any sensation from the needle entry. After this, the lip may be relaxed somewhat, maintaining visibility of the needle. Initially, deposit a small amount of solution slowly while observing and reassuring the patient. Then wait several seconds for the anesthetic to take effect near the injection site before continuing the injection.

Still maintaining proper needle direction, gently continue inserting the needle toward the periosteum target. Be careful to sense resistance when the needle tip touches the lining of the bone, at which time the needle is immediately withdrawn 1 to 2 mm.

Aspirate by slightly reversing the harpooned plunger a few millimeters by gentle backward movement of the thumb ring. Aspiration (negative pressure) verifies that the needle is not in a blood vessel. If blood appears in the cartridge, the aspiration is positive; immediately withdraw the needle 1 to 2 mm and aspirate again until blood does not appear.

If aspiration is negative, slowly deposit 1 ml (slightly more than half the cartridge) over the next 30 seconds, while continually observing and reassuring the patient. A rate of deposition of a minute for 1 ml is a good rule of thumb. Slow deposition is the most important safety procedure for the prevention of adverse reactions because of high blood levels of anesthetic or epinephrine. Aspiration is second in importance. Malamed[22] defines overly rapid deposition as taking less than 30 seconds for 1.8 ml (one cartridge). This fast rate separates tissue and is too rapid to allow diffusion along normal tissue planes. If the injection is intravascular, it can lead to serious adverse reactions. Also, it is painful or at least uncomfortable. Malamed states that a 1-minute rate for 1.8 ml of anesthetic (30 seconds for 1 ml, or half a cartridge) will not cause tissue damage and will not lead to serious overdose reactions, even if accidentally injected intravascularly.[22]

An important principle is to deposit the smallest volume that will provide effective anesthesia. One of the more common errors is to deposit so much anesthetic (with epinephrine) that overdose reactions may occur.

After deposition, gently withdraw the needle and resheath it. A one-handed procedure is recommended. Insert the needle partially into the propped sheath (remaining after the unsheathing procedure), upright the sheath on the tray or countertop, and seat the needle fully into the sheath (Fig. 10-7, A and B). The sheathed syringe is left propped for possible reuse or for later removal and disposal (see Fig. 10-7, C). Resheathing is extremely important in the prevention of a needlestick, which can cause cross-infection to the operator and other office personnel. The federal Occupational Safety and

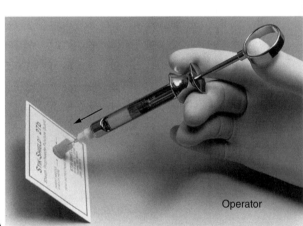

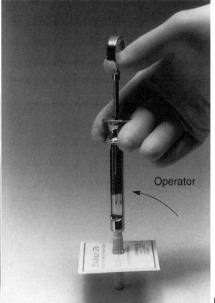

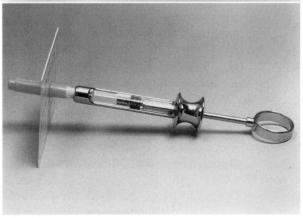

F I G. **10-7 A,** Behind the patient, the operator (or person who gave injection), using only the syringe-holding hand, inserts the needle partially into the sheath propped by prop/guard card, and then, **B,** uprights syringe and sheath upon the tray or countertop and presses the needle fully into sheath. **C,** Operator lays resheathed syringe propped by card on countertop.

Health Administration (OSHA) stipulates that needle resheathing should be a one-handed procedure.[31] It is also recommended that resheathing should be done by the same person who gave the injection; this eliminates the hazard of passing exposed needles.

Even though multiple injections using the same needle for a patient creates no infection control concerns, multiple uses are discouraged because the used needle and its lumen contents may be infectious to dental personnel if accidental needlestick occurs.

It is important that the patient be continually observed during and after the administration of local anesthesia. Never leave an anesthetized patient unattended and unobserved. Adverse reactions, if they occur, demand immediate attention by the dentist.

Disposal of the needle and cartridge. Proper disposal of the needle and cartridge is critical. Removal and disposal of the sheathed, used needle is done by the dental assistant, whose shield-protected hand carefully unscrews the sheathed needle from the syringe (see Fig. 10-7, *D*), and moves it away from the syringe (see Fig. 10-7, *E*). Avoid any tissue contact with the uncapped, exposed cartridge needle. If the needle hub is too tight to remove with controlled finger pressure alone, use a suture-needle holder (or similar instrument) to loosen the needle hub. Never manually recap the reverse end of the used needle. The assistant's hands should be gloved, preferably with utility gloves.

Disposal of the sheathed, used needle immediately follows its removal from the syringe. With the protective guard card still in place, convey it to a nearby sharps disposal container, laying the attached card on the orifice rim (see Fig. 10-7, *F*). Then, with thumb pressing on the plastic, push the sheathed needle out of the card into the container (see Fig. 10-7, *G*). The cartridge should

also be disposed of in the sharps container. The sharps container must be leakproof, hard-walled, and display an OSHA biohazard label.[31]

Emergency Procedures. The importance of taking pretreatment vital signs cannot be overemphasized. The patient's pretreatment blood pressure and pulse rate should be recorded in the chart. These vital signs are useful to uncover previously unknown cardiovascular problems and to serve as a baseline if an adverse reaction occurs during treatment. Adverse reactions occurring during or following administration of local anesthesia can lead to serious complications that require emergency procedures; foremost among these procedures are: (1) place the patient in a supine position (note the following exception), (2) summon medical assistance, (3) monitor vital signs, and (4) apply basic life support (open the airway, and use cardiopulmonary resuscitation [CPR] if needed). The supine position, with legs (only) slightly elevated increases the volume of circulating blood and aids in raising blood pressure. This procedure for the patient in syncope, or with syncopal symptoms, should relieve hypoxia of the brain and return him or her to or help maintain consciousness. However, the supine position should not be used when symptoms (e.g., fear, perspiration, weakness, pallor, palpitations) suggest an epinephrine overdose. In this case, a semierect or sitting position is best because it minimizes any further elevation in cerebral blood pressure.[22]

ANALGESIA (INHALATION SEDATION)

The most appropriate method of preventing pain is by blocking the nerve pathways capable of conducting nerve impulses. However, for those patients who have a low threshold of pain and are apprehensive (hyperresponders), raising the threshold by inhalation sedation

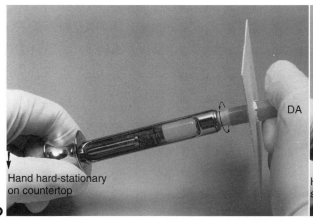
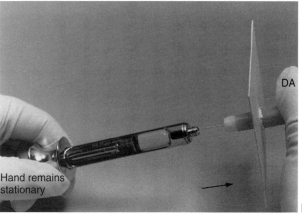

FIG. **10-7, cont'd D** through **G,** Dental assistant, after patient dismissal, holds the syringe stationary with the fingers of one hand at least 2 inches away from guard card as the fingers of the stronger hand unscrew (counterclockwise) the sheathed, used needle from the syringe **(D)** and **(E)** immediately move it (with reverse-end needle exposed) away from the syringe (distance from card to end of reverse-end needle is only 1 inch, and card will stop needle from sticking syringe-holding fingers, which are 2 inches or more away).

Continued

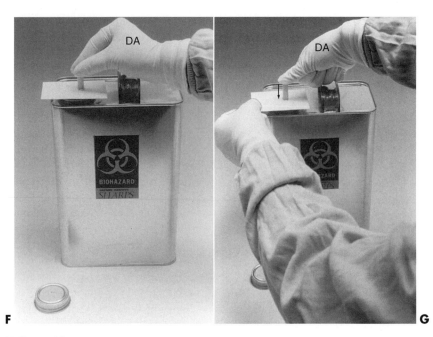

FIG. **10-7, cont'd** Then **(F)** the dental assistant continues to hold the sheathed needle and conveys it to a nearby (within a few feet) leakproof, hard-walled, OSHA biohazard-labeled container with a suitable size orifice, gently laying (on the rim) the guard card with the reverse-end needle down, and **(G)** steadies the card with fingers of one hand and presses (with the thumb of the other hand) the sheathed needle out of the card to free-fall into the container. The container should be kept upright, tightly closed between disposals of sharps, and out of the reach of children.

is an aid to be coupled with anesthesia by injection. The use of nitrous oxide and oxygen is one method of inhalation sedation.

For this, the reader is referred to a textbook on anesthesia that covers inhalation sedation in detail. The operator should understand that this method of pain control has definite limitations. Analgesia should not be thought of as general anesthesia in any stage or depth. It is simply a condition in which the pain threshold is elevated. With inhalation sedation the patient is conscious of surrounding activities.

HYPNOSIS

The fear of pain associated with dental procedures can sometimes be controlled by hypnosis. A favorable mental attitude may be established through suggestions of relaxation. Through hypnosis, the dentist and patient may derive certain benefits. The dentist has the opportunity to work on a more relaxed and cooperative patient and has better control over patient habits such as talking, rinsing, and oral tissue tension. The patient who is relaxed is less fatigued at the end of the appointment and has no specific recollection of having experienced discomfort.

Hypnosis has merit under certain circumstances and has produced satisfactory results for some practitioners when properly applied. However, before hypnosis is attempted, the operator must know how to recognize and cope with conditions associated with psychologic, emo-

tional, and mental factors and must be thoroughly familiar with all of the principles involved in hypnosis.

Hypnosis is not a way to eliminate all other accepted means of minimizing dental pain or discomfort, but it may well be a valuable adjunct in improving accepted procedures.[23] Also, posthypnotic suggestion has been found to be successful in alleviating certain noxious dental habits.

ISOLATION OF THE OPERATING FIELD

The goals of operating field isolation are moisture control, retraction, and harm prevention. Local anesthesia is also important in moisture control, as was previously discussed.

GOALS OF ISOLATION

Moisture Control. Operative dentistry cannot be executed properly unless the moisture in the mouth is controlled. Moisture control refers to excluding sulcular fluid, saliva, and gingival bleeding from the operating field. It also refers to preventing the handpiece spray and restorative debris from being swallowed or aspirated by the patient. The rubber dam, suction devices, and absorbents are varyingly effective in moisture control. These techniques and others are discussed in detail in this chapter. Generally, the rubber dam is the recommended technique for moisture control. However, Raskin et al[33] and Fusayama[14] have reported that achieving effective isolation is more important than the specific technique utilized.

Retraction and Access. The details of a restorative procedure cannot be managed without proper retraction and access. This provides maximal exposure of the operating site and usually involves maintaining an open mouth and depressing or retracting the gingival tissue, tongue, lips, and cheek. The rubber dam, high-volume evacuator, absorbents, retraction cord, and mouth prop are used for retraction and access. (Each of these is discussed later in this chapter.)

Harm Prevention. An axiom taught to every member of the health profession is, "Do no harm," and an important consideration of isolating the operating field is preventing the patient from being harmed during the operation.[15,17] Excessive saliva and handpiece spray can alarm the patient. Small instruments and restorative debris can be aspirated or swallowed. Soft tissue can be damaged accidentally. As with moisture control and retraction, a rubber dam, suction devices, absorbents, and occasional use of a mouth prop contribute not only to harm prevention but also to patient comfort and operator efficiency. Harm prevention is provided as much by the manner in which these devices are used as by the devices themselves.

Local Anesthesia. Local anesthetics play a role in eliminating the discomfort of dental treatment and controlling moisture. Use of these agents reduces salivation, apparently because the patient is more comfortable, less anxious, and less sensitive to oral stimuli, thus reducing salivary flow. Local anesthetics incorporating a vasoconstrictor also reduce blood flow, thus helping to control hemorrhage at the operating site.

RUBBER DAM ISOLATION

In 1864, S.C. Barnum, a New York City dentist, introduced the rubber dam into dentistry. Use of the rubber dam ensures appropriate dryness of the teeth and improves the quality of clinical restorative dentistry.[2,6,28]

The rubber dam is used to define the operating field by isolating one or more teeth from the oral environment. The dam eliminates saliva from the operating site and retracts the soft tissue. When the rubber dam is used, many procedures are facilitated because dryness is ensured during tooth preparation and restoration. Also, there are fewer interruptions to replace cotton rolls to maintain isolation. When excavating a deep carious lesion and risking pulpal exposure, use of the rubber dam is strongly recommended to prevent pulpal contamination from oral fluids.

Advantages. In general, the rubber dam is the most successful method of isolating the operating field. The advantages of the rubber dam are significant and become obvious as the operator gains proficiency. The advantages of isolation of the operating field are: (1) a dry, clean operating field, (2) improved access and visibility,

(3) potentially improved properties of dental materials, (4) protection of the patient and operator, and (5) operating efficiency. For best results, operative procedures require adequate isolation of the operating field.

Dry, Clean Operating Field. For most procedures, rubber dam isolation is the preferred method of obtaining a dry, clean, field. The operator can best perform procedures such as caries removal, proper tooth preparation, and insertion of restorative materials in a dry field. Teeth prepared and restored using rubber dam isolation are less prone to postoperative problems related to contamination from oral fluids. The time saved by operating in a clean field with good visibility may more than compensate for the time spent applying the rubber dam.[8]

Access and Visibility. The rubber dam provides maximal access and visibility. It controls moisture and retracts the soft tissue. Gingival tissue is retracted mildly to enhance access to and visibility of gingival aspects of the tooth preparation. The dam also retracts the lips, cheeks, and tongue. A black ("dark") rubber dam provides a dark, nonreflective background in contrast to the operating site. Because the dam remains in place throughout the operative procedure, access and visibility are maintained without interruption.

Improved Properties of Dental Materials. The rubber dam prevents moisture contamination of restorative materials during insertion and promotes improved properties of dental materials. Amalgam restorative material does not achieve its maximal physical properties if used in a wet field.[2] Bonding to enamel and dentin is unpredictable if the tooth substrate is contaminated with saliva, blood, or other oral fluids.[1,3,38] The dentist should provide the highest quality restoration possible by utilizing an appropriate operating environment.

Protection of the Patient and Operator. The rubber dam protects both patient and operator. It protects the patient from aspirating or swallowing small instruments or debris associated with operative procedures.[30] Immediate recovery of these items is facilitated by the rubber dam. A properly applied rubber dam protects the soft tissue from irritating or distasteful medicaments (e.g., etching agents). The dam also offers some soft tissue protection from rotating burs and stones.

Authors disagree on whether the rubber dam protects the patient from mercury exposure during amalgam removal.[5,21] However, there is agreement that the rubber dam is generally an effective infection control barrier for the dental office.[10,13,35]

Operating Efficiency. Use of the rubber dam allows for operating efficiency and increased productivity. Excessive patient conversation is discouraged. The rubber dam retainer (discussed later) helps to provide a moderate amount of mouth opening during the procedure. (For additional mouth-opening aids, see Mouth Props, later in this chapter.) Quadrant restorative procedures are facilitated. Many state dental practice acts permit the assistant to place the rubber dam, thereby saving the dentist time. Each of the rubber dam's advantages permits a more efficient operative procedure. The rubber dam can make things easier and more comfortable for the patient and create conditions that facilitate dental service of the highest possible quality. Smales concludes that there is no difference between the use of the rubber dam and cotton roll isolation; each relates to restoration quality and survival.[37] However, Christensen reports that use of a rubber dam increases both the quality and quantity of restorative services.[8]

Disadvantages. Rubber dam usage is low among private practitioners.[20,25] Time consumption and patient objection are the most frequently quoted disadvantages of the rubber dam. However, these concerns are reduced with the use of a simplified technique for application and removal. Usually, the rubber dam can be placed in 3 to 5 minutes. This is also the approximate time necessary for onset of anesthesia. After the dam is applied, most patients are more relaxed knowing that water spray and debris from the procedure are isolated from them. Jones and Reid have reported that use of the rubber dam was well accepted by patients and operators.[19]

Certain oral conditions may preclude the use of the rubber dam; these conditions include: (1) teeth that have not erupted sufficiently to support a retainer, (2) some third molars, and (3) extremely malpositioned teeth. In addition, patients suffering from asthma may not tolerate the rubber dam if breathing through the nose is difficult. Also, there are rare instances when the patient cannot tolerate a rubber dam because of psychologic reasons or latex allergy.[34] However, latex-free rubber dam material is currently available. Reports of patients disliking the rubber dam are usually the result of a lack of confidence of the dental team with its application.[16]

Materials and Instruments. The materials and instruments necessary for the use of the rubber dam are available from most dental supply companies.

Material. Rubber dam material, as with all rubber products, deteriorates over time, resulting in low tear strength. Therefore material that is reasonably new should be used. Dam material is available in 5 × 5 inch (12.5 × 12.5 cm) or 6 × 6 inch (15 × 15 cm) sheets. Sterile dam material is also available packaged as individual sheets. The thicknesses or weights available are thin (0.006 inch [0.15 mm]), medium (0.008 inch [0.2 mm]), heavy (0.010 inch [0.25 mm]), extra heavy (0.012 inch [0.30 mm]), and special heavy (0.014 inch [0.35 mm]). Both light and dark dam material are available, but the dark color is preferred for contrast. Green and blue colors are also marketed. (Fig. 10-8 illustrates rubber dam material.) Rubber dam material has a shiny and a dull side. Because the dull side is less light reflective, it is generally placed facing the occlusal of the isolated teeth. A thicker dam is more effective in retracting tissue and more resistant to tearing; it is especially recommended for isolating Class V lesions in conjunction with a cervical retainer. The thinner material has the advantage of passing through the contacts easier, which is particularly helpful when contacts are tight. Generally, dark, heavy, 6 × 6 inch sheets are recommended.

Holder. The rubber dam holder (frame) maintains the borders of the rubber dam in position. The Young holder is a U-shaped metal frame (Fig. 10-9) with small metal projections for securing the borders of the rubber dam. It is easily applied and comfortable for the patient. An optional adjustable neck strap (Fig. 10-10) may be placed behind the patient's neck and is attached to two hooks, one in the middle of each side of the frame. The neck strap is lightly tightened to snug the dam and frame to the face to maximize retraction and provide access to the operating site.

Retainer. The rubber dam retainer (clamp) consists of four prongs and two jaws connected by a bow (Fig. 10-11). The retainer is used to anchor the dam to the most posterior tooth to be isolated. Retainers are also used to retract gingival tissue. Many different sizes and

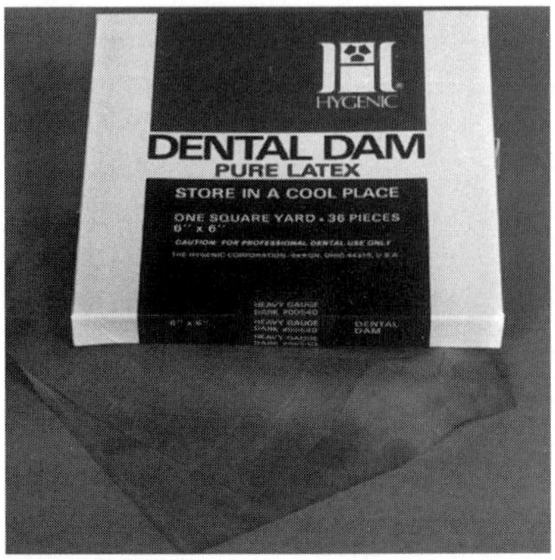

FIG. **10-8** Rubber dam material as supplied in sheets.

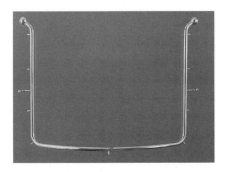

FIG. **10-9** The Young rubber dam frame (holder).

shapes are available, with specific retainers designed for certain teeth (Fig. 10-12). (Refer to Table 10-3 for suggested retainer applications.) Experience reduces the number of retainers necessary for most practitioners. When positioned on a tooth, a properly selected retainer should contact the tooth in four areas—two on the facial surface and two on the lingual surface (see Fig. 10-11). This four-point contact prevents rocking or tilting of the retainer. Movement of the retainer on the anchor tooth can injure the gingiva and tooth, resulting in postoperative soreness or sensitivity. The prongs of some retainers are gingivally directed (inverted) and are helpful when the anchor tooth is only partially erupted or when additional soft tissue retraction is indicated (Fig. 10-13). The jaws of the retainer should not extend beyond the mesial and distal line angles of the tooth because: (1) they may interfere with matrix and wedge placement, (2) gingival trauma is more likely to occur, and (3) a complete seal around the anchor tooth is more difficult to achieve.

Wingless and winged retainers are available (see Fig. 10-12). The winged retainer has both anterior and lateral wings (Fig. 10-14). The wings are designed to provide extra retraction of the rubber dam from the operating field and to allow attachment of the dam to the retainer before conveying the retainer (with dam) to the anchor tooth (see Fig. 10-29), after which the dam is removed from the lateral wings. A disadvantage of the winged retainer is that wings often interfere with the placement of matrix bands, band retainers, and wedges. Most opera-

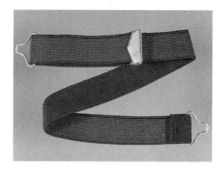

FIG. 10-10 Adjustable neck strap for use with the Young rubber dam frame.

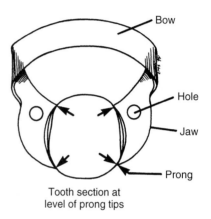

Bow

Hole

Jaw

Prong

Tooth section at
level of prong tips

FIG. 10-11 Rubber dam retainer. Note four-point prong contact *(arrows)* with tooth.

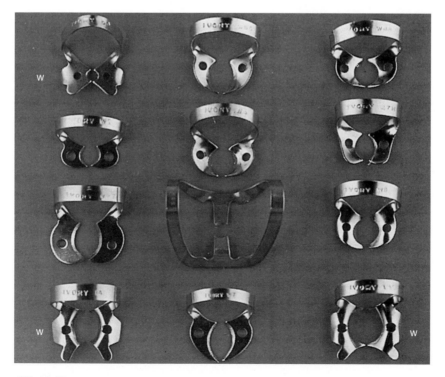

FIG. 10-12 Typical selection of rubber dam retainers. Note retainers with wings *(w)*.

TABLE 10-3	Suggested Retainers for Various Anchor Tooth Applications
RETAINER	APPLICATION
W56	Most molar anchor teeth
W7	Mandibular molar anchor teeth
W8	Maxillary molar anchor teeth
W4	Most premolar anchor teeth
W2	Small premolar anchor teeth
W27	Terminal mandibular molar anchor teeth requiring preparations involving the distal surface

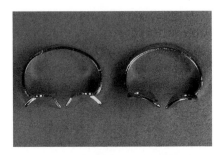

FIG. 10-13 Retainers with prongs directed gingivally are helpful when the anchor tooth is only partially erupted.

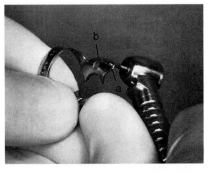

FIG. 10-14 Removing anterior wings (a) on molar retainer. Lateral wings (b) are for holding lip of stretched rubber dam hole.

tors prefer the wingless retainer. As seen in Fig. 10-14, the anterior wings can be cut away if they are not wanted.

The bow of the retainer (except the No. 212, which is applied after the rubber dam is in place) should be tied with dental floss (Fig. 10-15) approximately 12 inches (30.5 cm) in length before the retainer is placed in the mouth. For maximal protection the tie may be threaded through both holes in the jaws because the bow of the retainer could break. The floss allows retrieval of the retainer or its broken parts if they are accidentally swallowed or aspirated.

It is sometimes necessary to recontour the jaws of the retainer to the shape of the tooth by grinding with a mounted stone (Fig. 10-16).

A retainer usually is not required when the dam is applied for treatment of the anterior teeth, except for the cervical retainer for Class V restorations.

Punch. The rubber dam punch is a precision instrument having a rotating metal table (disk) with six holes of varying sizes and a tapered, sharp-pointed plunger (Fig. 10-17). Care should be exercised when changing from one hole to another. The plunger should be centered in the cutting hole so the edges of the holes are not at risk of being chipped by the plunger tip when the plunger is closed. Otherwise, the cutting quality of the punch will be ruined, as evidenced by incompletely cut holes. These holes tear easily when stretched during application over the retainer or tooth.

Retainer Forceps. The rubber dam retainer forceps is used both for placement and removal of the retainer from the tooth (Fig. 10-18).

Napkin. The rubber dam napkin, placed between the rubber dam and the patient's skin, has the following advantages:

1. It prevents skin contact with rubber to reduce the possibility of allergic reactions in sensitive patients.
2. It absorbs any saliva seeping at the corners of the mouth.

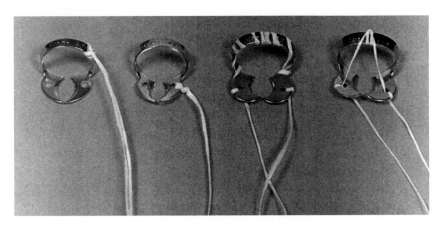

FIG. 10-15 Methods of tying retainers with dental floss.

3. It acts as a cushion.
4. It provides a convenient method of wiping the patient's lips on removal of the dam.

The rubber dam napkin adds to the comfort of the patient, particularly when the dam must be used for long appointments. Most operators use commercially available napkins that are soft, absorbent, and disposable (Fig. 10-19).

Lubricant. A water-soluble lubricant applied in the area of the punched holes facilitates the passing of the dam septa through the proximal contacts. A rubber dam lubricant is commercially available, but other lubricants, such as shaving cream or soap slurry, are also satisfactory. Applying the lubricant to both sides of the dam in the area of the punched holes aids in passing the dam through the contacts. Cocoa butter or petroleum jelly may be applied at the corners of the patient's mouth to prevent irritation. These two materials, however, are not satisfactory rubber dam lubricants because both are oil based and not easily rinsed from the dam once the dam is placed.

Modeling Compound. Low-fusing modeling compound is sometimes used to secure the retainer to the tooth to prevent retainer movement during the operative procedure. If used, the compound must not cover the holes in the retainer in order to have ready access to the retainer for rapid removal with forceps, if necessary.

Anchors (Other Than Retainers). Anchors other than retainers may be used. The proximal contact may be sufficient to anchor the dam on the tooth farthest from the posterior retainer (in the isolated field), thereby eliminating the need for a second retainer (see Placement of the Rubber Dam, *step 13*). To further secure the dam anteriorly or to anchor the dam on any tooth where a retainer is contraindicated, waxed dental tape (or floss) or a small piece of rubber dam material (cut from a sheet of dam) may be passed through the proximal contact. When dental tape is used, it should be passed through

the contact, looped, and passed through a second time (Fig. 10-20, *A*). The cut piece of dam material is first stretched, passed through the contact, and then released (Fig. 10-20, *B*). Once the anchor is in place, the tape, floss, or dam material should be trimmed to approximately 0.5 inch in total length to prevent interference with the operating site.

Hole Size and Position. Successful isolation of the teeth and maintenance of a dry, clean operating field largely depend on hole size and position in the rubber dam.[18] Holes should be punched by following the arch form, making adjustments for malpositioned or missing teeth. Most rubber dam punches have either five or six

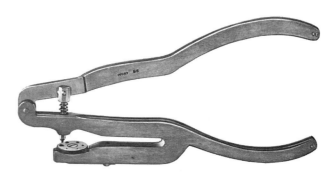

FIG. **10-17** Rubber dam punch.

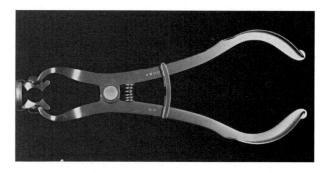

FIG. **10-18** Rubber dam retainer forceps engaging retainer.

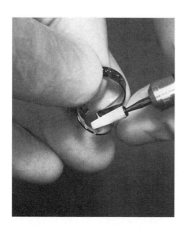

FIG. **10-16** Recontouring jaws of retainer with mounted stone.

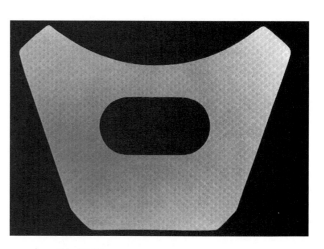

FIG. **10-19** Disposable rubber dam napkin.

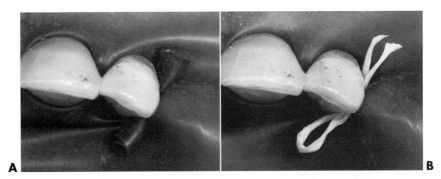

FIG. 10-20 **A,** Anchor formed from dental tape. **B,** Anchor formed from rubber dam material.

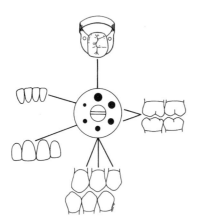

FIG. 10-21 Cutting table on rubber dam punch, illustrating use of hole size.

holes in the cutting table. Use the smaller holes for the incisors, canines, and premolars and the larger holes for the molars. The largest hole is generally reserved for the posterior anchor tooth (Fig. 10-21). The following guidelines and suggestions are helpful when positioning the holes:

- (Optional) Punch an identification hole in the upper left (that is, the patient's left) corner of the rubber dam for ease of location of that corner when applying the dam to the holder (see Fig. 10-23, *A*).
- When operating on the incisors and mesial surfaces of canines, isolate from first premolar to first premolar. Metal retainers usually are not required for this isolation (Fig. 10-22, *A*). If additional access is necessary after isolating the teeth as described, a retainer can be positioned over the dam to engage the adjacent nonisolated tooth, but care must be exercised not to pinch the gingiva beneath the dam (see Fig. 10-22, *B* and *C*). When operating on a canine, it is preferable to isolate from the first molar to the opposite lateral incisor. To treat a Class V lesion on a canine, isolate posteriorly to include the first molar to provide access for the cervical retainer placement on the canine.
- When operating on posterior teeth, it is beneficial to

isolate anteriorly to include the lateral incisor on the opposite side of the arch from the operating site. In this case the hole for the lateral incisor will be the most remote from the hole for the posterior anchor tooth. Anterior teeth may be included in the isolation to provide finger rests on dry teeth and better access and visibility for the operator and assistant.
- When operating on the premolars, punch holes to include two teeth distally, and extend anteriorly to include the opposite lateral incisor.
- When operating on the molars, punch holes as far distally as possible, and extend anteriorly to include the opposite lateral incisor.
- Isolation of a minimum of three teeth is recommended except when endodontic therapy is indicated, and in that case only the tooth to be treated is isolated. Obviously, the number of teeth to be treated as well as the tooth surface will influence the pattern of isolation.
- The distance between holes is equal to the distance from the center of one tooth to the center of the adjacent tooth, measured at the level of the gingival tissue. Generally, this is approximately $\frac{1}{4}$ inch (6.3 mm). When the distance between holes is excessive, the dam material is excessive and wrinkles between the teeth. Conversely, too little distance between holes causes the dam to stretch, resulting in space around the teeth and leakage. When the distance is correct, the dam intimately adapts to the teeth and covers and slightly retracts the interdental tissue.
- When the rubber dam is applied to the maxillary teeth, the first holes punched (after the identification hole) are for the central incisors. These holes are positioned approximately 1 inch (25 mm) from the superior border of the dam (Fig. 10-23, *A*), providing sufficient material to cover the patient's upper lip. For a patient with a large upper lip or mustache, position the holes more than an inch from the edge. Conversely, for a child or an adult with a small upper lip, the holes should be positioned less than an inch from the edge. Once the holes for the incisors are located, the remaining holes are punched.

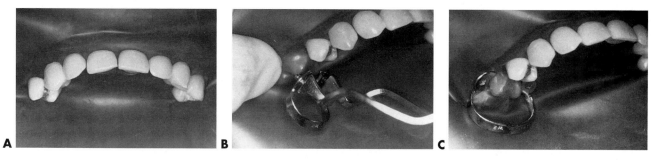

FIG. **10-22** **A,** Isolation for operating on incisors and mesial surface of canines. **B** and **C,** Increasing access by application of metal retainer over dam and adjacent non-isolated tooth.

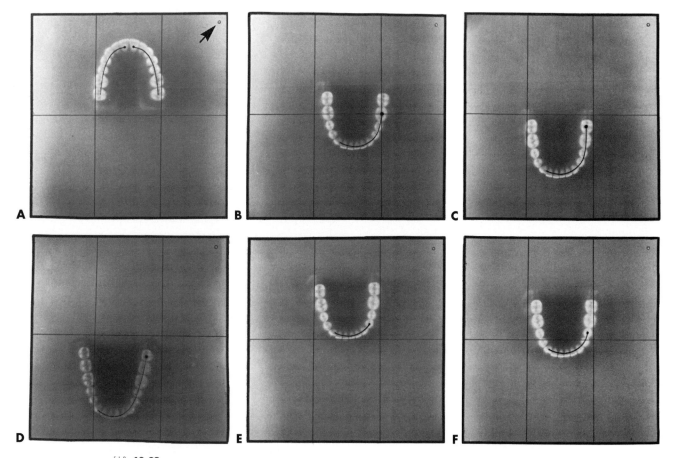

FIG. **10-23** Hole position. **A,** When maxillary teeth are to be isolated, the first holes punched are for central incisors, approximately 1 inch (2.5 cm) from superior border. **B,** Hole position when anchor tooth is mandibular first molar. **C,** Hole position when anchor tooth is mandibular second molar. **D,** Hole position when anchor tooth is mandibular third molar. **E,** Hole position when anchor tooth is mandibular first premolar. **F,** Hole position when anchor tooth is mandibular second premolar. Note the hole punched in each of these six representative rubber dam sheets for identification of the upper left corner (*arrow* in **A**).

- When the rubber dam is applied to the mandibular teeth, the first hole punched (after the identification hole) is for the posterior anchor tooth that is to receive the retainer. To determine the proper location, mentally divide the rubber dam into three vertical sections: left, middle, and right. If the anchor tooth is the mandibular first molar, punch the hole for this tooth at a point halfway from the superior edge to the inferior edge and at the junction of the right (or left) and middle thirds (Fig. 10-23, *B*). If the anchor tooth is the second or third molar, the position for the hole moves toward the inferior border and slightly toward the center of the rubber dam, as compared to the first molar hole just described (Fig. 10-23, *C* and *D*). If the anchor tooth is the first premolar, the hole is placed toward the superior border, compared with the hole for the first molar, and also toward the center of the dam (Fig. 10-23, *E*). The farther posterior the mandibular anchor tooth, the more dam material is required to come from behind the retainer over the upper lip. Fig. 10-24 illustrates the difference in the amount of dam required, comparing the first premolar and the second molar as anchor teeth. The distances may also be compared by noting the length of dam between the superior edge of the dam and the position of the hole for the posterior anchor tooth (see Fig. 10-23, *B* to *F*).

- When a cervical retainer is to be applied to isolate a Class V lesion, a heavier rubber dam is usually recommended for better tissue retraction, and the hole for the tooth should be punched slightly facial to the arch form to compensate for the extension of the dam to the cervical area. The farther gingivally the lesion extends, the further the hole must be positioned from the arch form. In addition, the hole should be slightly larger, and the distance between it and the holes for the adjacent teeth should be slightly increased (Fig. 10-25).
- When a thinner rubber dam is used, smaller holes must be punched to achieve an adequate seal around the teeth because the thin dam has greater elasticity.

Until these guidelines and suggestions related to hole position are mastered, the inexperienced operator may choose to use commercial products to aid in locating hole position (Fig. 10-26). A rubber stamp is available that imprints both permanent and primary arch forms on the rubber dam, and several sheets of dam material can be stamped in advance. A plastic template can also be used to mark hole position. Experience eliminates the need for

these aids. Accurate hole location is best achieved by noting the patient's arch form and tooth position. However, understanding the principles of hole punching is still helpful when using a stamp or template.

Placement. Before placing the rubber dam, the dental chair should be adjusted for optimal patient comfort and access for the operator and assistant. The patient's head and chest should not be lower than the feet. It may be necessary to remove debris and calculus from the teeth to be isolated.

Usually, administering the anesthetic precedes application of the rubber dam. This allows for the beginning of profound anesthesia and more comfortable retainer placement on the anchor tooth. Occasionally, the posterior anchor tooth in the maxillary arch may need to be anesthetized if it is remote from the anesthetized operating site.

The technique for application of the rubber dam is presented by numerous authors.[6,7,11,27] The step-by-step application and removal of the rubber dam using the maxillary left first molar for the posterior retainer and including the maxillary right lateral incisor as the anterior anchor is described and illustrated here. The procedure is described as if the operator and assistant are working together. However, application and removal of the rubber dam is often the responsibility of a single person, in which case that individual performs the described duties for both the operator and the assistant. Following the administration of the local anesthetic, many operators delegate rubber dam application to a second chairside assistant, permitting the operator to treat another patient.

When compared to the alternative procedures discussed in a later section, the illustrated procedure allows the retainer and dam to be placed sequentially. This provides for maximal visibility when placing the retainer, which reduces the risk of impinging gingival

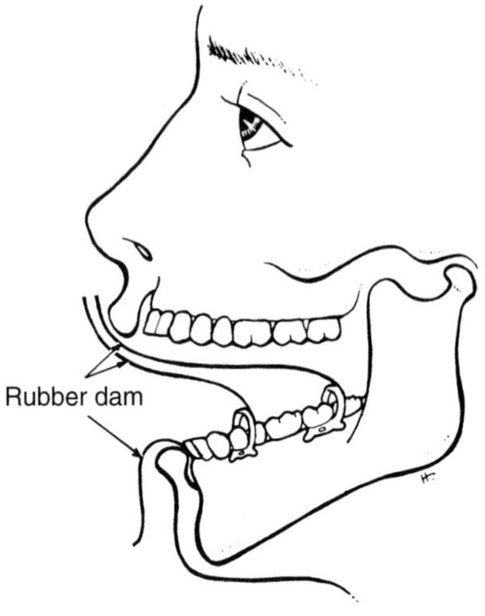

FIG. **10-24** The farther posteriorly the mandibular anchor tooth, the more dam material is required to come from behind retainer over upper lip.

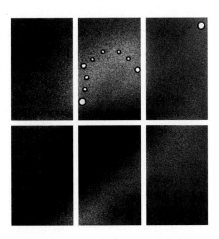

FIG. **10-25** Hole position for tooth (maxillary right canine) to receive cervical retainer is positioned facially to arch form.

tissue. For most operators this is a simpler procedure than placing the retainer and dam simultaneously. Isolating a greater number of teeth, as illustrated in this procedure, is indicated for quadrant operative procedures. For limited operative procedures, it is often acceptable to isolate fewer teeth. The general rule for limited isolation is to include one tooth posterior and two teeth anterior to the tooth (teeth) being operated on (Fig. 10-27).

The application procedure is described for right-handed operators. Left-handed users should substitute *left* where *right* is described. Each step number has a corresponding illustration.

Step 1: Testing and Lubricating the Proximal Contacts. The operator receives dental floss from the assistant to test the interproximal contacts and remove debris from the teeth to be isolated. Passing (or attempts to pass) floss through the contacts identifies any sharp edges of restorations or enamel that must be smoothed or removed to prevent tearing the dam. Using waxed dental tape may lubricate tight contacts to facilitate dam placement. Tight contacts that are difficult to floss but do not cut or fray the floss may be wedged apart slightly to permit placement of the rubber dam. A blunt hand instrument may be used for separation. For some clinical situations, the proximal portion of the tooth to be restored may need to be partially prepared to eliminate a sharp or difficult contact before the dam is placed.

Step 2: Punching the Holes. It is recommended that the assistant punch the holes after assessing the arch form and tooth alignment. However, some operators prefer to have the assistant prepunch the dam using holes marked by a template or a rubber dam stamp.

Step 3: Lubricating the Dam. The assistant lubricates both sides of the rubber dam in the area of the punched holes using a cotton roll or gloved fingertip to apply the lubricant. This facilitates passing the rubber dam through the contacts. The lips and especially the corners of the mouth may be lubricated with petroleum jelly or cocoa butter to prevent irritation.

Step 4: Selecting the Retainer. The operator receives (from the assistant) the rubber dam retainer forceps with the selected retainer and floss tie in position (*A*). The free end of the tie should exit from the cheek side of the retainer. Try the retainer on the tooth to verify retainer stability. If the retainer fits poorly, it is removed either for adjustment or selection of a different size.[32] (Retainer adjustment, if needed to provide stability, is presented in the previous section, Rubber Dam Retainer). Whenever the forceps is holding the retainer, care should be taken not to open the retainer more than necessary to secure it in the forceps. Stretching the retainer open for extended periods causes it to lose its elastic recovery. Retainers that have been deformed ("sprung"), such as the one shown in *B*, should be discarded.

Step 5: Testing the Retainer's Stability and Retention. If during trial placement the retainer seems acceptable, remove the forceps. Test the retainer's stability and retention by lifting gently in an occlusal direction with a fingertip under the bow of the retainer. An improperly fitting retainer will rock or be easily dislodged.

Step 6: Positioning the Dam Over the Retainer. Before applying the dam, the floss tie may be threaded through the anchor hole, or it may be left on the underside of the dam. With the forefingers, stretch the anchor hole of the dam over the retainer (bow first) and then under the jaws. The lip of the hole must pass completely under the jaws. The forefingers then may thin out, to a single thickness, the septal dam for the mesial contact of the retainer tooth and attempt to pass it through the contact, lip of the hole first. The septal dam must always pass through its respective contact in single thickness. If it does not pass through readily, it should be passed through with dental tape later in the procedure.

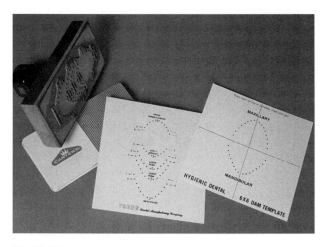

FIG. **10-26** Commercial products to aid in locating hole position.

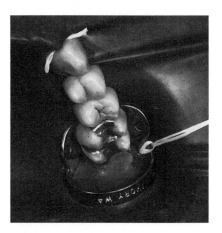

FIG. **10-27** Limited isolation for operating maxillary left second premolar.

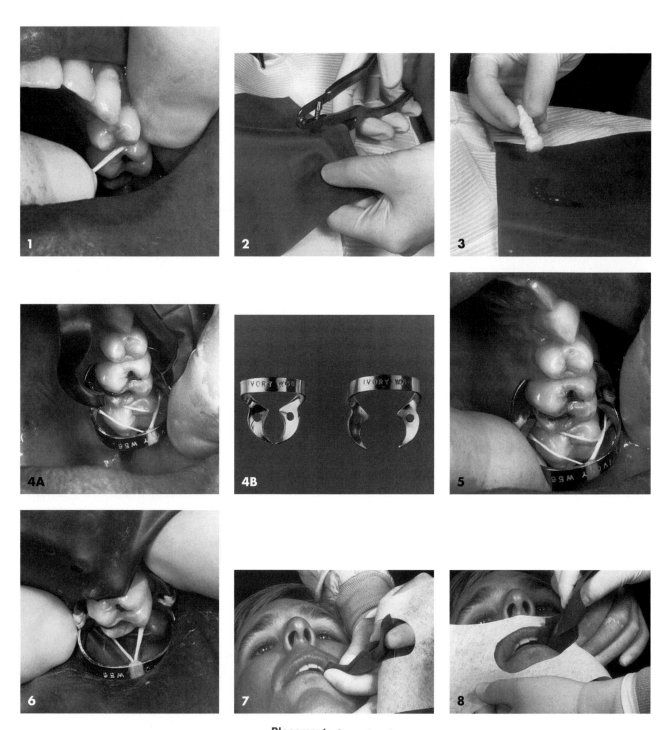

Placement. Steps 1 to 8.

Step 7: Applying the Napkin. The operator now gathers the rubber dam in the left hand while the assistant inserts the fingers and thumb of the right (or left) hand through the napkin's opening and grasps the bunched dam held by the operator.

Step 8: Positioning the Napkin. The assistant then pulls the bunched dam through the napkin and positions it on the patient's face. The operator helps by positioning the napkin on the patient's right side. The napkin reduces skin contact with the dam.

Step 9: Attaching the Frame. The operator unfolds the dam. (If an identification hole was punched, it is used to identify the upper left corner.) The assistant aids in unfolding the dam and, while holding the frame in place, attaches the dam to the metal projections on the left side of the frame. Simultaneously, the operator stretches

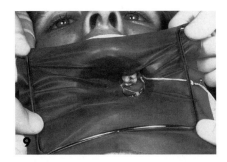
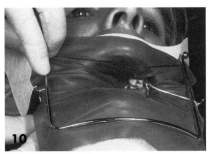
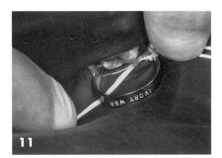

Placement. Steps 9 to 11.

and attaches the dam on the right side. The frame is positioned outside the dam. The curvature of the frame should be concentric with the patient's face. The dam lies between the frame and napkin. Either the operator or assistant attaches the dam along the inferior border of the frame. Attaching the dam to the frame at this time controls the dam to provide access and visibility. Secure the free ends of the floss tie to the frame.

Step 10 (Optional): Attaching the Neck Strap. The assistant attaches the neck strap to the left side of the frame and passes it behind the patient's neck. The operator then attaches it to the right side of the frame. Neck strap tension is adjusted to stabilize the frame and hold the frame (and periphery of the dam) gently against the face and away from the operating field. If desired, using soft tissue paper between the neck and strap may prevent contact of the patient's neck against the strap.

Step 11: Passing the Dam through Posterior Contact. If there is a tooth distal to the retainer, the distal edge of the posterior anchor hole should be passed through the contact (single thickness, with no folds) to ensure a seal around the anchor tooth. If necessary, use waxed dental tape to assist in this procedure (see *Step 15* for the use of tape). If the retainer comes off unintentionally as this is done or during subsequent procedures, passage of the dam through the distal contact anchors the dam sufficiently to allow easier reapplication of the retainer or placement of an adjusted or different retainer.

Step 12 (Optional): Applying Compound. If the stability of the retainer is questionable, low-fusing modeling compound may be applied. The assistant heats the end of a stick of compound in an open flame and tempers it by holding it in water for a few seconds. While the assistant holds the unheated end, the operator pinches off a sufficient amount to form a cone about ½ inch (12.7 mm) long.

The assistant should ensure dryness by directing a few short bursts from the air syringe on the occlusal surface of the tooth before compound placement. The operator positions the compound cone on the ball of the gloved forefinger, briefly resoftens the tip of the cone in the flame, and carries the compound to its place, cover-

ing the bow of the retainer and part of the occlusal surface of the tooth. The compound should not cover the holes in the jaws of the retainer. The compound will adhere to the tooth if the tooth is dry.

Step 13: Applying the Anterior Anchor (If Needed). The operator passes the dam over the anterior anchor tooth, anchoring the anterior portion of the rubber dam. Usually, the dam passes easily through the mesial and distal contacts of the anchor tooth if it is passed in single thickness starting with the lip of the hole. Stretching the lip of the hole and sliding it back and forth aids in positioning the septum. When the contact farthest from the retainer is minimal ("light"), an anchor may be required in the form of a double thickness of dental tape or a narrow strip of dam material that is stretched, inserted, and released (see Fig. 10-20, *A* and *B*). If the contact is open, a rolled piece of dam material may be used (as shown in Fig. 10-36).

Step 14: Passing the Septa Through the Contacts Without Tape. The operator passes the septa through as many contacts as possible without the use of dental tape by stretching the septal dam faciogingivally and linguogingivally with the forefingers. Each septum must not be allowed to bunch or fold. Rather, its passage through the contact should be started with a single edge and continued with a single thickness. Passing the dam through as many contacts as possible without using dental tape is urged because the use of tape always increases the risk of tearing holes in the septa. Slight separation (wedging) of the teeth is sometimes an aid when the contacts are extremely tight. Pressure from a blunt hand instrument (e.g., beaver-tail burnisher) applied in the facial embrasure gingival to the contact usually is sufficient to obtain enough separation to permit the septum to pass through the contact.

Step 15: Passing the Septa Through the Contacts With Tape. Use waxed dental tape to pass the dam through the remaining contacts. Tape is preferred over floss because its wider dimension more effectively carries the rubber septa through the contacts. Also, tape is not as likely to cut the septa. The waxed variety makes passage easier and decreases the chances for cutting

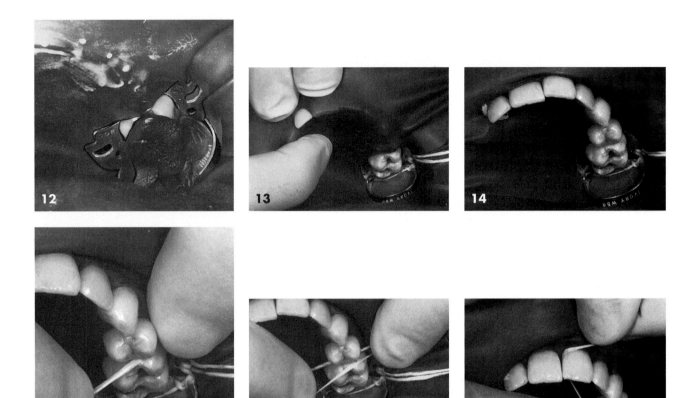

Placement. Steps 12 to 17.

holes in the septa or tearing the edges of the holes. The leading edge of the septum should be over the contact, ready to be drawn into and through the contact with the tape. As before, the septal rubber should be kept in single thickness with no folds. The tape should be placed at the contact on a slight angle. With a good finger rest on the tooth, the tape should be controlled so that it slides (not snaps) through the proximal contact, thus preventing damage to the interdental tissues. Once the leading edge of the septum has passed the contact, the remaining interseptal dam can be carried through more easily.

Step 16 (Optional): Technique for Using Tape. Often, several passes with dental tape are required to carry a reluctant septum through a tight contact. When this happens, previously passed tape should be left in the gingival embrasure until the entire septum has been successfully placed with subsequent passage of tape. This prevents a partially passed septum from being removed or torn. The double strand of tape is removed from the facial.

Step 17: Inverting the Dam Interproximally. Invert the dam into the gingival sulcus to complete the seal around the tooth and prevent leakage. Often, the dam inverts itself as the septa are passed through the contacts

as a result of the dam being stretched gingivally. The operator should verify that the dam is inverted interproximally. Inversion in this region is best accomplished with dental tape.

Step 18: Inverting the Dam Faciolingually. With the edges of the dam inverted interproximally, complete the inversion facially and lingually using an explorer or a beaver-tail burnisher while the assistant directs a stream of air onto the tooth. This is done by moving the explorer around the neck of the tooth facially and lingually with the tip perpendicular to the tooth surface or directed slightly gingivally. A dry surface prevents the dam from sliding out of the crevice. Alternatively, the dam can be inverted facially and lingually by drying the tooth while stretching the dam gingivally and then releasing it slowly.

Step 19 (Optional): Using a Saliva Ejector. The use of a saliva ejector is optional because most patients are able, and usually prefer, to swallow excess saliva. Furthermore, salivation is greatly reduced when profound anesthesia is obtained. If salivation is a problem, the operator or assistant uses cotton pliers to pick up the dam lingual to the mandibular incisors and cuts a small hole through which the saliva ejector is inserted. The hole should be positioned so that the rubber dam helps sup-

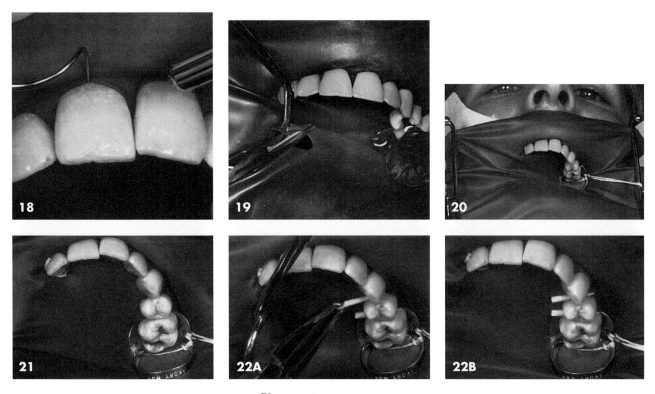

Placement. Steps 18 to 22.

port the weight of the ejector, preventing pressure on the delicate tissues in the floor of the mouth.

Step 20: Confirming a Properly Applied Rubber Dam. The properly applied rubber dam will be securely positioned and comfortable to the patient. The patient should be assured that the rubber dam does not prevent swallowing or closing the mouth (about halfway) when there is a pause in the procedure.

Step 21: Checking for Access and Visibility. Check to see that the completed rubber dam provides maximal access and visibility for the operative procedure.

Step 22: Inserting the Wedges. For proximal surface preparations (Classes II, III, and IV), many operators consider the insertion of interproximal wedges as the final step in rubber dam application. Wedges are generally round toothpick ends about ½ inch (12.7 mm) in length that are snugly inserted into the gingival embrasures from the facial or lingual embrasure, whichever is greater, using No. 110 pliers.

To facilitate wedge insertion, first stretch the dam slightly by fingertip pressure in the direction opposite wedge insertion (*A*), and then insert the wedge while slowly releasing the dam. This results in a passive dam under the wedge (i.e., the dam will not rebound the wedge) and prevents bunching or tearing of the septal

dam during wedge insertion. The inserted wedges appear in *B*.

Removal. Before removal of the rubber dam, rinse and suction away any debris that may have collected to prevent its falling into the floor of the mouth during the removal procedure. If a saliva ejector was used, remove it at this time. Each numbered step has a corresponding illustration.

Step 1: Cutting the Septa. Stretch the dam facially, pulling the septal rubber away from the gingival tissues and tooth. Protect the underlying soft tissue by placing a fingertip beneath the septum. Clip each septum with blunt-tipped scissors, freeing the dam from the interproximal spaces, but leave the dam over the anterior and posterior anchor teeth. To prevent inadvertent soft tissue damage, curved nose scissors are preferred.

Step 2: Removing the Retainer. Engage the retainer with retainer forceps. It is unnecessary to remove any compound, if used, because it will break free as the retainer is spread and lifted from the tooth. While the operator removes the retainer, the assistant releases the neck strap, if used, from the left side of the frame.

Step 3: Removing the Dam. Once the retainer is removed, release the dam from the anterior anchor tooth and remove the dam and frame simultaneously. While

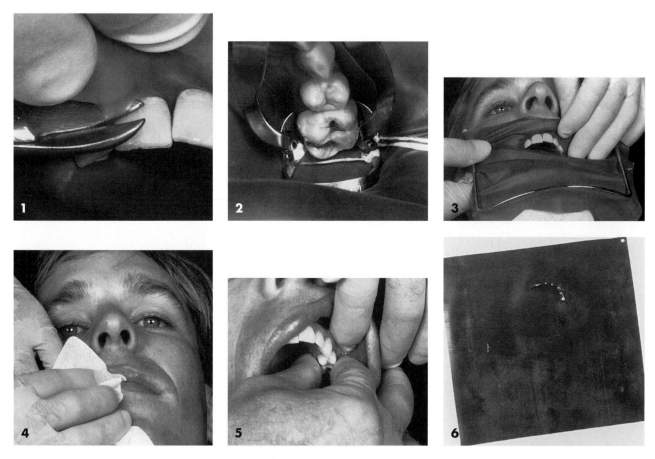

Removal. Steps 1 to 6.

doing this, caution the patient not to bite on newly inserted amalgam restorations until the occlusion can be evaluated.

Step 4: Wiping the Lips. Wipe the patient's lips with the napkin immediately after the dam and frame are removed. This helps to prevent saliva from getting on the patient's face and is comforting to the patient.

Step 5: Rinsing the Mouth and Massaging the Tissue. Rinse the teeth and mouth using air-water spray and the high-volume evacuator. To enhance circulation, particularly around the anchor teeth, massage the tissue around the teeth that were isolated.

Step 6: Examining the Dam. Lay the sheet of rubber dam over a light-colored flat surface or hold it up to the operating light to determine that no portion of the rubber dam has remained between or around the teeth. Such a remnant will cause gingival inflammation.

Alternative/Additional Methods and Factors. The procedure just detailed describes the method of sequentially placing the retainer and rubber dam on the anchor tooth. Some operators prefer alternative methods. In the hands of inexperienced operators, these alternative methods may not be as successful because of reduced visibility of the gingival tissues.

Applying the Dam and Retainer Simultaneously. The retainer and dam may be placed simultaneously to reduce the risk of the retainer being swallowed or aspirated before the dam is placed. This also solves the occasional difficulty of trying to pass the dam over a previously placed retainer, the bow of which is pressing against oral soft tissues.

In this method, first apply the posterior retainer to verify a stable fit. Remove the retainer and, with forceps still holding the retainer, pass the bow through the proper hole from the underside of the dam (the lubricated rubber dam is held by the assistant) (Fig. 10-28, *A*). The free end of the floss tie may remain on the underside of the dam, or it may be threaded through the anchor hole before the retainer bow is inserted. When using a retainer with lateral wings, place the retainer in the hole punched for the anchor tooth by stretching the dam to engage these wings (Fig. 10-29). Winged retainers are rarely used because the wings may interfere with subsequent procedures.

The operator grasps the handle of the forceps in the right hand and gathers the dam with the left hand to visualize clearly the jaws of the retainer and facilitate its placement (see Fig. 10-28, *B*).

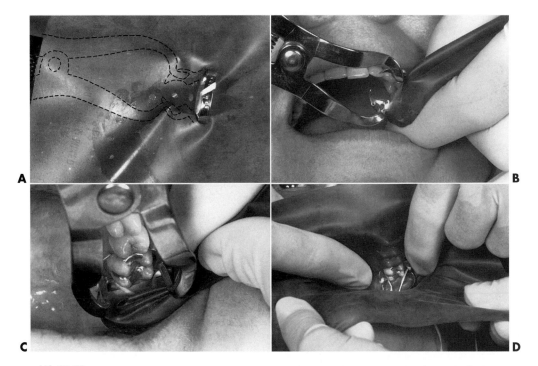

FIG. **10-28** **A,** Bow being passed through posterior anchor hole from underside of dam. **B,** Gathering dam to facilitate placement of retainer. **C,** Positioning retainer on anchor tooth. **D,** Stretching anchor hole borders over and under jaws of retainer.

The operator conveys the retainer (with dam) into the mouth and positions it on the anchor tooth. Care is necessary when applying the retainer to prevent the jaws from sliding gingivally and impinging on the soft tissue. The retainer should be opened slightly and moved occlusally when gingival tissue is trapped (see Fig. 10-28, C).

The assistant gently pulls the inferior border of the dam toward the chin while the operator positions the superior border over the upper lip. As the assistant holds the borders of the dam, the operator uses the second or middle finger of both hands, one finger facial and the other finger lingual to the bow, to pass the anchor hole borders over and under the jaws of the retainer (see Fig. 10-28, D). At this point, the application procedure continues as was previously described, beginning with Step 7.

Applying the Dam Before the Retainer. The dam may be stretched over the anchor tooth before the retainer is placed. The advantage of this method is not having to manipulate the dam over the retainer. The operator places the retainer, while the dental assistant stretches and holds the dam over the anchor tooth (Fig. 10-30). The disadvantage is the reduction in visibility of underlying gingival tissue, which may become impinged upon by the retainer.

Cervical Retainer Placement. The use of a No. 212 cervical retainer for restoration of Class V tooth preparations was recommended by Markley.[24] When punching the holes in the rubber dam, recall that the hole for

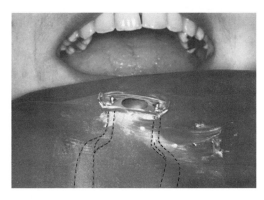

FIG. **10-29** Lip of hole for anchor tooth is stretched to engage lateral wings of retainer.

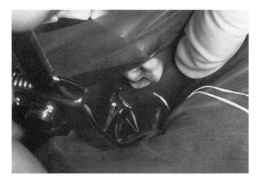

FIG. **10-30** Retainer applied after dam is stretched over posterior anchor tooth.

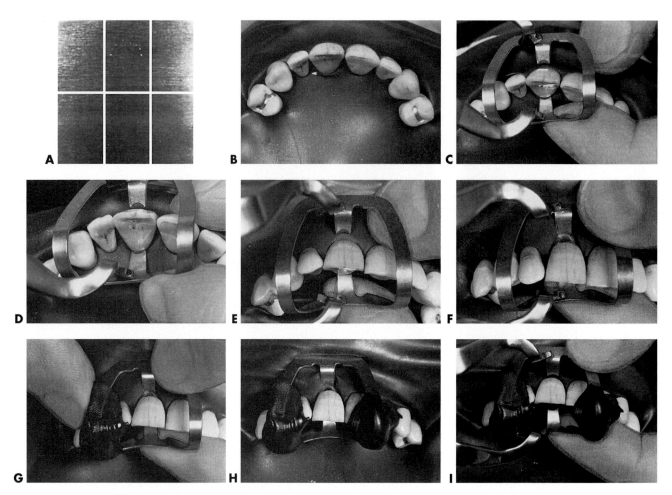

FIG. **10-31** Applying a cervical retainer. **A,** Hole for maxillary right central incisor is punched facial to arch form. **B,** Isolation is extended to include first premolars; metal posterior retainers are unnecessary. **C,** First, position lingual jaw touching height of contour, while keeping facial jaw from touching tooth; steady retainer with fingers of left hand using index finger under lingual bow and thumb under facial bow. **D,** Final position of lingual jaw after gently moving it apical of height of contour, with fingers continually supporting and guiding retainer and with facial jaw away from tooth. **E,** Stretch facial rubber apically by thumb to expose lesion and soft tissue, with forefinger maintaining position of lingual jaw and with facial jaw not touching. **F,** Facial jaw having apically retracted tissue and dam and in position against tooth 0.5 to 1 mm apical of lesion. Note that thumb has now moved from under facial bow to apply holding pressure, while index finger continues to maintain the lingual jaw position. **G,** Apply compound over and under bow and into the gingival embrasures, while fingers of left hand hold retainer's position. **H,** Application of retainer is completed by addition of compound to other bow and into gingival embrasures. Note that retainer holes are accessible to forceps for removal. **I,** Removal of retainer by ample spreading of retainer jaws before lifting from the site of the operation.

the tooth to receive this retainer for a facial cervical restoration should be positioned facially (a few millimeters) to the arch form (Fig. 10-31, *A*). Also, the distance to the adjacent holes should be increased approximately 1 mm on each side. If the cervical retainer is to be placed on an incisor, recall that isolation should be extended to include the first premolars, and that metal retainers usually are not needed to anchor the dam (see Fig. 10-31, *B*). If the cervical retainer is to be placed on a canine or a posterior tooth, remember to position the anchor tooth retainer sufficiently posterior so as not to interfere with

placement of the cervical retainer. If this is not possible, the anchor tooth retainer should be removed before positioning the cervical retainer.

Before positioning the cervical retainer, have a stick of low-fusing compound and a flame burner available. Engage the jaws of the cervical retainer with the forceps, spread the retainer sufficiently, and position the lingual jaw against the tooth at the height of contour (see Fig. 10-31, *C*). Gently move the jaw gingivally, depressing the dam and soft tissue, until the jaw of the retainer is positioned slightly apical of the height of contour (see

Fig. 10-31, *D*). Exercise care not to allow the lingual jaw to pinch the lingual gingiva or injure the gingival attachment. While positioning the lingual jaw, the index finger of the left hand (for a right-handed operator) should help in supporting and guiding the retainer jaw gingivally to the proper location.

While stabilizing the lingual jaw with the index finger, use the thumb of the left hand to pull the dam apically to expose the facial lesion and gingival crest (see Fig. 10-31, *E*). Position the facial jaw gingival to the lesion and release the dam held by the thumb. Next, move the thumb onto the facial jaw to secure it (see Fig. 10-31, *F*). Exercise care while positioning the facial jaw not to scar the enamel or cementum. The tip of each jaw should not be sharp and should conform to the contour of the engaged tooth surface. Do not position the jaw too close to the lesion because of the danger of collapsing carious or weak tooth structure. Such proximity would also limit access and visibility to the operating site. As a rule, the facial jaw should be 0.5 to 1 mm gingival to the anticipated location of the gingival margin of the completed tooth preparation. While maintaining the retainer's position with the fingers of the left hand, remove the forceps.

Often, the No. 212 retainer needs to be stabilized on the tooth with compound. If so, while the operator positions the retainer, the assistant heats and tempers the end of a stick of compound. Maintaining the retainer's position with the fingers of the left hand, the operator presses the softened compound under and over one bow. With a moistened thumb and forefinger, press the compound onto the incisal (occlusal) surface(s) and into the interproximal area(s), locking the compound in the embrasure(s) (see Fig. 10-31, *G*). The cervical area should be examined for adequate isolation and access before the compound hardens. If additional retraction is necessary, engage the retainer and move the facial jaw gingivally while the compound is soft. Cool the compound with air. Only after the compound has been cooled and hardened should the fingers of the left hand be removed from the retainer. Apply compound in a similar manner to the other bow of the retainer (see Fig. 10-31, *H*).

If the facial lip of the dam is not already inverted into the gingival sulcus, dry the tooth and tease the dam to proper position using a suitable blunt instrument. Continuous inversion provides coverage of soft tissue, slight retraction and some protection of marginal gingiva, and isolation from oral fluids.

If it is necessary to move the facial jaw gingivally during the operation subsequent to the initial placement of the retainer, the retainer is easily removed with the retainer forceps and reapplied. Using compound to stabilize a cervical retainer is recommended because the retainer may be inadvertently bumped out of place during the operative procedure. Also, it is a convenient resting place for the operator's fingers.

To remove the cervical retainer, engage it with the forceps, spread the jaws to free the compound support, and lift it incisally (occlusally), being careful to spread the retainer sufficiently to prevent the jaws from scraping the tooth or damaging the newly inserted restoration (see Fig. 10-31, *I*). Free the embrasures of any remaining compound before removing the rubber dam.

A modified No. 212 retainer is recommended, especially for treatment of cervical lesions with greatly extended gingival margins. The modified No. 212 retainer can be ordered, if specified, or the operator can modify an existing No. 212 retainer. The modification technique involves heating each jaw of the retainer in an open flame, and then bending it with No. 110 pliers from its oblique orientation to a more horizontal one. Allowing the modified retainer to bench-cool returns it to its original hardened state. (The principle involved in this modification is illustrated in Figure 21-18.)

Fixed Bridge Isolation. It is sometimes necessary to isolate one or more abutment teeth of a fixed bridge. Indications for fixed bridge isolation include restoration of an adjacent proximal surface and cervical restoration of an abutment tooth.

The technique suggested for this procedure is as follows.[4] The rubber dam is punched as usual except for providing one large hole for each unit in the bridge. Fixed bridge isolation is accomplished after the remainder of the dam is applied (Fig. 10-32, *A*). A blunted, curved suture needle with dental floss attached is threaded from the facial aspect through the hole for the anterior abutment and then under the anterior connector and back through the same hole on the lingual side (see Fig. 10-32, *B*). The needle's direction is then reversed as it is passed from the lingual side through the hole for the second bridge unit, then under the same anterior connector, and through the hole of the second bridge unit on the facial side (see Fig. 10-32, *C*). A square knot is then tied with the two ends of the floss, thereby pulling the dam material snugly around the connector and into the gingival embrasure. The free ends of the floss should be cut closely so they neither interfere with access and visibility nor become entangled in a rotating instrument. Each terminal abutment of the bridge is isolated by this method (see Fig. 10-32, *D*). If the floss knot on the facial aspect interferes with cervical restoration of an abutment tooth, the operator can tie the septum from the lingual. Removal of the rubber dam isolating a fixed bridge is accomplished by cutting the interseptal rubber over the connectors with scissors and removing the floss ties (see Fig. 10-32, *E*). As always, after dam removal the operator needs to verify that no dam segments are missing and massage the adjacent gingival tissue.

Substitution of a Retainer With a Matrix. When a matrix band must be applied to the posterior anchor tooth, the jaws of the retainer often prevent proper

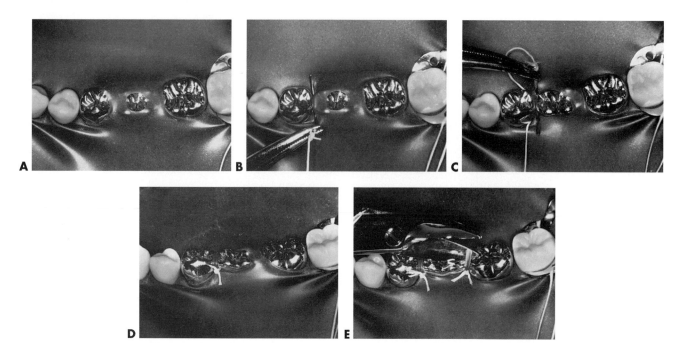

FIG. **10-32** Procedure for isolating a fixed bridge. **A,** Apply dam except in area of fixed bridge. **B,** Thread blunted suture needle from facial to lingual aspect through anterior abutment hole and then under anterior connector and back through same hole on lingual surface. **C,** Pass needle facially through hole for second bridge unit and then under the same connector and through the hole for the second unit. **D,** Tie off first septum. **E,** Cut posterior septum to initiate removal of dam.

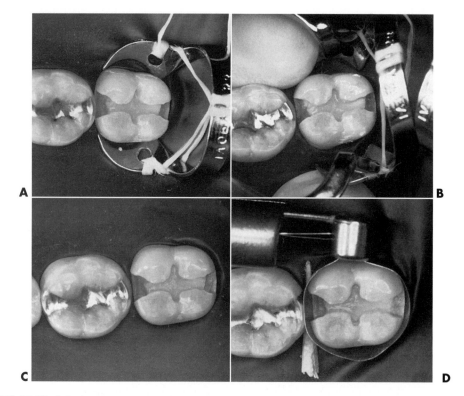

FIG. **10-33** Substituting retainer with matrix on terminal tooth. **A,** Completed tooth preparation of terminal tooth with retainer in place. **B,** Dentist and assistant stretch dam distally and gingivally as retainer is being removed. **C,** Retainer removed before placement of matrix. **D,** Completed matrix in place. To maximize access and visibility during insertion, the mouth mirror is used to reflect dam distally and occlusally.

positioning and wedging of the matrix (Fig. 10-33, *A*). Successful application of the matrix can be accomplished by substituting the retainer with the matrix. Fig. 10-33, *B* through *D*, illustrates this exchange on a mandibular right molar as the index finger of the operator depresses gingivally and distally the rubber dam adjacent to the facial jaw while the assistant similarly depresses the dam on the lingual side. After the matrix band is placed, the tension is released on the dam, allowing it to invert around the band. The matrix, unlike the retainer, has neither jaws nor bow, so there is a tendency for the dam to slip occlusally and over the matrix unless dryness is maintained.

The operator obtains access and visibility for insertion of the restorative material by reflecting the dam distally and occlusally with the mirror. However, care must be exercised not to stretch the dam so much that it is pulled away from the matrix, permitting leakage around the tooth or slippage over the matrix.

Following insertion, the occlusal portion is contoured before removing the matrix. To complete the procedure the operator has the choice of removing the matrix, replacing the retainer, and completing the contouring, or removing the matrix and rubber dam and completing the contouring. To maintain isolation throughout the procedure, it is preferable to replace the retainer before completing the contouring.

Variations with Age. The age of a patient often dictates changes in the procedures of rubber dam application. A few variations are described here.

Because young patients have smaller dental arches than adult patients, holes should be punched in the dam accordingly. For primary teeth, isolation is usually from the most posterior tooth to the canine on the same side. The sheet of rubber dam may be smaller (5 × 5 inch [12.5 × 12.5 cm]) for the young patient so that the rubber material does not cover the nose.

Some operators prefer to alter the procedure of application for a young patient. The unpunched rubber dam is attached to the frame, the holes are punched, the dam with the frame is applied over the anchor tooth, and the retainer is applied (Fig. 10-34). Since the dam is generally in place for shorter intervals than for the adult patient, the napkin might not be used.

The jaws of the retainers used on primary and young permanent teeth need to be directed more gingivally because of short clinical crowns or because the anchor tooth's height of contour is below the crest of the gingival tissue. The S.S. White No. 27 retainer is recommended for primary teeth. The Ivory No. W14 retainer is recommended for young permanent teeth.

Isolated teeth with short clinical crowns (other than the anchor tooth) may require ligation to hold the dam in position. Ligation is permissible but should be used only when necessary because of possible damage to gingival tissues. Ligatures should be removed first during the procedure of rubber dam removal. Generally, ligation is unnecessary if a sufficient number of teeth are isolated by the rubber dam. However, when ligatures are indicated, a surgeon's knot is used to secure the ligature (Fig. 10-35). Ligatures may be removed by teasing them occlusally with an explorer or by cutting them with a hand instrument or scissors.

A small piece of rubber dam material may be rolled, stretched, and placed into a diastema to serve as an anterior anchor (Fig. 10-36).

Errors in Application and Removal. Certain errors in application and removal can prevent adequate moisture control, reduce access and visibility, or cause injury to the patient.

Off-center arch form. A rubber dam punched off-center (off-center arch form) may not adequately shield the patient's oral cavity, allowing foreign matter to escape down the patient's throat. An off-center dam can

FIG. **10-34** On a child, the rubber dam is often attached to a frame before holes are punched. The dam is then positioned over the anchor tooth before a retainer is applied (as in Fig. 10-30).

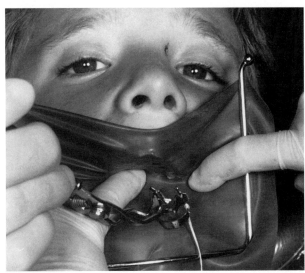

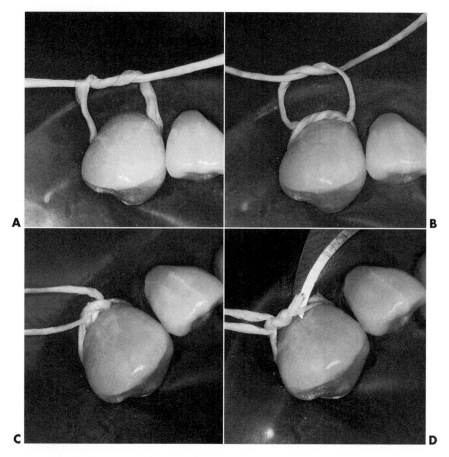

FIG. **10-35** Surgeon's knot. **A,** Dental tape is placed around tooth gingival to height of contour and a knot is tied by first making two loops with the free ends, followed by a single loop **(B). C,** Free ends are not cut but tied to frame to serve as a reminder that ligature is in place. **D,** To remove ligature, simply cut tape with scalpel blade, amalgam knife, or scissors.

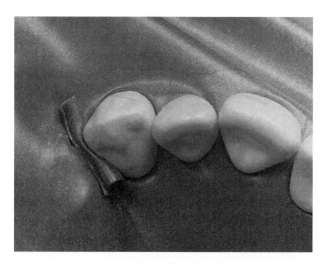

FIG. **10-36** A piece of rubber dam material may be rolled, stretched, and placed in diastema to serve as anterior anchor.

result in an excess of dam material superiorly that may occlude the patient's nasal airway (Fig. 10-37, *A*). If this happens, the superior border of the dam can be folded under or cut from around the patient's nose (see Fig. 10-37, *B* and *C*). Proper hole placement, however, will correctly position the dam. It is important to verify that the rubber dam frame has been applied so that its ends are not dangerously close to the patient's eyes.

Inappropriate distance between the holes. Inappropriate distance between the holes is a problem. Too little distance between holes precludes adequate isolation because the hole margins in the rubber dam are stretched and will not fit snugly around the necks of the teeth. Conversely, too much distance results in excess septal width causing the dam to wrinkle between the teeth, interfere with proximal access, and not provide adequate tissue retraction.

Incorrect arch form of holes. If the punched arch form is too small (incorrect arch form), the holes will be stretched open around the teeth, permitting leakage. If the punched arch form is too large, the dam will wrinkle around the teeth and thus may interfere with access.

Inappropriate retainer. An inappropriate retainer may: (1) be too small, resulting in occasional breakage when the jaws are overspread, (2) be unstable on the anchor tooth, (3) impinge on soft tissue, or (4) impede wedge placement. An appropriate retainer should maintain a stable four-point contact with the anchor tooth and not interfere with wedge placement.

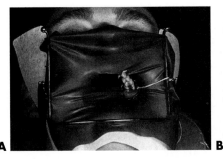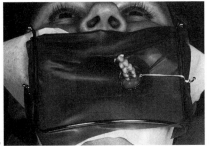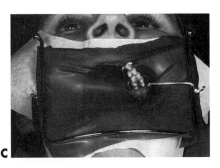

A **B** **C**

FIG. **10-37 A,** Inappropriately punched dam may occlude patient's nasal airway. **B,** Excess dam material along superior border folded under to proper position. **C,** Excess dam material cut from around patient's nose.

Retainer-pinched tissue. The jaws and prongs of the rubber dam retainer usually slightly depress the tissue, but they should not pinch or impinge on it.

Shredded or torn dam. Care should be exercised to prevent shredding or tearing the dam, especially during hole punching or passing the septa through the contacts. Moisture control is possible only if the dam is intact.

Incorrect location of hole for Class V lesion. If there is an incorrect location of the hole for a Class V lesion and the hole is not punched facial to the arch form, circulation in the interproximal tissue will be diminished because of the added pressure once the dam and cervical retainer are in place.

Sharp tips on No. 212 retainer. Sharp tips on a No. 212 retainer should be sufficiently dulled to prevent damaging the cementum.

Incorrect technique for cutting septa. During removal of the rubber dam an incorrect technique for cutting the septa may result in cut tissue or a torn septa. Stretching the septa away from the gingiva, protecting the lip and cheek with an index finger, and using curve-beaked scissors decreases the risk of cutting soft tissue or tearing the septa with the scissors as the septa are cut.

COTTON ROLL ISOLATION AND CELLULOSE WAFERS

Absorbents, such as cotton rolls and cellulose wafers (Fig. 10-38), can also provide isolation. Absorbents are isolation alternatives when rubber dam application is impractical or impossible. In conjunction with profound anesthesia, absorbents provide acceptable moisture control for most clinical procedures. Using a saliva ejector in conjunction with absorbents may further abate salivary flow. The assistant has the responsibility of keeping dry cotton rolls in the mouth. The assistant should change the cotton rolls when they become saturated. It is sometimes permissible to suction the free moisture from a saturated cotton roll in place in the mouth. This is done by placing the evacuator tip next to the end of the cotton roll while the operator secures the roll.

Several commercial devices for holding cotton rolls in position are available (Fig. 10-39). It is generally necessary to remove the holding appliance from the mouth to

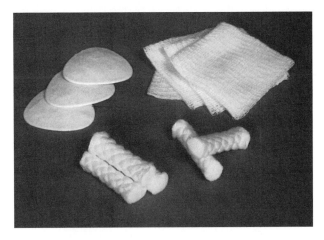

FIG. **10-38** Absorbents such as cotton rolls, cellulose wafers, and gauze sponges provide satisfactory dryness for short periods of time.

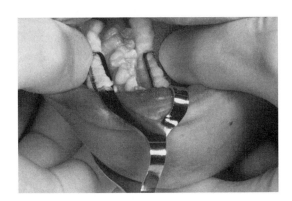

FIG. **10-39** A cotton roll holder in position.

change the cotton rolls. This is inconvenient and time consuming; consequently, they are not often used. An advantage of cotton roll holders is that they may slightly retract the cheeks and tongue from the teeth, which enhances access and visibility.

Placing a medium-sized cotton roll in the facial vestibule (Fig. 10-40) isolates the maxillary teeth. Placing a medium-sized cotton roll in the vestibule and a larger one between the teeth and the tongue (Fig. 10-41)

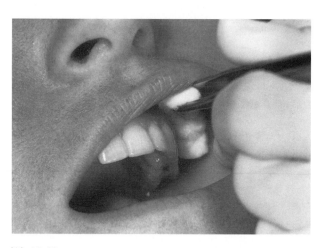

FIG. **10-40** Isolate maxillary posterior teeth by placing cotton roll in vestibule adjacent to teeth.

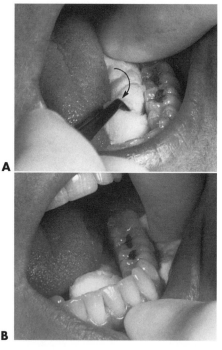

FIG. **10-41** **A,** Position large cotton roll between tongue and teeth by "rolling" it to place in direction of arrow. **B,** Properly positioned facial and lingual cotton rolls improve access and visibility.

isolates the mandibular teeth. While placement of a cotton roll in the facial vestibule is simple, placement on the lingual of mandibular teeth is more difficult. Lingual placement is facilitated by holding the mesial end of the cotton roll with operative pliers and positioning the cotton roll over the desired location. Use the index finger of other hand to push the cotton roll gingivally while twisting the cotton roll with the operative pliers toward the lingual of the teeth. The teeth are then dried with short blasts from the air syringe. Cellulose

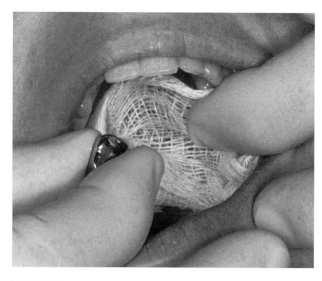

FIG. **10-42** A throat screen is used during try-in and removal of indirect restorations.

wafers may be used to retract the cheek and provide additional absorbency. After the cotton rolls or cellulose wafers are in place, the saliva ejector may be positioned. When removing cotton rolls or cellulose wafers, it may be necessary to moisten them using the air-water syringe to prevent inadvertent removal of the epithelium from the cheeks, floor of the mouth, or lips.

OTHER ISOLATION TECHNIQUES

Throat Shields. When the rubber dam is not being used, throat shields are indicated when there is danger of aspirating or swallowing small objects. This is particularly important when treating teeth in the maxillary arch. A gauze sponge (2 × 2 inch [5 × 5 cm]), unfolded and spread over the tongue and the posterior part of the mouth, is helpful in recovering small objects, such as an indirect restoration, should it be dropped (Fig. 10-42). Without a throat shield, it is possible for a small object to be aspirated or swallowed (Fig. 10-43).[29]

High-Volume Evacuators and Saliva Ejectors. When a high-speed handpiece is used, air-water spray is supplied through the head of the handpiece to wash the operating site and act as a coolant for the bur and tooth. High-volume evacuators are preferred for suctioning water and debris from the mouth (Fig. 10-44) because saliva ejectors remove water slowly and have little capacity for picking up solids. McWherter[26] showed that one type of evacuator would remove 1 pint (0.5 L) of water in 2 seconds, had a 75% to 95% pickup of water in air, and would remove 100% of solids during cutting procedures. A practical test for the adequacy of a high-volume evacuator is to submerge the evacuator tip in a 5-oz (150-ml) cup of water. The water should disappear in approximately 1 second.

The combined use of water spray or air-water spray and a high-volume evacuator during cutting procedures has the following advantages:

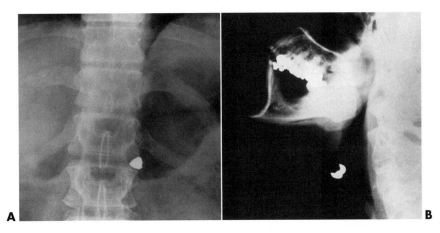

FIG. **10-43** **A,** Radiograph of swallowed casting in patient's stomach. **B,** Radiograph of casting lodged in patient's throat.

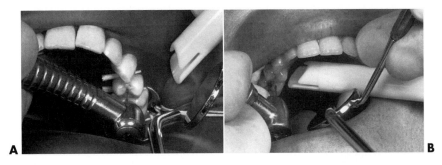

FIG. **10-44** Position of evacuator tip for maximal removal of water and debris in operating area. **A,** With rubber dam applied. **B,** With cotton roll isolation.

1. Cuttings both of tooth and restorative material, as well as other debris, are removed from the operating site.
2. A washed operating field improves access and visibility.
3. There is no dehydration of the oral tissues.
4. Without an anesthetic, the patient experiences less pain.
5. Pauses that are sometimes annoying and time consuming are eliminated.
6. Precious metals are more readily salvaged.
7. Quadrant dentistry is facilitated.

The assistant's responsibility is to place the evacuator tip as near to the tooth being prepared as possible. However, it should not obstruct the operator's access or vision. Also, the evacuator tip should not be so close to the handpiece head that the air-water spray is diverted from the rotary instrument (i.e., bur or diamond). The assistant should place the evacuator tip in the mouth before the operator positions the handpiece and mirror. The assistant usually places the tip of the evacuator just distal to the tooth to be prepared. For maximal efficiency the orifice of the evacuator tip should be positioned so it is parallel to the facial (lingual) surface of the tooth being prepared. The assistant's right hand holds the evacuator tip; the left hand manipulates the air-water syringe. (Hand positions are reversed if the operator is left-handed.) When the operator needs to examine the progress of tooth preparation, the assistant rinses and dry the tooth (teeth) using air from the syringe in conjunction with the evacuator.

Most patients do not require the use of saliva ejectors for removal of saliva because salivary flow is greatly reduced when the operating site is profoundly anesthetized. The dentist or assistant positions the saliva ejector if needed.

The saliva ejector removes saliva that collects on the floor of the mouth. It may be used in conjunction with sponges, cotton rolls, and the rubber dam. It should be placed in an area least likely to interfere with the operator's movements.

The tip of the ejector must be smooth and made from a nonirritating material. Disposable, inexpensive plastic ejectors that may be shaped by bending with the fingers are preferable because of improved infection control (Fig. 10-45). The ejector should be placed to prevent occluding its tip with tissue from the floor of the mouth. Some ejectors are designed to prevent suctioning of tissue. It also may be necessary to adjust the suction for each patient to prevent this occurrence. A Svedopter is a helpful device that serves as both a saliva ejector and a tongue retractor.

Retraction Cord. When properly applied, retraction cord often can be used for isolation and retraction in the direct procedures of treatment of accessible subgingival areas and in indirect procedures involving gingival margins. When the rubber dam is not used, is impractical, or is inappropriate, retraction cord, usually moistened with a noncaustic styptic (e.g., Hemodent, Premier Dental Products Company, King of Prussia, Pennsylvania), may be placed in the gingival sulcus to control sulcular seepage and/or hemorrhage. Most brands of retraction cord are available with and without the vasoconstrictor epinephrine, which also acts to control sulcular fluids. To achieve adequate moisture control, retraction cord isolation should be used in conjunction with salivation control by virtue of profound anesthesia of all tissues of the operating site. A properly applied retraction cord improves access and visibility and helps prevent abrasion of gingival tissue during tooth preparation. Retraction cord may help restrict excess restorative material from entering the gingival sulcus and provide better access for contouring and finishing the restorative material.

To use retraction cord, insert the cord after attaining profound anesthesia and before tooth preparation. When the proper cord is correctly inserted, its mild physical

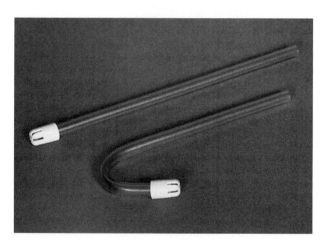

FIG. **10-45** Saliva ejectors.

and chemical (noncaustic styptic) effects achieve isolation from fluids (along with cotton roll use), provides access and visibility, and does not cause harm.

Choose a diameter of cord that can be gently inserted into the gingival sulcus and will produce lateral displacement (a few tenths of a millimeter) of the free gingiva ("opening" the sulcus) without blanching it (caused by ischemia due to pressure). The length of cord should be sufficient to extend approximately 1 mm beyond the gingival width of the tooth preparation. Use a thin, blunt-edged instrument blade or the side of an explorer to progressively insert the cord. To prevent displacement of previously inserted cord, the placement instrument should be moved slightly backward at each step as it is stepped along the cord (Fig. 10-46). Cord placement should not abuse the gingival tissue or damage the epithelial attachment. If ischemia of the gingival tissue is observed, the cord may need to be replaced with a smaller diameter cord. The objective is to obtain minimal yet sufficient lateral displacement of the free gingiva and not to force it apically. Cord insertion results in adequate apical retraction of the gingival crest in a short time.

Because of the delicate, thin dimension of the free gingiva on the facial aspect of anterior and premolar teeth, the smallest diameter cord is often used. If twisted cord is used, it may be helpful to separate the strands of the smallest cord to customize a still smaller cord. A second, usually larger, cord may be placed over (not beside) the first if additional retraction is necessary.

When a proximal crevice is involved, it may be helpful to insert a second, usually larger, cord over the initially inserted cord. This may be indicated when isolating for an impression to record adjacent gingival margins and the gingival papilla is difficult to retract.

In procedures for an indirect restoration (e.g., cast onlay), inserting the cord before removal of infected dentin and placement of any necessary liner assists in providing maximum moisture control. It also opens the sulcus in readiness for any beveling of the gingival margins. The cord may be removed before beveling, or it may be left in

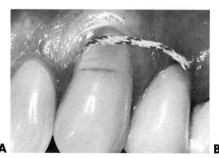
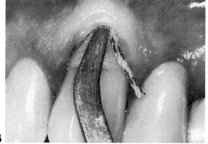
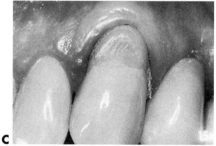

FIG. **10-46** Retraction cord placed in gingival crevice. **A,** Cord placement initiated. **B,** A thin, flat-bladed instrument is used for cord placement. **C,** Cord placed.

place during beveling. In either case, a cord should be reinserted and remain a few minutes before the impression to help ensure an open sulcus for the impression material to enter.

Inserting the cord as early as possible in the tooth preparation helps prevent abrasion of the gingival tissue, thereby reducing the potential for bleeding and allowing only minimal absorption of any medicament from the cord into the circulatory system. The cord may be moistened with a noncaustic styptic before insertion if bleeding of fragile tissue is anticipated. (Specific uses of retraction cord are detailed in subsequent technique chapters.)

Mirror and Evacuator Tip Retraction. A secondary function of the mirror and evacuator tip is to retract the cheek, lip, and tongue (Fig. 10-47). This is particularly important when a rubber dam is not used.

Mouth Props. A potential aid to restorative procedures on posterior teeth (for a lengthy appointment) is a mouth prop (Fig. 10-48, *A*). A prop should establish and maintain suitable mouth opening, thereby relieving the patient's muscles of this task, which often produces fatigue and sometimes pain. Moreover, with the use of a prop, the patient is relieved of the responsibility of maintaining mouth opening, thereby permitting added relaxation.

The ideal characteristics of a mouth prop are as follows:

1. It should be adaptable to all mouths.
2. It should be capable of being easily positioned, with no patient discomfort.
3. It should be easily adjusted, if necessary, to provide the proper mouth opening or improve its position in the mouth.
4. It should be stable once applied.
5. It should be easily and readily removable by the operator or patient in case of emergency.
6. It should be either sterilizable or disposable.

Mouth props of different designs and different materials are available. They are generally available either as block type or ratchet type (Fig. 10-48, *B* and *C*). Although the ratchet type is adjustable, its size and cost are disadvantages. The convenience and cost of the block type commend it for use in most operative procedures.

The use of a mouth prop may be beneficial to both the operator and patient. The most outstanding benefits to the patient are relief of responsibility of maintaining adequate mouth opening and relief of muscle fatigue and muscle pain. For the dentist, the prop ensures constant and adequate mouth opening and permits extended or multiple operations if desired.

Drugs. The use of drugs to control salivation is rarely indicated in restorative dentistry and is generally limited to atropine. As with any drug, the operator should be familiar with its indications, contraindications, and side effects. It is important to remember that atropine is contraindicated for nursing mothers and patients with glaucoma.[9]

SUMMARY

A thorough knowledge of the preliminary procedures addressed in this chapter reduces the physical strain on the dental team associated with daily dental treatment, reduces patient anxiety associated with dental procedures, and enhance moisture control, thereby improving the quality of operative dentistry.

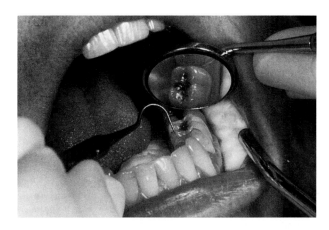

FIG. **10-47** Chairside assistant uses air syringe to dry teeth and to keep mirror free of debris.

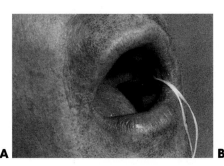
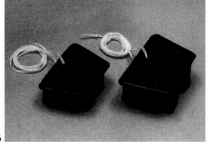
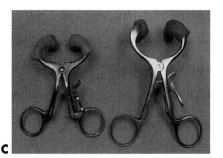

FIG. **10-48** Mouth props. **A,** Block-type prop maintaining mouth opening. **B,** Block-type prop. **C,** Ratchet-type prop.

REFERENCES

1. ADA Council on Dental Materials, Instruments, and Equipment: Posterior composite resins, *J Am Dent Assoc* 112:707-709, 1986.
2. Anusavice KJ, editor: *Phillips' science of dental materials,* ed 10, St Louis, 1996, Mosby.
3. Barghi N, Knight GT, Berry TG: Comparing two methods of moisture control in bonding to enamel: a clinical study, *Oper Dent* 16:130-135, 1991.
4. Baum L, Phillips RW, Lund MR: *Textbook of operative dentistry,* ed 3, Philadelphia, 1995, WB Saunders.
5. Berglund A, Molin M: Mercury levels in plasma and urine after removal of all amalgam restorations: the effect of using rubber dams, *Dent Mater* 13:297-304, 1997.
6. Black GL: *Operative dentistry,* ed 8, vol 2, Woodstock, Ill, 1947, Medico-Dental.
7. Brinker HA: Access—the key to success, *J Prosthet Dent* 28: 391-401, 1972.
8. Christensen GJ: Using rubber dams to boost quality, quantity of restorative services, *J Am Dent Assoc* 125: 81-82, 1994.
9. Ciancio SG, editor: *ADA guide to dental therapeutics,* ed 1, Chicago, 1998, American Dental Association.
10. Cochran MA, Miller CH, Sheldrake MA: The efficacy of the rubber dam as a barrier to the spread of microorganisms during dental treatment, *J Am Dent Assoc* 119:141-144, 1989.
11. Cunningham PR, Ferguson GW: The instruction of rubber dam technique, *J Am Acad Gold Foil Oper* 13: 5-12, 1970.
12. Dajani AS et al: Prevention of bacterial endocarditis: recommendations by the American Heart Association, *J Am Dent Assoc* 128:1142-1151, 1997.
13. Forrest WR, Perez RS: The rubber dam as a surgical drape: protection against AIDS and hepatitis, *Gen Dent* 37:236-237, 1989.
14. Fusayama T: Total etch technique and cavity isolation, *J Esthet Dent* 4:105-109, 1992.
15. Heling I, Sommer M, Kot I: Rubber dam—an essential safeguard, *Quintessence Int* 19:377-378, 1988.
16. Howard WW, Moller RC: *Atlas of operative dentistry,* ed 3, St Louis, 1981, Mosby.
17. Huggins DR: The rubber dam—an insurance policy against litigation, *J Indiana Dent Assoc* 65:23-24, 1986.
18. Ingraham R, Koser JR: *An atlas of gold foil and rubber dam procedures,* Buena Park, Calif, 1961, Uni-Tro College Press.
19. Jones CM, Reid JS: Patient and operator attitudes toward rubber dam, *ASDC J Dent Child* 55:452-454, 1988.
20. Joynt RB, Davis EL, Schreier PH: Rubber dam usage among practicing dentists, *Oper Dent* 14:176-181, 1989.
21. Kremers L et al: Effect of rubber dam on mercury exposure during amalgam removal, *Eur J Oral Sci* 107:202-207, 1999.
22. Malamed SF: *Handbook of local anesthesia,* ed 4, St Louis, 1997, Mosby.
23. Marcus HW: The role of hypnosis and suggestions in dentistry, *J Am Dent Assoc* 59:1149-1163, 1959.
24. Markley MR: Amalgam restorations for Class V cavities, *J Am Dent Assoc* 50:301-309, 1955.
25. Marshall K, Page J: The use of rubber dam in the UK: a survey, *Br Dent J* 169:286-291, 1990.
26. McWherter E: Modern method improvements and works simplification approach to clinical procedures of the washed field technic in dentistry, *Ark Dent J* 28:10, 1957.
27. Medina JE: The rubber dam—an incentive for excellence, *Dent Clin North Am* p. 255-264, March 1967.
28. Mosteller JH: Restoration of teeth with silver amalgam, *J Prosthet Dent* 11:288-297, 1961.
29. Nelson JF: Ingesting an onlay: a case report, *J Am Dent Assoc* 123:73-74, 1992.
30. Nimmo A et al: Particulate inhalation during the removal of amalgam restorations, *J Prosthet Dent* 63:228-233, 1990.
31. Occupational Safety and Health Administration: Bloodborne pathogens (Federal Register 56: Section 1910, 1030 [26 U.S.C. 653], 64175-64182), Washington, DC, 1991, Occupational Safety and Health Adminstration.
32. Peterson JE, Nation WA, Matsson L: Effect of a rubber dam clamp (retainer) on cementum and junctional epithelium, *Oper Dent* 11:42-45, 1986.
33. Raskin A, Setcos JC, Vreven J: Influence of the isolation method on the 10-year clinical behaviour of posterior resin composite restorations, *Clin Oral Investig* 25:148-152, 2000.
34. Roy A, Epstein J, Onno E: Latex allergies in dentistry: recognition and recommendations, *J Can Dent Assoc* 63:297-300, 1997.
35. Samaranayake LP, Reid J, Evans D: The efficacy of rubber dam isolation in reducing atmospheric bacterial contamination, *ASDC J Dent Child* 56:442-444, 1989.
36. Shugars DA et al: Musculoskeletal back pain among dentists, *Gen Dent* 32:481-485, 1984.
37. Smales RJ. Rubber dam usage related to restoration quality and survival, *Br Dent J* 174:330-333, 1993.
38. Straffon LH, Dennison JB, More FG: Three-year evaluation of sealant: effect of isolation on efficacy, *J Am Dent Assoc* 110: 714-717, 1985.
39. Sturdevant CM, Barton RE, Brauer, JC, editors: *The art and science of operative dentistry,* ed 1, New York, 1968, McGraw-Hill.

Introduction to Composite Restorations

THEODORE M. ROBERSON

HARALD O. HEYMANN

ANDRÉ V. RITTER

INTRODUCTION

The search for an ideal esthetic material for restoring teeth has resulted in significant improvements in both esthetic materials and techniques for using them. Composites and the acid-etch technique represent two major advances.[5,7,8,45] Adhesive materials that have stronger bonds to enamel and dentin further simplify restorative techniques.[4,42,43,51] The possibilities for innovative uses of esthetic materials are exciting and almost unlimited. Many of the specific applications of these materials are presented in Chapters 12 through 15; this chapter provides a general introduction to composite restorations, the predominant direct esthetic restorative material (Fig. 11-1).

Although these materials are referred to as *resin-based composites*, *composite resins*, and other things, this textbook refers to most direct esthetic restorations as *composites*. They are distinguished only from porcelain/ceramic or glass-ionomer esthetic restorations. There is also some information presented about various types of composites, including microfill, hybrid, flowable, and packable.

The choice of a material to restore carious lesions and other defects in teeth continues to be controversial. Tooth-colored materials, such as composite, are used in almost all types and sizes of restorations. Such restorations are accomplished with minimal loss of tooth structure, little or no discomfort, relatively short operating time, and modest expense to the patient when compared with esthetic porcelain crowns. However, when a tooth is significantly weakened by extensive defects (especially in areas of heavy occlusal function) and esthetics is of primary concern, the best treatment usually is a ceramic onlay or crown or a porcelain-fused-to-metal crown.

An interpretation of esthetics primarily is determined by an individual's perception and is subject to wide variations. What is pleasing for one patient may be completely unacceptable to another. For example, some people have no objection to gold or other types of metallic restorations in their front teeth, while most find these restorations unesthetic.

It is the dentist's responsibility to present all logical restorative alternatives to a patient, but the patient should be given an opportunity to help make the final decision regarding which alternative will be selected. Explaining the procedure and showing the patient color photographs and models of teeth that have been restored by various methods are helpful. Computer simulation of possible treatment outcomes, using computer imaging technology, is also helpful. Many patients are not aware that some teeth or some parts of the teeth are not visible during normal lip movements. For example, the patient in Fig. 11-2 does not show the gingival portion of the teeth, even with a broad smile. The deeply abraded cervical areas were restored with gold inlays, which have been in service for over 20 years with no esthetic detriments. Other examples of restoring anterior teeth with metal restorations are presented in the chapters on amalgam, cast metal, and direct gold (Chapters 18, 20, and 21).

Most people want their teeth to look natural, including areas of the dentition that normally do not show. As far back as 1959, Skinner[46] wrote, "The esthetic quality of a restoration may be as important to the mental health of the patient as the biological and technical qualities of the restoration are to his physical or dental health." Today, esthetic considerations are still primary factors for seeking dental treatment.

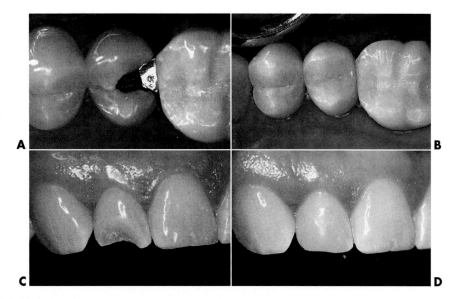

FIG. 11-1 Composite restorations. **A** and **B**, Class II composite restoration, before and after. **C** and **D**, Class IV composite restoration, before and after.

The lifespan of an esthetic restoration depends on many factors, including the nature and extent of the initial problem, the treatment procedure, the restorative material utilized, and the operator's skill, as well as patient factors such as oral hygiene, occlusion, and adverse habits. Since all direct esthetic restorations are bonded to tooth structure, the effectiveness of generating the bond is paramount for the success and longevity of such restorations. Failures can result from a number of causes, including trauma, improper tooth preparation, inferior materials, and misuse of dental materials. The dentist is responsible for performing or accomplishing each operative procedure with meticulous care and attention to detail. However, patient cooperation is of utmost importance in maintaining the clinical appearance and influencing the longevity of any restoration. Long-range clinical success requires that a patient be knowledgeable of the causes of dental disease and be motivated to practice

preventive measures, including a proper diet, good oral hygiene, and maintenance recall visits to the dentist.

This chapter primarily presents the properties and clinical uses of composite materials; they have largely replaced other types of tooth-colored materials used for esthetic restorations.

As is noted later, composite restorative materials now enjoy universal clinical application. They can be used almost anywhere in the mouth for any kind of restorative procedure. Naturally there are factors that must be considered for each specific application. The reasons for such expanded usage of these materials relate to improvements in both their ability to bond to tooth structure (enamel and dentin) and their physical properties. The possibility of bonding a relatively strong material (composite) to tooth structure (enamel and dentin) results in a restored tooth that is well sealed and regains much of its strength.[3,32]

TYPES OF ESTHETIC RESTORATIVE MATERIALS

Many esthetic restorative materials are available. To gain a full appreciation for available conservative esthetic materials, it is appropriate to review some of the tooth-colored materials, even though a few of these are no longer used. (These materials are presented in greater detail in Chapter 4.)

Fused Porcelain. The fused (baked) porcelain inlay, an indirect restoration, dates from 1908, when Byram described several designs of tooth preparations for its use.[9,11] Since the development of adhesive resin cements, there has been renewed interest in using fused porcelain for inlays and onlays in posterior teeth (Fig. 11-3) and veneers in anterior teeth (Fig. 11-4).[10,21,40,52] Many of these restorations are fabricated in a dental laboratory with materials and equipment similar to that used for other types of fused porcelain. However, sophisticated computer-aided design/computer-assisted machining (CAD/CAM) systems are available that also fabricate porcelain restorations chairside, eliminating the need for impressions, temporary restorations, laboratory procedures and costs, and additional appointments[31,35,36] (see Chapters 4 and 14).

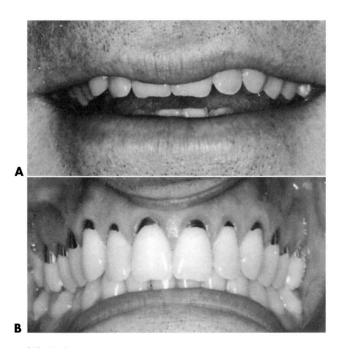

A

B

FIG. **11-2 A,** Many patients do not normally show gingival third of anterior teeth. **B,** Patient in **A** with gold cervical restorations.

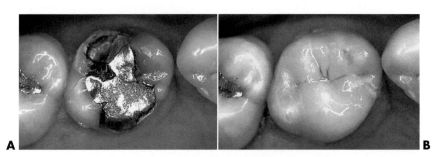

A   **B**

FIG. **11-3** Porcelain inlay. **A,** Before. **B,** After.

Silicate Cement. Silicate cement, the first translucent filling material, was introduced in 1878 by Fletcher in England.[11] It was used extensively to restore carious lesions in the anterior teeth for over 60 years. Silicate cement powder is composed of acid-soluble glasses, and the liquid contains phosphoric acid, water, and buffering agents. Although silicate cement is rarely used as a restorative material today, a practitioner still may encounter silicate restorations, especially in older patients.

Silicate cement was recommended for small restorations in the anterior teeth of patients with high caries activity.[54] By virtue of the high fluoride content and solubility of this restorative material, the adjacent enamel was thought to be rendered more resistant to recurrent caries. Tooth preparations for silicate cement were of the conventional type (boxlike form), and a butt joint was required at the cavosurface margin because the material was brittle and had poor edge strength. Mechanical retention was necessary in the tooth preparation because the material did not adhere to the tooth structure. A liner or base was required under the silicate cement to protect the pulp tissue from irritation due to the initial low pH of the material.

Tooth-matching ability, ease of manipulation, and an anticariogenic quality were favorable characteristics of silicate cement. It was also a good insulator, and its coefficient of thermal expansion approached that of enamel. Even though the average life of a silicate cement restoration was approximately 4 years,[39] some of these restorations have been reported to last for 10 years and longer in some patients.[17]

Failures of silicate cement are easy to detect because of their discoloration and loss of contour (Fig. 11-5). When examined with an explorer tip, silicate cement is rough and has the feel of ground glass. Old composite restorations may also exhibit a similar surface texture and discoloration (Fig. 11-6), but they are less subject to extensive ditching or loss of contour.

Acrylic Resin. Self-curing (chemically activated) acrylic resin for anterior restorations was developed in Germany in the 1930s, but it was not marketed until the late 1940s because of World War II.[38] Early acrylic materials were disappointing because of inherent weaknesses such as poor activator systems, high polymerization shrinkage, high coefficient of thermal expansion, and lack of abrasion resistance, resulting in marginal

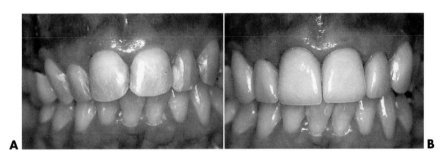

FIG. **11-4** Porcelain veneers. **A,** Before. **B,** After.

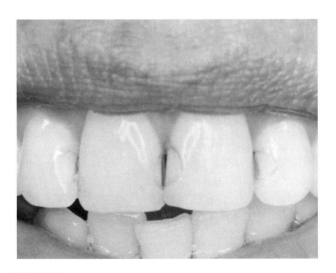

FIG. **11-5** Failed silicate cement restorations displaying discoloration and loss of contour.

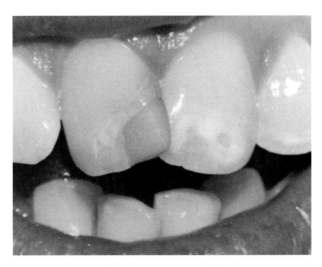

FIG. **11-6** Typical appearance of an old, extrinsically stained, and rough composite restoration.

leakage, pulp injury, recurrent caries, color changes, and excessive wear.[38,44] Improvements in these materials and their procedures reduced the severity and occurrence of some of these problems. Acrylic resin restorations are rarely used today, but, as with silicate cement restorations, may be seen in older patients.

The tooth preparation for acrylic resin usually was either the conventional type or beveled conventional type (described later for composites). As a restoration, acrylic resin was most successful in protected areas of teeth where temperature change, abrasion, and stress were minimal.[47] It was also used as an esthetic veneer on the facial surface of Class II and Class IV metal restorations and for facings in crowns and bridges. One of the current uses of acrylic resin is for making temporary restorations in operative and fixed prosthodontic indirect restoration procedures requiring two or more appointments. Satisfactory temporary restorations that are esthetic, comfortable, and adequately wear resistant can be made quickly with acrylic resin. Instructions for mixing acrylic resin must be followed carefully. When the powder and liquid are mixed, polymerization occurs at a rapid rate, resulting in some shrinkage and a slight rise in temperature as the material hardens.

As stated previously, several unfavorable physical properties prevented acrylic resin from being an ideal restorative material. Because of poor wear resistance, it would not maintain its contour in areas subject to abrasion or attrition. It was not indicated for high-stress areas because the material had low strength and would flow under load. Its high polymerization shrinkage and linear coefficient of thermal expansion caused microleakage and eventual discoloration at the margins as a result of percolation (Fig. 11-7).[38] This problem could be somewhat overcome by providing adequate internal retention

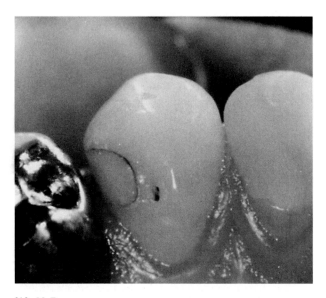

FIG. **11-7** Acrylic resin restoration displaying marginal discoloration after several years of service.

form in the tooth preparation, acid-etching the enamel, and inserting the material with a nonpressure technique.

The clinical appearance of an acrylic resin restoration is usually smooth and polished. When tested with an explorer tip, the material is relatively soft when compared to enamel. After a few years, a thin brown line may develop around the restoration, indicating microleakage (see Fig. 11-7). However, such discoloration of properly inserted restorations does not necessarily indicate recurrent caries and can be eliminated easily by a small-repair veneer restoration.

Composite. In an effort to improve the physical characteristics of unfilled acrylic resins, Bowen of the National Bureau of Standards (now called the National Institute of Standards Technology) developed a polymeric dental restorative material reinforced with silica particles.[5,16] The introduction of this filled resin material in 1962 became the basis for the restorations that are generically termed *composites.*

Composites are presently the most popular tooth-colored materials, having completely replaced silicate cement and acrylic resin. Basically, composite restorative materials consist of a continuous polymeric or resin matrix in which an inorganic filler is dispersed. This inorganic filler phase significantly enhances the physical properties of the composite (as compared to previous tooth-colored materials) by increasing the strength of the restorative material and reducing the linear coefficient of thermal expansion.[6] Composites possess linear coefficients of thermal expansion that are one half to one third the value typically found for unfilled acrylic resins and therefore nearer to that of tooth structure. (See Chapter 4 for details on composite components and properties.)

For a composite to have good mechanical properties, a strong bond must exist between the organic resin matrix and the inorganic filler. This bond is achieved by coating the filler particles with a silane coupling agent,[15] which not only increases the strength of the composite but also reduces its solubility and water absorption.[6]

Composites are usually divided into three types based primarily on the size, amount, and composition of the inorganic filler: (1) conventional composites, (2) microfill composites, and (3) hybrid composites. However, more recent changes in composite composition have resulted in several other hybrid type categories, including flowable and packable composites.

Conventional Composites. Conventional composites generally contain approximately 75% to 80% inorganic filler by weight. The average particle size of conventional composites in the 1980s was approximately 8 μm.[19] Because of the relatively large size and extreme hardness of the filler particles, conventional composites typically exhibit a rough surface texture. (This characteristic can be clearly seen in the scanning electron micrograph in Fig. 11-8.) The resin matrix wears at a faster rate than the filler particles, further roughening the surface. Unfortunately this type of surface texture causes the restoration to be more susceptible to discoloration from extrinsic staining (see Fig. 11-6). Conventional composites have a higher amount of initial wear at occlusal contact areas than do the microfill or hybrid types.

The composition of the inorganic filler in conventional composites also affects the degree of surface roughness. A "soft" or "friable" glass such as strontium or barium yields a smoother surface than those with a quartz filler. Also, when strontium or barium glasses are incorporated in sufficient amounts, the composite is made radiopaque. This is an important characteristic because caries around or under a composite restoration can be more easily interpreted when viewing a radiograph. It should be noted that most conventional composites currently have been supplanted by hybrid composites (see Hybrid Composites).

Microfill Composites. In the late 1970s the microfill, or "polishable," composites were introduced. These materials were designed to replace the rough surface characteristic of conventional composites with a smooth, lustrous surface similar to tooth enamel. Instead of containing the large filler particles typical of the conventional composites, the microfill composites contain colloidal silica particles whose average diameter ranges from 0.01 to 0.04 μm. As illustrated in the scanning electron micrograph in Fig. 11-9, this small particle size results in a smooth, polished surface in the finished restoration that is less receptive to plaque or extrinsic staining. However, because of the greater surface area per unit volume of these microfine particles, the microfill composites cannot be as heavily filled.[15] Typically, microfill composites have an inorganic filler content of approximately 35% to 60% by weight. Because these materials contain considerably less filler than do conventional or

hybrid composites, some of their physical and mechanical characteristics are somewhat inferior. Nonetheless, microfill composites are clinically very wear resistant. Also, their low modulus of elasticity may allow microfill composite restorations to flex during tooth flexure, thus better protecting the bonding interface. This feature may not have any effect on material selection for Class V restorations in general, but it may make microfill composites an appropriate choice for restoring Class V cervical lesions or defects where cervical flexure can be significant (e.g., bruxism, clenchers, stressful occlusion).[27]

Hybrid Composites. In an effort to combine the favorable physical and mechanical properties characteristic of conventional composites with the smooth surface typical of the microfill composites, the hybrid composites were developed. These materials generally have an inorganic filler content of approximately 75% to 85% by weight. The filler is typically a mixture of microfiller and small filler particles that results in a considerably smaller average particle size (0.4 to 1 μm) than that of conventional composites. Because of the relatively high content of inorganic fillers, the physical and mechanical characteristics are generally superior to those of conventional composites. Also, the presence of sub-micrometer–sized microfiller particles interspersed among the larger particles provides a smooth "patina-like" surface texture in the finished restoration. Hybrid composites currently are the predominant direct esthetic restorative materials used. They have almost universal clinical applicability and are the primary materials referred to as *composites* throughout this book.

Flowable Composites. Flowable composites have lower filler content and consequently inferior physical properties, such as lower wear resistance and strength, when compared to more heavily filled composites. Even

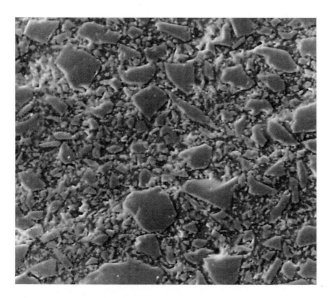

FIG. **11-8** Scanning electron micrograph of polished surface of a conventional composite (×300).

FIG. **11-9** Scanning electron micrograph of polished surface of a microfill composite (×300).

though manufacturers promote widespread usage of these products, they appear to be more appropriate for use in some small Class I restorations, as pit-and-fissure sealants, as marginal repair materials, or, more infrequently, as the first increment placed as a liner under hybrid or packable composites. While their ease of use, favorable wettability, and handling properties are popular features, clinical indications for their use are limited.

Packable Composites. Packable composites are designed to be inherently more viscous to afford a "feel" upon insertion, similar to that of amalgam. Because of increased viscosity and resistance to packing, some lateral displacement of the matrix band is possible. Currently there are no long-term clinical studies to equate packable composites' promoted benefits with improved clinical results when compared to hybrid composites. Their development is an attempt to accomplish two goals: (1) easier restoration of a proximal contact, and (2) similarity to the handling properties of amalgam. They do not completely accomplish either.

Glass Ionomer

Conventional Glass Ionomers. Glass ionomers were developed first by Wilson and Kent in 1972.[57] Like their predecessors, silicate cements, the original glass-ionomer restorative materials were powder/liquid systems. Glass ionomers enjoy the same favorable characteristics of silicate cements—they release fluoride into the surrounding tooth structure, yielding a potential anticariogenic effect, and possess a favorable coefficient of thermal expansion.[37,50] Unlike the silicate cements that have a phosphoric acid liquid, glass ionomers use polyacrylic acid, which renders the final restorative material less soluble.

Although conventional glass ionomers are relatively technique-sensitive regarding mixing and insertion procedures, they may be good materials for restoration of root-surface caries because of their inherent potential anticariogenic quality and adhesion to dentin. Similarly, glass ionomers may be indicated for other anterior restorations in patients exhibiting high caries activity. Because of their low resistance to wear and relatively low strength when compared to composite or amalgam, glass ionomers are not recommended for the restoration of occlusal areas of posterior teeth. Glass-ionomer cements also have been widely advocated for permanent cementation of crowns.

Like other cements, conventional glass-ionomer systems require hand mixing of a powder and liquid with a spatula. However, some glass ionomers are available in encapsulated forms that are mixed by trituration. The capsule containing the mixed material is subsequently placed in an injection syringe for easy insertion into the tooth preparation.

While fluoride-releasing materials have received much publicity and been very popular, one systematic review of numerous research articles on glass ionomers concluded that there was "no conclusive evidence for or against a treatment effect of inhibition of secondary caries by the glass ionomer restorations."[41]

Resin-Modified Glass Ionomers. In an effort to improve the physical properties and esthetic qualities of conventional glass ionomer cements, resin-modified glass ionomer (RMGI) materials have been developed (Table 11-1). RMGIs are probably best described as glass ionomers to which resin has been added. An acid-base setting reaction is present, similar to that of conventional glass-ionomer cements. This is the primary feature that distinguishes these materials from compomers (see the next section). Additionally, the resin component affords the potential for light-curing, auto-curing, or both. RMGIs are easier to use and possess better strength, wear resistance, and esthetics than conventional glass ionomers. However, their physical properties are generally inferior to those of composites, and their indications for clinical use are limited. Because they have the potential advantage of sustained fluoride release, they may be best indicated for Class V restorations in adults who are at high risk for caries and for Classes I and II restorations in primary teeth that will not require long-term service.[56]

Compomers (Polyacid-Modified Composites). Compomers are probably best described as composites to which some glass-ionomer components have been added. Primarily light-cured, they are very easy to use and have gained popularity because of their superb handling properties. Overall, their physical properties are superior to traditional glass ionomers and RMGIs but inferior to those of composites. Their indications for clinical use, therefore, are limited. Although compomers are capable of releasing fluoride, the release is not sustained at a constant rate and anticariogenicity is questionable.

IMPORTANT PROPERTIES

There are considerations regarding various properties of composites that must be understood if a successful composite restoration is to be done. These properties gener-

TABLE 11-1 Tooth-Colored Materials

CONVENTIONAL GLASS IONOMER	RESIN-MODIFIED GLASS IONOMER	COMPOMER	COMPOSITE
High fluoride release	←		Low fluoride release
Low strength	→		High strength
Poor esthetics	→		Excellent esthetics
Low wear resistance	→		High wear resistance

ally require that specific techniques be incorporated into the restorative procedure, either in the tooth preparation or the application of the material. The various property factors are presented here, with additional information provided primarily in Chapter 4 but also in Chapters 12, 13, 14, and 15.

Linear Coefficient of Thermal Expansion. The linear coefficient of thermal expansion (LCTE) is the rate of dimensional change of a material per unit change in temperature. The closer the LCTE of the material is to the LCTE of enamel, the less chance there is for creating voids or openings at the junction of the material and the tooth when temperature changes occur. The LCTE of improved composites is approximately three times that of tooth structure[13]; that for hybrid glass ionomer is 1.5 to 2 times that of tooth structure. Bonding a composite to etched tooth structure reduces the potential negative effects due to the difference between the LCTE of tooth structure and that of the material.

Water Absorption. Water absorption is the amount of water that a material absorbs over time per unit of surface area or volume. When a restorative material absorbs water, its properties change, and therefore its effectiveness as a restorative material is usually diminished. All of the available tooth-colored materials exhibit some water absorption. Materials with higher filler contents exhibit lower water absorption values.

Wear Resistance. Wear resistance refers to a material's ability to resist surface loss as a result of abrasive contact with opposing tooth structure, restorative material, food boli, and such items as toothbrush bristles and toothpicks. The filler particle size, shape, and content affect the potential wear of composites and other tooth-colored restorative materials. The location of the restoration in the dental arch and occlusal contact relationships also affect the potential wear of these materials.

Wear resistance of composite materials is generally good. While not yet as resistant as amalgam, the difference is becoming smaller.[12,34] A composite restoration offers stable occlusal relationship potential in most clinical conditions, particularly if the occlusal contacts are shared with those on natural tooth structure.

Surface Texture. Surface texture is the smoothness of the surface of the restorative material. Restorations in close approximation to gingival tissues require surface smoothness for optimal gingival health. The size and composition of the filler particles primarily determine the smoothness of a restoration, as does the material's ability to be finished and polished. While microfill composites offer the smoothest restorative surface, hybrid composites also provide surface textures that are both esthetic and compatible with soft tissues.

Radiopacity. Esthetic restorative materials must be sufficiently radiopaque, so that the radiolucent image of recurrent caries around or under a restoration can be more easily seen in a radiograph. Most composites contain radiopaque fillers, such as barium glass, to make the material radiopaque.

Modulus of Elasticity. Modulus of elasticity is the stiffness of a material. A material having a higher modulus is more rigid; conversely, a material with a lower modulus is more flexible. A microfill composite material with greater flexibility may perform better in certain Class V restorations than a more rigid hybrid composite.[27,28] This is particularly true for Class V restorations in teeth experiencing heavy occlusal forces, where stress concentrations exist in the cervical area. Such stress can cause tooth flexure that can disrupt the bonding interface.[30] Using a more flexible material such as a microfill composite allows the restorations to bend with the tooth, thereby better protecting the bonding interface. However, as noted, the elastic modulus of the material may be less significant with current bonding systems unless significant occlusal stress from bruxism, clenching, or other forms of stressful occlusion is present. Stressbreaking liners that possess a lower elastic modulus also can be used to better protect the bonding interface.

Solubility. Solubility is the loss in weight per unit surface area or volume due to dissolution or disintegration of a material in oral fluids, over time, at a given temperature. Composite materials do not demonstrate any clinically relevant solubility.

POLYMERIZATION OF COMPOSITE

Polymerization Shrinkage. Composite materials shrink while hardening. This is referred to as *polymerization shrinkage*. This phenomenon cannot be avoided, and there are important clinical procedural techniques that must be incorporated to help offset the potential problems associated with a material pulling away from the preparation walls as it hardens. Careful control of the amount and insertion point of the material and appropriate placement of etchant, primer, and adhesive on the prepared tooth structure to improve bonding reduces these problems.

Polymerization shrinkage usually does not cause significant problems with restorations cured in preparations having all-enamel margins. However, when a tooth preparation has extended onto the root surface, polymerization shrinkage can (and usually does) cause a *gap formation* at the junction of the composite and root surface.[18,53] This problem can be minimized with appropriate technique but probably not eliminated. The clinical significance of the gap is not fully known. The V-shaped gap occurs because the force of polymerization of the composite is greater than the initial bond strength of the composite to the dentin of the root. The V-shaped gap is probably composed of composite on the restoration side and hybridized dentin on the root side (Fig. 11-10).

An important clinical consideration regarding the effects of polymerization shrinkage is the configuration factor (C-factor). The C-factor is the ratio of bonded surfaces to the unbonded, or free, surfaces in a tooth

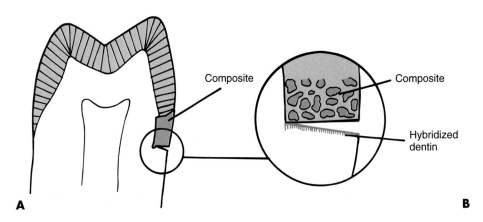

FIG. **11-10** Contraction gap. **A,** V-shaped gap on root surface. **B,** Restoration-side vector is composite; root-side vector is hybridized dentin.

preparation. The higher the C-factor, the greater is the potential for bond disruption from polymerization effects. For example, a Class IV restoration (one bonded surface and four unbonded surfaces) with a C-factor of 0.25 is at low risk for adverse polymerization shrinkage effects. However, a Class I restoration with a C-factor of five (five bonded surfaces, one unbonded surface) is at much higher risk of bond disruption associated with polymerization shrinkage, particularly along the pulpal floor[20,58] (Fig. 11-11).

Internal stresses can be reduced in restorations subject to potentially high disruptive contraction forces (e.g., Class I preparations with a high C-factor) by using: (1) "soft-start" polymerization instead of high-intensity light-curing, (2) incremental additions to reduce the effects of polymerization shrinkage, and (3) a stress-breaking liner, such as a filled dentinal adhesive or RMGI.

Method of Polymerization. The method of polymerization of a composite may affect the technique of insertion, direction of polymerization shrinkage, finishing procedure, color stability, and amount of internal porosity in the material. There are two polymerization methods: self-cured and light-cured using visible light. Self-cured materials require mixing two components, a catalyst and a base, which then react to cause the material to polymerize. Since the components are mixed, there is greater chance for air inclusion in the mixture and therefore greater internal porosity. Also, the working time to insert the self-cured material is restricted by the speed of chemical reaction and can result in the need for increased finishing time because limited contouring can be done before setting occurs. The color stability of self-cured materials also is less stable because of the eventual breakdown of the polymerization-initiating chemical ingredients, tertiary amines. Direction of polymerization shrinkage for self-cured materials is generally centralized (towards the center of the mass). It is theorized that this may help maintain marginal adaptation to prevent microleakage.

Light-cured materials require the use of curing light units or generators. The use of light sources may cause retinal damage unless appropriate precautions are taken to avoid direct, prolonged exposure to the light source. However, light-cured materials do provide increased working time during insertion of the material and therefore require less finishing time. They also exhibit greater color stability and less internal porosity. Effects of polymerization shrinkage can be partially compensated for by an incremental insertion (and curing) technique. However, there are also some clinical situations where positioning the light source close enough to the material is difficult or compromised. In spite of these disadvantages, almost all contemporary composites are of the light-cured type.

Interest continues in improving light-curing methods. In addition to the most common quartz/tungsten/halogen light-curing systems, plasma arc curing (PAC) and argon laser curing (Laser) systems are available for rapid polymerization of light-cured materials. The latter two systems provide high-intensity and high-speed curing when compared to the quartz/tungsten/halogen systems. However, they also significantly increase heat generation and polymerization shrinkage stresses and exhibit a narrow spectral output that may or may not coincide with the spectral requirements needed to cure the restorative material. Whether or not long-term clinical benefits will be identified for these systems is unknown.

In an effort to reduce polymerization shrinkage stresses, different curing mechanism are becoming available, primarily in quartz/tungsten/halogen light-curing units, with the intent of offering a slow or "soft-start" polymerization (see Chapter 4). Also, new light-curing systems using blue light-emitting diodes (LEDs) are being developed that are more efficient, cooler, more portable, and more durable than the systems noted previously.

All of these efforts are to develop a light-curing system that is consistent and faster and produces a stress-free cured material. These features will make light-

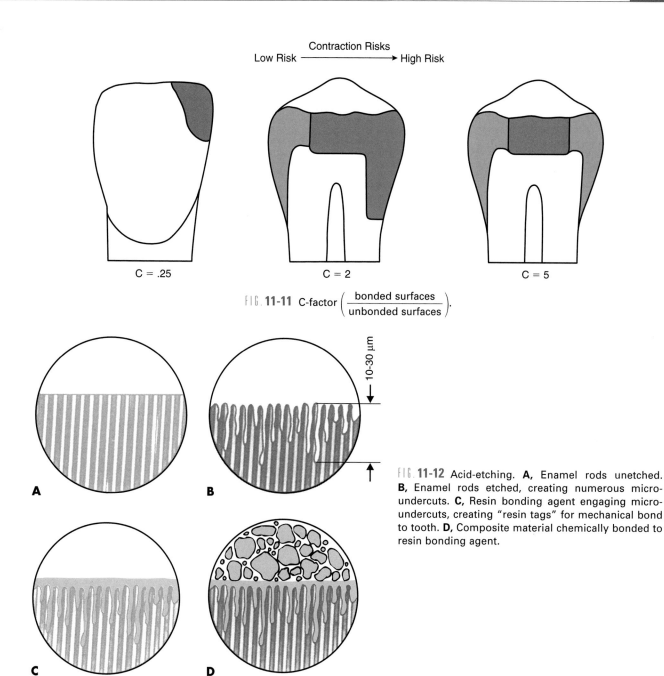

FIG. 11-11 C-factor $\left(\dfrac{\text{bonded surfaces}}{\text{unbonded surfaces}} \right)$.

FIG. 11-12 Acid-etching. **A,** Enamel rods unetched. **B,** Enamel rods etched, creating numerous micro-undercuts. **C,** Resin bonding agent engaging micro-undercuts, creating "resin tags" for mechanical bond to tooth. **D,** Composite material chemically bonded to resin bonding agent.

curing more successful and more economical and possibly result in restorations with better bonding and properties.

COMPOSITE RESTORATIONS

A composite restoration is placed as follows: (1) the fault is removed from the tooth, (2) the prepared tooth structure is acid-etched and primed (if preparation extends into dentin), (3) a fluid resin adhesive material is bonded to the etched and primed tooth structure, and (4) a stronger filled restorative material (composite) is bonded to the resin, contoured, and polished (Fig. 11-12). A successful composite restoration requires careful attention to technique detail, resulting in gaining

the maximum benefit of the material's properties and appropriate bonding of the material to the tooth (the main advantage of composite is its ability to bond to the tooth). The fundamental concepts of adhesion of a restorative material to tooth structure are presented in Chapter 5.

GENERAL CONSIDERATIONS FOR COMPOSITE RESTORATIONS

The following sections summarize some general considerations about all composite restorations. Information for specific clinical applications is presented in Chapters 12, 13, 14, and 15. In selecting a direct restorative material, practitioners usually choose between composite and amalgam. Consequently, some of the following information provides comparative analyses between those two materials.

INDICATIONS

Composite can be used for most clinical applications. Limiting factors for a specific clinical use are identified in later chapters. Generally, the indications for use are:

1. Classes I, II, III, IV, V, and VI restorations
2. Foundations or core buildups
3. Sealants and conservative composite restorations (preventive resin restorations)
4. Esthetic enhancement procedures
   - Partial veneers
   - Full veneers
   - Tooth contour modifications
   - Diastema closures
5. Cements (for indirect restorations)
6. Temporary restorations
7. Periodontal splinting

The American Dental Association[2] (ADA) has indicated the appropriateness of composites for use as pit-and-fissure sealants, preventive resins, initial Classes I and II lesions using modified conservative tooth preparations, moderate-sized Classes I and II restorations, Class V restorations, restorations of esthetically important areas, and restorations in patients allergic or sensitive to metals. The ADA does not support the use of composites in teeth with heavy occlusal stress, sites that cannot be isolated, or patients who are allergic or sensitive to composite materials. If composites are used as indicated, the ADA further states that "when used correctly in the primary and permanent dentition, *the expected lifetime of resin-based composites can be comparable to that of amalgam in Class I, Class II, and Class V restorations."*

Isolation Factors. For a composite restoration to be successful (i.e., to restore function, be harmonious with adjacent tissues, and be retained within the tooth), it must be appropriately bonded to the tooth structure (both enamel and dentin). Bonding to tooth structure requires an environment isolated from contamination by oral fluids or other contaminants; such contamination prohibits bond development. Therefore the ability to isolate the operating area (usually by a rubber dam or cotton rolls) is a major factor in selecting a composite material for a restoration. If the operating area can be isolated, a bonding procedure can be successfully done. This would include the use of a composite, a bonded amalgam, or a glass-ionomer restoration, as well as the bonding of an indirect restoration with an appropriate cementing agent. If the operating area cannot be totally protected from contamination, a nonbonded amalgam restoration may be the material of choice, because the presence of some oral fluids may not cause significant clinical problems with amalgam.

Occlusal Factors. Composite materials exhibit less wear resistance than amalgam; however, studies indicate that with contemporary composites, the wear resistance is not substantially different from that of amalgam.[12,34] For patients with either heavy occlusion, bruxism, or restorations that provide all of a tooth's occlusal contacts, amalgam, rather than composite, is usually the material of choice. Nevertheless, for most teeth experiencing normal occlusal loading and having occlusal contacts that are at least shared with tooth structure, composite restorations perform well. Factors that affect the wear resistance of a composite restoration include tooth location, width of the tooth preparation, and the type of contact from the opponent tooth on the composite surface.

Operator Ability and Commitment Factors. The tooth preparation for a composite restoration is relatively easy and less complex than that for an amalgam. However, tooth isolation; placement of etchant, primer, and adhesive on the tooth structure; and insertion, finishing, and polishing of the composite are more difficult than for an amalgam restoration. *The operator must pay greater attention to detail to successfully accomplish a composite restoration.* This requires both technical ability and knowledge of the material's use and limitations.

CONTRAINDICATIONS

The primary contraindications for use of composite as a restorative material relate to the factors presented in the preceding section—isolation, occlusion, and operator factors. If the operating site cannot be isolated from contamination by oral fluids, composite (or any other bonded material) should not be used. If all of the occlusion will be on the restorative material, composite may again not be the choice for use. However, both the need to strengthen remaining weakened unprepared tooth structure with an economical procedure (as compared to an indirect restoration) and the commitment to recall the patient routinely and in a timely manner may override any concern about excessive wear potential. Also, as discussed previously, composite restoration extensions on the root surface may exhibit gap formation at the junction of the composite and root. The long-term clinical effect of the gap is unknown. Any restoration that extends onto the root surface may result in less than ideal marginal integrity. For example, an amalgam exhibits a slight space at the margin until corrosion products better seal the area. Lastly, as stated previously, the operator must be committed to pursing those procedures, such as tooth isolation, which make bonded restorations successful. These additional procedures admittedly may make the procedures associated with successful bonded restorations more difficult and time consuming.

ADVANTAGES

Some advantages of composite restorations have already been stated, but the following list portrays the reasons composite restorations have become so popular, especially in comparison to nonbonded amalgam restorations. Composite restorations are:

1. Esthetic
2. Conservative of tooth structure removal (less extension; uniform depth not necessary; mechanical retention usually not necessary)
3. Less complex when preparing the tooth
4. Insulative, having low thermal conductivity
5. Used almost universally
6. Bonded to tooth structure, resulting in good retention, low microleakage, minimal interfacial staining, and increased strength of remaining tooth structure
7. Repairable

DISADVANTAGES

The primary disadvantages of composite restorations relate to potential gap formation and procedural difficulties. Following is a list of these and other disadvantages of composite restorations. Composite restorations:

1. May have a gap formation, usually occurring on root surfaces as a result of the forces of polymerization shrinkage of the composite material being greater than the initial early bond strength of the material to dentin
2. Are more difficult, time-consuming, and costly (compared to amalgam restorations) because:
   - Tooth treatment usually requires multiple steps.
   - Insertion is more difficult.
   - Establishing proximal contacts, axial contours, embrasures, and occlusal contacts may be more difficult.
   - Finishing and polishing procedures are more difficult.
3. Are more technique sensitive because the operating site must be appropriately isolated and the placement of etchant, primer, and adhesive on the tooth structure (enamel and dentin) is very demanding of proper technique
4. May exhibit greater occlusal wear in areas of high occlusal stress or when all of the tooth's occlusal contacts are on the composite material
5. Have a higher linear coefficient of thermal expansion, resulting in potential marginal percolation if an inadequate bonding technique is utilized

CLINICAL TECHNIQUE

INITIAL CLINICAL PROCEDURES

It is necessary that a complete examination, diagnosis, and treatment plan be finalized before the patient is scheduled for operative appointments (emergencies excepted). A brief review of the chart (including medical factors), treatment plan, and radiographs should precede each restorative procedure (see Chapter 9).

Local Anesthesia. Local anesthesia may be required for many operative procedures, as cited in Chapter 10. Profound anesthesia contributes to a more pleasant and uninterrupted procedure and usually results in a marked reduction in salivation. These effects of local anesthesia contribute to better operative dentistry, especially when placing bonded restorations.

Preparation of the Operating Site. If the planned composite procedure only requires minor or no tooth preparation, it may be necessary to clean the operating site with a slurry of pumice to remove plaque, pellicle, and superficial stains (Fig. 11-13). Calculus removal with appropriate instruments also may be needed. These steps create a site more receptive to bonding. Prophy pastes containing flavoring agents, glycerine, or fluorides act as contaminants and should be avoided to prevent a possible conflict with the acid-etch technique.

Shade Selection. Special attention should be given to matching the color of the natural tooth with the composite material. The shade of the tooth should be determined before the teeth are subjected to any prolonged drying, because dehydrated teeth become lighter in shade as a result of a decrease in translucency.

Normally, teeth are predominantly white, with varying degrees of grey, yellow, or orange tints. The color also varies with the translucency, thickness, and distribution of enamel and dentin and the age of the patient. Other factors such as fluorosis, tetracycline staining, and endodontic treatment also affect tooth color. With so many variables it is necessary to match the individual surface of the tooth to be restored. A cross-section of an anterior tooth (Fig. 11-14) illustrates why there are color zones. The incisal third *(w)* (mostly enamel) is lighter and more translucent than the cervical third *(y)* (mostly

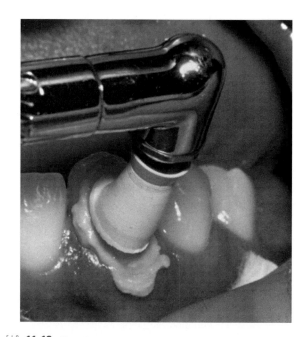

F I G. **11-13** Cleaning operating site with slurry of flour of pumice.

dentin), whereas the middle third *(x)* is a blend of the incisal and cervical colors.

Most manufacturers provide shade guides for their specific materials, which usually are not interchangeable with materials from other manufacturers. There are variations among the different manufacturers in the number of shades available. It should be noted, however, that most manufacturers also cross-reference their shades with those of the *VITA Shade Guide* (Vitazahnfabrik, Germany), a universally adopted shade guide. Also, most composite materials are available in enamel and dentin shades as well as translucent and opaque shades. The translucency of the composite material selected depends on the translucency of the tooth structure in the area of the tooth to be restored. Enamel shades are more translucent and typically are indicated for restoration of translucent areas such as incisal edges. Because of the popularity of bleaching, many manufactures also offer composites in very light shades.

Good lighting, either natural or artificial, is necessary when the color selection is made. Natural light is preferred for selection of shades. However, if no windows are present to provide natural daylight, color-corrected operating lights or ceiling lights are available to facilitate accurate shade selection. If the dental operating light is used, it should be moved away to decrease the intensity, thus allowing the effect of shadows to be seen.

In choosing the appropriate shade, hold the entire shade guide near the teeth to determine general color. Then select and hold a specific shade tab beside the area of the tooth to be restored (Fig. 11-15). The shade tab should be partially covered with the patient's lip or operator's thumb to create the natural effect of shadows. The cervical area of the tooth is usually darker than the incisal area. Make the selection as rapidly as possible, since physiologic limitations of the color receptors in the eye make it increasingly difficult to distinguish between similar colors after approximately 30 seconds. If more time is needed, the eyes should be rested by looking at a blue or violet object for a few seconds.[25,49] These are the complimentary colors of orange and yellow, which are the predominant colors in teeth. By looking at the complimentary color, the color receptors in the eye are revitalized and resensitized to perceiving minor variations in yellow and orange. Some dentists request that their assistants select or assist in shade selection. This practice not only saves time for the dentist, but the assistant, when adequately trained to select shades, may also feel a greater sense of responsibility and involvement. Final shade selection also can be verified by the patient with the use of a hand mirror.

Most teeth can be matched from manufacturers' basic shades, although some composites from different manufacturers do not match a *VITA Shade Guide* the same way. However, if additional shades are needed, they may be obtained by mixing two or more of the available shades together or by adding color modifiers, which may be available from the manufacturers. Record the shade on the patient's chart; however, since teeth darken with age, a different shade or material may be required if a replacement becomes necessary later. It is better to err on the barely perceptible darker side to allow for this age-related darkening. If bleaching (whitening) the teeth is contemplated, it should be done before any restorations are placed (see Bleaching in Chapter 15).

To be more certain of the proper shade selection, a small amount of material of the selected shade can be placed directly on the tooth, in close proximity to the area to be restored, and cured. This step may provide a more accurate assessment of the selected shade. If the shade is correct, an explorer is used to remove the cured material from the tooth surface. (A more comprehensive

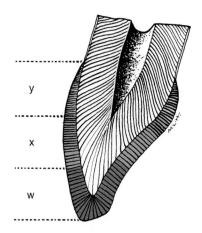

FIG. **11-14** Cross-section of anterior tooth showing three color zones. Incisal third *(w)* is a lighter shade and more translucent than gingival third *(y)*, whereas middle third *(x)* represents blending of incisal and gingival thirds.

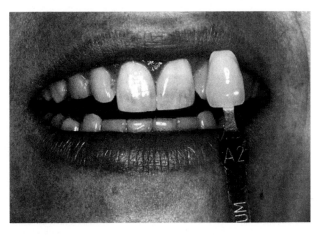

FIG. **11-15** Shade selection. Shade tab is held near the area to be restored.

review of factors affecting the esthetic considerations of tooth restoration is presented in Chapter 15.)

Isolation of the Operating Site. Complete instructions for the control of moisture are given in Chapter 10. Isolation for tooth-colored restorations can be accomplished with a rubber dam or cotton rolls, with or without a retraction cord. Regardless of the method, isolation of the area is imperative if the desired bond is to be obtained. Contamination of etched enamel or dentin by saliva results in a significantly decreased bond; likewise, contamination of the composite material during insertion results in degradation of physical properties.

Rubber Dam. A heavy rubber dam is an excellent means of acquiring superb access, vision, and moisture control. For proximal surface restorations, the dam should attempt to isolate several teeth mesial and distal to the operating site. This provides adequate access for tooth preparation, application of the matrix, and insertion and finishing of the material. If a lingual approach is indicated for an anterior tooth restoration, it is better to isolate all of the anterior teeth and include the first premolars to provide more access to the lingual area (Fig. 11-16). For Class V caries and other facial or lingual defects, it may be necessary to apply a No. 212 retainer (clamp), which may be stabilized with impression compound (Fig. 11-17). Stabilization with compound may be important to prevent movement of the retainer and subsequent injury to the tooth and soft tissue.

If a proximal restoration will involve all of the contact area and/or extend subgingivally, insert a wedge in the gingival embrasure after dam application and before tooth preparation. The wedge (1) depresses the interproximal soft tissue, (2) shields the dam and soft tissue from injury during the operative procedure, and (3) produces separation of the teeth to help compensate for the matrix thickness. Adequate preoperative wedging assists the eventual proximal contact restoration. Therefore this should occur whether or not a rubber dam is being used. Usually the wedge is inserted into the larger embrasure, facial or lingual, but this is at the discretion of the operator. Before placing the wedge from a facial approach, stretch the portion of the rubber dam that covers the interproximal papilla facially and gingivally (stretch lingually and gingivally if inserting the wedge from the lingual). Accomplish this by using a fingertip, first pressing firmly on the dam and underlying soft tissue near the teeth and then pulling the dam as the finger is moved slightly away from the teeth. While holding the dam in this stretched condition (Fig 11-18, *A*), begin the insertion of the wedge (see Fig 11-18, *B*); then, during the insertion, allow the stretched dam to slowly slide under the finger back to the normal position (see Fig. 11-18, *C*). This procedure helps to prevent catching the rubber dam (or even piercing it) with the tip of the wedge and decreases the tension of the stretched dam under the wedge (which may dislodge the wedge). (For additional details on isolation by rubber dam, see Chapter 10.)

Cotton Rolls (With or Without Retraction Cord). An alternate method of obtaining a dry operating field is the use of cotton roll isolation. With an experienced and careful dentist and dental assistant, cotton roll isolation results in an operating site conducive to accomplishing a successful composite (or any other) restoration. A cotton roll is placed in the facial vestibule directly adjacent to the tooth being restored. When restoring a mandibular tooth, a second, preferably larger, cotton roll should be placed adjacent to the tooth in the lingual vestibule. Easier placement of the lingual cotton roll is accomplished by holding the mesial end of the large cotton roll in the beaks of operative pliers and then twisting the handle of the pliers toward the tooth while using the index finger of the other hand to gently depress the cotton roll between the mandibular arch and the tongue. This more easily positions the cotton roll under the lateral border of the tongue.

When the gingival extension of a tooth preparation is to be positioned subgingivally, or near the gingiva, a retraction cord can be used to both temporarily retract the tissue and reduce seepage of tissue fluids into the

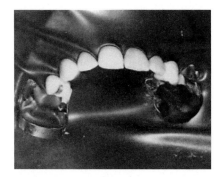

FIG. **11-16** Isolating anterior teeth with rubber dam. More access is provided for lingual instrumentation if premolars are included. Still more access may be provided by placing retainers over rubber dam and premolars.

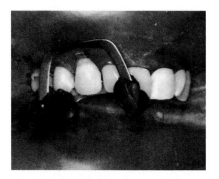

FIG. **11-17** Isolation of Class V preparation with rubber dam and No. 212 clamp. Impression compound stabilizes the retainer.

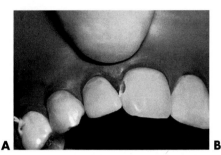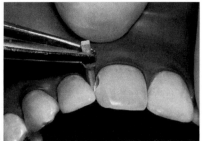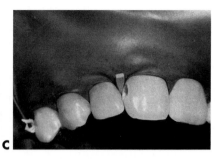

FIG. **11-18** Using triangular wood wedge to expose gingival margin of large proximal preparation. **A,** Dam is stretched facially and gingivally with fingertip. **B,** Insertion of wedge (dam is released during wedge insertion). **C,** Wedge in place.

operating site. If hemorrhage control is needed, the cord can first be saturated with a liquid astringent material.

Tissue retraction in Class V areas using a small-diameter cord is not difficult if properly done. A piece of cord approximately 0.5 to 1 mm in diameter (cords are usually available in various dimensions) and 8 to 10 mm long is usually sufficient, depending on the dimension of the involved gingival crevice. As noted, for controlling bleeding, the cord may be moistened with a small amount of astringent, such as Hemodent (Premier Dental Products Company, Norristown, Pennsylvania). A simple way to moisten the cord is to dip the closed beaks of sterilized cotton pliers (not the cord itself) into the bottle to pick up a small amount of liquid, then touch the cord with the tip of the beaks to transfer the liquid. Some operators prefer to place the cord in a dappen dish, wet it with a drop of Hemodent, and then blot it with a 2 × 2 inch (5 × 5 cm) gauze to remove excess liquid. Next, the cord may need to be twisted to distribute the liquid and make the cord more compact. However, many available cords are braided and do not require twisting. Now the cord may be tucked into the gingival crevice with the side of a No. 2 explorer, the end of an FP3 plastic instrument, or another suitable instrument, starting interproximally at one end of the cord (Fig. 11-19, *A*). Continue cord placement along the gingival margin (see Fig. 11-19, *B*) and slightly beyond the opposite extent of the proposed tooth preparation outline (see Fig. 11-19, *C*). If difficulty is encountered during placement, a "holding" instrument such as a periodontal probe or the blade of a suitable plastic instrument may be used to keep the submerged portion of the cord in the crevice during placement of the free end (see Fig. 11-19, *D*). As the tucking or packing procedure is continued, it may be necessary to follow with the holding instrument in a steplike manner. A slight backward vector to the insertion direction also helps keep the previously inserted cord in place. When additional tissue displacement is needed, a second cord may be placed on top of the first in the same manner. Remember that the cord is always inserted into the crevice and not on top of the gingiva. Any retraction cord placement must be done judiciously to avoid blunt

dissection of the gingival tissue or periodontal attachment. Also, do not overpack to cause ischemia of the gingiva (seen as blanching), which may result in tissue damage and recession. Gently insert the cord (with astringent) and in a few minutes the marginal gingiva will move laterally and apically approximately 0.5 mm away from the tooth preparation area. Do not leave any loose strands of the cord exposed, which may result in the cord catching a cutting instrument and being dislodged. Occasionally observe the displaced and retracted tissue during subsequent procedures to ascertain that tissue damage is not occurring.

Other Preoperative Considerations. When restoring posterior proximal surfaces, a preoperative wedge should be placed firmly into the gingival embrasure. This causes separation of the operated tooth from the adjacent tooth and creates some space to compensate for the matrix thickness that will be used later in the procedure. Preoperative wedging assists in reestablishing a proximal contact with a composite restoration. A complement for prewedging is the use of special matrices (Fig. 11-20).

Also, a preoperative assessment of the occlusion should be made. This should occur before rubber dam placement and should identify not only the occlusal contacts of the tooth or teeth to be restored, but also the occlusal contacts on adjacent teeth. Knowing the preoperative location of occlusal contacts is important both in planning the restoration outline form and establishing the proper occlusal contact(s) on the restoration. Remembering where contacts are located on adjacent teeth provides guidance in knowing when the restoration contacts are correctly adjusted.

TOOTH PREPARATION FOR COMPOSITE RESTORATIONS

Detailed descriptions of specific composite tooth preparations are presented in Chapters 6, 12, 13, and 15. As discussed in Chapter 6, the stages and steps of tooth preparation are appropriate for composite restorations and amalgam restorations, even though there may be some major differences. Basically, the tooth preparation for a composite restoration includes:

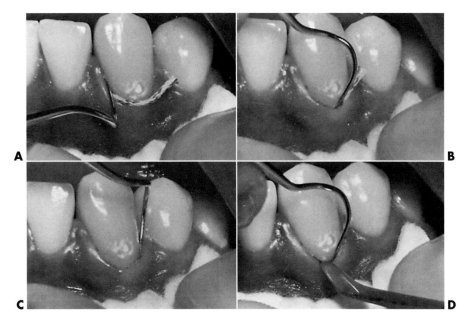

FIG. **11-19** Isolating Class V preparation with cotton roll and treated cord. **A,** One end of cord is tucked into gingival crevice with side of No. 2 explorer. **B,** Procedure is continued. **C,** Cord in place. **D,** Two instruments may be used to place cord in difficult cases. No. 2 explorer used to tuck, while small, blunt instrument used to hold cord in place.

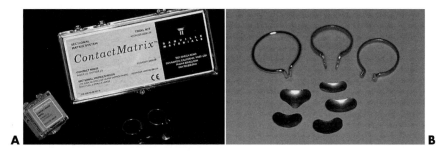

FIG. **11-20** New composite matrix systems. **A,** Contact matrix (Danville Materials). **B,** Composi-Tight Matrix System (Garrison Dental Solutions, Spring Lake, Michigan).

1. Removing the fault, defect, old material, or friable tooth structure
2. Creating prepared enamel margins of 90 degrees or greater (greater than 90 degrees usually preferable)
3. Creating 90-degree (or butt joint) cavosurface margins on root surfaces
4. Roughening the prepared tooth structure (enamel and dentin) with a diamond stone

These objectives can be met by producing a tooth preparation form significantly different from that for an amalgam restoration. Differences include:

1. Less outline extension (adjacent suspicious or at-risk areas [grooves or pits] may be "sealed" rather than restored)
2. An axial and/or pulpal wall of varying depth (not uniform)

3. Incorporation of an enamel bevel at some areas (the width of which is dictated by the need for secondary retention)
4. Tooth preparation walls being rough (to increase the surface area for bonding)
5. Use of a diamond stone (to increase the roughness of the tooth preparation walls)

The basic principles of tooth preparation must be followed for composite restorations. The tooth preparation should include removing (*outline form*) all of the caries, fault, defect, or old restorative material (when necessary) in the most conservative manner possible. The composite material must be retained within the tooth (*retention form*), but this primarily results from the micromechanical bonding of the composite to the roughened, etched, and primed enamel and dentin. In some instances, a dentinal retention groove or enamel bevel may be prepared to enhance the retention form. *Resistance form,* which keeps the tooth strong and protects it from fracture, is primarily accomplished by the strength of the micromechanical bond but may be increased, when necessary, by usual resistance form features such as flat preparation floors, boxlike forms, and floors prepared perpendicular to the occlusal forces. While the *caries removal* technique is the same as that presented in Chapter 6, *pulp protection* procedures are different for a composite restoration. Because the composite is bonded to the prepared tooth and the composite material is insulative, there is no need for any bases under composite restorations. However, a calcium hydroxide liner is still indicated when a pulpal exposure (or possible pulpal exposure) occurs.

Types of Composite Tooth Preparations. Tooth preparations for composite materials should be as conservative as possible. The extent of the preparation is usually determined by the size, shape, and location of the defect and whatever extensions are necessary to provide access for vision and instrumentation. Acid-etch techniques, effective bonding systems, and improved composites have significantly affected tooth preparation and expanded the ability to restore teeth.

The design of the tooth preparation to receive a composite restoration may vary depending on several factors. Five designs of tooth preparations for composite restorations are presented here, and sometimes they will be used in combination. The designs include: (1) conventional, (2) beveled conventional, (3) modified, (4) box-only, and (5) slot preparation designs. A discussion of general characteristics for each follows, with more detail in subsequent chapters.

Conventional. Conventional tooth preparations are those typical for amalgam restorations (as described in Chapters 16 to 19). Outline form is the necessary extension of external walls at an initial, limited, uniform dentinal depth, resulting in the formation of those walls in a butt joint junction (90 degrees) with the restorative material. In amalgam conventional tooth preparations, the butt joint marginal configuration and the retention grooves and coves in dentin are distinguishing features. These preparation designs were used extensively in the past for both amalgam and composite restorations and may be encountered when restoration replacement is indicated. It should be noted that the previous use of the conventional preparation for composites was not restricted to the root surface only. Fig. 11-21 illustrates models of old conventional tooth preparation designs for Classes III, IV, and V composite preparations.

The primary indications for conventional tooth preparation in composite restorations are: (1) preparations located on root surfaces (nonenamel areas) and (2) moderate to large Class I or Class II restorations. In the root areas, the butt joint design provides a better preparation configuration into which the groove and/or cove retention form can be placed, if deemed necessary (Fig. 11-22). This design facilitates a better seal between the composite and the dentin or cementum surfaces and enhances retention of the composite material in the tooth.

In moderate to large Class I or Class II composite restorations, there may be increased need for resistance form, which the conventional amalgamlike preparation design provides. An inverted cone diamond (similar in shape to a No. 245 bur) is used to prepare the tooth, resulting in a preparation design similar to that for amal-

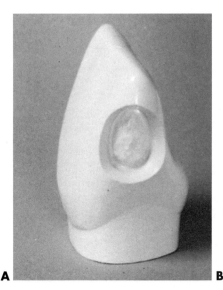 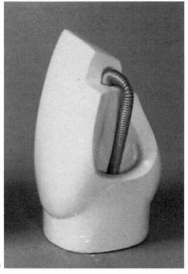 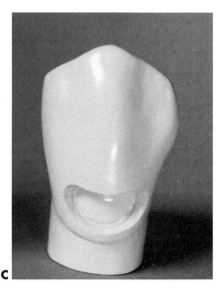

A   B   C

FIG. **11-21** Old conventional preparation designs for Class III **(A)**, Class IV **(B)**, and Class V **(C)** restorations. Butt joint marginal configuration and retention grooves in dentin characterized this preparation design. Currently this preparation design is used for root- surface restorations and large Class I and Class II restorations.

gam, but usually smaller in width and extensions and without prepared secondary retention form. The inverted cone diamond not only leaves the prepared tooth structure roughened, but also is conservative of the occlusal faciolingual extension. The butt joint marginal configuration between the tooth and the composite is not required (as it would be for amalgam). Thus the cavosurface angle in areas on the preparation periphery can be more flared (obtuse) than 90 degrees. The occlusal cavosurface angle is obtuse, yet provides for occlusally converging walls (Fig. 11-23).

Because of the similarity of the Class I or Class II conventional composite preparation to an amalgam tooth preparation, many operators prefer its use whether the Class I or Class II preparation is for a large posterior composite or for restoring a new, smaller carious lesion. It should be noted, however, that conservation of tooth structure is of paramount importance. Class I or Class II conventional composite preparations should be prepared with as little faciolingual extension as possible and should not routinely be extended into all pits and fissures on the occlusal surface where sealants may be otherwise indicated. Likewise, it should be remembered that the boxlike form increases the negative effects of the C-factor.

It is usually advantageous to use a diamond stone for preparing the tooth for a composite restoration. This results in a roughened prepared surface, which increases the surface area for bonding. Retention and marginal seal also are improved by beveling some enamel margins. Beveling increases favorable end-on etching of enamel prisms and increases the surface area for bonding. Because round diamonds or burs are typically used for Class III and Class IV preparations, a beveled or flared cavosurface margin results, and therefore few conventional preparation designs will occur for most anterior composite restorations of this type.

Beveled Conventional. Beveled conventional tooth preparations are similar to conventional preparations in that the outline form has external boxlike walls, but with some beveled enamel margins. The preparation also may be accomplished with a diamond stone. The principles of conventional outline form with the limited initial depth of the axial and pulpal walls are followed. *The beveled conventional preparation design typically is indicated when a composite restoration is being used to replace an existing restoration (usually amalgam) exhibiting a conventional tooth preparation design with enamel margins or to restore a large area.* This design is most typical for Classes III, IV, and V restorations. Usually all of the old material is removed, thereby providing increased bonding potential, not only to enamel but also to dentin. Sometimes the old restorative material may be only partially removed if the remaining material is judged acceptable (radiographically negative for caries, with symptomless tooth pulp). However, leaving old amalgam material

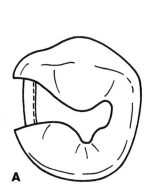
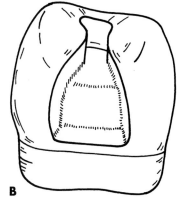

Axial wall depth 0.75 mm on root

Beveled or flared enamel margin

Retention groove

90-degree root-surface margin

FIG. **11-22** **A** and **B,** Combination preparation design for a Class III that extends onto root-surface. The root-surface portion is a conventional preparation design, utilizing butt joint marginal configuration and retention groove in dentin. The coronal portion is a beveled conventional design preparation.

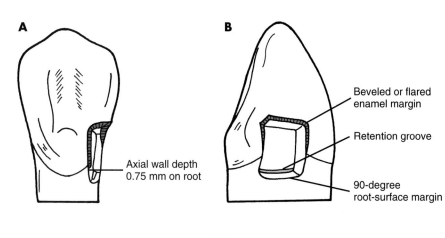

FIG. **11-23** Class II composite conventional tooth preparation. **A,** Occlusal view. **B,** Proximal view.

may result in a poor esthetic result because it may show through the overlying composite material. To facilitate better marginal sealing and bonding, some accessible enamel margins may be beveled and then acid-etched. Fig. 11-24 illustrates beveled conventional preparation designs for Classes III, IV, and V restorations.

As noted earlier, the advantage of an enamel bevel for a composite tooth preparation is that the ends of the enamel rods (exposed by beveling) are more effectively etched than otherwise occurs when only the sides of the enamel rods are exposed to the acid etchant (Fig. 11-25).[16,33] Also, the increase in etched surface area results in a stronger enamel-to-resin bond, which increases retention of the restoration and reduces marginal leakage and marginal discoloration.[55] Furthermore, incorporation of a cavosurface bevel may enable the restoration to blend more esthetically with the coloration of the surrounding tooth structure. Even recognizing these advantages, bevels are not usually placed on the occlusal surfaces of posterior teeth or other areas of potential heavy contact because a conventional preparation design already produces end-on etching of the enamel rods by virtue of the enamel rod direction on occlusal surfaces. Bevels also are not placed on proximal margins if such beveling results in excessive extension of the cavosurface margins. Therefore the beveled conventional preparation design is rarely used for posterior composite restorations.

Modified. Modified tooth preparations for composite restorations have neither specified wall configurations nor specified pulpal or axial depths; preferably, they have enamel margins. Unlike conventional preparations, modified preparations are not prepared to a uniform dentinal depth. Both the extension of the margins and the depth of a modified tooth preparation are dictated solely by the extent (laterally) and the depth of the carious lesion or other defects. The objectives of this preparation design are to remove the fault as conservatively as possible and rely on the composite bond to tooth structure to retain the restoration in the tooth. Modified tooth preparations conserve more tooth structure because retention is obtained primarily by micromechanical adhesion to the surrounding enamel and underlying dentin, rather than by preparation of retention grooves or coves in dentin.

Round burs or diamond stones may be used to prepare this type of preparation, resulting in a marginal design similar to a beveled preparation; however, less tooth structure is removed in the internal portions of the preparation. Often, the preparation appears to have been "scooped out" rather than having the distinct internal line angles characteristic of a conventional preparation design. Fig. 11-26 illustrates modified tooth preparation designs for Classes III, IV, and V preparations.

Modified preparations are primarily indicated for the initial restoration of smaller, cavitated, carious lesions usually sur-

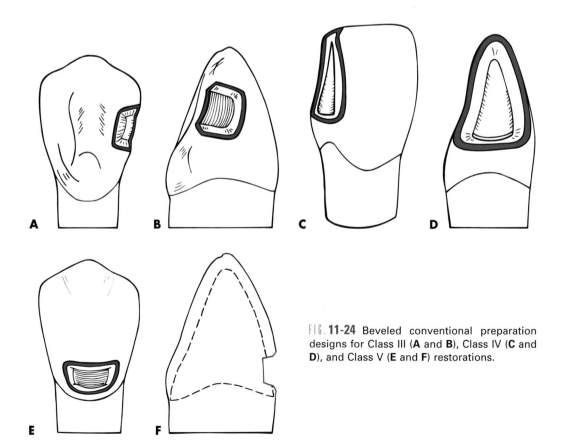

FIG. **11-24** Beveled conventional preparation designs for Class III (**A** and **B**), Class IV (**C** and **D**), and Class V (**E** and **F**) restorations.

rounded by enamel and for correcting enamel defects. However, they can be successful for larger restorations as well. For the restoration of large carious lesions, wider bevels or flares and retention grooves, coves, or locks may be indicated in addition to the retention afforded by the adhesive procedures.

Box-Only. Another modified design is the box-only tooth preparation (see Fig. 13-35). This design is indicated when only the proximal surface is faulty, with no lesions present on the occlusal surface. A proximal box is prepared with either an inverted cone or round diamond stone held parallel to the long axis of the tooth

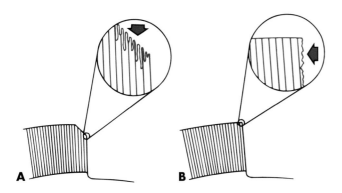

FIG. **11-25** Ends of enamel rods (**A**) are more effectively etched, producing deeper microundercuts than when only the sides of enamel rods are etched (**B**).

crown. The diamond is extended through the marginal ridge in a gingival direction. The initial proximal axial depth is prepared 0.2 mm inside the dentinoenamel junction (DEJ). The form of the box is dependent on which diamond is used—more boxlike with the inverted diamond, more scooped with the round diamond. The facial, lingual, and gingival extensions are dictated by the fault or caries. Caries excavation in a pulpal direction is done with a round bur or spoon excavator. Neither beveling nor secondary retention is usually indicated.

Facial/Lingual Slot. A third modified design for restoring proximal lesions on posterior teeth is the facial or lingual slot preparation (see Fig. 13-36). In this case, a lesion is detected on the proximal surface but the operator believes that access to the lesion can be obtained from either a facial or lingual direction, rather than through the marginal ridge from an occlusal direction. Usually a small round diamond stone is used to gain access to the lesion. The diamond is oriented at the correct occlusogingival height, and the entry is made with the diamond as close to the adjacent tooth as possible, thus preserving as much of the facial or lingual surface as possible. The preparation is extended occlusogingivally and faciolingually enough to remove the lesion. The initial axial depth is 0.2 mm inside the DEJ. The occlusal, facial, and gingival cavosurface margins are 90 degrees or greater. Caries excavation in a pulpal direction is done with a round bur or spoon excavator. This preparation

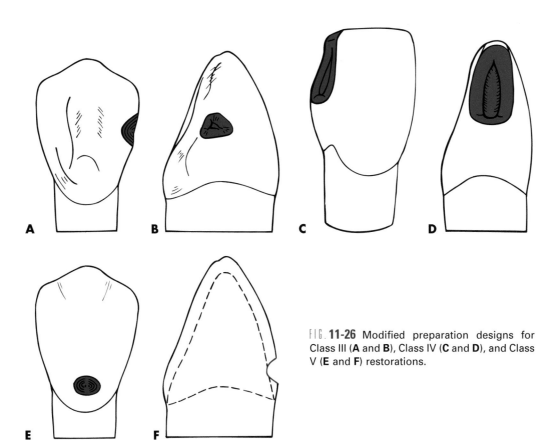

FIG. **11-26** Modified preparation designs for Class III (**A** and **B**), Class IV (**C** and **D**), and Class V (**E** and **F**) restorations.

is similar to a Class III preparation for an anterior tooth (see Chapter 12).

Pulpal Protection. As stated earlier, pulpal protection measures for composite restorations are indicated primarily for direct pulp cap procedures. While some would suggest the use of a resin-bonding agent on exposed pulps,[1,14,29] this textbook recommends the use of a calcium hydroxide liner on vital pulp exposures[48] (see Chapter 3). Also, because the composite material is insulative, retentive, and strong, the use of bases in deeply excavated preparations is unnecessary. Thus the placement of glass-ionomer types of materials as bases under composite restorations is not necessary for pulpal protection.

RESTORATIVE TECHNIQUE FOR COMPOSITE RESTORATIONS

Once the tooth preparation has been completed, the prepared tooth structure is readied for composite insertion and finishing. Treating the prepared tooth for bonding requires etching and then application of an adhesive if only enamel is prepared, or a primer and adhesive if the composite will be bonded to the dentin as well as the enamel.

Bonding systems are available in various forms, depending on the manufacturer. Components of one system usually are not interchangeable with another system. Following the manufacturer's directions is imperative for success. Likewise, effecting the bond in an acceptable clinical environment, free from moisture contamination, is a requirement.

Whether to place a matrix depends on the part of the tooth being restored, with most proximal surface restorations requiring a matrix. Whether to place a matrix before or after placement of the etchant, primer, and adhesive is dependent on factors presented in a subsequent section. Several options also are available for composite insertion into the tooth preparation, including injection of the composite or hand placement with an instrument. After insertion and curing of the material, the restoration is contoured and polished.

Preliminary Steps for Enamel and Dentin Bonding. The acid-etch technique requires that a very exacting sequence be followed if optimal results are to be obtained, including isolation from fluids (saliva and sulcular seepage) by using either a rubber dam or cotton rolls and/or retraction cord. Etching enamel affects both the prism core and prism periphery (Fig. 11-27). Etching dentin affects the intertubular and peritubular dentin, resulting in enlarging the tubular openings, removing much of the surface hydroxyapatite, and leaving an interconnected network of collagen fibrils.

Both liquid and gel etchants are available, most in concentrations of 32% to 37% phosphoric acid. Liquid etchants may be used when large surface areas are to be etched, such as when placing full veneers or sealants. However, thixotropic gels are preferred by most practitioners for the controlled application of etchant to preparation walls, including bevels and margins. The etchant gels can be placed carefully with brushes or endodontic paper points held in cotton pliers, but usually a syringe applicator is used to inject the gel etchant directly onto the prepared tooth structure (Fig 11-28). Etched surfaces must not be contaminated by mouth fluids; such contamination adversely affects the etch and requires repeating the etching procedure. For preparations involving the proximal area, a polyester matrix strip is placed between the teeth before the acid is applied to prevent inadvertently etching the adjacent tooth (Fig. 11-29).

If liquid etchants are used, they are applied with small cotton pellets, foam sponges, or special applicator tips or microbrushes (Fig. 11-30). The acid (liquid or gel) is gently applied to the appropriate surfaces to be bonded, keeping the excess to a maximum of 0.5 mm past the anticipated extent of the restoration. An etching

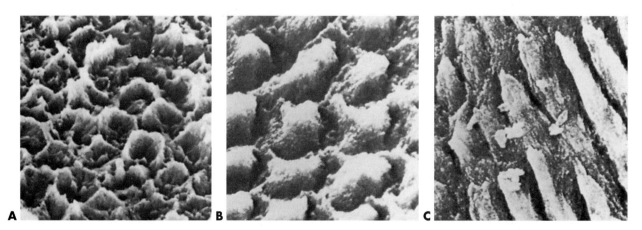

FIG. **11-27** Etching patterns of tooth enamel. **A,** Etching pattern characterized by removal of prism core. **B,** Etching pattern showing loss of prism periphery. **C,** Both etching patterns are evident. *(**B** and **C,** Courtesy Dr. Leon Silverstone.)*

time of 15 seconds for both dentin and enamel is considered sufficient. For enamel-only preparations, 30 seconds is considered optimal. The area is then rinsed with water for 5 seconds, starting on the adjacent tooth to prevent possible splashing of acid-rich water onto the patient, dentist, or assistant. If cotton rolls were used for isolation, they should be replaced at this time, making sure that the tooth preparation does not become contaminated with saliva. The area should be dried with clean, dry air from the air-water syringe if only enamel has been etched. Dried etched enamel should exhibit a ground glass or lightly frosted appearance. If this appearance is not evident, the enamel must be etched again for an additional 15 to 30 seconds. If both enamel and dentin have been etched, then the area must be left slightly moistened. This allows the primer and adhesive materials to more effectively penetrate the collagen fibrils to form a hybrid layer, which is the basis for the micromechanical bond to dentin. Overdrying etched dentin surfaces compromises dentin bonding as a result of the collapse of the collagen network in the etched dentin layer.[23,24,26] This collapse prevents optimal primer and adhesive penetration and compromises hybrid layer formation.

For application of a gel etchant, a brush, paper point, instrument, or syringe is used. The etchant is left untouched for 15 to 30 seconds. The area is then rinsed for approximately 5 seconds. Gel etchants are more easily applied with a small syringe. Various etchant syringes are available and provide the advantage of easier and more precise control of the etchant. (A typical etchant syringe is seen in Fig. 11-28.) If the patient has high caries activity, the enamel usually etches very easily. Enamel that is resistant to etching may require doubling or tripling the usual time. Care should be exercised not to etch adjacent teeth (see Fig. 11-29) or remote areas. Even though etched areas of enamel appear normal after several days, scanning electron microscopy has shown that etched enamel is not completely remineralized from salivary ions even after 90 days.[22] Once the area is etched and rinsed, it is dried if only enamel has been etched, but it is left moistened if dentin has been etched (see the preceding paragraphs).

Most dentin bonding systems rely on some type of dentin etching and priming to maximize micromechanical adhesion. Dentin etchants typically remove or solubilize the smear layer to achieve optimal adhesion to the underlying dentin. However, there is no one established regimen for dentin bonding because it may vary from one product to another. Dentin etchants and primers should be applied strictly in accordance with the manufacturer's instructions. Disposable brushes, microbrushes, or applicator tips are most frequently provided for primer and adhesive application (see Fig. 11-30).

Many enamel and dentin bonding systems etch enamel and dentin simultaneously, either with phosphoric acid or alternative etchants. Strict attention to the manufacturer's directions regarding use of the specific etchant is imperative to ensure optimal results.

If dentin walls have been dried, they may be rewetted with a water-saturated applicator tip or Gluma Desensitizer. The use of Gluma Desensitizer is especially

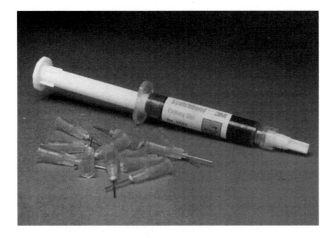

FIG. **11-28** Syringe used to dispense gel etchant.

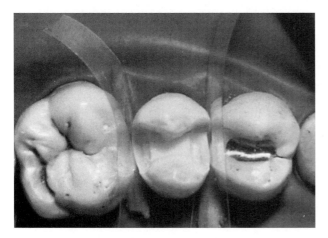

FIG. **11-29** Clear polyester strips applied (and wedged) before etching. Adjacent teeth protected from inadvertent etching.

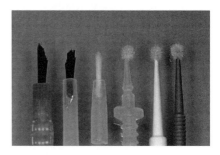

FIG. **11-30** Applicator tip or microbrush.

beneficial for Class II composite restorations (see Chapter 13). A shiny surface usually indicates a moist surface. Naturally, it is not desirable to have either excess rewetting agent pooled in the internal aspects of the preparation or dry spots on the prepared dentin.

Once the enamel (and dentin) is etched, rinsed, and left appropriately moist, the primer is applied to both surfaces. Most contemporary bonding systems combine the primer and adhesive into a single bottle, requiring only one application. If this is the case, it is applied to the moist, etched prepared surfaces. Application of primer to etched enamel does not result in any adverse effects on bond strength to the composite. Any contamination by saliva necessitates repeating the placement of etchant for a minimum of 10 seconds, followed again by appropriate primer and adhesive placement. (See Chapter 5 for a detailed description of adhesion philosophy and technique.)

Matrix Placement. A matrix is a device that may be applied to a prepared tooth before the insertion of the composite material. It fits around part or all of the tooth being restored and functions primarily to confine the restorative material on axial surfaces (usually the proximal) while assisting in the development of the appropriate axial contour. When a condensable (packable) restorative material is used, the matrix must be rigid enough to resist deformation from insertion forces (Fig. 11-31). Otherwise, the matrix may be more flexible, especially for anterior restorations (Fig. 11-32). The matrix should provide the appropriate proximal contact and contour and prevent major excess of the restorative material beyond the preparation margins on the proximal surface, especially the gingival margin. It should be relatively easy to apply and remove.

The matrix band may need to be altered (burnished) to have appropriate contour for the desired shape of the restoration. It should extend just above (occlusal to) the marginal ridge and below (gingival to) the gingival margin. It is held in place by a gingival wedge and, in some instances, also by a matrix retainer. Whether or not a matrix retainer is used, the wedge is placed into the gingival embrasure and is positioned (wedged) between the two adjacent teeth, below the prepared gingival margin, and exterior to (outside) the matrix material (Fig. 11-33). The wedge functions to: (1) separate the teeth (which helps to compensate for the thickness of the matrix material, as it relates to establishing a proximal contact), (2) hold the matrix in place, and (3) prevent or reduce any excess of restorative material at the gingival margin.

Numerous matrix systems are available. Usually a Tofflemire matrix system is used for most Class II restorations in posterior teeth, and a polyester strip is used for Classes III and IV restorations in anterior teeth. However, there are other matrix options presented in subsequent chapters. Likewise, there are different types of wedges. Triangular wooden wedges may be needed for tooth preparations with deeply extended gingival margins. However, the terminal half-inch of a round toothpick is the typical wedge selected for most uses in this textbook.

The placement of etchant, primer, and adhesive may or may not precede the application of a matrix. The exact sequence for applying the enamel/dentin etchant,

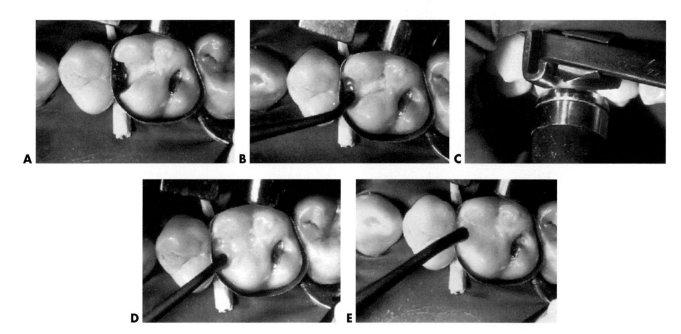

FIG. **11-31** Insertion of light-cured composite material, maxillary molar. **A,** A thin Tofflemire-type matrix is positioned and wedged. Bonding agent has been placed. **B** through **E,** Composite is placed and cured in small increments until preparation is slightly overfilled.

primer, bonding adhesive, and matrix is dependent on the operator. Some operators prefer matrix application first, followed by enamel/dentin etchant, primer, bonding adhesive, and finally composite. This sequence may provide the best isolation of the tooth preparation for maximum enamel and dentin adhesion. It also allows an assessment of any enamel fracture (upon insertion of the proximal wedge) before bonding to that area. If the matrix is applied first, care must be taken to avoid pooling of the bonding materials, especially the adhesive, along the junction of the matrix with the gingival margin. Placing the matrix first in the sequence is especially beneficial when the tooth preparation is deep gingivally.

Other operators prefer to complete all enamel and dentin etching, priming, and adhesive application before matrix placement. The primary reasons for this sequence are to minimize pooling potential and maximize the etching, priming, and adhesive placement at the cavosurface margins. Either sequence may be used as long as meticulous technique is followed.

Inserting the Composite. The composite restoration usually is placed in two stages. First, a bonding adhesive

is applied (if not already placed during enamel and dentin etching and priming procedures). Second, the composite restorative material inserted. With newer bonding systems the adhesive may be combined with another component of the system, usually the primer. Therefore, as always, etching and priming the prepared tooth structure and placing the bonding adhesive should be done according to the manufacturer's directions. As noted earlier, two types of composites exist: self-cured and light-cured. Self-cured composites are not used extensively because light-cured composites provide additional benefits such as less discoloration, less porosity, easy placement, and less required finishing. Because a light source must be applied to the light-cured composite to cause polymerization, it is important that the material be inserted into the tooth preparation in 1- to 2-mm thicknesses. This allows the light to properly polymerize the composite and may reduce the effects of polymerization shrinkage, especially along the gingival floor.

Either a hand instrument or syringe can be used for inserting self-cured or light-cured composites. Both methods and materials are presented in detail under insertion

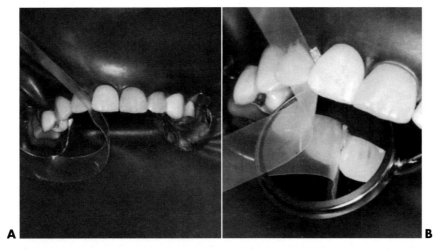

FIG. **11-32** Inserting and wedging polyester strip matrix. **A,** Strip with concave area next to preparation is positioned between teeth. **B,** Strip in position and wedge inserted.

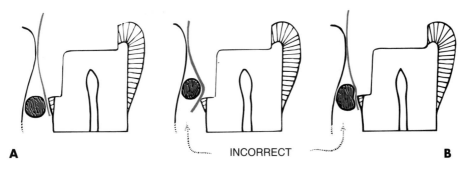

FIG. **11-33 A,** Correct wedge position. **B,** Incorrect wedge position.

instructions for specific restorations in the following chapters. The use of a hand instrument is a popular method for placing composites because it is easy and fast. In addition to the simplicity of hand instrument insertion, a smaller amount of composite material is required compared to the amount needed for the syringe method. A disadvantage of hand instrument insertion is that air can be trapped in the tooth preparation or incorporated into the material during the insertion procedure. Experience and care in insertion minimizes this problem.

The syringe technique is popular because it provides a convenient means for transporting the composite to the preparation and reduces the possibility of trapping air. Many manufacturers provide preloaded syringe compules with a light-cured composite (Fig. 11-34). The tips of the light-cured compules have covers that should be replaced when not using the material to keep it from being polymerized inadvertently by ambient light. The syringe technique can present a problem in small preparations with limited access because the syringe tip may be too large. When the preparation opening is questionable, an empty syringe tip should first be tried in the tooth preparation.

The injectability of composites varies because of differences in viscosity. Some microfill composites cannot be injected. Therefore this property of the material should be evaluated before clinical use.

Starting in the most remote area of an anterior tooth preparation, the composite is steadily injected, ensuring that the tip remains in the material while slowly withdrawing the syringe (Fig. 11-35). If the area is large, the light-cured composite is placed in 1- to 2-mm thicknesses, with each increment being cured per manufacturer's instructions. Usually a hand instrument is used to adapt the composite to the preparation after each syringe injection of material. When curing, the light tip is kept as close to the material as possible. If using a hand instrument insertion, a small amount of the composite is carried to the remote area of the preparation and condensed and cured; then more composite is placed and cured with care to adapt it well to the internal preparation walls. The preparation is filled to slight excess so that positive pressure can be applied by the matrix strip. Before the matrix strip is closed, any gross excess is removed with a hand instrument. The matrix strip is then closed and secured and the composite cured.

For Class II restorations it is also important to place and cure the composite incrementally to reduce the effects of polymerization shrinkage, especially along the gingival floor. For this reason, the first small increment should be placed along the gingival floor and should extend slightly up the facial and lingual walls (see Fig. 11-31, B). This increment should only be approximately 1 to 2 mm in thickness because it is the farthest increment from the curing light and is most critical in establishing a proper gingival seal. After the first increment is cured (see Fig. 11-31, C), subsequent additions are made and cured (usually not exceeding 2 mm in thickness at a time) until the preparation is filled to slight excess (see Fig. 11-31, D and E). The restoration can be contoured and finished immediately after the last increment is cured.

Following insertion and polymerization of the composite material, the matrix and wedges are removed, the restoration cured again from different angles (if light cured), and the restoration is examined for voids or lack of proximal contacts. If correction is needed, it should be accomplished at this time, because any additions will bond satisfactorily to the uncontaminated, oxygen-inhibited surface layer of the composite material.

Contouring the Composite. Contouring can be initiated immediately after a light-cured composite material has been polymerized or 3 minutes after the initial hardening of a self-cured material.

Good technique and experience in inserting a composite restoration significantly reduces the amount of finishing required. Usually a slight excess of material is

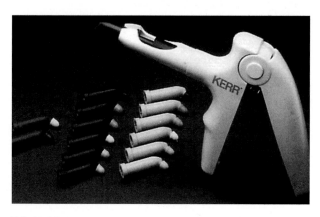

FIG. **11-34** Examples of pistol grip syringe and preloaded composite compule.

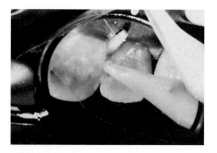

FIG. **11-35** Syringe injection of composite. Air entrapment is minimized by injecting composite starting in the remote corner of the preparation and by slowly withdrawing the tip while it is kept in the restorative material during injection. If light-cured, it should be injected and cured in 1- to 2-mm increments.

present that must be removed to provide the final contour and smooth finish. Coarse diamond instruments can be used for removing gross excess but are not generally recommended for finishing composites because of the high risk of inadvertently damaging adjacent tooth structure. They leave a rough surface on the restoration and tooth, as compared to finishing burs and discs. However, special fine-diamond finishing instruments are available commercially and can be used to obtain excellent results. Care must be exercised with all rotary instruments to prevent damage to the tooth structure, especially at gingival marginal areas (see Fig. 12-33).

Contouring the composite restoration requires skill and knowledge of correct dental anatomy. The contouring instruments are chosen based on the area being contoured (see Figs. 12-33, 13-19, and 13-43). Care must be taken to not injure the adjacent unprepared tooth structure while contouring the restoration. While accessible areas are relatively easily contoured, more inaccessible areas (interproximal contours and margins) are more difficult. Careful visual and tactile assessment of interproximal contours, contacts, and marginal integrity is necessary. Naturally, as a final step in contouring, the restoration's appropriate occlusal relationship must be developed. Specific contouring techniques for specific restorations are presented in the following chapters.

Polishing the Composite. Polishing the contoured composite restoration is done with very fine polishing discs, fine rubber points or cups, and/or composite polishing pastes. Specific details are presented in Chapters 12 to 15 (see Figs. 12-33, 13-19, and 13-43).

Microfill Composites. Although the same technique used for finishing composites generally applies to finishing microfill composites, certain differences do exist. Hybrid composites exhibit an opaque appearance during dry finishing, making the preparation margin easy to distinguish. Because microfill composites possess a surface luster similar to that of tooth enamel, it is more difficult to detect when the restoration has been finished back to the margin. Also, because less inorganic filler is present in microfill composites, finishing burs tend to clog and need periodic débridement.

Although conventional finishing techniques produce a smooth surface texture with microfill composites, a higher luster can be obtained by using discs, rubber points, or cups, all of which are specifically made for polishing these materials.

REPAIRING COMPOSITE RESTORATIONS

If a patient presents with a composite restoration that has a localized defect, a repair usually can be made. Easily accessible areas may be roughened with a diamond stone; the area is etched; primer may be applied if dentin is exposed; adhesive is applied; and finally the composite is inserted, contoured, and polished. If the defect is not easily accessible, a tooth preparation must be cre-

ated that exposes the defective area and a matrix may be necessary; placement of the etchant, primer, adhesive, and composite is then performed.

If a void is detected immediately after insertion of a composite restoration but before contouring is initiated, more composite can be added directly to the void area. These materials will bond because the void area has an oxygen-inhibited surface layer that permits composite additions. If, however, any contouring has occurred, the oxygen-inhibited layer may been removed or altered and the area must be re-etched and adhesive placed before adding more composite.

COMMON PROBLEMS: CAUSES AND POTENTIAL SOLUTIONS

The following list indicates the causes of common problems associated with some composite restorations, as well as potential solutions to those problems. The subsequent technique chapters refer back to these, because they describe specific composite procedures.

POOR ISOLATION OF THE OPERATING AREA

Causes of poor isolation of the operating area include:

- No rubber dam or leaking rubber dam
- Inadequate cotton roll isolation
- Careless technique
- Preparation so deep gingivally it cannot be isolated

Potential solutions for poor isolation of the operating area include:

- Better technique
- Use of matrix to help isolation
- Use of a nonbonded restorative material
- Repeat bonding procedures (if the area is contaminated)

WHITE LINE OR HALO AROUND THE ENAMEL MARGIN

The following factors cause microfracture of marginal enamel:

- Traumatic contouring or finishing techniques
- Inadequate etching and bonding of that area
- High-intensity light-curing, resulting in excessive polymerization stresses

Potential solutions include:

- Re-etch, prime, and bond the area
- Conservatively remove the fault and rerestore
- Use atraumatic finishing techniques (e.g., light intermittent pressure)
- Use slow-start polymerization techniques
- Leave as is

VOIDS

Causes of voids include:

- Mixing of self-cured composites
- Spaces left between increments during insertion
- Tacky composite pulling away from the preparation during insertion

Potential solutions include:

- More careful technique
- Repair of marginal voids by preparing the area and rerestoring

WEAK OR MISSING PROXIMAL CONTACTS (CLASSES II, III, AND IV)

Causes of weak and missing proximal contacts include:

- Inadequately contoured matrix band
- Inadequate wedging, both preoperatively and during the composite insertion
- Matrix band movement during composite insertion, or matrix band not in direct contact with the adjacent proximal surface
- A circumferential matrix being used when restoring only one contact
- Tacky composite pulling away from matrix contact area during insertion
- Matrix band too thick

Potential solutions include:

- Properly contour the matrix band
- Have matrix in contact with adjacent tooth
- Use firm preoperative and insertion wedging technique
- Use a matrix system that places matrix only around the proximal surface to be restored
- Use specially designed, triangular light-curing tips to help hold the matrix against the adjacent tooth while curing
- Use a hand instrument to hold the matrix against the adjacent tooth while curing the incremental placements of composite
- Be very careful with insertion technique

INCORRECT SHADE

Causes of an incorrect shade include:

- Inappropriate operator lighting while selecting the shade
- Selecting the shade after the tooth is dried
- Shade tab not matching the actual composite shade
- Wrong shade selected

Potential solutions include:

- Use natural light if possible
- Select the shade before isolating the tooth
- Preoperatively place some of the selected shade on the tooth and cure (then remove)
- Do not shine operating light directly on the area during shade selection
- Understand the typical zones of different shades for natural teeth

POOR RETENTION

Causes of poor retention include:

- Inadequate preparation form
- Contamination of operating area
- Poor bonding technique
- Intermingling of bonding materials from different systems

Potential solutions include:

- Prepare the tooth with appropriate bevels or flares and secondary retention feature, when necessary
- Keep the area isolated while bonding
- Follow the manufacturer's directions explicitly
- Do not intermingle bonding materials from different systems

CONTOURING AND FINISHING PROBLEMS

Causes of contouring or finishing problems include:

- Injuring adjacent unprepared tooth structure
- Overcontouring the restoration
- Undercontouring the restoration
- Ditching cementum
- Creating inadequate anatomic tooth form
- Dealing with difficult-to-see margins

Potential solutions include:

- Be careful with use of rotary instruments to not adversely affect adjacent tooth structure or teeth
- Have a proper matrix with appropriate axial and line angle contours
- Create embrasures to match the adjacent tooth embrasure form
- Do not use rotary instruments that leave roughened surfaces
- Use a properly shaped contouring instrument for the area being contoured
- Remember the outline form of the preparation
- View the restoration from all angles as it is contoured

CONTROVERSIAL ISSUES

Because the practice of operative dentistry is dynamic, constant changes are occurring. As new products and techniques are developed, their effectiveness cannot be assessed until appropriately designed research protocols have tested their worth. There are many such developments occurring at any time, many of which do not have the necessary documentation to prove their effectiveness, even though they receive very positive publicity. Several examples of such controversies follow.

LINERS AND BASES UNDER COMPOSITE RESTORATIONS

Various materials have been promoted as liners or bases under composite restorations. These include RMGIs, flowable composites, and compomers. Proponents of this approach do not promote these materials for pulp protection in the traditional sense, but as materials that provide a better seal for composite restorations when extended onto the root surface. These materials are suggested to not only improve the seal in that area (which would protect the pulp) but also to act as a stress breaker, to resist polymerization stresses placed on the composite restoration. This textbook does not recommend the use of any of these materials routinely for lining deeply extended composite restorations, although some merit for this technique may exist.

RETENTION IN CLASS V ROOT-SURFACE PREPARATIONS

This textbook recommends the use of retention grooves in composite tooth preparations when the operator feels additional retention form is necessary. However, it is likely that with the bonding systems available, retention groove placement is not always necessary.

WEAR PROBLEMS

This textbook recommends that occlusal factors be considered when selecting composite as a restorative material, especially in those clinical situations when it is anticipated there will be heavy occlusal forces or all of the occlusal contacts will be on the restoration only. However, the wear resistance of some composites is very similar to that of amalgam, and composite restorations should be successful for most occlusal patterns where occlusal contacts are shared with tooth structure.

GAP FORMATION SIGNIFICANCE

As discussed previously, the gap formation that usually occurs when composite is extended onto the root surface may not have any long-term clinical effects. With the two vectors of the V-shaped defect being primarily resin or composite, recurrent caries may not be a problem. However, how long the exposed hybridized resin layer on the root stays intact is unknown, and if it deteriorates in a short time, the area is left at risk to caries. Use of one of the proposed liner materials above may reduce the effect of gap formation.

SUMMARY

The use of composite restorations is increasing because of the benefits accrued from adhesive bonding to tooth structure, esthetic qualities, and almost universal clinical usage. When done properly, a composite restoration can provide excellent service for many years. However, composite restorations are more difficult and technique sensitive to operator ability than amalgam restorations. To effect the bond that provides the benefits, the operating site must be free from contamination and the material and bonding technique must be utilized properly.

Subsequent chapters provide additional information about the specific uses of composite as restorative material.

REFERENCES

1. Akimoto N et al: Biocompatibility of Clearfil Liner Bond 2 and Clearfil AP-X systems on nonexposed and exposed primate teeth, *Quintessence Int* 29(3):177-88, 1998.
2. American Dental Association Council on Scientific Affairs, ADA Council on Dental Benefit Programs: Statement on posterior resin-based composites, *J Am Dent Assoc* 130:1627-28, 1998.
3. Ausiello P et al: Fracture resistance of endodontically-treated premolars adhesively restored, *Am J Dent* 10:237-241, 1997.
4. Bowen RL: Adhesive bonding of various materials to hard tooth tissues: the effect of a surface active comonomer on adhesion to diverse substrates. V. *J Dent Res* 44:1369, 1965.
5. Bowen RL: Dental filling material comprising vinyl-silane treated fused silica and a binder consisting of the reaction product of bis-phenol and glycidyl acrylate, U.S. Patent No. 3,06,112, Nov. 27, 1962.
6. Bowen RL: Properties of a silica-reinforced polymer for dental restorations, *J Am Dent Assoc* 66:57, 1963.
7. Buonocore MG: A simple method of increasing the adhesion of acrylic filling materials to enamel surfaces, *J Dent Res* 34: 849, 1955.
8. Buonocore M, Wileman W, Brudevold F: A report on a resin composition capable of bonding to human dentin surfaces, *J Dent Res* 35:846, 1956.
9. Byram JQ: *Principles and practice of filling teeth with porcelain,* New York, 1908, Consolidated Dental Manufacturing Co.
10. Calamia JR: High-strength porcelain bonded restorations: anterior and posterior, *Quintessence Int* 20(10):717-726, 1989.
11. Charbeneau GT et al: *Principles and practice of operative dentistry,* ed 1, Philadelphia, 1975, Lea & Febiger.
12. Collins CJ, Bryant RW, Hodge K-LV: A clinical evaluation of posterior composite resin restorations: 8-year findings, *J Dent* 26(4):311-317, 1998.
13. Combe EC, Burke FJT, Douglas WH: Thermal properties. In Combe EC, Burke FJT, Douglas WH, editors: *Dental biomaterials,* Boston, 1999, Kluwer Academic Publishers.
14. Cox CF, Suzuki S: Re-evaluating pulp protection: calcium hydroxide liners vs. cohesive hybridization, *J Am Dent Assoc* 125: 823-831, 1994.
15. Craig, RG: Chemistry, composition, and properties of composite resins, *Dent Clin North Am* 25(2):219, 1981.
16. Craig RG, editor: *Restorative dental materials,* ed 11, St Louis, 2001, Mosby.

17. Davis WC: *Operative dentistry,* ed 5, St Louis, 1945, Mosby.
18. Ehrnford L, Derand T: Cervical gap formation in Class II composite resin restorations, *Swed Dent J* 8:15-19, 1984.
19. Farah JW, Dougherty EW: Unfilled, filled, and microfilled composite resins, *Oper Dent* 6(3):95, 1981.
20. Feilezer AJ, DeGee AJ, Davidson CL: Setting stress in composite resin in relation to configuration of the restoration, *J Dent Res* 66:1636-1639, 1987.
21. Friedman MJ: The enamel ceramic alternative: porcelain veneers vs metal ceramic crowns, *CDA Journal* 20(8):27-32, 1992.
22. Garberoglio R, Cozzani G: *In vivo* effect of oral environment on etched enamel: a scanning microscopic study, *J Dent Res* 58:1859, 1979.
23. Gwinnett AJ: Moist versus dry dentin: its effect on shear bond strength, *Am J Dent* 5:127-129, 1992.
24. Gwinnett AJ, Kanca JA: Micromorphology of the bonded dentin interface and its relationship to bond strength, *Am J Dent* 5:73-77, 1992.
25. Heymann HO: The artistry of conservative esthetic dentistry, *J Am Dent Assoc* (special issue):14E-23E, 1987.
26. Heymann HO, Bayne SC: Current concepts in dentin bonding: focusing on dentinal adhesion factors, *J Am Dent Assoc* 124(5):27-36, May 1993.
27. Heymann HO, Sturdevant JR, Bayne S, et al: Examining tooth flexure effects on cervical restorations: a two-year clinical study, *J Am Dent Assoc* 122:41-47, 1991.
28. Jorgensen KD, Matono R, Shimokobe H: Deformation of cavities and resin fillings in loaded teeth, *J Dent Res* 84:46-50, 1976.
29. Kanca J III: Replacement of a fractured incisor fragment over a pulpal exposure: a long-term case report, *Quintessence Int* 27(12):829-832, 1996.
30. Lee WC, Eakle WS: Possible role of tensile stress in the etiology of cervical erosive lesions of teeth, *J Prosthet Dent* 52(3):374-380, 1984.
31. Leinfelder KF, Isenberg BP, Essig ME: A new method for generating ceramic restorations: a CAD-CAM system, *J Am Dent Assoc* 118:703-707, 1989.
32. Liberman R et al: The effect of posterior composite restorations on the resistance of cavity walls to vertically applied loads, *J Oral Rehabil* 17:99-105, 1990.
33. Lorton L, Brady J: Criteria for successful composite resin restorations, *Gen Dent* 29(3):234, 1981.
34. Mair LH: Ten-year clinical assessment of three posterior resin composites and two amalgams, *Quintessence Int* 29:483-490, 1998.
35. Mormann WH et al: CAD-CAM ceramic inlays and onlays: a case report after 3 years in place, *J Am Dent Assoc* 120:517-520, 1990.
36. Mormann WH et al: Chairside computer-aided direct ceramic inlays, *Quintessence Int* 20:329-339, 1989.
37. Mount GJ: Adhesion of glass-ionomer cement in the clinical environment, *Oper Dent* 16:141-148, 1991.
38. Nelson RJ, Wolcott RB, Paffenbarger GC: Fluid exchange at the margins of dental restorations, *J Am Dent Assoc* 44:288, 1952.
39. Paffenbarger GC: Silicate cement: an investigation by a group of practicing dentists under the direction of the ADA research fellowship at the National Bureau of Standards, *J Am Dent Assoc* 27:1611, 1940.
40. Qualtrough AJE, Wilson NHF, Smith GA: The porcelain inlay: a historical view, *Oper Dent* 15:61-70, 1990.
41. Randall RC, Wilson NHF: Glass-ionomer restoratives: a systematic review of a secondary caries treatment effect, *J Dent Res* 78(2):628-637, 1999.
42. Reinhardt JW, Chan DC, Boyer DB: Shear strengths of ten commercial dentin bonding agents, *Dent Mater* 3(1)43-45, 1987.
43. Retief DH et al: Tensile bond strengths of dentin bonding agents to dentin, *Dent Mater* 2(2):72-77, 1986.
44. Seltzer S: The penetration of microorganisms between the tooth and direct resin fillings, *J Am Dent Assoc* 51:560, 1955.
45. Silverstone LM, Dogan IL, editors: *Proceedings of the international symposium on the acid etch technique,* St Paul, Minn, 1975, North Central Publishing.
46. Skinner EW: Comparison of the properties and uses of silicate cement and acrylic resin in operative dentistry, *J Am Dent Assoc* 58:27, 1959.
47. Sockwell CL: Clinical evaluation of anterior restorative materials, *Dent Clin North Am* 20:403, 1976.
48. Stanley HR: Criteria for standardizing and increasing credibility of direct pulp capping studies, *Amer J Dent* 11(special issue):S17-34, 1998.
49. Sturdevant CM et al: *The art and science of operative dentistry,* ed 1, New York, 1968, McGraw-Hill.
50. Swift EJ: Effects of glass ionomers on recurrent caries, *Oper Dent* 14:40-43, 1989.
51. Tagami J, Hosoda H, Fusayama T: Optimal technique of etching enamel, *Oper Dent* 13:181-184, 1988.
52. Taleghani M, Leinfelder KF, Lane J: Posterior porcelain inlays, *Compend Contin Educ Dent* 8(6):410-415, 1987.
53. Torstenson B, Brännström M: Composite resin contraction gaps measured with a fluorescent resin technique, *Dent Mater* 4:238-242, 1988.
54. Volker J, Bilkakis E, Melillo S: Some observations on the relationship between plastic filling materials and dental caries, *Tufts Dent Outlook* 18:4, 1944.
55. Welk DA, Laswell HR: Rationale for designing cavity preparations in light of current knowledge and technology, *Dent Clin North Am* 20(2):231, 1976.
56. Wilder AD et al: Effect of powder/liquid ratio on the clinical and laboratory performance of resin-modified glass-ionomers, *J Dent* 26(4):369-377, 1998.
57. Wilson AD, Kent BE: A new translucent cement for dentistry: the glass ionomer cement, *Brit Dent J* 132:133-135, 1972.
58. Yoshikawa T et al: Effects of dentin depth and cavity configuration on bond strength. *J Dent Res* 78(4):898-905, 1999.

12

Classes III, IV, and V Direct Composite and Other Tooth-Colored Restorations

THEODORE M. ROBERSON

HARALD O. HEYMANN

ANDRÉ V. RITTER

PATRICIA N.R. PEREIRA

CLASSES III, IV, AND V DIRECT COMPOSITE RESTORATIONS

This chapter presents information primarily about typical Classes III, IV, and V direct composite restorations (Fig. 12-1). Because Classes III and IV restorations involve only anterior teeth, an esthetic material such as composite is indicated almost always. Likewise, Class V restorations on anterior teeth usually require esthetic restorations. Although esthetic considerations also are valid for posterior restorations, many patients are not as concerned with esthetics in posterior teeth as they are in anterior teeth. However, the use of composite for any restoration provides benefits other than improved esthetics.

This chapter also presents information about any differences in these classes of restorations when a microfill composite or glass-ionomer type material is used.

PERTINENT MATERIAL QUALITIES AND PROPERTIES

The specific material qualities or properties that make composite the best material for most Classes III, IV, and V restorations relate to esthetics. In addition to esthetics, the other qualities presented in Chapter 11 apply as well. These include adequate strength and the benefits of being able to bond the composite to tooth structure, often resulting in less tooth structure removal during tooth preparation.

INDICATIONS

Almost all Class III and Class IV restorations are appropriately restored with composite. Most Class V restorations that are in esthetic prominent areas are also appropriately restored with composite or other tooth-colored materials. However, in all of these instances, the operating area must be able to be adequately isolated to attain an effective bond. Also, these classes of restorations are best suited for composite or other tooth-colored material usage when the tooth preparations have all-enamel margins.

CONTRAINDICATIONS

The contraindications for use of composite for these classes of restorations include: (1) an operating area that cannot be adequately isolated, (2) some Class V restorations in areas that are not esthetically critical, and (3) some restorations that extend onto the root surface. The extension onto the root surface (no marginal enamel) may be a contraindication, because for many extensions onto the root surface with composite restorations, a V-shaped gap (contraction gap) is formed between the root and the composite. This contraction gap[2,11] occurs because the force of polymerization shrinkage of the composite is greater than the initial bond strength of the composite to the dentin of the root. The V-shaped gap is composed of composite on the restoration side and hybridized dentin on the root side, as seen in Fig. 12-2. It is not known what the long-term clinical effects of these gaps may be. Regardless, it should be recognized that whenever a restoration extends onto the root surface, adverse effects may be associated with the restoration, no matter what restorative material is being used. For example, even high copper amalgam restorations will exhibit some marginal leakage, at least for a short period of time. Thus, any extension onto the root surface requires the best and most meticulous efforts of the operator to best insure a successful, long-lasting restoration.

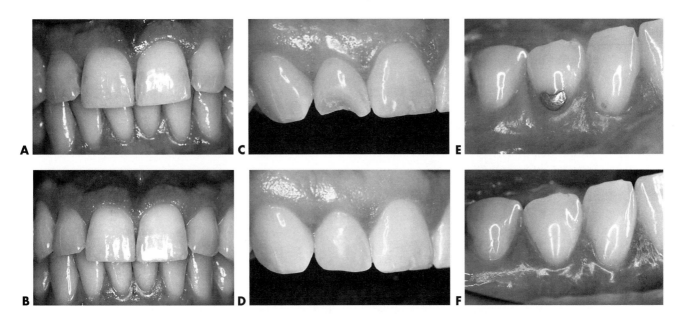

FIG. 12-1 Composite restorations before and after. **A** and **B,** Class III. **C** and **D,** Class IV. **E** and **F,** Class V.

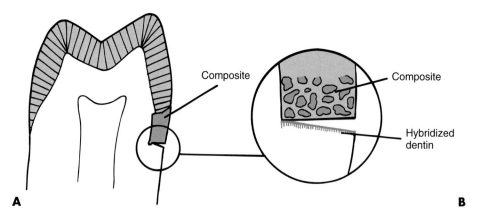

FIG. **12-2** Contraction gap. **A,** V-shaped gap on root surface. **B,** Restoration-side vector is composite; root-side vector is hybridized dentin.

ADVANTAGES

The advantages of using composite for these restorations are the same as those presented and discussed in Chapter 11.

DISADVANTAGES

Likewise, the disadvantages of using composites for Classes III, IV, and V restorations were presented and discussed in Chapter 11.

CLINICAL TECHNIQUE FOR DIRECT CLASS III COMPOSITE RESTORATIONS

INITIAL CLINICAL PROCEDURES

Chapters 10 and 11 presented information about procedures necessary before beginning the restoration: (1) Anesthesia may be necessary for patient comfort, and if used, will help decrease the salivary flow during the procedure. (2) Occlusal assessments should be made to help in properly adjusting the restoration's function and in determining the tooth preparation design. (3) The shade must be selected before the tooth dehydrates and experiences concomitant lightening. (4) The area must be isolated to permit effective bonding. (5) If the restoration will be large (including all of the proximal contact), prewedging the area will assist in the reestablishment of the proximal contact with composite.

TOOTH PREPARATION

Class III tooth preparations, by definition, are located on the proximal surfaces of anterior teeth. Such locations have been the predominant sites for the use of composite restorations in the past because of the typical need for esthetic restorations in anterior teeth. Because the bond of composite to enamel and dentin is so strong, most Class III composite restorations are retained only by the micromechanical bond from acid-etching and

resin bonding, so no additional preparation retention form is usually necessary. Using diamond stones for the tooth preparation leaves the prepared surfaces rougher, thereby increasing the surface area and the micromechanical retention. Sometimes a groove or cove may be necessary for Class III restorations that either extend onto the root surface or are very large. Usually, however, additional needed retention form can be achieved simply by increasing the surface area with a wider enamel bevel or flare along the margin.

When a proximal surface of an anterior tooth is to be restored and there is a choice between facial or lingual entry into the tooth, the lingual approach is preferable. A small carious lesion should be treated from the lingual approach unless such an approach would necessitate excessive cutting of tooth structure, such as in instances of irregular alignment of the teeth or facial positioning of the lesion.

The advantages of restoring the proximal lesion from the lingual approach include:

1. The facial enamel is conserved for enhanced esthetics.
2. Some unsupported, but not friable, enamel may be left on the facial wall of a Class III or Class IV preparation.
3. Color matching of the composite is not as critical.
4. Discoloration or deterioration of the restoration is less visible.

The indications for a facial approach include:

1. The carious lesion is positioned facially such that facial access would significantly conserve tooth structure.
2. The teeth are irregularly aligned, making lingual access undesirable.
3. Extensive caries extend onto the facial surface.
4. A faulty restoration that was originally placed from facial approach needs to be replaced.

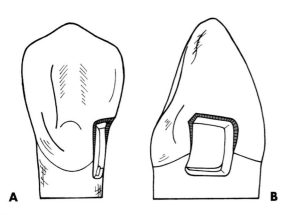

FIG. 12-3 **A** and **B,** Combination preparation design for a Class III lesion that extends onto root surface. The root-surface portion is a conventional tooth preparation design utilizing butt joint marginal configuration and retention groove in dentin. The coronal portion is a beveled conventional tooth preparation design.

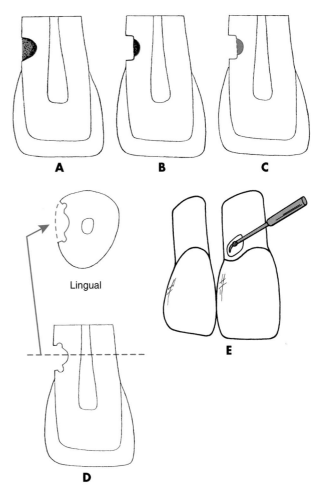

Lingual

FIG. 12-4 Class III conventional tooth preparation for a lesion entirely on root surface. **A,** Mesiodistal longitudinal section illustrating carious lesion. **B,** Initial tooth preparation. **C,** Tooth preparation with infected carious dentin removed. **D,** Retention grooves shown in longitudinal section, and transverse section through plane *cd* illustrates contour of axial wall and direction of facial and lingual walls. **E,** Preparing retention form to complete tooth preparation.

When both the facial and lingual surfaces are involved, use the approach that provides the best access for instrumentation.

It is expeditious to prepare and restore approximating carious lesions or faulty restorations on adjacent teeth at the same appointment. Usually one of the preparations will be larger (more extended outline form) than the other. When the larger outline form is developed first, the second preparation usually can be more conservative because of the improved access provided by the larger preparation. The reverse order would be followed when the restorative material is inserted.

Conventional Class III Tooth Preparation. The primary indication for this type of Class III preparation is for the restoration of root surfaces. Thus, it would be unusual to have an entire Class III preparation of the conventional type. More likely, only a portion of a tooth preparation—the portion on the root surface that has no enamel margin—would be prepared in this manner (Fig. 12-3). The design of the preparation then would be a combination of a modified or a beveled conventional preparation (as presented later) with a conventionally prepared root-surface area. The exception would be when all of a lesion, fault, or defective restoration is located on the root surface of a tooth, which would result in the entire preparation being the conventional type, exhibiting butt joint margins (Fig. 12-4). This preparation would be identical to the slot preparation for amalgam illustrated and described in Chapter 17.

When preparing the conventional portion of a preparation (on the root surface), the form of the preparation walls is the same as that of an amalgam preparation. The cavosurface margins exhibit a 90-degree cavosurface angle and provide butt joints between the tooth and the composite material. Thus the external walls are prepared perpendicular to the root surface. In this conventionally prepared area of the tooth, which is apical of the cervical line, the external walls will be entirely of dentin and cementum. These walls must be prepared to a sufficient depth pulpally to provide for the following: (1) adequate removal of the caries, old restorative material, or fault, and sometimes (2) the placement of retention grooves, if deemed necessary. This wall depth (depth to axial line angles) usually will be approximately 0.75 mm into dentin, assuming no additional caries excavation is required. Groove retention form may be necessary in nonenamel, root-surface preparations to both increase the retention of the material in the tooth and to optimize the seal of the composite to the root surface.

The crown areas of the preparation (where enamel margins are present) are prepared to have a beveled or flared marginal configuration (from either a beveled conventional or modified tooth preparation) and a pulpal depth dictated by either the extent of the existing restoration being replaced or the extent of the infected portion of the carious lesion. Typically the retention of the restorative material in the crown portion of the preparation would be provided by the bond afforded by etching the enamel and dentin surfaces, by priming the dentinal surfaces, and placing bonding adhesive to all prepared surfaces.

The specific design for the conventional Class III tooth preparation can be reviewed in Chapter 18 in the section on Class III tooth preparation for amalgam, but it is also presented for composite in the following paragraphs, which describe the stages and steps of this root-surface tooth preparation.

Using a No. 1/2, 1, or 2 round bur or diamond, prepare the outline form on the root surface, extending the external walls to sound tooth structure while extending pulpally to an initial depth of 0.75 mm, if, in a subsequent step, the preparation of retention grooves will be necessary. However, if no retention groove is anticipated, the initial depth will be only that which removes the caries or fault, although still no deeper at this stage than 0.75 mm. The bur or diamond at this limited depth may be touching dentin, previous restorative material, carious tooth structure, or air. Prepare the external walls perpendicular to the root surface, thus forming a 90-degree cavosurface angle. It is emphasized that during this step in tooth preparation, the instrument's cutting edges are moved to this limited, initial pulpal depth and no deeper. Any remaining infected dentin will be removed later.

The boxlike design may be considered a part of retention form; however, at this stage in tooth preparation the external walls may be retentive because of opposing wall parallelism or slight undercuts, or nonretentive because of slight divergence outwardly. If prepared with a diamond, the prepared walls also will be roughened.

If the preparation approach is from the facial, the opening may be enlarged to provide necessary access and visibility; if the approach is lingual, the access opening may be extended for the same reason. Once adequate access is achieved, remove all remaining infected dentin using round burs or small spoon excavators, or both. Remaining old restorative material on the axial wall should be removed if any of the following conditions are present: (1) the old material is amalgam and its color would negatively affect the color of the new restoration; (2) there is radiographic evidence of caries under the old material; (3) the tooth pulp was symptomatic preoperatively; (4) the periphery of the remaining restorative material is not intact (i.e., there is some breach in the junction of the material with the adjacent tooth structure, which may indicate caries under the material); or (5) the use of the underlying dentin is necessary to effect a stronger bond for retention purposes. If none of these conditions is present, the operator may elect to leave the remaining restorative material to serve as a base, rather than risk unnecessary: (1) excavation nearer to the pulp, or (2) irritation or exposure of the pulp. A calcium hydroxide liner would be indicated only for a direct or indirect pulp cap procedure as described in Chapters 4 and 6.

Groove retention may be necessary in root-surface preparations to better ensure that the restorative material is retained in the tooth. The retention groove created also may help in minimizing the potential negative effects of polymerization shrinkage (the composite pulling away from the margin) when inserting the composite incrementally. Additionally, this groove will enhance the marginal seal by resisting flexural forces (from tooth flexure) placed on the cervical portion of the restoration.

A continuous retention groove can be prepared in the internal portion of the external walls using a No. 1/4 round bur. A continuous groove is utilized when maximum retention need is anticipated. The groove is located 0.25 mm (half the diameter of the No. 1/4 round bur) from the root surface and is prepared to a depth of 0.25 mm (half the diameter of the No. 1/4 round bur). This groove is directed as the bisector of the angle formed by the junction of the axial wall and the external wall (see Fig. 12-4, D and E). For its entire length the groove should be parallel to the root surface. Use the side of the No. 1/4 round bur for cutting retention form whenever possible to control retention depth. When less retention need exists, the retention grooves may be omitted or placed only in the gingivoaxial and/or incisoaxial line angles. Lastly, clean the preparation of any visible debris and inspect for final approval.

Beveled Conventional Class III Tooth Preparation. The beveled conventional tooth preparation for composite restorations is indicated primarily for replacing an existing defective restoration in the crown portion of the tooth. However, it also may be used when restoring a large carious lesion for which the need for increased retention and/or resistance form is anticipated. The tooth preparation takes the shape of the existing restoration along with any extensions necessary to include recurrent caries, friable tooth structure, or defects. Any extensions required may be prepared with a modified tooth preparation design, as discussed in the next section. The beveled conventional preparation is characterized by external walls that are perpendicular to the enamel surface, with the enamel margin beveled. The axial line angles may or may not be of uniform pulpal depth, varying as the thickness of the enamel portion of the external walls varies. If part of the tooth to be restored is located on the root surface, a conventional cavosurface configuration should be used in this area as described earlier, resulting in a combination of two tooth preparation designs, a conventional type in the root portion, and a beveled conventional type in the crown portion.

The tooth preparation for the replacement restoration will have the same general form of the previous (old) tooth preparation (often the existing restoration will have utilized a conventional preparation design). Usually retention is obtained by bonding to the enamel and dentin and no groove retention is necessary. However, when replacing a large restoration or restoring a large Class III lesion, the operator may decide that retention form should be enhanced by placing groove (at gingival) and/or cove (at incisal) retention features in addition to the bonded tooth structure.

Lingual Access. Because indirect vision usually is required for the preferred lingual access for a tooth preparation, a clean, unscratched front surface mirror is recommended to provide a clear, undistorted view. Sometimes direct vision may be used to advantage by tilting the patient's head.

Use a round carbide bur (No. ½, 1, or 2) or diamond stone, the size depending on the extent of the caries or defective restoration, to prepare the outline form (Fig. 12-5). Before contacting the tooth, the cutting instrument is positioned for entry and rotated at high speed using air-water spray. The assistant directs air on the mirror surface and positions the evacuator tip near the operating site. The point of entry is within the incisogingival dimension of the carious lesion or defective restoration and as close to the adjacent tooth as possible, without contacting it (Fig. 12-6, *A*). Direct the cutting instrument perpendicular to the enamel surface, but at an entry angle that places the neck portion of the bur as far into the embrasure (next to the adjacent tooth) as possible; use light pressure and intermittent cutting (brush stroke) to gain access into the lesion. Incorrect entry overextends the lingual outline into potential stress areas (marginal ridges) and unnecessarily weakens the tooth (see Fig. 12-6, *B* and *C*). The same instrument may be used to enlarge the opening sufficiently to allow for the later described caries removal, completion of the preparation, and insertion of the restorative material (see Fig.12-6, *D*).

Extend the external walls to sound tooth structure during preparation of the outline form, but only to the initial limited prescribed depth. This extension should be as minimal as possible, dictated by the extent of caries and/or old restorative material on these walls. Unless absolutely necessary, do not: (1) include the proximal contact area, (2) extend onto the facial surface, or (3) extend subgingivally. The axial wall depth at this initial stage of tooth preparation is limited to 0.2 mm inside the dentinoenamel junction (DEJ) (if no retention groove will be used), which means it will be approximately 0.75 to 1.25 mm deep (the larger being incisally where enamel is thicker). The axial wall will be outwardly convex, following normal external tooth contour and the DEJ, both incisogingivally and faciolingually (Fig. 12-7, *A* and *B*). Usually the axial line angles should be positioned at an initial depth of 0.2 mm into dentin. However, if a retention groove is to be placed, the axial wall should be 0.5 mm into dentin at retention locations to prevent undermining enamel where the retention form is prepared. As noted previously when the preparation outline extends gingivally onto the root surface, the depth of the axial wall at the gingivoaxial line angle should be 0.75 mm, thus providing adequate dimension for composite strength, placement of a retention groove, and maintenance of strength of the gingival wall and margin. The axial depth should not be exceeded at this initial stage of tooth preparation even if the bur is cutting in air, caries, or old restorative material. Any remaining infected dentin or old, defective restorative material on the axial wall will be removed during the final tooth-preparation stage.

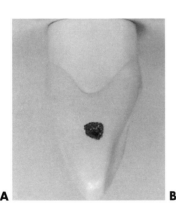
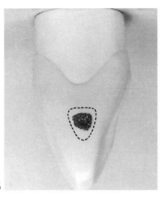
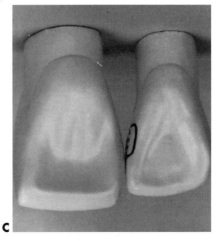

A   **B**   **C**

F I G. **12-5 A,** Small proximal carious lesion on mesial surface of maxillary lateral incisor. **B,** *Dotted line* indicates normal outline form dictated by shape of carious lesion. **C,** Extension (convenience form) required for preparing and restoring preparation from lingual approach when teeth are in normal alignment.

Prepare the enamel walls perpendicular to the external tooth surface. The gingival floor and lingual wall usually are finished with the same round cutting instrument that was used to prepare the outline form. If there is not an ample facial, lingual, or gingival embrasure space to avoid marring the adjacent tooth with the cutting instrument, use the 8-3-22 hoe to better finish those walls.

Once the outline form and initial axial wall depth have been established, the initial tooth preparation stage is completed and the final stage of tooth preparation begins. For most Class III restorations using the beveled conventional preparation, the preparation would be complete at this time except for placing an enamel bevel or flare.

Remove all remaining infected dentin using round burs or small spoon excavators, or both. Some undermined enamel can be left in nonstress areas, but very friable enamel at the margins should be removed. Re-

maining old restorative material on the axial wall should be removed if any of the conditions presented earlier are present. Apply a calcium hydroxide liner only if indicated.

If retention features (grooves or coves) are indicated (and usually they are not), prepare them along the gingivoaxial line angle and, sometimes, the incisoaxial line angle with a No. $\frac{1}{4}$ bur. Occasionally retention may be provided by undercuts left from caries removal. No purposeful attempt is made to provide retentive undercuts along the linguoaxial and facioaxial line angles because these areas usually are not needed to retain composites and might unnecessarily weaken the lingual and facial enamel walls and margins. Particular care must be exercised not to weaken the walls or incisal angles that are subject to masticatory forces.

If deemed necessary, prepare a gingival retention groove along the gingivoaxial line angle. Care should be

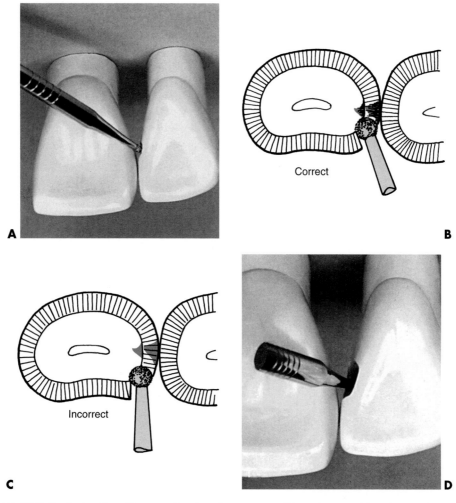

FIG. 12-6 Beginning Class III conventional tooth preparation (lingual approach). **A,** Bur or diamond is held perpendicular to enamel surface, and initial opening is made close to adjacent tooth at incisogingival level of caries. **B,** Correct angle of entry is parallel to enamel rods on mesiolingual angle of tooth. **C,** Incorrect entry overextends lingual outline. **D,** Same bur or diamond is used to enlarge opening for caries removal and convenience form while establishing initial axial wall depth.

exercised to prepare this groove approximately 0.2 mm inside the DEJ to a depth of 0.25 mm (half the diameter of the No. ¼ bur) so as not to undermine the enamel portion of the gingival wall. The depthwise direction of the groove is an angle that bisects the junction of the axial wall and external walls. Low handpiece speed with air coolant for this step provides better tactile sensation and vision. Start the gingival groove at the faciogingivoaxial point angle and extend along the gingivoaxial line angle to the linguogingivoaxial point angle. The lengthwise direction of the groove parallels the DEJ without undermining the adjacent enamel of its dentin support.

Prepare any necessary incisal retention cove with the No. ¼ bur at the axioincisal point angle with the bur oriented in a similar angle, 0.2 mm inside the DEJ, and 0.25 mm deep. Then extend it slightly into the facioaxial line angle where it fades out. Care should be exercised not to take away dentinal support from the enamel. It is emphasized that the incisal retention is directed facioincisopulpally, where possible, rather than incisopulpally. Sometimes this feature is critical in preserving the strength of a weak incisal corner of a tooth. The completed gingival retention groove and incisal retention cove for a large Class III beveled conventional tooth preparation are illustrated in Fig. 12-8.

The placement of incisal retention is not always as easy in the mouth as illustrated because of handpiece size and angulation problems caused by the anatomy of the maxilla and tooth positions. When teeth are rotated or abnormally aligned, additional extension of the incisal portion of the lingual wall may be necessary to provide the convenience form necessary to prepare the incisal retention with the No. ¼ bur. Also, extension of the bur out of the handpiece often enhances visibility and access in these circumstances. Another method is to use a bibeveled hatchet (i.e., 3-2-28) with delicate shav-

ing strokes in a facioincisopulpal direction, removing small amounts of dentin until the area is retentive. This is an excellent instrument for testing to see that the incisal retention is present, regardless of the method used to obtain the retention.

Class III beveled conventional tooth preparations are prepared as conventional preparations with the addition of a cavosurface bevel or flare of the enamel rather than a butt joint margin (Figs. 12-9, *A* and *B*, and 12-10). The cross-sectional view in Fig. 12-11 illustrates the cavosurface bevel that provides more surface area for end-on etching of the enamel rods. The cavosurface bevel or flare is best prepared with either a flame-shaped or round diamond instrument, resulting in an angle approximately 45 degrees to the external tooth surface

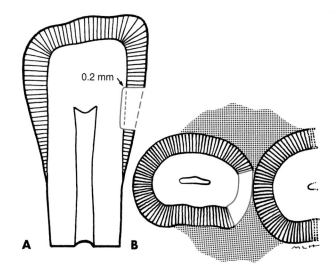

FIG. 12-7 Ideal initial axial wall preparation depth. **A,** Incisogingival section showing axial wall 0.2 mm into dentin. **B,** Faciolingual section showing facial extension and axial wall following contour of tooth.

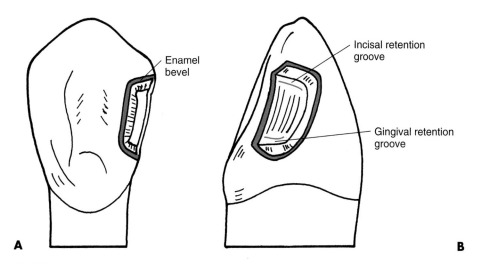

FIG. 12-8 Large beveled conventional Class III preparation. **A and B,** Beveled enamel walls and incisal and gingival retention grooves.

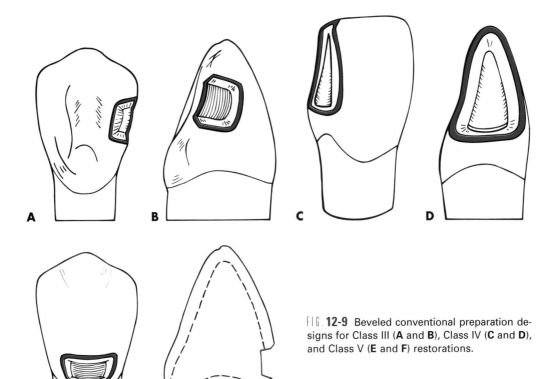

FIG. **12-9** Beveled conventional preparation designs for Class III (**A** and **B**), Class IV (**C** and **D**), and Class V (**E** and **F**) restorations.

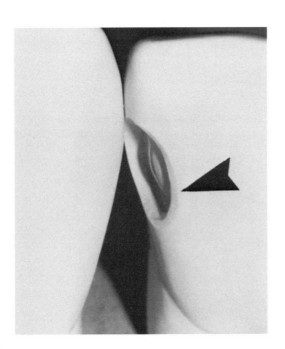

FIG. **12-10** Large Class III beveled conventional tooth preparation. Note cavosurface bevel *(arrow)*.

(Fig. 12-12). A bevel width of 0.25 to 0.5 mm is considered sufficient unless the operator elects to increase the retention form by preparing a wider bevel, which will increase the surface area to be etched and therefore the retention form. For moderate and large Class III beveled

conventional preparations, all accessible enamel margins usually are beveled, with the exception of the gingival margin. This margin is usually not beveled if little or no enamel is present or access is difficult for finishing procedures. If the preparation extends gingivally onto root structure, no bevel is placed on cementum, and the area is prepared as a conventional preparation. In addition, bevels may not be recommended on lingual surface margins that are in areas of centric contact or subjected to heavy masticatory forces because composite has less wear resistance than enamel for withstanding heavy attritional forces. Clean the preparation of any visible debris and inspect for final approval.

Facial Access. With a few exceptions, the same stages and steps of tooth preparation are followed as with lingual access. The procedure is simplified because direct vision is used and the lesion or faulty restoration is usually larger.

A large Class III lesion on the distal surface of a maxillary right central incisor is illustrated (Fig. 12-13, *A*). The rubber dam is placed after the anesthetic has been administered and the shade has been selected. A wedge is inserted in the gingival embrasure to depress the rubber dam and underlying soft tissue, thus improving gingival access (see Fig. 12-13, *B*). Using a No. 2 carbide bur or diamond stone rotating at high speed and with air-water spray, prepare the outline form with appropriate extension, as well as the initial, limited pulpal depth previously described in the lingual approach prepara-

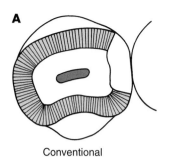
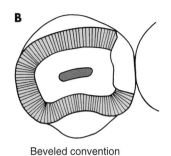

Conventional   Beveled convention

FIG. **12-11** **A,** Cross-section of facial approach Class III conventional tooth preparation with 90-degree cavosurface angle. **B,** Beveled conventional tooth preparation showing 45-degree cavosurface bevel on facial margin.

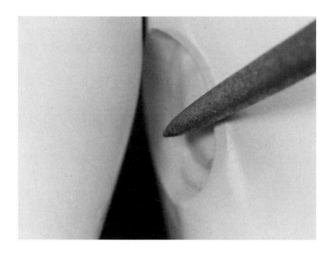

FIG. **12-12** Beveling. Cavosurface bevel is prepared with flame-shaped or round diamond resulting in an angle approximately 45 degrees to the external tooth surface.

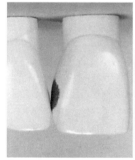
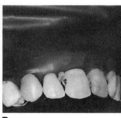
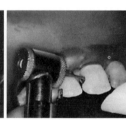
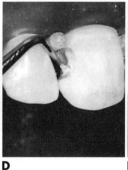
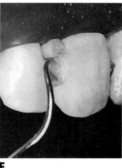

A   B   C   D   E

FIG. **12-13** Class III initial preparation (facial approach). **A,** Large proximal caries with facial involvement. **B,** Isolated area of operation. **C,** Entry and extension with No. 2 bur or diamond. **D,** Caries removal with spoon excavator. **E,** Explorer point removes caries at DEJ. This is a beveled conventional preparation if accessible margins are beveled (see Fig. 12-15).

tion (see Fig. 12-13, *C*). Some undermined enamel can be left if it is not in a high-stress area. Accessible enamel margins can be finished with the cutting instrument. Other walls may be completed with hand instruments, such as the 7-85-2½-6 or 12-85-5-8.

When a proximal carious lesion or faulty restoration extends onto both the facial and lingual surfaces, access may be accomplished from either a facial or lingual approach. An example of an extensive Class III initial tooth preparation that allows such choice is illustrated in Fig. 12-14. Recall that if the preparation extends gingivally onto root structure, no bevel is placed on cementum and the area is prepared as a conventional tooth preparation.

The final tooth preparation is accomplished by removing any remaining infected dentin with a round bur rotating at low speed or a small spoon excavator, or both (see Fig. 12-14, *D*). The point of a No. 2 explorer may be used for judiciously detecting and removing traces of caries at the DEJ (see Fig. 12-14, *E*). If old restorative material remains on the axial wall after preparing the outline form, follow the procedure previously described in the lingual access preparation. Apply a calcium hydroxide liner only if indicated for pulp protection. Prepare groove or cove retention, if indicated, using a No. ¼ bur, or undercuts remaining from caries removal may suffice. Bevel accessible enamel margins with a flame-shaped or round diamond instrument, resulting in an angle approximately 45 degrees to the external tooth surface. A bevel of 0.25 to 0.5 mm is considered sufficient. The completed Class III facial approach preparation is illustrated in Fig. 12-15. Final preparation procedures are cleaning and inspecting.

Modified Class III Tooth Preparation. A modified tooth preparation is the most used type of Class III tooth preparation. It is indicated for small and moderate lesions or faults and is designed to be as conservative as possible. The preparation design is dictated by the extent of the fault or defect and is prepared from a lingual approach when possible, with an appropriate size round bur or diamond instrument. No effort is made to produce preparation walls that have specific shapes or forms other than external angles of 90 degrees or greater. The extension axially also is dictated by the extent of the fault or carious lesion and usually will not be uniform in depth. Weakened, friable enamel is removed while preparing the cavosurface margins in a beveled or flared configuration with the round diamond. Usually no groove (or cove) retention form is indicated because the retention of the material in the tooth will result from the bond created between the composite material and the etched peripheral enamel. Thus, the preparation design appears to be "scooped" or concave (Fig. 12-16, A and B). Most initial composite restorations utilize the modified preparation design. Because a carious lesion that requires a restoration usually extends into dentin, many modified preparations will be prepared to an initial axial wall depth of 0.2 mm into dentin. However, no attempt is made to prepare distinct or uniform axial preparation walls, but rather, the objective is to include only the infected carious area as conservatively as possible by "scooping" out the defective tooth structure. Additional caries excavation (deeper than the initial

stage of 0.2 mm pulpal of the DEJ) or marginal refinement may be necessary later.

Begin the preparation from a lingual approach (if possible) by making an opening using a round carbide bur (No. ½, 1, or 2) or diamond instrument, the size depending on the extent of the lesion. Before contacting the tooth, the bur is positioned for entry and rotated at high speed using air-water spray. The assistant directs air on the mirror surface and positions the evacuator tip near the operating site. The point of entry is within the incisogingival dimension of the lesion or defect and as close to the adjacent tooth as possible without contacting it (see Fig. 12-6, A). Direct the cutting instrument perpendicular to the enamel surface, but at an entry angle that places the neck portion of the bur or diamond instrument as far into the embrasure (next to the adjacent tooth) as possible; use light pressure and intermittent cutting (brush stroke) to gain access into the preparation. Incorrect entry overextends the lingual outline into potential stress areas (marginal ridges) and unnecessarily weakens the tooth (see Fig. 12-6, B and C). The same instrument may be used to enlarge the opening sufficiently to permit, in subsequent steps, caries removal, completion of the preparation, and insertion of the restorative material (see Fig. 12-6, D).

No effort is made to prepare walls that are perpendicular to the enamel surface; in fact, for small preparations the walls may diverge externally from the axial depth in a scoop shape resulting in both (1) a beveled or flared marginal design and (2) conservation of internal tooth structure (Fig. 12-17). For larger modified preparations, the initial tooth preparation will still be prepared as conservatively as possible, but the preparation walls may not be as divergent from the axial wall. The term axial wall is used because in more extensive preparations at this initial preparation stage, an

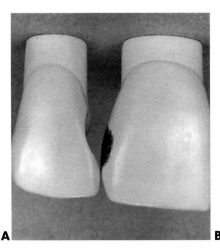
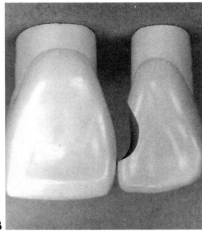
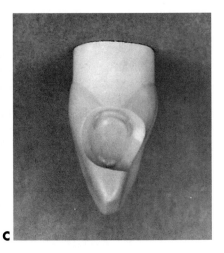

A   **B**   **C**

FIG. **12-14** Large Class III tooth preparation extending onto root surface. **A,** Facial view. **B,** Lingual view. **C,** Mesial view showing gingival and incisal retention. Tooth preparation is now ready for beveling of the enamel walls.

axial wall should be of limited depth, 0.2 mm internal of the DEJ (it may be in dentin, caries, or air). Subsequent beveling or flaring of accessible enamel areas may be required. However, *the objective of initial tooth preparation is* the same for both situations: *to prepare the tooth as conservatively as possible by extending the outline form only the amount necessary to include the peripheral extent of the lesion.* Note that sometimes the incorporation of an enamel bevel or flare also may be used to extend the final outline form to include the carious lesion (Fig. 12-18).

Extensions should be minimal, including only that tooth structure that is necessary because of the extent of the caries or defect. Some undermined enamel can be left in nonstress areas, but very friable enamel at the margins should be removed. If possible, the outline form should not: (1) include the entire proximal contact area, (2) extend onto the facial surface, or (3) be extended subgingivally.

Usually the axial wall will not be uniform in depth, but must provide access for the removal of infected dentin and the application of the etchant, primer, bonding adhesive, and composite. If the preparation outline extends gingivally onto the root surface, the gingival wall should form a cavosurface angle of 90 degrees and the depth of the gingivoaxial line angle should be 0.75 mm for reasons discussed previously. This depth should not be exceeded in this initial stage of tooth preparation.

When completed, the initial stage for the modified tooth preparation extends the outline form to include all of the fault unless it is anticipated that the incorporation of an additional enamel bevel will complete that objective. Small preparations will typically have a beveled or flared marginal configuration from the initial tooth preparation. Therefore, there may be little to do in the final tooth preparation stage for these preparations. If infected dentin remains (deeper than the initial axial wall

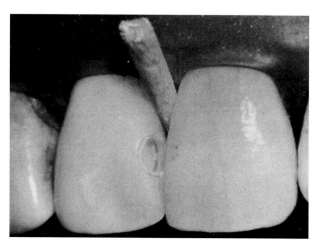

FIG. **12-15** Completed Class III beveled conventional tooth preparation (facial approach).

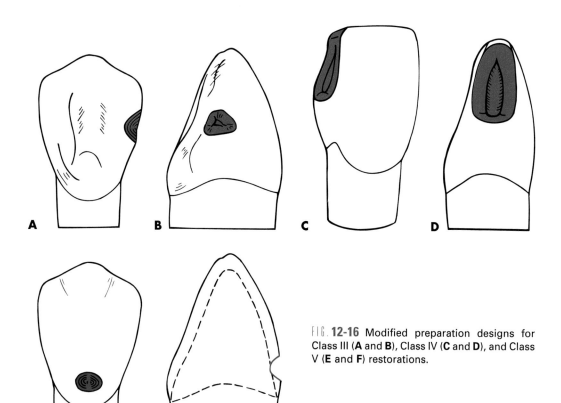

FIG. **12-16** Modified preparation designs for Class III (**A** and **B**), Class IV (**C** and **D**), and Class V (**E** and **F**) restorations.

depth), remove it by using suitably sized round burs and/or small spoon excavators. If indicated, place a calcium hydroxide liner over only the deepest portion of the excavated area, so that a maximum of dentinal surface is still exposed for bonding the restorative material.

Larger preparations that are extended into dentin may require additional beveling or flaring of the accessible enamel walls to enhance retention. Bevel these enamel margins with a flame-shaped or round diamond instrument. Prepare the bevel by creating a 45-degree angle to the external surface and to a width of 0.25 to 0.5 mm. Recall that if the gingival floor has been extended gingivally to a position where the remaining enamel thickness is minimal or nonexistent, the bevel is omitted from this area to preserve the remaining enamel margin. Likewise, a bevel on the lingual enamel margin of a maxillary incisor may be precluded because of the presence of occlusal contact, for reasons previously noted. Thus, final tooth preparation steps for a modified tooth preparation are, when indicated: (1) removal of infected dentin, (2) pulp protection, (3) bevel placement

on accessible enamel margins, and (4) final procedures of cleaning and inspecting.

RESTORATIVE TECHNIQUE

Etching, Priming, and Placing Adhesive. The etching, priming, and adhesive placement steps are accomplished with strict adherence to the manufacturer's directions for the particular bonding system being used. If the bonding will be to enamel only, a separate priming step is not necessary. However, if the bonding system combines the primer and adhesive components, placing this "one-bottle" type bonding material on etched enamel surfaces does not adversely affect the bond strength. If dentin is being bonded, it is important that the dentin be left in a slightly moistened state after etching and before primer application. (For a review of bonding methods, see Chapters 4 and 5.)

The usual technique for etching, priming, and adhesive placement is as follows. First, the proximal surface of the adjacent unprepared tooth should be protected from inadvertent etching by placing a polyester strip. Then a gel etchant is applied to all of the prepared tooth structure, approximately 0.5 mm beyond the prepared margins onto the adjacent unprepared tooth (Fig. 12-19). The etchant is typically left undisturbed for 15 to 30 seconds (30 seconds for enamel-only preparations and 15 seconds when dentin is involved). The area is then washed to remove the etchant. If dentin is exposed, rather than air-dry the rinsed area, it is better to use a damp cotton pellet, a disposable brush, or a paper tissue to remove the excess water. The dentin surface should remain moist, as evidenced by a glistening appearance. Neither areas of overdrying or pooling of excess water should be allowed (see Chapter 11).

The primer is applied to all of the prepared tooth structure with a microbrush or other suitable applicator

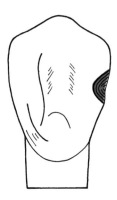

FIG. **12-17** Drawing of a small, scoop-shaped Class III modified tooth preparation.

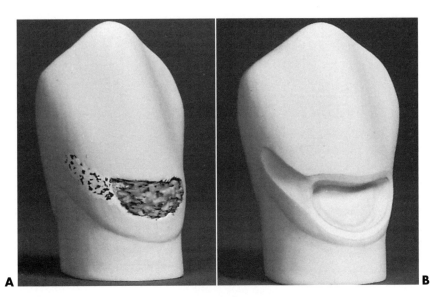

FIG. **12-18** **A,** Decalcified area extending mesially from cavitated Class V lesion. **B,** Completed beveled conventional Class V preparation with conservative mesial extension.

tip (Fig. 12-20). The manufacturer's directions will specify how long to apply the primer, how long it should be cured, and whether or not to apply additional coats. In all cases, the dentin should be uniformly shiny following primer application, as evidence of sufficient coating. If dry spots remain, an additional coat or coats of primer are indicated.

If the bonding system does not combine the primer and adhesive, the bonding adhesive is applied next. Another microbrush or applicator tip is used to place the adhesive on all of the tooth structure that has been etched and primed. Every effort should be made to prevent the adhesive from pooling in remote areas of the preparation. Once applied, the adhesive is polymerized with the curing light as directed. Because these materials are resin based, they generally exhibit an oxygen-inhibited layer on the surface, following polymerization. The composite material will bond directly to the cured adhesive unless the oxygen-inhibited layer is contaminated. Therefore the application of the adhesive and the composite should occur in a timely manner.

Matrix Application. A matrix is a device that is applied to a prepared tooth before the insertion of the restorative material. Its purposes include confining the restorative material excess and assisting in the development of the appropriate axial tooth contours (see Chapter 11 for other matrix objectives).

The matrix is usually applied and stabilized by a wedge (and compound if necessary) before application of the enamel/dentin etchant, primer, and bonding adhesive (the bonding system). Placing the matrix first provides an opportunity to assess that the gingival cavosurface tooth structure is sound and not fractured because of wedge insertion. However, care must be taken to avoid pooling of these bonding materials if the matrix is applied first. If any portion of the preparation remains in contact with the adjacent tooth, the matrix should be placed before etchant, primer, and adhesive use.

Not only will a matrix aid in placing, confining, and contouring the composite restorative material, but also it may aid in isolating the tooth preparation, thereby enhancing the effectiveness of the enamel/dentin bonding system (if done after matrix application). A proper matrix also reduces the amount of excess material, thereby minimizing the finishing time. A properly contoured and wedged matrix is a prerequisite for a restoration involving the entire proximal contact area.

A matrix for the proximal surface of an anterior tooth should be made of a thin material, such as polyester or metal, that can be easily contoured. There are two main types of matrices: (1) a clear polyester strip matrix and (2) a compound-supported metal matrix. The compound-supported matrix is seldom used for Class III restorations and will be described as an alternative matrix system only for Class IV restorations.

A properly contoured polyester strip matrix is used for most Class III and Class IV preparations. Because the proximal surface of a tooth is usually convex incisogingivally and the strip may be flat, it is necessary to shape the strip to conform with the desired tooth contour. One way to contour a polyester strip is by drawing it across a hard, round object such as the rounded, back end of operating pliers (Fig. 12-21). The amount of convexity placed in the strip depends on the size and contour of the anticipated restoration. Several pulls of the strip with

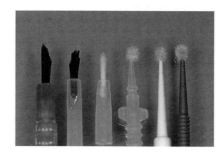

FIG. **12-20** Applicator tip or microbrush

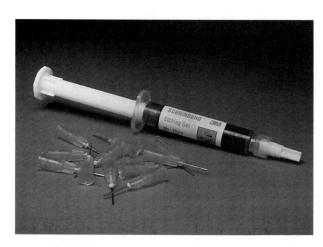

FIG. **12-19** Syringe used to dispense gel etchant.

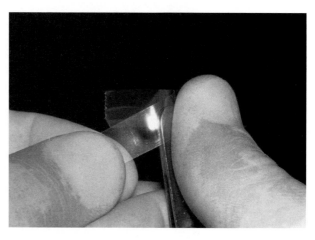

FIG. **12-21** Contouring polyester strip matrix by drawing it over rounded back end of operating pliers.

heavy pressure across the rounded end of the operating pliers may be required to obtain enough convexity. Some strip dispensers provide this convexity as the strip is dispensed (Fig. 12-22). Position the contoured strip between the teeth so that the convex area conforms to the desired tooth contour (Fig. 12-23, *A*). Extend the matrix strip at least 1 mm beyond the prepared gingival and incisal margins. Sometimes the strip will not slide through or is distorted by a tight contact or preparation margin. In such instances, a wedge is lightly positioned in the gingival embrasure before the strip is inserted. Once the strip is past the binding area, it may be necessary to loosen the wedge to place the strip past the gingival margin (between the wedge and margin). Then reinsert the wedge tightly (see Fig. 12-23, *B*).

A wedge is needed at the gingival margin to: (1) help hold the strip in position, (2) provide slight separation of the teeth, and (3) help prevent a gingival overhang of the composite material. A wedge is required when all of the proximal contact is involved because the wedge must separate the teeth sufficiently to compensate for the thickness of the matrix if the completed restoration is to properly contact the adjacent tooth.

Several types of commercial wedges are available in assorted sizes. A triangular-shaped wedge (in cross-section)

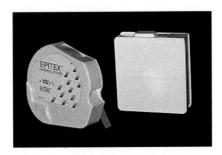

FIG. **12-22** Polyester strip matrix dispenser.

is indicated for preparations with margins that are deep in the gingival sulcus. An end of a round wooden toothpick approximately ⅜ inch (9 mm) long usually is an excellent wedge. The wedge is kept as short as possible to avoid conflict with access during insertion of the restorative material.

Place the wedge, using No. 110 pliers, from the facial approach for lingual access preparations (and vice versa for facial access), just apical to the gingival margin. When isolation is accomplished with the rubber dam, wedge placement may be aided by a small amount of water-soluble lubricant on the tip of the wedge. The rubber dam is first stretched gingivally (on the side from which the wedge is inserted) and then released gradually during wedge insertion (Fig. 12-24). Subsequently, a trial opening and closing of the matrix strip is helpful. It must open enough for access to insert the bonding materials and composite, and close sufficiently to ensure proper contour. It may be necessary to shorten the wedge or insert it from the opposite embrasure to optimize access. Wedge placement may result in fracture of the proximal cavosurface tooth structure. If this occurs, retreatment of that area with the bonding materials must occur.

Inserting and Curing the Composite. The composite restoration usually is placed in two stages: first, a bonding adhesive is applied (if not already placed during enamel and dentin treatment procedures) and then the composite restorative material is inserted. The free-flowing bonding adhesive engages the numerous microundercuts produced in the etched enamel as well as bonds to the etched and primed dentin to provide micromechanical retention. When the composite material is added, a chemical bond occurs with the bonding adhesive, thus forming a strong attachment between the tooth and the composite. If used in conjunction with enamel etching and dentin etching/priming, along with

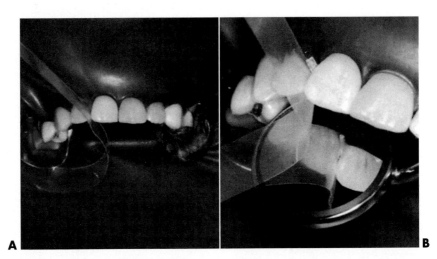

FIG. **12-23** Inserting and wedging polyester strip matrix. **A,** Strip with concave area next to preparation is positioned between teeth. **B,** Strip in position and wedge inserted.

a bonding adhesive, most composite restorations produce an effective seal.[9]

Recall that two types of composites exist: self-cured and light-cured. Even though most restorative composites used are the light-cured type, there are some indications for using self-cured composites, albeit more as cementing agents than restorative materials. For self-cured composites, both the bonding adhesive and composite are supplied in individual containers of a catalyst and a base. Whereas additional shades of the composite base material are available, the catalyst usually remains the same. Items needed for mixing include a disposable plastic spatula, applicator tips or microbrushes, mixing pads, and operating pliers.

Because the mixing and application of the bonding adhesive and then the mixing and insertion of composite should follow a reasonably rapid sequence, the materials are dispensed in advance. Equal amounts of the composite catalyst and base (pastes) are placed on the pad first because they do not have a tendency to run together. The setting time can be controlled by varying the proportion of catalyst and base. Variations as great as 2:1 of either catalyst or base to the other can be tolerated without an appreciable effect on the physical properties. However, it is always best to follow the manufacturer's instructions because of variations from one brand to another. The total amount of material dispensed depends on the size of the preparation and method of insertion. This material is expensive, and needless waste often occurs. A new disposable plastic spatula is used to remove the pastes from the jars. To prevent cross-contamination of the contents in the jars, it is important to use one end of a new spatula for dispensing the catalyst paste and the other end for base paste. This same spatula is placed adjacent to the pad so that it will be available for mixing.

The bonding adhesive is dispensed last and mixed first. It is a liquid with low surface tension and has a tendency to run together. Usually one drop of each component (catalyst and base) is dispensed onto a second mixing pad, leaving a space of $\frac{1}{4}$ inch (6 mm) between the drops. The applicator tip (or microbrush) is used to stir the components of the bonding adhesive together for 5 seconds. It should be quickly blotted against a paper towel to remove excess and the bonding adhesive immediately applied to the etched enamel and etched and primed dentin with a microbrush or applicator tip.

The composite material is mixed next with the same disposable plastic spatula that was used to dispense the materials. An assistant can mix the composite while the operator is mixing and applying the bonding adhesive. To initiate mixing, one paste is picked up with the spatula and placed on top of the other. With a wiping and folding motion, the catalyst and base are blended together for 30 seconds to obtain a homogeneous mixture. A stirring motion should be avoided because of the tendency to incorporate air into the mixture. Approximately 1 minute of working time remains for insertion of the material into the preparation. The self-cured material may be inserted with a syringe or hand instrument, as described later.

The use of a hand instrument is a good method for placing composites because it is easy and fast. In addition to the simplicity of hand instrument insertion, a smaller amount of composite material is required, as compared to the amount needed for the syringe method. A disadvantage of hand instrument insertion is that air can be trapped in the preparation and/or incorporated into the material during the insertion procedure. Experience and care in insertion, which is described later, will minimize this problem.

An example of a syringe used for injecting self-cured composites is shown in Fig. 12-25 with its disposable tip and stopper. Black tips that are impervious to light penetration also are available for storing and injecting light-cured composite. The syringe technique is popular because it provides a convenient means for transporting the composite to the preparation and reduces the possibility of trapping air. Many manufacturers produce preloaded syringe tips with a light-cured composite (Fig. 12-26) and most are color coded for easy shade identification.

The syringe technique may present a problem in small tooth preparations with limited access because the syringe tip may be too large. When the preparation access is questionable, an empty syringe tip can first be tried

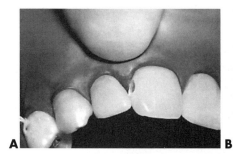
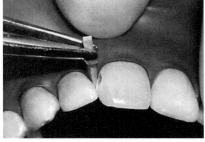
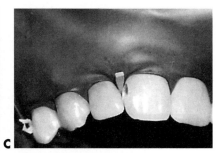

FIG. **12-24** Using a triangular wood wedge to expose gingival margin of large proximal preparation. **A,** Dam is stretched facially and gingivally with fingertip. **B,** Insertion of wedge (dam is released during wedge insertion). **C,** Wedge in place.

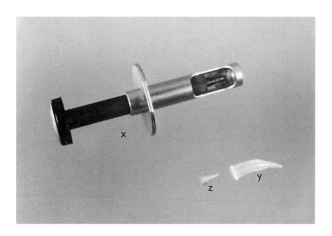

FIG. **12-25** Composite injection syringe *(x)* with disposable tip *(y)* and stopper *(z)*. Used for injection of self-cured composites.

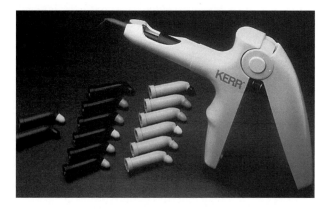

FIG. **12-26** Examples of pistol grip syringe and preloaded composite compule.

into the preparation to verify access and, if not possible, hand-instrument insertion should be used.

The injectability of composites varies because of differences in viscosity and inorganic filler. Some microfill composites cannot be injected. Therefore this property of the material should be evaluated before clinical use.

Insertion of Self-Cured Composites. The matrix is in place as previously described. Whenever possible, tilt the patient's head for direct vision, but most of the time indirect vision is required. With the mirror, hold the lingual portion of the strip away from the preparation opening to reflect light and to provide a clear view for inserting the composite (Fig. 12-27). Leave the facial end of the strip free.

With self-cured composites, the time interval between mixing and polymerization is very short. Therefore mixing and application of materials must be carefully coordinated for optimal results. Everything must be in a "ready-to-go" position before mixing is initiated. Materials are inserted in two steps: bonding adhesive first and composite material second.

The mesial surface of a maxillary left lateral incisor serves as an example for a hand instrument insertion procedure (Fig. 12-28, *A*). If not already applied, mix the previously dispensed bonding adhesive with an applicator tip and blot against a paper towel to remove excess that would flood the preparation. During application, cover the entire preparation (etched enamel and etched/primed dentin) with the bonding adhesive. It is not necessary to wait for the bonding adhesive to set before placing the composite, because the outer surface of the bonding adhesive does not harden in the presence of air. If placement of the composite is delayed, this sticky

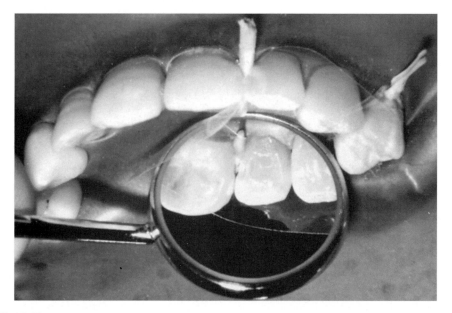

FIG. **12-27** Mirror is used to hold lingual portion of strip away from preparation, reflect light, and provide a clear view for insertion of composite.

film need not be removed, because it will polymerize when air is excluded by the composite that is subsequently placed over it.

Mix the composite material as previously described. Most self-cured composite restorations require approximately 4½ minutes for the complete procedure: 30 seconds for mixing, 1 minute for insertion, and 3 minutes undisturbed time for final setting. Insert the mixed composite in two stages. First, pick up a small amount (approximately one half the preparation size) on the blade end of the hand instrument (Fig. 12-29) and wipe into the tooth preparation (see Fig. 12-28, *B*). Then use the plugger end to press the material into the retentive areas. If the composite has a tendency to stick to the instrument, a sparing amount of bonding adhesive can be used as a lubricant. This is easily obtained by touching the tip of the instrument to the bonding material left on the mixing pad or on the applicator tip. Apply a second increment of composite to completely fill the preparation and provide a slight excess so that positive pressure can be applied with the matrix strip. Remove quickly any gross excess with the blade of the insertion instrument or an explorer tine before closing the matrix.

Set the mirror aside, and close the lingual end of the strip over the composite and hold with the index finger. Next, close the facial end of the strip over the tooth with the thumb and index finger of the other hand, tightening the gingival aspect of the strip ahead of the incisal portion. The matrix can be held in this manner until polymerization is complete, or the thumb of the first hand can be placed over the facial of the strip to hold it without movement during final polymerization (see Fig. 12-28, *C*). This latter maneuver frees the other hand for testing the hardening of the unused composite remaining on the mixing pad. After the composite hardens, remove the wedge and matrix strip before finishing the restoration.

A self-cured composite also may be inserted with a syringe. For this technique, mix the bonding adhesive and apply with an applicator tip in the usual manner. Following mixing of the composite, fill the syringe tip by pressing the large open end of the tip repeatedly into the composite mixture ("cookie-cutting") and then insert the stopper to force the material forward. Quickly place the filled syringe tip into the barrel of the injection syringe, and engage the plunger and press to extrude some of the composite out of the tip.

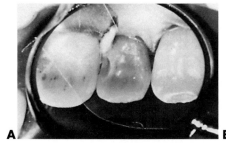
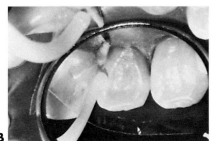
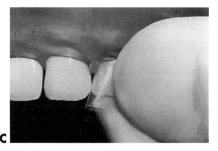

FIG. **12-28** Hand instrument insertion of composite. **A,** Class III lingual approach tooth preparation is to be restored. **B,** Composite is wiped into tooth preparation with blade end of hand instrument. **C,** Matrix strip is closed and held until composite is polymerized.

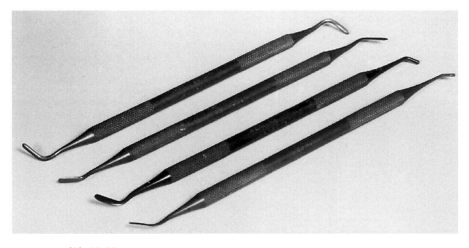

FIG. **12-29** Anodized aluminum insertion instruments for composite.

Starting in the most remote area of the preparation, steadily inject the composite, being sure that the tip remains in the composite, while slowly withdrawing the syringe to prevent air entrapment (Fig. 12-30). Fill the preparation to slight excess so that positive pressure can be applied by the matrix strip. Before the matrix strip is closed, remove any gross excess with a hand instrument. Close and secure the matrix strip as described previously.

If the tooth preparation has a facial access, hold the polyester strip on the lingual aspect of the tooth to be restored with the index finger while the thumb reflects the facial end out of the way. If the wedge protrudes enough to interfere with access, shorten and/or reposition it.

Mix and apply the bonding adhesive as previously described. Follow the same insertion technique with a hand instrument or syringe for the facial approach as with the lingual approach. The procedure is simplified because direct vision can be used.

Insertion of Light-Cured Composites. Most composite materials used for restorative purposes are the light-cured type. Many types of visible light units and brands of light-cured composites are commercially available. Light-cured materials usually include an enamel/dentin bonding system and numerous syringes or self-contained syringe tips (compules) of various shades of composite. No mixing of the visible light-cured materials is necessary unless a shade modification is desired. The operator should not dispense either the bonding adhesive or the composite until they are ready to be used. Both of these materials will begin to harden when exposed to daylight or other lights in the operatory.

The mesial surface of a maxillary left lateral incisor is used to demonstrate facial insertion of a light-cured composite. The matrix strip is contoured, placed interproximally, and wedged at the gingival margin. Secure the lingual aspect of the strip with the index finger while the thumb reflects the facial portion out of the way (Fig. 12-31, *A*). Light-cured materials do not have to be mixed and are not dispensed until ready for use.

Apply the bonding adhesive to the etched enamel and etched/primed dentin with a small foam sponge, microbrush, or applicator tip (see Fig. 12-31, *B*). Distribute this material evenly. Cure the bonding adhesive with the visible light source for 10 to 20 seconds, with the tip near the preparation, but not touching the tooth. Now insert the composite by hand instrument or syringe. Light-cured composites are available in two forms: a threaded syringe for hand instrument insertion or a self-contained compule that is placed into an injection syringe for syringe insertion. If a hand instrument is to be used for insertion, the knurled knob on the back of the syringe is rotated to force material out the other end. An instrument is used to cut off an amount that will restore the preparation, and it is then placed onto a paper pad. The insertion of the composite is then as described for self-cured composites. The material on the paper pad should be protected from ambient light, to prevent premature setting.

If the composite is to be injected directly into the preparation, the selected compule is placed into the injection syringe, the protective cap on the compule removed, and the composite injected into the preparation as described previously. The protective cap should be replaced when the compule is not being used to protect the material from exposure to ambient light.

Once the material has been inserted, cure it through the strip for 20 seconds (see Fig. 12-31, *C*). Do not touch the strip with the tip of the light initially because it could distort the contour of the restoration. Then re-

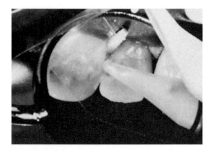

FIG. **12-30** Syringe injection of composite. Air entrapment is minimized by injecting composite starting in remote corner of preparation and by slowly withdrawing tip while it is kept in restorative material during injection. If light-cured, the composite should be injected and cured in 1 to 2 mm increments.

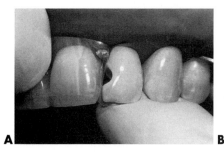 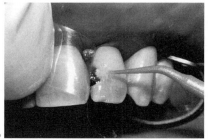 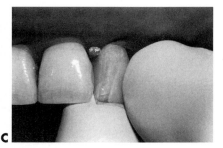

A   B   C

FIG. **12-31** Insertion of light-cured composite. **A,** Lingual aspect of strip is secured with index finger while facial portion is reflected away for access. Bonding adhesive is applied (**B**) and cured. **C,** Following insertion of composite, matrix strip is closed and material is cured through strip.

move the index finger and light-cure on the lingual surface an additional 20 seconds. Longer exposure to the light usually is required for the polymerization of dark and opaque shades. If the restoration is undercontoured, more composite can be added to the previously placed composite and cured. No etching or bonding adhesive is required between layers if the surface has not been contaminated and the oxygen-inhibited layer remains. With large restorations, it is better to add and cure the composite in several increments to reduce the effects of polymerization shrinkage and to ensure more complete curing in remote regions.

Adjacent proximal tooth preparations should be restored one at a time. Techniques have been suggested for inserting two approximating restorations simultaneously, but these procedures may result in matrix movement, poor adaptation, open contact, overhangs, and faulty contours (Fig. 12-32).

If there are two adjacent preparations, restore the preparation with the least access first. Once the matrix strip has been placed and wedged, apply the bonding adhesive and cure . Again, depending on the individual circumstance and operator, insert the composite with either a hand instrument or syringe. If there is too much convexity present on the first proximal restored, the excess must be removed before the second restoration is inserted. If too little contour is present, more material is added to correct the contour. The first restoration should be contoured completely before the second one is started.

Because the second tooth preparation will have been contaminated, it will need to be cleaned, etched, and primed before the adhesive and composite are inserted. During these procedures, a strip should be in place to protect the first restoration and tooth.

Contouring and Polishing the Composite. Good technique and experience in inserting composites significantly reduce the amount of finishing required. Usually a slight excess of material is present that must be removed to provide the final contour and smooth finish. Coarse diamond instruments can be used to remove gross excess, but they generally are not recommended for finishing composites because of the high risk of inadvertently damaging contiguous tooth structure. They also leave a rough surface on the restoration and tooth, as compared to finishing burs and discs. However, special fine diamond finishing instruments are available commercially that can be used to obtain excellent results if the manufacturer's instructions are followed. Care must be exercised with all rotary instruments to prevent damage to the tooth structure, especially at the gingival marginal areas.

Facial Areas. A flame-shaped carbide finishing bur or polishing diamond is recommended for removing excess composite on facial surfaces (Fig. 12-33, *A*). Use medium speed with light intermittent brush strokes and

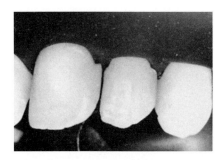

FIG. **12-32** Adjacent restorations, restored simultaneously and displaying faulty contours and gingival overhangs.

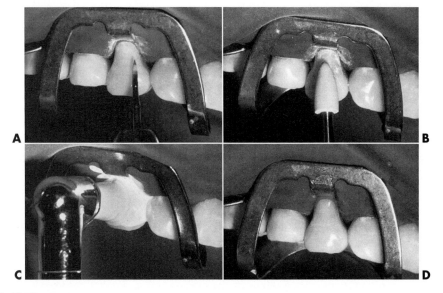

FIG. **12-33** Finishing and polishing. **A,** Flame-shaped finishing bur removing excess and contouring. Rubber polishing point **(B)** and aluminum oxide polishing paste **(C)** used for final polishing. **D,** Completed restoration.

an air coolant for contouring. Final finishing and polishing are achieved with a rubber polishing point (see Fig. 12-33, *B*) and, sometimes, an aluminum oxide polishing paste (see Fig. 12-33, *C* and *D*).

For some locations commercially available abrasive discs (degree of abrasiveness depends on the amount of excess to be removed) mounted on a mandrel specific to the disc type, in an angle handpiece at low speed, can be substituted for or used after the finishing bur or diamond (Fig. 12-34, *A*). An example of a disc system known as Sof-Lex (3M-ESPE, St. Paul, Minnesota) is available for contouring and polishing. These discs are flexible and are produced in several diameters and abrasive textures. Also, Pop-On discs and mandrels (3M-ESPE, St. Paul, Minnesota) are available. This unique design provides a much smaller metal center and allows the disc to be placed on, and removed from, the mandrel without the need for proper orientation. Thin discs with small diameters, such as Super Snap discs (Shofu Dental Corporation, Menlo Park, California), will fit into embrasure areas more easily and are especially useful in contouring and polishing gingival areas. Regardless of the type of disc used, discs are used sequentially from coarse to fine grit, thereby generating a smooth surface.

These discs are rotated at low speed. The external enamel surface should act as a guide for proper contour. A constant shifting motion will aid in contouring and preventing the development of a flat surface. Final polishing is done with a fine grit disc or suitable rubber points or cups. Use rotary instruments very carefully in gingival locations to prevent inadvertent and undesirable removal of tooth structure (see more information in the Class V section).

Lingual Areas. Lingual excess of composite is removed and a smooth surface is produced using a round or oval 12-bladed carbide finishing bur or diamond at medium speed with air coolant and light intermittent pressure (see Fig. 12-34, *B*). The appropriate size and shape used is dependent on the amount of excess and shape of the lingual surface. White stones in various shapes and sizes also may be used for final finishing of the lingual surface.

Proximal and Embrasure Areas. The proximal surface contours and margins should be assessed visually and tactilely with an explorer and dental floss. The floss is positioned below (gingival to) the gingival margin and "shoe-shined" as it is pulled occlusally. If the floss catches or frays, additional finishing is indicated. A sharp gold finishing knife, amalgam knife (Scaler 34/35), or No. 12 surgical blade mounted in a Bard-Parker handle (see Fig. 12-34, *C*) is well suited for removing excess material from the gingival proximal area. The instrument should be moved from the tooth to the restoration or along the margins, using light shaving strokes, keep-

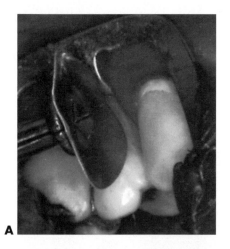

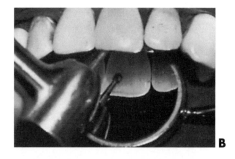

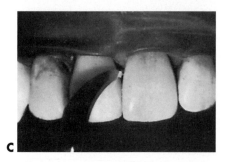

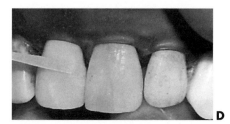

FIG. **12-34** Finishing composites. **A,** Abrasive disc mounted on mandrel can be used for finishing when access permits. **B,** Round carbide finishing bur is well suited for finishing lingual surfaces. **C,** No. 12 surgical blade in Bard-Parker handle can be used for removing interproximal excess. **D,** Abrasive strip should be curved over area to be finished.

ing a portion of the cutting edge on the external enamel surface as a guide to prevent overreduction. If a large amount of composite is removed with one stroke or in the wrong direction, it may fracture inside the tooth preparation and warrant a repair, because the irregular void created may collect plaque and debris and invite discoloration or recurrent caries. Using the secondary cutting edges on the heel aspect of the gold knife or amalgam knife blade in a scraping-pull mode is often preferred over using the primary cutting edge in the shaving mode. The knife blade design having these secondary edges in an arc is very helpful.

A No. 12 surgical blade in a Bard-Parker handle also may be used because the curved shape of the blade and the thin diameter make this instrument ideal for removing gingival overhangs. Gently shave away the excess to avoid removing a large chunk of material unintentionally.

Special carbide finishing burs (Esthetic Trimmers, Brasseler USA, Savannah, Georgia) and carbide hand instruments (Carbide Carvers, Brasseler USA, Savannah, Georgia) can be used for removing excess and opening embrasure areas. Caution must be taken with all instruments not to remove too much contour or to produce a "ledged" contact (a ledge bordering the contact area). All carbide instruments are made of carbon steel and may leave gray marks on the restoration. This discoloration is superficial and is easily removed during the final finishing by abrasive strips or discs (see Fig. 12-34, *D*).

Further contouring and finishing of proximal surfaces can be completed with abrasive finishing strips as well. Some strips have two different types of abrasives (medium and fine) on opposing ends of the strip, with a small area between where no abrasive is present to allow easy and safe insertion of the strip through the contact area. The medium grit is usually zirconium silicate, and the fine grit is generally aluminum oxide. Diamond coated thin metal strips also are commercially available and come in various grits as well. Different widths of the strips are available. A narrow width is usually more appropriate for contouring because it allows more versatility for finishing specific areas. Wide strips tend to flatten the proximal contour, remove too much material at the contact areas, and extend too far gingivally. This results in a poor contour and a weak or absent contact, which must be corrected.

The strip should not be drawn back-and-forth across the restoration in a "sawing" manner. Rather, it should be curved over the restoration and tooth surface in a fashion similar to that used with a shoe-shine cloth, concentrating on areas that need attention (see Fig. 12-34, *D*). To open the lingual embrasure or round the marginal ridge, the lingual part of the strip is held against the composite with the index finger of one hand, while the other end of the strip is pulled facially with the other hand.

Contouring and finishing the proximal surface, including the gingival margin, also develops the general embrasure form around the proximal contact. Further embrasure-form development is accomplished with additional use of flame-shaped 12-bladed carbide finishing burs, diamonds, the amalgam knife, or the No. 12 surgical blade.

Occlusion. Remove the rubber dam if one was used. Evaluate the occlusion by having the patient close lightly on a piece of articulating paper and slide the mandibular teeth over the restored area. If excess composite is present, remove only a small amount at a time and recheck with articulating paper. It is sometimes appropriate to recontour the adjacent and/or opposing natural teeth, although care must be taken not to remove that tooth's centric or functional contact or injudiciously remove too much tooth structure or restorative material.

CLINICAL TECHNIQUE FOR DIRECT CLASS IV COMPOSITE RESTORATIONS

INITIAL CLINICAL PROCEDURES

The same initial procedure considerations presented earlier are appropriate for Class IV restorations. The preoperative assessment of the occlusion is even more important for Class IV restorations because it may influence the tooth preparation extension (placing margins in noncontact areas) and retention and resistance form features (heavy occlusion requires increased retention and resistance form). Thus, occlusal factors may dictate a more conventional tooth preparation form, with more resistance form features (boxlike, flat floors, and walls and floors parallel to the long axis and perpendicular to the occlusal forces) and secondary retention form features (grooves and wider bevels).

Also, proper shade selection may be more difficult for large Class IV restorations that do not have normal dentin colorations. Use of separate translucent or opaque shades of composite may be necessary. Also, the use of a microfill composite as a veneer over a hybrid composite core may provide improved esthetic results. Specific information for esthetic considerations is presented in Chapter 15.

Because it is likely that the proximal contact must be restored, prewedging before tooth preparation will benefit the effort to restore the contact. Finally, for large Class IV lesions or fractures, isolation of the area may be difficult and extension onto the root surface may affect the preparation design.

TOOTH PREPARATION

The Class IV composite restoration has provided the profession with a conservative treatment to restore fractured (Fig. 12-35), defective, or cariously involved anterior teeth when, previously, a porcelain crown may have been the treatment of choice. A brief description of the three types of tooth preparations is presented. However, the conventional tooth preparation design has minimal clinical Class IV application except in those areas that have margins located on root surfaces. The beveled conventional tooth preparation usually is indicated for large Class IV restorations, while the modified tooth preparation is indicated for smaller Class IV needs. If a large amount of tooth structure is missing, groove retention form may be indicated even when the preparation periphery is entirely in enamel. Also, to provide additional retention in high stress areas, the enamel bevels may be increased in width to provide greater surface area for etching, resulting in a stronger bond between the composite and the tooth. Last, to provide appropriate resistance form, the preparation walls may need to be prepared in such a way as to resist occlusal forces. This often requires proximal facial and lingual preparation walls that form 90-degree cavosurface angles, which are subsequently beveled, and a gingival floor prepared perpendicular to the long axis of the tooth. This boxlike form may provide greater resistance to fracture of the restoration and tooth from masticatory forces.

Conventional Class IV Tooth Preparation. As previously noted, there are few indications for this tooth preparation form except for any portion(s) of the restoration extending onto the root. The typical conventional preparation design with 90-degree cavosurface margins is included in the following section on beveled conventional tooth preparations. Remember, however, any portion of any Class IV restoration that extends onto the root requires a 90-degree cavosurface margin and possible groove retention form, regardless of whether either a beveled conventional or modified preparation design is used for the portion of the preparation in the crown of the tooth.

Beveled Conventional Class IV Tooth Preparation. The beveled conventional Class IV tooth preparation is indicated for restoring large proximal areas that also include the incisal surface of an anterior tooth. In addition to the etched enamel margin, retention of the composite restorative material in beveled conventional Class IV tooth preparations may be obtained by groove or other shaped undercuts, dovetail extensions, threaded pins, or a combination of these. All of these features would be part of the final stage of tooth preparation. Gingival and incisal retentive undercuts may be indicated in large Class IV preparations and are similar to those used in the Class III preparation in which rounded undercuts are placed in the dentin along line angles and into point angles wherever possible, without undermining the enamel (see Fig. 12-9, *C* and *D*). An arbitrary dovetail extension onto the lingual surface of the tooth may enhance both the restoration's strength and retention, but it is less conservative and therefore not used often. Incisal and gingival retention and dovetail extension are illustrated in Fig. 12-36.

Although pin retention is sometimes necessary, the use of pins in composite restorations is discouraged for several reasons: (1) the placement of pins in anterior teeth involves the risk of perforation either into the pulp or through the external surface; (2) pins do not enhance the strength of the restorative material;[1] and (3) some pins may corrode because of microleakage of the restoration, resulting in significant discoloration of the tooth and restoration (Fig. 12-37). Despite these disadvantages, when a large amount of tooth structure is missing, pin retention may be necessary to retain the composite restoration.

A maxillary right central incisor is illustrated in Fig. 12-38, *A*. It has large defective Class III restoration and a fractured mesioincisal corner, which upon removal ne-

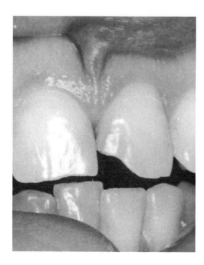

FIG. **12-35** Mesioincisal angle fractured on central incisor.

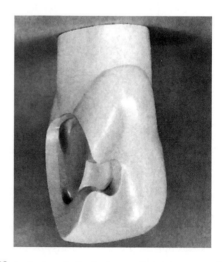

FIG. **12-36** Incisal and gingival retention grooves and dovetail extension in a large Class IV beveled conventional tooth preparation before beveling.

cessitates a Class IV restoration. Class IV beveled conventional tooth preparations are characterized by an outline form that occurs when the preparation walls are prepared as much as possible perpendicular or parallel to the long axis of the tooth. This results in a design that provides greater resistance to biting forces that could cause fracture of the tooth or restorative material. Using an appropriate size round carbide bur or diamond instrument at high speed with air-water coolant, prepare the outline form. Remove all weakened enamel and establish the initial axial wall depth at 0.5 mm into dentin (because groove retention form will likely be utilized). Prepare the walls as much as possible parallel and perpendicular to the long axis of the tooth.

Excavate any remaining infected dentin as the first step of final tooth preparation. If necessary, apply a calcium hydroxide liner. Bevel the cavosurface margin of all accessible enamel margins of the preparation. The bevel is prepared at a 45-degree angle to the external tooth surface with a flame-shaped or round diamond instrument (see Fig. 12-38, B). The width of the bevel should be 0.25 to 2 mm, depending on the amount of tooth structure missing and the retention perceived necessary. Retention form is provided primarily by the micromechanical bonding of the composite to the enamel and dentin. Additional retention may be obtained by increasing the width of the enamel bevels or placing retention undercuts. If retention undercuts are deemed necessary, prepare a gingival retention groove using a No. ¼ round bur. It is prepared 0.2 mm inside the DEJ at a depth of 0.25mm (half the diameter of the No. ¼ bur)

and at an angle bisecting the junction of the axial wall and gingival wall. This groove should extend the length of the gingival floor and slightly up the facioaxial and linguoaxial line angles (see Fig. 12-38, C). No retentive undercut is usually needed at the incisal area, where mostly enamel exists. Fig. 12-38, D, illustrates the completed Class IV beveled conventional tooth preparation.

Modified Class IV Tooth Preparation. The modified Class IV preparation for composite is indicated for small or moderate Class IV lesions or traumatic defects. The objective of the tooth preparation is to remove as little tooth structure as possible, while removing the fault and providing for appropriate retention and resistance

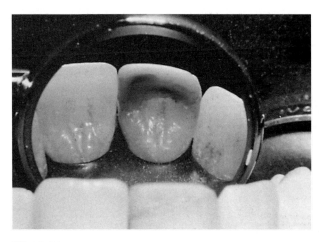

FIG. **12-37** Tooth and restoration discoloration caused by microleakage and subsequent corrosion of pin.

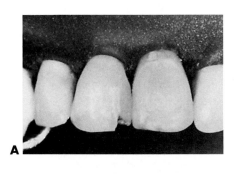
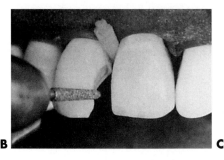
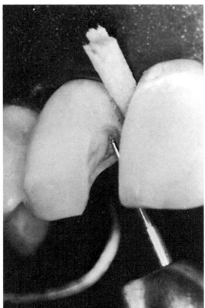
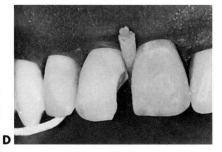

FIG. **12-38** Class IV beveled conventional tooth preparation. **A,** Large defective Class III restoration with resulting fractured incisal angle. **B,** Beveling cavosurface. **C,** Gingival retention groove. **D,** Completed Class IV beveled conventional tooth preparation.

forms. Remove any existing lesion or defective restoration with a suitable size round bur or diamond instrument and prepare the outline form to include weakened, friable enamel. Usually little or no initial tooth preparation is indicated for fractured incisal corners, other than roughening the fractured tooth structure. The cavosurface margins are prepared with a beveled or flared configuration similar to that previously described. The axial depth is dependent on the extent of the lesion, previous restoration, or fracture, but initially no deeper than 0.2 mm inside the DEJ. Usually no groove or cove retention form is indicated. Instead, the retention is obtained primarily from the bonding strength of the composite to the enamel and dentin (see Fig. 12-16, C and D). The treatment of teeth with minor traumatic fractures requires less preparation than the beveled conventional example. If the fracture is confined to enamel, adequate retention usually can be attained by simply beveling sharp cavosurface margins in the fractured area with a flame-shaped diamond instrument followed by bonding (Fig. 12-39).

RESTORATIVE TECHNIQUE

Etching, Priming, and Placing Adhesive. The etching, priming, and placement of adhesive techniques are the same as described for the Class III composite restoration. Also, the same considerations presented previously are appropriate for whether or not the matrix is placed before or after the etching, priming, and adhesive placement.

Matrix Application. The polyester strip matrix also can be used for most Class IV preparations, although the strip's flexibility makes control of the matrix somewhat difficult. This may result in an overcontoured or undercontoured restoration and/or open contact. Also, composite material will extrude incisally, but this excess can be easily removed when contouring and finishing.

Creasing (folding) the matrix at the position of the lingual line angle helps reduce the potential undercontouring (rounding) of that area of the restoration. The matrix is positioned and wedged as described for the Class III composite. Gingival overhangs and open contacts are common with any matrix techniques that do not employ gingival wedging. A commercially available preformed plastic or celluloid crown form is usually too thick and therefore is not recommended as a matrix.

If the operator does not have sufficient experience in using the more flexible polyester strip matrix, the compound-supported matrix may be necessary for large Class IV preparations. To ensure correct proximal contour, a nonyielding compound-supported metal matrix that provides an access area for insertion of the restorative material may be used. A Class IV tooth preparation, facial approach, serves as an example for the application of this type of matrix (Fig. 12-40, A). Cut a piece of dead-soft metal matrix material (Dead Soft Metal Matrix, DenMat Corporation, Santa Maria, California) (.0015 inch [0.04 mm] thick and ⅜ inch [8 mm] wide) to a length of ⅝ inch (16 mm). Then orient, trim, and adjust this strip so that the facial edge protrudes just flush with the facial surface of the tooth (vice versa for lingual access) and the gingival and incisal edges extend beyond the preparation margins at least 1 mm (see Fig. 12-40, B). For facial access the lingual portion of the strip is adapted to the lingual surface of the tooth and a wedge is placed from the facial or lingual embrasure, whichever is greater (see Fig. 12-40, C and D). Burnish proximal contour into the strip with the side of a No. 2 explorer or the back of a Black spoon excavator. An optional wedge technique is the use of a toothpick that is positioned while having a small amount of softened impression compound on its tip (Fig. 12-40, E).

Soften more impression compound over a Bunsen burner and form a small cone. Lightly flame the base and attach to the gloved index finger. Without delay, soften the cone tip over the flame and then press over the lingual area and into the gingival embrasure. It is helpful to hold the matrix strip against the adjacent contact area with a burnisher while the compound is applied. Observe the adaptation of the matrix to the lingual preparation margin through the open facial access and, if needed, correct the proximal contour using the back of a spoon excavator while the compound is still moldable (Fig. 12-40, F). If the compound has hardened,

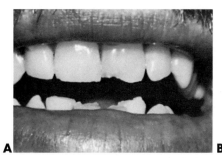
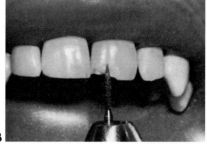
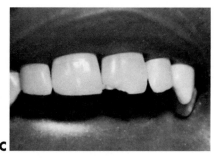

A   **B**   **C**

FIG. **12-39** Class IV modified tooth preparation. **A,** Minor traumatic fracture. **B,** Fractured enamel is roughened with flame-shaped diamond instrument. **C,** Completed Class IV modified tooth preparation.

it may be necessary to soften the compound by using a warmed burnishing instrument on the preparation side of the strip. Also, if a small amount of compound is pressed between the matrix strip and the adjacent tooth, the compound is easily repositioned correctly by the application of a warm burnisher on the preparation side of the matrix in the contact area. It is best to always do this to ensure that the strip is touching the adjacent tooth at contact area. This precaution, coupled with the separation by the wedge, better assures proper contour and proximal contact of the restoration after removal of the matrix. Any compound that may contact the composite during insertion should be removed because it may cause discoloration.

Ample opening is left in the completed matrix to insert the enamel/dentin bonding material and composite from the facial approach as illustrated in Fig. 12-40, G. If a Class IV preparation is to be filled from lingual approach, the position of the matrix is reversed.

Inserting and Curing the Composite. For most Class IV preparations a polyester strip matrix is used as previously described. Following application of the bonding adhesive (if not already applied), insert the composite either with a hand instrument or syringe as described earlier for Class III restorations. Light-cured composite is inserted and cured in 1- to 2-mm increments. Care must

be taken when closing the strip not to pull with excessive force because the soft material will be extruded incisally and result in an undercontoured restoration. If this happens, add composite to restore proper contour and contact.

A compound-supported matrix as previously described may be necessary for large Class IV tooth preparations. When restoring with a self-cured composite, insertion is best accomplished by injecting the material with a syringe. Care must be taken to provide a slight excess of material at the exposed margins to ensure proper contour of the restoration after finishing. A light-cured composite also can be used with a compound-supported matrix for a Class IV restoration. After the bonding adhesive has been applied and cured, insert the composite and cure in increments to ensure complete polymerization and to possibly reduce the effects of polymerization shrinkage. Insertion is best accomplished with a hand instrument, although a syringe can be used. Because light-cured composites possess the advantage of an extended working time, the material can be manipulated and shaped to a considerable degree before curing. Following polymerization, remove the supporting compound and strip. To ensure optimal polymerization, then cure the restoration from both facial and lingual directions.

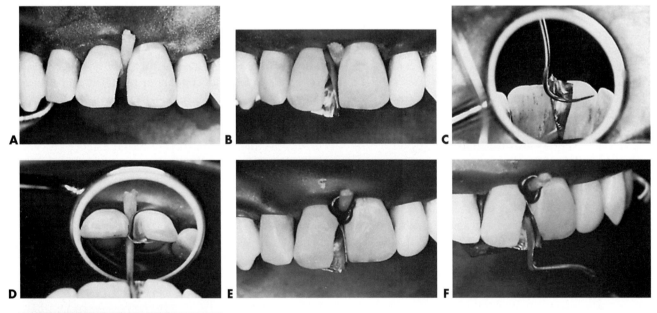

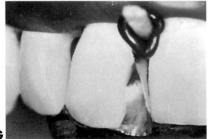

FIG. **12-40** Compound-supported metal matrix. **A,** Class IV tooth preparation to be restored. **B,** Dead-soft metal matrix strip is positioned interproximally. **C,** Metal matrix strip is adapted to lingual margin of tooth preparation. Note that strip extends over lingual margin but does not cover all of lingual surface of the tooth. **D,** Proximal contour of matrix is inspected incisally. **E,** Toothpick having a small amount of softened impression compound on its tip is positioned interproximally. **F,** Compound is applied from lingual approach to matrix and tooth; the back of a warmed spoon excavator can then be used from facial approach to make any necessary corrections to lingual and proximal contours of matrix strip. **G,** Finished compound-supported matrix with facial access.

Contouring and Polishing the Composite. Contouring and finishing the Class IV composite is similar to that described for a Class III composite, except more difficult. The primary difference is the involvement of the incisal corner and edge of the tooth. Contouring and polishing this part of the restoration requires similar procedural steps and close assessment of the incisal edge length and thickness. Also, the potential occlusal relationship may be greater and require more adjustment and refinement.

Thus the facial, lingual, and proximal areas will be contoured and finished as described previously.

CLINICAL TECHNIQUE FOR CLASS V COMPOSITE RESTORATIONS

The clinical indications for using composite for restoring Class V areas relate to all the benefits of bonded composite restorations. However, because isolation of the operating site may be very difficult in cervical areas, esthetically prominent teeth may be more appropriate for composite use than nonesthetic areas. Microfill composites may be selected for restoring Class V defects because their composition results in: (1) increased restoration smoothness, and (2) restoration flexibility when the tooth undergoes cervical flexure. It is thought the microfill composite restoration can flex, rather than debond, when the tooth flexes under heavy occlusal forces.[3]

INITIAL CLINICAL PROCEDURES

Anesthesia is usually necessary when restoring a Class V lesion. Before the tooth preparation is initiated, select the shade of the composite material, as previously discussed, and then isolate the operating area. During shade selection remember that the tooth is darker in the cervical third. Isolation may be achieved by a rubber dam and No. 212 retainer or with a cotton roll(s) and retraction cord as previously described in Chapter 10. Often cotton roll and/or retraction cord isolation is used.

TOOTH PREPARATION

Class V tooth preparations, by definition, are located in the gingival one third of the facial and lingual tooth surfaces. Because of esthetic considerations, composite materials most frequently are used for the restoration of Class V lesions in anterior teeth. Numerous factors must be taken into consideration in material selection, including esthetics, caries activity, access to the lesion, moisture control, and patient age. In fact, increased patient age is particularly important when considering the treatment of Class V root-surface lesions (see Chapter 9).

As stated in Chapter 1, the older adult component of the U.S. population will continue to increase. Furthermore, older adults will retain more of their teeth and experience gingival recession as they age. With more older adults having more root surfaces exposed, the prevalence of root caries and/or cervical erosion or abrasion defects will increase. Therefore the number of indicated Class V restorations also will increase. Because most of these restorative needs will involve root surfaces, careful consideration should be given to the restorative material to be used. The consideration for use of materials other than composite is intensified when it is realized that the older patient may present other factors that further complicate the use of composite on the root surfaces. These factors would include decreased salivary function, decreased motivation and ability for homecare, increased difficulty in adequately isolating the operating area, and increased difficulty in performing the operative procedure because of the patient's physical or medical problems. In spite of these concerns, the use of composite as a restorative material for Class V lesions will still predominate in areas of esthetic concern. Subsequently, the various tooth-preparation options are presented.

Conventional Class V Tooth Preparation. The conventional Class V tooth preparation for composite is indicated for that portion of a carious lesion or defect entirely or partially on the facial or lingual root surface of a tooth. The preparation form would be similar to that described in Chapter 18 (Class V Amalgam). The features of the preparation include a 90-degree cavosurface angle; uniform depth of the axial line angles; and, sometimes, groove retention form.

Because many Class V carious lesions or defects will have some enamel at the incisal (occlusal) and possibly the mesial and/or distal margins, the conventional composite tooth preparation design is indicated only for the portion of the lesion or defect extending onto the root surface. The enamel marginal areas are prepared using either a beveled conventional or modified preparation design as described in the following sections of this chapter. However, occasionally a Class V lesion/defect is located entirely on the root of the tooth requiring the use of a conventional preparation design exclusively. The following description of a conventional tooth preparation pertains to such a restoration that is located entirely on the root surface of a tooth (Fig. 12-41, A).

A tapered fissure carbide bur (No. 700, 701, or 271) or similarly shaped diamond is used at high speed with air-water spray. If access interproximally or gingivally is limited, a No. 1 or No. 2 round bur or diamond may be used to prepare the tooth. When a tapered fissure bur or diamond is used, make entry at a 45-degree angle to the tooth surface by tilting the handpiece distally; however, as the cutting progresses distally, maneuver the handpiece to thereafter maintain the bur's long axis perpendicular to the external surface of the tooth during preparation of the outline form, which should result in 90-degree cavosurface margins. At this initial tooth preparation stage, the extensions in every direction are to sound tooth structure, except the axial depth should only be 0.75 mm (see Fig. 12-41, B). The tip of the bur may be rotating in air, caries, or old restorative material

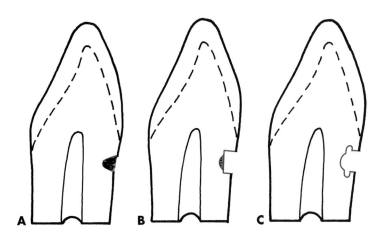

FIG. **12-41** Conventional Class V tooth preparation. **A,** Lesion entirely on root surface. **B,** Initial tooth preparation with 90-degree cavosurface margins and axial wall depth of 0.75 mm. **C,** Remaining infected dentin excavated and incisal and gingival retention form prepared.

while establishing this initial depth. Any infected dentin remaining on this initial axial wall will be removed during the final stage of tooth preparation. Any old restorative material remaining may or may not be removed according to the concepts stated previously. The 0.75 mm axial wall depth will provide adequate external wall width for: (1) strength of the preparation wall; (2) strength of the composite; and (3) placement of a retention groove, if necessary. When the desired distal extension is obtained, move the bur mesially, incisally (occlusally), and gingivally for indicated extensions, while maintaining the proper initial depth and keeping the bur's long axis perpendicular to the root surface. The axial wall should follow the original contour of the facial surface, which is convex outward mesiodistally and sometimes occlusogingivally. The outline form extension of the mesial, distal, occlusal (incisal), and gingival walls is dictated by the extent of the caries, defect, or old restorative material indicated for replacement (sometimes the new material will abut a still satisfactory, old restoration). All of the external preparation walls of a Class V conventional tooth preparation are visible when viewed from a facial position (outwardly divergent walls).

Final tooth preparation for the conventional preparation consists of the following steps: (1) removing remaining infected dentin or old restorative material (if indicated) on the axial wall; (2) applying a calcium hydroxide liner, only if necessary; and (3) sometimes preparing groove retention form.

If retention grooves are necessary, they are prepared with a No. ¼ bur along the full length of the gingivo-axial and incisoaxial (occlusoaxial) line angles. These grooves are prepared 0.25 mm in depth into the external walls and next to the axial wall at an angle that bisects the junction between the axial wall and the gingival or occlusal (or incisal) wall. This should leave, between the groove and the margin, sufficient remaining wall dimension (0.25 mm) to prevent fracture (see Fig. 12-41, C). It is helpful while preparing the grooves to observe that this remaining wall dimension is equal to half the di-

ameter of the bur head (which is 0.5 mm). Clean the preparation, if indicated, and inspect for final approval.

Beveled Conventional Class V Tooth Preparation. The beveled conventional Class V tooth preparation has beveled enamel margins and is indicated either for: (1) the replacement of an existing, defective Class V restoration that initially used a conventional preparation or (2) for a large, new carious lesion. The beveled conventional Class V preparation initially will exhibit 90-degree cavosurface margins (that subsequently will be beveled) and an axial wall that is uniform in depth (see Fig. 12-9, E and F). The axial depth into dentin is only 0.2 mm when groove retention is judged unnecessary and 0.5 mm when a retention groove is planned and the margin is still in enamel. However, groove retention usually is not indicated when the periphery of the tooth preparation is located in enamel. Many of these larger preparations will be a combination of beveled enamel margins and 90-degree root-surface (nonenamel) margins, with the root-surface areas having groove retention. Thus they are combined beveled conventional and conventional preparations. As stated previously, for the preparation portion on the root surface, the depth of the axial wall should be 0.75 mm.

The advantages of the beveled conventional tooth preparation as compared to the conventional tooth preparation are: (1) increased retention due to the greater surface area of etched enamel afforded by the bevel, (2) decreased microleakage due to the enhanced bond between the composite and the tooth, and (3) decreased need for groove retention form (and consequently less removal of tooth structure).

The typical outline form for a Class V lesion in enamel is seen in Fig. 12-42. Prepare the outline form as described in the preceding section with the initial axial wall depth only 0.2 mm into dentin when groove retention is unnecessary (Fig. 12-43).

Complete the following steps of final tooth preparation: (1) remove any remaining infected dentin, and, if indicated, remove any old restorative material; (2) apply a calcium hydroxide liner, but only if necessary; (3) usually prepare a gingival retention groove if either the gingival margin is located on the root surface or the preparation is large enough to warrant groove retention form; and (4) bevel the enamel margins. The bevel on the enamel margin is accomplished with a flame-shaped or round diamond instrument, resulting in an angle approximately 45 degrees to the external tooth surface and prepared to a width of 0.25 to 0.5 mm. A completed beveled conventional Class V preparation is shown in Fig. 12-44.

An even more conservative approach may be used when extending the outline form of beveled conventional Class V preparations. Fig. 12-18, *A*, illustrates a path of a decalcified enamel lesion (in enamel only) having a broken, rough surface that extends mesially and/or distally from the cavitated lesion (or failing existing restoration). After preparation of the cavitated le-

sion (or failing restoration), extend the margins of the preparation to include these areas of decalcification by using a round diamond instrument to prepare the cavosurface margin in the form of a chamfer, extended only in the enamel to a depth that removes the defect. A completed beveled conventional preparation of this type is illustrated in Fig. 12-18, *B*.

When a large Class V carious lesion or faulty restoration extends onto the root surface, the gingival wall is prepared in the same manner as a conventional Class V tooth preparation (i.e., butt joint, usually with a dentinal retention groove). The depth of the initial preparation on the root surface should be only 0.75 mm. Only the enamel cavosurface margins are beveled. A completed combination of a Class V beveled conventional with a conventional tooth preparation extending onto the root surface is illustrated in Fig. 12-45.

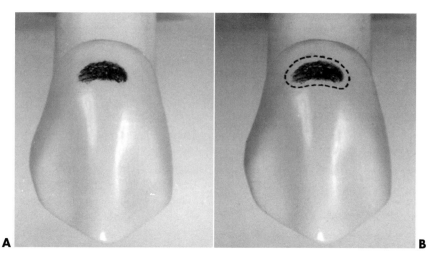

A   **B**

FIG. **12-42 A,** Class V caries. **B,** Typical outline form.

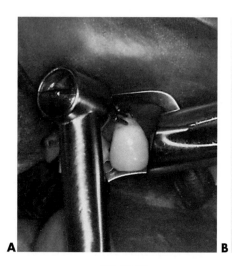
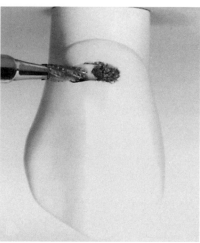
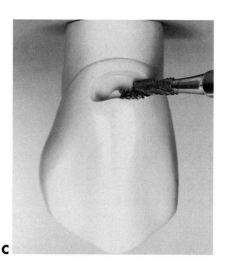

A   **B**   **C**

FIG. **12-43** Initiating a beveled conventional Class V tooth preparation. **A,** Operating position and equipment. Entry with No. 701 bur or tapered diamond held at 45-degree angle to tooth surface. **B,** As cutting proceeds distally (0.2 mm into dentin), bur shank is held perpendicular to enamel surface. **C,** Mesial extension, keeping bur shank perpendicular to surface and maintaining initial depth.

Modified Class V Tooth Preparation. The modified Class V tooth preparation is indicated for the restoration of small and moderate Class V lesions or defects. The objective is to restore the lesion or defect as conservatively as possible. Therefore, there is no effort to prepare the walls as butt joints and usually no groove retention is incorporated. The lesion or defect is "scooped" out, resulting in a preparation form that may have a divergent wall configuration and an axial surface that usually is not uniform in depth (see Fig. 12-16, *E* and *F*). Class V modified preparations are ideal for small enamel defects or small, but cavitated lesions that are largely or entirely in enamel (Fig. 12-46, *A*). These include decalcified and hypoplastic areas located in the cervical one third of the teeth.

After the usual preliminary procedures, prepare initial tooth preparation with a round or elliptical diamond instrument (see Fig. 12-46, *B*), eliminating all of the enamel lesion or defect. The preparation is only extended into dentin when the defect warrants such extension, and at this initial stage is prepared no deeper than 0.2 mm into dentin (because no groove retention form will be used). No effort is made to prepare 90-degree cavosurface margins.

If infected dentin remains, it is removed with a round bur or spoon excavator. Apply a calcium hydroxide liner, but only if indicated. The completed preparation with etched enamel and etched and primed dentin can be seen in Fig. 12-46, *C*.

Class V Tooth Preparation for Abrasion/Erosion Lesions. Class V modified tooth preparations also are used to restore abraded or eroded cervical areas. Abrasion, in the form of a notch, often V-shaped, is a loss or wearing away of tooth structure due to mechanical forces, such as strenuous toothbrushing with a hard bristle toothbrush or abrasive toothpaste.[6] Erosion, often a saucer-shaped notch, occurs primarily as a result of chemical dissolution (e.g., sustained exposure to citric acid [juices] or vomitus).[4] Idiopathic erosion or abfraction may occur as a result of flexure of the cervical area under heavy occlusal stress, beginning with microfrac-

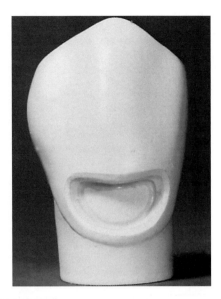

FIG. **12-44** Completed large beveled conventional Class V preparation.

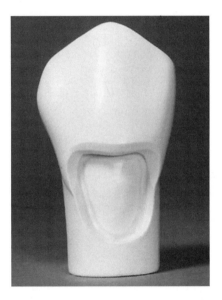

FIG. **12-45** Completed Class V tooth preparation extending onto the root; crown portion beveled conventional design; root portion conventional design.

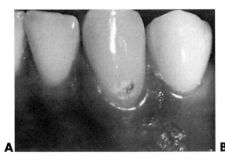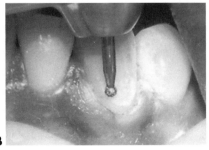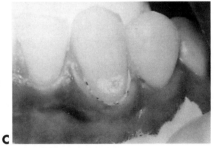

FIG. **12-46** Modified Class V tooth preparation. **A,** Small cavitated Class V lesion. **B,** Surrounding enamel defect is prepared with round diamond instrument. **C,** Completed modified tooth preparation after acid-etching.

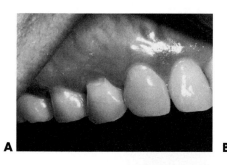
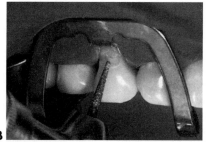
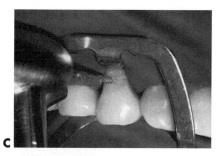

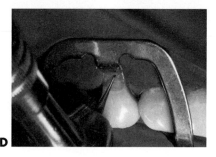
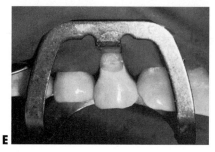

FIG. **12-47** Class V tooth preparation for abrasion/erosion lesions. **A,** Preoperative notched lesion. **B** through **D,** Beveling the enamel margin, roughening the internal walls, and placing retention groove. **E,** Completed preparation with etched enamel.

ture of the thin enamel tooth structure occlusal of the cementoenamel junction, which, when combined with abrasive toothbrushing, could produce a "notched" defect.[5] These notches are progressive, enlarging with time if the causative factor is not eliminated.

When notching occurs (Fig 12-47, *A*) the operator first must decide, with input from the patient, whether or not the area needs to be restored. This decision is based on the considerations discussed in the following sections.

Caries. If caries is present, the defect should be restored unless the lesion is incipient and very superficial. For the incipient root-caries lesion, treatment may consist only of minor recontouring of the area (cementoplasty) and application of a topical fluoride or bonding adhesive. (Most erosion and abrasion notches are not carious.)

Gingival Health. If the notched defect is determined to be causing gingival inflammation (i.e., plaque retention) and/or further gingival recession is anticipated, the notched defect should be restored. (Usually, however, gingival health is excellent, with the notching having occurred after gingival recession.)

Esthetics. If the notched area is in an esthetically critical position, the patient may elect to have the area restored with a tooth-colored restoration.

Sensitivity. If the notched area is very sensitive, application of a dentin bonding agent or desensitizing agent may, at least temporarily, reduce or eliminate the sensitivity. Continuing sensitivity may require restoration of the area.

Pulp Protection. If the notched area is very large and deep pulpally, the restoration of the defect may be indi-

cated to avoid further defect development that may cause a pulpal exposure.

Tooth Strength. If the notched area is very large or deep, the strength of the tooth at the cervical area may be compromised. Placement of a bonded restoration will eliminate further progression of the defect and may restore some of the lost strength.

The tooth preparation for a Class V abrasion or erosion area usually requires only roughening of the internal walls with a diamond instrument; beveling or flaring all enamel margins; and, sometimes, placing a retention groove in nonenamel areas (see Fig. 12-47, *A* through *C*). If necessary, prepare the root-surface cavosurface margins to approximately 90 degrees. Often the inherent form of an abraded/eroded lesion will result in no need for further preparation of root-surface cavosurface margins. Although success may be obtained without placement of the groove retention form, greater restoration retention may be provided when the retentive groove is utilized. Moreover, greater resistance to marginal leakage results from groove placement, because this retentive feature assists in resisting the effects of polymerization shrinkage and tooth flexure.[7] The completed preparation with etched enamel is seen in Fig. 12-47, *E*.

Tooth Preparation for Aberrant Smooth Surface Pit Fault. Occasionally a tooth surface that normally is smooth will have a pit in the enamel (Fig. 12-48, *A*). Most aberrant pit faults in enamel are restored best with use of a modified preparation. For such a preparation for an aberrant pit fault, the outline form (includes extensions and depth) is dictated by the extent of the fault and/or caries lesion. Faults existing entirely in enamel

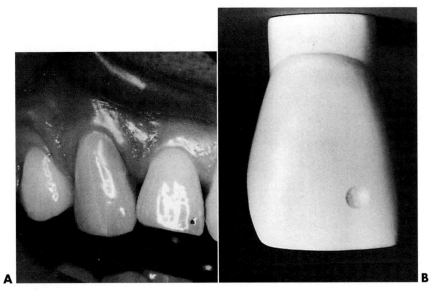

FIG. **12-48** **A,** Faulty pit on facial surface of maxillary incisor. **B,** Modified tooth preparation for enamel pit defect.

are prepared with an appropriately sized round diamond instrument by merely eliminating the defect (see Fig. 12-48, *B*). Adequate retention is obtained by etching the enamel (the first step in applying restorative materials). When the defect includes carious dentin, the infected portion is removed also, leaving a flared enamel margin.

RESTORATIVE TECHNIQUE

No matrix is needed for restoring preparations for which the contour can be controlled as the composite restorative material is being inserted, such as in the Class V restoration. This is especially true when using a light-cured material that has an extended working time, which permits the operator to initiate contouring of the restoration in the unpolymerized state.

Etching, Priming, and Placing Adhesive. The etching, priming, and placement of adhesive techniques are the same as previously described.

Inserting and Curing the Composite. A self-cured or light-cured composite can be inserted with a hand instrument or syringe. Self-cured composites are seldom used for Class V restorations because of the advantages of light-cured composites. In spite of that, the following describes the use of self-cured composites for Class V restorations. Recall that microfill composites also may be recommended for Class V restorations.

Because no matrix is used, care must be exercised to avoid having excess bonding adhesive because it tends to act as a lubricant within the preparation, and makes insertion more difficult. Wipe a small portion of mixed self-cured composite into the preparation with the blade of the hand instrument and vibrate to place with the plugger end. The tip can be lubricated with a sparing amount of bonding adhesive. Usually a second increment is needed and sufficient to slightly overfill the preparation. Remove the excess first at the gingival cavosurface margin with the tine of a No. 2 explorer or the blade of a composite instrument, the tip of which is on unprepared tooth structure, gingival to the prepared margin. If the composite begins to harden before contouring is complete, further contouring should not be attempted at this stage.

A light-cured material is recommended for most Class V preparations because of the extended working time and control of contour before polymerization. Less finishing is usually required. This feature is particularly valuable when restoring large preparations or preparations with margins located on cementum, because rotary instrumentation can easily damage contiguous tooth structure.

The restoration of an abrasion/erosion lesion (Fig. 12-49, *A*) will illustrate proper insertion technique for a light-cured material. Following etching and priming steps for enamel and dentin (per manufacturer's instructions), place a thin layer of bonding adhesive and cure (see Fig. 12-49, *B*). Then insert the composite incrementally with a hand instrument or syringe (see Fig. 12-49, *C*). Fill deep preparations having retentive undercuts in at least two increments. First, insert a small amount of material in the retentive undercuts and cure. Second, fill the outer portion of the preparation and shape the material as close to the final contour as possible. An explorer or blade of a composite instrument is useful in

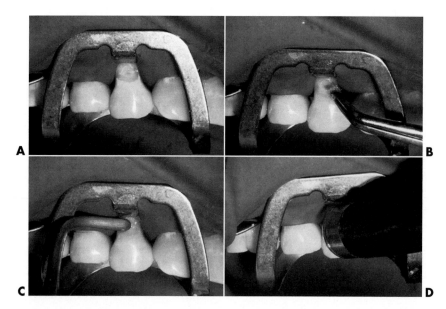

FIG. **12-49** Restoration of abrasion/erosion lesion. **A,** Tooth preparation. **B,** Bonding adhesive applied. **C,** Material inserted incrementally. **D,** Restoration cured with visible light source.

removing excess material from the cervical margin and obtaining the final contour. Then apply the light source for polymerization (see Fig. 12-49, *D*). The restoration should require very little finishing.

Contouring and Polishing the Composite. A flame-shaped carbide finishing bur or polishing diamond is recommended for removing excess composite on the facial surface of a Class V composite (see Fig. 12-33, *A*). Use medium speed with light intermittent brush strokes and an air coolant for contouring. Final finishing and polishing are achieved with a rubber polishing point (see Fig. 12-33, *B*) or cup and, sometimes, an aluminum oxide polishing paste (see Fig. 12-33, *C* and *D*).

For some locations, abrasive discs, as stated earlier, (degree of abrasiveness depends on the amount of excess to be removed) mounted on an appropriate mandrel in an angle handpiece at low speed can be used (see Fig. 12-34, *A*). The disc is rotated at low speed. The external enamel surface should act as a guide for proper contour. A constant shifting motion will aid in contouring and preventing the development of a flat surface. A fine-grit disc is used for final polishing.

Use rotary instruments very carefully in gingival locations (especially on the root surface) to prevent inadvertent and undesirable removal of tooth structure (usually cementum and dentin). Finely pointed rotary instruments (finishing burs or diamonds) are difficult to use to remove gingival margin excess. Because of the convexity that typically exists in this area, a more rounded rotary instrument (a fine diamond) may remove the excess with less potential to damage the unprepared root surface. Likewise, sandpaper or polishing discs used on the root

surface can cause ditching of the cementum if not used correctly.

MICROFILL COMPOSITE RESTORATIONS

Microfill composites are indicated primarily for small Class III, Class V, and partial veneer restorations. They are not typically used for Class I or Class II restorations because, even though some may have good wear resistance, they may have a greater tendency to fracture under occlusal load. The advantage of the microfill composite is that it is very esthetic, very smooth, and tends to flex with the tooth when used in abfracture lesions.

The disadvantage of these materials is that because of decreased filler amount, their physical properties are usually not as good as hybrid composites.

CLINICAL TECHNIQUE

The clinical technique for a microfill composite is very similar to a composite restoration. The initial considerations, tooth preparation, and most of the restorative technique are similar. The differences are that the microfill composite, because it is more viscous, is not as injectable as other composites, and contouring and finishing procedures are slightly different.

Although generally the same technique used for finishing conventional and hybrid composites apply to finishing microfill composites, certain differences do exist. Conventional and hybrid composites exhibit an opaque appearance during dry finishing, making the preparation margin easy to distinguish. Because microfill composites possess a surface luster similar to that of tooth enamel, it is more difficult to detect when the restoration has been finished back to the margin. Also, because less inorganic filler is present in microfill composites, finishing burs tend to clog and need periodic débridement.

Although conventional finishing techniques produce a smooth surface texture with microfill composites, a higher luster can be attained by using various discs, rubber points, or cups that are specifically made for polishing these materials.

GLASS-IONOMER RESTORATIONS

As noted earlier, glass ionomers possess the favorable quality of releasing fluoride when exposed to the oral environment.[8,10] This property may render glass-ionomer restorations more resistant to recurrent caries. Because of this potential anticariogenic quality, glass ionomer may be the material of choice for restoring root-surface caries in patients with high caries activity and where esthetics is not as critical. (See Chapter 4 for types of glass ionomers and compomers.)

Both self-cured and light-cured versions of glass ionomers are available. Resin-modified, light-cured glass ionomers are preferred because of both the extended working time and their improved physical properties and esthetic qualities. Also, resin-modified, light-cured glass ionomers tend to be more resistant to dehydration and cracking during setting than are conventional self-cured versions.

Conventional glass ionomers are not as esthetic as composite restorations, and glass ionomers are not usually recommended for use in areas of significant esthetic concern. However, resin-modified, light-cured versions of glass ionomers and compomers (poly-acid–modified composites) contain some resin and possess improved esthetic qualities, as well as other improved physical properties. In fact, these types of materials may be used in some esthetically demanding areas.

Because of their limited strength and wear resistance, glass ionomers are indicated generally for the restoration of low stress areas (not for typical Classes I, II, or IV restorations), where caries activity potential is of significant concern. In addition to glass ionomers being indicated for root-surface caries in Class V locations, slot-like preparations in either Classes II or III cervical locations (not involving the proximal contact) may be restored with glass ionomers if access permits.

The restoration of root-caries lesions in older patients or those with high caries activity is the primary indication for the use of glass ionomer. Notched cervical defects of idiopathic erosion, or abrasion origin (or any combination) also are well-suited for restoration with glass ionomers, if esthetic demands are not critical. The tooth preparations for either of these clinical indications are the same as previously described for composite restorations (see Figs. 12-41, 12-45, and 12-47). Older patients and those with high caries activity who have gingival recession also may experience carious lesions on the proximal root surfaces. Gingival recession sometimes provides access to this type of carious lesion from the facial or lingual direction, allowing a slot preparation to be used. The same slot preparation design used for amalgam is used for glass ionomers. (The reader is referred to the section on slot preparations in Chapters 13 and 17 and Fig. 12-4 for specific details.) With the exception of the matrix utilized (if needed), slot preparations for Classes II and III restorations are restored in a similar manner to a Class V preparation.

CLINICAL TECHNIQUE

Following preparation of the tooth, deeply excavated areas (within 0.5 mm of the pulp) may need protection with a calcium hydroxide liner. Most conventional glass-ionomer systems require etching the dentinal surfaces to remove the smear layer, thereby effecting improved adhesion of the glass ionomer to the dentin. To etch the dentin, a mild acid such as 10% polyacrylic acid is placed in the preparation for approximately 20 seconds, followed by rinsing and removal of excess water, leaving the dentin moist. It should be noted that not all glass-ionomer systems require dentin etching. Additionally, some resin-modified glass ionomers and all compomers use an intermediary bonding agent to facilitate bonding. Each glass-ionomer and compomer system should be used strictly according to the manufacturer's specific instructions.

Most conventional glass-ionomer systems are quite technique sensitive. Original glass ionomers usually required carefully mixing a powder and liquid within 30 seconds to optimize powder incorporation (higher powder/liquid ratio). Encapsulated versions for triturator mixing are available also. Such systems are recommended because they optimize and simplify the mixing procedure and facilitate insertion through direct injection into the preparation.

Self-cured glass-ionomer material should be placed into the preparation in slight excess and quickly shaped with a composite instrument. Clear plastic cervical matrices also are available for providing contour to the restoration. If a conventional type of glass ionomer is used, place a thin coat of light-cured resin bonding agent on the surface immediately after placement to prevent dehydration and cracking of the restoration during the initial setting phase. As noted earlier, new light-cured hybrid type glass ionomers are more resistant to dehydration and do not typically require this step. If a resin-modified, light-cured glass ionomer is used, cure for a minimum time of 40 seconds.

Conventional versions of glass ionomers ideally require a polymerization period of 24 hours before final contouring and finishing. However, most resin-modified,

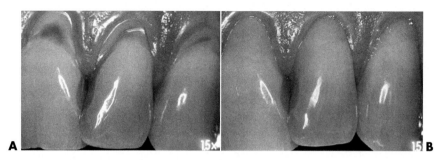

FIG. **12-50** Glass-ionomer cement. Three typical light-cured glass-ionomer restorations are shown before **(A)** and after **(B)** treatment.

light-cured glass ionomers available can be contoured and finished immediately after light-curing. (The manufacturer's recommendations should be followed to optimize clinical performance of the material.) Once the material has set, the matrix, if used, is removed and the gross excess is shaved away with either a No. 12 surgical blade in a Bard-Parker handle or other appropriately shaped knives or scalers. As much as possible of the contouring and finishing should be accomplished with hand instruments, while striving to preserve the smooth surface that occurs upon setting. If rotary instrumentation is needed, care must be taken not to dehydrate the surface of the restoration. Micron finishing diamonds used with a petroleum lubricant to prevent desiccation are ideal for contouring and finishing conventional glass ionomers. Also, flexible abrasive discs used with a lubricant can be very effective. A fine grit aluminum oxide polishing paste applied with a prophy cup is used to impart a smooth surface. Three typical resin-modified, light-cured glass-ionomer restorations are shown before and after treatment in Fig. 12-50, *A* and *B*.

SUMMARY

This chapter presents techniques and rationales for the use of composite and other tooth-colored materials for Classes III, IV, and V restorations. It should be apparent that composite is the material of choice for most Class III and Class IV restorations and most esthetically demanding Class V restorations. When done correctly, composite restorations provide excellent dental treat-

ment in those clinical situations. Common problems, potential solutions, and repair techniques for these types of restorations were presented in Chapter 11.

REFERENCES

1. Dilts WE, Podshadley A, Neiman R: Effect of pins on some physical characteristics of composite resins, *J Am Dent Assoc* 87:595, 1973.
2. Ehrnford L, Derand: Cervical gap formation in Class II composite resin restorations, *Swed Dent J* 8:15-19, 1984.
3. Heymann HO et al: Examining tooth flexure effects on cervical restorations: a two-year clinical study, *J Am Dent Assoc* 122: 41-47, 1991.
4. Jaärvinen VK, Rytömaa II, Heinonen OP: Risk factors in dental erosion, *J Dent Res* 70(6):942-947, 1991.
5. Lee WC, Eakle WS: Possible role of tensile stress in the etiology of cervical erosive lesions of teeth, *J Prosthet Dent* 52(3): 374-380, 1984.
6. Mair LH: Wear in dentistry: current terminology, *J Dent* 20: 140-144, 1992.
7. Monteiro S Jr et al: Evaluation of materials and techniques for restoration of erosion areas, *J Prosthet Dent* 55:434-442, 1986.
8. Mount GJ: Adhesion of glass-ionomer cement in the clinical environment, *Oper Dent* 16:141-148, 1991.
9. Silverstone LM, Dogan IL, editors: *Proceedings of the international symposium on the acid etch technique,* St Paul, Minn, 1975, North Central Publishing.
10. Swift EJ Jr: Effects of glass ionomers on recurrent caries, *Oper Dent* 14:40-43, 1989.
11. Torstenson B, Brännström M: Composite resin contraction gaps measured with a fluorescent resin technique, *Dent Mater* 4:238-242, 1988.

Classes I, II, and VI Direct Composite and Other Tooth-Colored Restorations

THEODORE M. ROBERSON

HARALD O. HEYMANN

ANDRÉ V. RITTER

PATRICIA N.R. PEREIRA

CLASSES I, II, AND VI COMPOSITE RESTORATIONS

This chapter presents information about typical Classes I, II, and VI composite restorations (Fig. 13-1). Posterior composite restorations were introduced in the mid-1960s.[20,21] Because of the improved physical properties of composite and bonding systems,[4,14,26,29,30] studies continuously reported encouraging results for their use in posterior teeth.[5,6,18,19] Further improvements have demonstrated that many Class I and Class II restorations are now indications for composite use. In fact, the American Dental Association (ADA)[2] has indicated the appropriateness of composites for use as pit-and-fissure sealants, preventive resins, and Classes I and II restorations for both initial and moderately sized lesions, using modified conservative tooth preparations. If composites are used as recommended, the ADA further states that "when used correctly in the primary and permanent dentition, the expected lifetime of resin-based composites can be comparable to that of amalgam in Class I, Class II, and Class V restorations."[1]

Before presenting the technique for Classes I and II composite restorations, the following sections provide reasons for their increased usage. This chapter also presents information and techniques for other treatment modalities involving the direct restoration of occlusal surfaces of posterior teeth. These include pit-and-fissure sealants, preventive resin or conservative composite restorations, Class VI restorations, extensive Class II restorations, and foundations.

PERTINENT MATERIAL QUALITIES AND PROPERTIES

As presented in Chapter 11, composite is a material that has sufficient strength for Class I and Class II restorations. It is insulative and therefore does not require pulpal protection with bases. Because composite is bonded to the enamel and dentin, tooth preparations for composite can be very conservative. A composite restoration not only is retained well in the tooth, but also strengthens the remaining unprepared tooth structure. Classes I and II composite restorations also have all the other bonding benefits presented in Chapter 11.

INDICATIONS

The following clinical indications are for composite restorations in Classes I and II.

1. Small and moderate restorations, preferably with enamel margins
2. Most premolar or first molar restorations, particularly when esthetics is considered
3. A restoration that does not provide all of the occlusal contacts
4. A restoration that does not have heavy occlusal contacts
5. A restoration that can be appropriately isolated during the procedure
6. Some restorations that may serve as foundations for crowns
7. Some very large restorations that are used to strengthen remaining weakened tooth structure (for economic or interim use reasons)

CONTRAINDICATIONS

Classes I and II composites may be contraindicated for restorations in the following instances:

1. When the operating site cannot be appropriately isolated
2. With heavy occlusal stresses
3. With all the occlusal contacts only on composite
4. In restorations that extend onto the root surface (see next paragraph.)

The extension onto the root surface (no marginal enamel) may be a contraindication for a composite restoration. For many extensions onto the root surface with composite

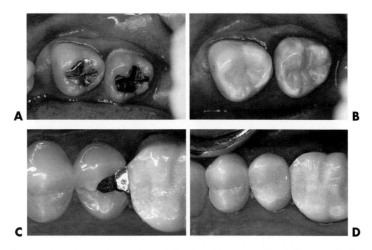

FIG. **13-1** Composite restorations. **A** and **B,** Class I composite, before and after. **C** and **D,** Class II composite, before and after.

restorations, a V-shaped gap (contraction gap) is formed between the root and the composite.[9,28] This contraction gap occurs because the force of polymerization shrinkage of the composite is greater than the initial bond strength of the composite to the dentin of the root. The V-shaped gap is probably composed of composite on the restoration side and hybridized dentin on the root side, as seen in Fig. 13-2. It is not known what the long-term clinical effects of these gaps may be. Regardless, it should be recognized that whenever a restoration extends onto the root surface there may be negative effects for the restoration no matter what restorative material is being used. For example, even high copper amalgam restorations will exhibit some marginal leakage, at least for a short period of time. Thus any extension onto the root surface requires the best and most meticulous efforts of the operator to best ensure a successful, long-lasting restoration.

ADVANTAGES

The advantages of composite as a Class I or Class II restorative material are:

1. Esthetics
2. Conservative tooth structure removal
3. Easier, less complex tooth preparation
4. Economics (compared to crowns and indirect tooth-colored restorations)
5. Insulation
6. Bonding benefits
   • Decreased microleakage
   • Decreased recurrent caries
   • Decreased postoperative sensitivity
   • Increased retention
   • Increased strength of remaining tooth structure[3,16]

DISADVANTAGES

The disadvantages of Class I and Class II composite restorations are:

1. Material related
   • Greater localized wear[7,17]
   • Polymerization shrinkage effects
   • Linear coefficient of thermal expansion (LCTE)[8]
   • Biocompatibility of some components unknown

2. Require more time to place
3. More technique sensitive
   • Etching, priming, adhesive placement
   • Inserting composite
   • Developing proximal contacts
   • Finishing and polishing
4. More expensive than amalgam restorations

This chapter presents the techniques for treating the occlusal and proximal areas of posterior teeth with composite and other directly placed tooth-colored materials. The least invasive treatments are presented first, followed by progressively more involved methods of treatment. Consequently, first the rationale and technique for pit-and-fissure sealants, preventive resin or conservative composite restorations, and Class VI composite restorations are presented. Next, the typical Class I and Class II composite restorations are presented, followed by more extensive Class II restorations, including composite foundations.

PIT-AND-FISSURE SEALANTS, PREVENTIVE RESIN AND CONSERVATIVE COMPOSITE RESTORATIONS, AND CLASS VI COMPOSITE RESTORATIONS

As detailed in Chapter 9, before any treatment is rendered, a thorough diagnosis must be made and many factors assessed. In assessing the occlusal surfaces of posterior teeth, the primary decision is whether or not a cavitated lesion exists. This decision is based on a radiographic and clinical examination. Remember from Chapters 3, 6, and 9 that explorers must be used very judiciously in the detection of caries, otherwise the explorer tine may actually cause a cavitation, possibly resulting in the necessity to restore rather than remineralize the lesion. The clinical examination is better focused on visual assessments. Therefore the following questions about occlusal surfaces should be addressed:

1. Is there chalkiness of the tooth structure at the base of the pit or groove?
2. Is there softening in the tooth structure at the base of the pit or groove?

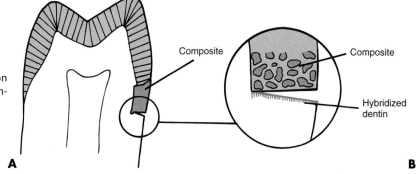

FIG. **13-2** Contraction gap. **A,** V-shaped gap on root surface. **B,** Restoration-side vector is composite; root-side vector is hybridized dentin.

A

B

3. Is there brown-gray discoloration radiating peripherally from the pit or groove?
4. Is there radiolucency beneath the enamel surface on the radiograph?
5. Is the patient at high risk for caries?

The interpretation of the answers to these assessments may indicate demineralized, decalcified, undermined, or carious tooth structure. Such information is critical in determining the course of treatment. When no cavitated carious lesion is diagnosed, the treatment decision is either to pursue no treatment or place a pit-and-fissure sealant, particularly if the surface is a high risk for future caries. If a small carious lesion is detected and the adjacent grooves and pits, although sound at the present time, are at risk to caries in the future, a preventive resin restoration (PRR) or conservative composite restoration (CCR) (which combines a small Class I composite with a sealant) may be the treatment recommendation. Before any of these treatments are initiated, the operator must be certain that no interproximal (Class II) caries or fault exists.

PIT-AND-FISSURE SEALANTS

As noted earlier in Chapters 2, 3, and 6, pits and fissures typically result from an incomplete coalescence of enamel and are particularly prone to caries. By using a low-viscosity fluid resin, these areas can be sealed, following acid-etching of the walls of the pits and fissures and a few millimeters of surface enamel bordering these faults.

Long-term clinical studies indicate that pit-and-fissure sealants provide a safe and effective method of preventing caries.[25,27] Sealants are most effective in children when they are applied to the pits and fissures of permanent posterior teeth immediately upon eruption of the clinical crowns. Adults also can benefit from the use of sealants if the individual experiences a change in caries susceptibility because of a change in their diet or medical condition (see Chapter 3).

Sealant materials (self-cured and light-cured) are based on urethane dimethacrylate or Bis-GMA resins. Tints frequently are added to sealants to produce color contrast for visual assessment.

Clinical studies also show that sealants can be applied even over small, cavitated lesions, with no subsequent progression of caries.[12,22] However, it is recommended that sealants be used for the prevention of caries rather than for the treatment of existing carious lesions. Therefore a recent bitewing radiograph should be made and evaluated before sealant placement, to ensure no dentinal caries is evident. Only caries-free pits and fissures or incipient lesions in enamel not extending to the dentinoenamel junction (DEJ) currently are recommended for treatment with pit-and-fissure sealants.

Indications for Sealants. The indications for sealants have been presented in ADA[1] and Public Health[15] publications. Both sources indicate that, regardless of age, caries risk of an individual should be the major factor for selecting teeth for sealant application. Sealants may be indicated for either preventive or therapeutic uses, depending on the patient's caries risk, tooth morphology, or presence of incipient enamel caries.

Clinical Technique. Because materials and techniques vary, it is important to follow the manufacturer's instructions for the sealant material being used. A standard method for applying sealants to posterior teeth is presented. Each quadrant is treated separately and may involve one or more teeth. The following discussion deals with a fissure present on a mandibular first permanent molar (Fig. 13-3, A). The tooth is isolated by a rubber dam (or cotton rolls). *The isolation of the area is critical to the success of the sealant.* Because sealant placement in younger patients is more common, the molar teeth are often not fully erupted, and therefore isolation is difficult. If proper isolation cannot be obtained, the bond of the sealant material to the occlusal surface will be compromised, resulting in either loss of the sealant or recurrent caries under the sealant. The area is cleaned with a slurry of pumice on a bristle brush (see Fig. 13-3, B). Bristles reach into faulty areas better than a rubber prophy cup, which tends to burnish debris and pumice into the pits and fissures. The tooth is rinsed thoroughly while the explorer tip is used carefully to help remove residual pumice or additional debris. After the area is dried, a liquid acid etchant (35% to 50% phosphoric acid) may be placed on the occlusal surface with a small sponge, brush, or applicator tip for 30 seconds. Gel etchants, traditionally used for most restorative procedures, may have less ability to effectively penetrate into the pits and fissures. Laser cleaning and etching is an alternative to traditional techniques, but lasing units are not yet widely available in general practice. Likewise, air abrasion techniques also are being advocated for preparing the pits and grooves before sealant placement, but their effectiveness has not yet warranted their additional expense.

Next, the tooth is rinsed with water for 20 seconds while the area is evacuated, and then dried of all visible moisture. The properly acid-etched enamel surface has a lightly frosted appearance (see Fig. 13-3, C). Fluoride-rich, resistant enamel may need to be etched longer. Any brown stains that originally may have been in the pits/fissures may still be present and should be allowed to remain. The self-cured sealant is mixed and applied with a small applicator provided in the sealant kit. The sealant is gently teased to place, to avoid entrapping air, and it should slightly overfill all pits and fissures. Some operators prefer light-cured sealants, which also work well. After polymerization of the sealant, the rubber dam is removed, and the occlusion is evaluated using articulating paper. If necessary, a round 12-bladed carbide finishing bur or white stone is used to remove the

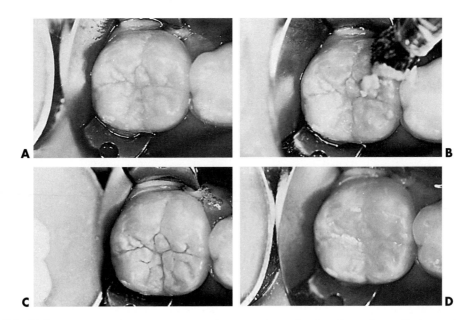

FIG. **13-3** Steps in application of sealant. **A,** Fissure in occlusal surface of mandibular molar with area isolated by rubber dam. **B,** Cleaning surface with pumice and bristle brush. **C,** Properly etched surface with lightly frosted appearance. **D,** Sealant inserted and finished. *(Courtesy of Dr. William Vann, Jr.)*

excess. The surface usually does not require further polishing (see Fig. 13-3, *D*).

CONSERVATIVE COMPOSITE AND PREVENTIVE RESIN RESTORATIONS

When restoring small pits and fissures on an unrestored tooth, an ultraconservative, modified preparation design is recommended. This design allows for restoration of the lesion or defect with minimal removal of tooth structure and often may be combined with the use of composite or sealant to seal radiating noncarious fissures or pits that are at high risk for subsequent caries activity (Fig. 13-4). Originally referred to as a preventive resin restoration,[23,24] this type of ultraconservative restoration is termed a conservative composite restoration (CCR) at the University of North Carolina. An accurate diagnosis is essential before restoring the occlusal surface of a posterior tooth. The critical factor in this clinical assessment is whether or not the suspicious pit or fissure is cavitated, therefore requiring restorative intervention (see Chapter 3). After deciding that cavitation has occurred, it usually must be determined whether to use amalgam or composite. Important factors related to this decision include: (1) ability to isolate the tooth or teeth, (2) occlusal relationship, (3) esthetics, and (4) operator ability. Usually, a CCR is the treatment of choice for the small occlusal restoration. The advantages of composite over amalgam for such restorations are: (1) conserving tooth structure, (2) enhancing esthetics, (3) bonding tooth structure together, (4) sealing the prepared tooth structure, and (5) including other suspicious areas

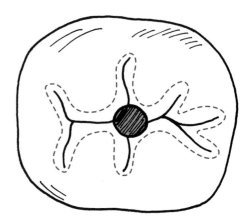

FIG. **13-4** Conservative composite restoration (CCR). Dotted line indicates area to be sealed around central pit tooth preparation.

on the occlusal surface with either the composite restorative material or a sealant material. Composite should not be used if the area cannot be properly isolated (resulting in an inadequate bond), or the operator does not have the ability to place a composite restoration satisfactorily.

Sometimes, if a definitive diagnosis of caries cannot be made, an exploratory preparation of the suspicious area is performed with a small bur or diamond. This approach is particularly indicated in patients at high risk for caries. The objective of this procedure is to explore suspicious pits or grooves with a very small bur or diamond to determine the extent of the suspected fault. As the tooth preparation is deepened, an assess-

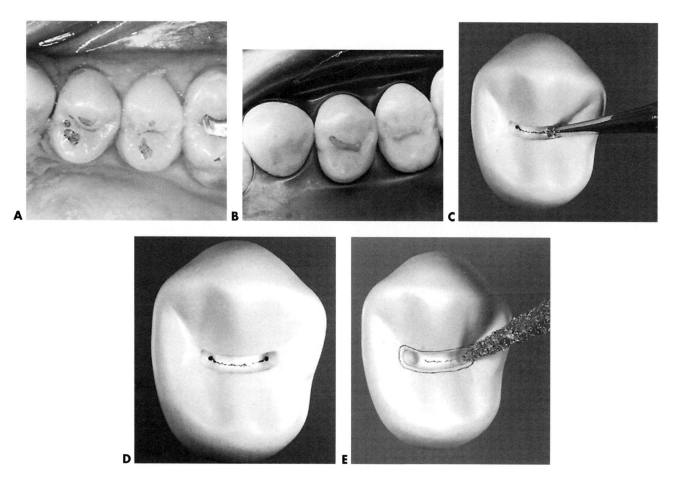

FIG. **13-5** Class I modified tooth preparation. **A** and **B,** Clinical examples of fissures and final exploratory tooth preparations. **C,** Preparation is made with a No. ½ bur or diamond. **D,** Initial extensions. Pit remnants remain. **E,** Carious pits excavated and preparation roughened.

ment is made in the suspicious areas whether or not to continue the preparation toward the DEJ. If the suspicious fault is removed or found to be sound at a shallow preparation depth, the area is restored with composite as described below. If the suspicious area is found to be carious, the preparation depth is continued until all of the caries is removed. The prepared area is then restored with composite.

A maxillary premolar may have a fissure in the occlusal surface as illustrated in the clinical example in Fig. 13-5, *A.* Although every effort should be made to determine the presence of a cavitated lesion, if this diagnosis cannot be made, an exploratory preparation may be considered. Fig. 13-5, *B* through *D,* shows the initial, exploratory tooth preparation of the fissure, using a No. ½ or No. 330 bur or diamond. The initial depth is kept in enamel at approximately 1 mm. The occlusal extension is complete when either the occlusal aspect of the fissure terminates or the opposite pit area is reached. Any pulpally directed remnants of pits and fissures are tested with a sharp explorer. If they are still defective as evidenced by a soft feel or "stick" of the explorer, the same bur is used to extend the preparation pulpally into

these areas. It is not necessary to extend the preparation in a pulpal direction if only a hard, dark line remains that cannot be penetrated by a sharp explorer, and the radiograph is negative for dentinal caries. If necessary, the preparation is completed by using a flame-shaped diamond instrument to flare the cavosurface margin (see Fig. 13-5, *E*). This flare may be widened to include any terminal ends of fissures. If no radiating fissures exist, the flaring is not necessary because of the enamel rod direction in this area, especially if steep cuspal inclines are present. The completed tooth preparation on a maxillary premolar is illustrated in Fig. 13-5, *F.*

CLASS VI COMPOSITE RESTORATIONS

One of the most conservative indications for a directly placed posterior composite is a small faulty developmental pit located on a cusp tip. Fig. 13-6, *A,* is an example of a Class VI fault on the facial cusp tip of a maxillary premolar and the occlusion in the area is minimal. Usually no anesthesia is required because the fault is entirely in enamel. The tooth is isolated with a cotton roll.

The typical Class VI tooth preparation should be as small in diameter and as shallow in depth as possible.

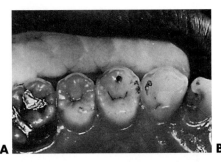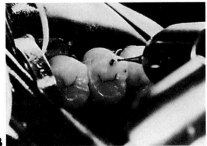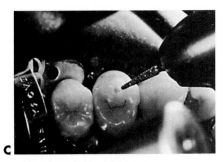

FIG. **13-6** Class VI tooth preparation for composite restoration. **A,** Class VI preparation on the facial cusp tip of maxillary premolar. **B,** Entry with small round bur or diamond. **C,** Preparation roughened with diamond, if necessary.

Enter the faulty pit with a small, round bur (No. ¼ or No. ½) or diamond oriented perpendicular to the surface and extend pulpally to eliminate the lesion (see Fig. 13-6, *B*). Visual examination and probing with an explorer often reveals that the fault is limited to enamel because the enamel in this area is quite thick. If the preparation is not already completed at this stage, complete the preparation using either a flame-shaped or round diamond instrument to roughen the prepared surfaces (see Fig. 13-6, *C*). If a faulty restoration or extensive caries is present on the cusp tip, a round bur of appropriate size is used for excavating remaining infected dentin. Stains that appear through the translucent enamel should be removed, otherwise they may be seen after the composite restoration is completed. Some undermined, but not friable, enamel may be left and bonded to the composite.

CLINICAL TECHNIQUE FOR DIRECT CLASS I COMPOSITE RESTORATIONS

INITIAL CLINICAL PROCEDURES

The same general procedures as described previously regarding anesthesia and shade selection are necessary before beginning a Class I composite restoration (see Chapters 10, 11, and 12). However, an assessment of the preoperative occlusal relationship of the tooth to be restored should be made. This information will not usually contraindicate the use of composite as the restorative material unless all occlusal contacts will occur solely on the restoration. Isolation of the operating area is not usually a problem, but must be ensured for a successful restoration.

TOOTH PREPARATION

The three typical composite preparations (conventional, beveled conventional, and modified) also may be considered for Class I and Class II composite restorations, although the beveled conventional design would rarely be used. When there is need to provide increased resistance form (resistance to fracture of the tooth or compos-

ite), the more amalgam-like conventional preparation form may be indicated. This would be most necessary for large preparations or restorations subjected to heavy occlusal forces. The conventional beveled design, conventional preparation design, or some combination of the two provides boxlike form, some flat walls that are perpendicular to occlusal forces, and strong tooth and restoration marginal configurations. All of these features help resist potential fracture.

Small-to-moderate restorations may use modified tooth preparations, which usually do not provide the characteristic resistance form features previously listed. Instead, the modified preparation typically utilizes more flared cavosurface forms without uniform or flat pulpal or axial walls. Usually a more rounded, and perhaps smaller, cutting instrument is used for the modified preparation, in an attempt to be as conservative as possible in the removal of tooth structure.

Various cutting instruments may be used for Class I and Class II tooth preparations, the size generally dictated by the size of the lesion or fault, and the shape dependent on retention and resistance forms needed. Usually, however, a diamond instrument is preferred because it roughens the prepared tooth structure, which increases the prepared surface area and retention of the composite to the tooth.

Composite restorations are indicated for most Class I restorations in premolars and first molars. The larger the restoration, the more concern about wear, although wear resistance of composite is sufficient for most posterior restorations. Also, the further the tooth position posteriorly, the more difficult is the isolation of the operating area, and the less is the esthetic need. Both of these factors reduce the indication for a composite restoration.

If the occlusal portion of the restoration is expected to be extensive, the more boxlike preparation design may be preferred, resulting in greater retention and resistance to fracture. This form is generated by any flat-tipped bur or diamond. However, inverted cone cutting instruments with rounded corners (Fig. 13-7) may be preferred because they: (1) provide flat floors, (2) result

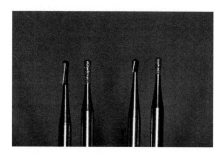

FIG. **13-7** Inverted cone composite preparation instruments.

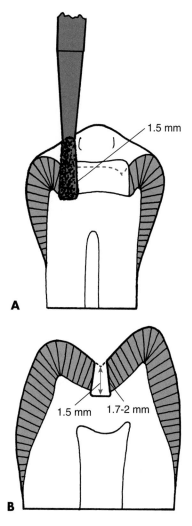

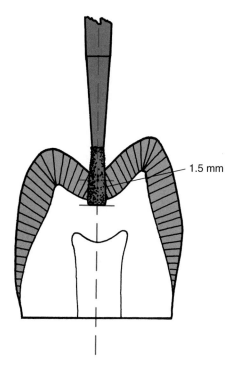

FIG. **13-8** Entry cut. Diamond held parallel to long axis of crown. Initial pulpal depth 1.5 mm from central groove.

FIG. **13-9** Initial pulpal depth. Once central groove removed, facial and lingual wall measurements will usually be greater than 1.5 mm. (The steeper the wall, the greater the height.) **A,** 1.5 mm depth from central groove. **B,** Approximately 1.75 to 2 mm facial or lingual wall heights.

in occlusal marginal configurations that are more representative of the strongest enamel margin, (3) enhance retention form by creating preparation walls that generally converge occlusally, and (4) result in a more conservative faciolingual preparation width.

While the boxlike form may provide the previously stated benefits, it also may increase the negative effects of the C-factor. Therefore the operator must carefully consider all of these issues in selecting the tooth preparation design.

When using the inverted cone cutting instrument, the tooth is prepared similarly to that described for a Class I amalgam in Chapter 17. The objective of the tooth preparation is to remove all of the caries or fault as conservatively as possible. Because the composite will be bonded to the tooth structure, other less-involved, or at-risk areas, can be sealed as part of the conservative preparation techniques. Thus sealants may be combined

with the typical Class I composite restoration, as described already.

Conventional Class I Tooth Preparation. For the large Class I composite tooth preparation, enter the tooth in the distal pit area of the faulty occlusal surface, with the inverted cone diamond, positioned parallel to the long axis of the crown. When it is anticipated that the entire mesiodistal length of a central groove will be prepared, it is easier to enter the distal portion first, and then transverse mesially. This technique permits better vision to the operator during the preparation. Prepare the pulpal floor to an initial depth of 1.5 mm, as measured from the central groove (Fig. 13-8). Once the central groove area is removed, the facial or lingual measurement of this depth will be greater, usually about 1.75 mm, but this depends on the steepness of the cuspal inclines (Fig. 13-9). Normally this initial depth is approximately 0.2 mm inside (internal to) the DEJ. The diamond is moved mesially (Fig. 13-10) to include other remaining faults, following the central groove, as well as any fall and rise of the DEJ (Fig. 13-11). Facial and lingual extension and width are dictated by the caries, old restorative material, or fault. Preserve the strength of the cuspal and marginal ridge areas as much as possible. Even though the final bonded composite restoration will help restore some of the strength of weakened, unprepared facial, lingual, mesial, or distal tooth structure, the outline form should be as conservative as possible in these areas. Extensions toward cusp tips should be as minimal as possible. Extensions into marginal ridges should result in approximately a 1.6-mm thickness of remaining tooth structure (measured from the internal extension to the proximal height of contour) for premolars and approxi-

mately 2 mm for molars (Fig. 13-12). These limited extensions help preserve the dentinal support of the marginal ridge enamel and cusp tips.

As the diamond is moved along the central groove, the resulting pulpal floor is usually flat (as a result of the shape of the tip of the diamond) and follows the rise and fall of the DEJ. If extension is required toward the cusp tips, the same approximate 1.5-mm depth is maintained, usually resulting in the pulpal floor rising occlusally (Fig. 13-13). The same uniform depth concept is also appropriate when extending a facial or lingual groove radiating from the occlusal surface. Once a groove extension is through the cusp ridge, the diamond prepares the facial (or lingual) portion of the faulty groove at an axial depth of 0.2 mm inside the DEJ, and gingivally to include all of the fault (Fig. 13-14). Either the side or the tip of the diamond may be used for the facial or lingual surfaced extension.

After extending the outline form to sound tooth structure, if any caries or old restorative material remains on the pulpal floor, it should be removed with the diamond or a round bur according to the descriptions presented in Chapters 11 and 12. Even though the occlusal margin does not have a beveled or flared form (because of the shape of the diamond instrument), it is left as prepared. No attempt is made to place additional beveling on the occlusal margin because it may result in thin composite in areas of heavy occlusal contact. Also, the inverted cone diamond results in occlusal walls that converge occlus-

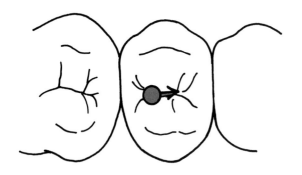

FIG. 13-10 Diamond is moved mesially to include all faults.

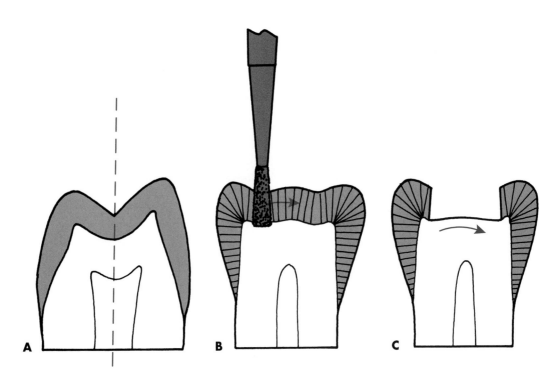

FIG. 13-11 Mesiodistal initial pulpal depth preparation follows DEJ. A, Mesiodistal cross-section of premolar. B, Move cutting instrument mesially. C, Follow contour of DEJ.

ally, thereby enhancing retention form. Because of the occlusal surface enamel rod direction, the ends of the enamel rods are already exposed by the preparation, which further reduces the need for occlusal bevels. The marginal form of a groove extension on the facial or lingual surface may be beveled with the diamond, resulting in a 0.25- to 0.5-mm width bevel at a 45-degree angle to the prepared wall (Fig. 13-15).

The larger Class I composite tooth preparation is primarily a conventional design. However, if a facial or lingual groove is included, it usually is beveled, and the resulting preparation design would be a combination of conventional and beveled conventional. Also it should be reemphasized that only the cavitated carious lesion is prepared in the manner described above. After the fault is removed, adjacent less-involved or at-risk areas should

be included more conservatively with sealants or minimally invasive preparations. A diamond may be used to roughen and/or include such adjacent areas. These will then either be sealed or restored with a small amount of composite when the conventionally prepared area is restored.

Although large, extensive posterior composite restorations may have some potential disadvantages when used routinely, "real world" dentistry sometimes necessitates esthetic treatment alternatives that may provide a needed service to the patient. Often patients simply cannot afford a more permanent esthetic restoration, or they may possess dental or medical conditions that preclude their placement. In such instances, large posterior composite restorations sometimes can be used as a reasonable alternative when more permanent options are not possible or realistic. Most extensive Class I and Class II composite restorations utilize a conventional tooth preparation design.

Modified Class I Tooth Preparation. Minimally involved Class I lesions or faults may be restored with composite using modified tooth preparations. These preparations are less specific in form, having a scooped-out appearance. Typically they are prepared with a small round or inverted cone diamond. The initial pulpal depth is still 1.5 mm or approximately 0.2 mm inside the DEJ, but may not be uniform (i.e., the pulpal floor is not necessarily flat throughout its length). If a round diamond is used, the resulting cavosurface margin angle may be more flared (obtuse) than if an inverted cone diamond were used (Fig. 13-16).

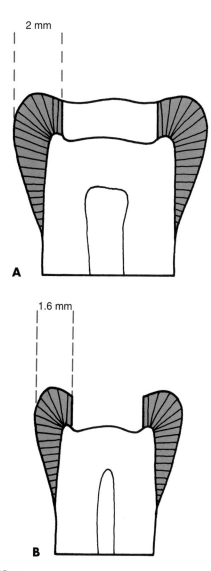

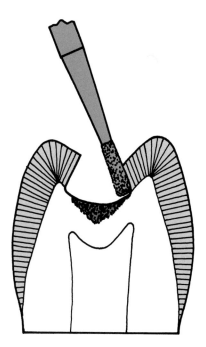

FIG. **13-12** Mesiodistal extension. Preserve dentin support of marginal ridge enamel. **A,** Molar. **B,** Premolar.

FIG. **13-13** Faciolingual extension. Maintain initial 1.5-mm pulpal depth up cuspal inclines.

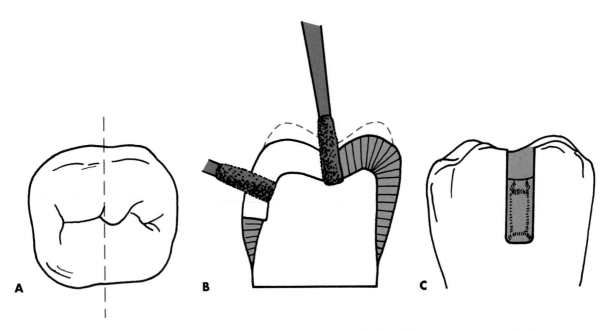

FIG. **13-14** Groove extension. **A**, Cross-section through facial and lingual groove area. **B**, Extension through cusp ridge at 1.5 mm initial pulpal depth; facial wall depth is 0.2 mm inside the DEJ. **C**, Facial view.

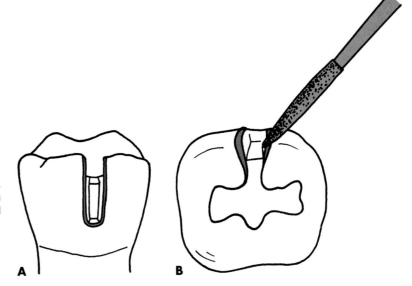

FIG. **13-15** Beveling a facial groove extension. Coarse diamond creates a 0.5-mm bevel width at a 45-degree angle. **A**, Facial view. **B**, Occlusal view.

Mandibular premolars often have two separate faulty occlusal pits located in areas of minimal function as illustrated in Fig. 13-17, *A*. Assuming a diagnosis of active caries, conservative restorations are indicated. The outline form for the tooth preparation of each pit (see Fig. 13-17, *B*) is similar to the Class VI modified preparation previously described with the use of a small diamond. Any shallow fissure that extends laterally from the pit is incorporated in the preparation by an extended cavosurface bevel or flare. This extended bevel or flare is similar to an enameloplasty procedure as described in Chapters 6 and 17. However, the entire bevel or flare becomes part of the final tooth preparation (a difference from enameloplasty for amalgam preparations), which is subsequently etched and restored with a posterior composite. Small radiating fissures also may be optionally filled with sealant.

RESTORATIVE TECHNIQUE

Etching, Priming, and Placing Adhesive. Etching, priming, and placement of adhesive techniques are the same as described previously. Remember that overdrying etched dentin may compromise dentin bonding.[10,11,13] Water may be used for rewetting needs, but other aqueous solutions containing glutaraldehyde and/or hydroxyethyl methacrylate (HEMA) (see Chapters 4 and 5)

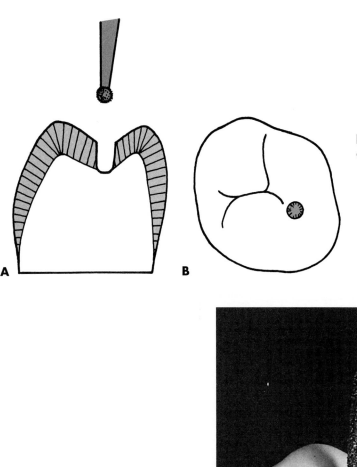

FIG. **13-16** Modified Class I tooth preparation using round diamond. **A,** Faciolingual cross-section. **B,** Occlusal view.

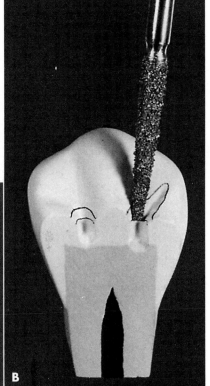

FIG. **13-17** Class I pit preparations for composite restorations. **A,** Two small, faulty pits are often present on a mandibular first premolar. **B,** Preparations are accomplished with coarse diamond as conservatively as possible. Note extension to include fissure.

may be even more beneficial when using one-bottle adhesive systems. No matrix usually is necessary for Class I composite restorations, even when facial and lingual surface grooves are included. However, if the operator deems a matrix necessary for a groove extension composite restoration, a Barton matrix as described in Chapter 17 may be used.

Inserting and Curing the Composite. A two-step procedure (enamel/dentin bonding adhesive, if not already applied, followed by the composite material) usually is necessary with a light-cured composite material.

The composite should not be dispensed until ready to use because it may begin to polymerize from the ambient light in the operatory. Because of variations in materials, each manufacturer's specific instructions should be followed.

The enamel/dentin bonding agents (including primers and adhesives) are placed over the entire preparation (etched enamel and dentin) with a microbrush, foam sponge, or applicator tip, in accordance with the manufacturer's instructions. The adhesive is polymerized with a visible light source, as recommended by the

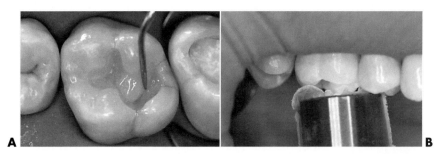

FIG. **13-18** Class I composite incremental insertion **(A)** and curing **(B)**.

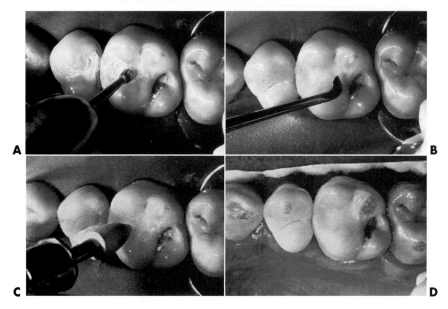

FIG. **13-19** Contouring and polishing Class I composite. **A,** Round or oval carbide 12-bladed finishing bur used to remove excess and develop anatomic form. **B,** Carbide carver. **C,** Rubber point polishes surface. **D,** Completed restoration.

manufacturer. Composite insertion hand instruments or a syringe may be used to insert the composite material. If a syringe is used, the tip on the compule must be kept covered when not in use to prevent premature hardening of the material. Small increments of composite material are added and successively cured (Fig. 13-18). It is important to place (and cure) the composite incrementally to maximize the polymerization depth of cure and possibly to reduce the effects of polymerization shrinkage. For this reason, the first small increment should be placed in the most remote area of the preparation. This increment should only be approximately 1 to 2 mm in thickness and should be cured with a light exposure of 20 to 40 seconds. Subsequent additions are made and cured (1 to 2 mm in thickness at a time) until the preparation is filled to slight excess. The restoration can be contoured and finished immediately after the last increment is cured.

Contouring and Polishing the Composite. Contouring can be initiated immediately after a light-cured composite material has been polymerized, or 3 minutes after the initial hardening of a self-cured material. The occlusal surface is shaped with a round or oblong, 12-bladed carbide finishing bur or similarly shaped finishing diamond. Special carbide-tipped carvers (Carbide Carvers, Brasseler USA, Savannah, Georgia) are useful for removing composite excess along occlusal margins. Finishing is accomplished with appropriate polishing cups and/or points after the occlusion is adjusted as necessary (Fig. 13-19).

CLINICAL TECHNIQUE FOR DIRECT CLASS II COMPOSITE RESTORATIONS

INITIAL CLINICAL PROCEDURES

The same general procedures as described previously are necessary before beginning a Class II composite restoration. However, several aspects of those activities need emphasis. First, an assessment of the expected tooth preparation extensions (outline form) should be made and a decision rendered on whether or not an enamel periphery will exist on the tooth preparation. The expected presence of an enamel periphery strengthens the choice of composite as the restorative material. If the preparation is expected to extend onto the root surface, composite is not necessarily contraindicated as the restorative material, but it must be recognized that potential problems with both isolation of the operating area and gap formation exist. Good technique and proper use of the material may reduce these potential problems.

Second, an assessment of the preoperative occlusal relationship of the tooth to be restored must be made. The presence of heavy occlusal contacts should not necessarily contraindicate composite as the choice for restorative material, but it may indicate that wear may be more of a consideration, necessitating timely recall appointment assessments.

Last, preoperative wedging in the gingival embrasure of the proximal surfaces to be restored should occur. Placing wedges (after rubber dam application, if utilized) before tooth preparation, begins the separation of the teeth, which may be beneficial in the reestablishment of the proximal contact with the composite restoration.

TOOTH PREPARATION

The tooth preparation for a Class II composite restoration may be either a conventional or modified preparation design. The modified design is for smaller restorations, generally using smaller diamond instruments and resulting in a preparation form that is more rounded, less boxlike, and less uniform in extension or depth. It is described later. The other predominant preparation design is similar to the conventional preparation for an amalgam restoration as described in Chapter 17. It is used for moderate to very large Class II composite restorations, generally using an inverted cone diamond. The design results in a preparation form that is more boxlike, has more uniform pulpal and axial depths, and has some preparation walls prepared perpendicular to occlusal forces (to enhance resistance form). However, unlike conventional amalgam tooth preparations, the conventional tooth preparation for composite does not usually incorporate secondary retention features; does not require 90-degree composite margins, is usually more conservative in extensions; and is left with roughened, rather than smooth, preparation walls.

Both preparation designs have the same objectives: (1) to remove the fault, defect, caries, or old material; (2) to remove friable tooth structure; and (3) to have cavosurface angles of 90 degrees or greater. The tooth preparation has two components, the occlusal step portion (similar to that already described for Class I composite tooth preparations) and a proximal box portion. Only faulty, carious, or defective tooth structure is included in the outline form. Remember that on the occlusal surface, less-involved or at-risk pits and grooves adjacent to the tooth preparation may be included with

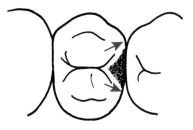

FIG. **13-20** Preoperative visualization of facial and lingual proximal box extensions. Arrows indicate desired extensions.

a sealant or other more conservative preparation, rather than extending to include such areas as part of the original tooth preparation.

Conventional Class II Tooth Preparation

Occlusal Step. The occlusal portion of the Class II preparation is prepared similarly as described for the Class I preparation. The primary differences are related to technique of incorporating the faulty proximal surface(s). Preoperatively, the proposed facial and lingual proximal extensions should be visualized, thus permitting a more conservative connection between the occlusal and proximal portions of the preparation (Fig. 13-20). Initial occlusal extension toward the involved proximal surface should go through the marginal ridge area at initial pulpal floor depth, exposing the DEJ. The DEJ serves as a guide for preparing the proximal box portion of the preparation.

Use a No. 330 or No. 245 shaped diamond to enter the pit opposite the faulty proximal surface. The diamond is positioned parallel with the long axis of the tooth crown. Remember that if only one proximal surface is being restored, the opposite marginal ridge dentinal support should be maintained. This may require using the proximal side of the diamond to include the faulty pit near the marginal ridge of the unaffected proximal surface, especially in smaller teeth (Fig. 13-21). Remember also that the entire central groove area may not need to be included, and only the faulty areas are prepared.

Prepare the pulpal floor with a diamond to a depth of 1.5 mm, as measured from the central groove. Once the central groove is removed, the facial or lingual measurement of this depth will be greater, usually about 1.75 mm, dependent on the steepness of the cuspal inclines. The diamond is then moved toward the affected proximal surface, including all faults facially and/or lingually as it transverses the central groove. However, every effort should be made to keep the faciolingual width of the preparation as narrow as possible. The initial depth is maintained during the mesiodistal movement, but follows the rise and fall of the underlying DEJ. The pulpal floor is relatively flat in a faciolingual plane, but may rise and fall slightly in a mesiodistal plane (Fig. 13-22). If caries is still present in enamel on the pulpal floor at the initial depth of 1.5 mm, then the pulpal floor is

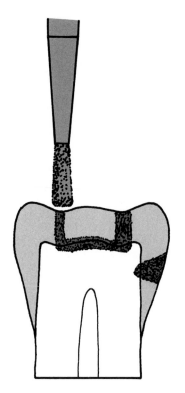

FIG. **13-21** For small teeth, use side of diamond to include faulty pit, maintaining dentin support of noninvolved marginal ridge enamel.

extended 0.2 mm inside the DEJ. If caries remains in the dentin, it is removed as part of final tooth preparation.

Because the facial and lingual proximal extensions of the faulty proximal surface were visualized preoperatively, the occlusal extension toward that proximal surface begins to widen facially and lingually to connect to those points. Care is taken to preserve cuspal areas as much as possible during these extensions. At the same time, the diamond extends through the marginal ridge to within 0.5 mm of the adjacent tooth. This exposes the proximal DEJ and also protects the adjacent tooth (Fig. 13-23). At this time, the occlusal portion of the preparation is complete, except for possible additional pulpal floor caries excavation. The occlusal walls generally converge occlusally because of the inverted shape of the diamond. This results in the occlusal cavosurface marginal form being representative of the strongest enamel margin (an obtuse angle). Also the occlusal walls and pulpal floor are left in a roughened state because of the diamond instrument. This increases the surface area for bonding.

Proximal Box. Typically, caries develops on a proximal surface immediately gingival to the proximal contact. The extent of the carious lesion or amount of old restorative material are two factors that dictate the facial, lingual, and gingival extension of the proximal box of the preparation. Other factors are discussed in Chap-

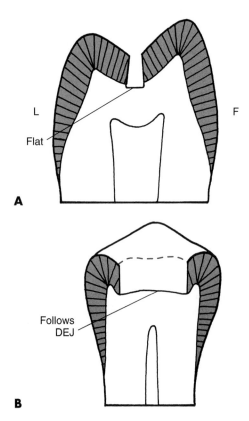

FIG. **13-22** Pulpal floor. **A,** Flat in a faciolingual plane. **B,** Follows DEJ in a mesiodistal plane.

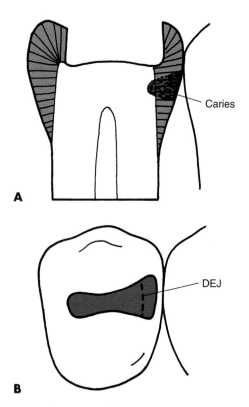

FIG. **13-23** Occlusal extension into faulty proximal. **A** and **B,** Extension exposes DEJ but does not hit adjacent tooth. Facial and lingual extensions as preoperatively visualized.

ter 6. Although it is not required to extend the proximal box beyond contact with the adjacent tooth (i.e., provide clearance with the adjacent tooth), it may simplify the preparation, matrix, composite insertion, and contouring procedures. However, if all of the fault can be removed without extending the proximal preparation beyond the contact, the restoration of the proximal contact with the composite (a major difficulty) will be simplified (Fig. 13-24).

Once the diamond has extended through the marginal ridge, be careful not to cut the adjacent tooth, the proximal ditch cut is initiated. Hold the diamond over the DEJ with the tip of the diamond positioned to create a gingivally directed cut that will be 0.2 mm inside the DEJ (Fig. 13-25). For a No. 245 diamond instrument with a tip diameter of 0.8 mm, this would require one fourth of the diamond's tip positioned over the dentin side of the DEJ (the other three fourths of the tip over the enamel side). The diamond is then extended facially, lingually, and gingivally to include all of the fault, caries, or old material. The faciolingual cutting motion follows the DEJ and therefore is usually in a slightly convex arc outward (see Fig. 13-25). During this entire cutting, the diamond is held parallel to the long axis of the tooth crown. The facial and lingual margins are extended as necessary and should result in at least a 90-degree margin, more obtuse being acceptable as well. If the preparation is conservative, use a smaller, thinner diamond instrument to complete the facial and lingual wall formation, avoiding contact with the adjacent tooth (Fig. 13-26). The gingival floor is prepared flat (due to the tip of the diamond) with an approximately 90-degree cavosurface margin. Gingival extension should be as minimal as possible, trying to maintain an enamel margin.

The axial wall should be 0.2 mm inside (internal to) the DEJ and have a slight outward convexity. For large carious lesions, additional axial wall (or pulpal floor) caries excavation may be necessary later, during final tooth preparation (Fig. 13-27).

At this point, the initial tooth preparation is complete. If no infected dentin remains and no proximal beveling is indicated, the final preparation also is considered complete at this time (Fig. 13-28). Because the composite will be retained in the preparation by micromechanical retention, no secondary preparation retention features are necessary. If an inverted cone diamond has been used, the facial and lingual occlusal walls will be convergent occlusally, adding to retention form. No bevels are placed on the cavosurface margins, especially the occlusal margins. A bevel placed on an occlusal margin would result in thin composite on the occlusal surface in areas of potentially heavy contact. This could result in fracture or wear of the composite in these areas. Beveled composite margins also may be more difficult to finish.

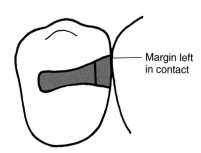

FIG. **13-24** Proximal wall may be left in contact with adjacent tooth.

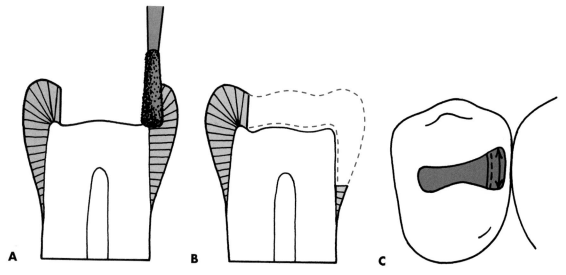

FIG. **13-25** Proximal ditch cut. **A,** Diamond positioned so gingivally directed cut will create axial wall 0.2 mm inside the DEJ. **B,** Faciolingual direction of axial wall preparation follows DEJ. **C,** Axial wall 0.2 mm inside DEJ.

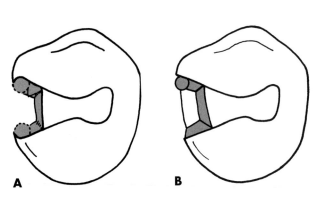

FIG. **13-26** Using smaller diamond to prepare cavosurface margin areas of facial and lingual proximal walls. **A,** Facial and lingual proximal margins undermined. **B,** Using smaller diamond instrument.

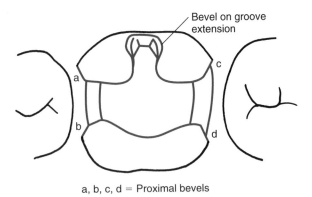

a, b, c, d = Proximal bevels

FIG. **13-29** Placing proximal bevels on extensive Class II tooth preparations. Diamond used to create bevel, width dependent on retention need.

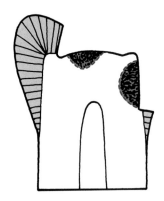

FIG. **13-27** Proximal extension. Try to maintain enamel margin on gingival floor. Any remaining infected axial wall (or pulpal floor) dentin will be excavated as part of final tooth preparation (as indicated by the dotted lines).

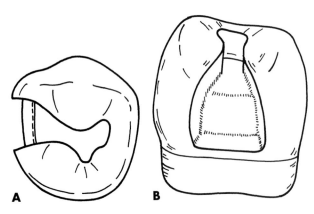

FIG. **13-28** Final conventional Class II composite tooth preparation. **A,** Occlusal view. **B,** Proximal view.

Usually, bevels are not placed on facial and lingual walls of the proximal box. However, bevels can be placed on the proximal facial and lingual margins if the proximal box is already wide faciolingually and if it is determined that additional retention form may be nec-

essary (Fig. 13-29). Such bevels will increase the surface area and expose enamel rod ends, thereby improving retention. Proximal bevels should not be placed if excessive extension of the margins is required.

A bevel is not usually placed on the gingival cavosurface margin, although it may be necessary to remove any unsupported enamel rods at the margin because of the gingival orientation of the enamel rods. For most Class II preparations, this margin is already approaching the DEJ, and therefore the enamel is thin. Care is taken to maintain any enamel in this area to result in a preparation with all-enamel margins. If the preparation extends onto the root surface, more attention must be focused on keeping the area isolated during the bonding technique, but no differences in tooth preparation are required. The preparation portion on the root should have: (1) a 90-degree cavosurface margin, (2) an axial depth of approximately 0.75 to 1 mm, and (3) usually no secondary retention form. If the gingival floor is extended onto the root surface, the axial depth of 0.75 to 1 mm must be obtained by either deepening the entire axial wall or orienting the diamond inclination more in a proximal direction (Fig. 13-30).

Usually, the only remaining final tooth preparation procedure that may be necessary is additional excavation of infected dentin on either the pulpal floor or axial wall. If necessary, a round bur or appropriate spoon excavator is used to remove any remaining infected dentin.

Thus the conventional Class II composite tooth preparation is similar to that for amalgam, except no secondary retention features are incorporated, the extensions are less, and there is no requirement for a 90-degree composite margin, unless the preparation is extended onto the root surface.

Fig. 13-31, *A*, illustrates an esthetic problem seen on the mesiofacial corner of a maxillary first premolar as a result of extensive recurrent caries and/or existing faulty restoration. The preoperative occlusion assessment indicates the facial cusp of the opposing man-

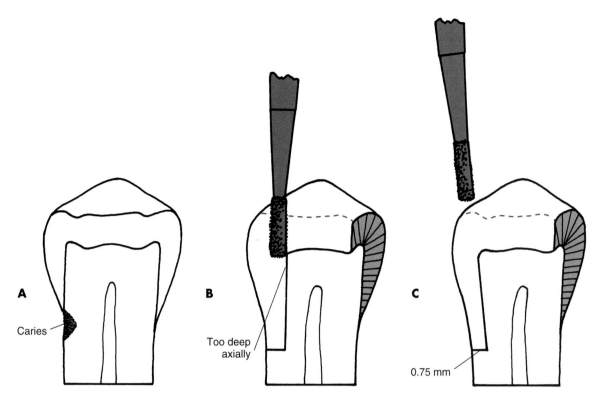

FIG. 13-30 Axial wall extension onto root surface. A, Caries below CEJ. B, Axial wall too deep when prepared with diamond in same axis. C, Diamond tilted toward adjacent tooth to create approximate 0.75- to 1-mm axial wall depth on root surface.

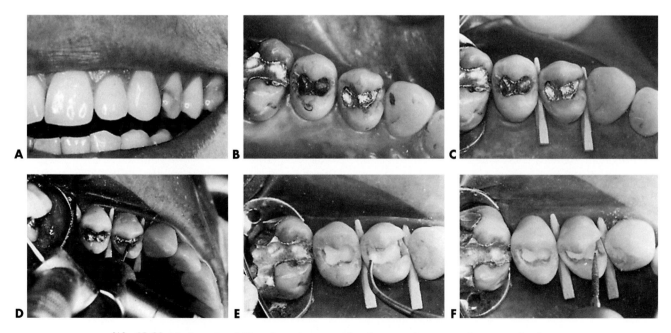

FIG. 13-31 Mesioocclusal Class II tooth preparation for posterior composite restoration in maxillary first premolar. A, Esthetic problem is caused by caries and existing amalgam restoration. B, In this patient the mesial marginal ridge is not a centric holding area. C, Early wedging after rubber dam placement. D, Inverted cone bur or diamond is used for initial tooth preparations on both premolars. E, After extensive caries is excavated, a calcium hydroxide liner is inserted (use of newer dentin bonding systems would favor having no liner except for excavations within 0.5 mm of pulp. F, Preparations are completed, if necessary, by roughening the prepared tooth structure with diamond instrument.

dibular premolar (which usually occludes on the mesial marginal ridge of the maxillary premolar) does not contact that area on this tooth (see Fig. 13-31, *B*). The existing occlusal amalgam on the maxillary second premolar also is determined to have extensive recurrent caries and will be replaced with a composite during the same appointment.

After the operator cleans the teeth, administers local anesthetic, selects the shade of composite, and isolates the area (preferably with a rubber dam), a wedge is placed in the gingival embrasure (see Fig. 13-31, *C*). Early wedging helps in separating the teeth, to compensate later for the thickness of the matrix band, thereby fulfilling one of several requirements for a good proximal contact for the composite restoration. The lack of pressure against the matrix during placement of composite, compared to pressure of amalgam during its condensation, presents the need, not only for increased separation by early wedge insertion, but also for alertness of the operator to verify matrix contact with the adjacent tooth before composite placement. The wedge also depresses and protects the rubber dam and gingival tissue when the proximal area is prepared. An additional, further tightening (insertion) of the wedge during tooth preparation may be helpful. The presence of the wedge during tooth preparation may serve as a guide to help prevent overextension of the gingival floor.

Recall that a conservative conventional tooth preparation is recommended for most Class II composite restorations because of the need for adequate resistance form. A No. 245 bur or diamond is used to remove the existing amalgam restorations and to prepare the mesial surface of the first premolar in a conservative manner (see Fig. 13-31, *D*). A smaller diamond may be more appropriate if the lesion is smaller.

A notable difference in the initial Class II preparation design for a composite restoration compared to that for an amalgam, is the axial wall depth. When preparing the proximal box for a composite restoration, the axial wall initial depth usually is limited to a depth of 0.2 mm into dentin. This means that the tip of the No. 245 bur or diamond would be cutting approximately one fourth in dentin and three fourths in enamel to be most conservative. (The diameter of the No. 245 bur's tip end is 0.8 mm.) This decreased pulpal depth of the axial wall occurs because retention locks will not be used; therefore the decreased depth provides greater conservation of tooth structure. The occlusal walls may converge occlusally (due to the inverted shape of the No. 245 bur or diamond) and the proximal walls may be parallel or convergent occlusally. Preparing convergent proximal walls will provide additional retention form when needed.

With a round bur or spoon excavator, remove any remaining infected dentin and also any stains that show through the mesiofacial enamel. In this example, a liner of calcium hydroxide was applied over the deeply excavated area (see Fig. 13-31, *E*). Because of the removal of the amalgam and extensive caries, many areas of the enamel are unsupported by dentin, but not friable. This undermined, but not friable enamel is not removed. If the No. 245 bur has been used, roughen the accessible prepared walls with a diamond. If a diamond has been used for the preparation, the prepared walls are already sufficiently roughened. At this time, the tooth preparation is complete (see Fig. 13-31, *F*).

For molars the same principles are followed for Class II conventional tooth preparations. Moderate caries exists on the mesial of a maxillary first molar (Fig. 13-32, *A*). Isolation is achieved with a rubber dam. Early wedging with a short segment of a wooden toothpick initiates tooth separation, which is critical to subsequently establishing a tight proximal contact (see Fig. 13-32, *B*). Preparation walls are extended to sound tooth structure and infected dentin is excavated (see Fig. 13-32, *C*) as described previously.

If a composite restoration is satisfactorily bonded to the preparation walls, such as in preparations in which all margins are enamel, there should be little or no potential for microleakage, and no need for a liner. However, a calcium hydroxide base (0.5 to 1 mm thick) is indicated to treat a near exposure of the pulp (within 0.5 mm of the pulp), a possible microexposure, or an actual exposure

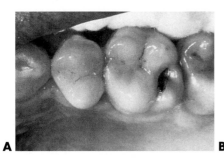
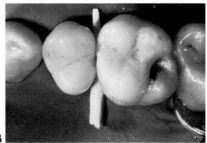
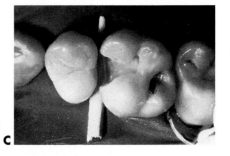

A **B** **C**

FIG. **13-32** Mesioocclusal Class II tooth preparation for posterior composite restoration in a maxillary molar. **A,** Carious lesion exists on mesial of maxillary molar in esthetically critical area. **B,** Rubber dam isolation and early wedging. **C,** Preparation walls are extended to nonfriable tooth structure and infected dentin excavated.

(see Chapter 3). Usually neither a liner nor a base is indicated in Class II tooth preparations for composite (Fig. 13-33). Actually, it is desirable not to cover any portion of the dentinal walls with a liner, unless necessary, because the liner would decrease dentin bonding potential.

Modified Class II Tooth Preparation. For small, initial restorations, an even more conservative preparation design may be used. A small round or inverted cone diamond may be used for this preparation to scoop out the carious or faulty material. This scooped appearance occurs on both the occlusal and proximal portions. The pulpal and axial depths are dictated only by the depth of the lesion and are not necessarily uniform. The proximal extensions likewise are dictated only by the extent of the lesion, but may require the use of another diamond with straight sides to prepare walls that are 90 degrees or greater (Fig. 13-34). The objectives are to conservatively remove the fault, create 90-degree cavosurface margins or greater, and remove friable tooth structure.

Another modified design is the box-only tooth preparation (Fig. 13-35). This design is indicated when only the proximal surface is faulty, with no lesions on the occlusal surface. A proximal box is prepared with either an inverted cone or round diamond, held parallel to the long axis of the tooth crown. The diamond is extended through the marginal ridge in a gingival direction. The axial depth is prepared 0.2 mm inside the DEJ. The form of the box is dependent on which diamond is used, the more boxlike with the inverted cone, and the more scooped with the round diamond. The facial, lingual, and gingival extensions are dictated by the fault or caries. No beveling or secondary retention is indicated.

A third modified design for restoring proximal lesions on posterior teeth is the facial or lingual slot preparation (Fig. 13-36). Here a lesion is detected on the proximal surface but the operator believes that access to the lesion can be obtained from either a facial or lingual direction, rather than through the marginal ridge in a gingival direction. Usually a small round diamond is used to gain access to the lesion. The diamond is oriented at the correct occlusogingival position and the entry is made with the diamond as close to the adjacent tooth as possible, thus preserving as much of the facial or lingual surface as possible. The preparation is extended occlusally, facially, and gingivally enough to remove the lesion. The axial depth is 0.2 mm inside the DEJ. The occlusal, facial, and gingival cavosurface margins are 90 degrees

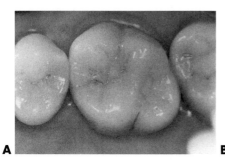
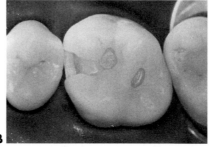
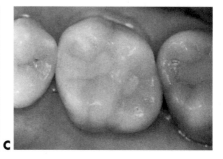

FIG. **13-33** Shallow mesioocclusal Class II tooth preparation for composite restoration, requiring no liner. **A,** Mesial caries exists preoperatively. **B,** Conservative tooth preparation. **C,** Completed restoration.

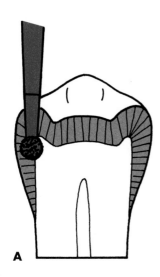
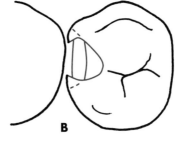
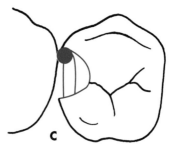

FIG. **13-34** Modified Class II composite tooth preparation. **A,** Round or oval, small inverted cone diamond used. **B** and **C,** Facial, lingual, and gingival margins may need undermined cavosurface enamel (indicated by dotted lines) removed with straight-sided thin and flat-tipped diamond.

or greater. This preparation is similar to a Class III preparation for an anterior tooth.

RESTORATIVE TECHNIQUE

Etching, Priming, and Placing Adhesive. The etching, priming, and adhesive placement techniques are as described previously.

Matrix Application. Undoubtedly one of the most important steps in restoring posterior teeth with directly placed composite is the selection and proper placement of the matrix. Unlike amalgam, which can be condensed to improve the proximal contact development, posterior composites are almost totally dependent on the contour and position of the matrix for establishing appropriate proximal contacts. Care must be exercised in placing a matrix for a Class II restoration because it is difficult to obtain good proximal contacts on posterior teeth when composite material is used. Early wedging and retightening of the wedge during tooth preparation aid in achieving sufficient separation of the teeth to compensate for the thickness of the matrix band. Before placing the composite material, the matrix band (strip) must be in absolute contact with (touching) the adjacent contact area.

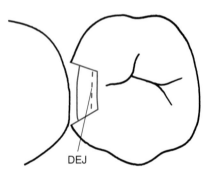

DEJ

FIG. **13-35** Box-only Class II composite preparation.

Recall that the matrix may be placed before or after the etching and priming treatment of the prepared tooth structure. There are potential advantages and disadvantages for either sequence (see Chapter 12). Generally the matrix is applied before the etching, priming, and adhesive placement.

An ultrathin metal matrix band is preferred for the restoration of a Class II composite, because it is thinner than a typical metal or polyester matrix and can be contoured better than a clear polyester matrix. Furthermore, a metal matrix offers greater resistance to condensation, which is especially important when a more viscous or packable composite is used. No significant problems are experienced in placing and curing composite material when using a metal matrix as long as small incremental additions (less than 2 mm each) are used (each increment cured before placing the next).

A Tofflemire matrix can be used for restoring a two-surface tooth preparation but must be sufficiently wedged to compensate adequately for the two thicknesses of matrix band (Fig. 13-37, *A*). An ultrathin (0.001 inch) universal metal matrix band (HO Bands, Young Dental Company, Earth City, Missouri) should be used in the Tofflemire retainer to aid in obtaining a good proximal contact. Before placement, the metal matrix band for posterior composites should be burnished on a paper pad to impart proper proximal contour to the band (the same as a matrix for amalgam).

If the Tofflemire matrix band is open excessively along the lingual margins of the preparation (usually because of the contour of the tooth), a "tinner's joint" can be used to close the matrix band. This joint is made by grasping the lingual portion of the matrix band with No. 110 pliers and cinching the band tightly together above the height of contour of the tooth (Fig. 13-38, *D*). The gathered matrix material can be easily folded to one

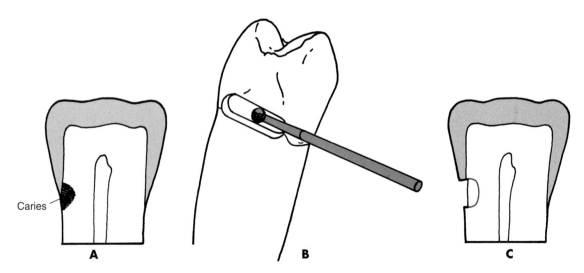

Caries

A   **B**   **C**

FIG. **13-36** Facial/lingual slot preparation. **A,** Cervical caries on proximal surface. **B,** Round diamond enters tooth from accessible embrasure, oriented to the occlusogingival middle of the lesion. **C,** Slot preparation (lingual view).

side with a large amalgam condenser. By closing the open portion of the matrix band, significant time and effort are saved when contouring and finishing the restoration.

A customized, compound-supported metal matrix is an excellent matrix for a two-surface posterior composite restoration because it is easier to obtain a good proximal contact when the wedge must compensate for only one thickness of metal matrix material. The materials needed for this matrix are shown in Fig. 13-39. A short length of thin, dead-soft or stainless steel metal matrix material

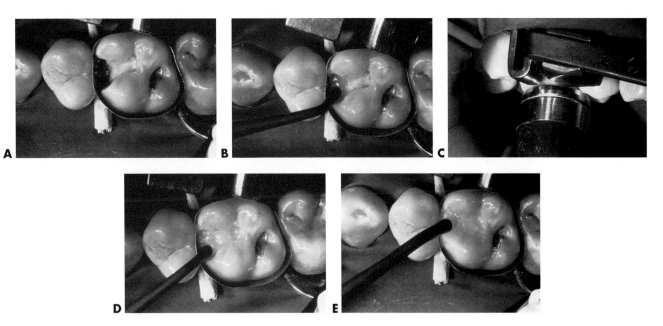

FIG. **13-37** Insertion of light-cured composite material, maxillary molar. **A,** A thin Tofflemire-type matrix is positioned and wedged. Bonding system has been placed. **B to E,** Composite is placed and cured in small increments until preparation is slightly overfilled.

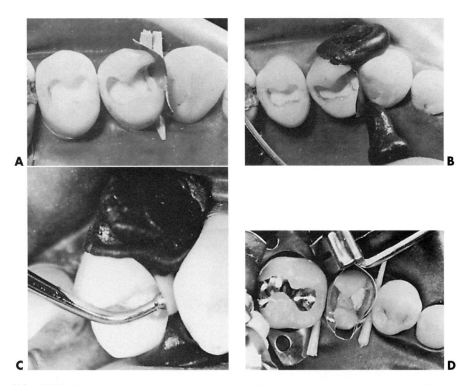

FIG. **13-38** Placement of proximal matrix for posterior composite restoration shown in Fig. 13-31. **A,** Strip matrix positioned and wedged for two-surface preparation. **B and C,** Compound cones are softened and applied to matrix while a burnisher is used to stabilize the strip against adjacent tooth. **D,** Tofflemire matrix positioned and contoured for three-surface preparation.

(Dead Soft Metal Matrix, DenMat Corporation, Santa Maria, California) is cut, contoured, and burnished. Commercial, precontoured types (Palodent Matrix, Palodent Company, Portola Valley, California; Composi-Tight Matrix, Garrison Dental Solutions, Spring Lake, Michigan) also are available. The small compound cones are made by softening green stick compound over a Bunsen burner as described in Chapter 17. The initial wedge placed during tooth preparation is removed, the matrix positioned, and a new wedge placed (see Fig. 13-38, A). It is helpful to hold the strip against the adjacent tooth with a burnisher while the matrix is stabilized with the softened, compound cones (see Fig. 13-38, B and C). If additional contouring is needed, it can be accomplished with the back side of a warmed Black's spoon excavator.

When both proximal surfaces are involved, a Tofflemire retainer with an ultrathin, burnishable matrix band is used. The band is contoured, positioned, wedged, and shaped as needed for proper proximal contacts and embrasures (see Fig. 13-38, D). The use of compound to help support a matrix of this type is generally not necessary because heavy condensing forces are not used when the posterior composite material is inserted.

Clear polyester matrices are available and may be used for the restoration of very small Class II prepara-

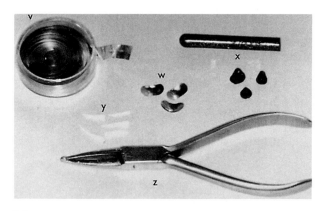

FIG. **13-39** Materials for application of compound-supported matrix on two-surface preparations: thin, dead-soft strip metal (v) or preformed matrices (w), green stick compound and cones (x), wooden wedges (y), and No. 110 pliers (z).

tions. Care must be taken to properly contour the polyester matrix strip, as described in Chapter 12, to impart sufficient convexity into the polyester band. Precontoured polyester matrices also are available for use in light-weight Tofflemeire retainers (Teledyne Water Pik, Fort Collins, Colorado) or as part of a unique circumferential matrix system called the Translite Auto Matrix System (Dentsply/Caulk, Milford, Delaware). Clear polyester matrices are typically thicker than metal matrices and must be firmly wedged to compensate for this additional thickness. Clear polyester matrices are not recommended for larger posterior composite restorations because they cannot be contoured as well as metal matrices and they do not provide adequate resistance to condensation if a viscous composite is used.

However, other matrix systems have been developed for Class II composite restorations. The primary benefit promoted by their manufacturers is a simpler method for establishing an appropriate composite proximal contact. Several of the available systems are shown in Fig. 13-40.

Inserting and Curing the Composite. A two-step procedure (applying the enamel/dentin bonding adhesive, if not already applied, then the posterior composite material) is followed with either self-cured (seldom used) or light-cured composite materials. A light-cured system is used for restoring the Class II preparation illustrated on the maxillary first molar shown in Fig. 13-37 and the maxillary left premolars in Fig. 13-41. These materials should not be dispensed until ready to use, because they will begin to polymerize from the ambient light in the operatory. Because of variations in materials, each manufacturer's specific instructions should be followed.

The enamel/dentin bonding adhesive is placed over the entire preparation (etched and primed enamel and dentin) with a microbrush, foam sponge, or applicator tip in accordance with the manufacturer's instructions. The adhesive is polymerized with a visible light source, usually for 20 seconds.

Composite insertion hand instruments or a syringe may be used to insert the composite material (Fig. 13-42). The first type of syringe (y) (Centrix Inc., Milford, Connecticut) shown can be used with a clear plastic tip for

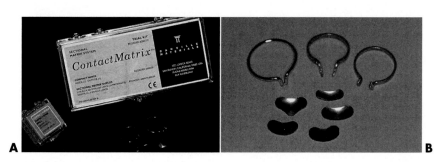

A   **B**

FIG. **13-40** New composite matrix systems. **A,** Contact Matrix (Danville Materials). **B,** Composi-Tight Matrix System (Garrison Dental Solutions, Spring Lake, Michigan).

self-cured composites or with a black or orange tip for light-cured composites. The second syringe (z) (Dentsply/ Caulk, Milford, Delaware) is designed by the manufacturer for use with preloaded compule tips. The tips on both types must be kept covered when not in use to prevent premature hardening of light-cured materials.

Following matrix and adhesive placement, small increments of composite material are added and successively cured (see Fig. 13-37). It is important to place (and cure) the composite incrementally to maximize the curing potential and, possibly, reduce the effects of polymerization shrinkage. For this reason, the first small increment should be placed along the gingival floor and should extend slightly up the facial and lingual walls (see Fig. 13-37, B). This increment should only be approximately 1 to 2 mm in thickness because it is the farthest increment from the curing light and is most critical in establishing a proper gingival seal. This first increment should be cured with a light exposure of 20 to 40 seconds (see Fig. 13-37, C). Subsequent additions are made and cured (usually not exceeding 2 mm in thick-

ness at a time) until the preparation is filled to slight excess (see Fig. 13-37, D and E). The restoration can be contoured and finished immediately after the last increment is cured. Another clinical example is illustrated in Fig. 13-41. Light-cured composites work very well for the restoration of posterior teeth because of extended working time and the ease of incremental placement (and cure). However, if a light-cured composite is not available, a self-cured composite can be used.

Contouring and Polishing the Composite. Contouring can be initiated immediately after a light-cured composite material has been polymerized, or 3 minutes after the initial hardening of a self-cured material. The occlusal surface is shaped with a round or oval, 12-bladed carbide finishing bur (Figs. 13-43, A, and 13-44, A) or finishing diamond. Special carbide-tipped carvers are useful for removing composite excess along occlusal margins (see Fig. 13-43, B). Excess composite is removed at the proximal margins and embrasures with a flame-shaped, 12-bladed carbide finishing bur (see Figs. 13-43, C, and 13-44, B) or finishing diamond and abrasive discs (see

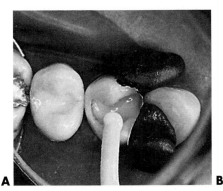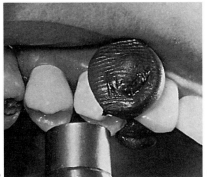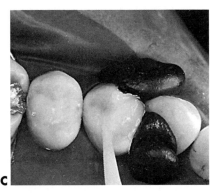

FIG. **13-41** Insertion of light-cured composite material, maxillary premolar. **A** to **C**, Compound-supported matrix has been positioned, wedged, and reinforced. Composite is inserted and cured in small increments until preparation is slightly overfilled.

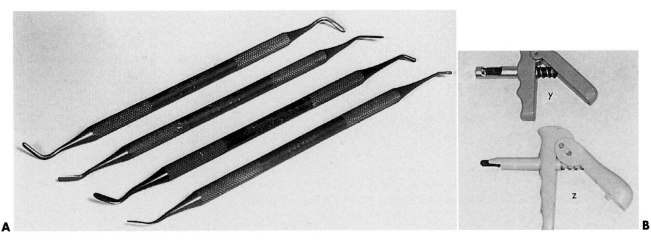

FIG. **13-42** Insertion instruments for composite. **A**, Anodized aluminum instruments. **B**, Two types of injection syringes: Centrix (y) and Caulk (z).

Fig. 13-44, *C*). Any overhangs at the gingival area are removed with a sharp amalgam knife, gold knife, or a No. 12 surgical blade mounted in a Bard-Parker handle. These instruments are used with light shaving strokes to remove the excess (see Fig. 13-44, *D*). Narrow finishing strips may be used to smooth the gingival proximal surface (see Fig. 13-43, *D*). Care must be exercised to maintain the position of the finishing strips gingival to the proximal contact area to avoid inadvertent opening of the contact.

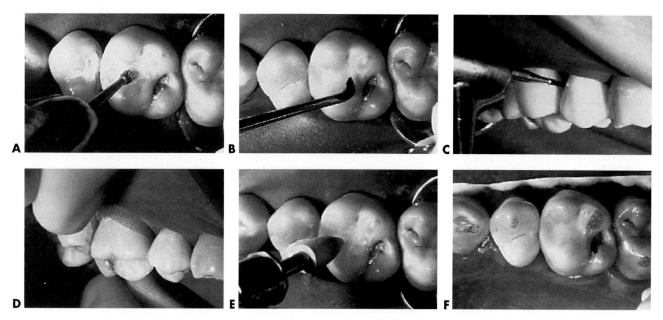

FIG. **13-43** Contouring and finishing posterior composite restoration. **A,** Round (or oval), 12-bladed carbide finishing bur is used to contour occlusal surface. **B,** Carbide-tipped carver is useful for removing excess composite along occlusal margins. **C,** Flame-shaped carbide finishing bur is used to contour proximal areas. **D,** Narrow finishing strip smoothes proximal areas. **E,** Abrasive rubber point is used to smooth occlusal surfaces. **F,** Completed posterior composite restoration with articulation marks.

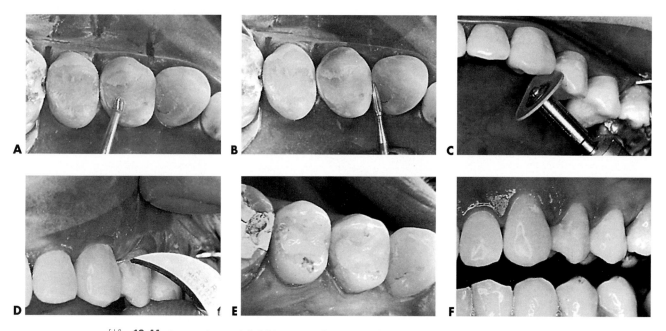

FIG. **13-44** Contouring and finishing posterior composite restoration. (**A, B,** and **E** are mirror views.) **A,** Occlusal surface shaped with round (or oval), 12-bladed carbide finishing bur. **B** and **C,** Proximal areas are shaped with flame-shaped finishing bur and abrasive discs. **D,** Removing excess material at gingival area with a No. 12 blade (Bard-Parker handle). **E** and **F,** Occlusal and facial views after rubber dam removal, occlusal adjustments, and final polishing.

The rubber dam (or other means of isolation) is removed and the occlusion is evaluated for proper contact. Further adjustments are made if needed, and the restorations are finished with fine, rubber abrasive points, cups, and/or discs (see Fig. 13-43, *E*). The restored teeth are illustrated in Figs. 13-43, *F,* and 13-44, *E* and *F*.

CLINICAL TECHNIQUE FOR EXTENSIVE CLASS II COMPOSITE RESTORATIONS AND FOUNDATIONS

When very large restorations are required, it usually indicates that: (1) most of the occlusal contacts will be restored by the restorative material, (2) the extensions will be onto the root surface, and (3) the area will probably be difficult to isolate. All three of these conditions increase the concerns of using composite as the restorative material. However, composite may be the material selected for either very large Class II restorations, or foundations that will serve under indirect restorations. Very large Class II preparations may be indicated when economic factors prevent the patient from selecting a more expensive indirect restoration. The ability to strengthen the weakened tooth structure with a bonded restoration sometimes makes this procedure a logical choice. This type of restoration also may be indicated as an interim restoration, while waiting to determine the pulpal response, or whether or not the restoration will function appropriately. Composite also may be considered for use as a foundation for indirect restorations (primarily crowns) when the operator determines that insufficient natural tooth structure remains to provide adequate retention and resistance form for the crown. Thus the tooth is first restored with a large restoration and then prepared for a crown. Parts of the axial and/or occlusal surfaces of the crown preparation may then be composite, rather than tooth structure.

It should be noted that amalgam may be the restorative material of choice for both of these procedures, because of its known wear resistance, strength, and track record in serving as both of these types of restorations. Amalgam restorations used for these purposes can also be bonded, providing the following: (1) a good dentinal seal, (2) additional retention form, and (3) reinforcement of the remaining weakened tooth structure, although the extent of the perceived advantages is largely unknown. Large Class II amalgam restorations and amalgam foundations are presented in Chapter 19. Whether a composite or bonded amalgam restoration is selected, the area must be kept isolated from moisture contamination during the bonding procedure, or a clinical failure is likely, especially considering the increased size of the restoration.

In addition to the tooth preparation form, the primary retention form for a very large Class II composite restoration is the micromechanical bonding of the composite to the enamel and dentin. However, secondary retention features usually are incorporated into the large preparation because of: (1) the increased amount of missing tooth structure; (2) the decreased amount of tooth structure available for bonding; and, therefore, (3) the increased concern for retaining the composite in the tooth. These may include grooves, coves, locks, slots, or pins. Increased retention form also may be accomplished by including otherwise sound areas of the remaining tooth structure (e.g., facial or lingual grooves), or making wider bevels or flares on accessible enamel margins, both of which increase the surface area for bonding.

The primary differences for these very large preparations include the following: (1) some or all of the cusps may be capped, (2) extensions in most directions will be greater, (3) more secondary retention features will be used, and (4) more resistance form features will be used. A cusp must be capped if the operator believes it will likely fracture if left in a weakened state. Capping a cusp usually is indicated when the occlusal outline form extends more than two thirds the distance from a primary groove to a cusp tip. An operator may sometimes choose to ignore this general rule when using a bonded restoration because the bonding strengthens the remaining weakened unprepared tooth structure.

If the tooth has had endodontic treatment, the pulp chamber can be opened, and extensions made several millimeters into each treated canal (Fig. 13-45). These areas are etched and primed, adhesive is placed, and composite is inserted and cured incrementally. Because of the increased surface area for bonding and the mechanical retention from extensions into the canals, usually fewer secondary retention features are incorporated into the tooth preparation.

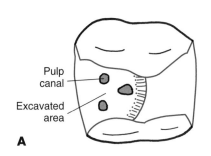

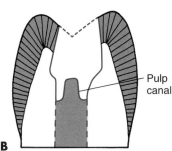

Pulp canal

Excavated area

Pulp canal

FIG. 13-45 Preparation extension into pulp chamber and canal for endodontically treated tooth. **A,** Occlusal view. **B,** Proximal view.

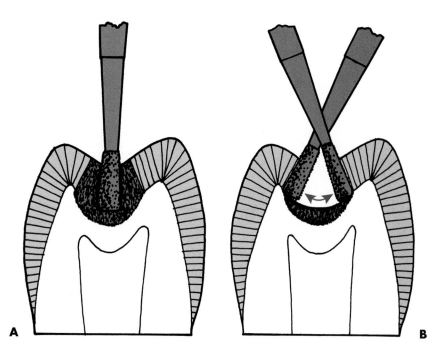

FIG. **13-46** Extensive caries facially and lingually. **A,** After initial entry cut at correct initial depth (1.5 mm), caries remains facially and lingually. **B,** Orientation of diamond must be tilted as instrument is extended facially or lingually to maintain a 1.5-mm depth.

CLINICAL TECHNIQUE

The inverted cone diamond is used to prepare the occlusal surface. As already indicated, usually the occlusal outline form is extensive. When moving the diamond from the central groove area toward a cuspal prominence, the 1.5-mm pulpal depth should be maintained, if possible. This creates a pulpal floor, which rises occlusally as it is extended either facially or lingually (Fig. 13-46). If a cusp must be capped, the side of the diamond can first be used to make several depth cuts in the remaining cuspal form to serve as a guide for cusp reduction. Cusps should be capped as early in the tooth preparation procedure as possible, providing more access and visibility for the preparation. The depth cut is made with the diamond held parallel to the cuspal incline (from cusp tip to central groove) and approximately 1.5 mm in depth. For a large cusp, several depth cuts can be made. Then the diamond is used to join the depth cuts and extend to the remainder of the cuspal form (Fig. 13-47). The reduced cusp will have a relatively flat surface that may rise and fall with the normal mesial and distal inclines of the cusp. It also should provide enough clearance with the opposing tooth to result in approximately 1.5 to 2 mm of composite material to restore form and function. The cusp reduction should be blended in with the rest of the occlusal step portion of the preparation.

The proximal boxes (usually both would be involved in a large restoration or foundation) are prepared as described previously. The primary difference is that they may be much larger, that is, more extension in every di-

rection. The extent of the lesion may dictate that a proximal box extend around the line angle of the tooth to include faulty facial or lingual tooth structure. Once the outline form has been established (the margins extended to sound tooth structure), the preparation is carefully assessed for additional retention form needs.

Retention form can be enhanced by the placement of grooves, locks, coves, or slots. Pins can be used, but not as effectively esthetically as the other potential secondary retention forms. All such retention form features must be placed entirely in dentin, thereby not undermining and weakening any adjacent enamel. At times, bevels may be placed on available enamel margins to enhance retention form, even occlusal areas. Additionally, for extensive Class II restorations or foundations, arbitrary inclusion of uninvolved facial or lingual grooves may be considered for preparation, thereby increasing the bonding surface area. Retention form for foundations must be placed far enough inside the DEJ (approximately 1 mm) to remain after the crown preparation is done subsequently. Otherwise, the potential retentiveness may be lost for the foundation (Fig. 13-48).

Fig. 13-49 illustrates an example of a very extensive Class II modified tooth preparation. A maxillary first premolar is badly discolored from a large, faulty, corroded amalgam restoration and caries (see Fig. 13-49, *A*). Esthetic and economic factors resulted in the decision to replace the amalgam with a composite restoration, rather than an indirect restoration. The preparation is shown with all of the old amalgam and infected dentin removed, leaving the facial and lingual enamel

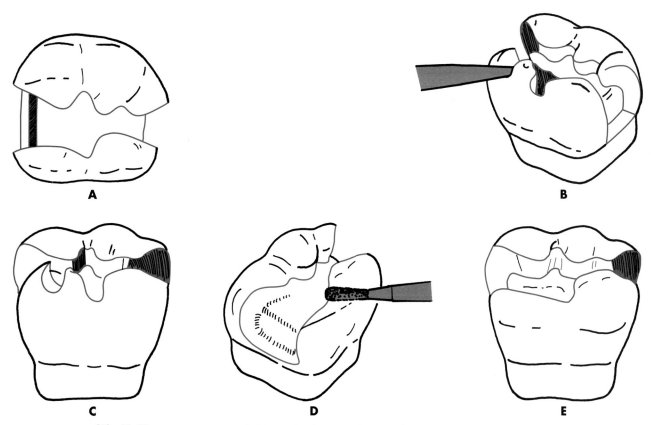

FIG. **13-47** Cusp reduction. **A,** Initial outline form weakens mesiolingual cusp enough to require capping. **B,** Depth cuts made. **C,** Depth cuts. **D,** Cusp reduction prepared. **E,** Vertical wall maintained between reduced and unreduced cusps.

wall severely weakened (see Fig. 13-49, *B*). After placement of a calcium hydroxide liner over the deeply excavated area (see Fig. 13-49, *C*), a diamond was used to reduce the severely undermined enamel of the lingual cusp approximately 1.5 mm and place a reverse bevel with a chamfered margin on the lingual surface (see Fig. 13-49, *D*). The same instrument was used to reduce the facial cusp 0.75 mm and place a slight counterbevel. This extensive tooth preparation has been observed to be successful, but not from controlled clinical research studies. The completed restoration is shown in Fig. 13-50, *C,* and, after 5 years of service, in Fig. 13-50, *D* and *E.*

Matrix placement is more demanding for these large restorations because more tooth structure is missing and more margins may be subgingival. Proper burnishing of the matrix band to effect appropriate axial contours is important. It also may be necessary to modify the matrix band to provide more subgingival extension in some areas and prevent extrusion of the composite from the matrix band-retainer junction.

Typical etching and priming techniques are followed. Because much of the composite bond will be to dentin, proper technique is very important. Placement of the adhesive (if a separate step) is accomplished as previously described, and the composite is inserted incrementally. The composite is first placed in 1- to 2-mm increments

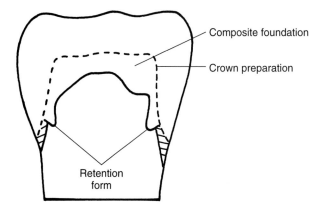

FIG. **13-48** Retention form for foundations must be internal to eventual crown preparation.

into the most gingival areas of the proximal boxes. Each increment is cured as directed. It may be helpful to use a hand instrument to hold the matrix against the adjacent tooth while curing the composite. This may assist in restoring the proximal contact. Fig. 13-51 shows the matrix placement and composite insertion for the tooth prepared in Fig. 13-49.

Contouring the large composite is also more difficult because of the number of surfaces that may be involved and the amount of composite present. Physiologic contours

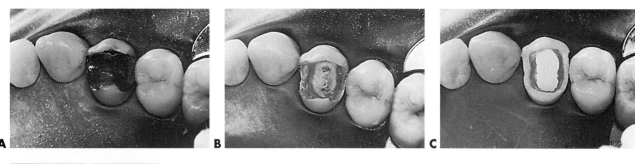

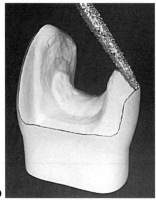

FIG. **13-49** Mesioocclusodistal Class II extensive modified tooth preparation for composite restoration. **A,** Esthetics and cost are factors in decision to replace faulty restoration with posterior composite. **B,** Amalgam and infected dentin removed. **C,** Calcium hydroxide liner inserted. **D,** Diamond used to reduce severely undermined lingual cusp and place bevel.

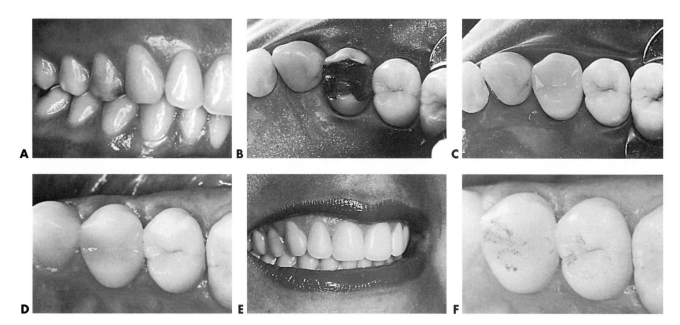

FIG. **13-50** Preoperative and postoperative views of posterior composite restoration. (**A** and **E** are mirror views.) **A** and **B,** Preoperative facial and occlusal views. **C,** After inserting and polishing composite restoration. Occlusal (**D**) and facial (**E**) views after 5 years of service. **F,** Occlusion marked with articulating paper at 5-year recall appointment.

and contacts are necessary for restorations, but they are less important for foundations that will only be present for a very short period of time before the crown preparation is done. Because of the extensiveness of these restorations, a careful assessment of the contours should be made from all angles. Once contouring is completed, the occlusion is adjusted as necessary and the restoration is polished. Because these very large restorations may stretch the limits of composite restorations, the patient should be on a frequent recall regimen. Fig. 13-50 illustrates the contouring, polishing, and 5-year recall of the extensive tooth preparation in Fig. 13-49.

Many dentists prefer to use self-cured composites for foundations and core build-ups. Without the need for

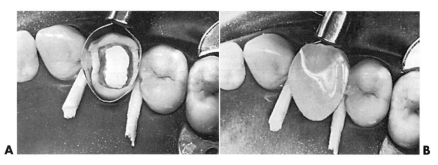

FIG. **13-51 A,** Self-cured composite will be inserted into the three-surface preparation shown with matrix in place. **B,** Injected composite was covered by matrix strip and held under pressure during polymerization.

light activation, the composite can be placed in bulk, which can save considerable time. The composite core is typically placed following application of an enamel/dentin adhesive. Most current adhesives contain the primer and bonding agent in one solution (see Chapter 5). Unfortunately, almost none of the "one-bottle" adhesives provide an acceptable bond of self-cure composite to tooth structure. While the reason for this is not completely understood, some investigators believe that acidic monomers in the adhesives can interfere with the activators (tertiary amines) in the self-cure composite. If the activator does not function properly, the composite at the adhesive interface will not polymerize thoroughly and will not bond to the adhesive or the underlying tooth structure. Some manufacturers have introduced optional chemical catalysts that can be mixed with the adhesive to reduce or prevent this problem.

SUMMARY

This chapter has presented the rationale and technique for composite use in the treatment of the occlusal and proximal surfaces of posterior teeth. This chapter and textbook emphasize the use of composite as the restorative material for many Class I and Class II restorations. Although greater emphasis has been placed on the use of composite in posterior teeth, this emphasis is not due to concerns for the use of amalgam as a restorative material. As later chapters demonstrate, amalgam restorations are still strongly recommended in this textbook. Regardless, many Class I and Class II lesions are best restored with composite. Typical problems, solutions, and repair techniques for composite restorations are presented in Chapter 11.

REFERENCES

1. American Dental Association: Intervention: pit and fissure sealants, *J Am Dent Assoc* 126:17S-18S, 1995.
2. American Dental Association Council on Scientific Affairs, ADA Council on Dental Benefits and Programs: statement on posterior resin-based composites, *J Am Dent Assoc*130: 1627-1628, 1998.
3. Ausiello P et al: Fracture resistance of endodontically-treated premolars adhesively restored, *Am J Dent* 10:237-241, 1997.
4. Barnes DM et al: A 5- and 8-year clinical evaluation of a posterior composite resin, *Quintessence Int* 22:143-151, 1991.
5. Bayne SC et al: Clinical longevity of ten posterior composite materials based on wear (abstract no. 630), *J Dent Res* 70:344, 1991.
6. Bayne SC et al: Long term clinical failures in posterior composites (abstract no. 32), *J Dent Res* 68:185, 1989.
7. Collins CJ, Bryant RV, Hodge KL: A clinical evaluation of posterior composite resin restorations: 8-year findings, *J Dent* 26(4):311-317, 1998.
8. Combe EC, Burke FJT, Douglas WH: Thermal properties. In Combe EC, Burke FJT, Douglas WH, editors: *Dental biomaterials*, Boston, 1999, Kluwer Academic.
9. Ehrnford L, Derand T: Cervical gap formation in Class II composite resin restorations, *Swed Dent J* 8:15-19, 1984.
10. Gwinnett AJ: Moist versus dry dentin: its effect on shear bond strength, *Am J Dent* 5:127-129, 1992.
11. Gwinnett AJ, Kanca JA: Micromorphology of the bonded dentin interface and its relationship to bond strength, *Am J Dent* 5:73-77, 1992.
12. Handelman SL et al: Clinical radiographic evaluation of sealed carious and sound tooth surfaces, *J Am Dent Assoc* 113: 751-754, Nov 1986.
13. Heymann HO, Bayne SC: Current concepts in dentin bonding: focusing on dentinal adhesion factors, *J Am Dent Assoc* 124(5):27-36, May 1993.
14. Heymann HO et al: Two-year clinical study of composite resins in posterior teeth, *Dent Mater* 2:37-41, 1986.
15. Kumar J, Siegal MD: Workshop on guidelines for sealant use: recommendations, *J Pub Health Dent* 55(No. 5; special issue):263-273, 1995.
16. Liberman R et al: The effect of posterior composite restorations on the resistance of cavity walls to vertically applied loads, *J Oral Rehabil* 17:99-105, 1990.
17. Mair LH: Ten-year clinical assessment of three posterior resin composites and two amalgams, *Quint Internat* 29:483-490, 1998.
18. Mazer RB, Leinfelder KF: Clinical evaluation of a posterior composite resin containing a new type of filler particle, *J Esthet Dent* 1:66-70, 1988.
19. Mazer RB, Leinfelder KF: Evaluating a microfill posterior composite resin: a five year study, *J Am Dent Assoc* 123(4):33-38, 1992.
20. McCune RJ, Cvar JF, Ryge G: Clinical comparison of anterior and posterior restorative materials (abstract no. 482), *Int Assoc Dent Res* 161, March 1969.
21. McCune RJ et al: Clinical comparison of posterior restorative materials (abstract no. 546), *Int Assoc Dent Res* 175, March 1967.

22. Mertz-Fairhurst EJ et al: Cariostatic and ultraconservative sealed restorations: six year results, *Quintessence Int* 23(12): 827-838, 1992.

23. Simonsen RJ: Preventive resin restoration, *Quintessence Int* 9(1):69-76, 1978.

24. Simonsen RJ: Preventive resin restorations: three year results, *J Am Dent Assoc* 100(4):535-539, 1980.

25. Simonsen RJ: Retention and effectiveness of a single application of white sealant after 10 years, *J Am Dent Assoc* 115: 31-36, July 1987.

26. Sturdevant JR et al: Five-year study of two light-cured posterior composite resins, *Dent Mater* 4:105-110, 1988.

27. Swift EJ Jr: The effect of sealants on dental caries: a review, *J Am Dent Assoc* 116:700-704, May 1988.

28. Torstenson B, Brannstrom M: Composite resin contraction gaps measured with a fluorescent resin technique, *Dent Mater* 4:238-242, 1988.

29. Wilder AD, May KN, Leinfelder KF: Three-year clinical study of UV-cured composite resins in posterior teeth, *J Prosthet Dent* 50(1):26, 1983.

30. Wilson NHF et al: Five-year findings of a multiclinical trial for a posterior composite, *J Dent* 19:153-159, 1991.

14

Classes I and II Indirect Tooth-Colored Restorations

EDWARD J. SWIFT, JR.

JOHN R. STURDEVANT

ANDRÉ V. RITTER

CLASSES I AND II INDIRECT RESTORATIONS

The previous three chapters describe directly placed tooth-colored composite restorations. Teeth also can be restored using indirect techniques, in which restorations are fabricated outside of the mouth. Most indirect restorations are made on a replica of the prepared tooth in a dental laboratory by a trained technician. Tooth-colored indirect systems include laboratory-processed composites or ceramics such as porcelain fired on refractory dies or hot pressed glasses. In addition, at least one chairside computer-aided design/computer-assisted manufacturing (CAD/CAM) system is currently available and is used to fabricate ceramic restorations (Fig. 14-1). This chapter reviews the indications, contraindications, advantages, disadvantages, and the clinical technique for Class I and Class II indirect tooth-colored restorations.

INDICATIONS

The indications for Classes I or II indirect tooth-colored restorations relate to a combination of esthetic demands and size of the restoration and include the following:

- *Esthetics*—Indirect tooth-colored restorations are indicated for Class I or Class II restorations located in areas of esthetic importance for the patient.
- *Large defects or previous restorations*—Indirect tooth-colored restorations should be considered for restoration of large Class I or Class II defects or replacement of large existing compromised restorations, especially those that are wide faciolingually and require cusp coverage. Large preparations are best restored with adhesive restorations that strengthen the remaining tooth structure.[4,34] The contours of large restorations are more easily developed when using indirect techniques. Indirect tooth-colored restorative materials are more durable than direct composites, especially in regard to maintaining occlusal surfaces and occlusal contacts.[7,49] The wear resistance provided by indirect materials is especially important in large posterior restorations that involve most or all of the occlusal contacts.[52] However, without sufficient bulk, an extensive indirect ceramic or composite restoration may fracture under occlusal loading, particularly in the molar region.[13]
- *Economic factors*—Some patients desire the best dental treatment available, regardless of cost. For these patients, indirect tooth-colored restorations may be indicated not only for large restorations, but also for moderate-sized restorations that might otherwise be restored with a direct restorative material (usually composite).

CONTRAINDICATIONS

Contraindications for indirect tooth-colored restorations include:

- *Heavy occlusal forces*—Ceramic restorations may fracture when they lack sufficient bulk or are subject to excessive occlusal stress, as in patients who have bruxing or clenching habits. Heavy wear facets or a lack of occlusal enamel are good indicators of bruxing and clenching habits (Fig. 14-2).
- *Inability to maintain a dry field*—Despite some research suggesting that modern dental adhesives can counteract certain types of contamination,[16,17] adhesive techniques require near-perfect moisture control to ensure successful long-term clinical results.
- *Deep subgingival preparations*—Although this is not an absolute contraindication, preparations with deep subgingival margins should be avoided. These margins are difficult to record with an impression and are difficult to finish. Additionally, bonding to enamel margins is greatly preferred, especially along gingival margins of proximal boxes.[20]

ADVANTAGES

The advantages of indirect tooth-colored restorations are similar to those of direct composite restorations (excluding cost and time) (see Chapter 11). Indirect tooth-colored restorations have the following additional advantages:

- *Improved physical properties*—A wide variety of high-strength tooth-colored restorative materials, including

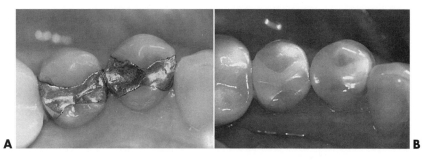

FIG. **14-1 A,** Defective mesioocclusodistal (MOD) amalgam restorations on mandibular premolars were replaced with CAD/CAM ceramic inlays. **B,** Ceramic inlays after 12 years of clinical service.

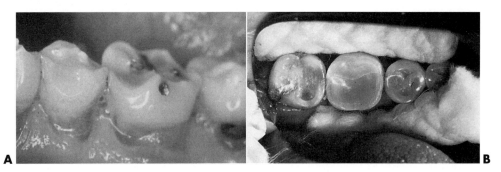

FIG. **14-2 A,** Clenching and bruxing habits can cause extensive wear of occlusal surfaces. This patient is not a good candidate for ceramic inlays. **B,** Example of a fractured inlay in a patient with heavy occlusion.

laboratory-processed and computer-milled composites and ceramics, can be used with indirect techniques. Indirect restorations have better physical properties than direct composite restorations because they are fabricated under relatively ideal laboratory conditions. Also, while CAD/CAM restorations are generally fabricated chairside, the materials themselves are manufactured under very nearly ideal industrial conditions.[56]

- *Variety of materials and techniques*—Indirect tooth-colored restorations can be fabricated with either composites or ceramics using various laboratory processes or CAD/CAM methods.
- *Wear resistance*—Ceramic restorations are more wear-resistant than direct composite restorations, an especially critical factor when restoring large occlusal areas of posterior teeth. Laboratory-processed composite restorations wear more than ceramics, but less than direct composites in laboratory studies.[7,49,55,59]
- *Reduced polymerization shrinkage*—Polymerization shrinkage and its consequential stresses are still a major shortcoming of direct composite restorations. With indirect techniques, the bulk of the preparation is filled with the indirect tooth-colored restoration, and stresses are reduced because very little composite cement is used during cementation. Although shrinkage of composite in thin bonded layers can produce relatively high stress,[18] studies indicate that indirect composite restorations have fewer marginal voids, less microleakage, and less postoperative sensitivity than direct composites.[12,14,47,58]
- *Ability to strengthen remaining tooth structure*—Tooth structure weakened by caries, trauma, and/or preparation can be strengthened by adhesively bonding indirect inlays and onlays.[8,58] The reduced polymerization shrinkage stress obtained with the indirect technique is also desirable when restoring such weakened teeth.
- *More precise control of contours and contacts*—Indirect techniques usually provide better contours (especially proximal contours) and occlusal contacts than

direct restorations because of the improved access and visibility outside the mouth.

- *Biocompatibility and good tissue response*—Ceramic materials are considered the most chemically inert of all materials. They are biocompatible and generally are associated with a good soft tissue response.[2,27] The pulpal biocompatibility of the indirect techniques is related more to the adhesive composite cements (see Chapter 4) rather than the ceramic materials used.
- *Increased auxiliary support*—Most indirect techniques allow the fabrication of the restoration to be totally or partially delegated to dental laboratory technicians. Such delegation allows for more efficient use of the dentist's time.

DISADVANTAGES

The following are disadvantages of indirect tooth-colored restorations:

- *Increased cost and time*—Most indirect techniques require two patient appointments, plus fabrication of a temporary restoration. These factors, along with laboratory fees, contribute to the greater cost of indirect restorations as compared to direct restorations. However, while indirect tooth-colored inlays and onlays are more expensive than direct restorations (amalgams or composites), they are usually less costly than more invasive esthetic alternatives, such as all-ceramic or porcelain-fused-to-metal (PFM) crowns.
- *Technique sensitivity*—Restorations made using indirect techniques require a high level of operator skill. A devotion to excellence is necessary during preparation, impression, try-in, cementation, and finishing the restoration. Diligence is required during all stages of the process to obtain a high-quality restoration.
- *Brittleness of ceramics*—A ceramic restoration can fracture if the preparation does not provide adequate thickness to resist occlusal forces and/or if the restoration is not appropriately supported by the cement medium and the preparation. Fractures can occur either during try-in or after cementation, especially in

patients who generate unusually high occlusal forces.

- *Wear of opposing dentition and restorations*—Ceramic materials can cause excessive wear of opposing enamel and/or restorations.[1,32] Recent improvements in ceramics have reduced this problem, but ceramics, particularly if rough and unpolished, can wear opposing teeth and restorations.

- *Resin-to-resin bonding difficulties*—Laboratory-processed composites are highly cross-linked, so few double bonds remain available for chemical adhesion of the composite cement.[44] Therefore the composite restoration must be mechanically abraded and/or chemically treated to facilitate adhesion of the cement.[48,50,54] The bond between the indirect composite restoration and the composite cement is the weak link in the system. However, bonding of composite cements to properly treated ceramic restorations is *not* a problem.[43]

- *Short clinical track record*—Indirect bonded tooth-colored restorations have become relatively popular only in recent years and are still not placed by many practitioners. Few controlled clinical trials are available, so the long-term durability of these restorations, although expected to be good, is not particularly well documented.[6,21,23,25,28,32,42,57,60]

- *Low potential for repair*—Indirect restorations, particularly ceramic inlays/onlays, are difficult to repair in the event of a partial fracture. If the fracture occurs in the restoration, an indirect composite inlay or onlay can be repaired using an adhesive system and a light-cured restorative composite. The bond strengths of indirect composite repair and direct composite repair appear to be equivalent.[24] When a partial fracture occurs in a ceramic inlay/onlay, repair is usually not a definitive treatment. The actual procedure (mechanical roughening, etching with hydrofluoric acid, and application of a silane coupling agent before restoring with an adhesive and composite) is relatively simple. However, because ceramic inlays/onlays are indicated in areas where occlusal wear, esthetics, and resistance are important, direct composite repairs are not suitable because that composite will be exposed to a challenging environment.

- *Difficult intraoral polishing*—Indirect composite restorations can be polished intraorally with the same instruments/materials used to polish direct composites. Ceramics, on the other hand, are more difficult to polish after they have been cemented because of either (1) limited access or (2) lack of appropriate instrumentation (see the later section Finishing and Polishing Procedures).

LABORATORY-PROCESSED COMPOSITE INLAYS AND ONLAYS

The physical properties of composite restorations are improved when the composite is free of voids, and the resin matrix is maximally polymerized. Generating dense, well-cured restorations is best accomplished in the dental laboratory using devices that polymerize the composite under pressure, vacuum, inert gas, intense light, heat, or a combination of these conditions.[15,19,38,40] Several commercial systems use these techniques to optimize the physical properties of their composite materials.

Laboratory-processed composite inlays and onlays are more resistant to occlusal wear than direct composites, particularly in occlusal contact areas.[7] However, they are less wear-resistant than ceramic restorations.[29] They offer easy adjustment, low wear of the opposing dentition, good esthetics, and potential for repair.[30] Processed composite restorations are indicated when: (1) maximum wear resistance is desired from a composite restoration, (2) achievement of proper contours and contacts would otherwise be difficult, and (3) a ceramic restoration is not indicated because of cost or concerns about wear of the opposing dentition. Regarding the latter, the indirect composite would likely cause less wear of the opposing dentition than a similar ceramic restoration.

A clinical trial on indirect composite inlays compared the performance of a heat- and pressure-cured microfill composite (Concept [Ivoclar Vivadent, Amherst, New York], which is no longer available) and gold restorations over 7 years.[13] Statistically, there was no difference between the two materials. However, the failure rate of the composite inlays in molars approached 50%, indicating that the composite material was better suited for use in premolars.

Several more complex laboratory-processed composites have been introduced recently. These are often called *polymer glasses, filled polymers,* or *ceramic-optimized resins (ceromers).* Manufacturers of these materials have recommended their use not only for inlays and onlays and some single-unit crowns, but also, with fiber reinforcement, for splints and short-span fixed partial dentures.

Although each manufacturer's system has unique aspects, the fabrication steps for one representative system can be summarized as follows:

1. The indirect composite restoration is initially formed on a replica of the prepared tooth (Figs. 14-3 and 14-4).
2. The composite is built up in layers, polymerizing each layer with a brief exposure to a visible light-curing unit (Fig. 14-5).
3. After it is built to full contour, the restoration is coated with a special gel to block out air and thus prevent formation of an oxygen-inhibited surface layer.
4. Final curing is accomplished by inserting the inlay into an ovenlike device that exposes the composite to additional light and heat (Fig. 14-6).
5. The cured composite inlay is trimmed, finished, and polished in the laboratory (Figs. 14-7 and 14-8).

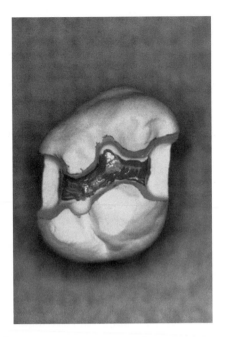

FIG. **14-3** Die prepared for making laboratory-processed composite inlay.

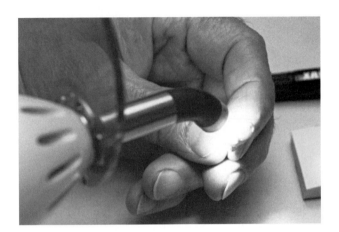

FIG. **14-5** Curing composite with curing light.

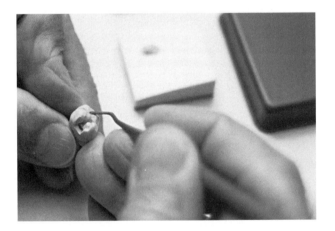

FIG. **14-4** Composite is added incrementally to form the inlay.

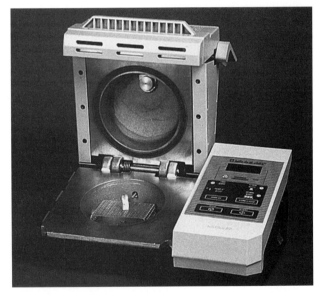

FIG. **14-6** Example of a curing device for additional polymerization. *(Courtesy of Kerr Corporation.)*

CERAMIC INLAYS AND ONLAYS

Ceramic inlays and onlays have become popular not only because of patient demand for esthetic, durable restorative materials, but also because of recent improvements in materials, fabrication techniques, and bonding systems. Among the ceramic materials used are feldspathic porcelain, hot pressed ceramics, and machinable ceramics designed for use with CAD/CAM systems.[39] The physical and mechanical properties of ceramics come closer to matching those of enamel than do composites. They have excellent wear resistance and a coefficient of thermal expansion very close to that of tooth structure. Some other physical properties of representative ceramics are shown in Table 14-1.

Feldspathic Porcelain Inlays and Onlays. Dental porcelains are partially crystalline minerals (feldspar, silica, alumina) dispersed in a glass matrix.[3] Porcelain restorations are made from finely ground ceramic powders that are mixed with distilled water or a special liquid, shaped into the desired form, then fired and fused together to form a translucent, material that looks like tooth structure. Currently, many ceramic inlays and onlays are

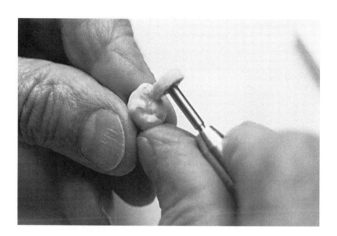

FIG. **14-7** Finishing composite inlay on die.

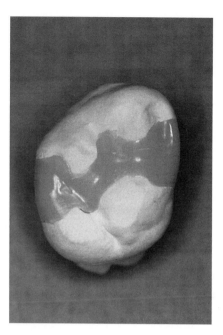

FIG. **14-8** Composite inlay, polished and ready for delivery.

TABLE 14-1 Mechanical Properties of Representative Ceramic Materials

CERAMIC	TYPE	ELASTIC MODULUS (GPa)	HARDNESS (GPa)	FRACTURE TOUGHNESS (MPa·m½)
Vita VMK 68	Sintered powder; leucite-reinforced	57.3	6.93	0.84
Optec HSP	Sintered powder; leucite-reinforced	64.9	6.67	1.29
IPS Empress	Hot pressed; leucite-reinforced	69.8	6.57	1.29
Dicor MGC	CAD/CAM material with fluormica plates	73.5	3.72	1.39

From Seghi RR, Denry IL, Rosenstiel SF: Relative fracture toughness and hardness of new dental ceramics, *J Prosthet Dent* 74(2):145-150, 1995.

fabricated in the dental laboratory by firing dental porcelains on refractory dies. The fabrication steps for fired ceramic inlays and onlays can be summarized as follows:

1. After tooth preparation, an impression is made and a "master" working cast is poured of die stone (Fig. 14-9).
2. The die is duplicated and poured with a refractory investment capable of withstanding porcelain firing temperatures. The duplication method must result in the master die and the refractory die being accurately interchangeable (Fig. 14-10).
3. Porcelain is added into the preparation area of the refractory die and fired in an oven. Multiple increments and firings are necessary to compensate for sintering shrinkage (Fig. 14-11).
4. The ceramic restoration is recovered from the refractory die, cleaned of all investment, and seated on the master die and working cast for final adjustments and finishing (Fig. 14-12).

Many dental laboratories use this technique to fabricate ceramic inlays and onlays because of its low start-up cost. The ceramic powders and investments are relatively inexpensive, and the technique is compatible with most existing ceramic laboratory equipment such as firing furnaces. The major disadvantage of this technique is its technique sensitivity. Although some technicians can routinely fabricate these restorations with excellent marginal integrity, many dentists complain of problems with fit and strength. Inlays and onlays fabricated with this technique must be handled very gently during try-in to avoid fracture. Even after cementation, the incidence of fracture is rather high for this type of ceramic restoration.[57]

Hot Pressed Glass Ceramics. In 1968, it was discovered that certain glasses could be modified with nucleating agents and, upon heat treatment, be changed into ceramics with organized crystalline forms. Such "glass-ceramics" were stronger, had a higher melting point than noncrystalline glass, and had variable coefficients of thermal expansion.[35] At first, these glass-ceramics were primarily developed for cookware and other heat-resistant products. In 1984, the glass-ceramic material Dicor (Dentsply International, York, Pennsylvania) was patented and rapidly became a popular ceramic for dental restorations. A major disadvantage of Dicor was its translucency, which necessitated external application of all shading.

Dicor restorations were made using a lost-wax, centrifugal casting process. Newer leucite-reinforced glass-ceramic systems also use the lost-wax method, but the material is heated to a high temperature and pneumatically pressed, rather than centrifuged, into a mold. Although some studies indicate that hot pressed ceramics are not significantly stronger than fired feldspathic porcelains,[9,10] they do appear to provide better clinical service.[21,32]

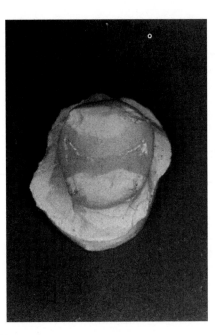

FIG. 14-11 Dental porcelains are added and fired in increments until inlay is the correct shape.

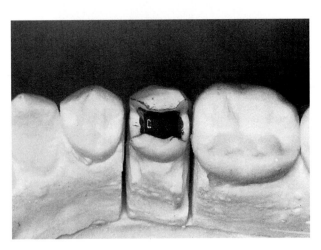

FIG. 14-9 Master cast for MOD ceramic inlay. Die spacer is usually applied to axial walls and pulpal floor before duplication.

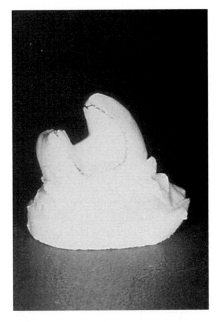

FIG. 14-10 Master die is impressed, then a duplicate die is poured with refractory investment.

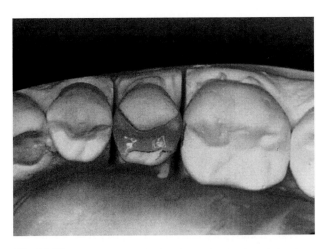

FIG. 14-12 Inlay is cleaned of all investment, then seated on master die for final adjustments and finishing. Ceramic inlay is now ready for delivery. (Courtesy of Dr. G. Sheen.)

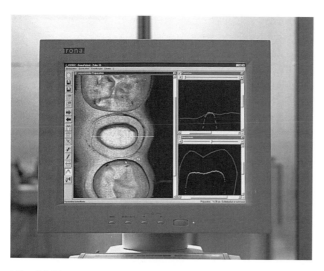

FIG. 14-20 The restoration is designed on the computer screen by drawing position of gingival margins and proximal contacts. *(Courtesy of Sirona USA.)*

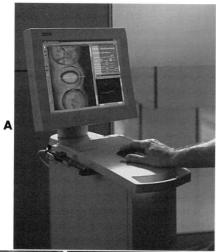

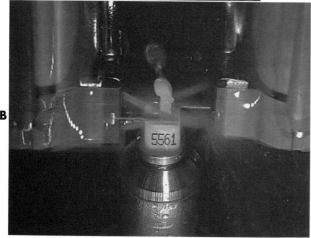

FIG. 14-21 **A,** Computer-driven software controls two small, diamond-coated milling devices that cut the restoration out of a block of high-quality ceramic. **B,** The ceramic block rotates as the diamond cutting instruments move as needed to generate the restoration. *(Courtesy of Sirona USA.)*

quality ceramic or composite in a matter of minutes (Fig. 14-21). The restoration is removed from the milling device, ready for try-in and cementation.

The CEREC systems are designed to be used chairside, which eliminates the need for a conventional impression, temporary restoration, and multiple appointments. In addition to the speed of these systems, a major advantage is the quality of the restorative material. Manufacturers make blocks of "machinable ceramics" or "machinable composites" specifically for computer-assisted milling devices. Because these materials are fabricated under ideal industrial conditions, their physical properties have been optimized.

The major disadvantages of CAD/CAM systems are high cost and the need for extra training. However, CAD/CAM technology is changing rapidly, with each new generation of devices having more capability, accuracy, and ease of use.[36,51]

CLINICAL PROCEDURES

Many of the clinical procedures described are common to both laboratory-fabricated and CAD/CAM restorations. Some specific procedural details for CAD/CAM restorations are described in the sections CAD/CAM Techniques and Clinical Procedures for CAD/CAM Inlays and Onlays.

TOOTH PREPARATION

Preparations for specific types of indirect tooth-colored inlays and onlays may vary because of differences in fabrication steps for each commercial system and variations in the physical properties of the restorative materials. (By definition, an onlay caps all cusps; an inlay may cap none, or may cap all but one cusp.) Before beginning any procedure, the clinician should have decided what type of restoration is indicated, according to the factors discussed in the previous sections in this chapter. If the clinician is not familiar with the technique, it is helpful to consult the manufacturer's literature and, if necessary, the dental laboratory to ensure the best results.

As a first clinical step, the patient should be anesthetized and the area isolated with rubber dam, preferentially. The compromised restoration (if present) is at this point completely removed, and/or all the caries is excavated. The walls are then restored to a more nearly ideal form with a light-cured glass-ionomer liner/base or a composite restorative material.

Preparations for indirect tooth-colored inlays and onlays basically are meant to provide adequate thickness for the restorative material and at the same time a passive insertion pattern with rounded internal angles and well-defined margins. All margins should have a 90-degree butt-joint cavosurface angle to ensure marginal strength of the restoration. All line and point angles, internal and external, should be rounded to avoid stress concentrations in the restoration and tooth, thereby reducing the potential for fractures (Figs. 14-22, 14-23, and 14-24).[5,30]

The carbide bur or diamond used for tooth preparation should be a tapering instrument that creates occlusally divergent facial and lingual walls (Fig. 14-25). Gingival-occlusal divergence allows for passive insertion and removal of the restoration (see Fig. 14-22). The junction of the sides and tip of the cutting instrument should have a rounded design to avoid creating sharp, stress-inducing internal angles in the preparation. Although the optimal gingival-occlusal divergence of the preparation is unknown, it should be greater than the 2° to 5° per wall recommended for cast metal inlays and onlays. Divergence can be increased because the tooth-colored restoration will be adhesively bonded and because very little pressure can be applied during try-in and cementation. Throughout preparation, the cutting instruments used to develop vertical walls are oriented to a single path of draw, usually the long axis of the

tooth crown. The occlusal step should be prepared 1.5 to 2 mm in depth. Most composite and ceramic systems require that any isthmus and any groove extension be at least 1.5 mm wide to decrease the possibility of fracture of the restoration. Facial and lingual walls should be extended to sound tooth structure and should go around the cusps in smooth curves. Ideally, there should be no undercuts that would prevent the insertion or removal of the restoration. Small undercuts, if present, can be blocked out using a glass-ionomer liner. The pulpal floor should be smooth and relatively flat. Following removal of extensive caries or previous restorative material from any internal wall, the wall is restored to more nearly ideal form with a light-cured glass-ionomer liner/base.

The facial, lingual, and gingival margins of the proximal boxes should be extended to clear the adjacent tooth by at least 0.5 mm. These clearances will provide adequate access to the margins for impression material and for finishing and polishing instruments. For all walls, a 90-degree cavosurface margin is desired because com-

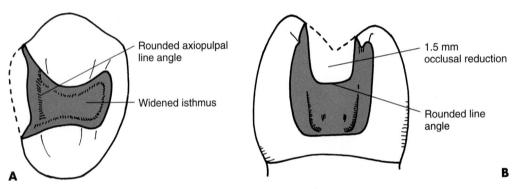

FIG. 14-22 **A,** Mesioocclusal (MO) inlay preparation for tooth-colored inlay in maxillary first premolar (occlusal view). Isthmus should be at least 1.5 to 2 mm wide to prevent inlay fracture. Axiopulpal line angle should be rounded to avoid seating errors and to lower stress concentrations.[5,30] **B,** MOD inlay preparation for tooth-colored inlay in maxillary first premolar (proximal view). Pulpal floor should be prepared 1.5 mm in depth, and axiopulpal line angles should be rounded. Interproximal margins should be extended to allow at least 0.5-mm clearance of contact with neighboring tooth. Gingival margins in enamel are greatly preferred.

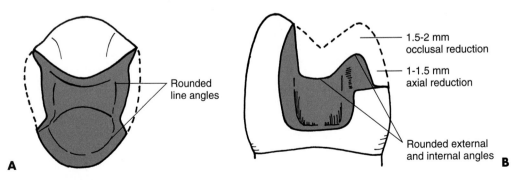

FIG. 14-23 **A,** MODL inlay preparation on maxillary first premolar (occlusal view). **B,** MODL inlay preparation on maxillary first premolar, proximal view. The lingual cusp has been reduced and the lingual margin extended beyond any possible contact with opposing tooth by preparing a "collar." Working cusps require 1.5 to 2 mm of occlusal reduction. All internal and external line angles are rounded.

posite and ceramic inlays are fragile in thin cross-section. The gingival margin should be extended as minimally as possible because margins in enamel are greatly preferred for bonding and because deep gingival margins are difficult to impress and to isolate properly during cementation. When a portion of the facial or lingual surface is affected by caries or other defect, it may be necessary to extend the preparation (with a gingival shoulder) around the transitional line angle to include the defect. The axial wall of the shouldered extension should be prepared to allow for adequate restoration thickness.

When extending through or along cuspal inclines to reach sound tooth structure, a cusp usually should be capped if the extension is two thirds or greater than the distance from any primary groove to the cusp tip (see Figs. 14-23 and 14-24). If cusps must be capped, they should be reduced 1.5 to 2 mm and should have a 90-degree cavosurface angle. When capping cusps, especially centric holding cusps, it may be necessary to prepare a shoulder to move the facial or lingual cavosurface margin away from any possible contact with the opposing tooth, either in maximum intercuspal position or during functional movements. Such contacts directly on margins can lead to premature deterioration of marginal integrity. The axial wall of the resulting shoulder should be sufficiently deep to allow for adequate thickness of the restorative material and should have the same path of draw as the main portion of the preparation.

During preparation, stains on the external walls, such as those often left by corrosion products of old amalgam restorations, should be removed. (This comment does not apply to stained, noncarious dentin on pulpal and axial walls, of course.) Such stains could appear as black or gray lines at the margin after cementation. It is especially critical to generously round all line and point angles, internal and external, to avoid areas of stress concentrations that could later lead to fracture of the restoration.

IMPRESSION

Most tooth-colored indirect inlay/onlay systems require an impression of the prepared tooth and the adjacent teeth as well as interocclusal records, which allow the restoration to be fabricated on a working cast in the laboratory (see Chapter 20).

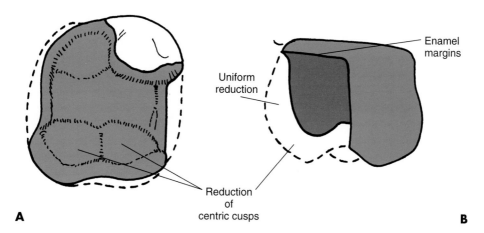

A

B

FIG. **14-24** MODFL inlay preparation on maxillary right first molar. Distofacial, mesiolingual, and distolingual cusps are reduced. **A,** Occlusal view. **B,** Facial view.

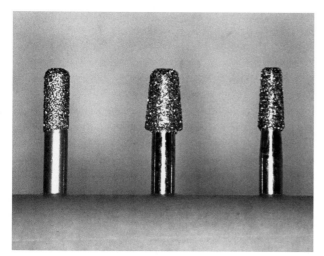

FIG. **14-25** Typical diamond instruments used for ceramic inlay/onlay tooth preparation.

TEMPORARY RESTORATION

A provisional restoration is necessary when using indirect systems that require two appointments. The temporary protects the pulp-dentin complex in vital teeth, maintains the position of the prepared tooth in the arch, and protects the soft tissues adjacent to prepared areas. The temporary restoration can be made using conventional techniques and acrylic resins or bis-acryl composite materials (see Chapter 20). Care should be taken to avoid the bonding of the temporary material to the preparation at this phase of the procedure. A lubricant of some sort may be applied to the preparation if desired, especially if a resin-based material was used to block out undercuts and level the walls of the preparation. Temporary restorations for PFM and cast gold restorations typically are cemented with eugenol-based temporary cements. However, eugenol is believed to interfere with resin polymerization,[41] and could potentially reduce the adhesion of the permanent composite cement to tooth structure. Although some studies report this does not occur if the tooth is pumiced before cementation of the permanent restoration,[45] use of a noneugenol temporary cement is recommended. For exceptionally nonretentive preparations, or when the temporary phase is expected to last longer than 2 to 3 weeks, zinc phosphate cement can be used to increase retention of the temporary restoration.

CAD/CAM TECHNIQUES

Clinical procedures for CAD/CAM systems such as the CEREC differ somewhat from the procedures previously described. Tooth preparations for CAD/CAM inlays must reflect the capabilities of the CAD software and hardware and the CAM milling devices that fabricate the restorations. One example of how preparations are modified when using the CEREC system pertains to undercuts. Laboratory-fabricated indirect systems require the preparation to have a path of draw that allows insertion and removal of the restoration without interferences from undercuts. However, the CEREC system automatically "blocks out" any undercuts during the optical impression (Fig. 14-26). Occlusally convergent walls can result in a more conservative preparation along the occlusal aspect, especially when replacing old amalgam restorations, which were prepared with such undercuts for retention. Care should be taken, however, not to allow excessive undercuts especially at the base of the cusps. These undercut areas eventually will be filled with the composite cement, and these materials lack the properties to act as "dentin replacement." Also, large undercuts may result in undetected internal voids during cementation, which could lead to dramatic failures. The facial and lingual walls of the proximal boxes should be prepared without undercuts and with draw to avoid excessively wide composite cement lines.

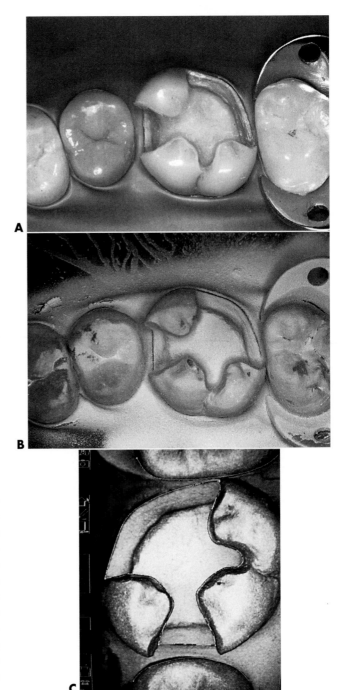

FIG. 14-26 A, MODF inlay preparation for ceramic inlay on maxillary first molar. B, Preparation coated with special powder for capture with optical impression by CEREC device. C, Optical impression. Any internal undercuts would be blocked out by the CEREC device.

Using the CEREC system, an experienced dentist can prepare the tooth, fabricate an inlay, and deliver it in approximately 1 hour (Fig. 14-27). This system eliminates the need for a conventional impression, temporary restoration, and multiple patient appointments.

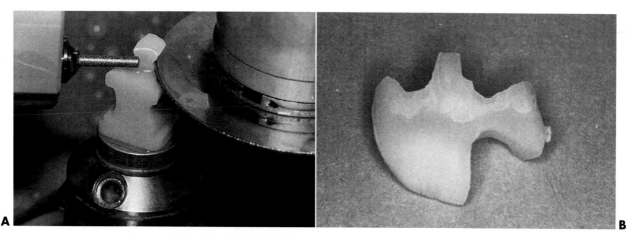

FIG. **14-27 A,** CEREC inlay being milled. **B,** Completed inlay.

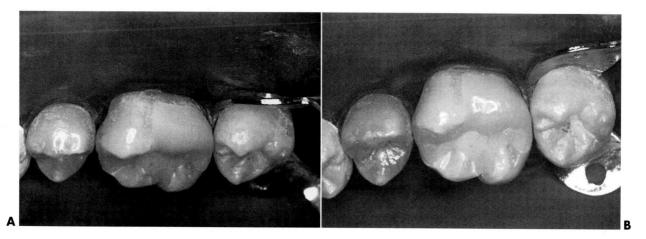

FIG. **14-28 A,** Initial try-in of CEREC inlay. Proximal contacts are too tight and must be adjusted. **B,** Inlay seated after contact adjustment. Proximal surfaces of the inlay must be polished before cementation.

TRY-IN AND CEMENTATION

The try-in and cementation of tooth-colored inlays/onlays are more demanding than that for cast metal restorations because of: (1) the relatively fragile nature of the ceramic or composite material, (2) the requirement of near-perfect moisture control, and (3) the use of composite cements. The ceramic or composite inlay is relatively fragile until it is bonded in place with composite cement. Very little pressure should be applied to the restoration during try-in. Because of this fragility, occlusal evaluation and adjustment are delayed until after cementation.

Preliminary Steps. The use of the rubber dam should be strongly considered to prevent moisture contamination of the conditioned tooth and/or restoration surfaces during cementation, as well as to improve access and visibility during restoration delivery. After removing the temporary restoration, all the temporary cement is cleaned from preparation walls.

Restoration Try-in and Proximal Contact Adjustment. The inlay or onlay is placed into the preparation using very light pressure to evaluate its fit. If the restoration does not seat completely, the most likely cause is an overcontoured proximal surface (Fig. 14-28). Using the mouth mirror where needed, the embrasures should be viewed from the facial, lingual, and occlusal aspects to determine where the proximal contour needs adjustment to allow final seating of the restoration, while simultaneously producing the correct position and form of the contact. Passing thin dental floss through the contact(s) will reveal the tightness and position, thus signifying to the experienced operator the degree and location of excess contact (see Chapter 20). Articulating papers also can be successfully used to identify overtight proximal contacts. Abrasive disks are used to adjust the proximal contour and contact relationship. While adjusting the intensity and location of the proximal contacts, successively finer grits of abrasive disks are used to polish the proximal surfaces because they will be inaccessible for polishing after cementation.

If the proximal contours are not overcontoured, and the restoration still does not fit completely, the preparation should be checked again for residual temporary materials or debris. If the preparation is clean, internal and/or marginal interferences might also prevent the restoration from seating completely. Once these interferences have been identified through careful visual inspection of the margins and/or using "fit-checker" materials, they should be adjusted on the restoration, on the preparation, or both. Fortunately, these interferences are rare because contemporary impression materials and ceramic systems are very accurate, and the laboratory usually applies a die-spacer on the internal aspects of the preparation to avoid difficulties in seating the restoration. In the event of a significant discrepancy between the preparation and the inlay/onlay, a new impression must be taken.

Marginal fit is verified after the restoration is completely seated. Slight excesses of contour can be removed, if access allows, using fine-grit diamond instruments or 30-fluted carbide finishing burs. These adjustments are preferably done after the restoration is cemented, to avoid marginal fractures. Most indirect tooth-colored restorations have slightly larger marginal gaps than comparable gold restorations.[36,51]

Cementation. For proper adhesive bonding, the internal surface of the inlay/onlay must be treated before cementation. The techniques and materials vary, depending on the specific restorative system used.

For most laboratory-processed composite inlays/onlays, the resin matrix has been polymerized to such an extent that few bonding sites are available for the composite cement to chemically bond to the internal surfaces of the restoration. To improve the bond of the cement to the processed composite restoration, some systems require the use of a solvent to soften the internal surfaces of the restoration before cementation.[54] Other systems recommend sandblasting (air-abrading) the inside of the composite restoration with aluminum-oxide abrasive particles to increase surface roughness and surface area for bonding.[48,50]

For ceramic inlays and onlays, hydrofluoric acid is usually used to etch the internal surfaces of the restoration (Fig. 14-29).[22] Such acid-etching increases surface relief and therefore not only increases the surface area, but also results in micromechanical bonding of the composite cement to the ceramic restoration. Hydrofluoric acid–etching is usually done by the laboratory. However, the clinician should check the internal surface of the restoration to confirm the etching, which is evident by a white-opaque appearance similar to acid-etched enamel. Chairside ceramic etching is done with a 2-minute application of 10% hydrofluoric acid on the internal surfaces of the inlay/onlay. After etching, the ceramic

is treated with a silane coupling agent to facilitate chemical bonding of the composite cement.[31]

Clear plastic matrix strips may be applied in each affected proximal area and wedged (Fig. 14-30, *A*). Care should be taken to avoid interference of the wedges with the seating of the restoration. The inlay/onlay can be tried in again and checked for fit (see Fig. 14-30, *B*). The preparation surfaces are etched (Fig. 14-31, *A*) and treated with the components of an appropriate enamel/dentin bonding system (see Chapter 5). Typically, the final step of the bonding system (e.g., an unfilled resin) also is applied to the internal surfaces of the restoration previously etched and silanated. A dual-cure composite cement is mixed and inserted into the preparation with a paddle-shaped instrument or a syringe. The internal surfaces of the restoration also are coated with the composite cement (see Fig. 14-31, *B* and *C*), and the inlay is immediately inserted into the prepared tooth, using light pressure. A ball burnisher applied with a slight vibrating motion is usually sufficient to seat the restoration (see Fig. 14-31, *D*). Excess composite cement is removed with thin-bladed composite instruments, brushes, or an explorer (see Fig. 14-31, *E* and *F*). The operator must be careful not to remove composite from the marginal interface between the tooth and the inlay. The cement is now light-cured from occlusal, facial, and lingual directions for a minimum exposure of 60 seconds from each direction (see Fig. 14-31, *G*).[37]

FINISHING AND POLISHING PROCEDURES

After light-curing the cement, the plastic matrix strips and the wedges are removed, and the setting of the composite cement is verified. All marginal areas are checked with an explorer tine. Because wedges and matrix were used interproximally, these areas—which are difficult to finish—should feel quite smooth, with little if any com-

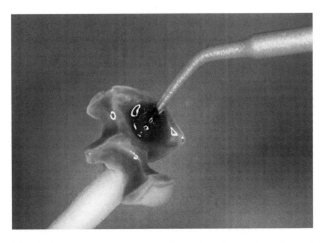

FIG. **14-29** Applying hydrofluoric acid to internal surface of ceramic inlay. After rinsing and drying, etched ceramic surfaces should have a "frosty" white appearance.

posite flash extending beyond the margins in a gingival direction.

For ceramic restorations, medium- or fine-grit diamond instruments are used initially to remove any excess composite cement back to the margin. Care must be taken to preserve the glazed surface of ceramic restorations as much as possible. Slender flame shapes are used inter-

proximally (Fig. 14-32, *A*), while larger oval or cylindric shapes are used on the occlusal surface. After using the fine-grit diamond instruments, 30-fluted carbide finishing burs are used to obtain a smoother finish (see Fig. 14-32, *B*).[26] For indirect composite restorations, finishing may be started with 12-fluted carbide finishing burs instead of diamonds.

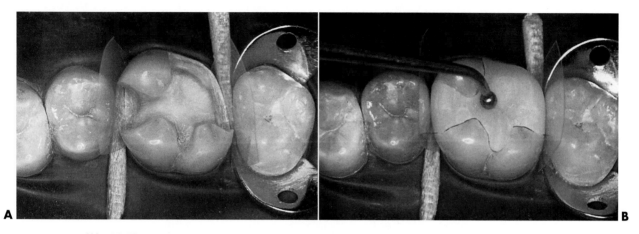

FIG. 14-30 **A,** Clear plastic matrix strips are applied and wedged before etching and cementation. **B,** The fit of the inlay is verified with the matrix and wedges in place.

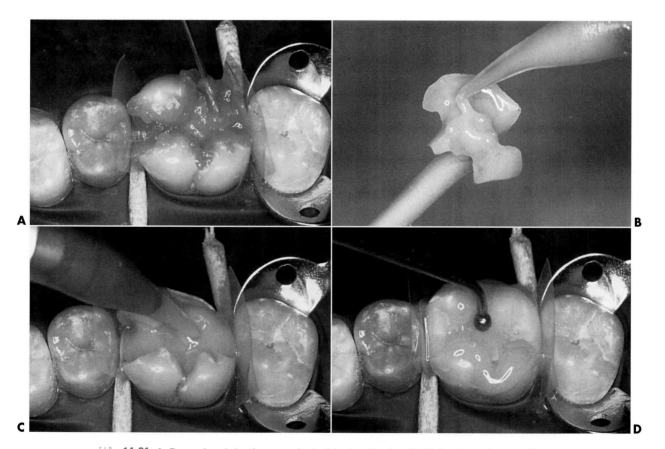

FIG. 14-31 **A,** Enamel and dentin are etched with phosphoric acid. **B,** Dual-cured composite cement is applied to inlay. **C,** After application of the adhesive system, cement is applied to the preparation. **D,** CEREC ceramic inlay is seated into preparation.

Continued

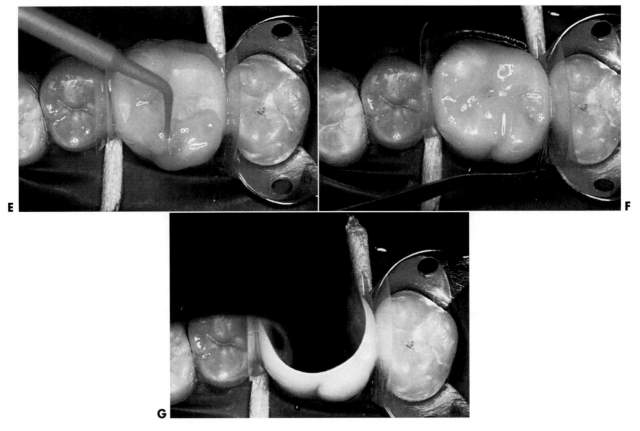

FIG. **14-31, cont'd** **E** and **F,** Before curing, excess composite cement is removed with explorer, brushes, and IPC carver. **G,** The composite cement is light-cured from occlusal, facial, and lingual directions.

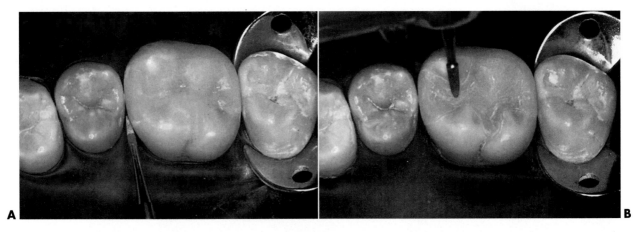

FIG. **14-32** **A,** Slender, fine-grit, flame-shaped, diamond instruments are used to remove flash along facial and lingual margins of CEREC ceramic inlay. **B,** 30-fluted finishing burs are used to smooth areas that were adjusted with diamonds.

Interproximally, a No. 12 surgical blade can be used to remove excess composite cement when access permits (Fig. 14-33, *A*). Abrasive strips of successively finer grits also can be used to remove slight interproximal excesses (see Fig. 14-33, *B*). Much care must be used to avoid damaging the gingiva or the root surfaces when using such instruments interproximally. With care and appropriate instrumentation, ceramic restorations can be polished to a surface smoother than glazed porcelain using the abrasive sequence shown in Table 14-2.[26] The same

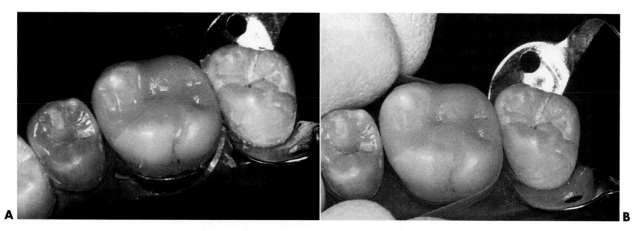

FIG. 14-33 A, Removing excess composite cement using a surgical blade. **B,** Smoothing the interproximal area with abrasive finishing strip.

TABLE 14-2	Instrumentation for Finishing and Polishing Ceramic Restorations

SEQUENCE	INSTRUMENTS
1	Medium- to fine-grit diamond instrument
2	30-fluted carbide burs
3	Rubber, abrasive-impregnated porcelain polishing points
4	Diamond polishing paste

fine-grit diamonds used to adjust margins may be used to adjust contour, followed by the use of 30-fluted carbide finishing burs. Further smoothing is accomplished with a series of rubber abrasive points and cups used at slow speed with air-water spray (Fig. 14-34, *A*). Final polishing of the ceramic restoration may be achieved by applying a diamond polishing paste with a bristle brush or another suitable instrument (see Fig. 14-34, *B*). Ceramic restorations properly polished with this series of instruments have a remarkably beautiful, smooth surface (see Fig. 14-34, *C*).

After all excess composite cement has been removed, marginal integrity has been verified, and the restoration has been polished as needed, the rubber dam is removed. The occlusion is now checked and adjusted if necessary. With good occlusal records and careful laboratory work, little if any correction should be necessary. Premature occlusal contacts can be adjusted using fine-grit diamond instruments, followed by 30-fluted carbide finishing burs, if the adjustments are made in the restoration.

In selected cases, the occlusion can be adjusted on the opposing dentition. This is only feasible if such adjustment is done to correct the occlusal plane of the opposing teeth, or to reduce a pronounced cusp present on the tooth opposing the restoration to avoid occlusal trauma.

After occlusal adjustments are completed, the restoration must be repolished in all areas where corrections have been made, especially in areas of ceramic restorations where the glaze may have been disrupted. Indirect composite inlays and onlays can be polished using the same instrumentation and materials used for direct composites (see Chapter 13).

CLINICAL PROCEDURES FOR CAD/CAM INLAYS AND ONLAYS

When delivering a CAD/CAM inlay, more adjustments are usually necessary when trying-in, finishing, and polishing. The original CEREC system milled the occlusal surface relatively flat without any significant surface detail, and did not take into account the opposing occlusion. The newer CEREC 2 and 3 systems are able to mill in occlusal contours in a variety of manners. They can extrapolate existing contours beyond the cavosurface margin to the central groove, or they can build the surface up to the level of a scanned wax bite. The neighboring teeth, in particular the marginal ridges and cusp heights, also can be used as references for the design of the occlusal surface of a CAD/CAM restoration. If the preoperative contours of the tooth were satisfactory, the system can reproduce them in the restoration. When adjusting the occlusion of a CAD/CAM inlay, it may be necessary to use medium-grit diamonds with air-water spray coolant for initial contouring of the occlusal surface, followed by the instrumentation previously discussed for finishing and polishing. An arch containing several CEREC CAD/CAM inlays is shown in Fig. 14-35.

COMMON PROBLEMS AND SOLUTIONS

The most common cause of failure of tooth-colored inlays and onlays is bulk fracture. If bulk fracture occurs, replacement of the restoration is almost always indicated.

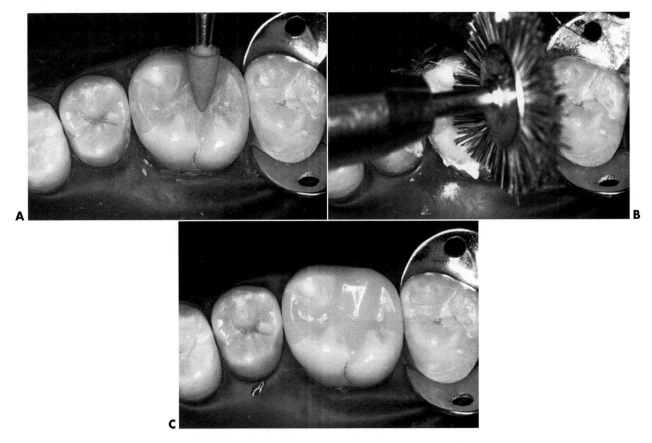

FIG. **14-34** Polishing sequence for ceramic inlays. **A,** After using fine-grit diamonds and 30-fluted carbide finishing burs to adjust contours and margins (as shown in Fig. 14-32), rubber abrasive points and cups of successively finer grits are used at slow speed. **B,** Final polish imparted by porcelain polishing paste applied with bristle brush. **C,** Occlusal view of polished ceramic inlay.

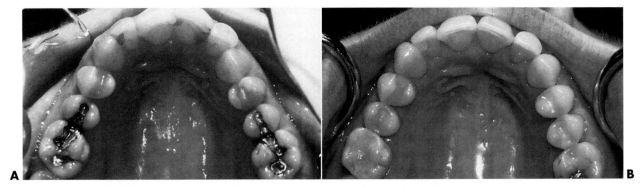

FIG. **14-35 A,** Preoperative view. **B,** Postoperative view of maxillary arch containing several CEREC inlays.

REPAIR OF TOOTH-COLORED INLAYS AND ONLAYS

Minor defects in indirect composite and ceramic restorations can be repaired with relative ease. Of course, before initiating any repair procedure, the operator should determine whether replacement rather than repair is the appropriate treatment. If repair is deemed to be the appropriate treatment, the dentist should attempt to identify the cause of the problem and correct it if possible. For example, a small fracture due to occlusal trauma may indicate that some adjustment of the opposing occlusion is required.

For both composite and ceramic inlays, the repair procedure is initiated by mechanical roughening of the involved surface. While a coarse diamond may be used, a better result is obtained with the use of air-abrading or grit-blasting with aluminum oxide particles and a special intraoral device.[50,53]

For ceramic restorations, the initial mechanical roughening is followed by brief (typically 2 minutes) application of 10% hydrofluoric acid gel. Hydrofluoric acid etches the surface, creating further microdefects to facilitate mechanical bonding. Although many indirect composites contain etchable glass filler particles, hydrofluoric acid treatment of composites is neither necessary nor recommended.[53,54] However, a brief application of phosphoric acid may be used to clean the composite surface after roughening.

The next step in the repair procedure is application of a silane coupling agent. Silanes mediate chemical bonding between ceramics and resins and also may improve the predictability of resin-resin repairs.[31] The manufacturer's guidelines should be followed when using silanes, as they can differ substantially from one particular product to another.

After the silane has been applied, a resin-bonding agent is applied and light-cured. A composite of the appropriate shade is placed, cured, contoured, and polished (see Chapter 13).

SUMMARY

Advances in ceramic, composite, and adhesive technology have resulted in the development of a variety of tooth-colored indirect restorations. These offer an excellent alternative to direct composite restorations, especially for large restorations, and are more conservative than full-coverage restorations. However, because the clinical procedures are relatively technique-sensitive, proper case selection, operator skill, and attention to detail are critical to success.

REFERENCES

1. Al-Hiyasat AS, Saunders WP, Smith GM: Three-body wear associated with three ceramics and enamel, *J Prosthet Dent* 82(4):476-481, 1999.
2. Anusavice KJ: Development and testing of ceramics for dental restorations. In Fischman G, Clare A, Hench J, editors: *Bioceramics: materials and applications*, Westerville, OH, 1995, The American Ceramic Society.
3. Anusavice KJ, editor: *Phillips' science of dental materials*, ed 10, Philadelphia, 1996, WB Saunders.
4. Ausiello P et al: Fracture resistance of endodontically-treated premolars adhesively restored, *Am J Dent* 10(5):237-241, 1997.
5. Banks RG: Conservative posterior ceramic restorations: a literature review, *J Prosthet Dent* 63(6):619-626, 1990.
6. Berg NG, Derand T: A 5-year evaluation of ceramic inlays (CEREC), *Swed Dent J* 21(4):121-127, 1997.
7. Burgoyne AR, Nicholls JI, Brudvik JS: In vitro two-body wear of inlay-onlay composite resin restoratives, *J Prosthet Dent* 65(2):206-214, 1991.
8. Burke FJT, Wilson NHF, Watts DC: The effect of cuspal coverage on the fracture resistance of teeth restored with indirect composite resin restorations, *Quintessence Int* 24(12):875-880, 1993.

9. Cattell MJ, Clarke RL, Lynch EJ: The transverse strength, reliability and microstructural features of four dental ceramics—part I, *J Dent* 25(5):399-407, 1997.
10. Cattell MJ, Clarke RL, Lynch EJ: The biaxial flexure strength and reliability of four dental ceramics—part II, *J Dent* 25(5):409-414, 1997.
11. DeLong R, Sasik C, Pintado MR, Douglas WH: The wear of enamel when opposed by ceramic systems, *Dent Mater* 5(7):266-271, 1989.
12. Dietschi D et al: Marginal adaptation and seal of direct and indirect Class II composite resin restorations: an in vitro evaluation, *Quintessence Int* 26(2):127-138, 1995.
13. Donly KJ, Jensen ME, Triolo P, et al: A clinical comparison of resin composite inlay and onlay posterior restorations and cast-gold restorations at 7 years, *Quintessence Int* 30(3):163-168, 1999.
14. Douglas WH, Fields RP, Fundingsland J: A comparison between the microleakage of direct and indirect composite restorative systems, *J Dent* 17(4):184-188, 1989.
15. Eldiwany M, Powers JM, George LA: Mechanical properties of direct and post-cured composites, *Am J Dent* 6(5):222-224, 1993.
16. El-Kalla IH, Garcia-Godoy F: Saliva contamination and bond strength of single-bottle adhesives to enamel and dentin, *Am J Dent* 10(2):83-87, 1997.
17. Feigal RJ, Hitt J, Splieth C: Retaining sealant on salivary contaminated enamel, *J Am Dent Assoc* 124(3):88-97, 1993.
18. Feilzer AJ, deGee AJ, Davidson CL: Increased wall-to-wall curing contraction in thin bonded layers, *J Dent Res* 68(1):48-50, 1989.
19. Ferracane JL, Condon JR: Post-cure heat treatments for composites: properties and fractography, *Dent Mater* 8(5):290-295, 1992.
20. Ferrari M et al: Influence of tissue characteristics at margins on leakage of Class II indirect porcelain restorations, *Am J Dent* 12(3):134-142, 1999.
21. Fradeani M, Aquilano A, Bassein L: Longitudinal study of pressed glass-ceramic inlays for four and a half years, *J Prosthet Dent* 78(4):346-353, 1997.
22. Giordano RA: Dental ceramic restorative systems, *Compendium* 17(8):779-782, 1996.
23. Gladys S et al: Clinical and semiquantitative marginal analysis of four tooth-coloured inlay systems at 3 years, *J Dent* 23(6):329-338, 1995.
24. Gregory WA et al: Physical properties and repair bond strength of direct and indirect composite resins, *J Prosthet Dent* 68(3):406-411, 1992.
25. Hayashi M, Tsuchitani Y, Miura M et al: Six-year clinical evaluation of fired ceramic inlays, *Oper Dent* 23(6):318-326, 1998.
26. Haywood VB et al: Polishing porcelain veneers: an SEM and specular reflectance analysis, *Dent Mater* 4(3):116-121, 1988.
27. Hench LL: Bioceramics: from concept to clinic, *J Amer Ceram Soc* 74(7):1487-1570, 1991.
28. Heymann HO et al: The clinical performance of CAD-CAM-generated ceramic inlays: a four-year study, *J Am Dent Assoc* 127(8):1171-1181, 1996.
29. Hudson JD, Goldstein GR, Georgescu M: Enamel wear caused by three different restorative materials, *J Prosthet Dent* 74(6):647-654, 1995.
30. Jackson RD: Indirect resin inlay and onlay restorations: a comprehensive clinical overview, *Practical Perio Aesthet Dent* 11(8):891-900, 1999.
31. Jardel V et al: Correlation of topography to bond strength of etched ceramic, *Int J Prosthodont* 12(1):59-64, 1999.

32. Krämer N et al: IPS Empress inlays and onlays after four years—a clinical study, *J Dent* 27(5):325-331, 1999.

33. Krejci I et al: Wear of ceramic inlays, their enamel antagonists, and luting cements, *J Prosthet Dent* 69(4):425-430, 1993.

34. Liberman R et al: The effect of posterior composite restorations on the resistance of cavity walls to vertically applied occlusal loads, *J Oral Rehabil* 17(1):99-105, 1990.

35. MacCulloch WT: Advances in dental ceramics, *Br Dent J* 124(8):361-365, 1968.

36. Mormann WH, Schug J: Grinding precision and accuracy of fit of CEREC 2 CAD-CIM inlays, *J Am Dent Assoc* 128(1):47-53, 1997.

37. Myers ML, Caughman WF, Rueggeberg FA: Effect of restoration composition, shade, and thickness on the cure of a photoactivated resin cement, *J Prosthodont* 3(3):149-157, 1994.

38. Powers JM, Eldiwany M, Ladd GD: Effects of post-curing on mechanical properties of a composite, *Am J Dent* 6(5):232-234, 1993.

39. Qualtrough AJ, Piddock V: Ceramics update, *J Dent* 25(2):91-95, 1997.

40. Reinhardt JW, Boyer DB, Stephens NH: Effects of secondary curing on indirect posterior composite resins, *Oper Dent* 19(6):217-220, 1994.

41. Rosenstiel SF, Gegauff AG: Effect of provisional cementing agents on provisional resins, *J Prosthet Dent* 59(1):29-33, 1988.

42. Roulet J-F: Longevity of glass ceramic inlays and amalgam—results up to 6 years, *Clin Oral Investig* 1(1):40-46, 1997.

43. Roulet J-F, Söderholm KJM, Longmate J: Effects of treatment and storage conditions on ceramic/composite bond strength, *J Dent Res* 74(1):381-387, 1995.

44. Ruyter, IE: Types of resin-based inlay materials and their properties, *Int Dent J* 42(3):139-44, 1992.

45. Schwartz R, Davis R, Hilton TJ: Effect of temporary cements on the bond strength of a resin cement, *Am J Dent* 5(3):147-150, 1992.

46. Seghi RR, Denry IL, Rosenstiel SF: Relative fracture toughness and hardness of new dental ceramics, *J Prosthet Dent* 74(2):145-150, 1995.

47. Shortall AC et al: Marginal seal comparisons between resin-bonded Class II porcelain inlays, posterior composite restorations, and direct composite resin inlays, *Int J Prosthodont* 2(3):217-223, 1989.

48. Shortall AC, Baylis RL, Wilson HJ: Composite inlay/luting resin bond strength—surface treatments, *J Dent* 24(1/2):129-135, 1996.

49. Söderholm KJM, Richards ND: Wear resistance of composites: a solved problem?, *Gen Dent* 46(3):256-263, 1998.

50. Stokes AN, Tay WM, Pereira BP: Shear bond strengths of resin cement to post-cured hybrid composites, *Dent Mater* 6(6):370-374, 1993.

51. Sturdevant JR, Bayne SC, Heymann HO: Margin gap size of ceramic inlays using second-generation CAD/CAM equipment, *J Esthet Dent* 11(4):206-214, 1999.

52. Sturdevant JR et al: Five-year study of two light-cured posterior composite resins, *Dent Mater* 4(3):105-110, 1988.

53. Swift EJ et al: Treatment of composite surfaces for indirect bonding, *Dent Mater* 8(3):193-196, 1992.

54. Tate WH, DeSchepper EJ, Powers JM: Bond strength of resin cements to a hybrid composite, *Am J Dent* 6(4):195-198, 1993.

55. Taylor DF et al: Pooling of long-term clinical wear data for posterior composites, *Am J Dent* 7(3):167-174, 1994.

56. Thompson JY, Bayne SC, Heymann HO: Mechanical properties of a new mica-based machinable glass ceramic for CAD/CAM restorations, *J Prosthet Dent* 76(6):619-623, 1996.

57. van Dijken JW, Hoglund-Aberg C, Olofsson AL: Fired ceramic inlays: a 6-year follow-up, *J Dent* 26(3): 219-225, 1998.

58. Wendt SL: Microleakage and cusp fracture resistance of heat-treated composite resin inlays, *Am J Dent* 4(1):10-14, 1991.

59. Wendt SL, Leinfelder KF: The clinical evaluation of heat-treated composite resin inlays, *J Am Dent Assoc* 120(2):177-181, 1990.

60. Zuellig-Singer R, Bryant RW: Three-year evaluation of computer-machined ceramic inlays—influence of luting agent, *Quintessence Int* 29(9):573-582, 1998.

15

Additional Conservative Esthetic Procedures

HARALD O. HEYMANN

CHAPTER OUTLINE

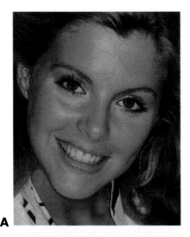

A

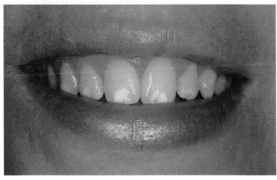

B

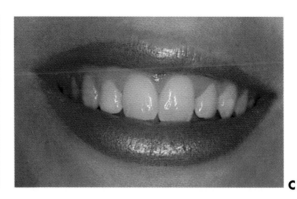

C

FIG. **15-1** Examples of conservative esthetic procedures. **A,** A beautiful radiant smile is one of the greatest assets a person can have. **B,** The appearance of this aspiring young model was marred by hypocalcified areas of the maxillary anterior teeth. **C,** A simple treatment consisted of removing part of the discolored enamel, acid-etching the preparations, and restoring with direct-composite partial veneers. *(Courtesy of Dr. C. L. Sockwell.)*

Significant improvements in tooth-colored restorative materials and adhesive techniques have resulted in numerous conservative esthetic treatment possibilities. Although restorative dentistry has enjoyed the distinction of being a blend of art and science, conservative esthetic *dentistry* truly emphasizes the *artistic component.* As Dr. Ronald E. Goldstein states, "Esthetic dentistry is the art of dentistry in its purest form."[15] As with many forms of art, conservative esthetic dentistry provides a means of artistic expression that feeds on creativity and imagination. Dentists find performing conservative esthetic procedures to be most enjoyable, and patients appreciate the immediate esthetic improvements rendered, often without the need for local anesthesia.

One of the greatest assets a person can have is a smile that shows beautiful, natural teeth (Fig. 15-1). Children and teenagers are especially sensitive about unattractive teeth. When teeth are discolored, malformed, crooked, or missing, there is often a conscious effort to avoid smiling and patients try to "cover up" the teeth. Correction of these types of dental problems can produce dramatic changes in appearance, which often result in improved confidence, personality, and social life.

The restoration of a smile is one of the most appreciated and gratifying services a dentist can render. In fact, the positive psychologic effects of improving a patient's smile often contribute to an improved self-image and enhanced self-esteem. These improvements make conservative esthetic dentistry particularly gratifying for

the dentist and represent a new dimension of dental treatment for patients.

This chapter presents conservative esthetic procedures in the context of their clinical applications. The principles and clinical steps involved in adhesive bonding for the treatment alternatives discussed in this chapter are similar to those described earlier (see Chapters 11 to 14). Only specific conservative esthetic clinical procedures or variations from previously described techniques are presented in this chapter.

ARTISTIC ELEMENTS

Regardless of the result desired, certain basic artistic elements must be considered to ensure an optimally esthetic result. In conservative esthetic dentistry these include:

- Shape or form
- Symmetry and proportionality
- Position and alignment
- Surface texture
- Color
- Translucency

Some or all of these elements are common to virtually every conservative esthetic dental procedure; therefore a basic knowledge and understanding of these artistic elements is required to attain esthetic results consistently.

FIG. **15-2** Cosmetic contouring. **A,** Anterior teeth before treatment. **B,** By reshaping teeth, a more feminine, youthful appearance is produced.

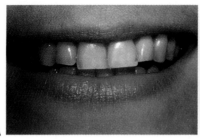
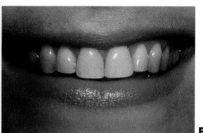

A

B

SHAPE OR FORM

The shape of teeth largely determines their esthetic appearance. To achieve optimal dental esthetics, it is imperative that natural anatomic forms be achieved. Therefore a basic knowledge of normal tooth anatomy is fundamental to the success of any conservative esthetic dental procedure.

When viewing the clinical crown of an incisor from a facial (or lingual) position, the crown outline is trapezoidal. However, subtle variations in shape and contour produce very different appearances. For instance, rounded incisal angles, open incisal and facial embrasures and softened facial line angles typically characterize a youthful, feminine smile. A more *masculine smile,* or a smile characteristic of an older individual having experienced attrition due to aging, typically exhibits incisal embrasures with more closed and prominent (i.e., less rounded) incisal angles. Frequently, minor modification of existing tooth contours, sometimes referred to as *cosmetic contouring,* can effect a significant esthetic change (see Alterations of Shape of Natural Teeth). Reshaping enamel by rounding incisal angles, opening incisal embrasures, and reducing prominent facial line angles can produce a more feminine, youthful appearance (Fig. 15-2).

Significant generalized esthetic changes are possible when treating all the anterior teeth (and also, occasionally, first premolars) visible in the patient's smile. This fact is particularly true when placing full-coverage facial restorations, such as *veneers* (see Veneers). With this treatment method, the dentist can produce significant changes in tooth shapes and forms to yield a variety of different appearances.

Although less extensive, restoring an individual tooth rather than all anterior teeth simultaneously may, in fact, require greater artistic ability. Generalized restoration of all anterior teeth with full facial veneers affords the dentist significant control of the contours generated. When treating an isolated tooth, however, the success of the result is largely determined by how well the restored tooth esthetically matches the surrounding natural teeth. The contralateral tooth to that being restored should be closely examined for subtle characterizing features, such as developmental depressions, embrasure form, prominences, or other distinguishing characteristics of form. A high degree of realism must be reproduced artfully to achieve optimal esthetics when restoring isolated teeth or areas.

Illusions of shape also play a significant role in dental esthetics. The border outline of an anterior tooth (i.e., facial view) is primarily two-dimensional (i.e., length and width). However, the third dimension of depth is critical in creating illusions, especially those of apparent width and length.

Prominent areas of contour on a tooth typically are highlighted with direct illumination, making them more noticeable, whereas areas of depression or diminishing contour are shadowed and less conspicuous. By controlling the areas of light reflection and shadowing, full facial coverage restorations (in particular) can be esthetically contoured to achieve various desired illusions of form.

Moreover, the *apparent size of a tooth* can be changed by altering the position of facial prominences or heights of contour without changing the actual dimension of the tooth. For example, when compared with normal tooth contours (Fig. 15-3, *A*) a tooth can be made to appear narrower by positioning the mesiofacial and distofacial line angles closer together (see Fig. 15-3, *B*). Developmental depressions also can be positioned closer together to enhance the illusion of narrowness. In like manner, greater apparent width can be achieved by positioning the line angles and developmental depressions further apart (see Fig. 15-3, *C*).

Although more difficult, the apparent length of teeth also can be changed by illusion. When compared with normal tooth contours (Fig. 15-4, *A*), a tooth can be made to appear shorter by emphasizing the horizontal elements, such as gingival perikymata, and by positioning the gingival height of contour further incisally (see Fig. 15-4, *B*). Slight modification of the incisal area, achieved by moving the incisal height of contour further gingivally, also enhances the illusion of a shorter tooth. The opposite tenets are true for increasing the apparent length of a tooth. The heights of contour are moved further apart incisogingivally, and vertical elements, such as developmental depressions, are emphasized (see Fig. 15-4, *C*).

Used in combination these illusionary techniques are particularly valuable for controlling the apparent di-

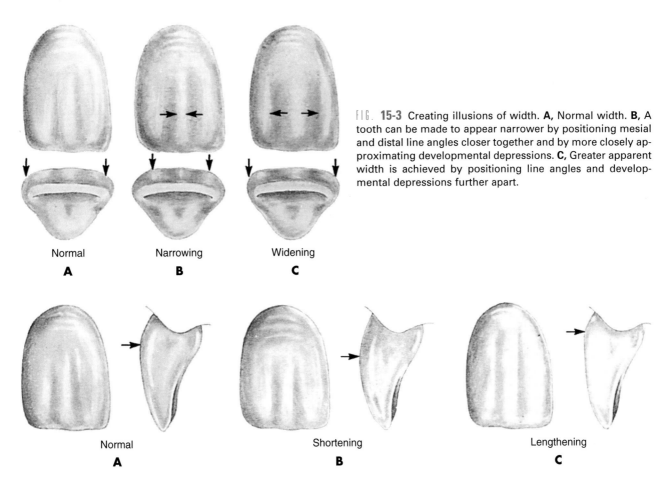

Normal Narrowing Widening
A **B** **C**

FIG. **15-3** Creating illusions of width. **A,** Normal width. **B,** A tooth can be made to appear narrower by positioning mesial and distal line angles closer together and by more closely approximating developmental depressions. **C,** Greater apparent width is achieved by positioning line angles and developmental depressions further apart.

Normal Shortening Lengthening
A **B** **C**

FIG. **15-4** Creating illusions of length. **A,** Normal length. **B,** A tooth can be made to appear shorter by emphasizing horizontal elements and by positioning the gingival height of contour further incisally. **C,** The illusion of length is achieved by moving the gingival height of contour gingivally and by emphasizing vertical elements, such as developmental depressions.

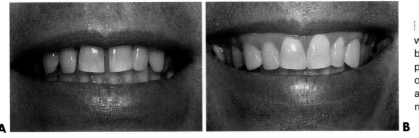

A **B**

FIG. **15-5** Controlling apparent tooth size when adding proximal dimension. **A,** Teeth before treatment. **B,** By maintaining original positions of the facial line angles (see areas of light reflection), increased widths of teeth after composite augmentations are less noticeable.

mension of teeth in procedures that result in an actual increased width of the teeth, such as *diastema* (i.e., spaces) *closure* (see Correction of Diastemas). By contouring the composite additions in such a way that the original positions of the line angles are maintained, the increased widths of the restored teeth are less noticeable (Fig. 15-5). Furthermore, if full facial coverage restorations are placed in conjunction with a diastema closure, vertical elements can be enhanced and horizontal features deemphasized to control further the apparent dimension of the teeth.

SYMMETRY AND PROPORTIONALITY

The overall esthetic appearance of a human smile is largely governed by the symmetry and proportionality of the teeth that constitute the smile. Asymmetric teeth or teeth that are out of proportion to the surrounding teeth disrupt the sense of balance and harmony essential for optimal esthetics. Assuming the teeth are of normal alignment (i.e., rotations or faciolingual positional defects are not present), dental symmetry can be maintained if the sizes of the contralateral teeth are equivalent. A dental caliper should be used in conjunction with

FIG. **15-6** Diastema closure. **A,** Teeth before composite additions. **B,** Symmetric and equal contours are achieved in the final restorations.

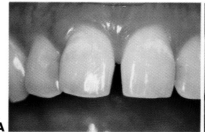
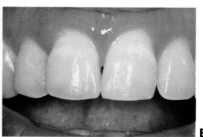

FIG. **15-7** The rule of the golden proportion. **A,** The exact ratios of proportionality. **B,** The anterior teeth of this patient are in "golden proportion" to one another.

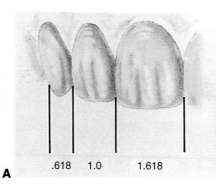

.618   1.0   1.618

A

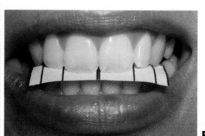

B

any conservative esthetic dental procedure that will alter the mesiodistal dimension of the teeth. This recommendation is particularly true for procedures such as diastema closure or other procedures involving augmentation of proximal surfaces with composite. By first measuring and recording the widths of the interdental space and the teeth to be augmented, the appropriate amount of contour to be generated with composite resin addition can be determined (Fig. 15-6). In this manner, symmetric and equal tooth contours can be generated (see Correction of Diastemas).

When dealing with restorations involving the midline, particular attention also must be afforded to incisal and gingival embrasure form; the mesial contours of both central incisors must be mirror images of one another to ensure an optimally symmetric and esthetic result.

In addition to being symmetric, anterior teeth must be in proper proportion to one another to achieve maximum esthetics. The quality of proportionality is relative and varies greatly depending on other factors (e.g., tooth position, tooth alignment, arch form, configuration of the smile). However, one long-accepted theorem of the relative proportionality of maxillary anterior teeth typically visible in a smile involves the concept of the *golden proportion*.[30] Originally formulated as one of Euclid's elements, it has been relied upon through the ages as a geometric basis for proportionality in the beauty of art and nature.[4] Based on this formula a smile, when viewed from the front, is considered to be esthetically pleasing if each tooth in that smile (starting from the midline) is approximately 60% of the size of the tooth immediately mesial to it. The exact proportion of

the smaller tooth to the larger tooth is 0.618 (Fig. 15-7, *A*). It must be emphasized that these proportions are based on the *apparent sizes* of the teeth when viewed straight on and not the actual sizes of the individual teeth. In a typical esthetically pleasing smile, the maxillary anterior teeth are generally in golden proportion to one another (see Fig. 15-7, *B*). Although this theorem is not the absolute determinant of dental esthetics, it does provide a practical and proven guide for establishing proportionality when restoring anterior teeth.

Currently there is no scientific basis for determining the proper proportions of individual anterior teeth. However, an accepted theorem for achieving esthetically pleasing central incisors maintains that the ideal width-to-length ratio should be 0.75:0.8.[7] This ratio represents the ideal proportions needed to optimize the esthetic result. Because the central incisors are the dominant focal point in dental composition, the dentist must avoid narrow, elongated, or short-and-wide contours.

POSITION AND ALIGNMENT

The overall harmony and balance of a smile depend largely on proper position of teeth and their alignment in the arch. Malposed or rotated teeth disrupt the arch form and may interfere with the apparent relative proportions of the teeth. Orthodontic treatment of such defects should always be considered, especially if other positional or malocclusion problems exist in the mouth. However, if orthodontic treatment is either impractical or unaffordable, *minor positional defects* often can be treated with composite augmentation or full facial veneers indirectly made from composite or porcelain. It

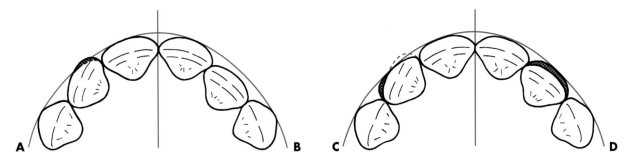

FIG. 15-8 Position and alignment. **A,** A minor rotation is first treated by reducing enamel in the area of prominence. **B,** The deficient area is restored to proper contour with composite. **C,** Maxillary lateral incisor is in slight linguoversion. **D,** Restorative augmentation of facial surface corrects malposition.

must be emphasized that only those problems that can be conservatively treated without significant alteration of the occlusion or gingival contours of the teeth should be treated in this manner.

Minor rotations can be corrected by reducing the enamel in the area of prominence and augmenting the deficient area with composite material (Fig. 15-8, *A* and *B*). Care must be taken to restrict all recontouring of prominent areas to enamel. If the rotation is to be treated with an indirectly fabricated composite or porcelain veneer, an intraenamel preparation is recommended with greater reduction provided in the area of prominence. This allows subsequent restoration to appropriate physiologic contours.

Malposed teeth are treated in a similar manner. Teeth in mild linguoversion can be treated by augmentation with full facial veneers either placed directly with composite or made indirectly from processed composite or porcelain (see Fig. 15-8, *C* and *D*). Care must be exercised to maintain physiologic gingival contours that do not impinge on tissue or result in an emergence profile of the restoration that is detrimental to gingival health. Furthermore, a functional incisal edge should be maintained by appropriate contouring of the restoration (an excessively wide incisal edge should be avoided). If the occlusion allows, limited reduction of enamel on the lingual aspect can be accomplished to reduce the faciolingual dimension of the incisal portion of the tooth. However, lingual areas participating in protrusive functional contact should not be altered. It should be pointed out that individual teeth that are significantly displaced facially (i.e., facioversion) are best treated orthodontically.

SURFACE TEXTURE

The character and individuality of teeth are largely determined by the *surface texture* and characteristics that exist. Realistic restorations closely mimic the subtle areas of stippling, concavity, and convexity that are typically present on natural teeth. Young teeth characteristically exhibit significant *surface characterization,* whereas teeth in older individuals tend to possess a smoother

surface texture caused by abrasional wear. However, even in older patients, restorations that are devoid of surface characterizations are rarely indicated.

The surfaces of natural teeth typically break up light and reflect it in many directions. Consequently, anatomic features (e.g., developmental depressions, prominences, facets, gingival perikymata) should be closely examined and reproduced to the extent that they are present on surrounding surfaces. The restored areas of teeth should reflect light in a similar manner to unrestored adjacent surfaces. In addition, as alluded to earlier, by controlling areas of *light reflection and shadowing* various desired illusions also can be created.

COLOR

Color is undoubtedly the most complex and least understood artistic element. It is an area in which numerous interdependent factors exist, all of which contribute to the final esthetic outcome of the restoration. Therefore, although complex, a basic knowledge of color is imperative to producing consistently esthetic restorations.

Dentists must understand the coloration of natural teeth to accurately and consistently select appropriate shades of restorative materials. Teeth are typically composed of a multitude of colors. A *gradation of color* usually occurs from gingival to incisal, with the gingival region being typically darker because of thinner enamel. The use of several different shades of restorative material may be required to esthetically restore a tooth. Exposed root surfaces are particularly darker (i.e., dentin colored) because of the absence of overlying enamel. Furthermore, in most individuals, *canines are slightly darker in coloration* than are the incisors.

Young patients with thick enamel characteristically exhibit lighter teeth. Moreover, patients with darker complexions usually will appear to have lighter teeth because of the contrast that exists between the teeth and surrounding facial structures. In fact, female patients can enhance the apparent lightness of their teeth simply by using a darker shade of makeup or lipstick. By increasing the contrast between the teeth and the

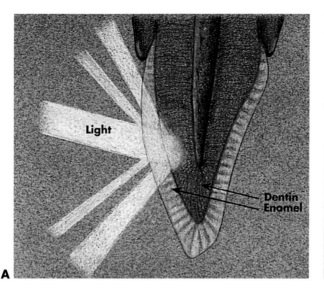
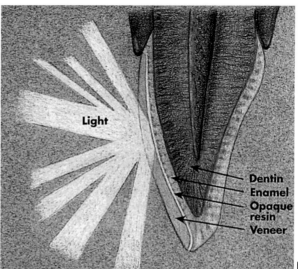

FIG. 15-9 Translucency and light penetration. **A,** Light normally penetrates deeply through the enamel and into dentin before being reflected outward. This affords lifelike esthetic vitality. **B,** Light penetration is limited by opaquing resin media under veneers. Esthetic vitality is compromised.

surrounding facial tissues, the illusion of lighter teeth can be created.

Color changes associated with aging also occur, primarily owing to wear. As the facial enamel is worn away, the underlying dentin becomes more apparent, resulting in a darker tooth. Incisal edges are often darker because of thinning of the enamel or exposure of the dentin because of normal attrition. Cervical areas also tend to darken because of abrasion.

An understanding of normal tooth coloration enhances the dentist's ability to create a restoration that appears natural. However, several clinical factors also must be considered to enhance the color-matching quality of the restoration. It should be recognized that many shade guides for composite materials are inaccurate. Not only are they often composed of a material dissimilar to that of the composite, they do not take into consideration color changes that occur from batch to batch or changes caused by aging of the composite. *Accurate shade selection* is best attained by applying and curing a small amount of the composite restorative material in the area of the tooth anticipated for restoration. Shade selection also should be determined *before isolating the teeth* to avoid color variations that can occur as a result of drying and dehydration of the teeth.

Problems in *color perception* also complicate selection of the appropriate shade of restorative material. Various light sources produce different perceptions of color. This phenomenon is referred to as *metamerism*.[41] Even the color of the surrounding environment influences what is seen in the mouth. Color perception also is influenced by the physiologic limitations of the eye. For example, upon extended viewing of a particular tooth site, the eyes experience color fatigue, resulting in a loss of sensitivity to yellow-orange shades.[37] By looking away at a blue object

or background (i.e., the complementary color), the eyes quickly recover and are once again able to distinguish subtle variations in yellow-orange hues. Because of the many indirect factors that influence color perception, it is recommended that the dentist, assistant, and especially the patient all be involved in shade selection.

TRANSLUCENCY

Translucency also affects the esthetic quality of the restoration. The *degree of translucency is related to how deeply light penetrates into the tooth or restoration before it is reflected outward.* Normally light penetrates through the enamel into dentin before being reflected outward (Fig. 15-9, *A*). This affords the lifelike *esthetic vitality* characteristic of normal, unrestored teeth. Shallow penetration of light often results in a loss of esthetic vitality. This phenomenon is a common problem encountered when treating severely intrinsically stained teeth, such as those affected by tetracycline, with direct or indirect veneers. Although opaque resin media can mask the underlying stain, a loss of esthetic vitality usually results because of reduced light penetration (see Fig. 15-9, *B*). Indirect veneers of processed composite or porcelain fabricated to include inherent opacity also may experience this problem.

Illusions of translucency also can be created to enhance the realism of a restoration. Color modifiers (also referred to as *tints*) can be used to achieve apparent translucency and tone down bright stains or characterize a restoration. A maxillary right central incisor with intrinsic yellow staining caused by trauma to the tooth warranted restoration (Fig. 15-10). When bleaching treatments were unsuccessful, a direct composite veneer was used. After an intraenamel preparation and acid-etching, a blue color modifier (the complementary color of yellow) was applied to the prepared facial surface to

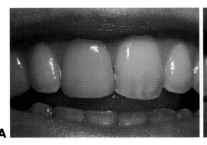
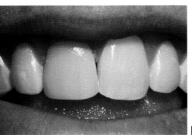

FIG. **15-10** Use of internally placed color modifiers. **A,** Maxillary right central incisor exhibits bright intrinsic yellow staining as a result of calcific metamorphosis. **B,** Color modifiers under direct-composite veneer reduce brightness and intensity of stain and simulate vertical areas of translucency.

reduce the brightness and intensity of the underlying yellow tooth. Additionally, a gray and violet mixture of color modifiers was used to simulate vertical areas of translucency. (The final restoration is shown in Fig. 15-10, *B.*) *Color modifiers* also can be incorporated in the restoration to simulate *maverick colors, check lines,* or *surface spots for further characterization.*

CLINICAL CONSIDERATIONS

Although an understanding of basic artistic elements is imperative to esthetic restorations, certain clinical considerations must be addressed concomitantly to ensure the overall quality of the restoration. In addition to being esthetic, restorations also must be *functional.* As Dr. Peter Dawson states, "Esthetics and function go hand in hand. The better the esthetics, the better the function is likely to be and vice versa."[11]

The *occlusion must always be assessed before any conservative esthetic procedure.* Anterior guidance, in particular, must be maintained and occlusal harmony ensured when treating areas involved in occlusion.

Another requirement of all conservative esthetic restorations is that they possess *physiologic contours* that promote good gingival health. Particular care must be taken in all treatments to finish gingival areas of the restoration adequately and to remove any gingival excess of material. *Emergence angles* of the restorations must be physiologic and not impinge on gingival tissues.

CONSERVATIVE ALTERATIONS OF TOOTH CONTOURS AND CONTACTS

Many unsightly tooth contours and diastemas can be corrected or greatly improved by several conservative methods. Often these procedures can be incorporated into routine restorative treatment. The objective is to improve esthetics, yet preserve as much healthy tooth structure as possible, consistent with acceptable occlusion and health of the surrounding tissue. These procedures include reshaping natural teeth, correcting embrasures, and closing diastemas.

ALTERATIONS OF SHAPE OF NATURAL TEETH

Some esthetic problems can be corrected very conservatively without the need for tooth preparation and restoration. Consideration always should be given to re-shaping and polishing the natural teeth to improve their appearance and function (Fig. 15-11). In addition, the rounding of sharp angles also can be considered a prophylactic measure to reduce stress and to help prevent chipping and fractures of the incisal edges.

Etiology. Attrition of the incisal edges often results in closed incisal embrasures and very angular incisal edges (see Fig. 15-11, *A*). Anterior teeth, especially maxillary central incisors, often are fractured in accidents. Other esthetic problems that often can be corrected or improved by reshaping the natural teeth include *attrition and abnormal wear from habits* (e.g., biting fingernails, holding objects with the teeth).

Treatment. Consultation and examination are necessary before any changes are made in the shape of a tooth or teeth. Photographs, study models, line drawings, and esthetic imaging devices enable the patient to envision the potential improvement before any changes are made.

As noted earlier, cosmetic contouring to achieve *youthful, feminine characteristics* often includes rounding incisal angles, reducing facial line angles, and opening incisal embrasures. The opposite characteristics are typically considered more *masculine features.* However, cosmetic reshaping to smooth rough incisal edges and improve symmetry is equally beneficial to both women and men.

The patient must understand what is involved and want to have the alteration made. If reshaping is desired, it is helpful to mark the outline of the areas to be reshaped on the teeth in the mouth with a pencil or alcohol-marking pen (see Fig. 15-11, *B*). By marking the anticipated areas for enamel reshaping, the patient is provided some indication of what the postoperative result may look like (see Fig. 15-11, *C*). If available, esthetic imaging using a computer also can be used to illustrate the possible result before treatment.

Because all reshaping is restricted to enamel, anesthesia is not required. A cotton roll is recommended for isolation. Diamond instruments and abrasive discs and points are used for contouring, finishing, and polishing (see Fig. 15-11, *D* and *E*). Through careful reshaping of appropriate enamel surfaces, a more esthetic smile (characterized by youthful, feminine features) is attained. Rounded incisal edges also will be less likely to chip or fracture (see Fig. 15-11, *F*).

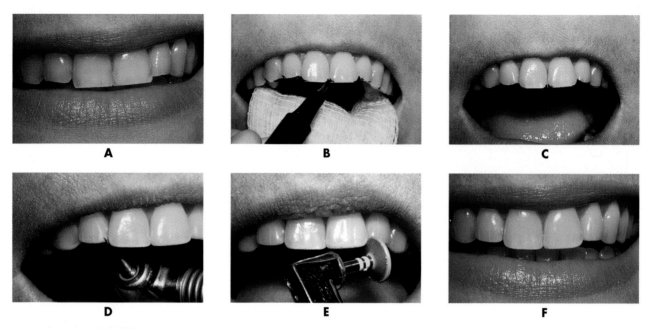

FIG. **15-11** Reshaping natural teeth. **A,** Maxillary anterior teeth with worn incisal edges. **B,** Areas to be reshaped are outlined. **C,** Outlined areas give the patient an idea of what the final result will look like. **D,** A diamond instrument is used to reshape incisal edges. **E,** A rubber abrasive disc is used to polish incisal edges. **F,** Reshaping results in more youthful, feminine smile.

FIG. **15-12** Irregular incisal edges. **A,** Central incisors have rough, fractured incisal edges. **B,** Esthetic result is obtained by recontouring incisal edges.

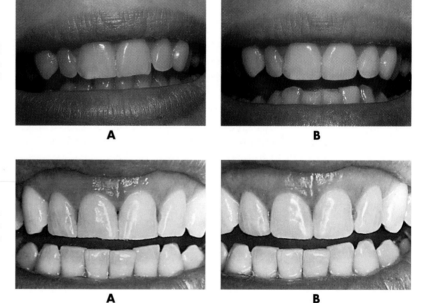

FIG. **15-13** Loss of incisal embrasures from attrition. Before (**A**) and after (**B**) recontouring teeth to produce a more youthful appearance and improve resistance to fracture.

A second example involves irregular, fractured incisal surfaces of the maxillary central incisors (Fig. 15-12, *A*). An esthetic result can be accomplished by slightly shortening the incisal edges and reshaping both teeth to a symmetric form. Again, photographs, line drawings, esthetic imaging, or marking the outline on the teeth in the mouth enables the patient to envision the potential improvement before any changes are made. Protrusive function always should be evaluated to prevent inadvertent elimination of this occlusal contact. Conserva-

tive treatment consists of using diamond instruments and abrasive discs and points for contouring and polishing the central incisors. (The finished result is illustrated in Fig. 15-12, *B*.)

As some patients grow older or have bruxing habits, the incisal surfaces often wear away, leaving sharp edges that chip easily. There is also an accompanying loss of the incisal embrasures (Fig.15-13, *A*). To lessen the chance of more fractures and to create a more youthful smile, the incisal embrasures are

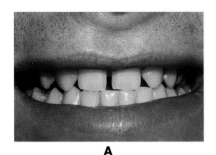
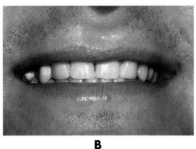

FIG. **15-14** Closing incisal embrasures. **A,** Maxillary canines moved to close spaces left by missing lateral incisors. Mesial incisal embrasures are too open. **B,** Canines reshaped to appear like lateral incisors.

opened and the incisal angles of the teeth are rounded (see Fig. 15-13, *B*).

ALTERATIONS OF EMBRASURES

Etiology. Anterior teeth can have embrasures that are too open as a result of the shape or position of the teeth in the arch. For example, when the permanent lateral incisors are congenitally missing, the canines and posterior teeth may drift mesially or the space may be closed orthodontically. The facial surface and cusp angle of some canines can be reshaped to appear like lateral incisors. However, in many instances the mesioincisal embrasures remain too open (Fig. 15-14, *A*).

Treatment. Composite can be added to establish an esthetic contour and correct the open embrasures. Evaluation of the occlusion before restoration determines if the addition will be compatible with functional movements. The patient should understand the procedures involved and want to have the change made. Line drawings, esthetic imaging, or photographs of similar examples are often helpful in explaining the procedure and allaying patient concerns. Another patient aid involves adding ivory-colored wax or composite to the teeth (unetched) to temporarily fill the embrasure to simulate the final result.

Preliminary procedures include cleaning the involved teeth, selecting the shade, and isolating the area. Local anesthesia is not usually required, because the preparation does not extend subgingivally and involves only enamel. A coarse, flame-shaped diamond instrument is used to remove overly convex enamel surfaces (if present) and to roughen the enamel surface area to be augmented with composite material. It may be necessary to place a wedge and use an abrasive strip to prepare the proximal surface. The final contour of the restoration should be envisioned before the preparation is made so that all areas to be bonded are adequately roughened.

A polyester strip is inserted to protect the adjacent tooth during acid-etching. After etching, rinsing, and drying, the contoured strip is positioned. A light-cured composite material is inserted, and the strip is closed during polymerization. The incisal embrasures of both canines are corrected, and both restorations are finished

by routine procedures (see Fig. 15-14, *B*). The occlusion should be evaluated to assess centric contacts and functional movements, and any adjustments or corrections should be made if indicated.

CORRECTION OF DIASTEMAS

Etiology. The presence of *diastemas* between the anterior teeth is an esthetic problem for some patients (Fig. 15-15, *A* through *Q*). Before treatment, a diagnosis of the cause is made, including an evaluation of the occlusion. Probably the most frequent site of a diastema is between the maxillary central incisors. A prominent labial frenum with nonelastic fibers extending proximally often prevents the normal approximation of erupting central incisors.[16] Other causative factors include congenitally missing teeth, undersized or malformed teeth, interarch tooth size discrepancies (i.e., Bolton discrepancy), supernumerary teeth, and heredity. Diastemas also may result from other problems, such as tongue thrusting, periodontal disease, or posterior bite collapse. Again, *diastemas should not be closed without first recognizing and treating the underlying cause.* Treating the cause may correct a diastema.

Treatment. Traditionally diastemas have been treated by surgical, periodontal, orthodontic, and prosthetic procedures. These types of corrections can be impractical or unaffordable and often do not result in permanent closure of the diastema. In carefully selected cases, a more practical alternative is use of the acid-etched technique and composite augmentation of proximal surfaces (see Figs. 15-5 and 15-6). It is emphasized that all treatment options (including no treatment) should be considered before resorting immediately to composite augmentation. Line drawings, photographs, computer imaging, models with spaces filled, or direct temporary additions of ivory-colored wax or composite material on the natural teeth (unetched) are important preliminary procedures.

The correction of a diastema between the maxillary central incisors is described and illustrated (see Fig. 15-15). After the teeth are cleaned and the shade selected, a Boley gauge or other suitable caliper is used to measure the width of the diastema and the individual teeth (see

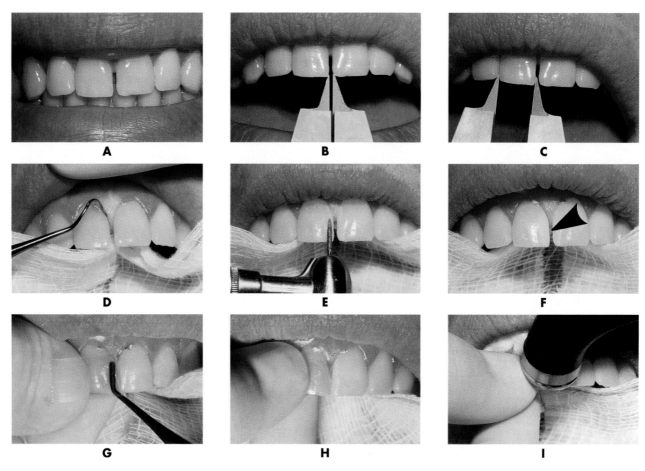

FIG. **15-15** Diastema closure. **A,** Esthetic problem created by space between central incisors. **B** and **C,** Interdental space and size of central incisors measured with caliper. **D,** Teeth isolated with cotton rolls and retraction cord tucked into gingival crevice. **E,** A diamond instrument is used to roughen enamel surfaces. **F,** Etched enamel surface indicated by arrow. **G,** Composite inserted with composite instrument. **H,** Matrix strip closed with thumb and forefinger. **I,** Composite addition is cured. *Continued*

Fig. 15-15, *B* and *C*). Occasionally, one central incisor will be wider, requiring a greater addition to the narrower tooth. Assuming the incisors are of equal width, symmetric additions can be ensured by using half of the *total* measurement of the diastema to gauge the width of the first tooth restored. Cotton rolls, instead of a rubber dam, are recommended for isolation because of the importance of relating the contour of the restoration directly to the proximal tissue. Usually the restoration must begin below the gingival crest to appear natural and to be confluent with the tooth contours.

With cotton rolls in place, a gingival retraction cord of an appropriate size is tucked in the gingival crevice of each tooth from midfacial mesially to midlingual (see Fig. 15-15, *D*). The cord retracts the soft tissue and prevents seepage from the crevice. In some instances the retraction cord may need to be inserted for one tooth at a time to prevent strangulation of the interproximal tissues during preparation and restorative procedures. To enhance retention of the composite, a coarse, flame-shaped diamond instrument is used to roughen the proximal surfaces, extending from the facial line angle to the lingual line angle (see Fig. 15-15, *E*). More extension may be needed to correct facial or lingual contours, depending on the anatomy and position of the individual tooth. The enamel is acid-etched approximately 0.5 mm past the prepared, roughened surface. The acid should not be allowed to flow into the gingival crevice. After rinsing and drying, the etched enamel should display a lightly frosted appearance (see Fig. 15-15, *F*). A 2 × 2 inch (5 × 5 cm) gauze is draped across the mouth and tongue to prevent inadvertent contamination of the etched preparations by the patient. After both preparations are completed, the teeth are restored one at a time.

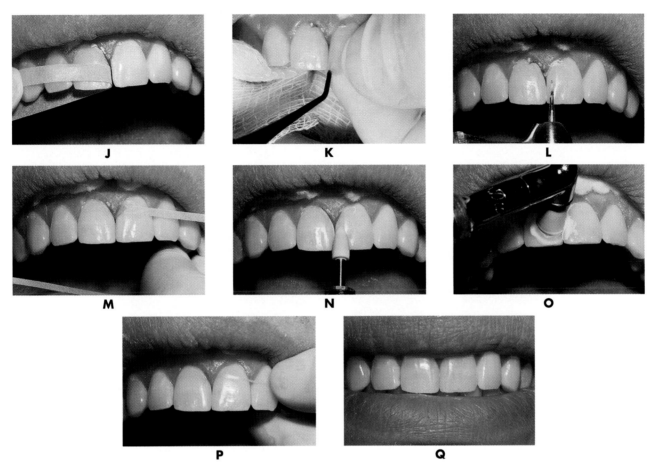

FIG. **15-15, cont'd** Diastema closure. **J,** Finishing strip used to finalize contour of first addition. **K,** A tight contact is attained by displacing the second tooth being restored in a distal direction with thumb and forefinger while holding matrix in contact with adjacent restoration. **L,** Flame-shaped finishing bur used to contour restoration. **M,** Finishing strip used to smooth subgingival areas. **N,** Restoration is polished with rubber abrasive point. **O,** Final luster attained with polishing paste applied with prophy cup. **P,** Unwaxed floss used to detect any excess composite. **Q,** Diastema closed with symmetric and equal additions of composite.

A polyester strip is contoured and placed proximally, with the gingival aspect of the strip extending below the gingival crest. Additional contouring may be required to produce enough convexity in the strip. (For contouring a polyester strip see Chapter 12.) In most cases a wedge cannot be used. The strip is then held (with the index finger) on the lingual aspect of the tooth to be restored, while the facial end is reflected for access. A light-cured composite is used for the restoration. After the resin-bonding agent is applied, the composite material is inserted with a hand instrument (see Fig. 15-15, *G*). Careful attention is given to pressing the material lingually to ensure confluence with the lingual surface. The matrix is then gently closed facially, beginning with the gingival aspect (see Fig. 15-15, *H*). Care must be taken not to pull the strip too tightly, because the resulting restoration may be undercontoured faciolingually or mesiodistally

or both. The light-cured composite material is polymerized with the light from both facial and lingual directions for a *minimum* of 20 seconds from each direction for a total of 40 seconds (see Fig. 15-15, *I*). Initially it is better to overcontour the first restoration slightly to facilitate finishing it to an ideal contour.

When polymerization is complete, the strip is removed. Contouring and finishing are achieved with appropriate carbide-finishing burs, fine diamonds, or abrasive discs (see Fig. 15-15, *L*). Finishing strips are invaluable for finalizing proximal contours (see Fig. 15-15, *J* and *M*). Final polishing is deferred until the contralateral restoration is completed. It is imperative for good gingival health that the cervical aspect of the composite addition be immaculately smooth and continuous with the tooth structure. *Overhangs must not be present.* Removal of the gingival retraction cord will facilitate in-

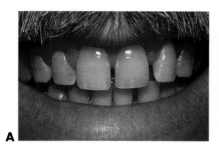
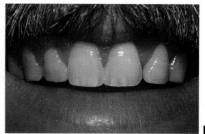

FIG. **15-16** Multiple diastemas occurring among maxillary anterior teeth. **A,** Before correction. **B,** Appearance after diastemas are closed with composite augmentation.

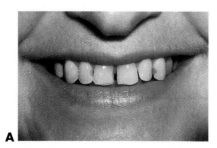
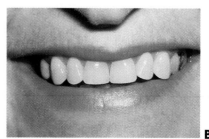

FIG. **15-17** **A** and **B,** Diastema closure and cosmetic contouring. Significant esthetic improvement is achieved by replacing defective Class III restorations and closing diastemas with conservative-composite additions and cosmetically reshaping the teeth.

spection and smoothing of this area. Flossing with a length of unwaxed floss will verify that the gingival margin is correct and smooth if no fraying of the floss occurs (see Fig. 15-15, *P*). *It is important that the correct mesiodistal dimension of the first tooth be established before the second tooth is restored.*

After etching, rinsing, and drying, the second restoration is completed. A tight proximal contact can be attained by displacing the second tooth being restored in a distal direction (with thumb and index finger), while holding the matrix in contact with the adjacent restoration (see Fig. 15-15, *K*). Contouring is accomplished with a 12-fluted carbide bur and finishing strips (see Fig. 15-15, *L* and *M*). Articulating paper should be used to evaluate the patient's occlusion to ensure that the restorations are not offensive in centric or functional movements; adjustments can be made with a carbide finishing bur or abrasive discs. Final polishing is achieved with rubber polishing points or polishing paste applied with a prophy cup in a low-speed handpiece (see Fig. 15-15, *N* and *O*). Again, unwaxed floss is used to detect any excess material or overhang (see Fig. 15-15, *P*). The esthetic result is seen in Fig. 15-15, *Q*.

Multiple diastemas among the maxillary anterior teeth are shown in Fig. 15-16, *A*. Closing the spaces by orthodontic movement was considered; however, be-cause the teeth were undercontoured mesiodistally, the spaces were filled by etching the teeth and bonding composite to the proximal surfaces. The teeth are shown after treatment (see Fig. 15-16, *B*). A similar case is illustrated in Fig. 15-5.

When defective Class III restorations or proximal caries exist, it is recommended that they be restored with the same composite used for closing the diastema. Often these restorations can be restored at the same time the diastema is closed with composite additions (Fig. 15-17).

Occasionally, diastemas are simply too large to esthetically close with composite augmentation alone (Fig. 15-18, *A*). Closing a large space of this magnitude with composite would merely create an alternative esthetic problem, excessively large central incisors, which would further exacerbate the existing discrepancy in proportionality among the anterior teeth. In such cases, large spaces are best redistributed orthodontically among the anterior teeth so that symmetric and equal composite additions can be made to both the central and lateral incisors (see Fig. 15-18, *B* and *C*). This approach involving *space distribution* results in improved *proportionality* among the anterior teeth (see Artistic Elements). The final result, right after completion, is shown in Fig. 15-18, *D*.

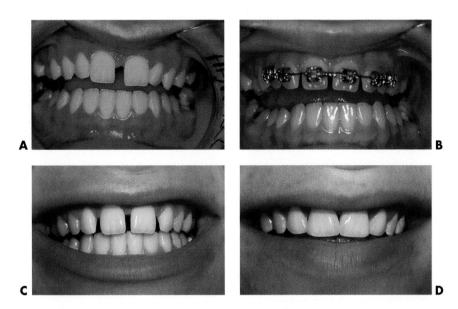

FIG. 15-18 Space distribution. **A,** Midline diastema too large for simple closure with composite additions. **B** and **C,** Space distributed among four incisors with orthodontic treatment. **D,** Final result after composite additions.

CONSERVATIVE TREATMENTS FOR DISCOLORED TEETH

One of the most frequent reasons patients seek dental care is discolored anterior teeth. Even patients with teeth of normal color request whitening procedures. Treatment options include removal of surface stains, bleaching, microabrasion or macroabrasion, veneering, and placement of porcelain crowns. Many dentists recommend porcelain crowns as the best solution for badly discolored teeth. If crowns are properly done with the highly esthetic ceramic materials currently available, they have great potential for being esthetic and long lasting. On the other hand, there are increasing numbers of patients who do not want their teeth "cut down" for crowns and are electing an alternative, conservative approach, such as veneers, that preserves as much of the natural tooth as possible. This treatment is performed with the understanding that the corrective measures may be less permanent.

Discolorations are classified as *extrinsic* or *intrinsic*. Extrinsic stains are located on the outer surfaces of the teeth, whereas intrinsic stains are internal. The etiology and treatment of extrinsic and intrinsic stains are discussed in the following sections.

EXTRINSIC DISCOLORATIONS

Etiology. Stains on the external surfaces of teeth (referred to as *extrinsic discolorations*) are quite common and may be the result of a number of causes. In young patients, stains of almost any color can be found and are usually more prominent in the cervical areas of the teeth

(Fig. 15-19, *A*). These stains may be related to remnants of Nasmyth's membrane, poor oral hygiene, existing restorations, gingival bleeding, plaque accumulation, eating habits, or the presence of chromogenic microorganisms.[21] In older patients, stains on the surfaces of the teeth are more likely to be brown, black, or gray and occur on areas adjacent to the gingival tissue. Poor oral hygiene is a contributing factor, but coffee, tea, and other types of chromogenic food or medications can produce stains (even on plaque-free surfaces). Tobacco stains also are observed frequently. Existing restorations may be discolored for the same reasons.

An example of one of the most interesting and unusual types of external staining is illustrated in Fig. 15-19, *B*. In Southeast Asia, some women traditionally dye their teeth with betel nut juice to match their hair and eyes as a sign of beauty.[13] Slices of lemon are held in contact with the teeth before applying the betel nut juice to make the staining process more effective. This example was probably one of the first applications of the acid-etching technique. A weak acid, such as that found in citrus fruits, is known to cause rapid decalcification of the enamel.

Treatment. Most surface stains can be removed by routine prophylactic procedures (Fig. 15-20, *A* through *C*). However, some superficial discolorations on tooth-colored restorations and decalcified areas on the teeth cannot be corrected by such cleaning. Conservative correction may be accomplished by mild microabrasion or by surfacing the thin, outer, discolored layer with a flame-shaped, carbide finishing bur or

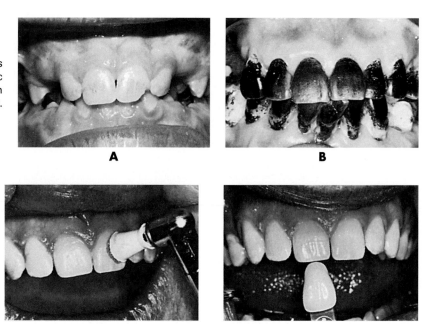

FIG. **15-19** Extrinsic stains. **A,** Surface stains on facial surfaces in young patient. **B,** Exotic decoration of anterior teeth by etching with citrus fruit juice and applying black pigment. *(Courtesy of Dr. Jeff Burkes.)*

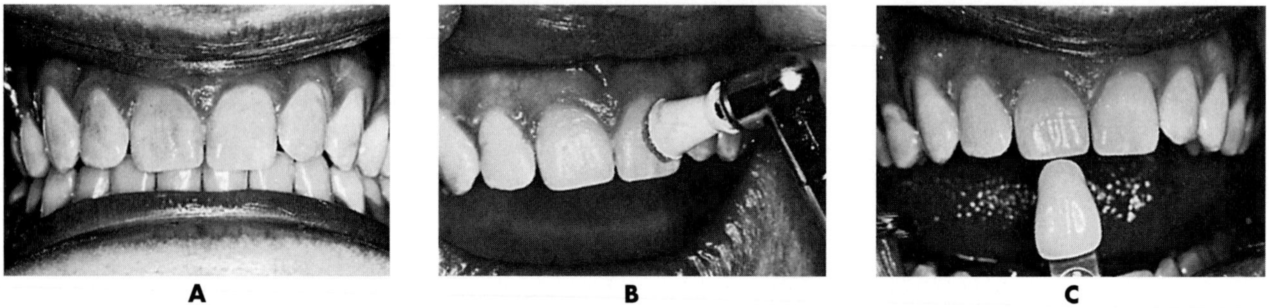

FIG. **15-20** Treatment of surface stains. **A,** Tobacco stains. **B,** Pumicing teeth with rubber cup. **C,** Shade guide used to confirm normal color of natural teeth.

diamond instrument (i.e., macroabrasion), followed by polishing with abrasive discs or points to obtain an acceptable result. (See the subsequent sections on Microabrasion and Macroabrasion for details of clinical technique.)

INTRINSIC DISCOLORATIONS

Etiology. *Intrinsic discolorations* are caused by deeper internal stains or enamel defects; these stains are more complicated to treat than external types. Teeth with vital or nonvital pulps and root canal–treated teeth can be affected. *Vital teeth* may be discolored at the time the crowns are forming, and the abnormal condition usually involves several teeth. Causative factors include hereditary disorders, medications (particularly tetracycline preparations), excess fluoride, high fevers associated with early childhood illnesses, and other types of trauma.[21] The staining may be located in enamel or in dentin. Discolorations restricted to dentin may still show through the enamel. Discoloration also may be *localized* or *generalized*, involving the entire tooth.

Various preparations of the antibiotic drug *tetracycline* can cause the most distracting, generalized type of intrinsic discoloration (Fig. 15-21, *A*).[6] The severity of the staining depends on the dose, duration of exposure to the drug, and the type of tetracycline analog used. Different types of tetracycline's induce different types of discoloration, varying from yellow-orange to dark blue-gray. Dark blue-gray, tetracycline-stained teeth are considerably more difficult to treat than are those with mild yellow-orange discolorations. Staining from tetracycline-type drugs most frequently occurs at an early age and is

caused by ingestion of the drug concomitant with the development of the permanent teeth. However, studies indicate that permanent teeth in adults also can experience a graying discoloration as a result of long-term exposure to minocycline, a tetracycline analog.[6]

The presence of excess fluoride in drinking water and other sources at the time the teeth are forming can result in another type of intrinsic stain called *fluorosis*, and it usually is generalized. Because of the high fluoride content in the enamel, fluorosed teeth may be difficult to treat with acid-etching and resin-bonding procedures.

Localized areas of discoloration may occur on individual teeth because of enamel or dentin defects induced during tooth development. High fevers and other forms of trauma can damage the tooth during its development, resulting in unesthetic hypoplastic defects. Additionally, localized areas of dysmineralization or the failure of the enamel to properly calcify can result in hypocalcified *white spots*. After eruption, poor oral hygiene also can result in decalcified white spots. Poor oral hygiene during orthodontic treatment frequently results in these types of decalcified defects. However, white or discolored spots with intact enamel surface (i.e., surface not soft) are often evidence of intraoral remineralization, and such spots are not indications for invasive treatment (unless for esthetic concerns). Additionally, caries, metallic restorations, corroded pins, and leakage or secondary caries around existing restorations can result in various types of intrinsic discoloration.

As noted earlier, aging effects also can result in yellowed teeth. As patients grow older, the tooth enamel becomes thinner because of wear and, thus, allows the

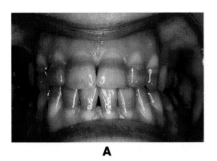
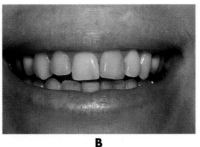

A   **B**

FIG. **15-21** Intrinsic stains. **A,** Staining by tetracycline drugs. **B,** Staining of maxillary left central incisor from tooth trauma and degeneration of the pulp.

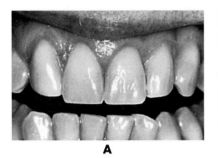
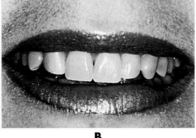

A   **B**

FIG. **15-22** Illusion of a lighter appearance of teeth by use of darker makeup. **A,** Before. **B,** After.

underlying dentin to become more apparent. This results in a yellowing effect, depending on the intrinsic color of the dentin. Additionally, the permeability of teeth usually allows the infusion (over time) of significant organic pigments (from chromogenic foods, drinks, and tobacco products) that produce a yellowing effect.

Nonvital teeth also can become discolored intrinsically. These stains usually occur in individual teeth after eruption has taken place. The pulp may become infected or degenerate as a result of trauma, deep caries, or irritation from restorative procedures. If these teeth are properly treated by root canal therapy, they usually will retain their normal color. If treatment is delayed, discoloration of the crown is more likely to occur. The degenerative products from the pulp tissue will stain the dentin and will be readily apparent because of the translucency of the enamel (see Fig. 15-21, *B*). Trauma resulting in calcific metamorphosis (i.e., calcification of the pulp chamber, root canal, or both) also can produce significant yellowing of the tooth. This condition is extremely difficult to treat (see Fig. 15-10).

Treatment. Many persons have definite esthetic problems from intrinsic stains, whereas others worry needlessly about the overall color of their teeth. In the latter instance, the dentist must decide if the color of the teeth can be improved enough to justify treatment even though the patient insists on having something done. For example, persons with light complexions may believe that their teeth are too dark, when actually they are normal in color (Fig. 15-22, *A*). Positioning a shade tab from a shade guide of tooth colors next to such teeth often will demonstrate to the patient that the color of their teeth is well within the normal range of shades. As stated, a suntan, darker makeup, or darker lipstick will

usually make teeth appear much whiter by increasing the contrast between the teeth and the surrounding facial features (see Fig. 15-22, *B*).

The patient should be told that many discolorations can be corrected or greatly improved through conservative methods such as bleaching, microabrasion or macroabrasion, or veneering. Mild discolorations are best left untreated, bleached, or treated conservatively with microabrasion or macroabrasion, because no restorative material is as good as the healthy, natural tooth structure. Moreover, the *patient should be informed that the gingival tissue will never be as healthy when adjacent to restorative material as when next to normal tooth structure.*

Color photographs of previously treated teeth with intrinsic staining (i.e., before and after treatment) are excellent adjuncts to help the patient make an informed decision. Esthetic imaging with modern computer simulation of the postoperative result also can be an effective educational tool. Patients appreciate knowing what the cause of the problem is, how it can be corrected, how much time is involved, and what the cost will be. They also should be informed of the life expectancy of the various treatment alternatives suggested. For example, vital bleaching usually will result in tooth lightening for only 1 to 3 years, whereas an etched porcelain veneer should last 10 to 15 years or longer. With continuous improvements in materials and techniques, a much longer lifespan may be possible with any of these techniques. The clinical longevity of esthetic restorations also is enhanced in patients who exhibit good oral hygiene, proper diet, a favorable bite relationship, and little or no contact with agents that cause discoloration or deterioration.

Correction of intrinsic discolorations caused by failing restorations entails replacement of the faulty portion or the entire restoration. Correction of discolorations caused by carious lesions requires appropriate restorative treatment. Conservative treatment methods are covered in the chapters on composite, amalgam, and cast restorations. Esthetic inserts for metal restorations are described later in this chapter. For the other types of intrinsic discolorations previously discussed, detailed treatment options are presented in the following three sections.

BLEACHING TREATMENTS

The lightening of the color of a tooth through the application of a chemical agent to oxidize the organic pigmentation in the tooth is referred to as *bleaching.* In keeping with the overall conservative philosophy of tooth restoration, consideration first should be given to bleaching anterior teeth when intrinsic discolorations are encountered. Bleaching techniques may be classified as to whether they involve vital or nonvital teeth, and whether the procedure is performed in the office, or with some outside the office component. Bleaching of nonvital teeth was first reported in 1848, whereas in-office bleaching of vital teeth was first reported in 1868.[22] By the early 1900s, in-office vital bleaching had evolved to include the use of heat and light for activation of the process. Although there are reports of a 3% ether and peroxide mouthwash used for bleaching in 1893, the "dentist prescribed–home applied" technique (also referred to as nightguard vital bleaching) for bleaching vital teeth outside the office began around 1968.[23]

Most bleaching techniques use some form or derivative of hydrogen peroxide in different concentrations and application techniques. The mechanism of action of bleaching teeth with hydrogen peroxide is considered to be oxidation of organic pigments, although the chemistry is not well understood. Bleaching generally has an approximate lifespan of 1 to 3 years, although the change may be permanent in some situations.

With all bleaching techniques, there is a transitory decrease in the potential bond strength of composite when it is applied to the bleached, etched enamel. This reduction in bond strength results from residual oxygen or peroxide residue in the tooth that inhibits the set of the bonding resin, precluding adequate resin tag formation in the etched enamel. However, *no loss of bond strength is noted if the composite restorative treatment is delayed at least 1 week after cessation of any bleaching.*[44]

NONVITAL BLEACHING PROCEDURES

The primary indication for nonvital bleaching is to lighten teeth that have undergone root canal therapy. This discoloration may be a result of bleeding into the dentin from trauma before root canal therapy, degradation of pulp tissue left in the chamber after such therapy, or staining from restorative materials and cements placed in the tooth as a part of the root canal treatment. Most posterior teeth that have received root canal ther-

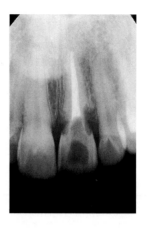

FIG. **15-23** Radiograph revealing the presence of extensive cervical resorption.

apy require cast restorations that encompass the tooth to prevent subsequent fracture. However, anterior teeth needing restorative treatment and that are largely intact may be restored with composite rather than with partial or full coverage restorations without significantly compromising the strength of the tooth.[40] This knowledge has created a resurgence in the use of nonvital bleaching techniques.

Nonvital bleaching techniques include an in-office *thermocatalytic technique* and an out of the office technique referred to as *walking bleach.* (See the following sections for details of these two techniques.)

Although nonvital bleaching is quite effective, there is a slight potential (i.e., 1%) for a most deleterious side effect termed *cervical resorption* (Fig. 15-23).[20] This sequela requires prompt and aggressive treatment. In animal models, cervical resorption has been observed most when using a thermocatalytic technique with high heat.[33] Therefore the "walking bleach" technique or an in-office technique that does not require the use of heat is preferred for nonvital bleaching. To reduce the possibility of resorption, immediately after bleaching, a paste of calcium hydroxide powder and sterile water is placed in the pulp chamber as described in the following sections.[28] Also, sodium perborate alone, rather than in conjunction with hydrogen peroxide, may be used as the primary bleaching agent. Although sodium perborate may bleach more slowly, it is safer and less offensive to the tooth.[27] Periodic radiographs should be made after bleaching to screen for cervical resorption, which generally has its onset in 1 to 7 years.[29]

In-Office Nonvital Bleaching Technique. The in-office bleaching for nonvital teeth is historically a *thermocatalytic technique* involving the placement of 35% hydrogen peroxide liquid into the débrided pulp chamber and acceleration of the oxidation process by placement of a heating instrument into the pulp chamber.

A more recent technique uses 35% hydrogen peroxide pastes or gels that require no heat. This technique is frequently the preferred in-office technique for bleaching nonvital teeth. In both techniques, it is imperative that a sealing cement (polycarboxylate or light-cured glass-

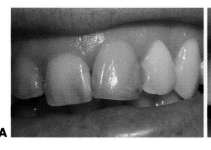 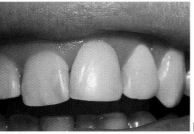

FIG. **15-24** Indication for bleaching root canal–filled tooth. **A,** Before. **B,** After intracoronal, nonvital bleaching.

ionomer cement is recommended) be placed over the exposed root canal filling before application of the bleaching agent to prevent leakage and penetration of the bleaching material in an apical direction.

"Walking" Bleach Technique. Before beginning the "walking bleach" technique, evaluate the potential for occlusal contact on the area of the root canal access opening. Place a rubber dam to isolate the discolored tooth and remove all materials in the coronal portion of the tooth (i.e., access opening). Remove gutta-percha (to approximately 2 mm apical of the clinical crown) and enlarge the endodontic access opening sufficiently to ensure complete débridement of the pulp chamber. Next, place a polycarboxylate or a light-cured glass-ionomer cement liner to seal the gutta-percha of the root canal filling from the coronal portion of the pulp chamber. After this seal has hardened, trim any excess material from the seal so that the discolored dentin is exposed peripherally. Using a cement spatula with heavy pressure on a glass slab, blend one drop of saline with enough sodium perborate to form a creamy paste. Caution must be exercised in handling the material, because 35% hydrogen peroxide is a potent oxidizer and will chemically burn tissue upon contact. Should tissue be inadvertently contacted by the bleaching material, the affected area should be rinsed with copious amounts of water. *To eliminate any risks associated with the hydrogen peroxide, water or saline may be mixed with sodium perborate to form the bleaching paste (although bleaching results are more slowly attained).*

Use a spoon excavator or similar instrument to fill the pulp chamber (with the bleaching mixture) to within 2 mm of the cavosurface margin, avoiding contact with the enamel cavosurface margins of the access opening. Use a cotton pellet to blot the mixture and then place a temporary sealing material (e.g., Intermediate Restorative Material [IRM] or Cavit) to seal the access opening. The area should remain isolated for approximately 5 minutes after closure to evaluate the adequacy of the seal of the temporary restoration. If bubbles appear around the margins of the temporary material indicating leakage, the temporary restoration must be replaced. If no bubbles appear, remove the rubber dam and check the occlusion to assess the presence or absence of contact on the temporary restoration.

The bleaching mixture is very active for 24 hours, after which little potential for harm to tissue exists. The mixture may be changed every 3 to 5 days, and usually one to three treatments are required to achieve optimal tooth lightening. If sodium perborate is used alone, it should be changed weekly. Upon successful bleaching of the tooth, rinse the chamber and fill it to within 2 mm of the cavosurface margin with a paste consisting of calcium hydroxide powder in sterile saline. (Keep the enamel walls and margins clean and free of the calcium hydroxide paste). Reseal the access opening with a temporary restorative material in a manner previously described and allow the calcium hydroxide material to remain in the pulp chamber for 2 weeks. Afterward, remove the temporary restorative material, rinse away the calcium hydroxide, and dry the pulp chamber. Next, etch the enamel and dentin and restore the tooth with a light-cured composite (Fig. 15-24).

Occasionally. a tooth that has been bleached by the "walking bleach" technique and sealed with a composite restoration will subsequently discolor. In this instance the alternative treatment option should be an attempt to bleach the tooth externally with one of the external bleaching techniques (see Vital Bleaching Procedures).

VITAL BLEACHING PROCEDURES

Generally, the indications for the different vital bleaching techniques are similar, with patient preference, cost, compliance, and difficulty in removing certain discolorations dictating the choice of treatment or combination of treatments. Indications for vital bleaching include intrinsically discolored teeth from aging, trauma, or drug ingestion. Alternative treatment options for a failed, nonvital, "walking bleach" procedures are the external vital bleaching techniques. Vital bleaching also is often indicated before and after restorative treatments to harmonize shades of the restorative materials with the natural teeth.

Teeth exhibiting yellow or orange intrinsic discoloration appear to respond best to vital bleaching, whereas teeth exhibiting bluish-gray discolorations often are considerably more difficult to treat in this manner. Other indications for external bleaching include single teeth that have darkened from trauma but are still vital or have a poor endodontic prognosis because of the absence of a radiographically visible canal (i.e., calcific metamorphosis). Brown fluorosis stains also are often responsive to treatment, but white fluorosis stains are not effectively resolved (although they can be made less obvious if the surrounding tooth structure can be significantly whitened).

Vital bleaching techniques include an in-office technique referred to as *power bleaching*[12] and an outside-the-office alternative that is a dentist prescribed–home applied technique (i.e., *nightguard vital bleaching*).[25] These techniques may be used separately or in combination with one another. (Details are provided in subsequent sections.)

Overall, vital bleaching has proven to be safe and effective when performed by, or under the supervision of, a dentist. With short-term treatment there does not appear to be any appreciable effect on existing restorative materials, either in loss of material integrity or in color change, with one exception: polymethylmethacrylate (PMMA) restorations experience a yellow-orange discoloration upon exposure to carbamide peroxide. For this reason, temporary crowns should be made from Bisacryl materials rather than PMMA crown and bridge resin if exposure to carbamide peroxide is anticipated.

Because hydrogen peroxide has such a low molecular weight, it easily passes through the enamel and dentin. This characteristic is thought to account for the mild tooth sensitivity occasionally experienced during treatment. However, this effect is transient, and no long-term harm to the pulp has been noted.

Often the choice for the dentist is whether to use an in-office bleaching technique or the dentist prescribed–home applied technique. The *advantages of the in-office vital bleaching technique* are that (although it uses very caustic chemicals) it is totally under the dentist's control, the soft tissue is generally protected from the process, and it has the potential for bleaching teeth more rapidly. *Disadvantages* primarily relate to the cost, the unpredictable outcome, and the unknown duration of the treatment. The features that warrant concern and caution include the potential for soft-tissue damage to patient and provider, the discomfort of a rubber dam, and the potential for posttreatment sensitivity. The *advantages of the dentist prescribed–home applied technique (i.e., nightguard vital bleaching)* are the use of a lower concentration of peroxide (generally 10% to 15% carbamide peroxide), the ease of application, minimal side effects, and lower cost because of the reduced chair time required for treatment. The *disadvantages* are the reliance on patient compliance, the longer treatment time, and the (unknown) potential for soft-tissue changes with excessively extended use.

In-Office Vital Bleaching Technique. In-office vital bleaching requires excellent rubber dam technique and careful patient management. Place Vaseline or cocoa butter on the patient's lips and gingival tissues before application of the rubber dam. Isolate the anterior teeth (and sometimes the first premolars) with a heavy rubber dam to provide maximum retraction of tissue and an optimal seal around the teeth. Ensure a good seal of the dam by either ligation of the dam with waxed dental tape or the use of a sealing putty or varnish. Etching of the teeth with 37% phosphoric acid, previously considered a required part of this technique, now is considered unnecessary.[17] Place a 35% hydrogen peroxide–soaked gauze or a gel or paste form of hydrogen peroxide on the teeth. Instruct the patient to note any sensations of burning of the lips or gingiva that would indicate a leaking dam and the need to terminate treatment. The oxidation reaction of the hydrogen peroxide can be accelerated by applying heat with either a heating instrument (2 minutes per tooth) set at the maximum tolerance of the patient, or with an intense light (30 minutes per arch). Use of a CO_2 laser to heat the bleaching mixture and accelerate the bleaching treatment currently is not recommended according to a recent report of the American Dental Association, because of the potential for hard- or soft-tissue damage.[1]

Upon completion of the treatment, rinse the teeth, remove the rubber dam, and caution the patient about postoperative sensitivity. A nonsteroidal, analgesic and antiinflammatory drug may be administered if sensitivity is anticipated.

Bleaching treatments are generally rendered weekly for two to six treatments, with each treatment lasting 30 to 45 minutes. Patients may experience transient sensitivity of teeth between appointments, but again, no long-term adverse pulpal effects have been reported. Because the enamel is not acid-etched, there is no need to polish the teeth posttreatment, nor is it essential to provide a fluoride treatment.

Dentist Prescribed–Home Applied Technique. The dentist prescribed–home applied technique (i.e., nightguard vital bleaching) is much less labor intensive and requires substantially less in-office time. An alginate impression of the arch to be treated is made and poured in cast stone. The impression should be made free of bubbles on or around the teeth by wiping alginate onto the teeth and adjacent gingival areas before inserting the impression. After appropriate infection control procedures, rinse the impression vigorously and then pour with cast stone. *Incomplete rinsing of the impression may cause a softened surface on the stone,* which may result in a nightguard (bleaching tray) that is slightly too small and irritates tissue. Trim the cast around the periphery to eliminate the vestibule and thin the base of the cast palatally (until a hole is produced). Generally, the cast must be lifted from the table of the cast-trimming machine to remove the vestibule successfully without damaging the teeth. Allow the cast to dry and block out any significant undercuts using a block-out material (e.g., putty, clay, light-activated spacer material).

The nightguard is formed on the cast using a heat vacuum–forming machine. After the machine has warmed up for 10 minutes, a sheet of 0.020 to 0.035 inch (0.75 to 1.5 mm) soft vinyl nightguard material is inserted and allowed to soften by heat until it sags approximately 1 inch. Close the top portion of the machine slowly and gently and allow the vacuum to form the heat-softened material around the cast. After sufficient time for adaptation of the material, turn off the machine and allow the material to cool.

Next, use scissors or a No. 11 surgical blade in a Bard-Parker handle to trim in a smooth, straight cut about 3 to 5 mm from the most apical portion of the gingival crest of the teeth (facially and lingually). This excess material is removed first. Remove the horseshoe-shaped nightguard from the cast. Trim the facial edges of the nightguard in a scalloped design, following the outline of the free gingival crest and using sharp, curved scissors. Scalloping of the lingual surface is optional, because the bleaching material is applied primarily to the facial aspects of the teeth. Alternatively (on the lingual), the nightguard may be trimmed apically to within 2 mm of the free gingival crest in a smooth, horseshoe-shaped configuration. This scalloped design is preferred because it allows the tray to cover only the teeth and prevents entrapment of the bleaching material between the gingival tissue and the nightguard. The nightguard is completed and ready for delivery to the patient (Fig. 15-25).

Insert the nightguard into the patient's mouth and evaluate it for adaptation, rough edges, or blanching of tissue. A properly fitting nightguard is shown in Fig. 15-26. Further shortening (i.e., trimming) may be indicated in problem areas. Evaluate the occlusion on the nightguard with the patient in maximum intercuspa-

tion. If the patient is unable to obtain a comfortable occlusion because of premature posterior tooth contacts, trim the nightguard to exclude coverage of the terminal posterior teeth as needed (to allow optimal tooth contact in maximum intercuspation). In addition, if no lingual scalloping is done, the edges of the guard on the palate should terminate in grooves or valleys where possible, rather than on the heights of soft-tissue contours (e.g., in the area of the incisive papilla).

A 10% to 15% carbamide peroxide–bleaching material generally is recommended for this bleaching technique. Commercial bleaching products are available as both clear gels and white pastes. Carbamide peroxide degrades into 3% hydrogen peroxide (active ingredient) and 7% urea. Bleaching materials containing carbopol are recommended because it thickens the bleaching solution and extends the oxidation process. Based on numerous research studies, carbamide peroxide bleaching materials appear to be *safe and effective when administered by or under the supervision of a dentist.*[24]

Instruct the patient in the application of the bleaching gel or paste into the nightguard. A thin bead of material is extruded into the nightguard along the facial aspects corresponding to the area of each tooth to be bleached. Usually only the anterior 6 to 8 teeth are bleached. The clinician should review proper insertion of the nightguard with the patient. After inserting the nightguard, excess material is wiped from the soft tissue along the edge with a soft-bristled toothbrush. No excess material should be allowed to remain on the soft tissue because of the potential for gingival irritation. The patient should be informed not to drink liquids or rinse during treatment, and to remove the nightguard for meals and oral hygiene.

Although no one treatment regimen is best for all patients; most patients prefer an overnight treatment approach. If the nightguard is worn at night, a single application of bleaching material at bedtime is indicated. In the morning, the patient should remove the nightguard, clean it under running water with a toothbrush, and store it in the container provided. Total treatment time using an overnight approach is usually 1 to 2 weeks. If patients cannot tolerate overnight bleaching, the bleaching time and frequency can be adjusted to accommodate the patient's comfort level. In addition, in

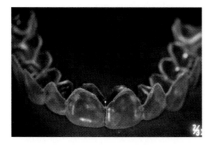

FIG. **15-25** Vacuum-formed clear-plastic nightguard used for vital bleaching (i.e., scalloped version).

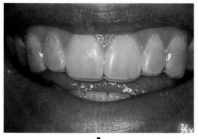

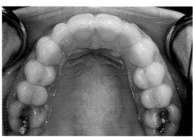

FIG. **15-26** Nightguard for vital bleaching. **A** and **B,** Clear-plastic nightguard properly seated and positioned in the mouth (scalloped on facial, unscalloped on lingual).

A

B

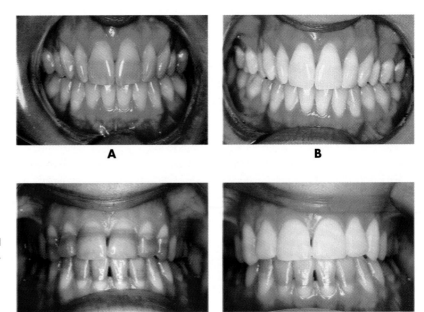

FIG. **15-27** Nightguard vital bleaching. **A,** Before bleaching treatment. **B,** After.

FIG. **15-28** Bleaching tetracycline-stained teeth. **A,** Before nonvital bleaching. **B,** After. *(Courtesy of Dr. Wayne Mohorn.)*

these cases, tolerance to the nightguard and bleaching material generally are improved if the patient gradually increases wearing time each day.

If either of the two primary side effects occurs (i.e., sensitive teeth or irritated gingiva) the patient should reduce or discontinue treatment immediately and contact the dentist so that the cause of the problem can be determined.

It is recommended that *only one arch be bleached at a time,* beginning with the maxillary arch. Bleaching the maxillary arch first allows the untreated mandibular arch to serve as a constant standard for comparison. Moreover, restricting the bleaching to one arch at a time reduces the potential for occlusal problems that could potentially occur if the thickness of two mouth guards were interposed simultaneously. Fig. 15-27 illustrates a typical case before and after treatment with nightguard vital bleaching.

Tetracycline-stained teeth typically are much more resistant to bleaching. Therefore teeth stained with tetracycline require prolonged treatment times up to several months before any results are observed. Often, tetracycline-stained teeth are unresponsive to the procedure, especially if the stains are blue-gray in color. Tetracycline-stained teeth may approach but never seem to achieve the appearance of normal teeth. A single tetracycline-stained tooth with previous endodontic therapy or a different pulp size may respond differently from other teeth in the arch to the bleaching technique.

Because bleaching tetracycline-stained teeth is difficult, some clinicians advocate intentional endodontic therapy, with the use of an intracoronal nonvital bleaching technique to overcome this problem (Fig. 15-28). Although the esthetic result appears much better than that obtained from external bleaching, this approach in-

volves all the inherent risks otherwise associated with root canal treatment. External bleaching techniques offer a safer alternative, even though they may not be as rapid or effective. Veneers or full crowns are alternative esthetic treatment methods for difficult tetracycline-stained teeth but involve irreversible restorative techniques (see Indirect Veneer Techniques).

No one bleaching technique is effective in every situation, and all successes are not equal. Often with vital bleaching, a combination of the in-office technique and the dentist prescribed home-applied technique will have better results than either technique used alone.

MICROABRASION AND MACROABRASION

Microabrasion and macroabrasion represent conservative alternatives for the reduction or elimination of *superficial* discolorations. As the terms imply, the stained areas or defects are abraded away. These techniques do result in the physical removal of tooth structure and, therefore, are indicated only for stains or enamel defects that *do not extend beyond a few tenths of a millimeter in depth.* If the defect or discoloration remains after treatment with microabrasion or macroabrasion, a restorative alternative is indicated.

MICROABRASION

In 1984 McCloskey reported the use of 18% hydrochloric acid swabbed on teeth for the removal of superficial fluorosis stains.[35] Subsequently, in 1986, Croll modified the technique to include the use of pumice with the hydrochloric acid to form a paste applied with a tongue blade.[10] This technique is called *microabrasion* and involves the surface dissolution of the enamel by the acid along with the abrasiveness of the pumice to remove superficial stains or defects. Since that time, Croll further modified the technique, reducing the concentration of the acid to approximately 11% and increasing the abrasiveness of the paste using silicon carbide particles (in a water-soluble gel paste) instead of pumice.[9] This product, marketed as Prema compound (Premier Dental Products Co., Box 111, Norristown, PA 19404), represents an improved and safer means for the removal of superficial stains or defects. It should be emphasized that this technique involves the physical removal of tooth structure and does not remove stains or defects through any bleaching phenomenon.

Before treatment the clinician should evaluate the nature and extent of the enamel defect or stain and differentiate between the nonhereditary developmental dysmineralization (i.e., abnormal mineralization) defects (e.g., white or light brown fluoretic enamel, and the idiopathic white or light-brown spot) versus the incipient carious lesion (see Examination of Teeth and Restorations in Chapter 9, Nomenclature in Chapter 6, and Histopathology of Caries in Chapter 3).

Incipient carious lesions are usually located near the gingival margin. These lesions have a smooth surface (i.e., macroappearance), and they appear opaque or chalky white when dried but are less visible when hydrated.

Incipient caries is reversible if treated immediately. Changing the oral environment by oral hygiene and dietary adjustments will allow remineralization to occur. If, however, the carious lesion has progressed to have a slightly roughened surface, microabrasion coupled with a remineralization program is an initial option. If unsuccessful this can be followed by a restoration. Cavitation of the enamel surface is an indication for restorative intervention. As the location of smooth surface enamel caries nears the cementoenamel junction (CEJ), the enamel is too thin to permit microabrasion or macroabrasion (see Macroabrasion) as a treatment option.

The *developmental discolored spot* (opaque white or light brown) is the result of an unknown, local traumatic event during amelogenesis and is, therefore, termed *idiopathic*. Its surface is intact, smooth, and hard. It is usually located in the incisal (occlusal) half of the enamel, which contributes to the unsightly appearance. The patient (or patient's parents) must be informed that an accurate prognosis for microabrasion cannot be given but that microabrasion will first be applied. If unsuccessful because of the depth of the defect exceeding 0.2 to 0.3 mm, then the tooth will be restored with a tooth-colored restoration.

Surface discolorations because of fluorosis also can be removed by microabrasion if the discoloration is within the 0.2- to 0.3-mm removal depth limit.

Fig. 15-29, *A*, shows young patient with fluorosis stains on teeth Nos. 8 and 9. A rubber dam is placed to isolate the teeth to be treated and to protect the gingival

tissues from the acid in the Prema paste or compound. Protective glasses should be worn by the patient to shield the eyes from any splatter. The Prema paste is applied to the defective area of the tooth with a special rubber cup that has fluted edges (see Fig. 15-29, *B* and *C*). The abrasive compound can be applied with either the side or the end of the rubber cup. A 10× gear reduction, low-speed handpiece (similar to that used for placing pins) is recommended for application of the Prema compound to reduce the possibility of removing too much tooth structure and to prevent spatter. Moderately firm pressure is used in applying the compound.

For small, localized, idiopathic white or light-brown areas, a hand application device is also available for use with the Prema compound (see Fig. 15-29, *D*). Periodically, the paste is rinsed away to assess defect removal. The facial surface also is viewed with a mirror from the incisal aspect to determine how much tooth structure has been removed. Care must be taken not to remove excessive tooth structure. The procedure is continued until the defect is removed or until it is deemed imprudent to continue further (see Fig. 15-29, *E*). The treated areas are polished with a fluoride-containing prophy paste to restore surface luster (see Fig. 15-29, *F*). Immediately following treatment, a topical fluoride is applied to the teeth to enhance remineralization (see Fig. 15-29, *G*). Results are seen in Fig. 15-29, *H*.

MACROABRASION

An alternative technique for the removal of localized, superficial white spots (not subject to conservative, remineralization therapy) and other surface stains or defects is called *macroabrasion*. Macroabrasion simply uses a 12-fluted composite finishing bur or a fine grit finishing diamond in a high-speed handpiece to remove the defect (Fig. 15-30, *A* and *B*). Care must be taken to use light, intermittent pressure and to carefully monitor removal of tooth structure to avoid irreversible damage to the tooth. Air-water spray is recommended, not only as a coolant, but also to maintain the tooth in a hydrated state to facilitate assessment of defect removal. Teeth that possess white spot defects are particularly susceptible to dehydration resulting in other apparent white spots that are not normally seen when the tooth is hydrated. Dehydration exaggerates the appearance of white spots and makes defect removal difficult to assess.

After removal of the defect or upon termination of any further removal of tooth structure, a 30-fluted composite-finishing bur is used to remove any facets or striations created by the previous instruments (see Fig. 15-30, *C*). Final polishing is accomplished with an abrasive rubber point (see Fig. 15-30, *D*). The results are seen in Fig. 15-30, *E*.

Comparable results can be achieved with either microabrasion or macroabrasion. However, advantages and disadvantages exist with each. Microabrasion has

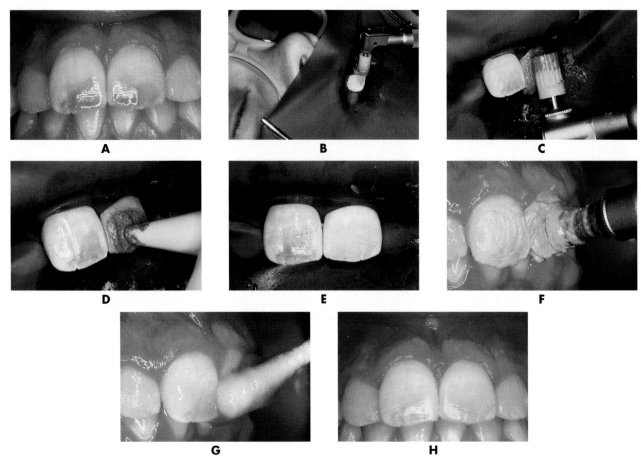

FIG. **15-29** Microabrasion. **A,** Young patient with unesthetic fluorosis stains on central incisors. **B** and **C,** Prema compound applied with special rubber cup with fluted edges. Protective glasses and rubber dam are needed for safety of patient. **D,** Hand applicator for applying Prema compound. **E,** Stain removed from left central incisor after microabrasion. **F,** Treated enamel surfaces polished with prophylactic paste. **G,** Topical fluoride applied to treated enamel surfaces. **H,** Final esthetic result. *(Courtesy of Dr. Ted Croll.)*

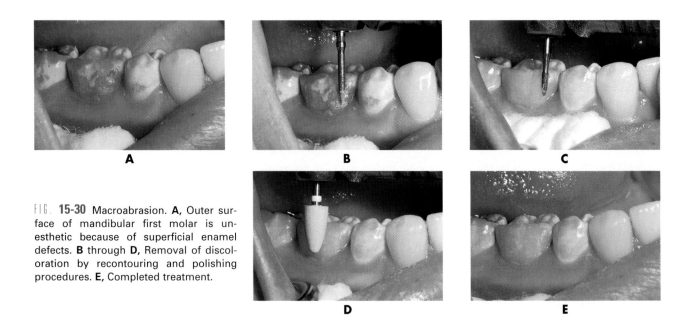

FIG. **15-30** Macroabrasion. **A,** Outer surface of mandibular first molar is unesthetic because of superficial enamel defects. **B** through **D,** Removal of discoloration by recontouring and polishing procedures. **E,** Completed treatment.

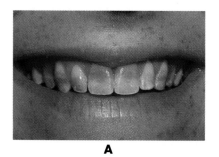
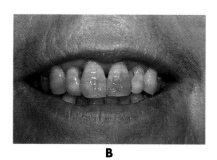
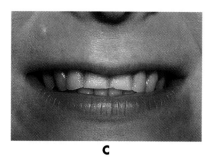

A **B** **C**

FIG. **15-31** Clinical examples of indications for treatment with veneers include teeth affected by: **A,** tetracycline drug staining; **B,** fluorosis or enamel hypoplasia; and **C,** acid-induced erosion (e.g., lemon-sucking habit).

the advantage of ensuring better control of the removal of tooth structure. High-speed instrumentation as used in macroabrasion is technique sensitive and can have catastrophic results if the clinician fails to use extreme caution. However, macroabrasion is considerably faster and does not require the use of a rubber dam or special instrumentation. Defect removal is also easier with macroabrasion compared with microabrasion if an air-water spray is used during treatment to maintain hydration of the teeth. Nonetheless, microabrasion is recommended over macroabrasion for the treatment of superficial defects in children because of better operator control and superior patient acceptance.

To accelerate the process a combination of macroabrasion and microabrasion also may be considered. Gross removal of the defect is accomplished with macroabrasion, followed by final treatment with microabrasion.

VENEERS

A veneer is a layer of tooth-colored material that is applied to a tooth to restore localized or generalized defects and intrinsic discolorations (see Figs. 15-33, 15-34, 15-37, and 15-41). Typically, veneers are made of chairside composite, processed composite, porcelain, or pressed ceramic materials. Common indications for veneers include teeth with facial surfaces that are malformed, discolored, abraded, eroded, or have faulty restorations (Fig. 15-31).

Two types of esthetic veneers exist: (1) partial veneers and (2) full veneers (see Fig. 15-31). *Partial veneers* are indicated for the restoration of localized defects or areas of intrinsic discoloration (see Figs. 15-1 and 15-31, *A* and *B*). *Full veneers* are indicated for the restoration of generalized defects or areas of intrinsic staining involving the majority of the facial surface of the tooth (see Figs. 15-34, 15-35, 15-37, 15-38, and 15-41). However, several important factors, including patient age, occlusion, tissue health, position and alignment of the teeth, and oral hygiene, must be evaluated before pursuing full veneers as a treatment option. Furthermore, if full veneers are done, care must be taken to provide proper physiologic contours, particularly in the gingival area, to favor good

gingival health. An example of poorly contoured veneers is seen in Fig. 15-31, *C;* severe gingival irritation exists around the overcontoured veneers.

Full veneers can be accomplished by a direct or an indirect technique. When a small number of teeth are involved or when the entire facial surface is not faulty (i.e., partial veneers), directly applied composite veneers can be completed for the patient in one appointment with chairside composite. Placing direct-composite full veneers is very time consuming and labor intensive. However, for cases involving young children, a single discolored tooth, or when economics or patient time are limited, precluding a laboratory-fabricated veneer, the direct technique is a viable option.

Indirect veneers require two appointments but typically offer three advantages over directly placed full veneers:

1. Indirectly fabricated veneers are much less sensitive to operator technique. Considerable artistic expertise and attention to detail are required to achieve esthetic and physiologically sound direct veneers consistently. Indirect veneers are made by a laboratory technician and are typically more esthetic.
2. If multiple teeth are to be veneered, indirect veneers usually can be placed much more expeditiously.
3. Indirect veneers typically will last much longer than direct veneers, especially if they are made of porcelain or pressed ceramic.

Some controversy exists regarding the extent of tooth preparation that is necessary and the amount of coverage for veneers (Fig. 15-32). Some operators prefer to etch the existing enamel and apply the veneer to the entire existing facial surface without any tooth preparation. The perceived advantage of this method is that, in the event of failure or if the patient does not like the veneer, it can be removed (thus being reversible). However, several significant problems exist with this approach. First, to achieve an esthetic result, the facial surface of such a restoration must be overcontoured, thus appearing and feeling unnatural. An overcontoured veneer frequently

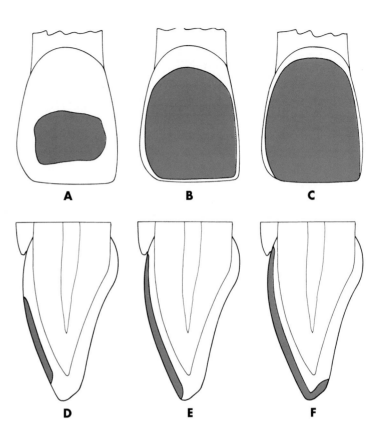

FIG. **15-32** Three types of veneers. **A,** Facial view of partial veneer that does not extend subgingivally or involve incisal angle. **B,** Full veneer with window preparation design that extends to gingival crest and terminates at the facioincisal angle. **C,** Full veneer with incisal-lapping preparation design extending subgingivally that includes all of incisal surface. (Note that subgingival extension is only indicated for preparation of darkly stained teeth and is not considered routine.) **D** to **F,** Cross-sections of the three types of veneers in **A** through **C.**

results in gingival irritation with accompanying hyperemia and bleeding caused by bulbous and impinging gingival contours. Second, the veneer is more likely to be dislodged when no tooth structure is removed before the etching and bonding procedures are done. If the veneer is lost, it can be replaced. However, the patient may live in constant fear that it will happen again, possibly creating an embarrassing situation.

The reversibility of these veneers may seem desirable and appealing to patients from a psychologic standpoint; however, few patients who elect to have veneers wish to return to the original condition. In addition, removing full veneers with no damage to the underlying unprepared tooth is exceedingly difficult, if not impossible. To achieve esthetic and physiologically sound results consistently, *an intraenamel preparation is usually indicated*. The only exception is in cases where the facial aspect of the tooth is significantly undercontoured because of severe abrasion or erosion. In these cases, mere roughening of the involved enamel and defining of the peripheral margins are indicated.

Intraenamel preparation (or the roughening of the surface in undercontoured areas) before placing a veneer is *strongly recommended* for the following reasons:

1. To provide space for opaque, bonding, or veneering materials for maximal esthetics without overcontouring
2. To remove the outer, fluoride-rich layer of enamel that may be more resistant to acid-etching

3. To create a rough surface for improved bonding
4. To establish a definite finish line

Establishing an intraenamel preparation with a definite finish line is of particular importance when placing indirectly fabricated veneers. Accurate positioning and seating of an indirectly made veneer are significantly enhanced if an intraenamel preparation is present.

Another controversy involves the *location of the gingival margin* of the veneer (see Fig. 15-32). Should it terminate short of the free gingival crest at the level of the gingival crest or apical of the gingival crest? The answer depends on the individual situation. *If the defect or discoloration does not extend subgingivally, then the margin of the veneer should not extend subgingivally.* The only logical reason for extending the margin subgingivally is if the area is carious or defective, warranting restoration, or if it involves significantly dark discoloration that presents a difficult esthetic problem. Clinicians should remember that *no restorative material is as good as normal tooth structure, and the gingival tissue is never as healthy when it is in contact with an artificial material.*

Two basic preparation designs exist for *full veneers:* (1) a *window preparation* and (2) an *incisal, lapping preparation* (see Fig. 15-32). A window preparation is recommended for most direct and indirect composite veneers. This intraenamel preparation design preserves the functional lingual and incisal surfaces of the maxillary anterior teeth, protecting the veneers from significant occlusal stress. A window preparation design also is recom-

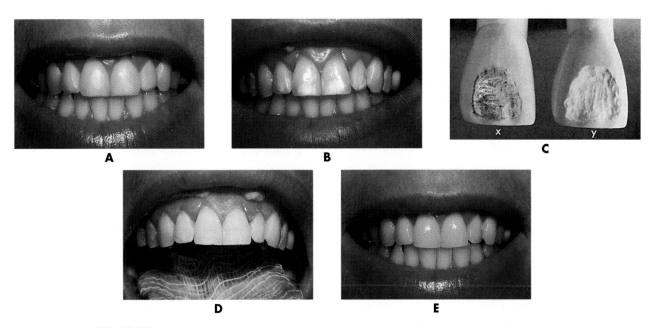

FIG. **15-33** Direct partial veneers. **A,** Patient with overcontoured direct full veneers. **B,** After removal of old veneer, localized white spots are evident. **C,** Models illustrate fault (*x*) and cavity preparation (*y*). The chamfered margins are irregular in outline. **D,** Intraenamel preparations for partial-veneer restorations. **E,** Conservative esthetic result of completed partial veneers.

mended for indirectly fabricated porcelain veneers if the patient exhibits significant occlusal function (as evidenced by wear facets on the lingual and incisal surfaces). This design is particularly useful in preparing maxillary canines in a patient with canine-guided lateral guidance. By using a window preparation, the functional surfaces are better preserved in enamel (see Fig. 15-43, *B* and *C*). This design reduces the potential for accelerated wear of the opposing tooth that could result if the functional path involved porcelain on the lingual and incisal surfaces, as with an incisal lapping design.

An incisal lapping preparation is indicated when the tooth being veneered needs lengthening or when an incisal defect warrants restoration. Additionally, the incisal lapping design is frequently used with porcelain veneers (see Fig. 15-43, *B* and *C*), because it not only facilitates accurate seating of the veneer upon cementation, but it also allows for improved esthetics along the incisal edge.

The preparation and restoration of a tooth with a veneer should be carried out in a manner that will provide optimal function, esthetics, retention, physiologic contours, and longevity. All of these objectives should be accomplished without compromising the strength of the remaining tooth structure. If the veneer becomes chipped, discolored, or worn, it can usually be repaired or replaced.

Darkly stained teeth, especially those discolored by tetracycline, are much more difficult to veneer with full veneers than teeth with generalized defects, but normal coloration. The difficulty is further compounded when the cervical areas are badly discolored

(see Fig. 15-35, *A*). Usually only the six maxillary anterior teeth require correction, because they are the most noticeable when a person smiles or talks. However, the maxillary first premolars (and to a lesser extent, second premolars) also are included if they, too, are noticeably apparent upon smiling.

Discolored mandibular anterior teeth are rarely indicated for veneers, because the facioincisal portions are thin and usually subject to biting forces and attrition. Therefore veneering lower teeth is discouraged if the teeth are in normal occlusal contact, because it is exceedingly difficult to achieve adequate reduction of the enamel to totally compensate for the thickness of the veneering material. Also, if porcelain veneers are placed, they may accelerate wear of the opposing maxillary teeth because of the abrasive nature of the porcelain. Fortunately, in most cases, the lower lip hides these teeth, and esthetics is not as much of a problem. Most patients are satisfied with the conservative approach of veneering only the maxillary anterior teeth.

DIRECT VENEER TECHNIQUES

Direct Partial Veneers. Small localized intrinsic discolorations or defects that are surrounded by healthy enamel are ideally treated with direct partial veneers (see Fig. 15-1, *B* and *C*). All too often, practitioners place full veneers when only partial veneers are indicated.

The four anterior teeth in Fig. 15-33, *A*, illustrate the clinical technique for placing partial veneers. These defects can be restored in one appointment with a light-cured composite. Preliminary steps include cleaning, shade selection, and isolation with cotton rolls or rubber

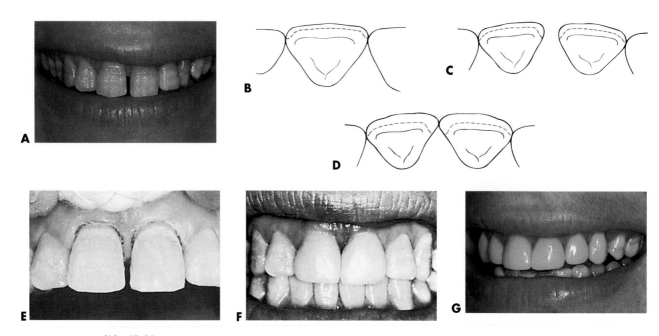

FIG. **15-34** Direct full veneers using light-cured composite. **A,** Enamel hypoplasia of maxillary anterior teeth. **B,** Drawing illustrates typical preparation of facial surface for direct full veneer. **C,** Preparation is extended onto mesial surface to provide for closure of diastema. **D,** Direct full veneers restore proximal contact. **E,** Etched preparations of central incisors. **F,** Veneers completed on maxillary central incisors. **G,** Treatment completed with placement of full veneers on remaining maxillary anterior teeth.

dam (see Chapters 10 and 11). Anesthesia is usually not required unless the defect is very deep, extending into dentin.

Fig. 15-33, *A,* shows four anterior teeth that received direct composite veneers with no enamel preparation for the restoration of developmental white spot lesions and the white spots that still show through the veneers (see Fig. 15-33, *A*). Upon removal of the defective veneers the localized white spots are evident (see Fig. 15-33, *B*). Models illustrating proper preparation are seen in Fig. 15-33, *C.* The outline form is dictated solely by the extent of the defect and should include all discolored areas. The clinician should use a coarse, elliptical or round diamond instrument with air-water coolant to prepare the tooth to a depth of about 0.5 to 0.75 mm (see Fig. 15-33, *D*). After preparation, etching, and restoration of the defective areas (as described in the following paragraph), the finished partial veneers are seen (see Fig. 15-33, *E*).

Usually it is not necessary to remove all of the discolored enamel in a pulpal direction. However, the preparation must be extended peripherally to sound, unaffected enamel. Use of an opaquing agent for masking dark stains is described later in the chapter. However, in this example no opaque is needed because the remaining stain is light and can be adequately hidden by the use of an appropriate composite restorative material. If the entire defect or stain is removed, then a microfilled composite is recommended for restoring the preparation. If, however, a residual lightly stained area or white

spot remains in enamel, an intrinsically less translucent composite can be used rather than extending the preparation into dentin to eliminate the defect. Most composites filled primarily with radiopaque fillers (e.g., barium glass), are more optically opaque with intrinsic masking qualities (in addition to being radiopaque). Use of these types of composites for the restoration of preparations with light, residual stains is most effective and conserves tooth structure.

Chapter 12 describes procedures used to insert and finish the composite restorations (see Fig. 15-33, *E*). In this example, all restorations are of a light-cured microfill composite.

Direct Full Veneers. Extensive enamel hypoplasia involving all of the maxillary anterior teeth was treated by direct full veneers (Fig. 15-34, *A*). A diastema also exists between the central incisors. The patient desired to have both the hypoplasia and the diastema corrected; examination indicated a good prognosis. A direct technique was used with a light-cured microfill composite. Although all six teeth can be restored at the same appointment, it may be less traumatic for the patient and the dentist if the veneers are accomplished in two appointments. In this example, the central incisors were completed during the first appointment and the lateral incisors and canines were completed during a second appointment.

After the teeth are cleaned and a shade selected, isolate the area with cotton rolls and retraction cords. Prepare both central incisors with a coarse, rounded end diamond instrument. The window preparation is typically made to a depth roughly equivalent to half the thickness of the facial enamel, ranging from approximately 0.5 to 0.75 mm midfacially and tapering down to a depth of about 0.2 to 0.5 mm along the gingival margin, depending on the thickness of enamel (see Fig. 15-32). A heavy chamfer at the level of the gingival crest provides a definite preparation margin for subsequent finishing procedures. The margins are not extended subgingivally because these areas are not defective. The preparation for a direct veneer normally is terminated just facial to the proximal contact, except in the area of a diastema (see Fig. 15-34, B). To correct the diastema, the preparations are extended from the facial onto the mesial surfaces, terminating at the mesiolingual line angles (see Fig. 15-34, C and D). (See Correction of Diastemas for more complete instructions regarding restoration of this area.) The incisal edges were not included in the preparations in this example, because no discoloration was involved. In addition, preservation of the incisal edges better protects the veneers from heavy functional forces as noted earlier for window preparations.

The teeth should be restored one at a time. After etching, rinsing, and drying procedures (see Fig. 15-34, E), apply and polymerize the resin-bonding agent. Place the composite on the tooth in increments, especially along the gingival margin, to reduce the effects of polymerization shrinkage. Place the composite in slight excess to allow some freedom in contouring. It is helpful to inspect the facial surface from an incisal view with a mirror to evaluate the contour before polymerization. After the first veneer is finished, restore the second tooth in a similar manner (see Fig. 15-34, F). In this case the remaining four anterior teeth are restored with direct composite veneers (see Fig. 15-34, G) at the second appointment.

As noted earlier, *tetracycline-stained teeth* are much more difficult to veneer, especially if dark banding occurs in the gingival third of the tooth (Fig. 15-35, A). In this example, time was a factor for the patient so all six maxillary anterior teeth were veneered in one appointment by using a *direct technique*. Veneer margins were placed subgingivally because of the dark discoloration in this area. This may indicate (along with other possible indications) local anesthesia. Shade selection is more difficult because all of the anterior teeth are discolored. The posterior teeth usually have a more normal shade and can often be used as guides. To obtain a natural appearance, it is helpful to make the cervical third of the teeth one shade darker than the middle or incisal areas. Additionally, the canines should be one shade darker than the premolars and incisors.

After cleaning and shade determination, mark the gingival tissue level before isolation on the facial surfaces of the teeth to be veneered by preparing a

shallow groove with a No. $\frac{1}{4}$ round, carbide bur (see Fig. 15-35, B). Because the cervical areas are badly discolored and the gingival tissue covers much of the clinical crown, isolation and tissue retraction is accomplished with a heavy rubber dam and No. 212 cervical retainer (see Fig. 15-35, C). (For details on application of the cervical retainer, see Chapters 10, 12, and 18.) Only one tooth is prepared and restored at a time. The outline form includes all of the facial surface, extending approximately 0.5 to 1 mm cervical to the mark indicating the gingival tissue level and into the facial embrasures (but not including the contact areas). The incisal margin includes the facioincisal angle in this instance because the discoloration involves this area. As much well-supported enamel as possible should always remain at the incisal ridge (i.e., surface) to preserve strength, wear resistance, and functional occlusion on enamel.

Prepare the tooth with a coarse, tapered, rounded end diamond instrument (see Fig. 15-35, D) by removing approximately one half of the enamel thickness (0.3 mm in the gingival region to 0.75 mm in the midfacial and incisal regions). Recall that the enamel is thinner in the cervical area. Some operators prefer to first make depth cuts to gauge the overall reduction. Although one preparation and restoration is completed at a time, if all veneers are to be completed in one appointment the proximofacial line angles of the adjacent teeth can be reduced along with the tooth being prepared. This procedure makes the operation more efficient and helps prevent damage later to the embrasure area of the restored tooth as the adjacent area is prepared.

After etching, rinsing, and drying (see Fig. 15-35, E), apply a thin layer of light-cured, resin-bonding agent to the etched enamel surface and lightly thin with a brush to remove any excess. Next, to mask the discolored area, apply a layer of resin-opaquing agent (see Fig. 15-35, F). Resin-opaquing agents should be applied in thin layers (usually two), each layer being cured because of the difficulty in light penetration through the opaque material. This will ensure complete polymerization of this intermediate layer. Care should be taken not to allow the opaque material to remain on the cavosurface margin, because it will appear as a definite opaque line along the margin of the final restoration. A stippled surface can be obtained by dabbing the partially cured opaque with the tip of a brush. This texturing will help reflect light rays in many directions outward through the veneer and result in a more natural appearance.

Now apply a gingival shade of composite with a hand instrument, starting with enough material to cover the gingival third of the tooth. An explorer tine, which first is touched to a sparing amount of bonding agent to prevent it from sticking to the composite, is used to adapt the composite to the margin. Excess composite should not be allowed to remain beyond the margin. The gingival shade of the composite is feathered out at the

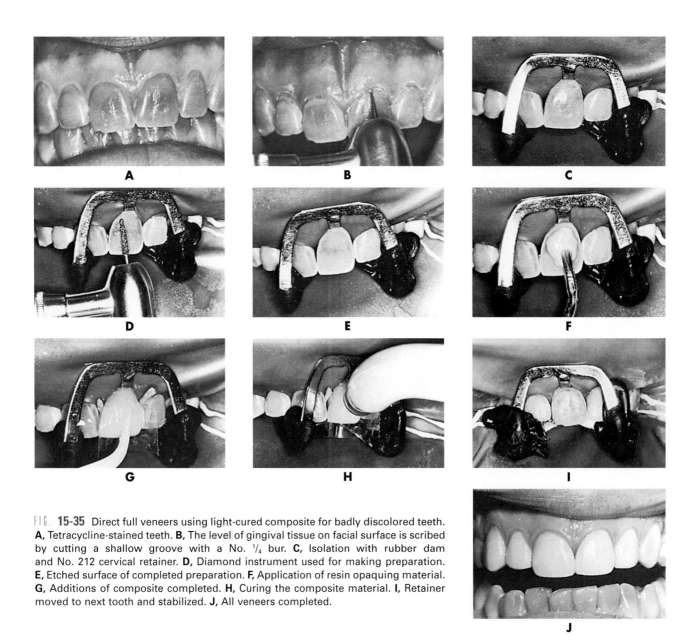

FIG. 15-35 Direct full veneers using light-cured composite for badly discolored teeth. A, Tetracycline-stained teeth. B, The level of gingival tissue on facial surface is scribed by cutting a shallow groove with a No. ¼ bur. C, Isolation with rubber dam and No. 212 cervical retainer. D, Diamond instrument used for making preparation. E, Etched surface of completed preparation. F, Application of resin opaquing material. G, Additions of composite completed. H, Curing the composite material. I, Retainer moved to next tooth and stabilized. J, All veneers completed.

middle third, smoothed (lightly stroking with a small disposable brush with fine bristles is helpful in smoothing the surface before curing), and cured.

Next, blend the incisal shade over the middle third and onto the incisal area to obtain proper contour and color (see Fig. 15-35, G). If the incisal area itself is very translucent, special translucent shades of composite are available from most manufacturers and are recommended for restoration of this area. In this clinical example the staining extended to the incisal edge, thus precluding significant translucency.

Evaluate the facial contour by inspecting from an incisal view with a mirror before the composite is polymerized (see Fig. 15-35, H). General contouring is done at this time, but final finishing is delayed until all six veneers are in place.

The No. 212 retainer is moved to the next tooth and stabilized with compound (see Fig. 15-35, I), and the steps for a direct veneer are repeated. This procedure is followed for each tooth until all veneers are placed, finished, and polished (see Fig. 15-35, J).

INDIRECT VENEER TECHNIQUES

Many dentists find that the preparation, placement, and finishing of several direct veneers at one time is too difficult, fatiguing, and time-consuming. Some patients become uncomfortable and restless during long appointments. In addition, veneer shades and contours can be better controlled when made outside of the mouth on a cast. For these reasons, indirect veneer techniques are usually preferable. Indirect veneers include those made of: (1) processed composite, (2) feldspathic porcelain, and (3) cast or pressed ceramic. Because of superior strength, durability, and esthetics, feldspathic porcelain is by far the most popular material for indirect veneering techniques used by dentists. Pressed ceramic veneers offer comparable qualities, but require exacting laboratory technique and a deeper tooth preparation depth; however, excellent laboratory support and the superb marginal fit of these veneers can minimize or eliminate this disadvantage.

Although two appointments are required for indirect veneers, chair time is saved because much of the work is done in the laboratory. Excellent results can be obtained when proper clinical evaluation and careful operating procedures are followed. Indirect veneers are attached to the enamel by acid-etching and bonding with either a light-cured, or dual-cured resin-bonding material.

Processed Composite Veneers. Composite veneers can be processed in a laboratory to achieve superior properties. Using intense light, heat, vacuum, pressure, or a combination of these, cured composites can be produced that possess improved physical and mechanical properties compared with traditional chairside composites. Additionally, indirectly fabricated composite veneers offer superior shading and characterizing potential and better control of facial contours.

Because their composition is similar to chairside composite, indirect composite veneers are capable of being bonded to the tooth with a resin-bonding medium. After acid-etching, a bonding agent is applied to the etched enamel as with any composite restoration. A fluid resin-bonding medium then is used to bond the veneer in place. A chemical bond is formed between the bonding agent and the bonding medium and, to a lesser extent, between the bonding medium and the processed composite veneer. Because laboratory processing results in a greater degree of polymerization, fewer bond sites remain in the processed composite for subsequent bonding to the bonding medium. Excellent mechanical retention occurs at the interface of the bonding medium and tooth from the roughened tooth surface resulting from preparation with a coarse diamond instrument and from tag formation into the etched enamel.

Although significant advantages exist over direct composite veneers, indirect veneers made of processed composites possess limited bond strength because of the reduced potential to form a chemical bond with the bonding medium (as noted earlier). Consequently it is necessary to provide additional micromechanical features through surface conditioning (acid-etching) or sandblasting to enhance retention.

Surface conditioning (i.e., acid-etching) with hydrofluoric acid of veneers made from a hybrid type of composite filled with barium glass and colloidal silica offers a significant improvement in bond strength.[43] Because this type of composite contains particles of barium glass, a relatively soft radiopaque filler, it can be sand-

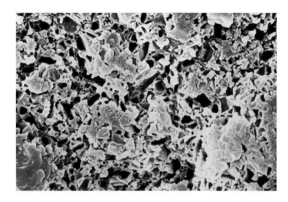

FIG. **15-36** Scanning electron micrograph (×5000) of sandblasted hybrid composite etched with mild concentration of hydrofluoric acid. *(Courtesy of Dr. James Hamilton.)*

blasted and etched in the laboratory with a mild concentration (i.e., 9% to 10%) of hydrofluoric acid to produce numerous areas of microscopic undercuts, similar to the phenomenon that occurs when enamel is etched (Fig. 15-36). By producing a surface capable of micromechanical bonding, *"etched composite"* veneers of this type can be strongly bonded to enamel without relying on significant chemical bonding. Most other types of processed composite veneers available today achieve enhanced bond strength from surface treatment with sandblasting alone.

Processed composite veneers are easily placed, finished, and polished. They also can be replaced or repaired easily with chairside composite (see Repairs of Veneers). For these reasons, indirect processed composite veneers are often recommended for placement in children and adolescents as interim restorations until the teeth have fully erupted and achieved their complete clinical crown length. At that time (i.e., 18 to 20 years of age), a more permanent alternative (e.g., porcelain or pressed ceramic veneers) can be pursued.

Indirect processed composite veneers also are indicated for placement in patients who exhibit significant wear of their anterior teeth caused by occlusal stress. Because of their somewhat lower cost, indirect processed composite veneers also offer an esthetic, affordable alternative to more costly porcelain or pressed ceramic types (when economics is the primary consideration). However, the patient must be told that processed composite veneers typically do not exhibit comparable clinical longevity.

The patient in Fig. 15-37, *A*, has six defective direct composite veneers that will be replaced with indirect processed composite veneers. Following shade selection, the teeth are isolated with bilaterally placed cotton rolls and gingival retraction cord . All existing defective Class III restorations or small carious lesions should be restored before preparation. *Multiple large existing restorations compromise the potential to bond the veneer to the tooth and may represent a contraindication.* Usually no

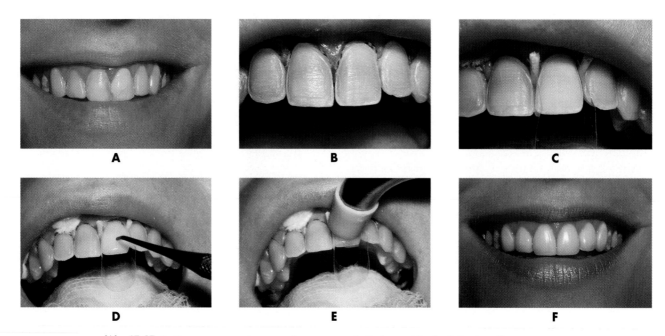

FIG. **15-37** Indirect processed composite veneers. **A,** Patient with six defective direct-composite veneers. **B,** Finished window preparations for indirect-processed composite veneers. **C,** Left central incisor isolated, etched, and ready for veneer bonding. **D,** Veneer is positioned and seated with blunt instrument or finger. **E,** Veneer-bonding medium is light-cured. **F,** Completed indirect-composite veneers.

anesthetic is required for intraenamel tooth preparations for veneers. In fact, the patient's response is important in judging preparation depth, especially in the gingival third of the tooth. If possible, the preparations should be restricted entirely to enamel.

A window preparation design (see Fig. 15-32, *E*) is recommended for most indirect processed composite veneers because of the limited bond strength of the composite veneer. An "incisal-lapping" design is used if the teeth require lengthening or if defects exist warranting involvement of the incisal edge (see Fig. 15-32, *F*).

The window preparation is made with a tapered, rounded end diamond instrument to a depth of approximately 0.5 to 0.75 mm midfacially, diminishing to a depth of 0.3 to 0.5 mm along the gingival margin, depending on enamel thickness. As noted earlier for direct composite veneers, the gingival margin should be positioned just at or slightly above the level of the gingival crest unless defects, caries, or dark discoloration warrant subgingival extension. Also, the interproximal margins should extend into the facial and gingival embrasures, without engaging an undercut, yet should be located just facial to the proximal contacts. The finished preparations are seen in Fig. 15-37, *B*.

Generally no temporary restorations are placed because the preparations are restricted to enamel. If a small amount of dentin is inadvertently exposed, a thin coat of a dentin-bonding agent or dentin desensitizer can be applied to the exposed dentin and cured to reduce the possibility of postoperative sensitivity. Patients always should be forewarned that the prepared teeth

will be slightly rough until the final veneer restorations are bonded.

An elastomeric impression is made of the preparations. If the gingival margins are well isolated and spaced from the retraction cord, the cord may be left in place during impression making. If, however, the margins are subgingival or close to the gingival tissue, better access for recording the gingival margin is afforded by cord removal just before injection of the impression material. It also is recommended that the lingual aspect of the gingival embrasures be blocked out with soft wax (see Fig. 15-43, *B*) if the gingival embrasures are open faciolingually. This step will prevent penetration and interlocking of the impression material through the gingival embrasure, which often results in torn impressions, especially along critical marginal areas.

A stone working cast is generated from the impression with individually removable dies to facilitate access to interproximal areas. Once the veneers are fabricated and returned, they should be closely inspected for fracture lines, chips along margins, or other significant defects that would preclude successful placement. Because the veneers are composed of composite, some intraoral recontouring is possible following bonding.

At the second appointment the teeth to be veneered are cleaned with a pumice slurry, the shade confirmed, and the operating site isolated. Frames are available that comfortably retract the lips for better access, if needed. Routine isolation is accomplished by the placement of cotton rolls and insertion of retraction cords. A 2 × 2 inch cotton gauze is placed across the back of the patient's mouth to protect against aspiration or swallowing of a veneer if inadvertently dropped (see Fig. 15-37, D).

The fit of each veneer is evaluated on the individual tooth and adjusted if necessary. All of the veneers should fit closely to the tooth at the gingival area. The veneers should be tried in place (both individually and collectively) to ensure the fit of adjacent seated veneers. Veneers should be tried in place only on *clean, dry teeth* to eliminate any potential for contamination. If accidental contamination occurs, the veneer should be thoroughly cleaned with alcohol or acid etchant, rinsed, and dried before bonding. On removal, each veneer is placed tooth side up (i.e., concave side facing upward) on an adhesive pad or palette. Some processed composites require that a priming agent be applied to the tooth side of the veneer according to the manufacturer's instructions. These priming agents are typically adhesion-promoting materials that increase the bond strength of the veneer to the resin-bonding medium. A thin layer of resin-bonding agent is applied (*but not cured*) to the tooth side of the veneer with a microbrush or small sponge. The veneers are stored under a jar lid or are placed in a container that is impervious to light to prevent premature curing of the bonding agent.

A light-cured, resin-bonding medium is recommended for bonding the veneer to the tooth. Shade selection of the bonding medium is determined once the fit of the individual veneers has been evaluated and confirmed. Shade selection is made by first placing a uniform layer of a selected shade of bonding medium, approximately 0.5 mm in thickness, on the tooth side of a single veneer. Typically, a central incisor veneer is used to facilitate shade determination of the bonding medium. The operatory light is turned away during shade assessment to prevent premature and inadvertent curing of the veneer to the tooth. The veneer is seated on a *clean, dry, unetched tooth,* the excess bonding medium removed with a brush, and the overall shade of the veneer evaluated. Following try-in, the veneer is quickly removed and stored under a jar lid or placed in a container that is impervious to light to prevent curing of the residual-bonding medium. If the shade of the bonding medium is determined to be appropriate, more of the same shade of bonding medium is added to the veneer just before bonding. If a different shade is deemed necessary, the existing shade is wiped from the inner aspect of the veneer with a disposable microbrush and a new shade of bonding medium is placed in the veneer. In the meantime, the assistant can remove residual-bonding medium of the previous shade from the tooth with a cotton pellet or brush. The veneer loaded with the new shade of resin-bonding medium is reseated and evaluated as previously described.

Water-soluble, try-in pastes that correspond to the same shades of bonding medium are also available with many veneer-bonding kits. These try-in pastes allow shade assessment without the concern for inadvertent premature curing of the bonding medium, because the try-in pastes are not capable of setting. After the try-in process with these try-in pastes, the veneers must be thoroughly cleaned according to the manufacturer's instructions to ensure that optimal bonding will occur. A light-cured or dual-cured bonding medium of the same shade is used for final cementation.

It should be emphasized that the inherent shade of the veneer, characterization, and internal opaquing must be accomplished during fabrication of the veneer itself. Some additional opaque can be incorporated into the resin-bonding medium at the time of bonding to achieve greater masking. Also, the overall shade of the veneer can be slightly modified by the shade of bonding medium selected. However, significant changes in shading or masking ability cannot be accomplished chairside.

The retraction cords are evaluated to ensure that they are adequately tucked into the gingival crevice. A technique for the individual placement of each veneer is recommended. The tooth used for try-in to assess shade of the bonding medium should be cleaned again with a slurry of pumice to remove any residual resin or try-in paste that may preclude proper acid-etching of the enamel.

Polyester strips are placed in the proximal areas of the first tooth to be restored. Wooden wedges can be used to secure the position of the strips, but care must be taken not to irritate the gingival papilla for risk of inducing hemorrhage. The acid etchant is artfully applied with a small microbrush, sponge, or syringe etchant applicator. Acid should not be allowed to flow onto the retraction cord or soft tissue. The prepared tooth (see Fig. 15-37, C) is ready for veneer bonding after acid-etching, rinsing, and drying. A thin layer of resin-bonding agent is applied to the etched enamel, lightly blown with air, *but not cured until placement of the veneer.* Premature curing of the bonding agent may preclude full seating of the veneer.

The selected shade of light-cured, resin-bonding medium is added to the tooth side of the veneer with enough material to cover the entire treated surface without entrapping air. The veneer is carefully placed on the appropriate tooth and lightly vibrated into place with a blunt instrument or light finger pressure (see Fig. 15-37, D). A microbrush is used to remove excess bonding medium. Proper seating of the veneer should be evaluated with a No. 2 explorer. With the veneer properly positioned and excess bonding medium removed, a visible light-curing unit is used to polymerize the material with a minimum exposure time of 40 to 60 seconds each from the facial and lingual directions for a total exposure of 80 to 120 seconds (see Fig. 15-37, E).

Excess of cured bonding resin remaining around the margins is best removed with a No. 12 surgical blade

FIG. **15-38 A** and **B,** Defective, discolored, direct-composite veneers are replaced with indirect composite veneers.

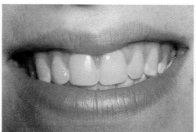
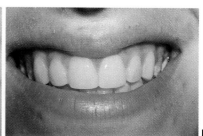

held in a Bard-Parker handle (see Fig. 15-40, *F*). Each veneer again should be tried in place immediately before bonding to ensure full seating in the presence of the already bonded adjacent veneer. New polyester strips are positioned for each tooth as the other veneers (one at a time) are placed in a similar manner.

Once the veneers are all bonded, only a minor amount of finishing is required at the marginal areas. Removal of the retraction cord at this time allows access and visibility for finishing gingival margins. This step is accomplished as previously described for composite restorations. Unwaxed floss always should be used to assess the final smoothness of interproximal areas. If incisal areas have been involved, protrusive excursions should be evaluated to ensure occlusal harmony in the restored areas. Patients also should be cautioned to avoid biting hard foods or objects to prevent fracturing the incisal edge, especially if an incisal-lapping design was used. The completed veneers (immediately after placement) are shown in Fig. 15-37, *F.* Another example of processed composite veneers is seen in Fig. 15-38.

Etched Porcelain Veneers. The most frequently used indirect veneer type is the etched porcelain (i.e., feldspathic) veneer. Porcelain veneers etched with hydrofluoric acid are capable of achieving high-bond strengths to the etched enamel via a resin-bonding medium[5,14,42] (This porcelain etching pattern can be seen in Fig. 15-39.) In addition to the high-bond strengths, etched porcelain veneers are highly esthetic, stain resistant, periodontally compatible, and appear to significantly outlast composite veneers. The incidence of cohesive fracture for etched porcelain veneers is much less than for direct or indirect composite veneers.

A patient has generalized discoloration of the anterior teeth and facial and incisal hypoplastic defects (Fig. 15-40, *A*). A midline diastema will be closed when porcelain veneers are placed. The procedures for preparation, impression, try-in, and cementation are the same as for indirect processed composite veneers, with a few exceptions. (See the previous section on indirect processed composite veneers for details of these basic techniques.)

Following cleaning, shade selection, and isolation of the teeth, the intraenamel preparations are made with a tapered, rounded end, diamond instrument. A hemipreparation, as shown on the maxillary left central in-

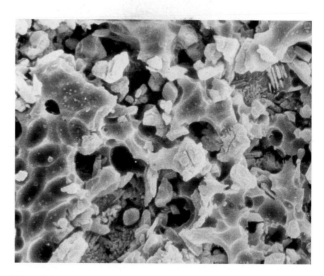

FIG. **15-39** Scanning electron micrograph (×1000) of feldspathic porcelain etched with hydrofluoric acid. *(Courtesy of Dr. Steven Bayne.)*

cisor (see Fig. 15-40, *B*) can be used to assess tooth reduction. Unlike with processed composite veneers, an incisal-lapping preparation design is generally used for porcelain veneers, especially if incisal defects warrant inclusion or the teeth need lengthening (see Fig. 15-32, *F*). As noted earlier, this preparation design facilitates seating of the veneer and enables the laboratory technician to produce a more esthetic incisal edge with the porcelain and resin margin located on the lingual surface. Because of the strength of the porcelain and excellent bond to enamel, incisal fractures are rarely encountered. Because of the presence of a midline diastema, the preparations on the mesials of both central incisors are extended to the mesiolingual line angles to allow subsequent restoration of the proximal contacts (see Fig. 15-34, *C* and *D*).

After the preparations are completed (see Fig. 15-40, *C*), an elastomeric impression is made. In most cases no temporary restorations are required, because the preparations are shallow and involve only the enamel. The patient should be instructed to avoid biting hard objects, keep the area clean with a soft bristled brush, and expect the possibility of some mild sensitivity to hot and cold.

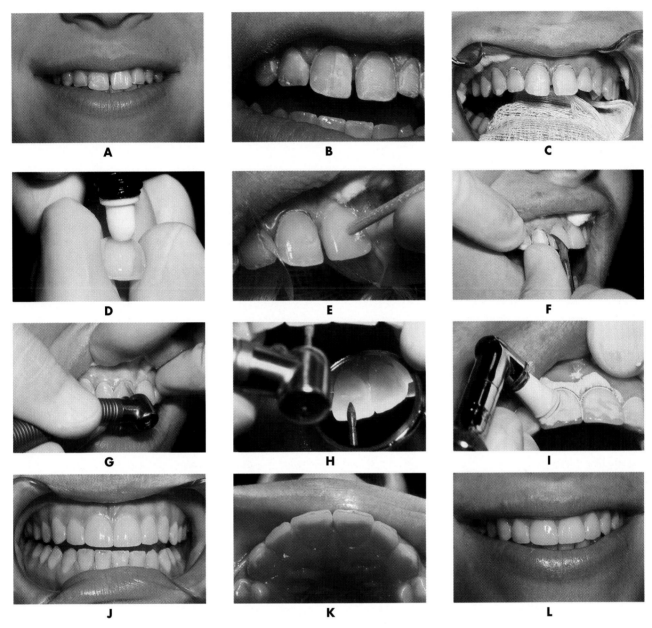

FIG. 15-40 Indirect etched porcelain veneers. **A,** Patient with generalized discoloration of the anterior teeth along with facial and incisal hypoplastic defects. **B,** A hemipreparation is often used to assess tooth reduction. **C,** Completed incisal-lapping veneer preparations. **D,** A thin layer of bonding medium is placed in the veneer. **E,** The etched porcelain veneer is carefully positioned and seated on the tooth. **F,** A No. 12 surgical blade in a Bard-Parker handle is ideal for removing excess cured bonding medium. **G,** A fine-diamond instrument is used to finish rough gingival margins. **H,** Lingual areas are best finished with an oval-shaped diamond instrument. **I,** A final surface luster is imparted through the use of porcelain-polishing paste. **J to L,** Completed etched porcelain veneers 18 months later.

Once fabricated by the laboratory, the porcelain veneers are returned to the dentist for cementation at the second appointment. The completed veneers must be inspected for cracks, overextended margins, and adequate internal etching (as evidenced by a frosted appearance). Marginal areas, in particular, should be inspected for proper etching so that an adequate seal will occur in these areas. Overextended marginal areas in-

terproximally may preclude full seating of adjacent veneers. These areas can be trimmed carefully with a micron-finishing diamond instrument or flexible abrasive disc. *However, unless severe or inaccessible, most minor overextensions should be trimmed only after bonding the veneer to the tooth because of the risk of fracturing the porcelain.*

After the prepared teeth are cleaned with a pumice slurry, rinsed, and dried, isolation is accomplished with

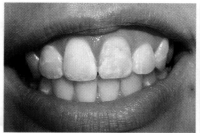
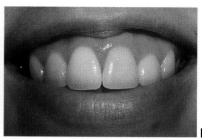

FIG. **15-41** **A** and **B**, Etched porcelain veneers. Generalized hypocalcification defects remaining after microabrasion are corrected with etched porcelain veneers.

a lip retractor (optional), cotton rolls, and retraction cords. Then the veneers are tried on the teeth to confirm proper contour and fit, and an appropriate shade of resin-bonding medium is selected. The only difference in this procedure for porcelain veneers from the composite veneers is the need to condition the internal surface of each veneer with a *silane primer* just before applying the resin-bonding agent. The silane acts as a *coupling agent*, forming a chemical bond between the porcelain and the resin.[3] It also improves wettability of the porcelain. The primary source of retention with porcelain veneers still remains the etched porcelain surface itself. Only a modest increase in bond strength results from silanation of the porcelain; however, it is recommended because it also may reduce marginal leakage and discoloration.

A technique is presented and recommended for applying the veneers *one at a time.* Polyester strips are placed interproximally to prevent inadvertent bonding to the adjacent tooth, followed by etching, rinsing, and drying procedures. It is recommended that the two central incisors be etched and their veneers bonded first, because of their critical importance esthetically. A resin-bonding agent is applied to the etched enamel and the tooth side of the silane-primed porcelain veneer. Next a thin layer (0.5 mm) of the selected shade of light-cured, resin-bonding medium is placed on the tooth side of the veneer, being careful not to entrap air (see Fig. 15-40, *D*). The first veneer is placed on the tooth and vibrated (carefully and lightly) into place with a blunt instrument or light finger pressure (see Fig. 15-40, *E*). The margins of the veneer are examined with a No. 2 explorer to verify accurate seating. Next, the excess resin-bonding medium is removed with a disposable microbrush, and the margins are once again evaluated before the veneer is exposed to the curing light. To ensure complete polymerization, the veneer should be cured for a minimum of 40 to 60 seconds each from facial and lingual directions for a total exposure time of 80 to 120 seconds. After positioning and bonding of the first veneer, the second veneer is positioned carefully and bonded in like manner, followed individually by the remaining veneers.

A No. 12 surgical blade in a Bard-Parker handle is ideal for removing excess cured resin-bonding medium remaining around the margins (see Fig. 15-40, *F*). Removal of the retraction cord at this time facilitates access and visibility to subgingival areas. If the marginal fit of the porcelain veneers is deemed acceptable and a favorable emergence angle exists, the marginal areas need only minimal finishing. This process is best accomplished with a bullet-shaped, 30-fluted carbide finishing bur (Midwest No. 9803 or Brasseler No. 7801) to remove any remaining excess resin-bonding medium.

If the porcelain margins are overextended beyond the cavosurface angles or the marginal areas are too bulbous, recontouring of these areas is required (especially along gingival margins) to ensure proper physiologic contours and gingival health. A fine diamond instrument is used to recontour these areas (see Fig. 15-40, *G*). Marginal areas should be confluent with surrounding unprepared tooth surfaces when assessed with a No. 2 explorer. Lingual areas are best finished with an oval-shaped diamond instrument (see Fig. 15-40, *H*). Because use of a diamond instrument breaks the glazed surface, a series of appropriate instruments is used to restore a smooth surface texture. First, a bullet-shaped, 30-fluted carbide finishing bur (Midwest No. 9803 or Brasseler No. 7801) is used to plane the porcelain surface and to remove the striations created by the diamond instruments. Studies show that the best results occur if the diamond instruments are used with air and water coolant, whereas the 30-fluted bur should be used dry.[26] Where access allows, the porcelain is smoothed and polished with a series of abrasive rubber, porcelain polishing cups and points (Brasseler, Dialite Porcelain Polishing Kit). Final surface luster is imparted through the use of a porcelain-polishing paste, applied either with a rubber prophy cup or a felt wheel (Fig. 15-40, *I*). This step is optional if a suitable polish has been attained with the polishing points and cups. The completed veneers are shown in Fig. 15-40, *J* to *L*. A similar example of a completed case using etched porcelain veneers is seen in Fig. 15-41.

Etched porcelain veneers also can be effectively used to restore malformed anterior teeth conservatively. Malformed lateral incisors are seen in Fig. 15-42, *A*. Incisal-lapping preparations that are extended well onto the lingual surface are used (see Fig. 15-42, *B*). The resulting restorations are virtually comparable to "three-quarter

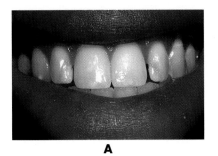
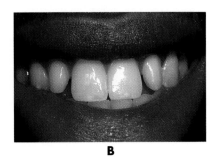
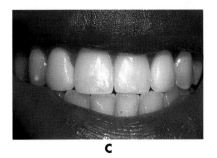

A   **B**   **C**

FIG. **15-42** Treatment of malformed teeth with porcelain veneer. **A,** Malformed lateral incisors. **B,** An incisal-lapping preparation much like a ¾ crown in enamel is used. **C,** Final esthetic results.

crowns" in porcelain. The final esthetic results are shown in Fig. 15-42, C. *Darkly discolored teeth* are more difficult to treat with porcelain veneers.

However, several modifications in the veneering technique can be used to enhance the final esthetic result. First, the most important difference in technique is that opaque porcelain is incorporated in the fabrication of the veneers to induce more inherent masking. If the veneers are not inherently opaque, little chance exists for adequate masking of a darkly stained tooth. Typically 5% to 15% opaque porcelain is required to achieve optimal masking. Exceeding 15% opaque porcelain dramatically reduces light penetration and results in a significant loss of esthetic vitality; the esthetic vitality or lifelike appearance of teeth depends on light penetration (see Translucency in the section on artistic elements). Second, a slightly deeper tooth preparation can be used to allow greater veneer thickness. However, the preparation should always be restricted to enamel to ensure optimal bonding of the veneer to the tooth. Even with improved dentin-bonding agents, the bonds to dentin are less predictable or durable than those to enamel because of the high variability and dynamic nature of dentin. Bonds to etched enamel are highly predictable and very durable.

Third, the laboratory can be instructed to use several coats of a die-spacing medium on the laboratory model to allow a slightly greater thickness of resin-bonding medium. The die-spacing medium must not be extended closer than 1 mm to the margins to ensure adequate positioning of the veneer to the preparation during try-in and bonding and to provide for a slight internal space. In a typical case, after preparation of the anterior teeth for etched porcelain veneers (Fig. 15-43, A), a window preparation design was used for the canines to preserve the functional occlusal path on tooth structure. An incisal-lapping preparation was used on the other teeth. An incisal view aptly illustrates the difference between the two designs (see Fig. 15-43, B). Soft wax is placed in the lingual embrasures to prevent interproximal tearing during impression-making procedures (see Fig. 15-43, B). Incisal and facial views of the completed veneers are seen in Fig. 15-43, C and D. A similar case of darkly discolored teeth showing prepared teeth and postoperative result is seen in Fig. 15-44, A and B.

Patients who possess darkly stained teeth always should be informed that although porcelain (or composite) veneers can result in improved esthetics, they may not entirely eliminate or mask very dark stains. Moreover, because of the limited thickness of the veneers and the absolute necessity of incorporating intrinsic opacity, the lifelike translucency or esthetic vitality of veneered teeth may never be comparable to that of natural, unaffected teeth (see Fig. 15-9, A and B). Full porcelain coverage with all-ceramic crowns may be indicated in some patients with severe discoloration because of the crown's greater capacity to restore esthetic vitality. Nonetheless, porcelain veneers are a viable option in most cases for the patient who desires esthetic improvement without significant tooth reduction.

Pressed Ceramic Veneers. Another esthetic alternative for veneering teeth is the use of pressed ceramics, such as IPS Empress. Unlike etched porcelain veneers that are fabricated by stacking and firing feldspathic porcelain, pressed ceramic veneers are literally cast using a lost wax technique. Excellent esthetics are possible using pressed ceramic materials for most cases involving mild-to-moderate discoloration. However, because of the more translucent nature of pressed ceramic veneers, *dark discolorations are best treated with etched porcelain veneers.* The clinical technique for placing pressed ceramic veneers, such as those made by IPS Empress, is not markedly different from that for feldspathic porcelain veneers (other than the need for a slightly greater tooth reduction depth).

The procedures for tooth preparation, try-in, and bonding of pressed veneers are the same as for etched porcelain veneers except that the marginal fit is often superior. For that reason, little marginal finishing is often necessary. Only the excess bonding medium needs to be removed. A typical case involving pressed ceramic veneers, showing before and after treatment views is seen in Fig. 15-45.

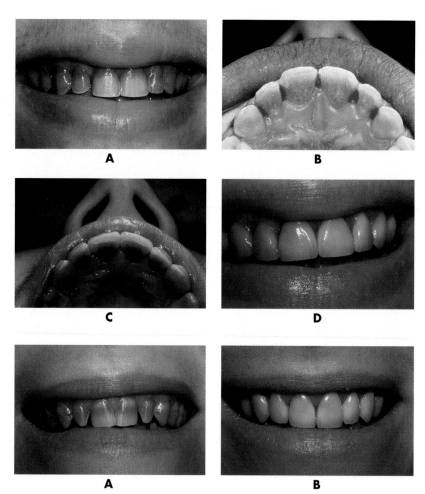

FIG. **15-43** Treatment of darkly discolored teeth with porcelain veneers. **A,** Tetracycline-stained anterior teeth (including first premolars) shown following preparation for etched porcelain veneers. **B,** Incisal view shows window preparation design on canines and incisal-lapping design on remaining prepared teeth. Soft wax is used to block out lingual embrasures to facilitate impression making. **C** and **D,** Incisal and facial views of completed etched porcelain veneers.

FIG. **15-44** Darkly stained teeth treated with porcelain veneers. Old, defective direct-composite veneers are seen. **A,** Before treatment. **B,** After.

VENEERS FOR METAL RESTORATIONS

Esthetic inserts (i.e., partial or full veneers) of a tooth-colored material can be placed on the facial surface of a tooth previously restored with a metal restoration. For new castings, plans are made at the time of tooth preparation and during laboratory development of the wax pattern to incorporate a *veneer into the cast restoration.* After such a casting has been cemented, the veneer can be inserted as described in the next section, except that the portion of mechanical retention of the veneer into the casting has been provided in the wax pattern stage.

Veneers for Existing Metal Restorations. Occasionally the facial portion of an existing metal restoration (amalgam or gold) is judged to be distracting (Fig. 15-46, *A*). A careful examination, including a radiograph, is required to determine that the existing restoration is sound before an esthetic correction is made. The size of the unesthetic area determines the extent of the preparation. Anesthesia is not usually required, because the preparation is in metal and enamel. Preliminary procedures consist of cleaning the area with pumice, selecting the shade, and isolating the site with a cotton roll. When the unesthetic metal extends subgingivally, the level of the gingival tissue is marked on the restoration

with a sharp explorer and a retraction cord is placed in the gingival crevice. Rubber dam isolation may be required in some instances.

A No. 2 carbide bur rotating at high speed with an air-water spray is used to remove the metal, starting at a point midway between the gingival and occlusal margins. The preparation is made perpendicular to the surface (a minimum of approximately 1 mm in depth), leaving a butt joint at the cavosurface margins. The 1-mm depth and butt joint should be maintained as the preparation is extended occlusally. All of the metal along the facial enamel is removed, and the preparation is extended into the facial and occlusal embrasures just enough for the veneer to hide the metal. *The contact areas on the proximal or occlusal surfaces must not be included in the preparation.* To complete the outline form the preparation is extended gingivally approximately 1 mm past the mark indicating the clinical level of the gingival tissue.

The final preparation should have the same features as those described for veneers in new cast restorations. Mechanical retention is placed in the gingival area with a No. $\frac{1}{4}$ carbide bur (using air coolant to enhance vision) 0.25 mm deep along the gingivoaxial and lin-

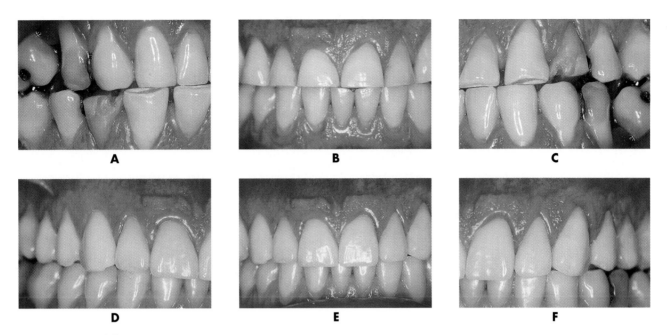

FIG. 15-45 Pressed ceramic veneers (IPS Empress). **A** through **C,** Before treatment, facial views. **D** through **F,** Esthetic result after completed veneers. *(Courtesy of Dr. Luiz N. Baratieri.)*

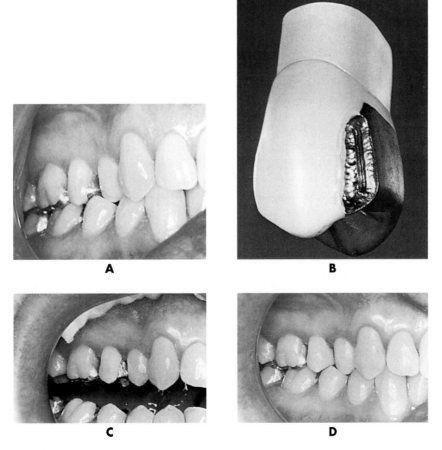

FIG. 15-46 Veneer for existing cast restoration. **A,** Mesiofacial portion of onlay is distracting to patient. **B,** Model of tooth and preparation. Note 90-degree cavosurface angle and retention prepared in gold and cavosurface bevel in enamel. **C,** Clinical preparation ready for composite resin. **D,** Completed restoration.

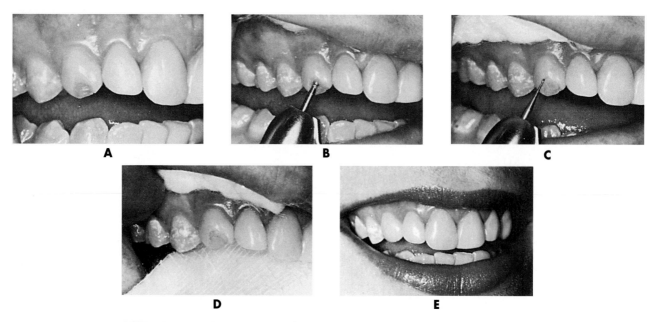

FIG. **15-47** Repairing veneer. **A,** Fractured veneer on maxillary canine. **B,** Preparation with round-diamond instrument. **C,** Undercuts placed in existing veneer with a No. ¼ bur. **D,** Completed preparation is shown isolated and etched. **E,** Veneer restored to original color and contour.

guoaxial angles. Retention and esthetics are enhanced by beveling the enamel cavosurface margin (approximately 0.5 mm wide) with the coarse, flame-shaped diamond instrument oriented at 45 degrees to the external tooth surface (see Fig. 15-46, *B*). After it is etched, rinsed, and dried, the preparation is complete (see Fig. 15-46, *C*). Adhesive resin liners containing 4-methyloxy ethyl trimellitic anhydride (4-META), capable of bonding composite to metal, also may be used but are quite technique sensitive.[8] Manufacturers' instructions should be followed explicitly to ensure optimal results with these materials. The composite material is inserted and finished in the usual manner (see Fig. 15-46, *D*).

REPAIRS OF VENEERS

Failures of esthetic veneers occur because of breakage, discoloration, or wear. Consideration should be given to conservative repairs of veneers if examination reveals that the remaining tooth and restoration are sound. It is not always necessary to remove all of the old restoration. The material most commonly used for making repairs is light-cured composite.

Veneers on Tooth Structure. Small chipped areas on veneers can often be corrected by recontouring and polishing. When a sizable area is broken, it can usually be repaired if the remaining portion is sound (Fig. 15-47, *A*).

For *direct composite veneers,* repairs ideally should be made with the same material that was used originally. After cleaning the area and selecting the shade, the operator should roughen the damaged surface of the veneer or tooth or both with a coarse, tapered, rounded end diamond instrument to form a chamfered cavosur-

face margin (see Fig. 15-47, *B*). Roughening with microetching (i.e., sandblasting) is also effective. For more positive retention, mechanical locks may be placed in the remaining composite material with a small, round bur (see Fig. 15-47, *C*). Acid etchant is applied to clean the prepared area and etch any exposed enamel that is then rinsed and dried (see Fig. 15-47, *D*). Next, a resin-bonding agent is applied to the preparation (i.e., existing composite and enamel) and polymerized. Composite is then added, cured, and finished in the usual manner (see Fig. 15-47, *E*).

Indirect processed composite veneers are repaired in a similar manner. However, to repair *porcelain veneers,* a mild hydrofluoric acid preparation, suitable for intraoral use, must be used to etch the fractured porcelain. Hydrofluoric acid gels are available in approximately 10% buffered concentrations that are intended for intraoral porcelain repairs. Although caution still must be taken when using hydrofluoric acid gels intraorally, the lower acid concentration allows for relatively safe intraoral use. Full-strength hydrofluoric acid should *never* be used intraorally for etching porcelain. Isolation of the porcelain veneer to be repaired should be accomplished with a rubber dam to protect the gingival tissues from the irritating effects of the hydrofluoric acid. The manufacturer's instructions must be followed regarding application time of the hydrofluoric acid gel to ensure optimal porcelain etching. A lightly frosted appearance, similar to that of etched enamel, should be seen if the porcelain has been properly etched. A *silane coupling agent* may be applied to the etched porcelain surface before the resin-bonding agent is applied. Composite ma-

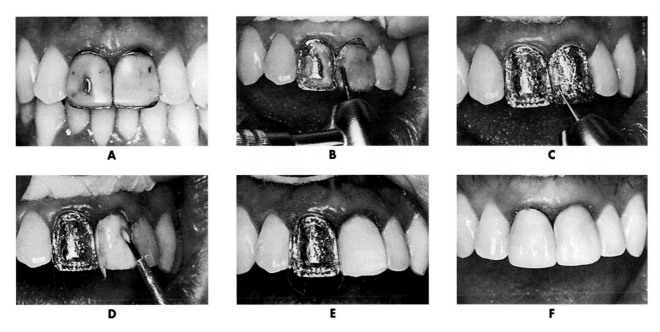

FIG. **15-48** Replacing faulty veneers in metal restorations with light-cured composite veneers. **A,** Acrylic resin veneers stained and worn after 18 years of service. **B,** Removal of existing veneers with a carbide bur. **C,** Mechanical retention is placed in metal with a No. 33½ bur. **D,** Masking agent (opaquing resin) is needed to cover metal surface. This material also may provide metal adhesion. **E,** Composite material is added and cured in the first preparation. The same steps are repeated for second veneer. **F,** Both veneers completed.

terial is then added, cured, and finished in the usual manner. Large fractures are best treated by replacing the entire porcelain veneer.

Faulty Veneers in Metal Restorations. Fig. 15-48, *A,* illustrates two faulty acrylic resin veneers on gold crowns that need replacing after 18 years because of wear and discoloration. The teeth are cleaned with a slurry of pumice and the shade selected before isolation by cotton rolls and retraction cords. With superficial wear or staining, part of the old restoration (silicate cement, acrylic, or composite) can be left to achieve some masking of the underlying metal. In this example, all of the old resin material is removed with an appropriate instrument, such as a No. 1558 carbide metal cutting bur (see Fig. 15-48, *B*). Both preparations are accomplished together. The outline of each preparation is extended gingivally by removing some of the gold. The operator should try to create a chamfered finish line. Retention is placed with a No. 33½ carbide bur in selected areas in the metal along the line angles approximately 0.25 mm deep (see Fig. 15-48, *C*). If available, a chairside air abrasion device, such as the Microetcher (Danville Engineering) unit, can be used to sandblast the preparation to enhance micromechanical retention. If not, the preparation can be roughened internally with a course diamond to enhance retention.

Although the preparations are done simultaneously, it is usually better to place the veneers one at a time. A light-cured composite is recommended because of the extended working time. Polyester strips are placed between the proximal surfaces. The preparation is cleaned with acid etchant for 30 seconds, then rinsed and dried to remove debris and obtain a clean, dry surface. In this instance, the acid is used only to clean the surface, not to etch the metal. Wedges placed in the gingival embrasure may help to establish proper contour of the matrix. A masking material (opaquing resin) is artfully placed with a small brush over the metal areas of the preparation by applying and curing successive thin layers (see Fig. 15-48, *D*). Adhesive resin liners containing 4-META (or other resin monomers capable of bonding to metal) also may be used to achieve additional retention and some masking. These materials should be placed directly over the prepared metal surface. Manufacturers' instructions should be followed closely to ensure optimal results with these materials because they are quite sensitive to proper technique.

Next, a small amount of composite material (i.e., gingival shade) is placed at the cervical area with a hand instrument, adapted with the tine of a No. 2 explorer, and cured with visible light. Now material of the preselected lighter shade is added to restore the middle and incisal portions; a small brush is helpful in smoothing the surface and obtaining the final contour before curing. Finishing is delayed except for removing any excess contour at the mesiofacial embrasure (see Fig. 15-48, *E*).

Evaluation of the width of the teeth can be achieved with a Boley gauge or another appropriate caliper. The second preparation is abraded, cleaned, and dried before the opaque or adhesive liner is added. Composite material is inserted and cured as described for the first veneer. The retraction cords are removed, and both restorations are finished together to obtain symmetric contours (see Fig. 15-48, *F*).

ACID-ETCHED, RESIN-BONDED SPLINTS

There are many causes for mobility of teeth: traumatic injury to the face, advanced periodontal disease, habits such as thumb sucking and tongue thrusting, and malocclusion. In addition, teeth often need stabilization and retention after orthodontic treatment. In the past, clinical procedures for the stabilization of teeth either involved extensive loss of tooth structure or were poor in appearance. A conservative and esthetic alternative has been made possible by using acid-etched, resin-bonded splints.

Certain criteria must be met when mobile teeth are splinted. Occlusal adjustment may be necessary initially. The splint should have a hygienic design so that the patient is able to maintain good oral hygiene. It also should allow further diagnostic procedures and treatment, if necessary. The acid-etched, resin-bonded splinting tech-

nique satisfies these criteria. Light-cured composites are recommended for splinting, because they afford extended working time for placement and contouring.

PERIODONTALLY INVOLVED TEETH

Loss of bone support allows movement of teeth, resulting in increased irritation to the supporting tissues and possible malpositioning of the teeth. Stabilizing mobile teeth is a valuable treatment aid before, during, and after periodontal therapy. Splinting the teeth aids in occlusal adjustment and tissue healing, thus allowing better evaluation of the progression and prognosis of treatment.

A resin-bonded splint via the acid-etch technique is a conservative and effective method of protecting the teeth from further injury by stabilizing them in a favorable occlusal relationship. If the periodontal problem is complicated by missing teeth, a bridge incorporating a splint design is indicated (see *Conservative Bridges*).

Techniques for Splinting Anterior Teeth. In short span segments subject to minimal occlusal forces, a relatively simple technique can be used for splinting periodontally involved teeth. Fig. 15-49, *A*, illustrates a maxillary lateral incisor that remains mobile because of

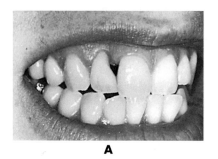 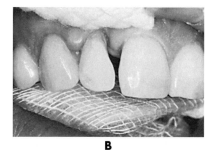 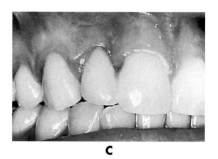

| A | B | C |

FIG. 15-49 Splinting and recontouring a mobile tooth using a light-cured composite. **A,** Maxillary right lateral incisor is mobile from lack of bone support. **B,** Preparations completed and etched. **C,** Splinted and recontoured tooth after 4 years.

FIG. 15-50 Splinting maxillary anterior teeth with composite only. **A,** All maxillary incisors are loose and need splinting. **B,** Preparation consists of roughening proximal surfaces and creating slight diastemas to provide bulk to the connector areas of the composite splint. **C,** Splint contoured and finished. **D,** Teeth and splint remain stable at 3-year recall.

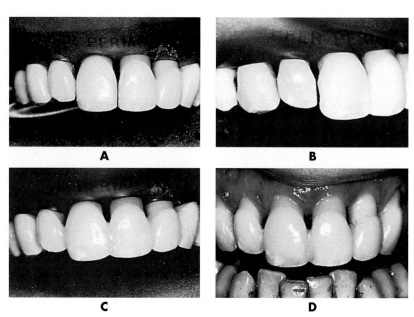

insufficient bone support even after occlusal adjustment and elimination of a periodontal pocket. Esthetic recontouring with composite augmentation can be accomplished along with the splinting procedure.

Anesthesia is generally not required for a splinting procedure when enamel covers the clinical crown. However, when root surfaces are exposed and extreme sensitivity exists, local anesthesia is necessary. The teeth are cleaned with a pumice slurry, and the shade of light-cured composite is selected. A cotton roll and retraction cords are used for isolation in this instance.

With a coarse, flame-shaped diamond instrument, the enamel on both teeth at the proximal contact area is reduced to produce an interdental space approximately 1 mm wide. This amount of space will enhance the strength of the splint by providing more bulk of composite material in the connector between the teeth. Other enamel areas of the tooth or teeth that need more contour are prepared by roughening the surface with a coarse diamond instrument. Where no enamel is present, such as on the root surface, a dentin-bonding agent is used following the manufacturer's instructions. Optionally, a mechanical lock is prepared with a No. $\frac{1}{4}$ round bur in the dentin at the gingivoaxial line angle of the boxlike preparation. After the prepared enamel surfaces are acid-etched, rinsed, and dried, a lightly frosted appearance should be observed (see Fig. 15-49, *B*).

The enamel- and dentin-bonding agent is applied, lightly blown with air, and polymerized. A hand instrument is used to place a small amount of composite material in the gingival area. Additional shaping with a No. 2 explorer will reduce the amount of finishing necessary later. It is helpful to add and cure the composite in small increments, building from the gingival toward the incisal aspect. Finishing is accomplished with round and flame-shaped carbide burs, fine diamonds, and polishing discs and points. The retraction cord is removed, and the occlusion is evaluated to assess centric contacts and functional movements. Instructions on brushing and flossing are reviewed with the patient. Results at 4 years are illustrated in Fig. 15-49, *C*.

Another indication for splinting periodontally involved teeth is illustrated in Fig. 15-50, *A*. All of the maxillary incisors are mobile from lack of periodontal support. Typically, the incisors are weaker than the canines because of the difference in root length. To stabilize the incisors, a composite splint must include all of the maxillary anterior teeth. The same procedures are followed as before, except that a rubber dam is used to isolate the teeth. After etching, rinsing, and drying procedures (see Fig. 15-50, *B*), a light-cured composite is inserted, polymerized, and finished (see Fig. 15-50, *C*). The completed splint is shown after 3 years of service (see Fig. 15-50, *D*).

Splinting also can be used when the mandibular incisors are mobile from severe bone loss. The same general steps are followed as with the maxillary teeth. However, if further reinforcement is deemed necessary, a stainless steel mesh, such as Splint-Grid (Ellman International Mfg., Hewlett, NY 11557), or a plasma-coated woven polyethylene strip, such as Ribbond (Ribbond Inc., Seattle, WA 98101) can be used to strengthen the splint (Figs. 15-51 and 15-52). Once the interproximal connectors are completed, the lingual surfaces are roughened and acid-etched. Bonding agent is applied and cured; a small amount of composite is placed onto the lingual surfaces (but not cured) to receive the auxiliary splinting strip. An appropriate length of splinting material (wire mesh or polyethylene-coated woven fabric) is cut and pressed into the uncured composite. Once adapted to the lingual surfaces, the composite is cured to hold the strip in place. Additional composite is used

FIG. **15-51** Periodontal splint of mobile mandibular incisors reinforced with wire mesh (Splint-Grid, Ellman International Mfg., Hwelett, NY 11557). **A,** Mobile periodontally involved teeth before treatment. **B,** Teeth isolated with rubber dam. **C,** Lingual view of completed splint. **D,** Facial view of splint after treatment.

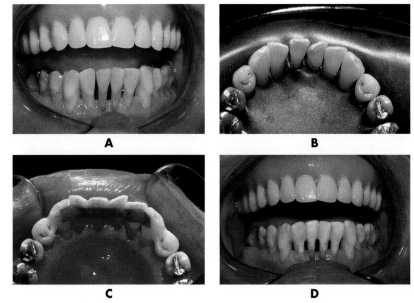

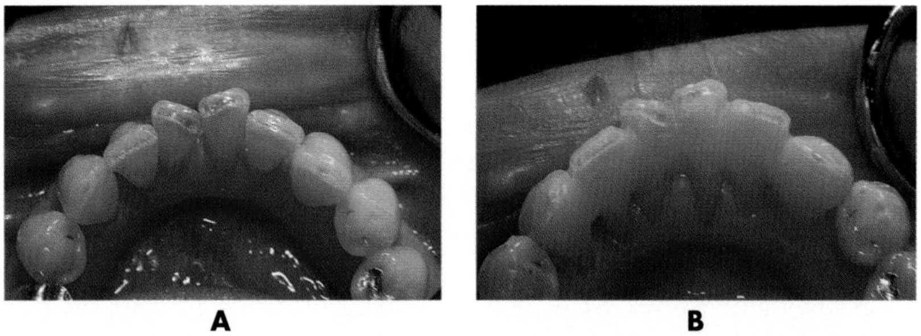

FIG. 15-52 Splinting of mobile mandibular incisors reinforced with a plasma-coated, polyethylene-woven strip (Ribbond, Ribbond Inc., Seattle, WA 98101). **A,** Mobile periodontally involved mandibular teeth before splinting. **B,** Lingual view of completed splint.

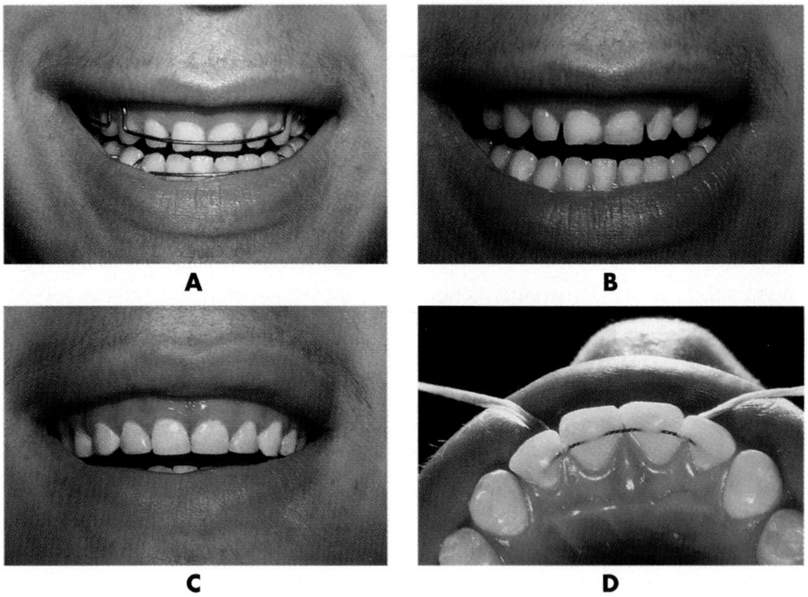

FIG. 15-53 Stabilizing teeth after orthodontic treatment. **A,** Patient with existing removable retainer. **B,** Residual spaces resulting from undersized teeth. **C,** Closure of spaces with composite additions is completed. **D,** Orthodontic wire is held in position with dental tape and bonded to place with composite.

to completely overlay the reinforcing material. Care must be taken to cover the wire mesh completely with composite to avoid rough, irritating edges. After finishing procedures, the rubber dam is removed and the occlusion is evaluated.

STABILIZATION OF TEETH AFTER ORTHODONTIC TREATMENT

After orthodontic treatment, teeth may require stabilization using either fixed or removable appliances. The latter method allows continued minor movements for final positioning of the teeth. Once this position is reached it is better to stabilize the teeth with a fixed retainer. Removable retainers tend to irritate the soft tissue. Also they may be damaged, lost, or not worn, which usually allows undesired movement of the teeth.

Fig. 15-53, *A,* shows a patient with a removable orthodontic retainer. Optimal positioning of the teeth has been achieved by orthodontic movement; however, stabilization of the teeth is required, and the unattractive spaces caused by undersized maxillary teeth need to be closed (see Fig. 15-53, *B*). A carefully planned appointment is required to accomplish the following: (1) remove any fixed orthodontic appliance, (2) add composite to close the diastemas, and (3) stabilize the teeth with a twisted stainless steel wire and composite.

Technique. After the orthodontic appliance is removed and routine procedures followed for closing the diastemas (see Fig. 15-53, *C*), the occlusion is carefully examined to determine the best position for locating the twisted wire, because it will be placed only on the lingual surfaces. A sufficient length of twisted stainless steel wire (i.e., 0.0175 inch [0.45 mm] in diameter) is adapted to the lingual surface of the anterior teeth. A stone cast is helpful for adapting the wire. The wire must rest against the lingual surfaces passively without tension or interference with the occlusion. In the mouth, waxed dental tape is used to position the wire against the teeth and hold it in place while occlusal excursions are evaluated. The wire will be attached only to the lingual fossa of each tooth. After the position of the wire has been determined it is removed, and the enamel in the fossae only (not the marginal ridges or embrasures) is etched, rinsed, and dried.

A light-cured composite is best used for attaching the fixed wire splint. The wire is repositioned and held in place with dental tape, while a sparing amount of resin-bonding agent is applied and lightly blown with air. After polymerization of the bonding agent, a small amount of composite material is placed to encompass the wire in each fossa and bond it to the enamel. The operator must be careful not to involve the proximal

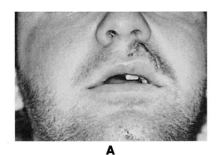 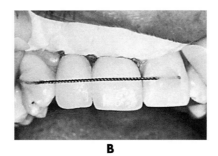 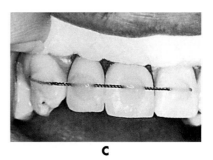

A **B** **C**

FIG. **15-54** Splinting avulsed teeth. **A,** Patient with traumatically avulsed maxillary right incisors. **B,** Orthodontic wire is positioned and bonded to adjacent uninvolved teeth with composite. **C,** Completed splint stabilizes repositioned incisors.

surfaces (see Fig. 15-53, *D*). After polymerization of the composite, the occlusion is evaluated and adjusted as needed for proper centric contacts and functional movements.

This unique splint allows some physiologic movement of the teeth, yet it holds them in the correct position. The splint should remain in place for at least 6 months to ensure stabilization. Longer retention may be necessary, depending on the individual situation and recommendations of the orthodontist.

AVULSED OR PARTIALLY AVULSED TEETH

Facial injuries often involve the hard and soft tissues of the mouth. The damage may range from lacerations of the soft tissue to fractures of the teeth and alveolar bone. There can be partial or complete avulsion of teeth. Maxillary central incisors are involved more often than other teeth. A thorough clinical examination of soft tissue, lips, tongue, and cheeks should be made for lacerations and embedded tooth fragments and debris. Radiographic examination is necessary to diagnose deeply embedded fragments or root fractures.

Treatment of soft-tissue lacerations should include lavage, conservative débridement, and suturing. Consultation with or referral to an oral surgeon may be necessary. A partially avulsed tooth is repositioned digitally and may or may not need splinting. *Traumatically avulsed teeth that are reimplanted immediately or within 30 minutes have a good prognosis for being retained.*[2,38] After 30 minutes the rate of success drops rapidly. Therefore the avulsed tooth should be repositioned as soon as possible. In the interim it should be placed in a moist environment, such as saliva (i.e., held in the cheek or under the tongue), milk, saline, or wet towel. The replacement of avulsed teeth has immediate psychologic value and maintains the natural space in the event that a fixed prosthesis is required later.

Technique. The maxillary right incisors that were completely avulsed in an accident (Fig. 15-54, *A*) are repositioned immediately. After the teeth are repositioned, radiographs reveal that no other complications exist. Isolation with cotton rolls or gauze is preferred to

use of a rubber dam, which could cause malpositioning of the loose teeth. The occlusion should be evaluated to ensure that the teeth are properly positioned.

The facial surfaces of the crowns are quickly cleaned with hydrogen peroxide, rinsed, and dried by blotting with a gauze or cotton roll or by lightly blowing with air. The dentist should avoid blowing air into areas of avulsion or deep wounds to prevent the possibility of air emboli. If a crown is fractured, any deeply exposed dentin should be covered with calcium hydroxide to protect the pulp. A *twisted orthodontic wire* (0.0195 inch [0.49 mm]) must be long enough to cover the facial (or lingual) surfaces of enough teeth to stabilize the loose teeth. The wire is adapted and the ends rounded to prevent irritation to the soft tissue. In an emergency a disinfected paper clip can be used as a temporary splint.

No preparation of the enamel surface is necessary other than that provided by acid-etching the enamel. The middle third of the facial surfaces are etched, rinsed, and dried of all visible moisture. Again, drying should be accomplished by blotting with a gauze or cotton roll and a light stream of air. A self-cured or light-cured composite may be used. The wire is positioned and held lightly in place, while the ends are attached with the composite material (see Fig. 15-54, *B*). Light pressure is applied to the repositioned teeth as the facial surfaces are bonded to the wire in succession (see Fig. 15-54, *C*). Care is exercised not to allow the composite to flow into the proximal areas. Once the teeth are stabilized, any fractured areas can be conservatively repaired by the acid-etch, resin-bond technique. Finishing is accomplished by a flame-shaped, carbide finishing bur and abrasive discs. The occlusion is evaluated carefully to ensure that no premature contacts exist.

The patient is advised to gently care for the involved teeth. Antibiotic therapy may be required if the alveolar bone is fractured or significant soft-tissue damage has occurred. Tetanus shots or boosters are advised if indicated by the nature of the accident; the patient's physician should be contacted regarding this need. Appointments are made for follow-up examinations on a weekly basis for the first month. The patient is alerted to the symptoms of pulpal necrosis and advised to call if a problem develops. If a root canal therapy is required, it is better accomplished with the splint in position.

Removal of the splint is accomplished in 4 to 8 weeks, provided recall visits have shown normal pulp test results and the teeth are asymptomatic. The wire is sectioned, and the resin material is removed with a flame-shaped, carbide finishing bur at high speed with air-water spray and a light, intermittent application. Abrasive discs are used to polish the teeth to a high luster.

CONSERVATIVE BRIDGES

In selected cases, conservative bridges can be made by acid-etching enamel and bonding a pontic to the adjacent natural teeth. These conservative bridges are classified according to the type of pontic: (1) natural tooth pontic; (2) denture tooth pontic; (3) pontic, either of porcelain-fused-to-metal pontic or all-metal pontic with metal retainers; and (4) all-porcelain pontic. Although the four types differ in the degree of permanency, they share a major advantage—conservation of natural tooth structure. In addition, they can be viable alternatives to conventional fixed bridges in circumstances where age, expense, or clinical impracticality are considerations.

It should be noted that because of the conservative preparation and bonded nature of all of these bridge types, *retention is never as strong as for a conventional bridge.* As part of informed consent, patients should be told of the potential, although remote, for swallowing or aspirating bonded bridges that are dislodged. Furthermore, to reduce the risk of dislodgement, patients should be cautioned not to bite hard foods or objects with bonded bridge pontics.

The ideal site for a conservative bridge is where the edentulous space is no wider than one or two teeth. Other considerations include bite relation, oral hygiene, periodontal condition, and extent of caries, defects, and restorations in the abutment teeth. Conservative bridges are especially indicated for young patients, because the teeth usually have large pulp chambers and short clinical crowns. Many older patients with gingival recession and mobile teeth are prime candidates because splinting can be incorporated with the bridge. More specific indications and clinical procedures for each of the four types of bridges are presented in the following sections.

NATURAL TOOTH PONTIC

The crowns of natural teeth (primarily incisors) often can be used as acid-etched, resin-bonded pontics. Considerations for this type of treatment occur when: (1) periodontally involved teeth warrant extraction, (2) teeth have fractured roots, (3) teeth are unsuccessfully reimplanted after avulsion, and (4) root canal treatment has been unsuccessful. However lost, the immediate replacement of a natural anterior tooth has great psychologic value for most patients, although the procedure may be temporary. Natural tooth pontics also can be placed as interim restorations until an extraction site heals if conditions require a conventional bridge or an implant.

Certain prerequisites must exist to ensure a successful result: (1) the extracted tooth and abutments must be in reasonably good condition, especially the pontic, because it may become brittle and more susceptible to fracture; (2) the abutment teeth should be fairly stable; and (3) the tooth to be replaced because a pontic must not participate in heavy centric or functional occlusion. Because of this third restriction, canines and posterior teeth are not usually good candidates for this procedure. If the adjacent teeth are mobile, it is frequently necessary to secure them by splinting with composite (see Acid-Etched, Resin-Bonded Splints).

Technique. A maxillary right central incisor must be extracted for periodontal reasons (Fig. 15-55, *A* and *B*). Before the tooth is extracted, a small, round bur is used to place a shallow identifying mark on the facial surface to indicate the level of the gingival crest. Following extraction, a 2 × 2 inch (5 × 5 cm) sponge is held in the space with pressure for hemorrhage control.

By using a separating disc or a diamond instrument, the extracted tooth is transversely cut a few millimeters apical to the identification mark. When pontic length is determined, shrinkage of the healing tissue underlying the pontic tip must be anticipated. The root end is discarded.

If the pulp canal and chamber have completely calcified, the next procedure is shaping and polishing the apical end of the natural tooth pontic as described in the following paragraphs. If the chamber is calcified as disclosed on the radiograph and the canal is nearly calcified, the canal is opened from the apical end by using a small round bur or diamond to the extent of the canal. The operator should be as conservative of tooth structure as possible, yet provide access for subsequent injection of composite material to fill the canal. A large chamber and canal are instrumented and débrided using conventional endodontic procedures with access from the apical end (see Fig. 15-55, *C*). Access is provided for subsequent injection of composite. Removal of the pulpal tissue in this manner prevents possible later discoloration of the tooth caused by degeneration products. Traditional lingual access for instrumentation is avoided to prevent weakening the pontic. Following these procedures the canal (and chamber, if present) is filled and closed with a self- or light-cured composite. Light-cured materials must be placed incrementally to ensure complete polymerization.

After the composite has been polymerized, the apical end is contoured to produce a bullet-shaped ovate design (see Fig. 15-55, *C*). This design provides adaptation of the pontic tip to the residual ridge, yet it allows the tissue side of the pontic tip to be cleaned with dental

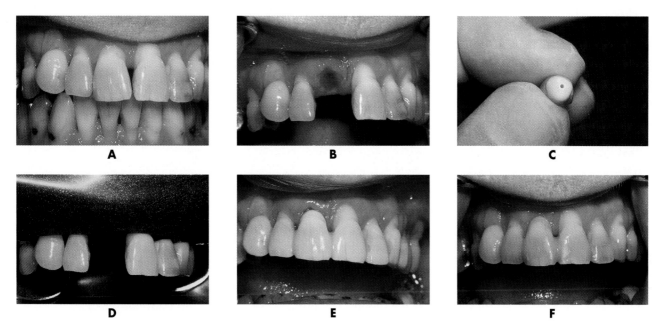

FIG. 15-55 Resin-bonded maxillary natural-tooth pontic. **A,** Preoperative photograph before extraction of periodontally involved maxillary right central incisor. **B,** Extraction site immediately following removal of incisor. **C,** Enlarged apical opening ready to be filled with composite. Pontic tip has been contoured to an ovate design. **D,** Abutment teeth isolated, roughened, and acid-etched. **E,** Immediate postoperative photograph of natural-tooth pontic bonded in place. **F,** Resin-bonded natural-tooth pontic with healed residual ridge 6 weeks later.

floss. It is also by far the most esthetic pontic tip design that can be used. While being contoured, the tip is occasionally evaluated by trying the pontic in the space. In the maxillary arch, passive contact between the pontic tip and the healed residual ridge is considered ideal for maximal phonetic and esthetic potential. However, in the mandibular arch (where esthetics is not generally a problem) the pontic tip is best shaped into the same bullet-shaped design but positioned as a hygienic pontic type that does not contact tissue (Fig. 15-56, *A*).

The pontic tip is smoothed and polished using a proper sequence of abrasive discs or polishing points. A polished pontic tip not only is easier to clean, but it also retains less plaque.

A rubber dam is usually needed for isolation of the region to prevent seepage of blood and saliva. Isolation using cotton rolls and gingival retraction cords is acceptable if hemorrhage has been controlled. Any carious lesions or faulty proximal restorations on involved proximal surfaces of both the pontic and the abutments are now restored with light-cured composite (preferably the same material to be subsequently used for the bridge connectors) by using modified preparation designs. It is recommended that the resulting restored surfaces be undercontoured rather than overcontoured to facilitate positioning of the natural tooth pontic.

Next, the involved proximal surfaces on both the abutment teeth and the pontic are roughened with a coarse, flame-shaped diamond instrument. Spaces of

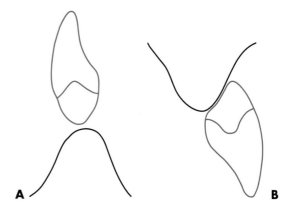

FIG. 15-56 Pontic tip design. **A,** Hygienic-type pontic with ovate or bullet-shaped tip. **B,** Modified ridge lap-type pontic with slight concavity conforming to residual ridge.

approximately 0.5 mm should exist between the pontic and the abutment teeth, because stronger connectors are provided by the additional bulk of composite material. Now the operator should acid-etch, rinse, and dry all prepared (i.e., roughened) surfaces (see Fig. 15-55, *D*).

A light-cured composite is preferred for bonding natural tooth pontics, because the extended working time allows the operator to contour the connectors before polymerization. First, the resin-bonding agent is applied to the etched surfaces of the pontic and lightly blown with air to remove the excess. Then it is polymerized by application of light, and the pontic is set

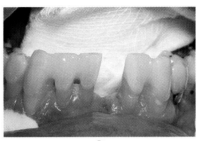
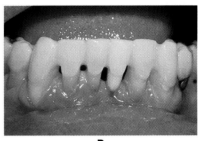

FIG. **15-57** Resin-bonded mandibular bridge splint using natural-tooth pontic. **A,** Anterior segment splinted with composite and abutment teeth isolated, roughened, and etched. **B,** Natural-tooth pontic bonded in place.

A   **B**

aside (ready for bonding in the mouth). Next, the bonding agent is applied to the etched surfaces of the abutment teeth and cured. Then a small amount of composite material is placed on the proximal contact areas of the natural tooth pontic, and the pontic is carefully inserted in the proper position in the mouth. The composite is shaped around the contact areas with an explorer tip. After final verification that the pontic position is correct, the composite is polymerized with light. Next, additional composite is applied in the proximal areas (more material is added on the lingual than on the facial surface), contoured, and cured. Adequate gingival embrasures must be provided to facilitate flossing and ensure gingival health. After sufficient material has been added and polymerized, the embrasure areas should be shaped and smoothed with carbide finishing burs or fine diamonds and polishing discs or points. The rubber dam is removed, and the occlusion is evaluated for centric contacts and functional movements. Heavy contacts on the pontic or the connector areas must be adjusted. The finished bridge immediately after bonding is illustrated in Fig. 15-55, *E.* The patient should return in 4 to 6 weeks for evaluation of the relationship of the pontic tip to the tissue. Passive contact should exist between the pontic tip and the underlying tissue to prevent ulceration. If tissue ulceration is present, the pontic must be removed, recontoured, and rebonded. The finished bridge and healed residual ridge appear in Fig. 15-55, *F.*

As stated earlier, abutment teeth that are mobile can often be splinted with composite to afford stability to periodontally involved teeth. The abutments are isolated, roughened, and acid-etched (Fig. 15-57, *A*). Because esthetics is not as critical, a hygienic pontic tip is recommended for mandibular incisors (see Fig. 15-56, *A*). The finished bridge splint is illustrated in Fig. 15-57, *B.*

DENTURE TOOTH PONTIC

An acrylic resin denture tooth can be used as a pontic for the replacement of missing maxillary or mandibular incisors by using the acid etch–resin bonding technique (Fig. 15-58, *A* through *H*). Although this type of bridge is sometimes used as an interim prosthesis and is called a *temporary bridge,* it can be a viable alternative to a conventional bridge and may last for years in some circumstances. As with the natural tooth pontic, the major contraindications to this type of resin-bonded bridge are abutment teeth that have extensive caries, restorations, mobility, or a pontic area that is subjected to heavy occlusal forces.

In the illustrated example, the permanent maxillary right lateral incisor is missing and the adjacent teeth are in favorable condition and position (see Fig. 15-58, *A*). Further examination reveals an ideal situation for a conservative bridge that uses a *denture tooth pontic.*

Technique. Although the entire procedure can be completed at chairside in one appointment, considerable time can be saved by an indirect technique. During the first appointment the shade (see Fig. 15-58, *B*) and mold of the denture tooth are selected, and alginate impressions are made. In the laboratory, stone casts are poured and the ridge area is relieved slightly and marked with a soft-lead pencil. As the pontic is trial positioned, the pencil markings will rub off onto its tip to facilitate contouring of this area (see Fig. 15-58, *C*). Contouring is best accomplished with acrylic burs and a Burlew wheel in a straight handpiece. The tissue side of the pontic should be contoured to a modified ridge lap configuration that is convex mesiodistally and slightly concave faciolingually (see Fig. 15-56, *B*). This type of design not only allows the pontic tip to adapt to the residual ridge, but it also allows for effective cleaning with dental floss. After it is contoured, the pontic tip should be smoothed and highly polished with pumice and an acrylic-polishing agent (see Fig. 15-58, *D*).

Because composite does not normally bond to acrylic resin, provisions must be made to facilitate a strong connection between the pontic and the adjacent teeth. One provision may be completed in the laboratory by preparing large Class III conventional preparations in the pontic that will mechanically retain the composite material. The outline of the preparations must be large enough to provide adequate surface area of the composite restoration for bonding to the adjacent teeth (see Fig. 15-58, *E* to *G*). An appropriately sized round bur (No. 2 or No. 4) is used to cut each preparation to a depth of approximately 1.5 mm and extend the outline approximately 0.5 mm past the contact areas into the gingival, incisal, and facial embrasures. Even more extension should be made into the lingual embrasure to

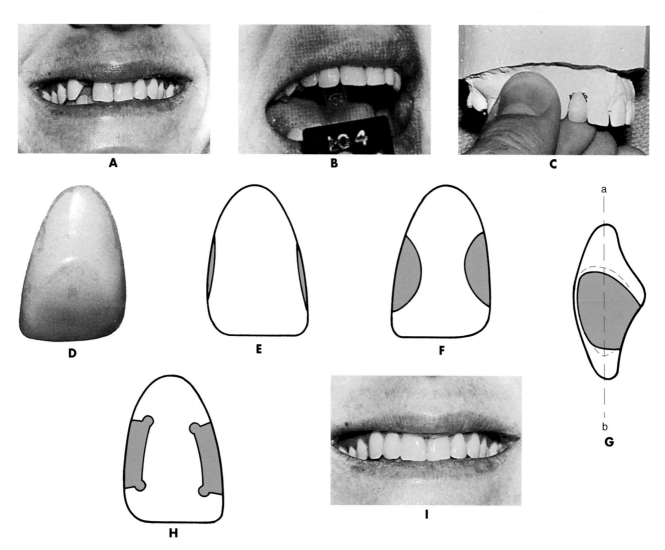

FIG. 15-58 Resin-bonded denture tooth pontic. **A,** Preoperative photograph showing missing maxillary lateral incisor. **B,** Shade and mould selection. **C,** Positioning pontic on working model while contouring. **D,** Contoured and polished pontic (lingual view). Outline form of Class III preparations: facial (**E**), lingual (**F**), and proximal (**G**) views. **H,** Cross-section of denture tooth (longitudinal section) in plane *ab* as seen in (**G**) showing mechanical-retention form incisally and gingivally as prepared with a No. ½ bur. **I,** Denture tooth pontic bonded in place with composite.

provide for bulk of composite material in the connector areas. The lingual extensions should not be connected, because this unnecessary step would unduly weaken the pontic.

Mechanical undercuts are placed at the incisoaxial and gingivoaxial line angles with a No. ½ bur to mechanically lock the composite material (to be inserted later in the technique) in the acrylic resin pontic (see Fig. 15-58, *G* and *H*).

During the next appointment, the pontic is tried in place to confirm that the shade and contours are correct. There should be approximately 0.5 mm of space between each proximal "contact" and the abutment tooth. The pontic is cleaned with acetone to remove dust and debris. Retention of the pontic by undercuts, as previously described, also can be augmented by a second

provision—the conditioning of the proximal aspects of the pontic with two applications of ethyl acetate, a polymer softener. A thin layer is applied in the Class III preparations and on the cavosurface areas and allowed to dry for 5 minutes. This process is repeated to ensure optimal bonding. The preparations are filled with the same light-cured composite material anticipated for bonding the pontic in place. The composite should be applied and cured in the retentive areas before the remainder of the preparation is filled. This step ensures complete polymerization. After the entire preparation is filled, it should be polymerized again with the light source. It is better to leave the contact areas slightly undercontoured for the pontic to fit easily between the abutment teeth. The pontic is set aside momentarily in a safe place.

Isolation of the abutment teeth should be accomplished with cotton rolls and retraction cords (rather than with a rubber dam) to better relate the pontic to the residual ridge area. Any caries or old restorations in the adjoining proximal areas of the abutment teeth should be removed at this time, and any indicated liners applied. The proximal surfaces of the abutment teeth are roughened with a coarse flame-shaped diamond instrument. This step is followed by acid-etching, rinsing, and drying. The resin-bonding agent is applied, lightly blown with air, and cured. Tooth preparations, if present, are restored with the same composite material. Care is taken not to overcontour the restoration or restorations.

The pontic is evaluated by positioning it temporarily in the edentulous space. If adjustments are made, the surfaces should be cleaned with acetone. Next, a small amount of composite is wiped onto the contact areas (mesial and distal) of the pontic, and the pontic is placed into the proper position between the abutment teeth. An explorer tip is helpful in placing the material evenly around the contact area. Care must be taken to place the pontic so that it lightly touches the ridge but does not cause tissue blanching. The composite material used to position the pontic is polymerized. It is helpful to add and cure the additional composite in small increments to obtain the correct contour and minimize finishing procedures. The facial, incisal, and gingival embrasures should be defined with a flame-shaped finishing bur or fine diamond and polished with appropriate discs or points. The lingual aspect of the bridge is contoured with a round finishing bur without defining lingual embrasures because this could weaken the connectors. The retraction cords are removed from the gingival crevice. Articulating paper is used to mark the occlusion, and any offensive contacts are removed. The final restoration is shown in Fig. 15-58, I.

PORCELAIN-FUSED-TO-METAL PONTIC OR ALL-METAL PONTIC WITH METAL RETAINERS

A stronger and more permanent type of acid-etched, resin-bonded bridge is possible by use of a cast metal framework.[31,39] In *anterior areas* where esthetics is a consideration, the design of the bridge includes a porcelain-fused-to-metal pontic with metal winged retainers extending mesially and distally for attachment to the proximal and lingual surfaces of the abutment teeth. In *posterior areas* where esthetics is not a critical factor, the bridge can have either a porcelain-fused-to-metal or an all-metal pontic.

The technique is more complicated and time consuming than the previously described methods, because it requires some initial tooth preparation, an impression, laboratory procedures, and a second appointment for etching and bonding. When compared with conventional bridges, resin-bonded bridges of this type offer five distinct advantages:

1. Anesthesia is usually not required.
2. Tooth structure is conserved (i.e., no dentin involvement).
3. Gingival tissues are not irritated because margins usually are not placed subgingivally.
4. An esthetic result can be obtained more easily.
5. The cost is less because not as much chair time is required and laboratory fees are lower.

Ideally this type of conservative bridge is used for short spans in the anterior or posterior areas with sound abutment teeth in good alignment. The most favorable occlusal relationship exists where little or no centric contact and only light functional contact are present. However, the teeth can be prepared and the bridge framework designed to withstand moderately heavy occlusal forces. Orthodontics may be required to improve tooth alignment. The bridge also can be extended to splint adjacent periodontally involved teeth. Crown-lengthening procedures are sometimes indicated for teeth with short clinical crowns.

Although minimal, some preparation of enamel of the abutment teeth is mandatory in the retainer area of the bridge to: (1) provide a definite path of insertion or seating or both, (2) enhance retention and resistance forms, (3) allow for the thickness of the metal retainers, and (4) provide physiologic contour to the final restoration. The importance of tooth preparation design cannot be overemphasized. The success of these types of bridges depends on preparation design. The bridges must be independently retentive by design and cannot rely solely on the bonding resin for retention. Preparation design for these types of bridges is much like that for a cast three-quarter crown; however, it is restricted to enamel.

The preparation for each abutment varies, depending on the individual tooth position and anatomy. Approximately the same amount of surface area should be covered on each abutment tooth. In some situations recontouring of the adjacent and opposing teeth may be indicated. The details of the preparations are described later.

Two primary types of resin-bonded bridges with metal retainers currently exist: (1) *Rochette*[39] and (2) *Maryland*.[31] Each type has advantages and disadvantages.

The Rochette type uses small countersunk perforations in the retainer sections for retention and is best suited for anterior bridges (Fig. 15-59, A).[39] Care must be exercised in placing the perforations to prevent weakening the framework. Perforations that are too large or too closely spaced will invite failure of the metal retainer by fracture. The perforations should be approximately 1.5 to 2 mm apart and have a maximum diameter of 1.5 mm on the tooth side. Each hole is countersunk so that the widest diameter is toward the outside of the retainer. When the bridge is bonded with a bonding medium, it is mechanically locked in place by micro-

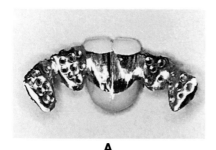
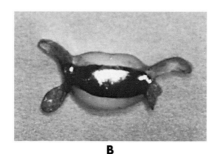
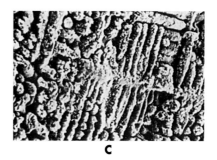

A   **B**   **C**

FIG. **15-59** Acid-etched, resin-bonded metal bridges. **A,** Rochette type. **B,** Maryland type. **C,** Scanning electron micrograph of etched metal surface. *(Courtesy of Dr. John Sturdevant.)*

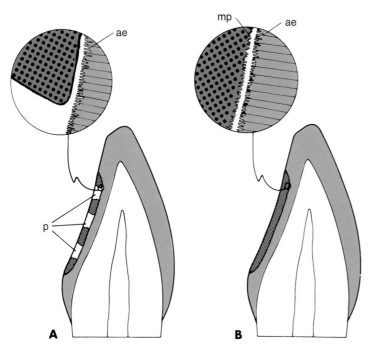

A   **B**

FIG. **15-60** Cross-sectional diagram of two types of resin-bonded bridges. **A,** In addition to acid-etching prepared enamel surfaces (*ae*), the Rochette type uses small countersunk perforations (*p*) in retainer section. **B,** In Maryland type, tooth side of framework is either etched to produce microscopic pores (*mp*) or bonded with no etching with an adhesive cement.

scopic undercuts in the etched enamel and the countersunk holes in the retainer (Fig. 15-60, *A*).

Advantages of this design include:

- It is easy to see the retentive perforations in the metal;
- If the bridge must be removed or replaced, the bonding medium can be cut away in the perforations to facilitate easy removal; and
- No metal etching is required.

Disadvantages of this design include:

- The perforations could weaken the retainers if improperly sized or spaced;
- The exposed resin-bonding medium is subject to wear; and
- It is not possible to place perforations in proximal or rest areas.

A second type of cast metal framework, commonly known as the Maryland bridge, is reported to have im-

proved bonding strength (see Fig. 15-59, *B*).[31,32] Instead of perforations, the tooth side of the metal framework is electrolytically or chemically etched, which produces microscopic undercuts (see Fig. 15-59, *C*). The bridge is attached with a self-cured, resin-bonding medium that locks into the microscopic undercuts of both the etched retainer and the etched enamel (see Fig. 15-60, *B*). It can be used for both anterior and posterior bridges. Although this design has been reported to be stronger, it is more technique sensitive because the retainers may not be properly etched or may be contaminated before cementation. Because the retentive features cannot be seen with the unaided eye, the etched metal surfaces must be examined under a microscope to verify proper etching (minimum magnification).

More recently, Maryland bridges are fabricated with no electrolytic etching of the surface and chemically bonded to the tooth either following a process called *silicoating* or with a 4-META or phosphate ester–containing, resin-bonding medium.[18,19] Recall that resin materials containing 4-META or other resin monomers are capable of

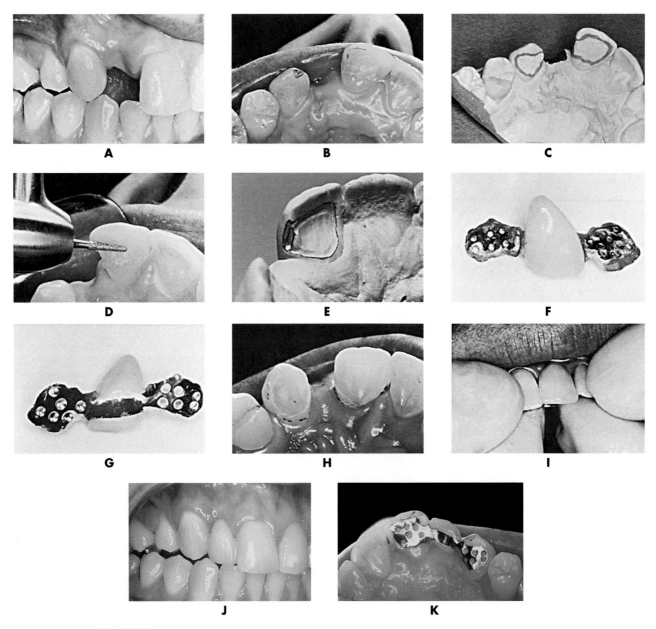

FIG. 15-61 Resin-bonded, porcelain-fused-to-metal maxillary anterior bridge. **A,** Congenitally missing maxillary lateral incisor. **B,** Occlusion marked with articulating paper. **C,** Model with outline of preparations. **D,** Preparing lingual surface with diamond instrument. **E,** Working cast shows proximal groove prepared (a second groove is on mesial of canine) to establish path of insertion for prosthesis and provide positional stability and increase retention form. Completed Rochette-type bridge from facial view (**F**) and lingual view (**G**). **H,** Teeth isolated with gingival-retraction cord and cotton rolls. Preparations are etched and ready for bonding. **I,** Holding bridge in place during polymerization. Bonded bridge: facial view (**J**) and lingual view (**K**).

strongly bonding to metal surfaces.[8,34] Surface roughening with microetching (i.e., sandblasting) is commonly used in conjunction with these adhesive cements. These types of Maryland bridges are referred to as *adhesion bridges* and differ only in the means of retention. The design of adhesion bridges is the same for this alternative Maryland bridge design.

Successes and failures have been observed with both bonded bridge designs. Because the procedures are technique sensitive, every step must be carefully followed.

Maxillary Anterior Bridge. In Fig. 15-61, *A,* a maxillary lateral incisor is congenitally missing, and the teeth on either side are sound. The occlusion is favorable, and there are no periodontal problems (see Fig. 15-61, *B*). The patient has been wearing a removable partial denture that is undesirable. Radiographs and study casts are made to complete the diagnosis and to facilitate preparation design. The outline of the proposed preparation is penciled on the cast to cover as much enamel surface as possible for maximal bonding area, but with the following two stipulations: (1) the lingual portions are extended neither subgingivally nor too far incisally, and (2) the proximal portions are not extended facially of the contact areas but enough to allow preparation of retention grooves (see Fig. 15-61, C and E).

Before tooth preparation, clean the teeth, select the shade of the pontic, and mark the occlusion with articulating paper to evaluate centric contact or contacts and functional movements. If adjustment or recontouring of the abutment teeth is indicated, it should be accomplished at this time. When a base metal alloy is used rather than high gold alloys for the bridge framework, less tooth structure is removed because the metal retainers can be made thinner. Base metal alloys have superior tensile strength.

Preparation. Make several depth cuts (0.3 to 0.5 mm) in the enamel with a small, round, coarse diamond instrument (1 to 1.5 mm in diameter). Join the depth cuts with the same instrument or a round diamond instrument (see Fig. 15-61, D). A large surface area (i.e., outline form) is desirable to obtain maximum bonding and strength of the bridge. A *shallow* groove is cut *in the enamel* of each proximal portion of the preparations with a small, tapered, cylindrical diamond instrument to establish a path of draw in an incisal direction. This feature provides a definite path of insertion and positional stability for the prosthesis during try-in and bonding (see Fig. 15-61, E). In addition, the retention of the bridge is improved because a shear force is required to unseat the bridge. Fig. 15-61, E, illustrates this groove on the working cut.

Make an elastomeric impression of the completed preparations and a bite registration. The patient continues to wear the partial denture as a temporary prosthesis. A small amount of self-curing acrylic resin is added to the mesial and distal portions of the removable partial denture tooth to maintain proximal relationships.

Laboratory Phase. The impression, bite registration, patient information, and instructions are sent to the dental laboratory. A perforated retention design (i.e., Rochette) is specified in this instance, although the other types could be used. The bridge is fabricated in the laboratory (porcelain contoured but unglazed and perforations prepared in the retainers).

Try-In Stage. During the initial try-in the bridge is examined for proper shade, contour, tissue compatibility, marginal fit, and occlusion. Adjustments are made, and the bridge is returned to the laboratory for corrections (if needed), glazing, and polishing of the metal framework. Fig. 15-61, F and G, shows the completed bridge from facial and lingual views.

Bonding Steps. The steps in bonding require an exacting coordination between the dentist and assistant. All of the equipment and materials needed for isolation, etching, and bonding must be available at the beginning of the appointment: prophylaxis angle handpiece, pumice slurry, a self-curing, resin-bonding medium kit with all accessories, plastic hand instrument, polyester strip, and cotton rolls. Alternatively, rubber dam isolation also can be used and is recommended, particularly for placement of posterior bonded bridges.

The abutment teeth are cleaned with pumice slurry, rinsed, dried, and isolated with cotton rolls. If the cervical area of the retainer is subgingival, insert a retraction cord in the gingival crevice to displace the tissue and prevent seepage. The bridge should be carefully tried in place to review the path of insertion and verify the fit. On removal, place it in a convenient location near where the resin-bonding medium will be mixed.

Artfully apply the etching gel for 30 seconds to the prepared enamel and slightly past the margins. The acid must not be allowed to flow onto the unprepared proximal areas of the abutment or adjacent teeth. After rinsing the teeth, dry them of all visible moisture (see Fig. 15-61, H). If a lightly frosted surface is not present, the etching procedure is repeated. It is emphasized that a *clean, dry* surface is absolutely essential. The slightest amount of saliva will contaminate the etched enamel and necessitate an additional 10 seconds of etching, followed by rinsing and drying. A rubber dam is preferred for isolation; however, cotton rolls and gingival retraction cord will provide adequate isolation in selected areas where salivary flow can be controlled.

The manufacturer's instructions for the bonding procedure should be read and followed. Usually equal parts of the resin-bonding medium (i.e., base and catalyst) are placed on one mixing pad, and equal parts of the bonding agent (i.e., base and catalyst) are placed on another mixing pad. The operator mixes the bonding agent with a small, foam sponge or brush and quickly paints a thin layer on the tooth side of the bridge and then onto the etched enamel. While the operator uses the air syringe to blow the excess bonding agent off the bridge and then the enamel, the assistant mixes the resin-bonding medium and places a thin layer on the tooth side of the bridge retainers. The bridge is positioned on the abutment teeth and held in place with a polyester strip over the lingual surface. The retainers are seated and held firmly in place with the index fingers positioned on the strip over the lingual retainers, and the thumbs are held on the facial aspect of the abutment teeth to equalize the pressure (see Fig. 15-61, I). The amount of resin-bonding medium at the facial and gingival embrasures is quickly inspected. Sometimes the assistant may need to add more resin-bonding medium or remove excess unpolymerized resin with an explorer or plastic instrument. Priority is given to the gingival embrasure, because later correction is more difficult in this area.

Finishing Procedure. After the resin-bonding medium has hardened, remove the polyester strip and inspect the lingual area. If voids are present, more resin is mixed and added. Additions will bond to the previously placed resin-bonding medium without additional

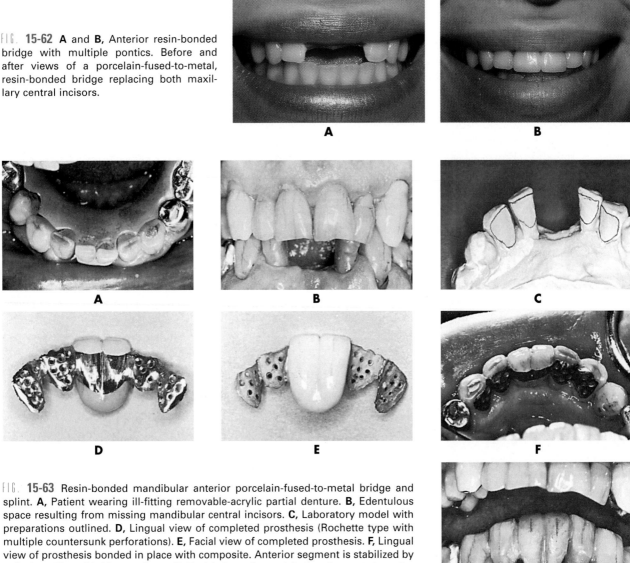

FIG. **15-62 A** and **B,** Anterior resin-bonded bridge with multiple pontics. Before and after views of a porcelain-fused-to-metal, resin-bonded bridge replacing both maxillary central incisors.

FIG. **15-63** Resin-bonded mandibular anterior porcelain-fused-to-metal bridge and splint. **A,** Patient wearing ill-fitting removable-acrylic partial denture. **B,** Edentulous space resulting from missing mandibular central incisors. **C,** Laboratory model with preparations outlined. **D,** Lingual view of completed prosthesis (Rochette type with multiple countersunk perforations). **E,** Facial view of completed prosthesis. **F,** Lingual view of prosthesis bonded in place with composite. Anterior segment is stabilized by splinting effect of bridge retainers. **G,** Facial view of porcelain-fused-to-metal pontics bonded in place.

surface treatment. Remove excess resin along the lingual margins with a discoid-cleoid hand instrument, evaluate the occlusion, and adjust if necessary. Contouring and polishing are accomplished in the usual manner with carbide finishing burs, fine diamonds, hand instruments, and discs. A completed Rochette-type bridge is shown in Fig. 15-61, *J* and *K*, as viewed from the facial and lingual aspects. When the bridge is complete, the patient is instructed in how to use a floss threader and dental floss to clean under the pontic and around the abutment teeth. Another example of an anterior resin-bonded bridge replacing both maxillary central incisors is seen in Fig. 15-62.

Mandibular Anterior Splint-and-Bridge Combination. An indication for a conservative bridge that incorporates a splint design of the porcelain-fused-to-metal framework is illustrated in Fig. 15-63. The mandibular central incisors were extracted because of advanced periodontal disease. The weak lateral incisors are stabilized by including the canines in a splint-and-bridge design. These teeth are caries free and have no restorations. An ill-fitting removable, partial denture was uncomfortable and did not support the adjacent teeth (see Fig. 15-63, *A* and *B*).

The preparations for the splint-and-bridge combination consist of removing approximately 0.3 mm of enamel on the lingual aspect of the lateral incisors and canines (as outlined on the laboratory cast) and preparing proximal retention grooves (see Fig. 15-63, *C*). The perforated design of the winged retainers was the Rochette type for ease of replacement or repair (see Fig. 15-63, *D* and *E*). The splint bridge is bonded by the method previously de-

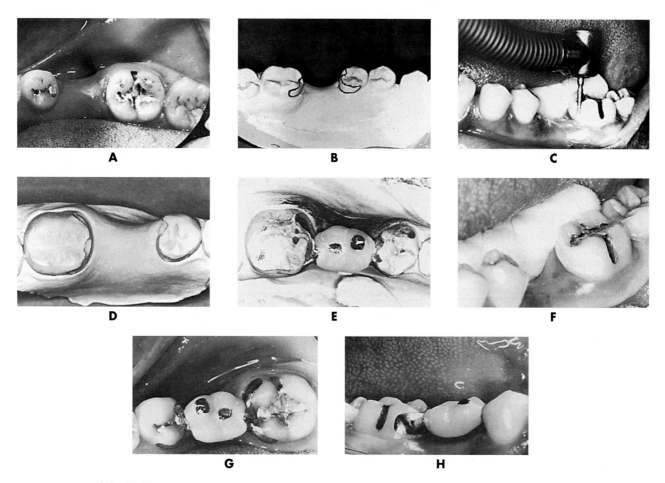

FIG. **15-64** Conservative mandibular posterior bridge with a combination metal and porcelain pontic. (**A**, **G**, and **H** are mirror views.) **A**, Missing mandibular first molar with occlusion identified by marks from articulating paper. **B**, Study model surveyed and outlines of the preparation marked with pencil. **C**, Preparation of axial surfaces with coarse, cylindric-diamond instrument. **D**, Laboratory model with margins outlined. **E**, Completed bridge on cast ready for try-in. Note centric contacts on metal to minimize wear of opposing teeth. **F**, Teeth cleaned, isolated, and etched. **G**, Occlusal view of bonded bridge. **H**, Facial view of bonded bridge.

scribed (see Fig. 15-63, *F* and *G*). Note that the gingival aspect of the pontic is free of tissue contact and has sufficient space for cleaning. A similar splint also can be achieved with a Maryland bridge design.

Mandibular Posterior Bridge with Metal-and-Porcelain-Pontic. In Fig. 15-64, *A*, a missing mandibular first molar needs to be replaced to maintain proper occlusal contacts and to preserve the integrity of the arch. A clinical examination with radiographs confirms that the abutment teeth are in good alignment and are sound and that the occlusion is favorable. Conservative amalgam restorations have been inserted to correct occlusal fissures on the abutment teeth. Impressions and a bite registration are made for study casts. An acid-etched, resin-bonded, cast metal bridge (Maryland type), including a porcelain pontic with metal, occlusal, centric stops will provide for optimal occlusal wear resistance and an acceptable esthetic result.

Use a surveyor to determine the most favorable path of draw, and mark the outline of the retainer area with a pencil (see Fig. 15-64, *B*). The occlusal rest areas will provide rigidity and resistance form to vertical forces, and the extensions on the facial and lingual surfaces will provide a "wrap-around" design for added retention and resistance against lateral forces. In this example the teeth have sufficient crown length to avoid subgingival margination.

Preparation. Prophylaxis, shade selection, and any needed occlusal adjustment are accomplished before the preparations are begun. As with the anterior teeth, some preparation is necessary to provide "draw," to increase retention and resistance forms, and to provide bulk to the retainers for strength without overcontouring. Preparation is minimal and involves only the enamel. Using the surveyed penciled cast as a reference, prepare the teeth with a coarse, tapered, rounded end diamond

FIG. **15-65 A** and **B**, Maryland-type, resin-bonded posterior bridge. A missing mandibular right first molar is conservatively replaced by a porcelain-fused-to-metal, resin-bonded bridge.

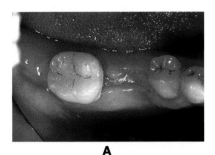

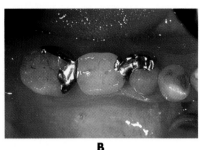

A   **B**

instrument (see Fig. 15-64, *C*). Prepare the occlusal rests with a round diamond instrument. Make an elastomeric impression and a bite registration for laboratory use.

Laboratory Phase. Include a sketch of the bridge design with the laboratory instructions. The nonperforated, etched metal design (Maryland) is specified in this instance because the "wings" will be very thin and other areas of the bridge will be inaccessible for placing perforations. It is helpful to the technician if the margins of the preparation are marked with an indelible pencil (see Fig. 15-64, *D*). Before any glazing of porcelain or polishing of framework or etching of metal, the bridge is returned to the dentist for the try-in stage (see Fig. 15-64, *E*).

Try-In Stage. Seat the bridge and evaluate for proper fit, occlusion, and color matching. After adjustments are made, the bridge is returned to the laboratory for corrections, final glazing, polishing of the metal framework, and etching or other metal treatment procedures. The etched metal must be examined under a microscope to ensure that proper etching of the metal has occurred.

Bonding Steps. Care must be exercised in handling the bridge, because *the etched area can be easily contaminated*. The bridge should not be tried in place (again) until the teeth are isolated and the enamel has been etched (see Fig. 15-64, *F*). Rubber dam isolation is preferred when bonding mandibular resin-bonded bridges. However, cotton roll isolation can be used with retraction cords if a rubber dam cannot be placed. Being careful not to touch or contaminate the etched metal, try-in the bridge to verify fit and path of draw. Everything must be "ready to go" as the manufacturer's instructions are followed for mixing and applying the bonding materials to the teeth and the bridge. Again, the preparations must be clean and dry to ensure proper bonding. Once the bridge is in place a polyester strip is placed over the pontic, and finger pressure is used to secure the bridge until polymerization is complete. After removal of the excess resin, the occlusion is evaluated. The occlusal and facial views are esthetic with only the centric contacts in metal (see Fig. 15-64, *G* and *H*). Another example of a posterior, resin-bonded, Maryland-type bridge is seen in Fig. 15-65.

Maxillary Bridge with Porcelain-Fused-to-Metal Pontic. Fig. 15-66, *A*, illustrates a space resulting from the extraction of a maxillary second premolar. As with the mandibular bridge, resistance to lateral forces must be provided by the design of the preparations and resulting prosthesis. However, because esthetics is more critical in the maxillary arch, the wraparound design used in the mandibular arch cannot be employed to as great an extent, especially in the area adjacent to the facial aspect of the pontic. Therefore, proximal grooves are prepared (in enamel) in the same occlusogingival orientation as the path of draw to provide additional resistance form to lateral forces. The lingual extensions and occlusal rests are prepared as described for the mandibular bridge (see Fig. 15-66, *B* and *C*). For retention, perforations in the retainer (e.g., Rochette design) are used in addition to acid-etching the preparations. Perforations are placed in the accessible lingual extensions. This design aids in removing the bridge if replacement becomes necessary (see Fig. 15-66, *D*). The etched preparations, which are ready for bonding, are illustrated in Fig. 15-66, *E*. The completed bonded bridge is illustrated in Fig. 15-66, *F*.

Mandibular Posterior Bridge with Metal Pontic. Fig. 15-67, *A*, illustrates a space between the mandibular premolars resulting from extraction of the permanent first molar at an early age and subsequent distal migration of the second premolar. Because esthetics was not a factor, an all-metal bridge (e.g., Maryland type) with a hygienically designed pontic was used. The steps are identical to those previously described for the mandibular posterior bridge with a porcelain-fused-to-metal pontic. The bridge is illustrated after several years of service (see Fig. 15-67, *B* and *C*).

ALL-PORCELAIN PONTIC

Improvements in dental porcelains along with the capacity to etch and bond strongly to porcelain surfaces have made all-porcelain pontics a viable alternative to pontics with metal, "winged" retainers (e.g., Maryland and Rochette bridges).[36] Although all-porcelain pontics are not as strong as pontics with metal retainers, far superior esthetic results can be achieved because no metal substructure or framework is present. Moreover, all-porcelain pontics often can be used when tooth anatomy precludes or restricts the preparation and placement of a metal, "winged" pontic. For example, long, pointed canines with proximal surfaces exhibiting little occlusogingival height often lack adequate areas

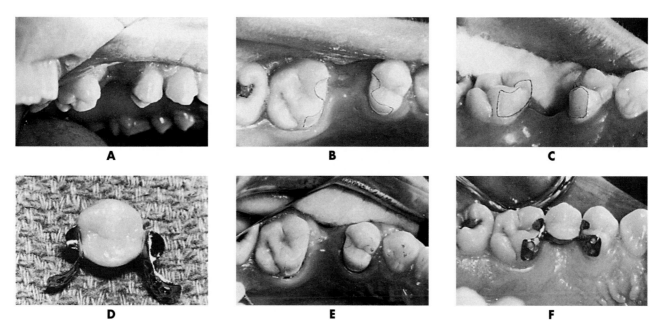

FIG. **15-66** Maxillary posterior resin-bonded bridge with porcelain-fused-to-metal pontic. **A,** Preoperative photograph (mirror view) of missing maxillary second premolar. Outlined final tooth preparations: occlusal (**B**) and lingual (**C**) views. **D,** Completed prosthesis. **E,** Etched preparations isolated and ready for bonding. **F,** Porcelain-fused-to-metal bridge bonded in place.

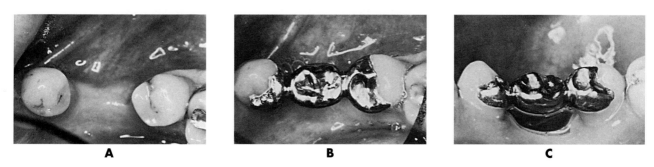

FIG. **15-67** Resin-bonded mandibular posterior all-metal bridge. **A,** Edentulous space resulting from loss of first molar and distal migration of second premolar. All-metal bridge with electrolytically etched retainers (Maryland type) bonded to place: occlusal view (**B**) and lingual view (**C**). Note non–tissue-contacting, hygienic-type pontic. *(Courtesy of Dr. William Sulik.)*

for the placement of retention grooves. Anterior teeth that are notably thin faciolingually also are not good candidates for metal, resin-bonded bridge retainers, and often are esthetic failures because of metal showing through the tooth. In both instances, custom-fabricated, etched porcelain pontics frequently can provide an esthetic, functional alternative.

All-porcelain pontics are particularly indicated for placement in adolescents and young adults, in whom virgin, unrestored teeth are often encountered. Because the teeth are not extensively prepared, this procedure is almost entirely reversible. This is a major benefit in young patients where all-porcelain pontics can be placed as interim restorations until implants or a more permanent prosthesis can be done at an older age. Again, because of their limited strength, all-porcelain pontics should be considered *provisional in nature,* similar to the natural tooth pontic and the acrylic denture tooth pontic.

Similar to the natural tooth and denture tooth pontics, certain prerequisites must exist to ensure a successful result. First, the abutment teeth must be in reasonably good condition with *proximal enamel surfaces* that are intact or contain very small composite restorations. Second, the abutment teeth should be stable with little mobility present. If the abutment teeth are mobile, it is frequently necessary to secure them as well by splinting with composite to adjacent teeth before placement of the bonded pontic (see Acid-Etched, Resin-Bonded Splints). Third, the pontic must not be placed in a position that will subject it to heavy centric or functional occlusal contacts. Because of these occlusion concerns, canines and posterior teeth are not usually good candidates for these types of resin-bonded bridges.

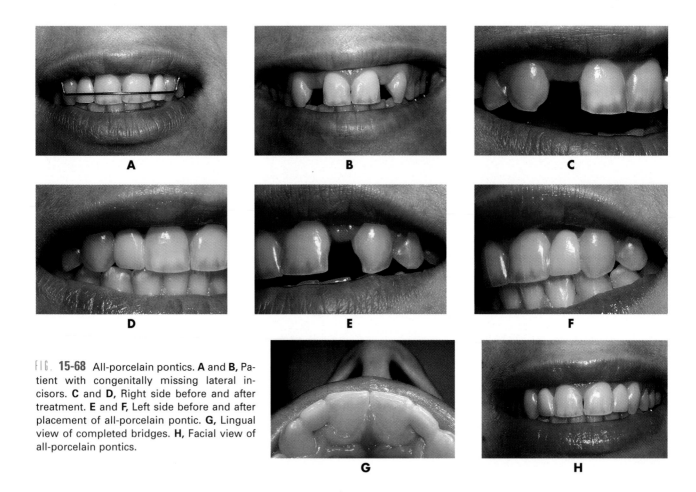

FIG. **15-68** All-porcelain pontics. **A** and **B,** Patient with congenitally missing lateral incisors. **C** and **D,** Right side before and after treatment. **E** and **F,** Left side before and after placement of all-porcelain pontic. **G,** Lingual view of completed bridges. **H,** Facial view of all-porcelain pontics.

Technique. Fig. 15-68, *A* and *B*, illustrates a typical case of congenitally missing lateral incisors in which tooth contours contraindicated the use of resin-retained bridges with metal retainers. The central incisors are very translucent and the mesial contours of the canines are deficient (see Fig. 15-68, *C* and *E*). After assessing centric and functional occlusion, it was determined that all-porcelain pontics could be placed without subjecting them to heavy occlusal forces. At the first appointment the involved abutments are cleaned with flour of pumice, and an accurate shade selection is made, noting any desired color gradients or characterizations.

No preparation of the teeth is recommended unless the proximal surfaces of the abutment teeth adjacent to the edentulous space are markedly convex. In such cases, slight flattening of the proximal surfaces with a diamond instrument will facilitate closer adaptation of the pontic to the abutment teeth; thereby increasing strength of the connectors. Otherwise, no retentive features are recommended for preparation in the abutment teeth; thus the connector areas will be entirely made of composite.

Bridge connectors composed of porcelain are subject to eventual fatigue fracture, after which repair is made more difficult. Studies show, in particular, that "veneer bridges" (i.e., all-porcelain pontics retained by adjacent

etched porcelain veneers) are the weakest design of all and should be avoided.[36] These types of bridges not only provide little bond strength to the pontic, but also needlessly cover adjacent, healthy facial tooth surfaces. All-porcelain pontics, which have connector areas consisting of the composite used for bonding to the abutment teeth, are much like extracted natural tooth pontics in this regard. This design feature allows for easy repair and replacement of the composite connector should a fracture in this area be encountered.

It should be noted that if high-strength ceramics are developed that are totally immune to crack propagation and cohesive fracture, retentive features prepared in the adjacent abutment teeth may be desired. These features, *prepared in enamel,* would consist of proximal grooves or boxes, depending on the faciolingual dimension of the proximal surfaces. In the absence of totally fracture-resistant ceramics, all-porcelain pontics are best placed with composite connectors for ease of repair and replacement.

An elastomeric impression is made from which a working cast is generated. A modified ridge lap pontic tip design as previously described (see Fig. 15-56, *A*) is recommended. An occlusal bite registration should be made and forwarded to the laboratory so that the occlusal relationship can be considered during fabrication of the all-porcelain pontic. Proximal surfaces of the pontics are etched with hydrofluoric acid. Note that *the area etched must include all areas anticipated for bonding to the composite-bonding medium.* The etched proximal surfaces should extend just beyond the lingual line angles so that additional composite can be placed in the lingual embrasure areas for additional connector strength.

At the next appointment, the teeth are isolated with cotton rolls. A 2 × 2 inch (5 × 5 cm) cotton gauze is placed across the back of the patient's mouth to act as a protective shield should the pontic be inadvertently dropped. A rubber dam is not recommended for this procedure, because it precludes accurate assessment of the adaptation of the pontic tip to the residual ridge.

Before the teeth dehydrate, the position of each pontic is tested in the edentulous space to assess the shade and relationship of the pontic tip to the residual ridge. The pontic tip should contact the residual ridge passively with no blanching of the underlying tissue evident. Spaces of approximately 0.3 to 0.5 mm should exist between the pontic and the abutment teeth, because stronger connectors are provided by the additional bulk of composite material. Care must be taken not to allow contamination of the etched pontic from saliva to occur during the try-in phase. If saliva contamination occurs, the etched proximal surfaces of the pontic must be cleaned thoroughly with alcohol and dried. Following try-in, all etched proximal surfaces of the porcelain pontics are primed with a suitable silane-coupling agent (see the manufacturer's instructions for the specific technique). The pontics are now ready for bonding.

Next, the involved proximal enamel surfaces of the abutment teeth are roughened with a coarse, flame-shaped diamond instrument. Thereafter, all prepared (i.e., roughened) enamel surfaces should be acid-etched, rinsed, and dried. Care must be taken to maintain clean, dry, uncontaminated etched surfaces until the pontic is positioned and bonded. The abutment teeth are now ready for bonding.

A light-cured composite is preferred for bonding all-porcelain pontics, because the extended working time allows the operator to initially contour the connectors before polymerization. First, apply the bonding agent to the etched surfaces of the porcelain pontic and the abutment teeth, and lightly blow with air to remove the excess. A 20-second application of light from the light-curing unit is used to polymerize the bonding agent on each etched surface.

A small amount of composite material is placed on the proximal contact areas of the natural tooth pontic, and the pontic is carefully inserted into the proper position in the edentulous space. A stent, or index, made from bite registration material or fast-setting plaster can be used to position the pontic, if desired. However, positioning by hand is recommended so that optimal gingival pressure can be maintained for best tissue adaptation. Shape the excess composite extruding from the connector areas around the contact areas with an explorer tip or small plugger end of a composite instrument. After final verification that the pontic position is correct, polymerize the composite with light for a minimum of 40 to 60 seconds each from facial and lingual directions (for a total of 80 to 120 seconds).

Next, additional composite is applied in the proximal areas (more material is added on the lingual surface than on the facial surface), contoured, and polymerized. Adequate gingival embrasures must be maintained to facilitate flossing and ensure good gingival health. After sufficient material has been added and polymerized, shape and smooth the embrasure areas with carbide finishing burs, fine diamonds, and polishing discs. Facial embrasures are defined for esthetics, but lingual embrasures are closed with composite to strengthen the connectors (see Fig. 15-68, *D, F,* and *G*).

Evaluate the occlusion centric contacts and functional movements. Heavy contacts on the pontic or the connector areas must be adjusted. The finished bridges (immediately after bonding) are illustrated in Fig. 15-68, *D* and *F* through *H.* As with all resin-bonded bridges, patients must be advised to avoid biting hard foods or objects to reduce the potential for dislodgement. Also, as noted earlier, *the patient must be advised as part of informed consent that although the chances are remote, the potential for dislodgement exists with the possibility of swallowing or aspirating the pontic.* This possibility exists for all resin-bonded bridges, and patients must be made aware of this hazard even though the risk is minimal.

ACKNOWLEDGMENTS

Portions of the section on artistic elements were reprinted with permission from Heymann HO: The artistry of conservative esthetic dentistry, *J Am Dent Assoc* 115(12E; special issue):14, 1987.

REFERENCES

1. American Dental Association Council on Scientific Affairs: Report on laser bleaching, *J Am Dent Assoc* 129(10):1484, 1998.
2. Andreasen JO: The effect of pulp extirpation or root canal treatment on periodontal healing after replantation of permanent incisors in monkeys, *J Endod* 7:245, 1981.
3. Bayne SC, Taylor DF, Zardiackas LD: *Biomaterials science,* Chapel Hill, NC, 1991, Brightstar.
4. Borissavlievitch M: *The golden number,* London, 1964, Alec Tiranti.
5. Calamia JR: Etched porcelain facial veneers: a new treatment modality based on scientific and clinical evidence, *NY J Dent* 53:255, 1983.
6. Carver CC, Heymann HO: Dental and oral discolorations associated with minocycline and other tetracycline analogs, *J Esthet Dent* 11(1):43, 1999.
7. Chiche GJ, Pinault A: *Esthetics of anterior fixed prosthodontics,* Chicago, 1994, Quintessence.
8. Cooley RL, Burger KM, Chain MC: Evaluation of a 4-META adhesive cement, *J Esthet Dent* 3(1):7, 1991.

9. Croll TP: Enamel microabrasion for removal of superficial dysmineralization and decalcification defects, *J Am Dent Assoc* 120:411, 1990.

10. Croll TP, Cavanaugh RR: Enamel color modification by controlled hydrochloric acid-pumice abrasion. Part 1: technique and examples, *Quintessence Int* 17:81, 1986.

11. Dawson PE: *Evaluation, diagnosis, and treatment of occlusal problems,* ed 2, St Louis, 1989, Mosby.

12. Feinman RA, Goldstein RE, Garber DA: *Bleaching teeth,* Chicago, 1987, Quintessence.

13. Flynn M: Black teeth: a primitive method of caries prevention in southeast Asia, *J Am Dent Assoc* 95(1):96, 1977.

14. Friedman MJ: The enamel ceramic alternative: porcelain veneers vs. metal ceramic crowns, *CDA J* 20(8):27, 1992.

15. Goldstein RE: *Esthetics in dentistry,* Philadelphia, 1976, JB Lippincott.

16. Graber TM, Vanarsdall RL: *Orthodontics: Current principles and techniques,* ed 3, St Louis, 2000, Mosby.

17. Hall DA: Should etching be performed as a part of a vital bleaching technique? *Quintessence Int* 22:679, 1991.

18. Hamada T, Shigeto N, Yanagihara T: A decade of progress for the adhesive fixed partial denture, *J Prosthet Dent* 54(1):24, 1985.

19. Hansson O: The Silicoater technique for resin-bonded prostheses: clinical and laboratory procedures, *Quintessence Int* 20(2):85, 1989.

20. Harrington GW, Natkin E: External resorption associated with bleaching of pulpless teeth, *J Endod* 5(11):344, 1979.

21. Hattab FN et al: Dental discolorations: an overview, *J Esthet Dent* 11(6):291, 1999.

22. Haywood VB: History, safety, and effectiveness of current bleaching techniques and applications of the nightguard vital bleaching technique, *Quintessence Int* 23:471, 1992.

23. Haywood VB: Nightguard vital bleaching: a history and products update: part 1, *Esthetic Dent Update* 2(4):63, 1991.

24. Haywood VB, Heymann HO: Nightguard vital bleaching: how safe is it? *Quintessence Int* 22:515, 1991.

25. Haywood VB, Heymann HO: Nightguard vital bleaching, *Quintessence Int* 20:173, 1989.

26. Haywood VB et al: Polishing porcelain veneers: an SEM and specular reflectance analysis, *Dent Mater* 4:116, 1988.

27. Holmstrup G, Palm AM, Lambjerg-Hansen H: Bleaching of discolored root-filled teeth, *Endod Dent Traumatol* 4:197, 1988.

28. Lado EA: Bleaching of endodontically treated teeth: an update on cervical resorption, *Gen Dent* 36:500, 1988.

29. Lado EA, Stanley HR, Weisman MI: Cervical resorption in bleached teeth, *Oral Surg* 55:78, 1983.

30. Levin EI: Dental esthetics and the golden proportion, *J Prosthet Dent* 40(3):244, 1978.

31. Livaditis G: Cast metal resin-bonded retainers for posterior tooth, *J Am Dent Assoc* 101:926, 1980.

32. Livaditis G, Thompson VP: Etched castings: an improved retentive mechanism for resin-bonded retainers, *J Prosthet Dent* 47(1):52, 1982.

33. Madison S, Walton R: Cervical root resorption following bleaching of endodontically treated teeth, *J Endod* 16:570, 1990.

34. Matsumura H, Nakabayashi N: Adhesive 4-META/MMA-TBB opaque resin with poly(methyl methacrylate)-coated titanium dioxide, *J Dent Res* 67(1):29, 1988.

35. McCloskey RJ: A technique for removal of fluorosis stains, *J Am Dent Assoc* 109:63, 1984.

36. Moore DL et al: Retentive strength of anterior etched porcelain bridges attached with composite resin: an in vitro comparison of attachment techniques, *Quintessence Int* 20(9):629, 1989.

37. Muia PJ: *The four dimensional tooth color system,* Chicago, 1982, Quintessence.

38. O'Riorden MW et al: Treatment of avulsed permanent teeth: an update, *J Am Dent Assoc* 105(6):1028, 1982.

39. Rochette AL: Attachment of a splint to enamel of lower anterior teeth, *J Prosthet Dent* 30(4):418, 1973.

40. Sorensen JA, Martinoff JT: Intracoronal reinforcement and coronal coverage: a study of endodontically treated teeth, *J Prosthet Dent* 51(4):780, 1984.

41. Sproull RC: Understanding color. In Goldstein RE: *Esthetics in dentistry,* Philadelphia, 1976, JB Lippincott.

42. Stangel I, Nathanson D, Hsu CS: Shear strength of the composite bond to etched porcelain, *J Dent Res* 66:1460, 1987.

43. Swift EJ et al: Treatment of composite surfaces for indirect bonding, *Dent Mater* 8:193, 1992.

44. Titley KC, Torneck CD, Ruse ND: The effect of carbamide-peroxide gel on the shear bond strength of a microfill resin to bovine enamel, *J Dent Res* 71(1):20, 1992.

16

Introduction to Amalgam Restorations

THEODORE M. ROBERSON

HARALD O. HEYMANN

ANDRÉ V. RITTER

AMALGAM

Dental amalgam is a metal-like restorative material composed of a mixture of silver-tin-copper alloy and mercury. The unset mixture is pressed (condensed) into a specifically prepared undercut tooth form and contoured to restore the tooth's form and function. Once the material hardens, the tooth is functional again, restored with a silver-colored restoration (Fig. 16-1). Dental amalgam is described in detail in Chapter 4. *In this text, dental amalgam is referred to as amalgam.* Amalgam has been the primary direct restorative material for over 150 years in the United States. It has been the subject of intense research but has been found to be safe and beneficial as a direct restorative material,[1,8] and many people have benefited from amalgam restorations, which restore a tooth in a very economical manner. The United States Public Health Service (USPHS) has stated, "In fact, hundreds of millions of teeth have been retained that otherwise would have been sacrificed because restorative alternatives would have been too expensive for many people."[10] Amalgam restorations also can be bonded to tooth structure. When an amalgam restoration is bonded, many of the benefits of bonding accrue.

HISTORY

Amalgam was introduced to the United States in the 1830s. Initially, amalgam restorations were made by dentists filing silver coins and mixing the filings with mercury, creating a putty-like mass that was placed into the defective tooth. As knowledge increased and research intensified, major advancements in the formulation and use of amalgam occurred. However, concerns about mercury toxicity were expressed in many countries about the use of amalgam; concerns reached major proportions in the early 1990s. The American Dental Association and the USPHS have issued many statements expressing their support for the use and safety of amalgam as a restorative material.[1,10]

CURRENT STATUS

Today, the popularity of amalgam as a direct restorative material has decreased,[4,11] in part because of concerns (valid or not) about its safety and environmental effects but primarily because of the recognized benefits and esthetics of composite as a restorative material. During the past 20 years, the number of amalgam restorations has decreased by approximately 60% in the United States.[1] Concerns about the use of amalgam restorations relate to poor esthetics, weakening of the tooth by removal of more tooth structure, recurrent caries, and lack of adhesive bonding benefits (unless the amalgam restoration is bonded).

Amalgam restorations are still well suited for restoring many defects in teeth. The ability to restore a tooth in a reasonably simple and economical manner has re-

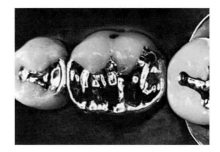

FIG. **16-1** Clinical example of an amalgam restoration.

sulted in the continued use of amalgam by many U.S. dentists, even though most dentists have also increased their use of composite. The most significant factor that may eventually lead to an even greater reduction in amalgam use in the United States will most likely be concern about disposal of amalgam from the dental office. Increased attention to mercury contamination of municipal water supplies has resulted in some communities passing regulations that have addressed this concern. Often these regulations have defined specific limits of allowable amounts of mercury that can be discharged in wastewater, including that from dental offices. Monitoring mercury levels in wastewater and installing equipment that will reduce these levels can be costly, although new filtration systems may prove relatively inexpensive.

Because of these environmental concerns about mercury contamination, the use of amalgam as a restorative material in many countries has already decreased. Legislation restricting and, in some cases, phasing out the use of amalgam has been implemented in Japan, Denmark, Canada, Sweden, and Germany.

Even with the concern about the disposal of mercury, this textbook advocates the continued use of amalgam as a direct restorative material. Research has demonstrated both the safety of the material and the success of restorations made from amalgam. While the scope of the clinical uses of amalgam presented in this textbook will be narrower than in the past, amalgam still is recognized as an excellent material for restoring many defects in teeth.

TYPES OF AMALGAM RESTORATIVE MATERIALS

Specific information about amalgam is presented in Chapter 4. For review purposes, the following types of amalgam are presented.

Low-Copper Amalgam. Low-copper amalgams were prominent before the early 1960s. When the setting reaction occurred, the material was subject to corrosion because a tin-mercury phase (gamma-two) formed. This corrosion led to rapid breakdown of the amalgam restorations. Subsequent research for improving amalgam led to the development of high-copper amalgam materials. Low-copper amalgams are used very little in the United States.

High-Copper Amalgam. High-copper amalgams are the materials predominantly used today in the United States. *In this textbook, unless otherwise specified, the term amalgam refers to a high-copper dental amalgam.* The increase in copper content to 12% or greater designates an amalgam as a high-copper type. The advantage of the added copper is that it preferentially reacts with the tin and prohibits the formation of the more corrosive phase (gamma-two) within the amalgam mass. This change in composition reduces or eliminates possible deleterious corrosion effects on the restoration. However, the reduction of the corrosion products reduces the formation of a corrosion layer at the amalgam-tooth interface, the formation of which sometimes aids in sealing the restoration.[2,14] These materials can provide satisfactory performance for more than 12 years.[13,15] High-copper materials can be either spherical or admixed in composition.

Spherical Amalgam. A spherical amalgam contains small, round alloy particles that are mixed with mercury to form the mass that is placed into the tooth preparation. Because of the shape of the particles, the material is condensed into the tooth preparation with little condensation pressure. This advantage is combined with its high early strength[25] to provide a material that is well suited for very large amalgam restorations, such as complex amalgams or foundations.

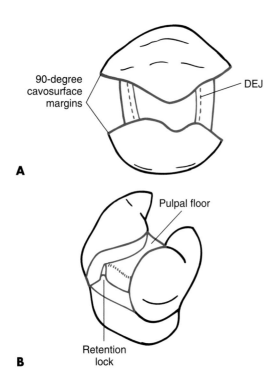

A

B

FIG. **16-2** **A** and **B**, Diagrams of Class II amalgam preparations illustrating uniform pulpal and axial wall depths, 90-degree cavosurface margins, and convergence of walls and/or prepared retention form.

90-degree cavosurface margins

DEJ

Pulpal floor

Retention lock

Admixed Amalgam. An admixed amalgam contains irregularly shaped and sized alloy particles, sometimes combined with spherical shapes, which are mixed to form the mass that is placed into the tooth preparation. The irregular shape of many of the particles makes a mass that requires more condensation pressure (which many dentists prefer) and permits this heavier condensation pressure to assist in displacing matrix bands to more easily generate proximal contacts.

New Amalgam Alloys. Because of the concern about mercury toxicity, many new compositions of amalgam are being promoted as mercury-free or low-mercury amalgam restorative materials. Alloys with gallium or indium or those using cold-welding techniques are presented as alternatives to mercury-containing amalgams. Unfortunately, none of these new alloys show sufficient promise to become a universal replacement for current amalgam materials.[21,22,26]

IMPORTANT PROPERTIES

The linear coefficient of thermal expansion (LCTE) of amalgam is 2.5 times greater than that of tooth structure,[7,28] yet it is closer than the LCTE of composite.[9] While the compressive strength of high-copper amalgam is similar to tooth structure, the tensile strength is lower,[6,19] making amalgam restorations somewhat subject to fracture. Usually, high-copper amalgam fracture is a bulk fracture, not a marginal fracture. All amalgams are brittle and have low edge strength. Therefore the amalgam material must have sufficient bulk (usually 1 to 2 mm, depending on the position within the tooth) and a 90-degree or greater marginal configuration.

Creep and flow relate to the deformation of a material under load over time. High-copper amalgams exhibit no clinically relevant creep or flow.[16,27] Because amalgam is metallic in structure, it is also a good thermal conductor. Therefore an amalgam restoration should not be placed in close proximity to the pulpal tissues of the tooth without the use of a liner and/or base between the pulp and the amalgam.

AMALGAM RESTORATIONS

Amalgam functions as a direct restorative material by easily being inserted into a tooth preparation and, once hardened, restoring the tooth to proper form and function. Amalgam restorations may be bonded or nonbonded.

Nonbonded amalgam restorations are still predominantly used, even though more bonded amalgam restorations are now being done. Both nonbonded and bonded amalgam restorations require a specific tooth preparation form into which the amalgam material is inserted (Fig. 16-2). The tooth preparation form must not only remove the fault in the tooth and remove weakened tooth structure, but it also must be formed to allow the amalgam material to function properly. The required tooth preparation form must allow the amalgam to: (1) possess a uniform specified minimum thickness for strength, (2) produce a 90-degree amalgam angle (butt joint form) at the margin, and (3) be mechanically retained in the tooth. Without this preparation form, the amalgam could possibly be dislodged or fracture. After sealing the prepared tooth structure, mixing, inserting, carving, and finishing the amalgam is relatively fast and easy (Fig. 16-3, *A*). For these reasons, it is a very user-friendly material that is less technique- or operator-sensitive than composite.

The use of bonded amalgam restorations has increased steadily (see Fig. 16-3, *B*). The mechanism of bonding an amalgam restoration is similar to that for bonding a composite restoration in some aspects, but it is different in others. For example, a bonded amalgam restoration, done properly, seals the prepared tooth structure and strengthens the remaining unprepared tooth structure. However, the retention gained by bonding may be minimal[12,29]; consequently, bonded amalgam restorations still require the same tooth preparation retention form as nonbonded amalgam restorations. It should also be noted that isolation requirements for a bonded amalgam restoration are the same as for a composite restoration.

Another amalgam technique gaining popularity is the use of light-cured adhesive as a sealer under the amalgam material (see Fig. 16-3, *C*). For this procedure, the prepared tooth structure is etched and primed and adhesive placed and cured before insertion of the amalgam. (Usually a one-bottle sealer material that combines the primer and adhesive is used.) This technique seals the dentinal tubules very effectively.[3,20]

USES

Because amalgam is not an esthetic restorative material, it is no longer used much in areas where esthetics is critical. Because of the benefits of conservative bonded composite restorations, amalgam is also not used as much for the restoration of small defects on molars and premolars. However, because of its strength and ease of use, amalgam provides an excellent means for restoring large defects[24] in nonesthetic areas, especially if it can be bonded. In fact, a recent review of almost 3500 four- and five-surface amalgams revealed successful outcomes at 5 years for 72% of the four-surface and 65% of the five-surface amalgams. This result compared somewhat favorably with the 5-year success rates for gold and porcelain crowns, which were 84% and 85% respectively.[18] Specific uses of amalgam as a direct restorative material are covered in subsequent chapters. Generally amalgams can be used for the following clinical procedures:

1. Classes I, II, and V restorations (Fig. 16-4)
2. Foundations (Fig. 16-5)
3. Caries control restorations (see Figs. 3-49 and 3-50)

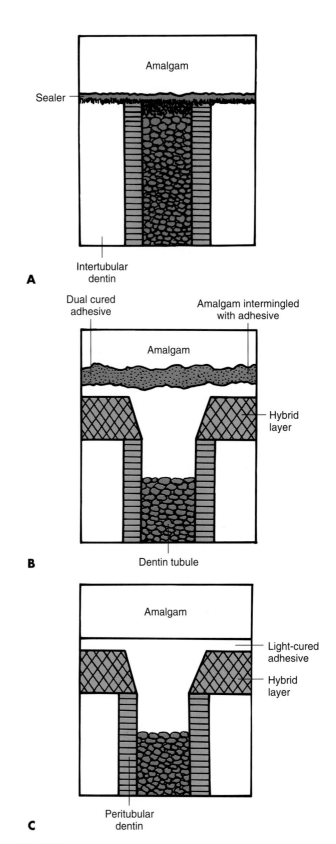

FIG. 16-3 Types of amalgam restorations. **A,** Conventional amalgam restoration. **B,** Bonded amalgam (amalgam intermingled with adhesive resin). **C,** Sealed amalgam (adhesive resin placed and cured before amalgam placement).

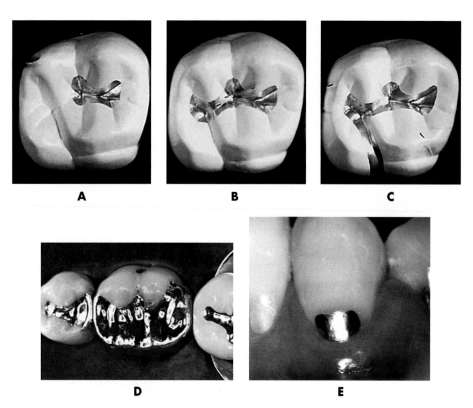

FIG. **16-4** Amalgam restorations. **A** to **C**, Class I. **D**, Class II. **E**, Class V.

HANDLING

Because of the concern about mercury, amalgam restorations require meticulous handling to avoid unnecessary mercury exposure to the environment, office, personnel, or patient. Proper mercury hygiene procedures are described in Chapter 4 and in the subsequent chapters on amalgam restorations.

GENERAL CONSIDERATIONS FOR AMALGAM RESTORATIONS

The following sections summarize general considerations about all amalgam restorations. Information for specific applications is presented in Chapters 17, 18, and 19. Because the typical direct restorative material decision is usually a choice between amalgam and composite, some of the following information involves a comparative analysis between these two materials.

INDICATIONS

Occlusal Factors. Amalgam has somewhat greater wear resistance than composite.[8,17] It therefore may be indicated in clinical situations that have heavy occlusal functioning. It also may be more appropriate when a restoration restores all of the occlusal contact for a tooth.

Isolation Factors. Unless an amalgam restoration is to be bonded, the isolation of the operating area is less critical than for a composite restoration. Minor contamination of an amalgam during the insertion procedure

may not have as adverse an effect on the final restoration as the same contamination would produce for a composite restoration. However, if an amalgam restoration is to be bonded, the isolation needs are the same as for composite.

Operator Ability and Commitment Factors. The tooth preparation for an amalgam restoration is very exacting. It requires a specific form with uniform depths and a precise marginal form. Many failures of amalgam restorations may be related to inappropriate tooth preparations. The insertion and finishing procedures for amalgam are much easier than for composite. However, if the amalgam restoration is to be bonded, the procedure is almost as demanding as that for a composite restoration.

Clinical Indications for Direct Amalgam Restorations. Because of the factors already presented, amalgam is most appropriately considered for:

1. Moderate to large Class I and Class II restorations (especially including those with heavy occlusion, that cannot be isolated well, or that extend onto the root surface) (see Fig. 16-4, *A* and *B*).
2. Class V restorations (including those that are not esthetically critical, cannot be well isolated, or are located entirely on the root surface) (see Fig. 16-4, *C*).
3. Temporary caries control restorations (including those teeth that are badly broken down and require a

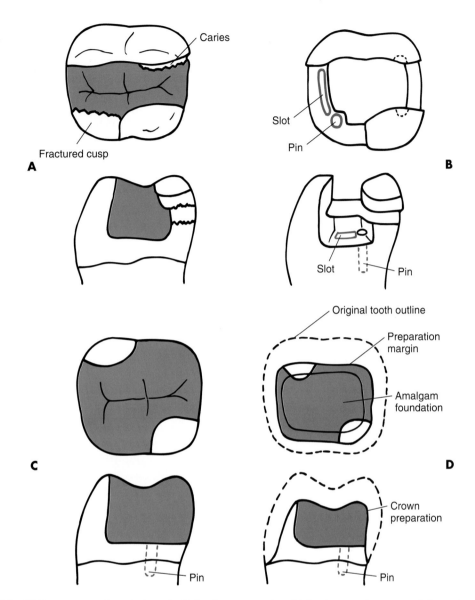

FIG. 16-5 Amalgam foundation. **A,** Defective restoration (defective amalgam, mesiolingual fractured cusp, mesiofacial caries). **B,** Tooth preparation with secondary retention and bonding, using pin and slot. **C,** Amalgam foundation placed. **D,** Tooth prepared for crown with amalgam foundation.

subsequent assessment of pulpal health before a definitive restoration) (see Chapter 3 and Figs. 3-49 and 3-50).

4. Foundations (including for badly broken-down teeth that will require increased retention and resistance form in anticipation of the subsequent placement of a crown or metallic onlay) (see Fig. 16-5).

CONTRAINDICATIONS

There are few indications for the use of amalgam for restorations in anterior teeth. Occasionally, a Class III amalgam restoration may be done if isolation problems exist. Likewise, in rare clinical situations, Class V amal-

gam restorations may be indicated in anterior areas where esthetics is not important. While esthetics is subject to wide variations in personal interpretation, most patients find the appearance of an amalgam restoration objectionable when compared to a composite restoration. Therefore the use of amalgam in more prominent esthetic areas of the mouth is usually avoided. These areas include anterior teeth, premolars, and, in some patients, molars. Because the tooth preparation for an amalgam is larger than for a composite, most small to moderate defects in posterior teeth should be restored with composite rather than amalgam. Use of composite in these situations results in conservation of tooth structure.

ADVANTAGES

Some of the advantages of amalgam restorations have already been stated, but the following list presents the primary reasons why amalgam restorations have been used successfully for many years:

1. Ease of use
2. High compressive strength
3. Excellent wear resistance
4. Favorable long-term clinical research results
5. Lower cost than for composite restorations
6. Bonded amalgams have "bonding" benefits:
   - Less microleakage
   - Less interfacial staining
   - Slightly increased strength of remaining tooth structure
   - Minimal postoperative sensitivity
   - Some retention benefits
   - Esthetic benefit of sealing by not permitting the amalgam to discolor the adjacent tooth structure

DISADVANTAGES

The primary disadvantages of amalgam restorations relate to esthetics and increased tooth structure removal during tooth preparation. The following is a list of these and other disadvantages of amalgam restorations:

1. Noninsulating
2. Nonesthetic
3. Less conservative (more removal of tooth structure during tooth preparation)
4. Weakens tooth structure (unless bonded)[5,23]
5. More technique sensitive if bonded
6. More difficult tooth preparation
7. Initial marginal leakage[7]

CLINICAL TECHNIQUE
INITIAL CLINICAL PROCEDURES

A complete examination, diagnosis, and treatment plan must be finalized before the patient is scheduled for operative appointments (emergencies excepted). A brief review of the chart (including medical factors), treatment plan, and radiographs should precede each restorative procedure. At the beginning of each appointment, the dentist should also carefully examine the operating site and assess the occlusion, particularly of the tooth (teeth) scheduled for treatment.

Local Anesthesia. Local anesthesia may be advocated for many operative procedures (as cited in Chapter 10). Profound anesthesia contributes to a comfortable and uninterrupted operation and usually results in a marked reduction in salivation. Because most amalgam tooth preparations are relatively more extensive, local anesthesia usually is necessary.

Isolation of the Operating Site. Complete instructions for the control of moisture are given in Chapter 10.

Isolation for amalgam restorations can be accomplished with a rubber dam or cotton rolls, with or without a retraction cord. Refer to Chapter 11 for a discussion of isolation techniques for composite restorations, which are the same for amalgam restorations.

Other Preoperative Considerations. A wedge placed preoperatively in the gingival embrasure is useful when restoring a posterior proximal surface. This step causes separation of the operated tooth from the adjacent tooth and may help protect the rubber dam and the interdental papilla.

Also, a preoperative assessment of the occlusion should be made. This step should occur before rubber dam placement and identify not only the occlusal contacts of the tooth to be restored, but also those contacts on opposing and adjacent teeth. Knowing the preoperative location of occlusal contacts is important both in planning the restoration outline form and in establishing the proper occlusal contacts on the restoration. Remembering the location of contacts on adjacent teeth provides guidance in knowing when the restoration contacts have been correctly adjusted and positioned.

For smaller amalgam restorations, it also is important to visualize the anticipated extension of the tooth preparation preoperatively. Since the tooth preparation requires specific depths, extensions, and marginal forms, the connection of the various parts of the tooth preparation should result in minimal tooth structure removal (i.e., as little as is necessary), thus maintaining as much strength of the cuspal and marginal ridge areas of the tooth as possible (Fig. 16-6). Therefore the projected facial and lingual extensions of a proximal box should be visualized before preparing the occlusal portion of the tooth, thereby reducing the chance of overpreparing the cuspal area while maintaining a butt joint form of the facial and/or lingual proximal margins.

TOOTH PREPARATION FOR AMALGAM RESTORATIONS

Detailed descriptions of specific amalgam tooth preparations are presented in Chapters 6, 17, 18, and 19. As discussed in Chapter 6, the stages and steps of tooth preparation are very important for amalgam tooth preparations.

For an amalgam restoration to be successful, numerous steps must be accomplished correctly. After an accurate diagnosis is made, a tooth preparation must be created that not only removes the defect (e.g., caries, old restorative material, malformed structure) but also leaves the remaining tooth structure in as strong a state as possible. Equally important is making the tooth preparation form appropriate for the use of amalgam as the restorative material. Because of amalgam's physical properties, it must: (1) be placed into a tooth preparation that provides for a 90-degree or greater restoration angle at the cavosurface margin (because of its limited edge strength), (2) have a minimum thickness of 0.75 to

2 mm (because of its lack of compressive strength), and (3) be placed into a prepared undercut form in the tooth in order to be mechanically retained (because of its lack of bonding to the tooth). After an appropriate tooth preparation, the success of the final restoration is dependent on proper insertion, carving, and finishing of the amalgam material.

Requirements. As indicated previously, appropriate tooth preparation for an amalgam restoration is dependent on both tooth and material factors. Those preparation features that relate specifically to the use of amalgam as the restorative material include the following and are subsequently discussed in more detail:

1. 90-degree or greater amalgam margin (butt joint form).
2. Adequate depth (thickness of amalgam).
3. Adequate mechanical retention form (undercut form).

Principles. The basic principles of tooth preparation must be followed for amalgam tooth preparations to ensure clinical success. The procedure is presented in two stages, academically, to facilitate student understanding of proper extension, form, and caries removal. The *initial stage*: (1) places the tooth preparation extension into sound tooth structure at the marginal areas (not pulpally or axially), (2) extends the depth (pulpally and/or axially) to a prescribed, uniform dimension, (3) provides an initial form that retains the amalgam in the tooth, and (4) establishes the tooth preparation margins in a form that results in a 90-degree amalgam margin once the amalgam is inserted. The *final stage* of tooth preparation removes any remaining defect (caries or old restorative material) and incorporates any additional preparation features (slots, pins, steps, amalgampins, or bonding) to achieve appropriate retention and resistance form. Even if the amalgam restoration is to be bonded, retention form must be provided by the features and shape of the tooth preparation. Amalgam bonding is an adjunct to mechanical retention form, *not* a substitute. As noted earlier, even if bonding an amalgam, adequate mechanical retention features still must be incorporated into the preparation.

The following subsections briefly describe certain aspects of tooth preparation that pertain to all amalgam restorations. The initial tooth preparation steps, although discussed separately, are performed at the same time. Thus, extension, depth, tooth preparation wall shape, and marginal configuration are accomplished simultaneously.

Initial Tooth Preparation Depth. All initial depths of a tooth preparation for amalgam relate to the dentino-enamel junction (DEJ), except in the following two instances: (1) when the occlusal enamel has been significantly worn thinner, and (2) when the preparation extends onto the root surface. The initial depth pulpally

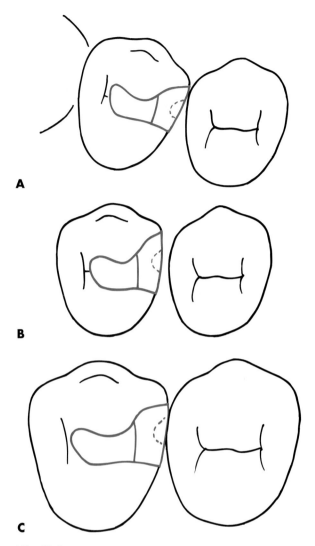

FIG. **16-6** Preoperative visualization of tooth preparation extensions when caries is present gingival to the mesial proximal contact and in the central groove area. **A,** Rotated tooth. **B,** Open proximal contact. **C,** Normal relationship.

will be 0.2 mm inside (internal to) the DEJ or 1.5 mm as measured from the depth of the central groove (Fig. 16-7), whichever results in the greatest thickness of amalgam. The initial depth of the axial wall will be 0.2 mm inside the DEJ when retention locks are not used and 0.5 mm inside the DEJ when retention locks are used (Fig. 16-8). The deeper extension allows placement of the retention locks without undermining marginal enamel. However, axial depths on the root surface should be 0.75 to 1 mm deep, providing room for a retention groove or cove while providing for adequate thickness of the amalgam.

Outline Form. The initial extension of the tooth preparation should be visualized preoperatively by estimating the extent of the defect, the preparation form requirements of the amalgam, and the need for adequate access to place the amalgam into the tooth. Because of the structure of enamel, enamel margins must be left in

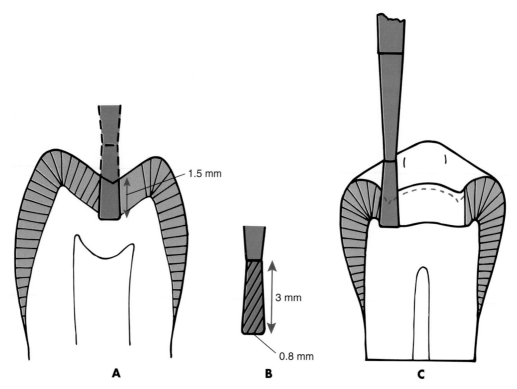

FIG. **16-7** Pulpal floor depth. **A**, Pulpal depth measured from central groove. **B**, No. 245 bur dimensions. **C**, Guides to proper pulpal floor depth: (1) one half the length of the No. 245 bur, (2) 1.5 mm, and/or (3) 0.2 mm inside (internal to) the DEJ.

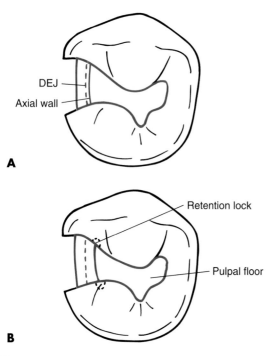

FIG. **16-8** Axial wall depth. **A**, No retention locks needed, axial depth 0.2 mm inside (internal to) DEJ. **B**, Retention locks needed, axial depth 0.5 mm inside (internal to) DEJ.

a form of 90 degrees or greater. Otherwise, the enamel is subject to fracture. For enamel strength, the marginal enamel rods should be supported by sound dentin. These requirements for enamel strength must be combined with marginal requirements for amalgam (90-degree butt joint) when establishing the periphery of the tooth preparation (see Fig. 17-48).

The preparation extension primarily is dictated by the amount of caries, old restorative material, or defect present. Adequate extension to provide access for the tooth preparation, caries removal, matrix placement, and amalgam insertion also must be considered. When making the preparation extensions, every effort should be made to preserve the strength of cusps and marginal ridges. Therefore, when possible, the outline form should be extended around cusps and avoid undermining the dentinal support of the marginal ridge enamel.

When viewed from the occlusal, the facial and lingual proximal cavosurface margins of a Class II preparation should be 90 degrees (i.e., perpendicular to a tangent drawn through the point of extension facially and lingually [Fig. 16-9]). In most instances, the facial and lingual proximal walls should be extended just into the facial or lingual embrasure. This extension

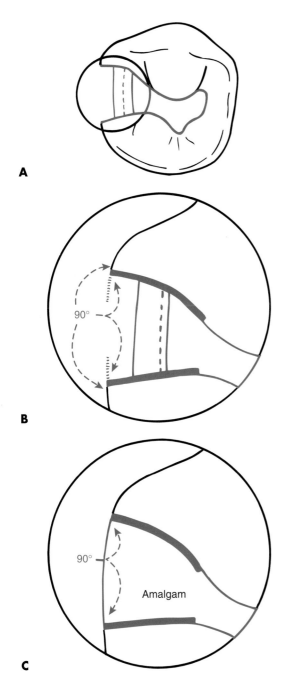

FIG. 16-9 Proximal cavosurface margins. **A**, Facial and lingual proximal cavosurface margins prepared at a right angle (90 degrees) to a tangent drawn through the point on the external tooth surface. **B**, 90-degree proximal cavosurface margin produces 90-degree amalgam margin. **C**, 90-degree amalgam margins.

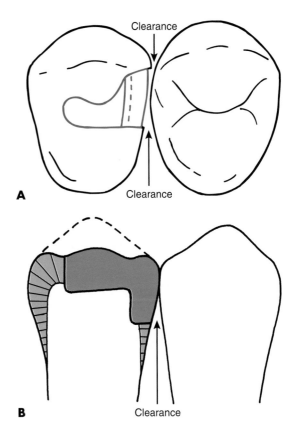

FIG. 16-10 Proximal box preparation clearance of adjacent tooth. **A**, Occlusal view. **B**, Lingual view of a cross-section through the central groove.

provides adequate access for performing the preparation (with decreased potential to mar the adjacent tooth), easier placement of the matrix band, and easier condensation and carving of the amalgam. Such extension provides clearance between the cavosurface margin and the adjacent tooth (Fig. 16-10). For the more experienced operator, extending the proximal margins beyond the proximal contact into the respective embrasure is not always necessary. Obviously the less the outline form is extended, the more conservative is the resulting preparation and the less tooth structure that is removed.

Factors dictating outline form are presented in greater detail in Chapter 6. They include caries, old restorative material, inclusion of all the defect, proximal and/or occlusal contact relationship, and need for convenience form.

Cavosurface Margin. Enamel must have a marginal configuration of 90 degrees or greater (a right or obtuse angle), while amalgam must have the same. If either have marginal angles less than 90 degrees, they are subject to fracture, because both are brittle structures. Preparation walls on vertical parts of the tooth (facial, lingual, mesial, or distal) should result in 90-degree enamel walls (representing a strong enamel margin; see Fig. 16-9) that meet the inserted amalgam at a butt joint (both enamel and amalgam having 90-degree margins). Preparation walls on the occlusal surface should be prepared to provide 90 degree or greater amalgam margins and usually have obtuse enamel margins (representing the strongest enamel margin; see Fig. 16-11). The 90-degree occlusal amalgam margin results from the amal-

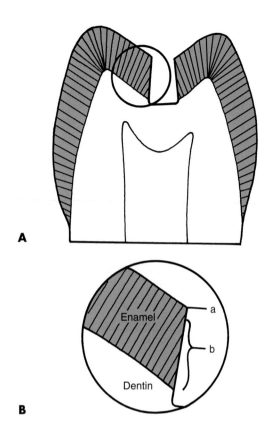

FIG. **16-11** Occlusal cavosurface margins. **A,** Tooth preparation. **B,** Occlusal margin representing the strongest enamel margin. *a,* Full-length enamel rods. *b,* Shorter enamel rods.

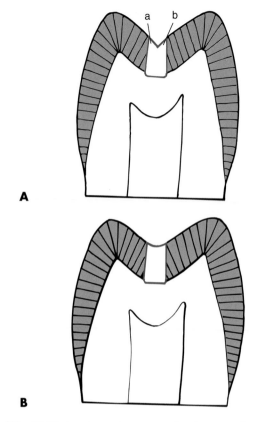

FIG. **16-12** Amalgam form at occlusal cavosurface margins. **A,** Amalgam carved too deep resulting in acute angles *a* and *b* and stress concentrations within the amalgam, both increasing the potential for fracture. **B,** Amalgam carved with appropriate anatomy, resulting in an amalgam margin close to 90 degrees, even though the enamel cavosurface margin is obtuse.

gam carving in the central groove area being more rounded (as depicted in Fig. 16-12).

Primary Retention Form. Retention form preparation features lock or retain the restorative material in the tooth. For composite restorations, micromechanical bonding provides most of the retention needed. However, for both nonbonded and bonded amalgam restorations, the amalgam must be mechanically locked inside the tooth. Amalgam retention form (Fig. 16-13) is provided by: (1) mechanical locking of the inserted amalgam into surface irregularities of the preparation (even though the desired texture of the preparation walls is smooth) to allow good adaptation of the amalgam to the tooth, (2) preparation of vertical walls (especially facial and lingual walls) that converge occlusally, (3) special retention features such as locks, grooves, coves, slots, pins, steps, or amalgampins that are placed during the final stage of tooth preparation, and (4) bonding of the amalgam to the tooth (optional). The first two of these are considered primary retention form features and are provided by the orientation and type of the preparation instrument. The remaining two are secondary retention form features and are discussed in a subsequent section. An inverted cone car-

bide bur (No. 245) provides the desired wall shape and texture (as seen in Fig. 16-7, *B*).

Primary Resistance Form. Resistance form preparation features help the restoration and tooth resist fracturing as a result of occlusal forces. Resistance features that assist in preventing the tooth from fracturing include: (1) maintaining as much unprepared tooth structure as possible (preserving cusps and marginal ridges), (2) having pulpal and gingival walls prepared perpendicular to occlusal forces, when possible, (3) having rounded internal preparation angles, (4) removing unsupported or weakened tooth structure, (5) placing pins into the tooth as part of the final stage of tooth preparation, and (6) bonding the amalgam in the tooth. The last two of these are considered secondary resistance form features and are discussed in a subsequent section. Resistance form features that assist in preventing the amalgam from fracturing include: (1) adequate thickness of amalgam (1.5 to 2 mm in areas of occlusal contact and 0.75 mm in axial areas), (2) marginal amalgam of 90 degrees or greater, (3) boxlike preparation form, which provides uniform amalgam thickness, and (4) rounded axiopulpal line angles in Class II tooth preparations. Many of these resistance form features can be achieved using

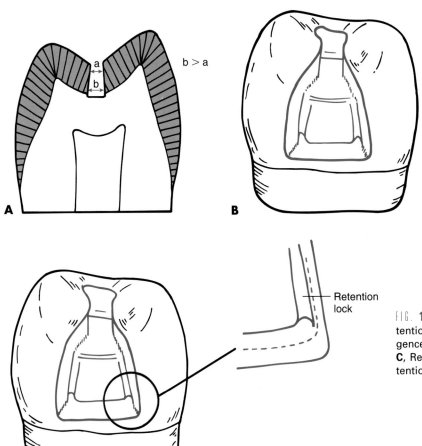

Retention
lock

FIG. **16-13** Typical amalgam tooth preparation retention form features. **A** and **B**, Occlusal convergence of prepared walls (primary retention form). **C**, Retention lock in proximal box (secondary retention form).

the No. 245 bur, which is an inverted cone design with rounded corners.

Convenience Form. Convenience form preparation features are those that make the procedure easier or the area more accessible. Convenience form may include arbitrary extension of the outline form so marginal form can be established, caries can be accessed for removal, matrix can be placed, and/or amalgam can be inserted, carved, and finished. Convenience form features also may include extending the proximal margins to provide clearance from the adjacent tooth and extension of other walls to provide greater access for caries excavation.

For simplification in teaching, these steps in the tooth preparation constitute what is referred to as the *initial stage of tooth preparation.* While each step is an important consideration, they are actually accomplished simultaneously. In academic institutions, assessing the tooth preparation after the initial preparation stage provides an opportunity to evaluate a student's knowledge and ability to properly extend the preparation and establish the proper depth. If the student were to excavate extensive caries before any evaluation, the attending faculty would not know whether the prepared depths were be-

cause of appropriate excavation or inappropriate overcutting of the tooth. The following factors constitute the *final stage of tooth preparation.*

Removal of Remaining Fault and Pulp Protection. If caries or old restorative material remains after the initial preparation, it should only be located in the axial or pulpal walls (the extension of the peripheral preparation margins should have already been to sound tooth structure). Chapter 6 addresses: (1) when to leave or remove old restorative material, (2) how to remove remaining caries, and (3) what should be done to protect the pulp. For most nonbonded amalgam restorations, a sealer is placed on the prepared dentin before amalgam insertion. The objective of the sealer is to occlude the dentinal tubules. (Use of liners and bases under amalgam restorations is addressed in Chapters 4 and 6.)

Secondary Resistance and Retention Form. If it is determined (from clinical judgment) that insufficient retention or resistance forms are present in the tooth preparation, then additional preparation is indicated. Many features that enhance retention form also enhance resistance form. Such features include the placement of grooves, locks, coves, pins, slots, or amalgampins. Bonding an amalgam also enhances retention and resistance

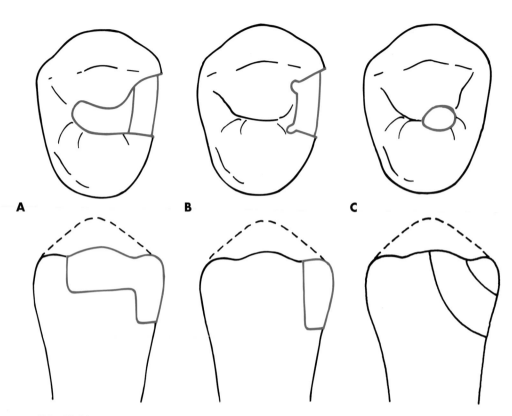

FIG. **16-14** Types of amalgam tooth preparations. **A,** Conventional. **B,** Box-only. **C,** Tunnel.

form, but it is not considered a substitute for mechanical retention. Usually the larger the tooth preparation, the greater the need for secondary resistance and retention forms.

Final Procedures. After the previous steps are performed, the tooth preparation should be viewed from all angles. Careful assessment should be made that all caries has been removed, depths are proper, margins provide for the correct amalgam and tooth preparation angles, and the tooth is cleaned of any residual debris.

Preparation Designs. The typical tooth preparation for amalgam is referred to as a *conventional tooth preparation.* Other types include box-only and tunnel preparations for amalgam restorations. Fig. 16-14 illustrates the various preparation designs. Appropriate details of specific tooth preparations are presented in subsequent chapters.

RESTORATIVE TECHNIQUE FOR AMALGAM RESTORATIONS

After the tooth preparation, the tooth must be readied for insertion of the amalgam. If the amalgam is not to be bonded, a sealer is placed on the prepared dentin. The sealer may be either a coating material or a polymerized resin adhesive (see Fig. 16-3). This step may occur before or after the matrix application. If the amalgam is to be bonded, the etching, priming, and adhesive placement procedures for the prepared tooth structure must be timed to coincide with the insertion of the amalgam. Therefore bonding an amalgam when using a matrix requires the etching, priming, and adhesive procedures to occur after the matrix is applied. It is important that the bonding adhesive be fluid and unset when the amalgam condensation occurs. This allows for intermingling of the resin with the amalgam particles during condensation, thus providing some mechanical retention between the restoration and the tooth via the set resin adhesive. Some adhesives also achieve chemical adhesion with the amalgam.

Matrix Placement. A matrix primarily is used when a proximal surface is to be restored. The objectives of a matrix are to: (1) provide proper contact, (2) provide proper contour, (3) confine the restorative material, and (4) reduce the amount of excess material. For a matrix to be effective, it should: (1) be easy to apply and remove, (2) extend below the gingival margin, (3) extend above the marginal ridge height, and (4) resist deformation during material insertion. Chapters 17, 18, and 19 describe matrix placement for specific amalgam restorations and illustrate some of the types of matrices available. It should be noted that when bonding an amalgam restoration, it might be necessary to coat the internal aspect of the matrix before its placement to prevent the bonded material from sticking to the matrix material.

In some clinical circumstances, a matrix may be necessary for Class I or Class V amalgam restorations. Examples of Class V matrices are shown in Chapter 18; examples of Class I matrices are shown in Chapter 17. It should also be noted that matrix application might be beneficial during tooth preparation to help protect the adjacent tooth from being damaged. The matrix, when used for this reason, would be placed on the adjacent tooth (teeth).

Mixing (Triturating) the Amalgam Material. The manufacturer's directions should be followed when mixing the amalgam material. Both the speed and time of mix are factors in the setting reaction of the material. Alterations in either may cause changes in the properties of the inserted amalgam.

Inserting the Amalgam. Manipulating the amalgam during insertion is described in Chapters 4, 17, 18, and 19. It is important to properly condense the material into the tooth preparation. Lateral condensation (facially and lingually directed condensation) is very important in the proximal box portions of the preparation to ensure confluence of the amalgam with the margins. Spherical amalgam is more easily condensed than admixed (lathe-cut) amalgam, but some practitioners prefer the handling properties of the admixed type. Both types are easily inserted.

As a general rule, smaller amalgam condensers are used first. This allows the amalgam to be properly condensed into the internal line angles and secondary retention features. Subsequently, larger condensers are used.

As stated previously, if the amalgam is to be bonded, the adhesive application and amalgam condensation must occur simultaneously. This permits intermingling of the resin (which also is bonding to the tooth structure) with the amalgam particles. When bonding an amalgam restoration, usually the priming/adhesive application for the prepared tooth structure is different than that for a composite restoration. The product manufacturer's directions must be followed. It is very important that the amalgam condensation occur before the adhesive polymerizes.

Once the amalgam is placed to slight excess with condensers, it should be pre-carve burnished with a large egg-shaped burnisher to finalize the condensation, remove excess mercury, and initiate the carving process.

Carving the Amalgam. The amalgam material selected for the restoration has a specific setting time. The insertion (condensation) and carving of the material must occur before the material has hardened so much as to be noncarvable. Once pre-carve burnishing has been done, the remainder of the accessible restoration must be contoured to achieve proper form and function. A nonbonded amalgam is relatively easy to carve. However, a bonded amalgam is more difficult because the excess polymerized adhesive resin accumulates at the margins and is harder to

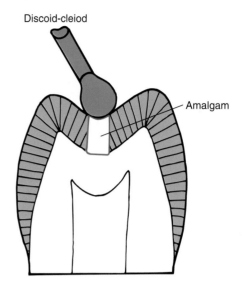

FIG. **16-15** Carving occlusal margins.

remove. Care must be taken to prevent breaking out chunks of amalgam when carving a bonded amalgam. Specific details are presented in Chapters 17 and 19.

Occlusal Areas. A discoid-cleoid instrument is used to carve the occlusal surface of an amalgam restoration. The rounded end (discoid) is positioned on the unprepared enamel adjacent to the amalgam margin and pulled parallel to the margin (Fig. 16-15). This removes any excess at the margin while not allowing the marginal amalgam to be overcarved (too much removed). The pointed end (cleoid) can be used to define the primary grooves, pits, and cuspal inclines. However, as presented earlier, an amalgam restoration is not carved with deep, acute grooves or pits because that may leave the adjacent amalgam material more subject to fracture. Once the pit and groove anatomy is initiated with the cleoid end of the instrument, the instrument is switched and the discoid end is used to smooth out the anatomic form. Some semblance of pits and grooves is necessary, however, to provide appropriate sluiceways for the escape of food from the occlusal table. Also it may be beneficial to be certain that the mesial and distal pits are carved to be inferior to the marginal ridge height, thus helping prevent food from being wedged into the occlusal embrasure. Having definite but rounded occlusal anatomy also helps result in a 90-degree amalgam margin on the occlusal surface (see Fig. 16-12, *B*).

For large Class II or foundation restorations, the initial carving of the occlusal surface should be rapid, concentrating primarily on the marginal ridge height and occlusal embrasure areas. These areas are developed with an explorer tip or carving instrument by mimicking the adjacent tooth. The explorer tip is pulled along the inside of the matrix band, creating the occlusal embrasure form. When viewed from the facial or lingual, the embrasure form created should be identical to that of the adjacent tooth, assuming the adjacent tooth has appropriate contour. Likewise the height of the amalgam marginal ridge should be the same as that of the adjacent tooth (see Figs. 17-94 and 17-103). If both of these areas are developed properly, the potential for fracture of the marginal ridge area of the restoration is significantly reduced. Placing the initial carving emphasis on the occlusal areas for a large restoration permits the operator to more quickly remove the matrix and carve any extensive axial surfaces of the restoration, especially the interproximal areas. Some of these areas may be relatively inaccessible and must be carved while the amalgam material is still not fully set. The remaining carving or contouring necessary on the occlusal surface can be done later and, if the amalgam is too hardened to carve, may require the use of rotary instruments in the handpiece.

Once the initial occlusal carving has occurred, the matrix is removed to provide access to the other areas of the restoration that require carving. Details of matrix removal are described in subsequent chapters.

Facial/Lingual Areas. Most facial and lingual areas are accessible and can be carved directly. A Hollenbeck carver is useful in carving these areas. The base of the amalgam knife (scaler 34/35) is also appropriate. For cervical areas, it is important to remove any excess and develop the proper contour of the restoration. Usually the contour will be convex; therefore care in carving this area is necessary. The convexity is developed by using both the occlusal and gingival unprepared tooth structure as guides for initiating the carving (see Fig. 18-41). The marginal areas are then blended together, resulting in the desired convexity and providing the physiologic contour that promotes good gingival health.

Proximal Embrasure Areas. The development of the occlusal embrasure already has been described. The amalgam knife (or scaler) is an excellent instrument for removing proximal excess and developing proximal contours and embrasures (see Figs.17-104 and 17-105). The knife is positioned below the gingival margin and excess is carefully shaved away. The knife is drawn occlusally to refine the proximal contour (below the contact) and the gingival embrasure form. The sharp tip of the knife also is beneficial in developing the facial and lingual embrasure forms. Care must be used to prevent carving away any of the desired proximal contact. If the amalgam is hardening, the amalgam knife must be used to shave, rather than cut the excess away. If a cutting motion is used, the possibility of breaking or chipping the amalgam is increased.

Developing a proper proximal contour and contact is very important for the physiologic health of the interproximal soft tissues. Likewise, developing a smooth proximal junction between the tooth and the amalgam is important. An amalgam overhang (excess of amalgam) can result in compromised gingival health. Voids at the cavosurface margins can result in recurrent caries.

The proximal portion of the carved amalgam can be evaluated by visual assessment (reflecting light into the contact area to confirm a proximal contact) and placement of dental floss into the area. If dental floss is used, it must be used judiciously, making sure that the contact area is not inadvertently removed. A piece of floss can be inserted through the contact and into the gingival embrasure area by initially wrapping the floss around the adjacent tooth and exerting pressure on that tooth rather than the restored tooth while moving the floss through the contact area. Once the floss is into the gingival embrasure area, it is wrapped around the restored tooth and moved occlusally and gingivally to both determine whether excess exists and smooth the proximal amalgam material. If excess material is felt along the gingival margin, the amalgam knife should be used again until a smooth margin is obtained.

Finishing the Amalgam Restoration. Once the carving is completed, the restoration is visualized from all angles and an assessment of the thoroughness of the carving is made. If a rubber dam was used, it is removed and the occlusal relationship of the restoration is assessed. Knowing the preoperative occlusal relationship of the restored and adjacent teeth is helpful in developing the appropriate contacts in the restoration; the tooth should be restored to appropriate occlusal contacts. Initially, the patient should be instructed to close very lightly, stopping when any contact is noted. At this point the operator should visually assess the occlusion. If spacing is seen between the adjacent teeth and their opposing teeth, the area of premature occlusal contact on the amalgam should be identified and relieved. Articulating paper is used to more precisely adjust the contacts until the proper occlusal relationship is generated. After the occlusion is adjusted, the discoid-cleoid can be used to smooth the accessible areas of the amalgam. A lightly moistened cotton pellet held in the operative pliers can be used to smooth the accessible parts of the restoration. If the carving and smoothing is done properly, no subsequent polishing of the restoration is needed and good long-term clinical performance will result.

Repairing an Amalgam Restoration. If an amalgam restoration fractures during insertion, the defective area must be reprepared as if it were a small restoration. Appropriate depth and retention form must be generated, sometimes entirely within the existing amalgam restoration. If necessary, another matrix must be placed. A new mix of amalgam can be condensed directly into the defect and will adhere to the amalgam already present if no intermediary material has been placed between the two amalgams. Therefore the sealer material can be placed on any exposed dentin, but it should not be placed on the amalgam preparation walls. If the amalgam has been bonded, carefully condition and apply adhesive to the exposed tooth structure in the preparation.

COMMON PROBLEMS: CAUSES AND POTENTIAL SOLUTIONS

The following is a list of common problems associated with amalgam restorations. It provides typical causes and potential solutions. Subsequent technique chapters may refer back to these.

POSTOPERATIVE SENSITIVITY

Causes of postoperative sensitivity include:

- Lack of adequate condensation, especially lateral condensation in the proximal boxes
- Lack of proper dentinal sealing with sealer or bonding system

Potential solutions include:

- Proper condensation technique
- Proper dentinal sealing technique

MARGINAL VOIDS

Causes of marginal voids include:

- Inadequate condensation
- Material pulling away or breaking from the marginal area when carving bonded amalgam

Potential solutions include:

- Proper condensation technique
- Careful carving of marginal areas, especially bonded amalgam restorations

MARGINAL RIDGE FRACTURES

Causes of marginal ridge fractures:

- Axiopulpal line angle not rounded in Class II tooth preparations
- Marginal ridge left too high
- Occlusal embrasure form incorrect
- Improper removal of matrix
- Overzealous carving

Potential solutions include:

- Proper rounding of axiopulpal line angles in Class II tooth preparations
- Creating marginal ridge height correctly, with both the adjacent tooth and occlusion
- Creating an occlusal embrasure form that mirrors the adjacent tooth

- Removing matrix correctly after defining the marginal ridge and embrasure forms

AMALGAM SCRAP AND MERCURY COLLECTION AND DISPOSAL

Causes of amalgam scrap and mercury collection and disposal problems include:

- Careless handling
- Inappropriate collection technique

Potential solutions include:

- Careful attention to proper collection and disposal
- Following the guidelines presented in Chapter 4

CONTROVERSIAL ISSUES

Because the practice of operative dentistry is dynamic, constant changes are occurring. As new products and techniques are developed, their effectiveness cannot be assessed until appropriately designed research protocols have tested their worth. Many such developments are occurring at any time, many of which do not have the necessary documentation to prove their effectiveness, even though they receive very positive publicity. Several examples of such controversies follow.

AMALGAM RESTORATION SAFETY

Chapter 4 specifically addresses this issue and presents facts that indicate amalgam restorations are safe. Likewise, the USPHS has reported the safety of amalgam restorations. Even recognizing these assessments, the mercury contained in current amalgam restorations still causes concerns, both legitimate and otherwise. Proper handling of mercury in mixing the amalgam mass, removal of old amalgam restorations, and amalgam scrap disposal are very important. Amalgam restorations have provided many millions of patients the opportunity to have teeth restored in an efficient, physiologic, and economic manner.

SPHERICAL OR ADMIXED AMALGAM

As presented earlier, both spherical and admixed amalgam types have beneficial qualities. Regardless of the advantage of one type versus the other, the choice usually is made by the dentist's preference on the handling characteristics of the material. Still, spherical materials have advantages in providing higher earlier strength and permitting the use of less pressure. Admixed materials, on the other hand, permit easier proximal contact development because of higher condensation forces.

BONDED AMALGAM RESTORATIONS

Sealing the underlying, prepared tooth structure is beneficial for any type of restoration. For an amalgam restoration, this can be accomplished without actually bonding the amalgam to the tooth. Nonbonded amalgams can have a sealed, prepared tooth structure through use of a sealer material (such as Gluma Desensitizer) or a cured resin adhesive placed before the amalgam insertion.

Bonded amalgams are indicated for large restorations that require additional retention features or strengthening of the remaining unprepared tooth structure. However, the amount of increased retention gained from bonding an amalgam is controversial. While recognizing some increase in retention is gained from bonding an amalgam, this textbook endorses the use of typical secondary retention form preparation features (e.g., grooves, locks, pins, slots) for large amalgam restorations that are bonded. Small to moderate amalgam restorations do not require bonding; in fact, many small to moderate restorations would be better indicated for composite restorations.

PROXIMAL RETENTION LOCKS

The need for proximal retention locks for all Class II amalgam tooth preparations is debatable. This textbook endorses the use of proximal retention locks for large amalgam restorations, while their use for smaller restorations is not deemed necessary. However, because correct placement of proximal retention locks is difficult, this book presents many illustrations of locks placed in smaller restorations, primarily to promote the operator gaining sufficient experience in their use.

SUMMARY

Amalgam is a very good restorative material. While there are some concerns about its use, it is a safe and effective direct restorative material. A successful amalgam restoration is still relatively easy to accomplish, and adherence to tooth preparation and material handling requirements will result in a successful restoration. Indications for the use of amalgam in posterior restorations have decreased in this textbook, but this is not because of problems with either amalgam as a material or as a restoration; it is because of the recognized benefits of bonded composite restorations.

REFERENCES

1. American Dental Association Council on Scientific Affairs: Dental amalgam: update on safety concerns, *J Am Dent Assoc* 129:494-503, 1998.
2. Ben-Amar A, Cardash HS, Judes H: The sealing of the tooth/amalgam interface by corrosion products, *J Oral Rehab* 22(2):101-104, 1995.
3. Ben-Amar A et al: Long term sealing properties of Amalgambond under amalgam restorations, *Amer J Dent* 7(3):141-143, 1994.
4. Berry TG et al: Amalgam at the new millennium, *J Am Dent Assoc* 129(11):1547-1556, 1998.
5. Boyer DB, Roth L: Fracture resistance of teeth with bonded amalgams, *Amer J Dent* 7(2):91-94, 1994.
6. Bryant RW: The strength of fifteen amalgam alloys, *Austral Dent J* 24(4):244-252, 1979.
7. Bullard RH, Leinfelder KF, Russell CM: Effect of coefficient of thermal expansion on microleakage, *J Am Dent Assoc* 116(7):871-874, 1988.
8. Collins CJ, Bryant RW, Hodge KL: A clinical evaluation of posterior composite resin restorations: 8-year findings, *J Dent* 26(4):311-317, 1998.
9. Combe EC, Burke FJT, Douglas WH: Thermal properties. In Combe EC, Burke FJT, Douglas WH, editors: *Dental biomaterials*, Boston, 1999, Kluwer Academic Publishers.
10. Corbin SB, Kohn WG: The benefits and risks of dental amalgam: current findings reviewed, *J Am Dent Assoc* 125:381-388, 1994.
11. Dunne SM, Gainsford ID, Wilson NH: Current materials and techniques for direct restorations in posterior teeth: silver amalgam: part 1, *Internat Dent J* 47(3):123-136, 1997.
12. Gorucu J, Tiritoglu M, Ozgunaltay G: Effects of preparation designs and adhesive systems on retention of class II amalgam restorations, *J Prosthet Dent* 78(3):250-254, 1997.
13. Letzel H et al: The influence of the amalgam alloy on the survival of amalgam restorations: a secondary analysis of multiple controlled clinical trials, *J Dent Res* 76(1):1787-1798, 1997.
14. Liberman R et al: Long-term sealing properties of amalgam restorations: an *in vitro* study, *Dent Mater* 5(3):168-170, 1989.
15. Mahler DB: The high-copper dental amalgam alloys, *J Dent Res* 76(1):537-421, 1997.
16. Mahler DB, Adey JD. Factors influencing the creep of dental amalgam, *J Dent Res* 70(11):1394-1400, 1991.
17. Mair LH: Ten-year clinical assessment of three posterior resin composites and two amalgams, *Quintessence Int* 29:483-490, 1998.
18. Martin JA, Bader JD: Five-year treatment outcomes for teeth with large amalgams and crowns, *Oper Dent* 22:72-78, 1997.
19. Murray GA, Yates JL: Early compressive and diametral tensile strengths of seventeen amalgam alloy systems, *J Pedodontics* 5(1):40-50, 1980.
20. Olmez A, Ulusu T: Bond strength and clinical evaluation of a new dentinal bonding agent to amalgam and resin composite, *Quintessence Int* 26(11):785-793, 1995.
21. Osborne JW: Photoelastic assessment of the expansion of direct-placement gallium restorative alloys, *Quintessence Int* 30(3):185-191, 1999.
22. Osborne JW, Summitt JB: Direct-placement gallium restorative alloy: a 3-year clinical evaluation, *Quintessence Int* 30(1):49-53, 1999.
23. Pilo R, Brosh T, Chweidan H: Cusp reinforcement by bonding of amalgam restorations, *J Dent* 26(5-6):467-472, 1998.
24. Plasmans P, Creugers N, Mulder J: Long-term survival of extensive amalgam restorations, *J Dent Res* 77(3):453-460, 1998.
25. Suchatlampong C, Goto S, Ogura H: Early compressive strength and phase-formation of dental amalgam, *Dent Mater* 14(2):143-151, 1995.
26. Venugopalan R, Broome JC, Lucas LC: The effect of water contamination on dimensional change and corrosion properties of a gallium alloy, *Dent Mater* 14(3):173-178, 1998.
27. Vrijhoef MM, Letzel H: Creep versus marginal fracture of amalgam restorations, *J Oral Rehab* 13(4):299-303, 1986.
28. Williams PT, Hedge GL: Creep-fatigue as a possible cause of dental amalgam margin failure, *J Dent Res* 64(3):470-475, 1985.
29. Winkler MM et al: Comparison of retentiveness of amalgam bonding gent types, *Oper Dent* 22(5):200-208, 1997.

17

Classes I, II, and VI Amalgam Restorations

ALDRIDGE D. WILDER, JR.

THEODORE M. ROBERSON

PATRICIA N.R. PEREIRA

ANDRÉ V. RITTER

KENNETH N. MAY, JR.*

*This author is inactive this edition. See the Acknowledgments.

INTRODUCTION TO CLASSES I, II, AND VI AMALGAM RESTORATIONS

Amalgam is used for the restoration of carious or fractured posterior teeth and in the replacement of failed restorations (see Chapter 16). If properly placed, an amalgam restoration will provide many years of service.[7,16,43,57,67,70] Currently, more posterior teeth are restored with amalgam than any other material. Understanding the physical properties of amalgam and the principles of tooth preparation is necessary to produce amalgam restorations that provide optimal service. The success of amalgam restorations depends on many factors. Unfortunately, although improved techniques and materials are available, amalgam failures occur. Much clinical time is spent replacing restorations that fail as a result of recurrent caries, marginal deterioration (i.e., ditching), fractures, or poor contours.[52,53] However, attention to detail throughout the procedure can significantly decrease the incidence of failures and extend the life of any restoration.[34,39,77] Many amalgam restorations are also replaced because of improper diagnosis.[3] Careful evaluation of existing amalgams is important because they have the potential to provide long-term clinical service and should not be replaced unless an accurate diagnosis is made.

This chapter presents the techniques and procedures that affect the quality and longevity of Classes I, II, and VI amalgam restorations (Fig. 17-1). Class I restorations restore defects on the occlusal surface of posterior teeth, the occlusal two thirds of the facial and lingual surface of molars, and the lingual surfaces of maxillary anterior teeth. Class II restorations restore defects that affect one or both of the proximal surfaces of the posterior teeth. Class VI restorations restore those rare defects affecting the cusp tips of posterior teeth or the incisal edges of interior teeth.

PERTINENT MATERIAL QUALITIES AND PROPERTIES

Pertinent material qualities and properties for Classes I, II, and VI amalgam restorations include:

- Strength
- Longevity
- Ease of use
- Clinically proven success

In addition, amalgam is the only restorative material with an interfacial seal that improves over time.[9,29,33] Amalgam may be used for almost any Class I, II, or VI restoration, but its specific indications are presented in the following section. (See Chapter 16 for a more detailed discussion of the pertinent material qualities and properties for amalgam.)

INDICATIONS

The following is a list of clinical indications for amalgam restorations in Classes I, II, and VI. Amalgam is indicated in:

- Moderate-to-large restorations
- Restorations that are not in highly esthetic areas of the mouth
- Restorations that have heavy occlusal contacts
- Restorations that cannot be well isolated
- Restorations that extend onto the root surface
- Foundations
- Abutment teeth for a removable partial denture
- Temporary or caries control restorations

CONTRAINDICATIONS

Although amalgam has no specific contraindications for use in Classes I, II, and VI restorations, the following is a list of general contraindications that may be considered. Amalgam may be contraindicated in:

- Esthetically prominent areas of posterior teeth
- Small-to-moderate Classes I and II restorations that can be well isolated
- Small Class VI restorations

ADVANTAGES

The primary advantages are the ease of use and the simplicity of the procedure. As noted in the following

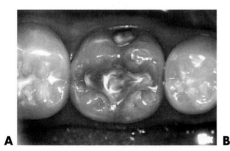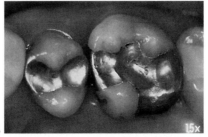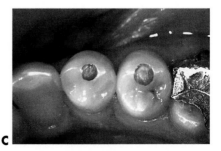

FIG. **17-1** Clinical examples of Classes I, II, and VI amalgam restorations. **A,** Class I amalgam in the occlusal surface of the first molar. **B,** Class II amalgams in a premolar and molar. **C,** Class VI amalgams in premolars.

sections, the placing and contouring of amalgam restorations are generally easier than that for composite restorations.[15] (The general advantages of amalgam restorations were presented in Chapter 16.)

DISADVANTAGES

The primary disadvantages of using amalgam for Classes I, II, and VI restorations are:

- More complex tooth preparation required for an amalgam restoration compared to a composite restoration
- Potential nonesthetic appearance

The general disadvantages of amalgam restorations were presented in Chapter 16.)

CLINICAL TECHNIQUE FOR CLASS I AMALGAM RESTORATIONS

As presented earlier, Class I refers to restorations on the occlusal surfaces of posterior teeth, the occlusal two thirds of facial and lingual surfaces of posterior teeth, and the lingual surfaces of anterior teeth. Although most small Class I restorations will be restored with a composite restoration, amalgam is still indicated in more extensive Class I restorations. This section describes the use of amalgam in both conservative and extensive Class I restorations.

CONSERVATIVE CLASS I AMALGAM RESTORATIONS

Conservative tooth preparation is recommended to protect the pulp,[24] preserve the strength of the tooth,[1,51] and reduce deterioration of the amalgam restoration.[6,66] This section describes conservative Class I tooth preparations for amalgam restorations. Although composite may be the restorative material of choice for most small Class I restorations, the following information describing the technique for a small, conservative Class I amalgam restoration is presented for several reasons. First, amalgam can be and has been successfully used for small Class I restorations. Second, the procedural description for a small, conservative Class I amalgam restoration more clearly and simply presents the basic information relating to the entire amalgam restoration technique, including tooth preparation and placement and contouring of the restoration. This basic procedural information then can be more easily expanded to describe extensive Class I restorations, which are better indications for use of amalgam. The maxillary first premolar is used for illustration in this section. Management of extensive occlusal caries and other Class I amalgam restoration are presented later in this chapter.

Initial Clinical Procedures. Generally, isolation of the operating site with the rubber dam is recommended.[2] The rubber dam can be applied in the few minutes nec-

essary for onset of profound anesthesia before initiating the tooth preparation. For a single maxillary tooth, where caries is not extensive, adequate moisture control may be achieved with cotton rolls and profound anesthesia. Rubber dam isolation is strongly recommended when removing deep caries judged to be less than a millimeter from the pulp. Moisture control is also necessary during amalgam condensation.[2] A preoperative assessment of the occlusal relationship of the involved and adjacent teeth is also necessary (see Chapter 10). (A more detailed review of the initial procedures for direct restorations, in general, and amalgam restorations, specifically, is presented in Chapters 10 and 16.)

Tooth Preparation. This section describes the specific technique for preparing the tooth for a conservative Class I amalgam restoration. It is divided into initial and final stages (see Chapter 6).

Initial Tooth Preparation. Initial tooth preparation is defined as establishing the outline form by extension of the external walls to sound tooth structure, while maintaining a specified, limited depth and providing resistance and retention forms (see Chapter 6).

The outline form for the Class I occlusal amalgam tooth preparation should include only the faulty, defective occlusal pits and fissures (in a way that sharp angles in the marginal outline are avoided). Occasionally the marginal outline for maxillary premolars is somewhat butterfly shaped, because of extension to include the developmental fissures facially and lingually. The ideal outline form for a very conservative amalgam restoration (Fig. 17-2, *A*) incorporates the following resistance form principles that are basic to all amalgam tooth preparations of occlusal surfaces. These principles allow the operator to position margins in areas that are sound and subject to minimal forces, while conserving structure to maintain the strength and health of the tooth.

Resistance principles include:

- Extending around the cusps to conserve tooth structure and prevent the internal line angles from approaching the pulp horns too closely
- Keeping the facial and lingual margin extensions as minimal as possible between the central groove and the cusp tips
- Extending the outline to include fissures, thereby placing the margins on relatively smooth, sound tooth structure
- Minimally extending into the marginal ridges (only enough to include the defect) without removing dentinal support
- Eliminating a weak wall of enamel by joining two outlines that come close together (i.e., less than 0.5 mm apart)
- Extending the outline form to include enamel undermined by caries (in some bonded amalgam restora-

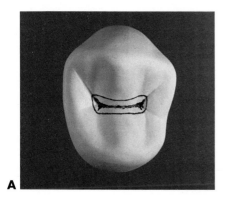
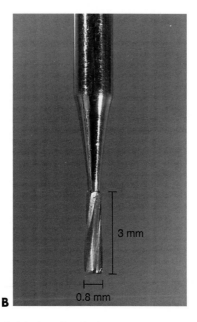
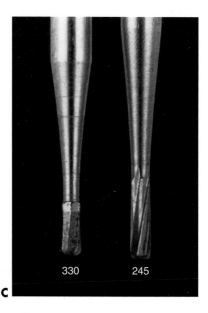

FIG. **17-2** Outline and entry. **A,** Ideal outline includes all occlusal pits and fissures. **B,** Dimensions of head of a No. 245 bur. **C,** No. 330 and No. 245 burs compared.

tions, weakened enamel may be strengthened by the bonding process)

- Using enameloplasty on the terminal ends of shallow fissures to conserve tooth structure
- Establishing an optimal, conservative depth of the pulpal wall

A No. 245 bur with a head length of 3 mm and a tip diameter of 0.8 mm or a smaller No. 330 bur is recommended to prepare the conservative Class I tooth preparation (see Fig. 17-2, *B* and *C*). The silhouette of the No. 245 inverted cone bur reveals sides slightly convergent toward the shank (this produces an occlusal convergence of the facial and lingual preparation walls, providing adequate retention form for the tooth preparation). The slightly rounded corners of the end of the No. 245 bur produce slightly rounded internal line angles that render the tooth more resistant to fracture from occlusal force.[80] The No. 330 bur is a smaller and pear-shaped version of the No. 245 bur. It is indicated for the most conservative amalgam preparations (see Fig. 17-2, *C*).

Begin the Class I occlusal tooth preparation by entering the deepest or most carious pit with a punch cut using the No. 245 carbide bur at high speed with air-water spray.[24] A punch cut is performed by orienting the bur so that its long axis parallels the long axis of the tooth crown (Fig. 17-3, *A* and *B*), and then the bur is inserted directly into the faulty pit. When the pits are equally faulty, enter the distal pit as illustrated. Entering the distal pit first provides increased visibility for the mesial extension. The bur should be positioned so that its distal aspect is directly over the distal pit, thereby minimizing extension into the marginal ridge (see Fig. 17-3, *C*).

The bur should be rotating when it is applied to the tooth and should not stop rotating until it is removed from the tooth. As the bur enters the pit, the proper depth of 1.5 mm (one half the length of the cutting portion of the bur) should be established. The 1.5 mm pulpal depth is measured at the central fissure (see Fig. 17-3, *D* and *E*). Depending of the cuspal incline, the depth of the prepared external walls will be 1.5 to 2 mm (see Fig. 17-3, *D* and *E*). The desired pulpal depth is usually 0.1 to 0.2 mm into dentin. The length of the blades of an unfamiliar entry bur should be measured before it is used as a depth gauge.

Distal extension into the distal marginal ridge to include a fissure or caries occasionally requires a slight tilting of the bur distally (no more than 10 degrees). This creates a slight occlusal divergence to the distal wall to prevent undermining the marginal ridge of its dentin support (Fig. 17-4, *A* through *C*). Because the facial and lingual prepared walls will converge, this slight divergence does not present any retention form concerns. For premolars, the distance from the margin of such an extension to the proximal surface usually should not be less than 1.6 mm or two diameters of the end of the No. 245 bur (see Fig. 17-4, *B*) measured from a tangent to the proximal surface (i.e., the proximal surface height of contour). For molars, this minimal distance is 2 mm. A minimal distal (or mesial) extension often does not require changing the orientation of the bur's axis from being parallel to the long axis of the tooth crown; thus the mesial and distal walls will be parallel to the long axis of the tooth crown (or slightly convergent occlusally).

While maintaining the bur's orientation and depth, extend the preparation distofacially or distolingually to include any fissures that radiate from the pit (see

FIG. **17-3** **A,** No. 245 bur oriented parallel to long axis of tooth crown for entry as viewed from lingual aspect. **B,** Bur positioned for entry as viewed from distal aspect. **C,** Bur positioned over more carious pit (distal) for entry. Distal aspect of bur is positioned over distal pit. **D,** Mesiodistal longitudinal section. Relationship of head of No. 245 bur to excised central fissure and cavosurface margin at ideal pulpal floor depth. **E,** Faciolingual longitudinal section. The dotted line indicates long axis of tooth and direction of bur.

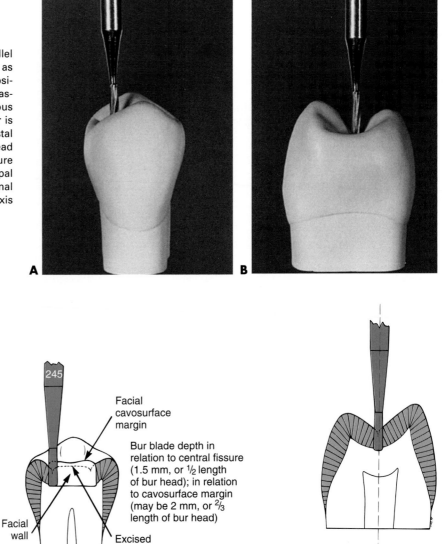

Fig. 17-4, *D*). Care should be taken not to undermine the marginal ridge. However, when these fissures require extensions of more than a few tenths of a millimeter, consideration should be given to changing to a smaller diameter bur, such as a No. 169L or No. 329, or to using enameloplasty. Both of these approaches conserve tooth structure and, hence, minimize weakening the tooth.

Continue to maintain the bur's orientation and depth and, with intermittent pressure, extend along the central fissure toward the mesial pit, following the DEJ. This may create a flat pulpal floor. However, the pulpal floor should follow the DEJ to maintain a more uniform pulpal floor depth (see Fig. 17-4, *E*). When the central fissure has minimal caries, one pass along the fissure at the prescribed depth provides the desired minimal width to the isthmus. Ideally the width of the isthmus need be no more than the diameter of the bur. It has been demonstrated that an isthmus width of one fourth the distance

between the cusp tips does not reduce the strength of the tooth.[41,90] As previously described for the distal margin, the orientation of the bur should not change as it approaches the mesial pit if the mesial extension is minimal. If the fissure extends farther onto the marginal ridge, the long axis of the bur should be changed to establish a slight occlusal divergence to the mesial wall if the marginal ridge would be otherwise undermined of its dentinal support. Fig. 17-5, *A* through *C*, illustrates the correct and incorrect preparation of the mesial and distal walls. It should be emphasized that minimal faciolingual width of the outline form and minimal occlusal convergence of the facial and lingual walls is desired. This is ideally achieved when the bur makes only one pass along the central fissure.

The remainder of any occlusal enamel defects is included in the outline, and the facial and lingual walls are extended, if necessary, to remove enamel

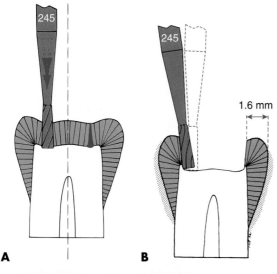

A

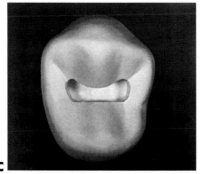

B

1.6 mm

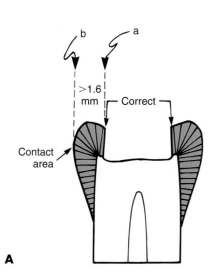

C

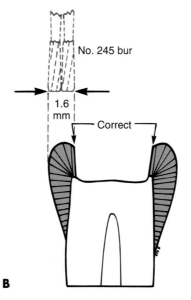

D

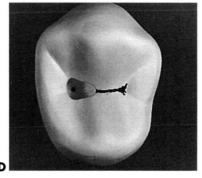

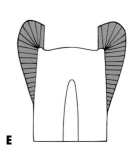

E

FIG. 17-4 **A,** Enter pit with punch cut to a depth of 1.5 to 2 mm or one half to two thirds the head length of bur. (The 1.5 mm depth is measured at central fissure; the measurement of same entry cut [but of prepared external wall] is up to 2.0 mm.) **B,** Incline bur distally to establish proper occlusal divergence to distal wall to prevent removal of dentin supporting marginal ridge enamel when pulpal floor is in dentin and distal extension is necessary to include a fissure or caries. For such an extension on premolars, the distance from margin to proximal surface (i.e., imaginary projection) must not be less than 1.6 mm (i.e., two diameters of end of bur). **C,** Occlusal view of initial tooth preparation that has mesial and distal walls that diverge occlusally. **D,** Distofacial and distolingual fissures that radiate from pit are included before extending along central fissure. **E,** Mesiodistal longitudinal section. Pulpal floors are generally flat but may follow the rise and fall of occlusal surface.

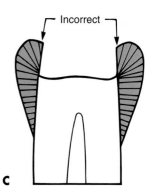

A

B

C

FIG. 17-5 Direction of mesial and distal walls is influenced by remaining thickness of marginal ridge as measured from mesial or distal margin (*a*) to proximal surface (i.e., imaginary projection of proximal surface) (*b*). **A,** Mesial and distal walls should converge occlusally when distance from *a* to *b* is greater than 1.6 mm. **B,** However, when operator judges that extension will leave only 1.6-mm thickness (two diameters of No. 245 bur) of marginal ridge (i.e., premolars) as illustrated here and in Fig. 17-4, *B* and *C*, the mesial and distal walls must diverge occlusally to conserve ridge-supporting dentin. **C,** Extending mesial or distal wall to two-diameter limit without diverging wall occlusally will undermine marginal-ridge enamel.

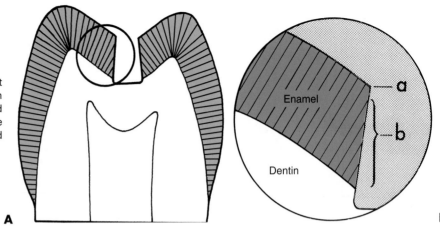

FIG. **17-6** **A** and **B,** Ideal and strongest enamel margin is formed by full-length enamel rods (*a*) resting on sound dentin supported on preparation side by shorter rods, also resting on sound dentin (*b*).

undermined by caries.[25] The strongest and ideal enamel margin should be made up of full-length enamel rods resting on sound dentin, supported on the preparation side by shorter rods, also resting on sound dentin (Fig. 17-6).

The conservative Class I tooth preparation should have an outline form with gently flowing curves and distinct cavosurface margins. For the conservative Class I preparation a faciolingual width of no more than 1 to 1.5 mm and a depth of 1.5 to 2 mm are considered ideal. The pulpal floor, depending on the enamel thickness, is usually in dentin (see Fig. 17-4, *C*). Such conservative preparation saves tooth structure, minimizing pulpal ir-ritation and leaving the remaining tooth crown as strong as possible.[26,40] Although conservation of tooth structure is very important, convenience form requires that the extent of the preparation provides adequate ac-cess and visibility.

This completes the initial tooth preparation for the Class I amalgam tooth preparation. Extension should ensure that all caries is removed from the peripheral dentinoenamel junction (DEJ). For initial tooth prepara-tion the pulpal floor should remain at the initial ideal depth, even if restorative material or caries remains (Fig. 17-7). The remaining caries (and usually the old restorative material) will be removed during final tooth preparation.

To summarize, primary resistance form is provided by:

- Sufficient area or areas of relatively flat pulpal floor in sound tooth structure to resist forces directed in the long axis of the tooth and provide a strong, stable seat for the restoration
- Minimal extension of external walls, which reduces weakening the tooth
- Strong, ideal enamel margins (defined and illustrated previously)
- Sufficient depth (i.e., 1.5 mm) to result in adequate thickness of the restoration, providing resistance to fracture and wear

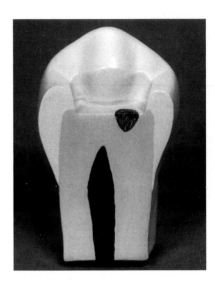

FIG. **17-7** Mesiodistal longitudinal section showing example when pulpal floor is in dentin and caries is exposed after ini-tial tooth preparation. Note also that the carious lesion is sur-rounded by sound dentin on the pulpal floor for resistance form.

The parallelism or slight occlusal convergence of two or more opposing, external walls provides the primary retention form.

Usually the No. 245 bur is used for extensions into the mesiofacial and distofacial fissures. During such exten-sions the remaining length of the fissure can be viewed in cross-section by looking at the wall being extended. When the remaining fissure is no deeper than one quar-ter to one third the thickness of the enamel, enamelo-plasty is indicated. Enameloplasty refers to eliminating the developmental fault by removing it with the side of a flame-shaped diamond stone, leaving a smooth surface (Fig. 17-8, *A* through *C*). This procedure fre-quently reduces the need for further extension into the fissures with the No. 245 bur, thereby conserving tooth structure. The extent to which enameloplasty should be used cannot be determined exactly until the process of

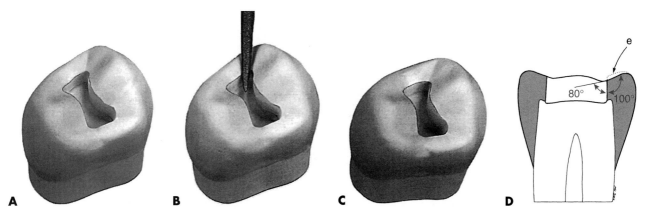

FIG. **17-8** Enameloplasty. **A,** Developmental fault at terminal end of fissure. **B,** Fine-grit diamond stone in position to remove fault. **C,** Smooth surface after enameloplasty. **D,** Cavosurface angle should not exceed 100 degrees, and marginal-amalgam angle should not be less than 80 degrees. Enamel external surface (*e*) before enameloplasty.

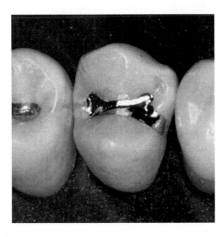

FIG. **17-9** Mesial fissure that cannot be eliminated by enameloplasty may be included in preparation if margins can be lingual of contact.

extending into the fissured area occurs, at which time the depth of the fissure into the enamel can be observed. The surface left by enameloplasty should meet the tooth preparation wall, preferably with a cavosurface angle no greater than approximately 100 degrees. This would produce a distinct margin for amalgam of no less than 80 degrees (see Fig. 17-8, *D*). During carving, amalgam should be removed from areas of enameloplasty. Otherwise, thin amalgam left in these areas may fracture because of its low edge strength. Thus enameloplasty does not extend the outline form for amalgam preparations.

If enameloplasty is unsuccessful in eliminating a mesial (or distal) fissure that extends to the crest of a marginal ridge or beyond, the operator has one of three alternatives:

1. Make no further change in the outline form
2. Extend through the marginal ridge when margins will be lingual to the contact (Fig. 17-9)

3. Include the fissure in a conservative Class II tooth preparation.

The first alternative usually should be strongly considered, except for patients at high risk for caries. Enameloplasty is not indicated if an area of centric contact is involved. In this case, the choices are either to consider the preparation completed (an option for patients at low risk for caries) or to extend the preparation to include the fissure as previously described.

Final Tooth Preparation. Final tooth preparation includes: (1) removal of remaining defective enamel and infected dentin on the pulpal floor; (2) pulp protection, where indicated; (3) procedures for finishing external walls; and (4) final procedures of cleaning and inspecting the prepared tooth. The use of desensitizers or bonding systems is considered the first step of the restorative technique.

Remaining enamel pit-and-fissure in the pulpal floor should be removed. If several enamel pit and fissure remnants remain in the floor, or if a central fissure remnant extends over most of the floor, deepen the floor with the No. 245 bur to eliminate the fault or faults or to uncover the caries to a maximal-preparation depth of 2 mm (Fig. 17-10). If the pit-and-fissure remnants are few and small, remove them with a suitably sized, round carbide bur (Fig. 17-11). Removal of the remaining infected dentin (i.e., caries that extends pulpally from the established pulpal floor) is best accomplished using a discoid-type spoon excavator or a slowly revolving, round carbide bur of appropriate size (Fig. 17-12, *A* and *B*). Using the largest instrument that fits the carious area is safest because it is least likely to penetrate the tooth uncontrollably. When removing infected dentin, stop the excavation when tooth structure feels hard or firm (i.e., the same feel as sound dentin). This often occurs before all lightly stained or discolored dentin is removed.[23] Ensure that caries is removed from the peripheral DEJ where it

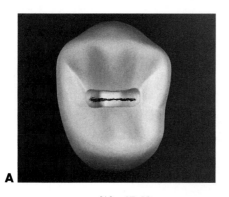
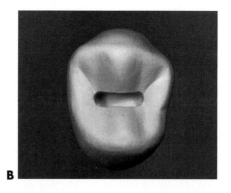
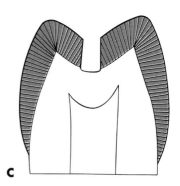

FIG. **17-10** Removal of enamel fissure extending over most of pulpal floor. **A,** Full-length occlusal fissure remnant remaining on pulpal floor after initial tooth preparation. **B** and **C,** Pulpal floor is deepened to maximal depth of 2 mm to eliminate the fissure or uncover dentinal caries.

FIG. **17-11** Removal of enamel pit and fissure and infected dentin that is limited to a few small pit-and-fissure remnants. **A,** Two pit remnants remain on pulpal floor after initial tooth preparation. **B,** Defective enamel and infected dentin have been removed.

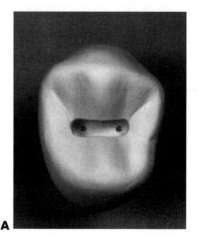
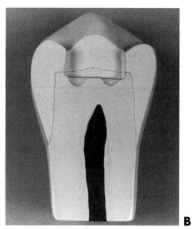

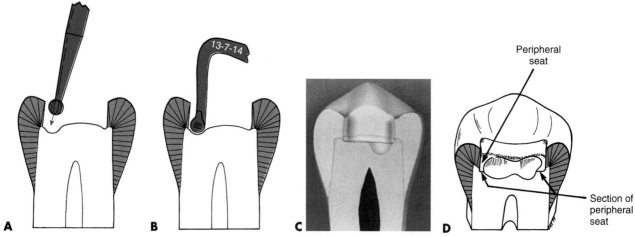

FIG. **17-12** Removal of dentinal caries is accomplished with round burs **(A)** or spoon excavators **(B)**. **C** and **D,** Resistance form may be improved with flat floor peripheral to excavated area or areas.

is less visible than on the pulpal floor. A caries-detecting solution may be helpful in determining adequate excavation. A sharp explorer or hand instrument is more reliable than a rotating bur in judging the adequacy of removal of infected dentin. However, these instruments should be used judiciously in areas of possible pulpal exposure.

The removal of carious dentin should not further affect resistance form because the periphery will not need further extension. In addition, it should not affect resistance form if the restoration will rest on a flat floor peripheral to the excavated area or areas. The flat floor should be at the previously described initial pulpal floor depth of 1.5 to 2 mm and in sound enamel or dentin (see

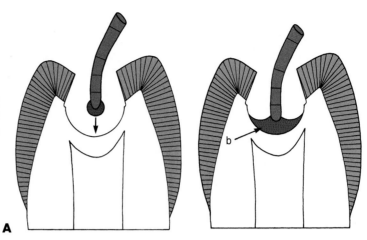

FIG. **17-13** Base application. **A,** Inserting RMGI with Williams periodontal probe. **B,** In moderately deep excavations a base (*b*) thickness of 0.5 to 0.75 mm is indicated.

Fig. 17-12, *C*). If a flat seat cannot be established around the entire circumference of the excavation or excavations, then an attempt could be made to establish flat seats at this depth with the No. 245 bur equally spaced around the periphery of the excavation to promote resistance form (see Fig. 17-12, *D*).

If the tooth preparation is of ideal or shallow depth, no liner or base is indicated. In deeper carious excavations (where the remaining dentin thickness is judged to be 0.5 to 1.0 mm),[31,32] place a thin layer (i.e., 0.5 to 0.75 mm) of a light-cured, resin-modified glass-ionomer (RMGI) base. The RMGI base insulates the pulp from thermal changes, bonds to the dentin, releases fluoride, and is strong enough to resist the forces of condensation.[22, 32] The RMGI is picked up on the tip of a cement-placing instrument or blunt-tipped periodontal probe and inserted in small increments. The RMGI should flow when it is touched to the dentin surface. It should be placed only over the deepest portion of the excavation. The entire dentin surface should not be covered (Fig. 17-13). Dentin peripheral to the liner should be available for bonding (if indicated) and for support of the restoration.[73] Use of liners and bases for even deeper excavations will be presented in a later section.

The external walls have already been finished during earlier steps in this conservative tooth preparation for amalgam. An occlusal cavosurface bevel is contraindicated in the tooth preparation for an amalgam restoration.[50] It is important to provide an approximate 90- to 100-degree cavosurface angle,[25] which should result in 80- to 90-degree amalgam at the margins (see Fig. 17-21, *F*). This butt joint margin of enamel and amalgam is the strongest for both. Amalgam is a brittle material with low edge strength and tends to chip under occlusal stress if its angle at the margins is less than 80 degrees.

Every completed tooth preparation should be inspected and cleaned before restoration. The tooth preparation should be free of debris after rinsing the tooth with the air-water syringe. Disinfectants are available for cleaning tooth preparations,[27,91] but are usually considered unnecessary. A cotton pledget or commercially available applicator tip moistened with water only is generally used.

Other Conservative Class I Amalgam Preparations. Several other conservative Class I amalgam preparations may be restored with composite, because of their small size and the maximal thickness of enamel available for bonding around their periphery. However, these preparations could be restored with amalgam. The preparations include:

- The facial pit of the mandibular molar
- The lingual pit of the maxillary lateral incisor
- The occlusal pits of the mandibular first premolar
- The occlusal pits and fissures of the maxillary first molar
- The occlusal pits and fissures of the mandibular second premolar

These preparations may be accomplished with a No. 245 bur or, if the lesion is very small, a No. 330 or 169L bur may be used. Depending on the extent of the caries and the angulation of the walls, retention grooves may be added with a No. ¼ or 33½ bur. Otherwise the techniques for these preparations are similar to those previously described. Examples of some of these types of preparations and restorations are illustrated in Figs. 17-14 to 17-19.

Restorative Technique

Placing a Sealer or Adhesive System. As stated previously, adhesives are not routinely used with conservative amalgam restorations. They are used more appropriately for larger restorations where bonding may increase the resistance and retention forms. However, a dentin desensitizer is placed in the preparation before amalgam condensation for nonbonded amalgam restorations (Fig. 17-20). It is recommended instead of traditional varnish to better seal the prepared dentin. The dentin desensitizer is rubbed onto the prepared tooth surface for 30 seconds, dried, and then the amalgam is condensed into place. Dentin desensitizer precipitates protein and forms lamellar plugs in the dentinal tubules.[75] These

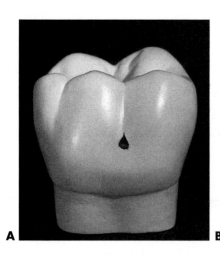
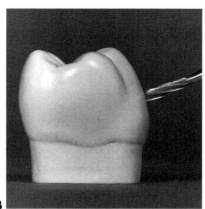
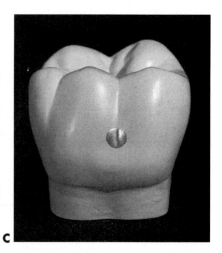

FIG. **17-14** Mandibular molar. **A,** Carious (or at risk for caries) facial pit. **B,** Position bur perpendicular to tooth surface for entry. **C,** Outline of restoration.

FIG. **17-15** Carious (or at risk for caries) lingual pit and fissure and restoration on maxillary lateral incisor.

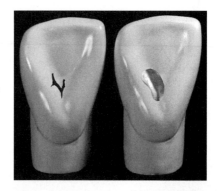

FIG. **17-16** Maxillary lateral incisor. **A,** Preoperative radiograph of dens in dente. **B,** Radiograph of restoration after 13 years. *(Courtesy of Dr. Ludwig Scott.)*

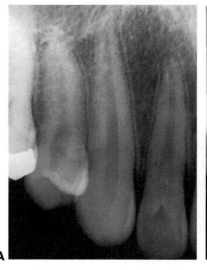
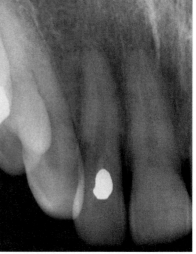

plugs are thought to be responsible for reducing dentin permeability and sensitivity. Dentin may not be totally sealed by a desensitizing agent, because no hybrid layer is formed. Because these desensitizing agents represent only a single component of an adhesive system (i.e., primers) the etching and adhesive steps of typical adhesive systems are omitted.

If amalgam adhesives are to be used, a separate desensitizing agent is usually unnecessary. Amalgam adhesives can increase the fracture resistance of the restored tooth[20, 64] and reduce microleakage.[5,47,63,76] However, no difference has been found between bonded and nonbonded amalgam restorations in vivo after 1 to 5 years.[8,19,48] In addition, there is concern about the long-

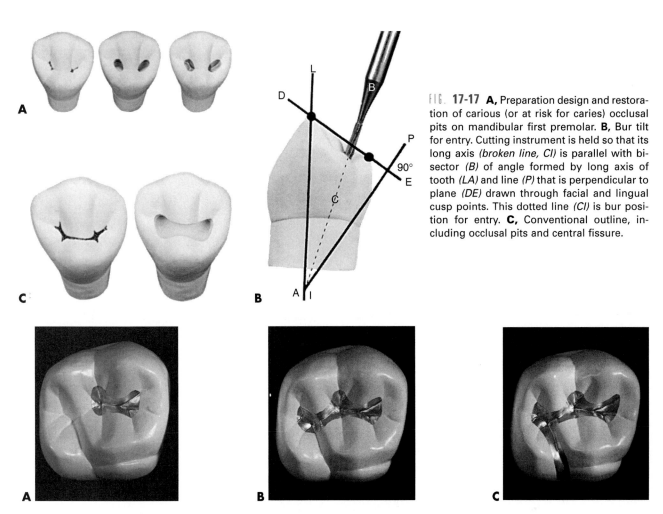

FIG. **17-17** **A,** Preparation design and restoration of carious (or at risk for caries) occlusal pits on mandibular first premolar. **B,** Bur tilt for entry. Cutting instrument is held so that its long axis *(broken line, CI)* is parallel with bisector *(B)* of angle formed by long axis of tooth *(LA)* and line *(P)* that is perpendicular to plane *(DE)* drawn through facial and lingual cusp points. This dotted line *(CI)* is bur position for entry. **C,** Conventional outline, including occlusal pits and central fissure.

FIG. **17-18** Maxillary first molar. **A,** Outline necessary to include mesial and central pits connected by fissure. **B,** Preparation outline extended from outline in **(A)** to include distal pit and connecting deep fissure in oblique ridge. **C,** Preparation outline extended from outline in **(B)** to include distal oblique and lingual fissures.

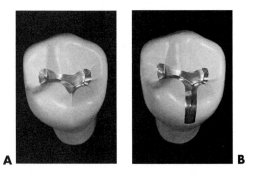

FIG. **17-19** Mandibular second premolar. **A,** Typical occlusal outline. **B,** Extension through lingual ridge enamel is necessary when enameloplasty does not eliminate lingual fissure.

term durability of the bonding resin[33,49] and about whether the bonding resin may interfere with the self-sealing capability of the amalgam.[44]

The application of the amalgam adhesive requires several steps: etching the preparation, rinsing, applying the primer and adhesive, and immediately condensing the amalgam, which permits the adhesive to interlock mechanically with the amalgam. The specific technique for use of amalgam adhesives is described later.

Placing a Matrix. Generally, matrices will not be necessary for a conservative Class I amalgam restoration except as specified in later sections.

Inserting the Amalgam. To promote mercury hygiene and minimize mercury exposure in the dental office, precautions should be taken to protect the patient and the dental staff.[11] When removing an amalgam restoration, a rubber dam should be in place and air-water spray and high-volume evacuation should be used. Air-water spray and high-volume evacuation should also be used when recontouring or polishing an amalgam restoration. Goggles and disposable facemasks should be worn to reduce hazards associated with flying particles and the inhalation of amalgam dust. Reusable amalgam capsules that allow mercury leakage during trituration should not be used. Amalgamators that

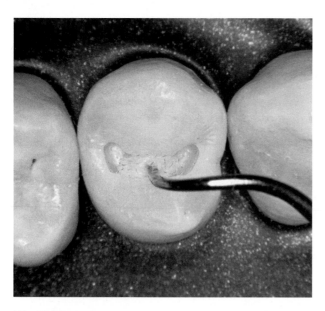

FIG. **17-20** Use explorer tip, applicator tip, or microbrush to apply the dentin desensitizer throughout tooth preparation.

completely enclose the arms and amalgam capsule during trituration should be used. Free mercury and amalgam scraps should be stored in an unbreakable, tightly closed container away from any source of heat. Because mercury vaporizes at room temperature, operatories should be well ventilated to minimize the mercury level in the air. An annual mercury assessment for personnel regularly employed in the dental office is encouraged. Disposal of scrap amalgam should be in accordance with local and state environmental standards.

Select an alloy certified by the American Dental Association (ADA). Because of its superior clinical performance, high-copper amalgam is recommended. Alloys are commercially available in powder, tablet, and preproportioned forms. Most operators prefer disposable capsules for: (1) consistency of mix because the alloy and mercury are preweighed and (2) their contribution to mercury hygiene. Preproportioned, disposable capsules are available in sizes ranging from 400 to 800 mg. Some precapsulated brands require activation of the capsules before trituration. Amalgam should be triturated (i.e., mixed) according to the manufacturer's directions. It is often necessary to make several mixes to complete the restoration, particularly for large preparations. Large tooth preparations often require two or more capsules. Empty the triturated amalgam into a Dappen dish or an amalgam well. It is not necessary to squeeze excess mercury (using an amalgam cloth) from the mix when using controlled mercury systems (Fig. 17-21, *A*). Correctly mixed amalgam should not be dry and crumbly. It will have a minimal, yet sufficient, "wetness" to aid in achieving a homogeneous and well-adapted restoration.[2]

The principle objectives during insertion of amalgam are to condense the amalgam to adapt it to the prepara-

tion walls and matrix and produce a restoration free of voids and have as low as possible mercury content in the restoration to improve strength and decrease corrosion. Condensation of amalgam that contains spherical particles requires larger condensers than are commonly used for admixed amalgam. Smaller condensers tend to penetrate a mass of spherical amalgam, resulting in little or no effective force to compact or adapt the amalgam within the preparation. In contrast, smaller condensers are indicated for the initial increments of admixed amalgam because it is more resistant to condensation pressure.

Before inserting the amalgam, review the outline of the tooth preparation to form a mental image that will aid later in carving the amalgam to the cavosurface margin and remembering the preoperative occlusal contact locations (see Fig. 17-21, *B*). Use an amalgam carrier to transfer amalgam to the tooth preparation. Increments extruded from the carrier should be smaller (often only half or less of a full-carrier tip) for a small preparation, particularly during the initial insertion. Use a flat-faced, circular or elliptic condenser to condense the amalgam over the pulpal floor of the preparation. Be careful to condense the amalgam into the pulpal line angles (see Fig. 17-21, *C*). The initial condenser should be small enough to condense into the line angles but large enough not to "poke holes" in the amalgam mass. Usually a smaller condenser is used while filling the preparation and a larger one for overpacking. Thoroughly condense each portion extruded from the carrier before placing the next increment. Each condensed increment should fill only one third to one half the preparation depth. Each condensing stroke should overlap the previous condensing stroke to ensure that the entire mass is well condensed. The condensation pressure required will depend on the amalgam used and the diameter of the condenser nib. Condensers with larger-diameter nibs require greater condensation pressure. The preparation should be overpacked 1 mm or more using heavy pressure (see Fig. 17-21, *D*). This will ensure that the cavosurface margins are completely covered with well-condensed amalgam. Final condensation over cavosurface margins should be done perpendicular to the external enamel surface adjacent to the margins.

Condensation of a mix should be completed within the time specified by the manufacturer (usually $2\frac{1}{2}$ to $3\frac{1}{2}$ minutes). Otherwise, crystallization of the unused portion will be too advanced to react properly (i.e., chemically bond) with the condensed portion. Discard the mix if it becomes dry, and quickly make another mix to continue the insertion.

Precarve burnishing is a form of condensation. As stated previously, tooth preparations should be overfilled with amalgam. To ensure that the marginal amalgam is well condensed before carving, the overpacked amalgam should be burnished immediately with a large burnisher,

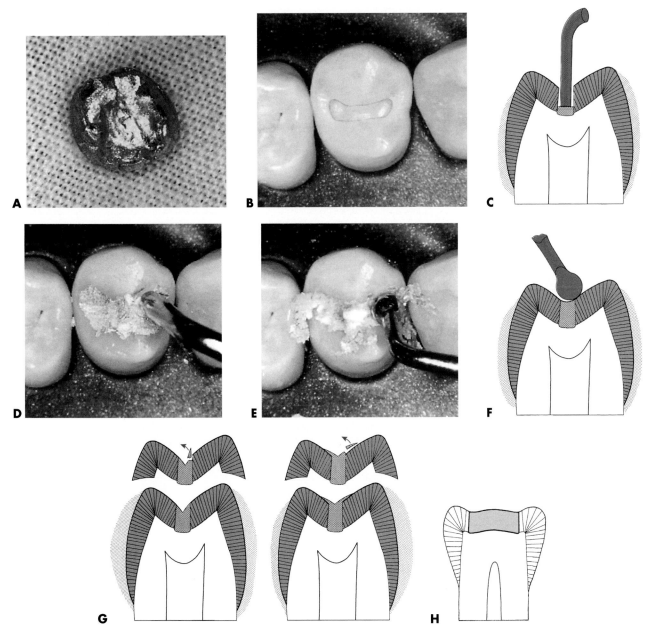

FIG. **17-21** Restoration of occlusal tooth preparation. **A,** Properly triturated amalgam is a homogeneous mass with slightly reflective surface. It flattens slightly if dropped on a table top. **B,** Operator should have a mental image of outline form of preparation before condensing amalgam to aid in locating cavosurface margins during carving procedure. **C,** Amalgam should be inserted incrementally and condensed with overlapping strokes. **D,** Tooth preparation should be overpacked to ensure well-condensed marginal amalgam that is not mercury rich. **E,** Precarve burnishing with large burnisher is a form of condensation. **F,** Carver should rest partially on external tooth surface adjacent to margins to prevent overcarving. **G,** Deep occlusal grooves invite chipping of amalgam at margins. Thin portions of amalgam left on external surfaces soon break away, giving the appearance that amalgam has grown out of preparation. **H,** Carve fossae slightly deeper than proximal marginal ridges.

using heavy strokes mesiodistally and faciolingually. To maximize its effectiveness, the burnisher head should be large enough that in the final strokes it will contact the cusp slopes but not the margins (see Fig. 17-21, *E*). Precarve burnishing produces denser amalgam at the mar-

gins of occlusal preparations restored with high-copper amalgam alloys and initiates carving.[4,46]

Contouring and Finishing the Amalgam. With care, carving may begin immediately after condensation. Sharp discoid-cleoid instruments of suitable sizes are

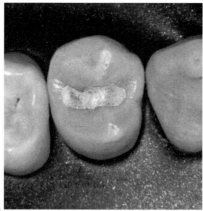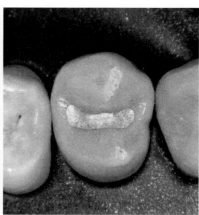

FIG. **17-22 A,** Undercarved amalgam with flash beyond the margins. Note that restoration outline is irregular and larger than preparation outline in Fig. 17-21, *B.* **B,** Correctly carved amalgam restoration.

A   **B**

recommended carvers. Use the larger discoid-cleoid instrument (No. 3-6) first, followed by the smaller instrument (No. 4-5) in regions not accessible to the larger instrument. All carving should be done with the edge of the blade perpendicular to the margins as the instrument is moved parallel to the margins. Part of the edge of the carving blade should rest on the unprepared tooth surface adjacent to the preparation margin (see Fig. 17-21, *F*). Using this surface as a guide helps to prevent overcarving the amalgam at the margins and to produce a continuity of surface contour across the margins.

Deep occlusal grooves should not be carved into the restoration, because these may thin the amalgam at the margins, invite chipping, and weaken the restoration (see Fig. 17-21, *G*). Undercarving leaves thin portions of amalgam (subject to fracture) on the unprepared tooth surface. Such margins give the appearance that the amalgam has expanded beyond the preparation. The thin portion of amalgam extending beyond the margin is referred to as *flash*. The mesial and distal fossae should be carved slightly deeper than the proximal marginal ridges (see Fig. 17-21, *H*).

After carving, the outline of the amalgam margin should reflect the contour and location of the prepared cavosurface margin, revealing a regular (i.e., not ragged) outline with gentle curves. It is important to recall the mental image of the preparation outline form. An amalgam outline that is larger or irregular is undercarved and requires further carving or finishing (Fig. 17-22). An amalgam restoration that is more than minimally overcarved (i.e., a submarginal defect greater than 0.2 mm) should be replaced.[72]

If total carving time is short enough, the smoothness of the carved surface may be improved by wiping with a small, damp ball of cotton held in the operating pliers. All shavings from the carving procedure should be removed from the mouth with the aid of the oral evacuator.

Some operators prefer to postcarve burnish the amalgam surface using a small burnisher when carving is completed. Postcarve burnishing is done by lightly rubbing the carved surface with a burnisher of suitable size and shape to improve smoothness and produce a satin (not shiny) appearance. Do not rub the surface hard enough to produce grooves in the amalgam. With high-copper amalgams, postcarve burnishing may improve the marginal integrity of high-copper amalgams,[54] but it is not recommended as a routine part of the procedure (although it may also improve the smoothness of the restoration).

Postcarve burnishing in conjunction with precarve burnishing of low-copper amalgams may serve as a viable substitute for conventional polishing.[55] Postcarve burnishing produces denser amalgam at the margins of occlusal preparations restored with low-copper amalgam.[36]

Next, the occlusion of the restoration must be evaluated. After completion of the carving and during the removal of rubber dam or cotton rolls, the patient is advised not to bite because of the danger of fracturing the restoration, which is weak at this stage. Even if the carving has been carefully accomplished, the restoration occasionally will be "high," indicating a premature occlusal contact. Whenever possible, visually inspect the contact potential of the restored tooth and assess the extent of closure. To ensure that the occlusion is correct, place a piece of articulating paper over the restoration and instruct the patient to close very lightly. If anesthesia is still present it may be difficult for the patient to tell when the teeth are in contact. High spots will be marked, which are then removed by additional carving. The process of light closure with articulating paper is repeated, and additional carving is accomplished until the patient can close the teeth to prerestoration occlusion. While carving, establish stable centric-holding contacts in correct locations (Fig. 17-23). These contacts should be perpendicular to the direction of occlusal load where possible. If the contact area is on an incline (not perpendicular to occlusal load), try, when carving away excess amalgam, either to remove the undesirable portion of the contact area (on an incline) or to carve a plateau perpendicular to the direction of load. Amalgam restorations carved out of occlusion may result in undesirable

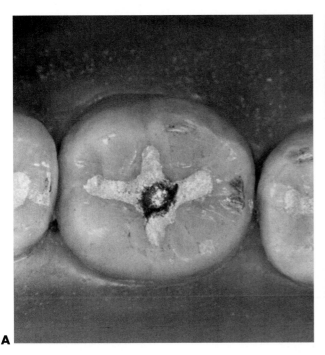
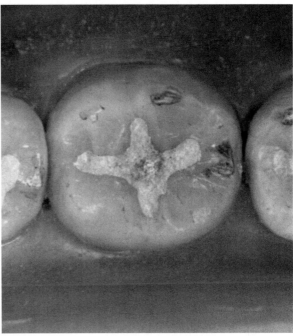

A   **B**

FIG. **17-23** Occluding the restoration. **A,** Heavy occlusal contacts on new amalgam should be avoided. Articulating paper will mark heavy contacts as dark areas, and it will mark very heavy contacts as dark areas with shiny centers. **B,** Amalgam should not be carved out of occlusion. Rather, it should have light occlusal contact or contacts as indicated by faint markings.

tooth movement. Finally, caution the patient to protect the restoration from any heavy biting pressure for several hours.

Most amalgams do not require further finishing and polishing. However, these procedures are occasionally necessary to: (1) complete the carving; (2) refine the anatomy, contours, and marginal integrity; and (3) enhance the surface texture of the restoration. Additional finishing and polishing procedures for amalgam restorations are not attempted within 24 hours of insertion, because crystallization is not complete.[2] If used, these procedures are often delayed until all of the patient's amalgam restorations have been placed, rather than finishing and polishing periodically during the course of treatment. An amalgam restoration is less prone to tarnish and corrosion if a smooth, homogeneous surface is achieved.[2,25] Polishing of high-copper amalgams is less important[10,17,56,82] than it is for low-copper amalgams, because high-copper amalgams are less susceptible to tarnish and marginal breakdown.[67,68]

During carving the margins are located and the desired contours and occlusion are developed. Finishing and polishing reduces the initial roughness of a carved restoration. These procedures must not leave the restoration undercontoured and must not alter the centric-holding contacts. The final anatomy of the polished restoration should be patterned after normal occlusal contours. After polishing is completed, the tip of an explorer should pass from the tooth surface to the restoration surface (and vice versa) without jumping or catching. There should be a

continuity of contour across the margin, which is a requirement of all restorations.

Begin any necessary finishing procedure by marking the occlusion with articulating paper and evaluating the margins with an explorer. If the occlusion can be improved or there is not a continuity of surface contour across the margins, a pointed, white, fused alumina stone or a green carborundum stone is used to correct the discrepancy (Fig. 17-24, *A*). The green stone is more abrasive than the white stone; the tip of either stone may be blunted on a diamond stone before use. This will help to prevent marring the center of the restoration while the margins are being adjusted. During surfacing of the amalgam, the stone's long axis is held at a right angle to the margins. Guard against reducing any centric-holding area. After the stone is used, the margins should be reevaluated with an explorer tine. If no discrepancy is detected, the area may be further smoothed using light pressure with a suitably shaped round finishing bur (see Fig. 17-24, *B*). A large, round finishing bur (comparable to a No. 4 or 6) is generally used for this finishing step. If the groove and fossa features are not sufficiently defined, a small round finishing bur may also accentuate them without reducing the centric-holding areas. The bur should be held perpendicular to the margin to allow the unprepared tooth structure to guide the bur and prevent unnecessary removal of amalgam (see Fig. 17-24, *C*). A smooth surface should be achieved before the polishing procedure is initiated. The finishing bur should remove the scratches

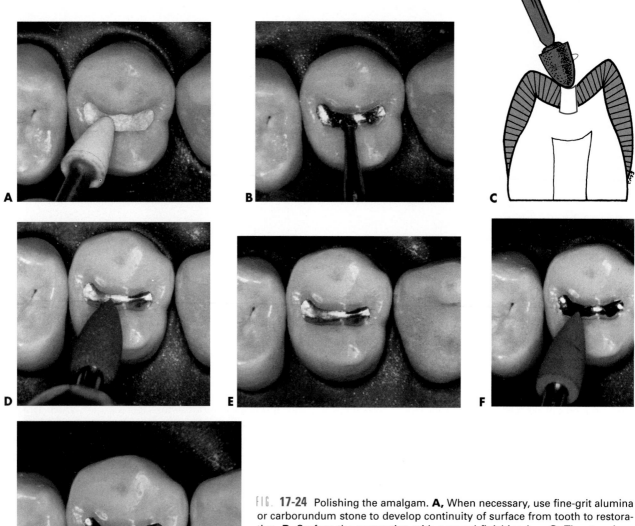

FIG. 17-24 Polishing the amalgam. **A,** When necessary, use fine-grit alumina or carborundum stone to develop continuity of surface from tooth to restoration. **B,** Surface the restoration with a round finishing bur. **C,** The stone's or bur's long axis is held at a right angle to the margin. **D,** Initiate polishing with coarse, rubber abrasive point at low speed. **E,** Point should produce smooth, satiny appearance. **F,** Obtain high polish with medium- and fine-grit abrasive points. **G,** Polished restoration.

from the green or white stone. However, often these scratches can be removed with only the use of a rubber abrasive point.

Initiate a polishing procedure by using a coarse, rubber abrasive point at low speed and air-water spray to produce an amalgam surface with a smooth, satiny appearance (see Fig. 17-24, *D* and *E*). If the amalgam surface does not exhibit this appearance after only a few seconds of polishing, the surface was too rough at the start. In this instance, resurfacing with a finishing bur is necessary, followed by the coarse, rubber abrasive point to develop the satiny appearance. It is important that

the rubber points be used at low speed or "stall out" speed for two reasons:

1. The danger of the point disintegrating at high speeds
2. The danger of elevating the temperature of the restoration and the tooth

An excessive temperature rise (i.e., above 140° F [60° C]) can cause irreparable damage to the pulp or restoration or both. When overheated, the surface of the amalgam will appear cloudy even though it may have a high polish. This cloudy appearance indicates that mercury has been

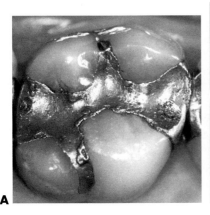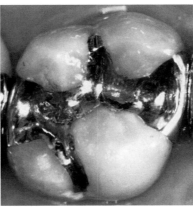

A　　　　　　　　　　　　　　　　　　　　**B**

FIG. **17-25 A,** Existing amalgam restoration exhibiting marginal deterioration and surface roughness. **B,** Same restoration after finishing and polishing.

brought to the surface, which results in corrosion of the amalgam and loss of strength.[2]

After polishing with the coarse, abrasive rubber point, there should be no deep scratches on the amalgam surface, only the moderately polished surface left by the rubber point. In addition, the contour from tooth to restoration should be continuous when tested by the explorer tip.

After the area is washed free of abrasive particles, a high polish may be imparted to the restoration with a series of medium- and fine-grit abrasive points (see Fig. 17-24, *F*). As with the more abrasive points, the finer abrasive points must be used at low speed. If a high luster does not appear within a few seconds, the restoration requires additional polishing with the more abrasive points. The system that is illustrated includes coarse-, medium-, and fine-grit rubber abrasive points. Using these points in sequence from coarse to fine will produce an amalgam surface with a brilliant luster (see Fig. 17-24, *G*). As an alternative to rubber abrasive points, final polishing may be accomplished using a rubber cup with flour of pumice followed by a high-luster agent, such as precipitated chalk.

Polishing of older, existing restorations is infrequently indicated. However, finishing may be indicated to improve the contour, margins, surface, or anatomy of older, existing restorations (Fig. 17-25, *A* and *B*). Occlusal contours of amalgam restorations that have expanded beyond the cavosurface margins or that were originally undercarved may be corrected with abrasive stones and finishing burs. Margins exhibiting minimal ditching may be refined and rough surfaces smoothed. Round finishing burs may be used to correct poorly defined anatomy.

EXTENSIVE CLASS I AMALGAM RESTORATIONS

Caries is considered extensive if the distance between infected dentin and the pulp is judged to be less than 1 mm or when the faciolingual extent of the defect is up the cuspal inclines. Obviously, extensive caries requires a more extensive restoration (which is a more typical in-

dicated use for amalgam). The use of amalgam in large Class I restorations provides good wear resistance and occlusal contact relationships. For very large Class I restorations, a bonding system may be used that improves both retention and resistance forms.

Initial Clinical Procedures. The rubber dam should be used for isolation of the operating site when caries is extensive. If caries excavation exposes the pulp, pulp capping may be more often successful if the site is isolated with a properly applied rubber dam. In addition, the dam will prevent moisture contamination of the amalgam mix during insertion.[2] Preoperative occlusal assessment and anesthetic administration are also factors to consider (see Chapters 10 and 16).

Tooth Preparation

Initial Tooth Preparation. In teeth with extensive caries, excavation of infected dentin and, if necessary, insertion of a liner may precede the establishment of outline, resistance, and retention forms. This approach protects the pulp as early as possible from any additional insult of tooth preparation. Normally, however, the procedure occurs as follows:

Using a No. 245 bur at high speed with air-water spray and oriented with its long axis parallel to the long axis of the tooth crown, prepare the outline, primary resistance, and primary retention forms. An initial depth of 1.5 to 2 mm (measured 1.5 mm at any pit or fissure and up to 2 mm on the prepared external walls) should be maintained. The preparation is extended laterally to remove all enamel undermined by caries by alternately cutting and examining the lateral extension of the caries. For caries extending up the cuspal inclines, it may be necessary to alter the bur's long axis to prepare a 90- to 100-degree cavosurface angle while maintaining the initial depth (Fig. 17-26). If not, a significantly obtuse cavosurface angle may remain (resulting in an acute, or weak, amalgam margin), or the pulpal floor may be prepared too deeply.

When extending the outline form, enameloplasty should be used when possible (as described previously). When the defect extends to one half the distance between the primary groove and a cusp tip, capping the cusp (i.e., reducing the cuspal tooth structure and restoring it with amalgam) may be indicated. When that distance is two thirds, cusp capping is usually required because of the risk of cusp fracture postoperatively. A Class I restoration that has either a wide faciolingual extension or a capped cusp may also be considered for adhesive bonding. Fig. 17-27 illustrates some examples of large Class I amalgam preparation outlines.

Final Tooth Preparation. Removal of remaining infected dentin is accomplished in the same manner as described previously for the conservative preparation. If a pulp exposure occurs, the operator must decide whether to apply a direct pulp cap of calcium hydroxide to the exposure or to treat the tooth endodontically. (For factors influencing this decision, see Caries Control Restoration in Chapter 3.)

For pulpal protection in very deep carious excavations (where the remaining dentin thickness is judged to be less than 0.5 mm), a thin layer (i.e., 0.5 to 0.75 mm) of a calcium hydroxide liner may be placed. The calcium hydroxide liner may stimulate secondary dentin forma-

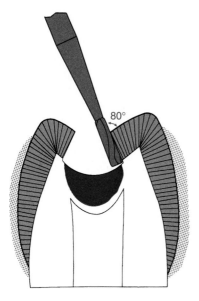

FIG. **17-26** Initial tooth preparation with extensive caries. When extending laterally to remove enamel undermined by caries, alter the bur's long axis to prepare a 90- to 100-degree cavosurface angle. A 100-degree cavosurface angle on the cuspal incline will result in an 80-degree marginal amalgam angle.

tion in an area where a microexposure is suspected. If used it is placed with the same instrument using the same technique as described for the RMGI liner. The calcium hydroxide liner should be placed only over the deepest portion of the excavation (nearest the pulp). A thin base of RMGI should then be used to cover the calcium hydroxide. As before, the entire dentin surface should not be covered (Fig. 17-28). Dentin peripheral to the RMGI base should be available for bonding, if desired. The RMGI liner is recommended to cover the calcium hydroxide to resist the forces of condensation, to avoid dissolution of the calcium hydroxide during acid-etching, and to seal the deeply excavated area.[22] Usually no secondary resistance or retention form features are necessary for extensive Class I amalgam preparations. Primary resistance form was obtained by extending the outline of the tooth preparation to include only undermined and defective tooth structure, while preparing strong enamel walls and allowing strong cuspal areas to remain. If the excavation of caries has removed most (or all) of the flat pulpal floor that was initially prepared, secondary resistance form may be indicated. If so, establish flat seats in dentin (0.2 mm inside the DEJ, at the pulpal wall level) that are somewhat equally spaced around the periphery of the excavation. Primary retention was obtained by the occlusal convergence of the enamel walls; secondary retention form may result from undercut areas that are occasionally left in dentin (and that are not covered by a liner) after removal of infected dentin. The external walls of the preparation are finished as described previously.

Restorative Technique. After any indicated liner or base is placed, regardless of the depth of the excavation, either a dentin desensitizer or adhesive system is used. The objective of the use of a dentin desensitizer is to better seal the prepared dentin. As described previously, it is used instead of varnish. It is rubbed into the dentin surface with an applicator tip for 30 seconds and dried. Light-curing is unnecessary.

Amalgam adhesives may be used with all amalgam restorations, but they are generally reserved for foundations and large amalgam restorations, particularly those with deep excavations, remaining weakened tooth structure, and capped cusps. Amalgam adhesives seal the dentin with an acid-resistant layer of resin-reinforced dentin called the *hybrid layer*. This is a multistepped pro-

FIG. **17-27** Examples of Class I amalgam tooth preparation outline forms. **A,** Occlusal outline form in the mandibular second premolar. **B,** Occlusolingual outline form in the maxillary first molar. **C,** Occlusofacial outline form in the mandibular first molar.

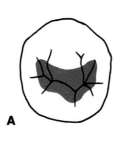

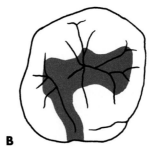

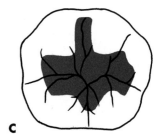

A   B   C

cedure that involves applying an etchant, primer, and adhesive to the prepared tooth surface. For a given product, the etchant and primer (or primer and adhesive) may be combined into a single component (i.e., bottle). Therefore the specific technique of amalgam adhesion is product specific and will involve two or more bottles. Currently no self-curing, all-in-one adhesive is commercially available. To understand the action of each bonding component, the general technique for amalgam adhesives will be presented as a three-step procedure (Fig. 17-29).

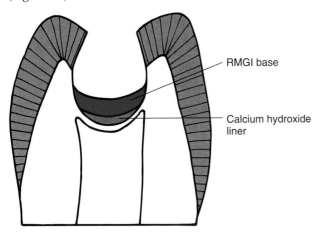

FIG. **17-28** Placement of Ca(OH)₂ liner and RMGI base.

RMGI base

Calcium hydroxide liner

When amalgam adhesives are used, varnish should not be used and dentin desensitizers are usually unnecessary. The adhesive itself serves as a desensitizer, reducing dentin permeability. Adhesives used with amalgam must be self-curing or dual curing, because it is impossible to light-cure an adhesive through the amalgam. Use only adhesives recommended for amalgam restorations by the manufacturer, and follow the technique instructions. The primer and adhesive components should not be dispensed in advance because the primer will volatilize (especially those containing acetone solvents) and the adhesive will set (because most are dual cured).

The preparation side of the matrix band should be waxed (i.e., lubricated) before placement to ensure that the bonded amalgam does not adhere to the band itself. The band may be lubricated with inlay wax.

Generally the etchant is applied for 15 to 30 seconds to enamel and dentin simultaneously and rinsed from the tooth preparation (see Fig. 17-29, *A*). The preparation should be only very briefly dried (i.e., about 1 sec), resulting in a moist dentin surface that is not visibly dry. The dentin preparation surface should be "glistening" in appearance (see Fig. 17-29, *B*). As an alternative to drying, the preparation may be blot dried with a damp cotton pellet. If the preparation is overdried, it may be rewetted with water or with a HEMA and glutaraldehyde-based

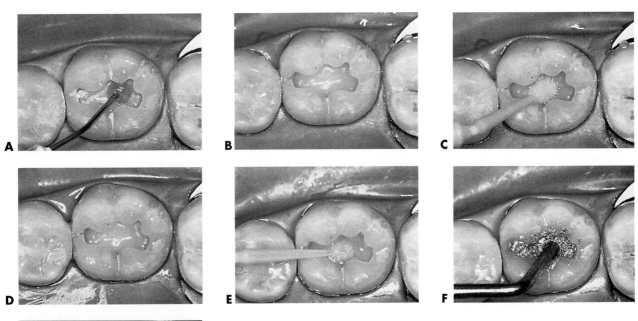

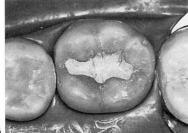

FIG. **17-29** Bonding technique. **A,** Etchant application. **B,** Moist preparation surface. **C,** Primer application. **D,** Primed preparation surface. **E,** Adhesive application. **F,** Amalgam condensation. **G,** Carved restoration.

desensitizer on an applicator tip. The primer should be applied using the technique described by the manufacturer (see Fig. 17-29, *C*). After primer application the preparation surface should be dried but not rinsed. After drying, the primed surface should be glossy in appearance. If it is not, the primer should be reapplied until the surface is glossy (see Fig. 17-29, *D*). Separate applicators should be used for the primer and adhesive components. Before mixing base and catalyst from the adhesive, the amalgam should be triturated and ready to be inserted in the preparation. Base and catalyst from the adhesive are mixed following the manufacturer's recommendations, and the mixture is usually applied to the preparation with an applicator tip or microbrush furnished by the manufacturer (see Fig. 17-29, *E*). The preparation should be lightly coated with adhesive. Excess adhesive should be removed with the applicator tip or microbrush (not with the air syringe, which may remove adhesive from some areas). Excess adhesive in the preparation encourages the formation of "barnacles" of set resin at the cavosurface margins (which will be discussed later in this section). After the adhesive is placed, amalgam should be condensed into the preparation immediately to facilitate the intermingling of amalgam and unset resin. Immediate condensation of amalgam is also important to ensure that amalgam adapts to the cavosurface margins and fills the retentive grooves before the adhesive resin sets. It is difficult to condense amalgam quickly enough into adhesive resin to avoid having a layer of resin at the margin that is visible radiographically (Fig. 17-30). The long-term effect of this radiographically visible resin interface is unknown. If it remains intact, it may be an advantage; if it hydrolyzes, the preparation may be subject to recurrent caries. The use of spherical amalgams is occasionally advocated with amalgam adhesives because they are more quickly condensed than admixed amalgams.

The trituration of the amalgam material is as described previously. However, the timing of amalgam condensation is critical if the restoration is being bonded (i.e., if the insertion of the adhesive resin is immediately followed by the amalgam condensation). The preparation is slightly overfilled and final condensation is enhanced by use of precarve burnishing. Carving the

extensive Class I restoration is often more complex, because more cuspal inclines are included in the preparation. Appropriate contours, occlusal contacts, and groove and fossa anatomy must be provided. Finishing and polishing indication and techniques are as described previously.

CLASS I OCCLUSOLINGUAL AMALGAM RESTORATIONS

Occlusolingual (OL) amalgam restorations may be used on maxillary molars when a lingual fissure connects with the distal oblique fissure and distal pit on the occlusal surface (Fig. 17-31). Composite may also be used as the restorative material, especially in smaller restorations.

Initial Clinical Procedures. After local anesthesia and evaluation of the occlusal contacts, the rubber dam is generally recommended for isolation of the operating (see Chapter 10). However, in most cases, typical Class I preparations can be adequately isolated with cotton rolls.

Tooth Preparation. The initial tooth preparation involves the establishment of the outline, primary resistance, primary retention forms, and initial preparation depth. The accepted principles of outline form (previously presented) are to be observed with special attention to the following:

- The tooth preparation should be no wider than necessary; ideally the mesiodistal width of the lingual extension should not exceed 1 mm, except for extension necessary to remove carious or undermined enamel or to include unusual fissuring.
- When indicated, the tooth preparation should be cut more at the expense of the oblique ridge rather than centering over the fissure (weakening the small distolingual cusp).
- Especially on smaller teeth, the occlusal portion may have a slight distal tilt to conserve the dentin support of the distal marginal ridge (Fig. 17-32).

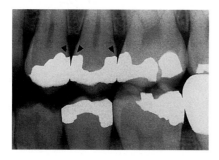

FIG. **17-30** Radiograph showing bonding adhesive at gingival margin (*arrows*).

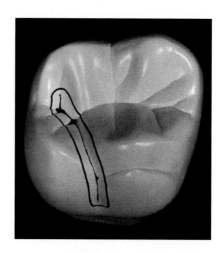

FIG. **17-31** Outline of margins for OL tooth preparation.

- The margins should extend as little as possible onto the oblique ridge, distolingual cusp, and distal marginal ridge.

These objectives help to conserve the dentinal support and strength of the tooth, and they aid in establish-

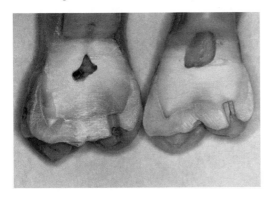

FIG. **17-32** Small distal inclination of bur on smaller teeth may be indicated to conserve dentinal support and strength of marginal ridge.

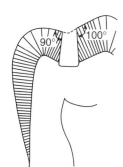

FIG. **17-33** Enamel cavosurface angles of 90 to 100 degrees are ideal.

ing an enamel cavosurface angle as close as possible to 90 degrees (Fig. 17-33). They also help to minimize marginal deterioration of the restoration by locating the margins away from enamel eminencies where occlusal forces may be concentrated.

Using the mirror for indirect vision and the high-speed handpiece with air-water spray, enter the distal pit with the end of the No. 245 bur (Fig. 17-34, *A*). The long axis of the bur usually should be parallel to the long axis of the tooth crown. Remember to conserve the dentinal support and strength of the distal marginal ridge and distolingual cusp, which may require directing the bur so that it cuts more of the tooth structure mesial to the pit rather than distal (e.g., 70:30 rather than 50:50). Penetrate to a depth of 1.5 to 2 mm as measured by the bur on the cut walls (1.5 mm at the fissure and up to 2 mm on the external walls) (see Fig. 17-34, *B*). At this depth the pulpal floor is usually in dentin. Once the entry cut is made (see Fig. 17-34, *C*), move the bur (maintaining the initial established depth) to include any remaining fissures facial to the point of entry (see Fig. 17-34, *D*). However, remember to use enameloplasty, if indicated. Next, at the same depth, move the bur along the fissure toward the lingual surface (see Fig. 17-34, *E*). As with Class I occlusal preparations, a slight distal inclination of the bur will occasionally be indicated (e.g., smaller teeth) to conserve the dentinal support and strength of the marginal ridge and the distolingual cusp. To ensure adequate strength for the marginal ridge, the distopulpal line angle should not approach the distal surface of the tooth closer than 2 mm. On large molars the bur position should remain parallel

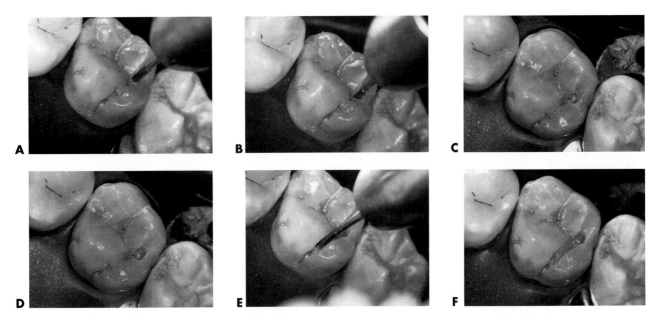

FIG. **17-34** OL tooth preparation. **A,** No. 245 bur positioned for entry. **B,** Penetrate to minimal depth of 1.5 to 2 mm. **C,** Entry cut. **D,** Remaining fissures facial to point of entry are removed with same bur. **E** and **F,** Cut lingually along fissure until bur has extended the preparation onto lingual surface.

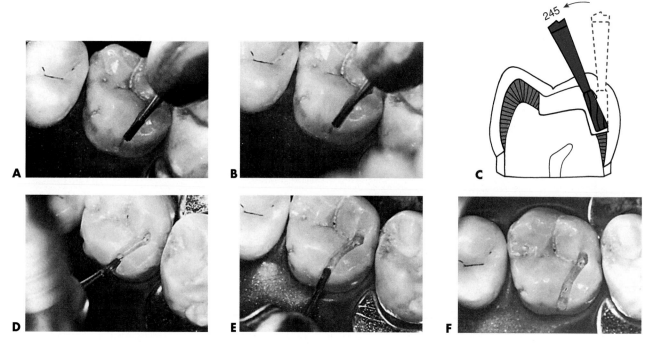

FIG. **17-35** OL tooth preparation. **A,** Position of bur to cut lingual portion. **B,** Initial entry of bur for cutting lingual portion. **C,** Alter inclination of bur to establish correct axial wall depth. **D** and **E,** Direct bur perpendicular to axial wall to accentuate mesioaxial and distoaxial line angles. **F,** Axial wall depth should be 0.2 to 0.5 mm inside the DEJ.

to the long axis of the tooth, particularly if the bur is off-set slightly mesial to the center of the fissure. Keeping the bur parallel to the long axis of the tooth creates a distal wall with slight occlusal convergence, providing favorable enamel and amalgam angles. Continue to move the bur lingually along the fissure, maintaining a uniform depth until the bur has extended the preparation onto the lingual surface (see Fig. 17-34, *F*). The pulpal floor should follow the contour of the occlusal surface and DEJ, which usually rises occlusally as the bur moves lingually.

The mesial and distal walls of the occlusal portion of the preparation should converge occlusally because of the shape of the bur. This convergence provides sufficient retention form to the occlusal portion of the preparation. If the slight distal bur tilt was required, the mesial and distal walls should still converge relative to each other (although the distal wall may be divergent occlusally, relative to the tooth's long axis). Thus occlusal retention form will usually be adequate.

Next, prepare the lingual portion. This may be accomplished by two techniques. In one technique the lingual surface is prepared with the bur's long axis parallel with the lingual surface (Fig. 17-35, *A* and *B*). The tip of the bur should be located at the gingival extent of the lingual fissure. Be careful to control the bur and not allow it to "roll out" onto the lingual surface, because this could "round over" or damage the cavosurface margin. Using the bur at high speed to prepare the lingual por-

tion usually prevents this occurrence. The facial inclination of the bur must be altered as the cutting progresses to establish the axial wall of the lingual portion at a uniform depth of 0.5 mm inside the DEJ (see Fig. 17-35, *C*). The axial wall should follow the contour of the lingual surface of the tooth. An axial depth of 0.5 mm inside the DEJ is indicated if retentive locks are required; an axial depth of 0.2 inside the DEJ is permissible if retentive locks are not required.

The No. 245 bur may be used with its long axis perpendicular to the axial wall to accentuate (i.e., refine) the mesioaxial and distoaxial line angles. This will also result in the mesial and distal walls converging lingually because of the shape of the bur (see Fig. 17-35, *D* and *E*). During this step the axial wall depth is not altered (see Fig. 17-35, *F*). The occlusal and lingual convergences usually provide sufficient preparation retention form; thus no retention locks are needed.

Keeping the bur perpendicular to the tooth surface, round the axiopulpal line angle (Fig. 17-36). Leaving a sharp line angle increases the possibility of fracture of the amalgam because of stress concentration. It also helps to ensure adequate preparation depth and amalgam thickness. Initial tooth preparation of the OL preparation is now complete. As mentioned previously, enameloplasty may be used to conserve tooth structure and limit extension.

The second technique is more difficult. In this case, the No. 245 bur is held perpendicular to the cusp ridge

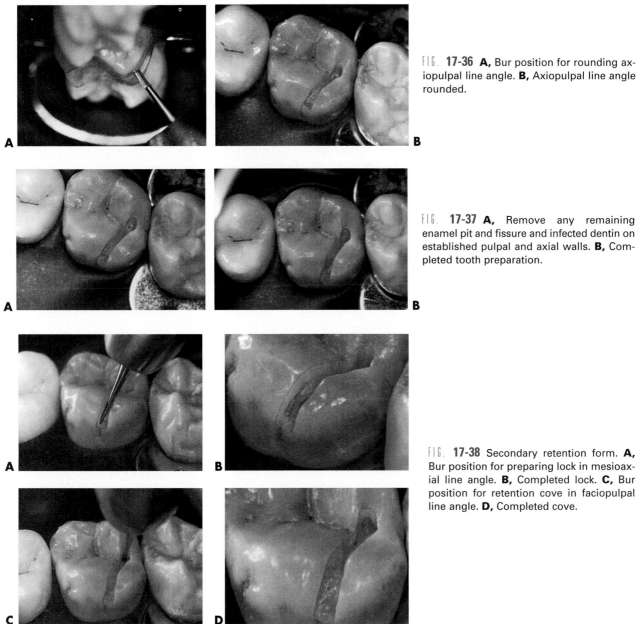

FIG. **17-36 A,** Bur position for rounding axiopulpal line angle. **B,** Axiopulpal line angle rounded.

FIG. **17-37 A,** Remove any remaining enamel pit and fissure and infected dentin on established pulpal and axial walls. **B,** Completed tooth preparation.

FIG. **17-38** Secondary retention form. **A,** Bur position for preparing lock in mesioaxial line angle. **B,** Completed lock. **C,** Bur position for retention cove in faciopulpal line angle. **D,** Completed cove.

and lingual surface as it extends the preparation from the occlusal surface gingivally (to include the entire fault). This technique also results in opposing preparation walls that converge lingually. Initiate final tooth preparation by removal of remaining caries on the pulpal and axial walls (Fig. 17-37, *A* and *B*) with a suitably sized round bur, a discoid-type spoon excavator, or both. Excavation of caries should not affect resistance form if flat pulpal wall seats are present or prepared in sound tooth structure peripheral to the excavated areas. As described previously, if necessary, place a liner or base or both in deep excavations for pulpal protection.

Additional retention in the lingual extension may be required if the extension is wide mesiodistally or if it was prepared without a lingual convergence. If additional retention is required, the No. ¼ or 169 bur can be used to prepare locks into the mesioaxial and distoaxial line angles (Fig. 17-38, *A*). If these angles are in enamel, the axial wall must be deepened to 0.5 mm axially of the DEJ (because the locks must be in dentin to not undermine enamel). The depth of the locks at the gingival floor is one half the diameter of the No. ¼ bur. The cutting direction for each lock is the bisector of the respective line angle. The lock is slightly deeper pulpally than the correctly positioned axial wall and is 0.2 mm pulpal to the DEJ. The locks should diminish in depth toward the occlusal surface, terminating midway along the axial wall (see Fig. 17-38, *B*). Test the adequacy of the lock by inserting the tine of an explorer into the lock and moving it lingually. The mesial or distal depth of the lock should prevent the explorer from being withdrawn directly to the lingual. (Refer to Secondary Resistance

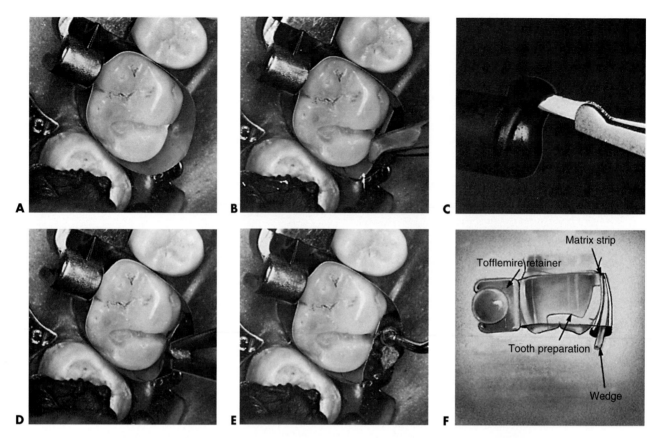

FIG. **17-39** Matrix for OL tooth preparation. **A,** Matrix band secured to tooth with Tofflemire retainer. **B,** Positioning small strip of stainless steel matrix material between tooth and band already in place. **C,** Covering wedge with softened compound. **D,** Inserting wedge and compound. **E,** Compressing compound gingivally, which adapts steel strip to lingual surface. **F,** Cross-section of tooth preparation and matrix construction.

and Retention Forms in this chapter for a description of placing retentive locks in the proximal boxes of Class II amalgam preparations; the techniques are similar.)

Extension of a facial occlusal fissure may have required a slight divergence occlusally to the facial wall to conserve support of the facial ridge. If so and if deemed necessary, the No. 33½ bur may be used to prepare a retention cove in the faciopulpal line angle (see Fig. 17-38, C and D). The tip of the No. 245 bur held parallel to the long axis of the tooth crown also might be used to prepare this cove. Be careful not to undermine the occlusal enamel (this retentive cove is recommended only if occlusal convergence of the mesial and distal walls of the occlusal portion is absent or inadequate). Finish the external walls as described previously, if necessary. Any irregularities at the margins may indicate weak enamel that may be smoothed by the side of the No. 245 bur rotating at slow speed.

Restorative Technique

Placing a Sealer or Adhesive System. As presented previously, after any indicated liner or base or both is placed, regardless of the depth of the excavation, either

a dentin desensitizer or dentin-bonding system is placed. A desensitizer is usually indicated in conservative preparations. A dentin-bonding system may be indicated in more extensive preparations. Either is used instead of varnish.

Placing a Matrix (if Necessary). Using a rigid matrix to support the lingual portion of the restoration during condensation is occasionally necessary. A matrix is helpful to prevent "land-sliding" during condensation and to ensure marginal adaptation and strength of the restoration. The Tofflemire matrix retainer is used to secure a matrix band to the tooth (as described later in this chapter). Because this type of matrix band does not intimately adapt to the lingual groove area of the tooth (Fig. 17-39, *A*), an additional step may be necessary to provide a matrix that is rigid on the lingual portion of the tooth preparation. If so, cut a piece of stainless steel matrix material (0.002 inch [0.05 mm] thick, ⁵⁄₁₆ inch [8 mm] wide) that will fit between the lingual surface of the tooth and the band already in place (see Fig. 17-39, *B*). Place the gingival edge of this segment of matrix material slightly gingival to the gingival edge of the band to

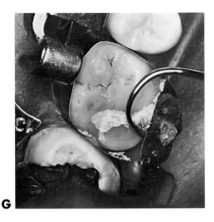 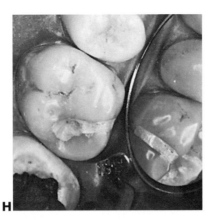 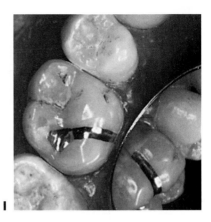

FIG. **17-39, cont'd G,** Using explorer to remove excess amalgam adjacent to lingual matrix. **H,** Carving completed. **I,** Polished restoration.

help secure the band segment. Break off approximately ½ inch (12.7 mm) of a round toothpick, while holding it with the No. 110 pliers. Heat the end of a stick of green compound and cover the end of the tooth-pick wedge (see Fig. 17-39, *C*). Immediately insert the compound-coated wedge between the Tofflemire band and the cut piece of matrix material (see Fig. 17-39, *D*). While the compound is still soft, use a suitable burnisher to press the compound gingivally, thereby securing the matrix tightly against the gingival cavosurface margin and the lingual surface of the tooth to provide a rigid, lingual matrix (see Fig. 17-39, *E* and *F*). A unique property of the lingual matrix is its ability to respond to needed change in contour by pressing a warmed, metal instrument against the band from the preparation side. The heat is transferred through the matrix material to the compound, which may then be reshaped to provide the proper contour. This matrix for the OL amalgam restoration is referred to as the *Barton matrix.* Occasionally the piece of strip matrix can be positioned appropriately by using only the wedge (not the compound).

Inserting the Amalgam. Insertion of the amalgam is accomplished as previously described for the Class I occlusal tooth preparation. Begin condensation at the gingival wall. If a matrix is not used, care must be taken to ensure that "landsliding" of the amalgam does not occur because two adjoining surfaces of the tooth are being restored. For this technique, the last increments of amalgam may be condensed on the lingual surface with the side of a large condenser. Its long, broadly rounded contour conforms to the rectangular shape for the lingual groove preparation. However, the operator must still be careful (when condensing the occlusal surface) not to fracture out the lingual amalgam. Another technique is to have the assistant secure the condensed lingual surface with a broad condenser nib while the operator completes the condensation of the occlusal surface.

Neither technique is as fail-safe as using a Barton matrix. Regardless of the technique used, the amalgam must be well condensed.

Contouring and Finishing the Restoration. When the preparation is sufficiently overfilled, carving of the occlusal surface may begin immediately with a suitable size, sharp discoid-cleoid instrument. All carving should be done with the edge of the blade perpendicular to the margin and with the blade moving parallel to the margin. To prevent overcarving, the blade edge should be guided by the unprepared tooth surface adjacent to the margin. Use an explorer to remove excess amalgam adjacent to the lingual matrix before matrix removal (see Fig. 17-39, *G*). After the occlusal carving is complete, loosen the Tofflemire retainer from the band and remove the retainer with No. 110 pliers. Push the free ends of the band one at a time, lingually and occlusally, through the proximal contacts. As the band is freed from the tooth, the compound, wedge, and the cut segment of steel matrix material may be lifted away from the tooth. Complete the carving on the lingual surface. Only slight excess should remain to carve away. With carving completed (see Fig. 17-39, *H*), remove the rubber dam and adjust the restoration for proper occlusion.

As stated previously, most amalgams do no require finishing and polishing. However, the procedure is described in the section on Conservative Class I Amalgam Restorations. Fig. 17-39, *I*, illustrates the polished OL restoration.

CLASS I OCCLUSOFACIAL AMALGAM RESTORATIONS

Occasionally mandibular molars exhibit fissures that extend from the occlusal surface through the facial cusp ridge and onto the facial surface. Although these may be restored with composite, restoration with amalgam is illustrated in Fig. 17-40.

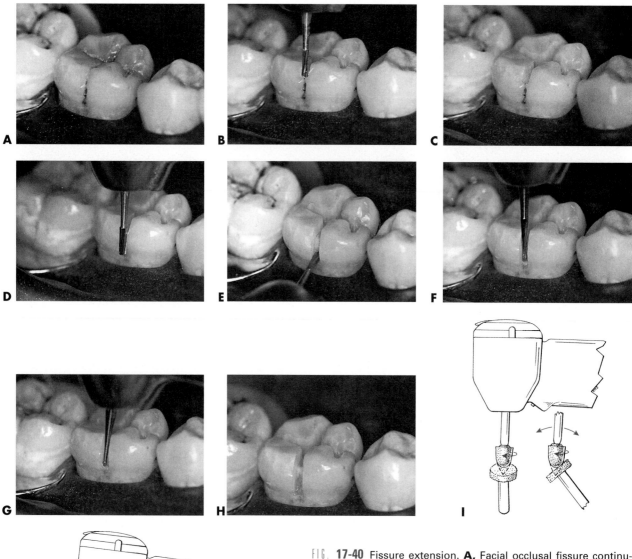

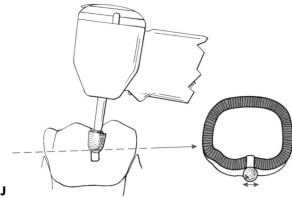

FIG. **17-40** Fissure extension. **A,** Facial occlusal fissure continuous with fissure on facial surface (fissures carious or at risk for caries). **B,** Extend through facial ridge onto facial surface. **C,** Appearance of tooth preparation following extension through ridge. **D,** Facial surface portion of extension is cut with side of bur. **E,** Sharpen line angles by directing bur from facial aspect. **F,** Sharpening line angles from occlusal direction with No. 169L bur. **G,** Ensuring retention form by preparing retention locks with No. ¼ round bur. **H,** Completed tooth preparation. **I,** Rubber polishing point may be trued and blunted on a coarse diamond wheel. **J,** Proper orientation of rubber point when polishing facial surface groove area.

CLASS II AMALGAM RESTORATIONS

Amalgam restorations that restore one or both of the proximal surfaces of the tooth may provide years of service to the patient when the: (1) tooth preparation is correct, (2) matrix is suitable, (3) operating field is isolated, and (4) restorative material is manipulated properly. Inattention to these criteria may produce inferior restorations prone to early failure. This section of the chapter deals with the principles, techniques, and procedures necessary to produce quality Class II amalgam restorations.

INITIAL CLINICAL PROCEDURES

As stated previously, local anesthesia is usually required. It controls pain from the tooth and adjacent soft tissues and usually reduces salivation, because the patient is less sensitive to stimulation of the oral tissues. In addition, the operator is more relaxed and efficient when the patient is comfortable (see Chapter 10.)

Occlusal contacts should be marked with articulating paper before tooth preparation. The operator should make a mental image of these contacts to serve as guide in tooth preparation and restoration. Any opposing "plunging cusp" or other pointed cusp may need to be recontoured to reduce the risk of fracture of the new restoration or the cusp from occlusal forces.

Before tooth preparation for amalgam, the placement of the rubber dam is generally recommended. It is especially beneficial when the restoration is large, when the caries is extensive, and when quadrant dentistry is practiced. The rubber dam can be applied in the time necessary for onset of profound anesthesia.

If the existing restoration has rough proximal contacts, the restoration may be removed before rubber dam application. However, infected carious dentin should be removed with the rubber dam in place, especially if a pulpal exposure is a possibility. Insertion of interproximal wedge or wedges is the last step in rubber dam application when Class II tooth preparations are scheduled. The wedges depress and protect the rubber dam and underlying soft tissue, separate the teeth slightly, and may serve as a guide to prevent gingival overextension of proximal boxes (see Chapter 10.)

If necessary to prevent friction between the septal dam and wedge during wedge insertion, stretch the dam slightly away from the teeth (i.e., wedge insertion side) and insert the wedge while slowly releasing the dam. This results in a passive dam under the wedge and tends to prevent bunching or tearing of the septal dam during wedge insertion. (Refer to Placement of the Rubber Dam, Step 22, in Chapter 10.)

TOOTH PREPARATION

Class II Amalgam Restorations Involving Only One Proximal Surface. This section introduces the principles and techniques of a Class II tooth preparation for an amalgam restoration involving a carious lesion on one proximal surface. For illustration, a mesioocclusal (MO) tooth preparation on a mandibular second premolar is presented. Although this restoration would typically use composite as the restorative material, the use of a small, conservative Class II amalgam restoration is presented to more clearly and simply provide the basic concepts of Class II amalgam tooth preparation and restoration.

Initial Tooth Preparation

Occlusal outline form (occlusal step). The occlusal outline form of a Class II tooth preparation for amalgam is similar to that for the Class I tooth preparation. Using high speed with air-water spray, enter the pit nearest the involved proximal surface with a punch cut using a No. 245 bur oriented as illustrated in Fig. 17-41, *A* and *B*. Entering the pit nearest the involved proximal surface

allows the mesial pit (in this case) not to be included if it is sound. The bur should be rotating when applied to the tooth and should not stop rotating until removed. Viewed from the proximal and lingual (facial) aspects, the long axis of the bur and the long axis of the tooth crown should remain parallel during cutting procedures. Proper depth of the initial entry cut is 1.5 to 2 mm (i.e., one half to two thirds the length of the cutting portion of a No. 245 bur), 1.5 mm as measured at the central fissure, and approximately 2 mm on the prepared external walls. The operator should measure and be familiar with each bur's dimensions to prevent being misled by various bur sizes. This pulpal depth is usually 0.1 to 0.2 mm into the dentin. While maintaining the same depth and bur orientation, move the bur to extend the outline to include the central fissure and the opposite pit (the distal pit in this example), if necessary (see Fig. 17-41, *C* and *D*). For the very conservative preparation, the isthmus width should be as narrow as possible[1,51] and no wider than one quarter the intercuspal distance.[41,51,74,90] Ideally it should be the width of the No. 245 bur. Narrow restorations provide a greater length of clinical service.[6,65] Generally the amount of remaining tooth structure is more important to restoration longevity than the restorative material used.[35] The pulpal floor should be prepared to a uniform (previously described) depth (and is usually flat). However, the pulpal floor of the preparation should follow the slight rise and fall of the DEJ along the central fissure in teeth with prominent triangular ridges.

Maintaining the bur parallel to the long axis of the tooth crown creates facial, lingual, and distal walls with a slight occlusal convergence, which provides favorable amalgam angles at the margins. It may be necessary to tilt the bur to diverge occlusally at the distal wall if extension of the distal margin would undermine the marginal ridge of its dentinal support (see Fig. 17-4, *B* and *C*). During development of the distal pit area of the preparation, extension to include any distofacial and distolingual developmental fissures radiating from the pit may be indicated. The distal pit area (in this example) provides dovetail retention form, which may prevent mesial displacement of the completed restoration. A dovetail feature is not required in the occlusal step of a single proximal surface preparation unless a fissure emanating from an occlusal pit indicates it. However, without a dovetail the occlusal step should not be in a straight direction, which may reduce retention form. This type of retention form is also provided by any extension of the central fissure preparation that is not in a straight direction from pit to pit (see Fig. 17-41, *E*). A dovetail outline form in the distal pit is not required if radiating fissures are not present.[69,85] Enameloplasty should be used where indicated to conserve tooth structure (see the discussion of enameloplasty earlier in the chapter).

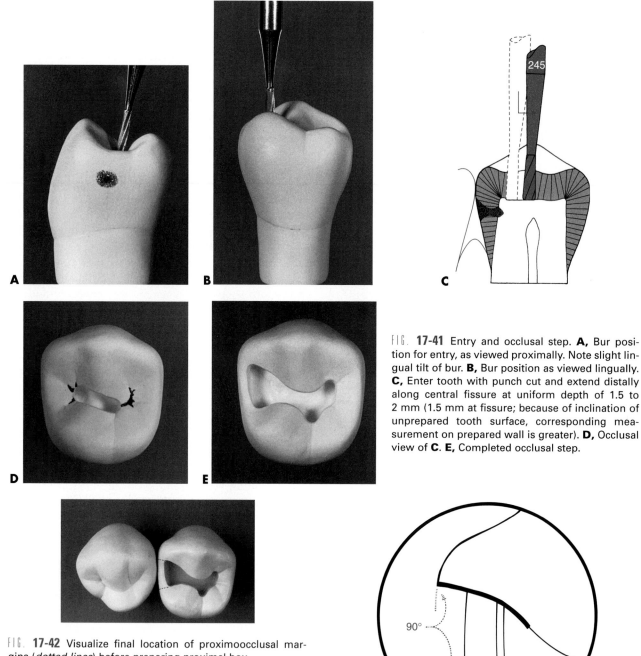

FIG. **17-41** Entry and occlusal step. **A,** Bur position for entry, as viewed proximally. Note slight lingual tilt of bur. **B,** Bur position as viewed lingually. **C,** Enter tooth with punch cut and extend distally along central fissure at uniform depth of 1.5 to 2 mm (1.5 mm at fissure; because of inclination of unprepared tooth surface, corresponding measurement on prepared wall is greater). **D,** Occlusal view of **C. E,** Completed occlusal step.

FIG. **17-42** Visualize final location of proximoocclusal margins (*dotted lines*) before preparing proximal box.

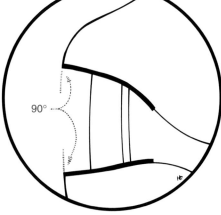

FIG. **17-43** Reverse curve in occlusal outline is usually created when mesiofacial enamel wall is parallel to enamel rod direction. Lingually, reverse curve is very slight, often unnecessary.

Before extending into the involved proximal marginal ridge (the mesial ridge in this example), visualize the final location of the facial and lingual walls of the proximal box relative to the contact area. This will prevent overextension of the occlusal outline form (i.e., occlusal step) where it joins the proximal outline form (i.e., proximal box). Fig. 17-42 illustrates visualization of the final location of proximoocclusal margins before preparing the proximal box. Viewed from the occlusal, Fig. 17-43 illustrates a *reverse curve* in the occlusal outline of a Class II preparation, which often results when developing the mesiofacial wall perpendicular to the enamel rod direction[74] and conserving the facial cusp structure. (Note that the ex-

tension is sufficient only to permit 90-degree amalgam at the mesiofacial margin and yet "curve" around the mesial portion of the facial cusp). Lingually, the reverse curve usually is minimal (if necessary at all) because the embrasure form is larger.

While maintaining the established pulpal depth and with the bur parallel to the long axis of the tooth crown, extend the preparation mesially, stopping approximately 0.8 mm (the diameter of the end of the bur) short of cutting through the marginal ridge into the contact area. The occlusal step in this region is made slightly wider faciolingually than in the Class I preparation because additional width is necessary for the proximal box. However, the proper depth of the occlusal portion of the preparation increases the strength of the restoration more than does faciolingual width (see Fig. 17-41, *E*, for an illustration of the completed occlusal outline form.) Although this extension includes part of the mesial marginal ridge, it also exposes the marginal-ridge DEJ. The location of the DEJ is an important guide in the development of the proximal preparation.

Proximal outline form (proximal box). Again visualize the desired final location of the facial and lingual walls of the proximal box or proximal outline form relative to the contact area. The objectives for extension of proximal margins are to:

- Include all caries, faults, or existing restorative material.
- Create 90-degree cavosurface margins (i.e., butt joint margins).
- Establish (ideally) not more than 0.5 mm clearance with the adjacent proximal surface facially, lingually, and gingivally.

The initial procedure in preparing the outline form of the proximal box is the isolation of the proximal (i.e., mesial) enamel by the proximal ditch cut. This is a very important procedure in conservative tooth preparation and is, therefore, presented in much detail. With the same orientation of the bur, position it over the DEJ in the pulpal floor next to the remaining mesial marginal ridge (Fig. 17-44, *A*). Allow the end of the bur to cut a ditch gingivally along the exposed DEJ, two thirds at the expense of dentin and one third at the expense of enamel. The 0.8-mm diameter bur end will cut approximately 0.5 to 0.6 mm into dentin and 0.2 to 0.3 mm into enamel. Pressure is directed gingivally and lightly toward the mesial surface to keep the bur against the proximal enamel, while the bur is moved facially and lingually along the DEJ. Extend the ditch gingivally just beyond the caries or the proximal contact, whichever is greater (see Fig. 17-44, *B*). Because dentin is softer and cuts more easily than enamel, the bur should be cutting away the dentin immediately supporting the enamel. The harder enamel acts to guide the bur, thus creating an axial wall that follows the faciolingual contour of the proximal surface and the DEJ (see Fig. 17-44, *D*).

As a guide for the facial and lingual extension of the ditch, visualize the completed mesiofacial and mesiolingual margins as right-angle projections of the facial and lingual limits of the ditch (see Fig. 17-44, *E*). When preparing a tooth with a small lesion, these margins should clear the adjacent tooth by only 0.2 to 0.3 mm.[74] A guide for the gingival extension is the visualization that the finished gingival margin will be only slightly gingival to the gingival limit of the ditch. This margin should clear the adjacent tooth by only 0.5 mm in a small tooth preparation (see Fig. 17-44, *F*).[69] Clearance of the proximal margins (i.e., mesiofacial, mesiolingual, gingival) greater than 0.5 mm is excessive unless indicated to include caries, undermined enamel, or existing restorative material (see Fig. 17-106 for conservative extension of proximal margins). The location of final proximal margins (i.e., facial, lingual, gingival) should be established with hand instruments (i.e., chisels, hatchets, trimmers) in conservative proximal box preparations. Otherwise, these margins may be overextended to achieve 90-degree cavosurface margins with the No. 245 bur (see Fig. 17-44, *E*). Extending gingival margins into the gingival sulcus should be avoided where possible because subgingival margins are more difficult to restore and may be a contributing factor to periodontal disease.[42,45,92]

The proximal ditch cut should be sufficiently deep into dentin (i.e., 0.5 to 0.6 mm) that retention locks, if deemed necessary, can be prepared into the axiolingual and axiofacial line angles without undermining the proximal enamel. If the proximal ditch cut is entirely in dentin, the axial wall usually will be too deep. Because the proximal enamel becomes thinner from occlusal to gingival, the end of the bur will come closer to the external tooth surface as the cutting progresses gingivally (see Fig. 17-44, *B*). Premolars may have proximal boxes that are shallower pulpally than molars, because premolars typically have thinner enamel. However, in the tooth crown the ideal dentinal depth of the axial wall of proximal boxes of premolars and molars should be the same (two thirds to three fourths the diameter of the No. 245 bur [or 0.5 to 0.6 mm]).[74] When extension places the gingival margin in cementum, the initial pulpal depth of the axiogingival line angle should be 0.7 to 0.8 mm (the diameter of the tip end of the No. 245 bur is 0.8 mm). The bur may shave the side of the wedge that is protecting the rubber dam and underlying gingiva (see Fig. 17-44, *C*).

The gingival depth of the proximal ditch may be measured by first noting the depth of the nonrotating bur in the ditch. Then, remove the bur from the preparation and hold it in the facial embrasure at the same level to observe the relationship of the end of the bur to the proximal contact. A calibrated periodontal probe may also be used.

The proximal ditch cut may be diverged gingivally to ensure that the faciolingual dimension at the gingival is greater than at the occlusal (see Fig. 17-44, *G*). However, the shape of the No. 245 inverted cone bur should provide this divergence. The gingival divergence

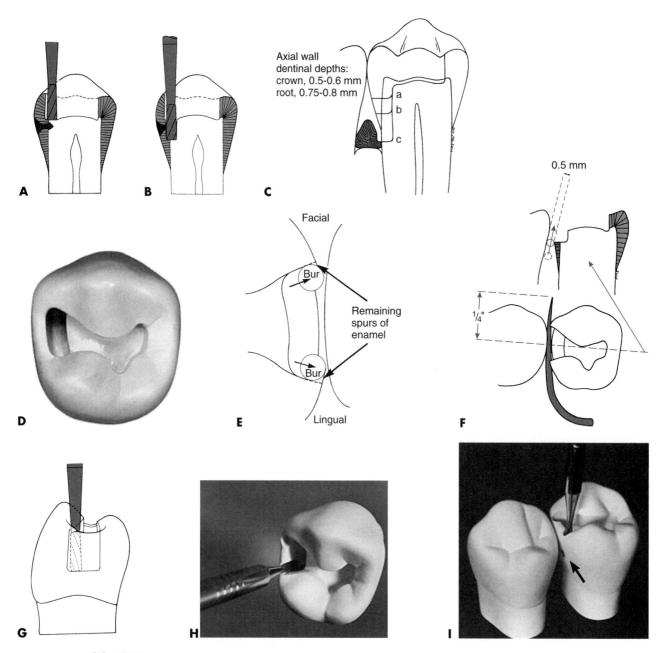

FIG. 17-44 Isolation of proximal enamel. **A,** Bur position to begin proximal ditch cut. **B,** Proximal ditch is extended gingivally to desired level of gingival wall (i.e., floor). **C,** Variance in pulpal depth of axiogingival line angle as extension of gingival wall varies: *a*, at minimal gingival extension; *b*, at moderate extension; *c*, at extension that places gingival margin in cementum, whereupon pulpal depth is 0.75 to 0.8 mm and bur may shave side of wedge. **D,** Proximal ditch cut results in axial wall that follows outside contour of proximal surface. **E,** Position of proximal walls (i.e., facial, lingual, gingival) should not be overextended with No. 245 bur, considering additional extension provided by hand instruments once remaining spurs of enamel are removed. **F,** When small lesion is prepared, gingival margin should clear adjacent tooth by only 0.5 mm. This clearance may be measured with side of explorer. The diameter of the tine of a No. 23 explorer is five tenths millimeter, ¼ inch (6.3 mm) from its tip. **G,** Faciolingual dimension of proximal ditch is greater at gingival than at occlusal level. **H,** To further isolate and weaken proximal enamel, bur is moved toward and perpendicular to proximal surface (parallel to direction of enamel rods). **I,** Side of bur may emerge slightly through proximal surface at level of gingival floor (*arrow*).

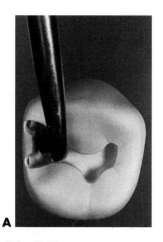
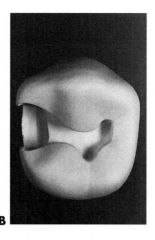
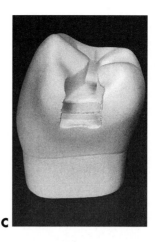

FIG. 17-45 Removing isolated enamel. **A,** Using spoon excavator to fracture out weakened proximal enamel. **B,** Occlusal view with proximal enamel removed. **C,** Proximal view with proximal enamel removed.

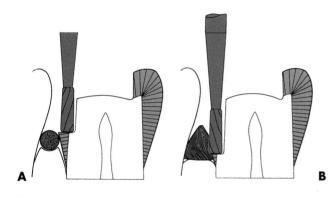

FIG. 17-46 Wedging. **A,** Round toothpick wedge placed in gingival embrasure protects gingiva and rubber dam during preparation of proximal box. **B,** Triangular wedge is indicated when deep gingival extension of proximal box is anticipated, because wedge's greatest cross-sectional dimension is at its base. Consequently, it will more readily engage the remaining clinical tooth surface.

contributes to retention form and provides for desirable extension of the facial and lingual proximal margins to include defective tooth structure or old restorative material at the gingival level, while conserving the marginal ridge and providing for 90-degree amalgam at the margins on this ridge.[51]

Occasionally, it is permissible not to extend the outline of the proximal box facially or lingually beyond the proximal contact to conserve tooth structure.[69] An example of this modification is a narrow proximal lesion where there is broad proximal contact in a patient with low risk for caries. If it is necessary to extend as much as a millimeter to break contact arbitrarily, leave the proximal margin in the contact. Usually it is the facial margin that is affected by this rule, which may not extend beyond the proximal contact into the facial embrasure.

In completing the proximal extensions, next make two cuts, one starting at the facial limit of the proximal ditch and the other starting at the lingual limit, extending toward and perpendicular to the proximal surface (until the bur is nearly through the enamel at contact level) (see Fig. 17-44, *H*). The side of the bur may emerge slightly through the surface at the level of the gingival floor (see Fig. 17-44, *I*). This weakens the remaining enamel by which the isolated portion is held. If this level is judged to be insufficiently gingival, additional

gingival extension should be accomplished using the isolated proximal enamel that is still in place to guide the bur. This prevents the bur from marring the proximal surface of the adjacent tooth. At this stage, however, the remaining wall of enamel often breaks away during cutting, especially when high speed is used. At such times, if additional use of the bur is indicated, a matrix band may be used around the adjacent tooth to prevent marring its proximal surface. The isolated enamel, if still in place, may be fractured out with a spoon excavator (Fig. 17-45) or by additional movement of the bur.

To protect the gingiva and the rubber dam when extending the gingival wall gingivally, a wooden wedge should already be in place in the gingival embrasure to depress the soft tissue and rubber dam.[51] A round toothpick wedge is preferred, unless a deep gingival extension is anticipated (Fig. 17-46, *A*). A triangular (i.e., anatomic) wedge is more appropriate for deep gingival extensions because the greatest cross-sectional dimension of the wedge is at its base; as the gingival wall is cut, the bur's end corner may slightly shave the wedge (see Fig. 17-46, *B*). (For wedge insertion, refer to Chapter 10.)

With the enamel hatchet (10-7-14), the bin-angle chisel (12-7-8), or both, cleave away any remaining undermined proximal enamel (Fig. 17-47, *A* and *B*), establishing

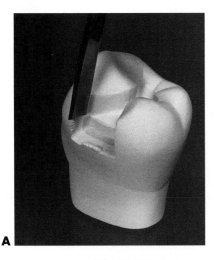
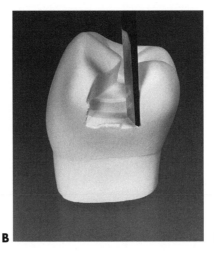
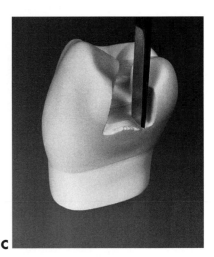

FIG. **17-47** Removing remaining undermined proximal enamel with enamel hatchet on facial proximal wall (**A**), lingual proximal wall (**B**), and gingival wall (**C**).

FIG. **17-48** Direction of mesiofacial and mesiolingual walls. **A,** Failure caused by weak enamel margin. **B,** Failure caused by weak-amalgam margin. **C,** Proper direction to proximal walls results in full-length enamel rods and 90-degree amalgam at preparation margin. Note also that retention locks have been cut 0.2 mm inside DEJ, and their direction of depth is parallel to DEJ.

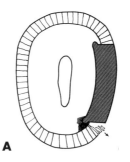
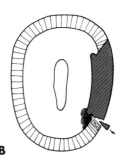
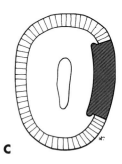

the proper direction to the mesiolingual and mesiofacial walls. Proximal margins having cavosurface angles of 90 degrees are indicated.[51] Cavosurface angles of 90 degrees ensure that no undermined enamel rods remain on the proximal margins and that the maximal edge strength of amalgam is maintained. Exercise care not to thrust the cutting edge against the gingival wall, because this can cause a craze line (i.e., fracture) that extends gingivally in the enamel, perhaps to the cervical line. Fig. 17-48 shows the importance of the correct direction of the mesiofacial and mesiolingual walls, dictated by enamel rod direction and physical properties of the amalgam. Again, ideally the mesiofacial and mesiolingual margins of the conservative preparation should clear the adjacent tooth by only 0.2 to 0.3 mm (see Figs. 17-60 and 17-106). If hand instruments were not used to remove the remaining spurs of enamel, the proximal margins would have undermined enamel. To create 90-degree facial and lingual proximal margins with the No. 245 bur, the proximal margins would have to be significantly overextended for an otherwise conservative preparation (see Fig. 17-44, *E*).

In addition, remove the weakened enamel along the gingival wall by using the enamel hatchet in a scraping motion (see Fig. 17-47, *C*). If the gingival cavosurface margin is in enamel, it will usually require a slight bevel, as described later. Ideally the minimal clearance of the completed gingival margin with the adjacent tooth is 0.5 mm.[69] This may be measured by passing an explorer tine of this diameter between the margin and adjacent tooth (see Fig. 17-44, *F*).

When the isolation of the proximal enamel has been properly executed, the proximal box can be completed easily with hand-cutting instruments. Otherwise, more cutting with rotary instruments may be indicated. High-speed equipment has reduced the use of hand instruments. However, the value of sharp hand-cutting instruments should not be underestimated.

When a rotary instrument is used in a proximal box after the proximal enamel is removed, there is a danger of the instrument either marring the adjacent proximal surface or "crawling out" of the box into the gingiva or across the proximal margins. The latter misfortune produces a rounded cavosurface angle, which, if not corrected, will result in a weak amalgam margin of less than 90 degrees. The danger of this occurring is markedly reduced when high-speed burs are used. When finishing enamel margins by rotary instrument, use intermittent application of the bur along with air coolant to improve vision.

Primary resistance form is provided by: (1) the pulpal and gingival walls being relatively flat and perpendicular to forces directed with the long axis of the tooth; (2) restricting extension of the walls to allow strong

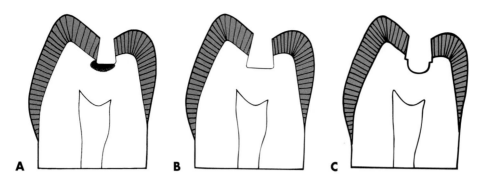

FIG. **17-49** Management of small-to-moderate size carious lesion on pulpal wall. **A,** Infected carious dentin extending beyond ideal pulpal wall position. **B,** Incorrect lowering of pulpal wall to include infected carious dentin. **C,** Correct extension facially and lingually beyond infected carious dentin. Note excavation below ideal pulpal wall level and facial and lingual seats are at ideal pulpal wall level.

cusps and ridge areas to remain with sufficient dentin support; (3) restricting the occlusal outline form (where possible) to areas receiving minimal occlusal contact;[66] (4) the reverse curve optimizing the strength of both the amalgam and tooth structure at the junction of the occlusal step and proximal box; (5) slightly rounding the internal line angles to reduce stress concentration in tooth structure (automatically created by bur design, except for the axiopulpal line angle); and (6) providing enough thickness of restorative material to prevent its fracture under mastication. Primary retention form is provided by the occlusal convergence of facial and lingual walls and by the dovetail design of the occlusal step, if present.

This completes the initial tooth preparation. Initial Class II tooth preparation is defined as extension of external walls at a specified limited depth to:

- Reach sound tooth structure
- Resist fracture of the tooth or restorative material from forces directed with the long axis of the tooth
- Retain restorative material in the tooth (see Chapter 6)

Axial and pulpal walls should be prepared to this ideal depth whether cutting in existing restorative material or caries. With proper outline form the pulpal and axial line angles should be in sound dentin.

After completing the initial tooth preparation, the adjacent proximal surface should be evaluated. An adjacent proximal restoration may require recontouring and smoothing to develop proper contact, contour, and embrasure form for the new restoration. This may be done with abrasive finishing strips or disks. Detection of caries would indicate restoration of the adjacent proximal surface or replacement of the existing restoration. If inadvertent minimal damage occurred to the adjacent proximal surface during initial tooth preparation, it should be corrected with abrasive strips and disks.

Final Tooth Preparation

Removal of any remaining defective enamel and infected carious dentin. Removing any remaining enamel pit and fissure and infected carious dentin on the pulpal wall in Class II preparations is accomplished in the same manner as in the Class I preparation. The presence of infected carious dentin on a portion of either the pulpal wall (floor) or axial wall does not indicate deepening the entire wall. Infected carious dentin is removed with a slowly revolving round bur of appropriate size or a discoid-type spoon excavator or both. Stop excavating when a hard or firm feel with an explorer or small spoon excavator is achieved. This often occurs before all of the stained or discolored dentin is removed. Removing any remaining enamel pit and fissure and infected carious dentin should not affect resistance form. To enhance good resistance form, the occlusal step should have pulpal seats at initial preparation depth, perpendicular to the long axis of the tooth in sound tooth structure and peripheral to the excavated area or areas (Fig. 17-49).

Any old restorative material (including base and liner) remaining should not be removed if there is no evidence of recurrent caries, if its periphery is intact, and if the tooth pulp is symptomless. This concept is particularly important if removal of all remaining restorative material may increase the risk of pulpal exposure.

Caries in the axial wall does not dictate extending the entire axial wall toward the pulp (Fig. 17-50). Recall that in initial tooth preparation, the facial, lingual, and gingival walls of the proximal box are extended as necessary until each wall is located in sound dentin. In all such extensions the pulpal depth of the axiofacial, axiolingual, and axiogingival line angles should never be altered because of the presence of caries in the axial wall "central" of these line angles. Infected carious dentin in the axial wall is then removed with suitably sized round burs or spoon excavators or both.

After completion of the minimal gingival extension (gingivoaxial line angle is in sound dentin), a remnant of the enamel portion of a carious lesion may remain on the gingival floor (wall), seen in the form of a decalcified (i.e., white, chalky) or faulty area bordering the margin (Fig. 17-51). This dictates extending part or the entire gingival floor gingivally to place it in sound tooth structure. Extension of the entire gingival wall to include a large carious lesion may place the gingival margin so deep that proper matrix application and (particularly) wedging are extremely difficult. Fig. 17-52, *A*, illustrates an outline form that extends gingivally in the central portion of the gingival wall to include caries that is deep gingivally, although leaving the facial and lingual gingival corners at a more occlusal position. This partial extension of the gingival wall will permit wedging of the matrix band where otherwise it may be difficult and damaging to the soft tissue. In this instance, the gingival wedge may not tightly support a small portion of the band. Special care must then be exercised by placing

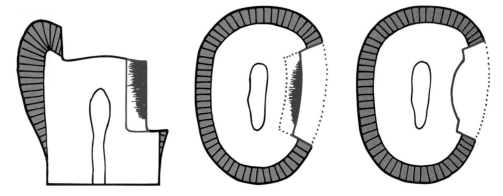

FIG. **17-50** Management of moderate-to-extensive size carious lesion. Infected carious dentin on axial wall does not call for preparing axial wall toward pulp as shown by dotted lines. Infected carious dentin extending pulpally of ideal axial wall position is removed with round bur.

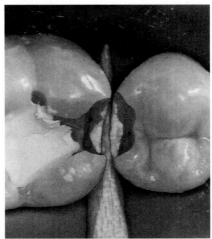

FIG. **17-51** Remnant of carious lesion bordering the enamel margin after insufficient gingival extension. Such a lesion indicates extending part or all of gingival floor gingivally to place it in sound tooth structure. *(Courtesy of Dr. C.L. Sockwell.)*

FIG. **17-52 A,** Outline form that permits extension of center portion of gingival wall to facilitate proper matrix construction and wedging in situations where caries extends deep gingivally. **B,** Outline form that permits partial wall extension facially and gingivally to conserve tooth structure.

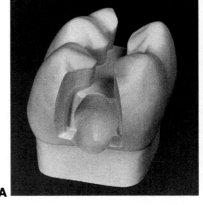

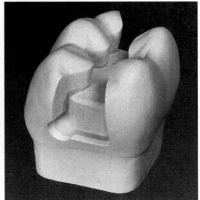

A

B

small amounts of amalgam in this area first and condensing lightly but thoroughly. In addition, care is exercised in carving the restoration in this area to remove any excess that may have extruded gingivally during condensation.

Fig. 17-52, *B*, illustrates a carious excavation facially and gingivally beyond the conventional margin position. Such minor variations from ideal preparation form permit conservation of tooth structure. A partial extension of a facial or lingual wall is permissible if: (1) the entire wall is not weakened, (2) the extension remains accessible and visible, (3) sufficient gingival seats remain to support the restoration, and (4) a butt joint fit at the amalgam and enamel margin (90-degree amalgam angle and 90-degree cavosurface angle) is possible.

Pulp protection. The reader is referred to this same step in tooth preparation in the previous section, Conservative Class I Amalgam Preparations.

Secondary resistance and retention forms. Secondary resistance form in final tooth preparation involves both resistance of the remaining tooth structure against fracture from oblique forces and resistance of restorative material against fracture. Restricting extensions of external walls provides the former; the latter is enhanced by using the gingival margin trimmer to bevel or round the axiopulpal line angle (Fig. 17-53), thereby increasing the bulk of and decreasing the stress concentration within the restorative material. Proximal retention locks (discussed later) may also increase the fracture resistance of the amalgam restoration.[14,28]

The use of retention locks in proximal boxes is controversial. It has been reported that proximal retention locks in the axiofacial and axiolingual line angles significantly strengthen the isthmus of a Class II restoration, and that these locks are significantly superior to axiogingival grooves in increasing the restoration's fracture strength.[59,60] However, others have suggested that retention locks located occlusal to the axiopulpal line angle provide more resistance than conventional

grooves.[84] It has also been reported that with high-copper amalgams, proximal retention locks are unnecessary in preparations that include dovetails.[62,83] However, the use of retention locks is recommended in tooth preparation with extensive proximal boxes.

Ideally secondary retention form for the occlusal and proximal portions of the preparation should be independent of each other. The occlusal convergence of the facial and lingual walls and the dovetail design (if needed) provide sufficient retention form to the occlusal portion of the tooth preparation. The occlusal convergence of the mesiofacial and mesiolingual walls offers retention in the proximal portion of the preparation against displacement occlusally. To enhance retention form of the proximal portion, proximal locks may be indicated to counter proximal displacement.[12,51,84,87] Many operators use proximal locks routinely to ensure that each portion of the tooth preparation is independently retentive. However, evidence suggests that retentive locks may not be needed in conservative, narrow proximal boxes.[87]

To prepare a retention lock, use a No. 169L bur with air coolant (to improve vision) and reduced speed (to improve tactile "feel" and control). The bur is placed in the properly positioned axiolingual line angle and directed (i.e., translated) to bisect the angle (Fig. 17-54, *A*) approximately parallel to the DEJ (Fig. 17-55). This positions the retention lock 0.2 mm inside the DEJ, thus maintaining the enamel support. The bur is tilted to allow cutting to the depth of the diameter of the end of the bur at the point angle and permit the lock to diminish in depth occlusally, terminating at the axiolinguopulpal point angle. In a similar manner prepare the facial lock in the axiofacial line angle. When the axiofacial and axiolingual line angles are less than 2 mm in length, reduce the tilt the bur slightly so that the proximal locks are extended occlusally to disappear midway between the DEJ and the enamel margin (see Fig. 17-54, *B* and *C*).

There are four characteristics or determinants of proximal locks: (1) position, (2) translation, (3) depth, and (4) occlusogingival orientation (see Fig. 17-55). Position refers to the axiofacial and axiolingual line angles of initial tooth preparation (0.2 mm axial to DEJ). It is important to note that the retention locks should be placed 0.2 mm inside the DEJ, regardless of the depth of the axial walls and axial line angles. Translation refers to the direction of movement of the axis of the bur. Depth refers to the extent of translation (i.e., 0.5 mm at gingival floor level). Occlusogingival orientation refers to the tilt of the No. 169L bur, which dictates the occlusal height of the lock, given a constant depth.

Some operators prefer using the No. ¼ bur to cut the proximal locks. The rotating bur is carried into the axiolinguogingival (or axiofaciogingival) point angle, and then moved parallel to the DEJ to the depth of the diameter of the bur. It is then drawn occlusally along the

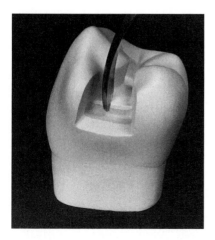

FIG. **17-53** Beveling axiopulpal line angle.

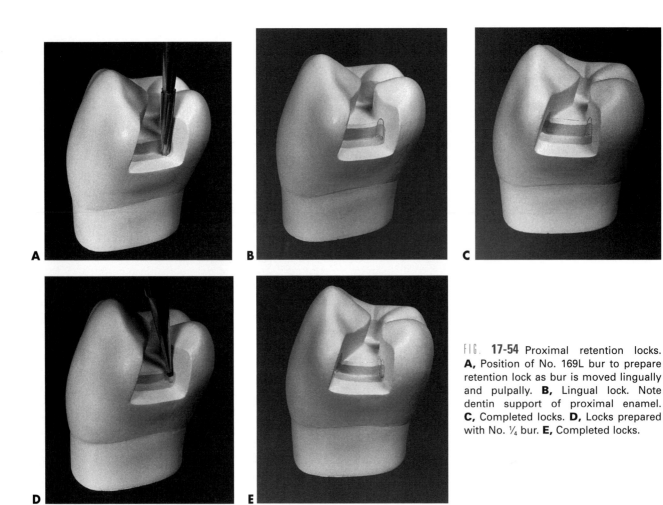

FIG. **17-54** Proximal retention locks. **A,** Position of No. 169L bur to prepare retention lock as bur is moved lingually and pulpally. **B,** Lingual lock. Note dentin support of proximal enamel. **C,** Completed locks. **D,** Locks prepared with No. 1/4 bur. **E,** Completed locks.

axiolingual (or axiofacial) line angle, allowing the lock to become shallower and to terminate at the axiolinguopulpal (or axiofaciopulpal) point angle (or more occlusally if the line angles are less than 2 mm in length) (see Fig. 17-54, *D* and *E*).

Regardless of the method used in placing the locks, extreme care is necessary to prevent the removal of dentin that immediately supports the proximal enamel. In addition, it is essential not to prepare the locks entirely in the axial wall (i.e., incorrect translation [moving the bur only in a pulpal direction]), because no effective retention is obtained and there is a risk of pulpal involvement.

An improperly positioned axiofacial or axiolingual line angle must not be used as a positional guide for the proximal lock. If the axial line angle is too shallow, the lock may undermine the enamel of dentinal support. If the line angle is too deep, preparation of the lock may result in exposure of the pulp. Retention locks should always be placed in the facial and lingual proximal walls (0.2 mm inside the DEJ), regardless of the depth of the axial wall.

Procedure for finishing external walls. The preparation walls and margins should not have unsupported enamel and marginal irregularities (if present, they re-

quire correction). It has been demonstrated that less marginal leakage occurs if the margins are straight and smooth.[37] No occlusal cavosurface bevel is indicated in the tooth preparation for amalgam. Ideally there should be a 90-degree cavosurface angle (maximum of 100 degrees) at the proximal margin. The occlusal line angle may be 90 to 100 degrees or greater. This angle aids in obtaining a marginal amalgam angle of 90 degrees (no less than 80 degrees). Clinical experience has established that this "butt joint" relationship of enamel and amalgam creates the strongest margin.[51] Amalgam is a brittle material and may fracture under occlusal stress if its angle at the margin is less than 80 degrees.

Use the mesial gingival margin trimmer (13-85-10-14, R and L) to establish a slight cavosurface bevel at the gingival margin (6 centigrades [or 20 degrees] declination gingivally) if it is in enamel. The bevel is angled no more than necessary to ensure full-length enamel rods forming the gingival margin, and it is no wider than the enamel (Fig. 17-56). When the gingival margin is positioned gingival to the cementoenamel junction (CEJ) on the tooth root, the bevel is not indicated.[51] (When beveling the gingival margin on the distal surface, use the distal gingival margin trimmer [3-95-10-14, R and L]. Alternatively, the side of an explorer tine may be used to

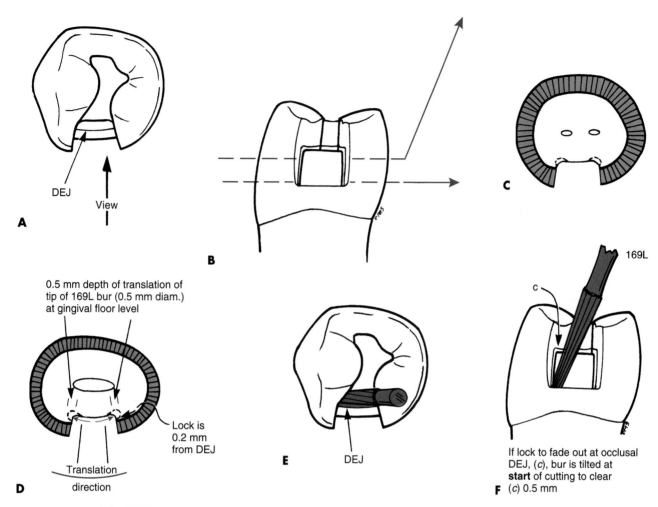

FIG. 17-55 Four characteristics of retentive locks. **A,** Occlusal view of MO preparation before placement of retention locks. **B,** Proximal view of MO preparation. **C** and **D,** Position, translation, and depth. **E** and **F,** Occlusogingival orientation.

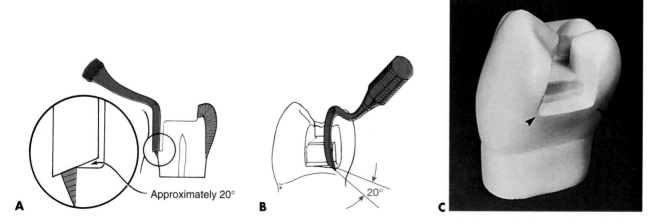

FIG. 17-56 **A,** Bevel of enamel portion of gingival wall is established with gingival margin trimmer to ensure full-length enamel rods forming gingival margin. **B** and **C,** Sharp angles at linguogingival and faciogingival corners are rounded by rotational sweep with gingival margin trimmer.

remove any friable enamel at the gingival margin. The tine is placed in the gingival embrasure apical to the gingival margin. With some pressure against the prepared tooth, the tine is moved occlusally across the gingival margin to "trim" the margin.

Final procedures: cleaning, inspecting, desensitizing, and bonding. Refer to the similar section in Conservative Class I Amalgam Restorations.

Variations of One Proximal Surface Tooth Preparations. The following sections prevent variations in tooth preparation for some conservative Class II amalgam restorations. However, in most clinical situations, the restoration presented would be restored with composite. If amalgam is used, the features presented should be considered in the tooth preparation portion of the procedure.

Mandibular first premolar. For the conservative Class II tooth preparation for amalgam on a mandibular first premolar, the conventional approach and technique must be modified because the morphologic structure of this tooth is different from the other posterior teeth (particularly because of the diminished size of the lingual cusp). For this tooth, as in all teeth, the principles of

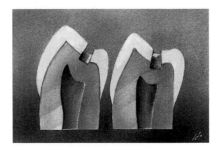

F I G. **17-57** When mandibular first and second premolars are compared, note differences in size of pulp chambers, lingual cusps, and direction of pulpal walls.

tooth preparation for amalgam must be correlated with the physical properties of the restorative material and the anatomic structure of the tooth. The relationship of the pulp chamber to the DEJ and the relatively small size of the lingual cusp are illustrated in Fig. 17-57 (this figure also illustrates the correct position of the pulpal wall and how it differs in direction as compared with the second premolar). Incorrect preparation of the central groove area could weaken the lingual cusp and excessive extension in a facial direction could approach or expose the facial pulp horn. Therefore when preparing the occlusal portion, tilt the bur slightly lingually to establish the correct pulpal wall direction (see Fig. 17-17, *B*).

In addition, the mandibular first premolar presents a variety of occlusal patterns, most of which exhibit a large transverse ridge of enamel. Often such a ridge has no connecting fissure between the mesial and distal pits, dictating a Class II preparation with an outline form that does not extend to, or across, the ridge (Fig. 17-58, *A*). If the opposite pit or proximal surface is faulty, it is restored with a separate restoration.

For a preparation that will not cross the transverse ridge, prepare the proximal box before the occlusal portion to prevent removing the tooth structure that will form the isthmus between the occlusal dovetail and the proximal box. Enter the pit adjacent to the involved proximal surface with the No. 245 bur. Immediately after the entry, direct the bur into the proximal marginal ridge and then pulpally (if necessary) until the proximal DEJ is visible. The bur axis for the proximal ditch cut should be parallel to the tooth crown, which is tilted slightly lingually for the mandibular posterior teeth. Isolate the proximal enamel, and complete the proximal box as previously described for the mandibular second premolar. Return the bur to the area of entry, and prepare the occlusal step with a dovetail, if needed. When

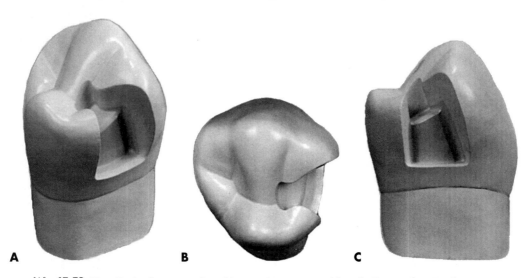

F I G. **17-58** Mandibular first premolar with sound transverse ridge. **A,** Two-surface tooth preparation that does not include opposite pit. **B,** Occlusal outline form. **C,** Proximal view of completed preparation.

preparing the occlusal portion, the bur is tilted slightly lingual to establish the correct pulpal wall direction (which maintains dentin support for the small lingual cusp and prevents encroachment on the facial pulp horn). Thus the primary difference in tooth preparation on this tooth, when compared with the preparation on other posterior teeth, is the facial inclination of the pulpal wall. Broaden the isthmus as necessary, but maintain the dovetail retention form, if required. Fig. 17-58, *B*, illustrates the correct occlusal outline form. Removing any remaining caries (if present) and inserting necessary liners or bases or both precede the placement of proximal locks and finishing of the enamel margins to complete the preparation (see Fig. 17-58, *C*).

Maxillary first molar. When mesial and distal proximal surface amalgam restorations are indicated on the maxillary first molar that has an unaffected oblique ridge, separate two-surface tooth preparations are indicated (rather than a mesioocclusodistal [MOD] preparation) because the strength of the tooth crown is significantly greater when the oblique ridge is intact.[51]

The MO tooth preparation is generally uncomplicated (Fig. 17-59, *A*). Extension into the enamel oblique ridge is avoided whenever possible to maintain the cross-splinting strength it provides to the tooth. Occasionally extension through the ridge and into the distal pit is necessary because of the extent of caries. The outline of this OL pit-and-fissure portion is similar to that of the Class I OL preparation. Fig. 17-59, *B* and *C*, illustrates a MO preparation extended to include the distal pit and the outline form that includes the distal oblique and lingual fissures.

When the occlusal fissure extends into the facial cusp ridge and it cannot be removed by enameloplasty, the defect should be eliminated by extension of the tooth preparation. Occasionally this can be accomplished by tilting the bur to create an occlusal divergence of the facial wall, while maintaining the dentin support of the ridge. If this fault cannot be eliminated without extending the margin to the height of the cusp ridge or undermining the enamel margin, extend the preparation facially through the ridge (see Fig. 17-59, *D*). The pulpal wall of this facial extension may have remaining enamel, but a depth of 1.5 to 2 mm is necessary to provide sufficient bulk of material for adequate strength. For the best esthetic results minimal extension of the proximal mesiofacial margin is indicated.

The distoocclusal (DO) tooth preparation may take one of several outlines, depending on the occlusal anatomy. The occlusal outline is determined by the pit-and-fissure pattern and by the amount and extension of caries. An extension onto the lingual surface to include a lingual fissure should be prepared only after the distolingual proximal margin is established. This may permit the operator to maintain more tooth structure between the distolingual wall and the lingual fissure extension, resulting in more strength of the distolingual cusp. It is accomplished by preparing the lingual fissure extension more at the expense of the mesiolingual cusp than the distolingual cusp. Nevertheless, the distolingual cusp on many maxillary molars (particularly maxillary second molars) may be weakened during such a distoocclusolingual tooth preparation because of the small cuspal portion remaining between the lingual fis-

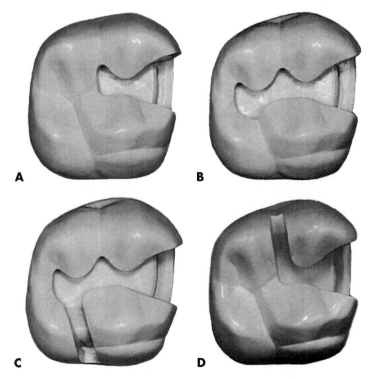

FIG. **17-59** Maxillary first molar. **A,** Conventional MO preparation. **B,** MO preparation extended to include distal pit. **C,** Mesioocclusolingual preparation, including distal pit and distal oblique and lingual fissures. **D,** MO preparation with facial fissure extension.

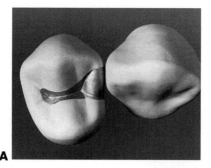
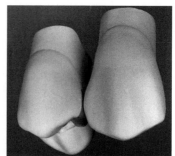

FIG. **17-60** To produce inconspicuous margin on maxillary first premolar, mesiofacial wall does not diverge gingivally and facial extension with a No. 245 bur should be minimal so that mesiofacial proximal margin of preparation will minimally clear the contact as margin is finished. **A,** Occlusal view. **B,** Facial view.

sure preparation and the distolingual proximal wall. In addition, caries excavation may weaken the cusp. Thus capping of the distolingual cusp is often necessary to provide proper resistance form. The procedure is described in a later section (see Fig. 17-70).

Maxillary first premolar. A Class II amalgam tooth preparation involving the mesial surface of a maxillary first premolar requires special attention because the mesiofacial embrasure is esthetically prominent. The occlusogingival preparation of the facial wall of the mesial box should be parallel to the long axis of the tooth instead of converging occlusally to minimize an unesthetic display of amalgam in the faciogingival corner of the restoration. In addition, the facial extension of the mesiofacial proximal wall should be minimal so that the mesiofacial proximal margin of the preparation will only minimally clear the contact as the margin is finished with an appropriate enamel hatchet or chisel (Fig. 17-60).

If the mesial proximal involvement (1) is limited to a fissure in the marginal ridge that is at risk for caries, (2) is not treatable by enameloplasty, and (3) does not involve the proximal contact, the proximal portion of the tooth preparation is prepared by extending through the fault with the No. 245 bur so that the margins are lingual to the contact. Often this means that the proximal box will be the faciolingual width of the bur and the gingival floor may be at the same depth as the pulpal floor. Retention form for this extension is provided by the slight occlusal convergence of the facial and lingual walls (see Fig. 17-9).

If proximal caries is limited to the mesiolingual embrasure, do not involve the mesial proximal contact in the tooth preparation. If only the lingual aspect of the mesial proximal contact is carious, the mesiofacial wall may be left in contact with the adjacent tooth (reducing the display of amalgam). A Class II tooth preparation involving the distal surface of the maxillary first premolar is similar to the preparation of the mandibular second premolar described earlier.

Box-only preparation. When restoring a small, cavitated, proximal lesion in a tooth with neither occlusal fissures nor a previously inserted occlusal restoration, a proximal box preparation without an occlusal step has been recommended.[1,51] To maximize retention, prepara-

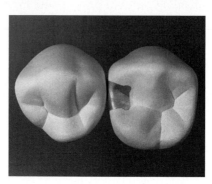

FIG. **17-61** Simple box restoration without occlusal step is permissible when restoring small proximal lesion in tooth without either occlusal fissures or previously inserted occlusal restoration and when involved marginal ridge does not support occlusal contact. Note that proximal locks extend to occlusal surface.

tions with facial and lingual walls that almost oppose each other are recommended. Therefore this type of preparation should be limited to a proximal surface with a narrow proximal contact (allowing minimal facial and lingual extensions). As in the typical preparation, the facial and lingual proximal walls converge occlusally. Retention locks are necessary in box-only preparations.[86] The proximal retention locks should have a 0.5-mm depth at the gingival point angle, tapering to a depth of 0.3 mm at the occlusal surface (Fig. 17-61).

Modifications in Tooth Preparation

Slot preparation for root caries. Older patients who have gingival recession exposing the cementum may experience caries on the proximal root surface that is appreciably gingival to the proximal contact (Fig. 17-62, *A*). Assuming that the contact does not need restoring, the tooth preparation is usually approached from the facial and has the form of a slot (see Fig. 17-62, *B*). A lingual approach is used when the caries is limited to the linguoproximal surface. Amalgam is particularly indicated for slot preparations if isolation is difficult.[9]

After anesthesia and isolation of the operating field, prepare the initial outline form from a facial approach with a No. 2 or No. 4 bur using high speed and air-water spray. Outline form extension to sound tooth structure is at a limited depth axially (i.e., 0.75 to 1 mm at the gingival aspect [if no enamel is present], increasing to

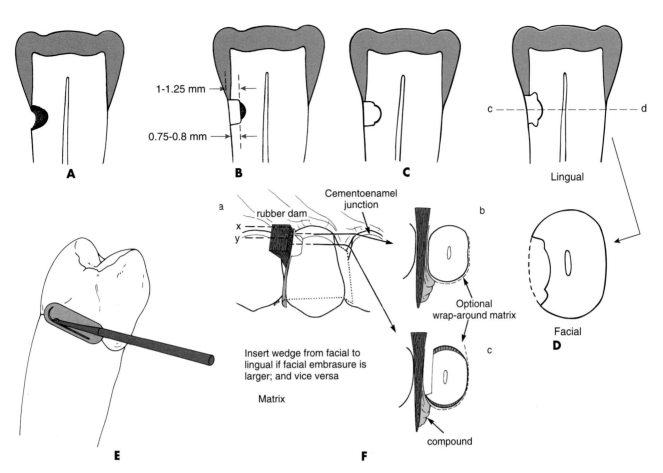

FIG. **17-62** Slot preparation. **A,** Mesiodistal longitudinal section illustrating carious lesion. Proximal contact is not involved. **B,** Initial tooth preparation. **C,** Tooth preparation with infected carious dentin removed. **D,** Retention grooves are shown in longitudinal section, and transverse section through plane *cd* illustrates contour of axial wall and direction of facial and lingual walls. **E,** Preparing retention form to complete tooth preparation. **F,** Matrix for slot preparation: *a,* Facial view of wedged matrix; *b,* Wedged matrix as viewed in transverse cross-section (*x*), gingival to gingival floor; *c,* Wedged matrix as viewed in transverse cross-section (*y*), occlusal to gingival floor.

1 to 1.25 mm at the occlusal wall [if margin in enamel]) (see Fig. 17-62, *B*). If the occlusal margin is in enamel, the axial depth should be 0.5 mm inside the DEJ. During this extension the bur should not remove any infected carious dentin from the axial wall deeper than the outline form initial depth. The remaining infected carious dentin (if any) will be removed during final tooth preparation (see Fig. 17-62, *C*). External walls should form a 90-degree cavosurface angle. With a facial approach, the lingual wall should face facially as much as possible. This will aid condensation of amalgam during its insertion. The facial wall must be extended to provide access and visibility or convenience form (see Fig. 17-62, *D*).

In final tooth preparation use the No. 2 or No. 4 bur to remove any remaining infected carious dentin on the axial wall. If indicated, apply a liner or base or both (as described for the Class I tooth preparation).

Prepare retention grooves with a No. 1/4 bur into the occlusoaxial and gingivoaxial line angles, 0.2 mm inside the DEJ or 0.3 to 0.5 mm inside the cemental cavosurface margin (see Fig. 17-62, *E*). The depth of these grooves is one half the diameter of the bur head (i.e., 0.25 mm), and the bur is directed to bisect the angle formed by the junction of occlusal (or gingival) and axial walls. Ideally the direction of the occlusal groove is slightly more occlusal than axial, and the direction of an gingival groove would be slightly more gingival than axial (as in the Class III amalgam preparation) (see Figs. 18-8 and 18-13).

Before application of the matrix, dentin should be desensitized or a bonding system applied (refer to the discussion of dentin desensitizers and bonding systems in Conservative Class I Amalgam Preparations). The matrix for inserting amalgam in a slot preparation for root caries is similar to that illustrated in Fig. 17-62, *F*.

For those instances where root caries encircles the tooth, the proximal areas can be restored as described previously. Subsequently, Class V preparations are

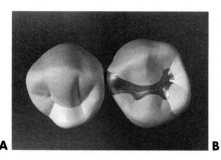
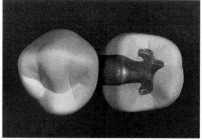
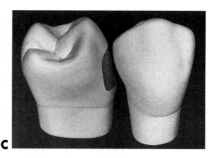

A   **B**   **C**

FIG. **17-63** Restoration outlines for rotated teeth. **A,** MO outline for mandibular premolar with 45-degree rotation. **B,** MO outline for mandibular premolar with 90-degree rotation. **C,** Slot preparation outline for restoration of a small mesial lesion involving proximal contact of mandibular premolar with 90-degree rotation.

prepared and abutted with the proximal restorations. The amalgam used to restore the proximals should be fully set (to avoid dislocation during preparation and during insertion of the Class V restorations). Alternatively, the Class V portions can be restored first. When the proximals are restored first, the mesial and distal walls of the Class V preparations would be in amalgam. Doing a circumferential restoration in segments allows proper condensation of amalgam. A full-coverage restoration is usually preferred if caries encircles the tooth cervically. These patients should be counseled to improve their oral hygiene and use fluoride rinses.

Rotated teeth. Tooth preparation for rotated teeth follows the same principles as for normally aligned teeth. The outline form for a MO tooth preparation on the rotated mandibular second premolar (Fig. 17-63, *A*) differs from normal in that its proximal box is displaced facially because the proximal caries involves the mesiofacial line angle of the tooth crown.

When the tooth is rotated 90 degrees and the "proximal" lesion is on the facial or lingual surface or orthodontic correction is declined or ruled out, the preparation may require an isthmus that includes the cuspal eminence (see Fig. 17-63, *B*). If the lesion is small, consideration should be given to the slot preparation. In this instance, the occlusal margin may be in the contact area or slightly occlusal to it (see Fig. 17-63, *C*).

Unusual outline forms. Outline forms should conform to the restoration requirements of the tooth and not necessarily to the classic example of a Class II tooth preparation. For example, as mentioned earlier, a dovetail feature is not required in the occlusal step of a single proximal surface preparation unless a fissure emanating from the occlusal step is involved in the preparation. Another example is an occlusal fissure that is segmented by coalesced enamel (as illustrated previously for mandibular premolars and maxillary first molars). This should be treated with individual amalgam restorations if the preparations are separated by approximately 0.5 mm or more of sound tooth structure (Fig. 17-64).[1,85]

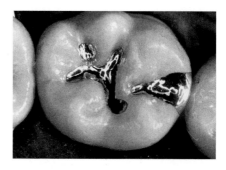

FIG. **17-64** Restoration of MO tooth preparation with central fissure segmented by coalesced enamel.

Adjoining restorations. It is permissible to repair or replace a defective portion of an existing amalgam restoration if the remaining portion of the original restoration retains adequate resistance and retention form. Adjoining restorations on the occlusal surface occur more often in molars because the dovetail of the new restoration can usually be prepared without eliminating the dovetail of the existing restoration. Where the two restorations adjoin, care should be taken that the outline of the second restoration does not weaken the amalgam margin of the first (Fig. 17-65, *A*). The intersecting margins of the two restorations should be at right angles as much as possible. The decision to adjoin two restorations implies that the first restoration, or a part of it, does not need to be replaced and assumes that the procedure for the single proximal restoration (when compared with a MOD restoration) is less complicated, especially in matrix application.

Occasionally, preparing an amalgam restoration in two or more phases is indicated, such as for a Class II lesion that is contiguous with a Class V lesion. Preparing both lesions before placing the amalgam introduces condensation problems that can be eliminated by preparing and restoring the Class II lesion before preparing and restoring the Class V lesion (see Fig. 17-65, *B*). For example, it is better to condense amalgam against a carious wall of the first preparation than to attempt condensation where no wall exists.

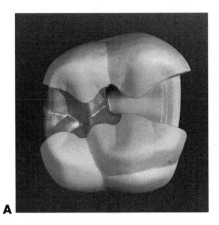
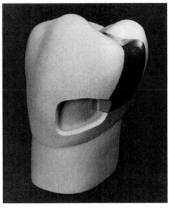

FIG. **17-65** Adjoining restorations. **A,** Adjoining MO tooth preparation with DO restoration so that new preparation does not weaken amalgam margin of existing restoration. **B,** Preparing and restoring Class II lesion before preparing and restoring Class V lesion contiguous with it will eliminate condensation problems that occur when both lesions are prepared before either is restored.

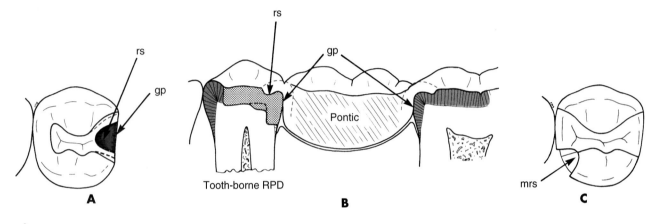

FIG. **17-66** Abutment teeth with Class II restorations designed for removable partial denture (RPD). **A,** Occlusal view showing location of rest seat *(rs)* and guiding plane *(gp)* for a tooth-borne RPD. **B,** Cross-sectional view illustrating deepened pulpal wall in area of rest seat *(rs)* to provide adequate thickness of amalgam. Note relationship of guiding planes *(gp)* to tooth-borne RPD. **C,** Occlusal view showing mesial rest seat *(mrs)* for tissue-borne (i.e., distal extension) RPD. **D,** Lingual view of tissue-borne RPD showing relationship of RPD to Class II restoration and edentulous ridge *(er)*.

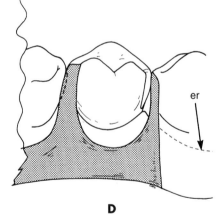

Abutment teeth for removable partial denture. When the tooth is an abutment for a planned removable partial denture, the occlusoproximal outline form adjacent to the edentulous region may need additional extension if a rest seat is planned, such as for the tooth-borne partial denture. This additional extension must be sufficient facially, lingually, and axially to allow preparing the rest seat in the restoration without jeopardizing its strength. The facial and lingual proximal walls and respective occlusal margins must be extended so that the entire rest seat can be prepared in amalgam without encroaching on the occlusal margins. If the rest seat is to be within the amalgam margins, it is recommended that

there be a minimum of 0.5 mm of amalgam between the rest seat and the margins (Fig. 17-66, *A*). The portion of the pulpal wall apical to the planned rest seat is deepened 0.5 mm so that the total depth of the axiopulpal line angle measured on the facial and lingual wall is 2.5 mm (see Fig. 17-66, *B*). However, a rest seat may involve both amalgam and enamel as illustrated on the mesiolingual of an abutment tooth, such as for a tissue-borne (i.e., distal extension) partial denture. In this case, no modification of the outline form of the tooth preparation is indicated (see Fig. 17-66, *C*). Fig. 17-66, *D*, illustrates the relationship of the tissue-borne removable partial denture with the abutment tooth (see Fig. 17-66, *C*).

Class II Amalgam Restorations Involving Both Proximal Surfaces.

Preparation and Restoration Factors. Perhaps the best indications for the use of amalgam restorations are moderate and large Class II defects that include both proximal surfaces and much of the occlusal surface. (Although Chapter 19 presents the technique for very extensive or complex Class II amalgam restorations, this section describes the use of amalgam for moderate and large Class II restorations.)

The principles of tooth preparation are the same for all amalgam restorations:

- A cavosurface marginal design that results in an approximate 90-degree amalgam margin
- Appropriate removal of tooth structure to provide for adequate strength of the amalgam
- Appropriate retention features

The tooth preparation techniques presented for a two-surface Class II restoration apply to larger Class II restorations as well. However, when the defect is large, certain modifications in tooth preparation may be necessary and the use of an amalgam-bonding system may be more strongly considered.

Occlusal extensions. Often a larger Class II defect will require greater extension of the occlusal surface outline form. This may require extending grooves that are fissured, capping cusps that are undermined, or extending the outline form up the cuspal inclines. These alterations can be accomplished easily by following the principles presented previously. Groove extension occurs at the same initial pulpal floor depth (i.e., 1.5 mm) but follows the DEJ as the groove is extended in a facial or lingual direction. Thus the pulpal floor of an extended groove will usually slightly rise occlusally as it extended toward the cusp ridge (see Fig. 17-35, *C*). If it is necessary to extend through the cusp ridge onto the facial or lingual surface, the preparation is accomplished as described for the OL Class I restoration.

If an occlusal outline form extends up a cuspal incline, the extension should also maintain the pulpal floor at the desired initial pulpal floor depth (i.e., 1.5 mm). This extension (and groove extension) will usually require some alteration in the orientation of the No. 245 bur: a slight lingual tilt when extending in a facial direction, and a slight facial tilt when extending in a lingual direction (see Fig. 17-26). Maintaining the correct pulpal floor depth preserves tooth structure and reduces the potential for pulpal encroachment. The prepared facial (or lingual) cavosurface margin should still result in a 90-degree amalgam margin.

When the occlusal outline form extends from a primary groove to within two thirds of the distance to a cusp tip, that cusp is usually sufficiently weakened so as to require replacement (see Fig. 6-27). Leaving the cusp

in a weakened state may be acceptable if the cusp is very large or, occasionally, if the amalgam is to be bonded (which will provide some reinforcement of the strength of the remaining cuspal structure). Routine preparations in some teeth may predispose some cusps for capping (i.e., reduction). The small distal cusp of mandibular first molars, the distolingual cusp of maxillary molars, and the lingual cusp of some mandibular premolars (especially first premolars) may be weakened when normal preparations of surrounding areas of the tooth are included.

Cusp reduction for an amalgam restoration should result in a uniform amalgam thickness over the reduced cusp of 1.5 to 2 mm. The thicker amount is necessary for functional cusps. These dimensions provide adequate strength for the amalgam. The cusp reduction should occur as early in the preparation as can be determined to provide better access and vision for completing the preparation (see Fig. 19-4). To reduce the cusp, orient the No. 245 bur parallel to the cuspal incline (lingual incline for facial cusp reductions and facial inclines for lingual cusp reduction) and make several depth cuts in the cusp (to a depth of 1.5 or 2 mm). The depth cuts will provide guides for the correct amount of cusp reduction. Without depth cuts, after the beginning reduction of the cusp the operator may no longer know how much more reduction is necessary. Use the bur to reduce the cusp, following the mesiodistal inclines of the cusp. This results in a uniform reduction. If only one of two facial (or lingual) cusps is to be capped, the cusp reduction should extend slightly beyond the facial (or lingual) groove area, provide the correct amount of tooth structure removal, and meet the adjacent, unreduced cusp to create a 90-degree cavosurface margin. This results in both adequate thickness and edge strength of the amalgam. Cusp capping reduces the amount of vertical preparation wall heights and, therefore, increases the need for the use of secondary retention features. Increased retention form may be provided by proximal box retention locks, but may require the use of pins or slots (as described in Chapter 19). If indicated, cusp capping increases the resistance form of the tooth.[30,61] It has been reported that the survival rate of cusp-covered amalgam restorations is 72% at 15 years.[78]

Proximal extensions. Larger Class II restorations will often require larger proximal box preparations. These may include not only increased faciolingual or gingival extensions, but also extension around a facial or lingual line angle. Large proximal box preparations also need secondary retention features (i.e., retention locks, pins, slots) for adequate retention form. Extensive proximal boxes are usually prepared the same as a more conservative proximal box, but may require modifications (see Figs. 17-72 and 19-8, *A*). For increased faciolingual extensions, it may be necessary to tilt the No. 245 bur to include proximal faults that are extensive gingival to the contact area. Tilting the bur (to the lingual when extending a facial proximal wall or to the facial when extending a facial wall) conserves more of the marginal ridge and cuspal tooth structure. Although this enhances preservation of some tooth structure strength, it results in a more occlusally convergent wall, which increases the difficulty of amalgam condensation in the gingival corners of the preparation.

When proximal extension around a line angle is necessary, it is usually associated with a reduction of the involved cusp (see Fig. 19-14). Such proximal extension is usually necessitated by a severely defective (or fractured) cusp or a cervical lesion that extends from the facial (or lingual) surface into the proximal area. Often these areas are included in the preparation by extending the gingival floor of the proximal box around the line angle, using the same criteria for preparation as the typical proximal box: (1) facial (or lingual) extension results in an occlusogingival wall that has a 90-degree cavosurface margin, and (2) axial depth is 0.5 mm inside the DEJ.

The increased dimensions of a large proximal box usually require the use of retention locks or other secondary retention form features (i.e., pins or slots). Secondary retention form features better ensure the retention of the amalgam within the preparation by resisting displacement of the amalgam in an proximal direction (and occasionally in a occlusal direction). Placement of retention locks may be more difficult because of the extent of the preparation and the amount of caries excavation that may be necessary. However, if the outline form is developed correctly, the axiofacial and axiolingual line angles will be correctly positioned and can be used as the location for retention lock placement. The retention locks are prepared as described previously.

When the proximal defect is extensive gingivally, isolation of the area, tooth preparation, matrix placement, and condensation and carving of the amalgam are more difficult. If the proximal box is extended onto the root surface, the axial wall depth is no longer dictated by the DEJ. Any root surface preparation for amalgam should result in an initial axial wall depth of approximately 0.8 mm. This axial depth provides appropriate strength for the amalgam, preserves the pulp integrity, and creates enough dimension for placement of retention locks of 0.5 mm depth, while preserving the strength of the adjacent, remaining marginal dentin and cementum. The extent of the preparation onto the root surface or the contour of the tooth or both may require that the bur be tilted toward the adjacent tooth when preparing the gingival floor of the proximal box (see Figs. 17-44, *C*, and 13-30, *A* through *C*). This may result in an axial wall that has two planes, the more gingival plane angled slightly internally. This may also cause more difficulty in retention lock placement. The more occlusal part of the axial wall may be overreduced if the bur is not tilted.

When it is determined that pins or slots are necessary for a Class II restoration, the axial depth is increased in pin or slot locations. Techniques for pin and slot placement are presented in Chapter 19.

Caries excavation and pulp protection. Larger Class II restorations will often require more extensive caries excavation and pulp protection procedures during tooth preparation. If the outline form is correct after the initial preparation, caries should only remain on the pulpal floor or axial wall or both. Initial tooth preparation may have removed all of the caries, defect, or old restorative material. If so, final tooth preparation will consist of only placement of secondary retention form features. If caries remains, the pulpal or axial wall or both must be excavated with a suitable technique (see Figs. 17-49 and 17-50). If extensive caries was the reason for doing the procedure, then excavation should be done with the area properly isolated, preferably with a rubber dam. Proper isolation may improve the success of an indirect or direct pulp-capping procedure, if necessary. Deep excavations indicate the increased need for pulp protection with a liner or base or both. If necessary, a calcium hydroxide liner or a RMGI base is placed as described previously (see Fig. 17-28).

Amalgam-bonding procedures. Because larger amalgam restorations have less remaining tooth structure and more amalgam material that must be retained in the tooth, they may require increased consideration of amalgam-bonding techniques (see Fig. 17-29). Although amalgam-bonding techniques improve sealing of the prepared tooth structure and strengthen the remaining unprepared tooth structure, their ability to increase retention form significantly is questionable. Therefore adequate secondary retention form must be used in the tooth preparation (in addition to the bonding technique).

Matrix placement. When a tooth preparation is extensive, matrix placement is more difficult. This is especially true for preparations that extend onto the root surface. Use of modified matrix bands and wedging techniques may be required (see Figs. 17-82, 17-83, 17-85, 17-87, 17-89, and 19-42 through 19-46). (Different types of matrix systems are presented in Chapter 19.)

Condensation and carving of the amalgam. Larger Class II preparations that extend around line angles, cap cusps, or extend onto the root surface require careful amalgam condensation and carving techniques. Condensation of amalgam is more difficult in areas where cusps have been capped, where slots or pins have been placed, where vertical walls are more convergent occlusally, and where the root surface is involved. For larger restorations, lateral condensation is important to produce a properly condensed restoration in the gingival corners; also, carving cusps and gingival areas is more difficult.

Examples of Moderate Class II Amalgam Tooth Preparations That Involve Both Proximal Surfaces

Mandibular second premolar. A moderate MOD tooth preparation in a mandibular second premolar is illustrated in Fig. 17-67. Note the similarity with the two-surface MO preparation.

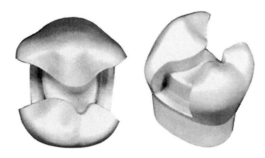

FIG. **17-67** MOD preparation on mandibular second premolar.

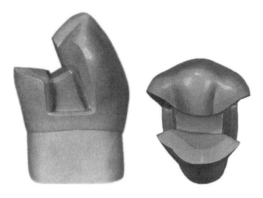

FIG. **17-68** Mandibular first premolar with lingual cusp reduced for capping.

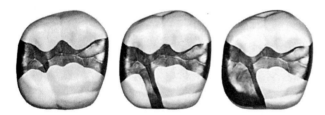

FIG. **17-69** Typical three- and four-surface restorations for maxillary first molar. (See Fig. 17-70 for preparation of distolingual cusp for capping.)

Mandibular first premolar. When a MOD amalgam tooth preparation is needed for the mandibular first premolar, the support of the small lingual cusp may be conserved by preparing the occlusal step more at the expense of tooth structure facial to the central groove than lingual. In addition, recall that the bur is tilted slightly lingually to establish the correct pulpal wall direction. Despite these precautions, the lingual cusp may need to be reduced for capping if the lingual margin of the occlusal step extends more than two thirds the distance from the central fissure to the cuspal eminence (Fig. 17-68). Special attention is given to such cusp reduction because retention is severely diminished when the cusp is reduced, eliminating the lingual wall of the occlusal portion. Depth cuts of 1.5 mm will aid the operator in establishing the correct amount of cusp reduction and conserving a small portion of the lingual wall in the occlusal step. It is acceptable when restoring diminutive nonfunctional cusps, such as the lingual cusp of a mandibular first premolar, to reduce the cusp only 0.5 to 1 mm and then restore the cusp to achieve an amalgam thickness of 1.5 mm. This procedure conserves more of the lingual wall of the isthmus for added retention form. (For the correct lingual tilt of the bur to establish the appropriate pulpal wall orientation, see Fig. 17-31.)

Maxillary first molar. The MOD tooth preparation of the maxillary first molar may require extending through the oblique ridge to unite the proximal preparations with the occlusal step. Cutting through the oblique ridge is indicated only if: (1) the ridge is undermined with caries, (2) it is crossed by a deep fissure, or (3) occlusal portions of the separate MO and DO outline forms leave less than 0.5 mm of tooth structure between them. The remainder of the outline form is similar to the two-surface outline forms described previously in this chapter. Fig. 17-69 illustrates several typical three- and four-surface restorations for this tooth. The procedure for reducing the distolingual cusp of a maxillary first molar for capping is illustrated in Fig. 17-70. Extending the facial or lingual wall of a proximal box to include the entire cusp is done (if necessary) to include weak or carious tooth structure or existing restorative material (Figs. 17-71 and 17-72).

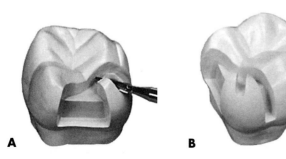
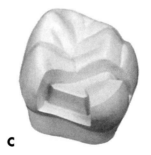
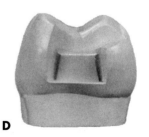

A   **B**   **C**   **D**

FIG. **17-70** Reduction of distolingual cusp of maxillary molar. **A,** Cutting depth gauge groove with side of bur. **B,** Completed depth gauge groove. **C** and **D,** Completed cusp reduction.

Maxillary second molar with caries on distal portion of facial surface. Close examination of the distal portion of the facial surface of the maxillary second molar may reveal decalcification or cavitation or both. When the enamel is only slightly cavitated (i.e., softened and rough), polishing with sandpaper discs may eliminate the fault. Careful brushing technique, daily use of fluoride (i.e., rinses, toothpaste), and periodic applications of a topical fluoride may prevent further breakdown. However, when decalcification is as deep as the DEJ and distal proximal caries is also present, the entire distofacial cusp may need to be included in a mesioocclusodistofacial (MODF) tooth preparation. The facial lesion may be restored separately, if it is judged that the distofacial cusp would not be significantly weakened if left unrestored (i.e., uncapped) by amalgam. In that case, the MOD preparation would be restored first, followed by preparation and restoration of the facial lesion. When such sequential preparations are contraindicated, the preparation outline (see Fig. 17-71) is extended gingivally to include the distofacial cusp (just beyond the caries) and mesially to include the facial groove. The No. 245 bur should be used to create a gingival floor (i.e., shoulder) perpendicular to the occlusal force when extending the distal gingival floor to include

the affected facial surface. Including the distofacial caries often indicates a gingival margin that follows the gingival tissue level. The width of the shoulder should be approximately 1 or 0.5 mm inside the DEJ, whichever is greater. Some resistance form is provided by the shoulder. A retention lock should be placed in the axiofacial line angle of this distofacial extension, similar to the locks placed in the proximal boxes. For additional retention, a slot may be placed (see Chapter 19).

Mandibular first molar. The distal cusp on the mandibular first molar may be weakened when positioning the distofacial wall and margin. Facial extension of the distofacial margin to clear the distal contact often places the occlusal outline in the center of the cusp. This dictates relocation of the margin to provide a sound enamel wall and 90-degree amalgam that is not on a cuspal eminence. When the distal cusp is small or weakened or both, extension of the distal gingival floor and distofacial wall to include the distal cusp places the margin just mesial to the distofacial groove. (In Fig. 17-72, compare the ideal distofacial extension [*A*] with that necessary to include the distal cusp [*B*].)

Capping the distal cusp is an alternative to extending the entire distofacial wall when the occlusal margin crosses the cuspal eminence (see Fig. 17-72, *C*). A minimal reduction of 2 mm should result in a 2-mm thickness of amalgam over the capped cusp (see Fig. 17-72, *D*). The cusp reduction should result in a butt joint between the tooth structure and the amalgam. Whenever possible, capping the distal cusp is more desirable than extending the distofacial margin because the remaining portion of the cusp helps in applying the matrix for the development of proper embrasure form. It also conserves tooth structure. The plane of the reduced cusp should parallel the facial (or lingual) outline of the unreduced cusp mesiodistally and the cuspal incline emanating from the central groove faciolingually.

RESTORATIVE TECHNIQUE

Placing a Sealer or Adhesive System. As stated previously, dentin desensitizers or dentin bonding systems are currently used in lieu of cavity varnish. Dentin

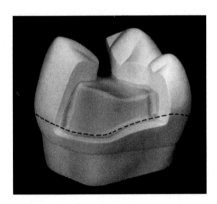

FIG. **17-71** MODF preparation of maxillary second molar showing extension to include moderate to extensive caries in distal half of facial surface. Outline includes distofacial cusp and facial groove. Dotted line represents soft-tissue level.

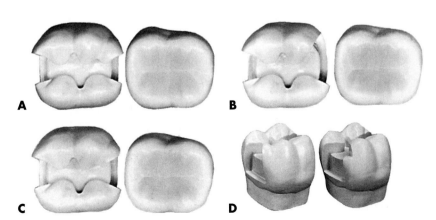

A   B   C   D

FIG. **17-72** Mandibular first molar. **A,** Ideal distofacial extension. **B,** Entire distal cusp included in preparation outline form. **C,** Capping of distal cusp is indicated when occlusal margin crosses cuspal eminence. **D,** *Left*, Distofacial view of distal cusp shown in **C** before reduction for capping; *right*, distal cusp after reduction. Reduction of 2 mm is necessary to provide for minimal 2-mm thickness of amalgam.

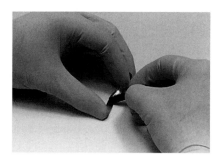

FIG. **17-73** Rubbing inlay wax on preparation side of matrix band.

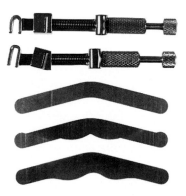

FIG. **17-74** Straight and contra-angled Universal (Tofflemire) retainers. Bands are available with varying occlusogingival measurements.

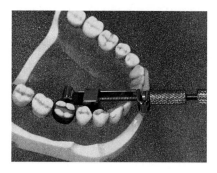

FIG. **17-75** Lingual positioning requires contra-angled Universal retainer.

desensitizers are used routinely in conservative Class I and II tooth preparations. Dentin bonding systems are usually reserved for more extensive tooth preparations with deep excavations, foundations, and teeth prone to fracture. Although dentin bonding systems may provide some adhesion of amalgam to tooth structure, they are not a substitute for conventional retention features and preparation resistance form.

If a dentin bonding system is indicated, it is recommended to lubricate the matrix band on the preparation side before applying the bonding system. This may be done by rubbing the preparation side of the burnished (i.e., precontoured) band with a stick of inlay wax (before the band and retainer are assembled) to leave wax film (Fig. 17-73). It is important to follow carefully the manufacturers' instructions regarding application of the bonding system components. Remember that amalgam must be condensed immediately into the preparation once the adhesive resin is applied. After matrix removal and before carving the proximal amalgam, check the gingival sulcus for any excess bonding resin, which, if present, must be removed. Refer to an earlier section for a more complete description of the indications and use of dentin desensitizers and dentin bonding systems. Often the sealer is applied after matrix placement. Bonding procedures always occur after the matrix placement.

Bonding the amalgam restoration to the tooth structure significantly reduces microleakage.[13,38,89] In addition, amalgam that is bonded to the tooth results in a restoration that is more resistant to displacement than conventionally placed amalgam retained with proximal grooves or dovetails.[81] It is not known whether microleakage, recurrent caries, or retention of the amalgam is a problem if the resin fatigues and breaks down. Long-term clinical trials are needed to assess these factors. A 5-year clinical evaluation reported no difference in Class II molar restorations using bonding systems and those using varnish.[79] However, bonding systems may decrease cuspal deflection[21] and increase the fracture strength of the tooth.[20]

Placing a Matrix. The primary function of the matrix is to restore anatomic contours and contact areas. Qualities of a good matrix include: (1) rigidity, (2) establish-

ment of proper anatomic contour, (3) restoration of correct proximal contact relation, (4) prevention of gingival excess, (5) convenient application, and (6) ease of removal. The following information presents the technique of placement for the Universal (Tofflemire), compound-supported, precontoured, and Automatrix systems.

Universal Matrix. The Universal matrix system (designed by B.R. Tofflemire) is ideally indicated when three surfaces (i.e., mesial, occlusal, distal) of a posterior tooth have been prepared (Fig. 17-74). It is commonly used also for the two-surface Class II restoration. A definite advantage of the Tofflemire matrix retainer is that it may be positioned on the facial or lingual aspect of the tooth. Lingual positioning, however, requires the contra-angled design of the retainer (which can be used on the facial aspect as well) (Fig. 17-75). The retainer and band are generally stable when in place. The retainer is easily separated from the band to expedite removal of the band. Matrix bands of various occlusogingival widths are available (see Fig. 17-74). A small Tofflemire retainer is available for use with the primary dentition. Even though the Universal retainer is a versatile instrument, it still does not meet all the requirements of the ideal retainer and band. The conventional, flat Tofflemire matrix band (unburnished) must be shaped (i.e., burnished) to achieve proper contour and contact.

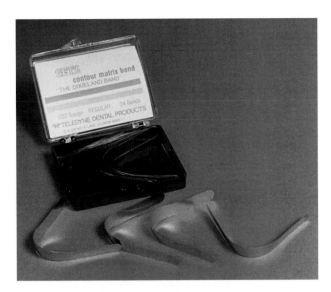

FIG. **17-76** Precontoured bands for Universal retainer.

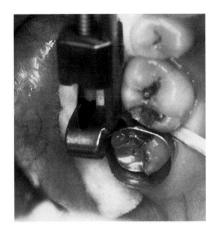

FIG. **17-77** Tofflemire retainer maintaining cotton roll in maxillary vestibule during condensation.

The uncontoured bands are available in two thicknesses, 0.002 (0.05 mm) and 0.0015 (0.038 mm) inch. Burnishing the thinner band to contour is more difficult, and the band is less likely to retain its contour when tightened around the tooth. Proximal surfaces restored using the Tofflemire matrix may require more carving than those restored with the compound-supported matrix (presented next). However, much less time is required for placement of the Tofflemire matrix.

Precontoured bands for the Universal retainer are commercially available and need little or no adjustment before placing in the retainer (Fig. 17-76). These bands are also simpler to use because they usually require little or no adjustment or modification after positioning around the tooth. Although precontoured bands are more expensive, they are generally preferred over the uncontoured bands. The difference in cost is justified because they require less chair time.

Moisture control during insertion of the amalgam is important for the success of the restoration. (Isolation procedures are discussed in Chapter 10.) When cotton roll isolation is used, the Tofflemire retainer will help to hold the cotton roll in place (Fig. 17-77).

The uncontoured band must be burnished before assembling the matrix band and retainer. Burnishing must occur in the areas corresponding to the proximal surface or surfaces to be restored once the band is positioned around the tooth. For example, if the mesial surface of the tooth is being restored, the area of the band corresponding to the mesial surface must be burnished. If the mesial and distal surfaces of the tooth are being restored, the areas corresponding to the mesial and distal surfaces must be burnished.

Burnishing means that the metal band has been deformed occlusogingivally with a suitable hand instrument to produce a rounded or convex surface that (when in place around the tooth) will produce a restoration that is symmetric in contour with the adjacent proximal surface (Fig. 17-78). The No. 26-28 burnisher is generally recommended for burnishing the band. The band should be placed on a resilient paper pad because contouring cannot occur on a hard, nonresilient surface. The smaller round burnisher tip should be used with firm pressure in back-and-forth, overlapping strokes along the length of the band, until the band is deformed occlusogingivally in the appropriate areas. Once the band is deformed, the larger egg-shaped end may be used to smooth the burnished band. If a convex surface is not obvious in burnished areas once the band is removed from the pad, it has not been adequately burnished. The band can be burnished with the larger egg-shaped burnisher only, but more work is required to do so. It is not necessary to burnish the entire length of the band. When a precontoured band is used, burnishing is unnecessary.

To prepare the retainer to receive the band, turn the larger of the knurled nuts counterclockwise until the locking vise is a short distance (¼ inch [6 mm]) from the end of the retainer (Fig. 17-79, *A*). Next, while holding the large nut, turn the smaller knurled nut counterclockwise until the pointed spindle is free of the slot in the locking vise (see Fig. 17-79, *B*). Fold the matrix band end to end, forming a loop (see Fig. 17-79, *C*). Notice that when the band is folded, the gingival edge has a smaller circumference than the occlusal edge. The band design accommodates the difference in tooth circumferences at the contact and gingival levels. Position the band in the retainer so that the slotted side of the retainer is directed gingivally to permit easy separation of the retainer from the band in an occlusal direction (later procedure). This is accomplished by placing the occlusal edge of the band in the correct guide channel (i.e., right, left, or parallel to the long axis of the retainer) depending on the location of the tooth. The two ends of the band are placed in the slot of the locking vise, and the smaller of the knurled nuts is turned clockwise to tighten the pointed spindle against the band (see Fig. 17-79, *D*). If proximal wedges were used during tooth preparation, remove them and slip the matrix band over the tooth (allowing the gingival edge of the band to be positioned at least 1 mm apical to the gingival margin). However, do not damage the gingival attachment. If needed, the larger of the knurled nuts may be turned counterclockwise to obtain a larger loop to fit over the tooth. Be careful not to trap rubber dam between the band and the gingival margin. If the dam material is trapped between the band and the tooth, stretch the septum of the dam and depress it gingivally to reposition the dam material. Next, turn the larger knurled nut clockwise to tighten the band slightly and use an explorer along the gingival margin to determine that the gingival edge of the band extends beyond the preparation. Once the band is correctly positioned, tighten the band securely around the tooth.

When one of the proximal margins is deeper gingivally, the Tofflemire MOD band may be modified to prevent damage to the gingival tissue or attachment on the more shallow side. A band may be trimmed for the shallow gingival margin, permitting the matrix to extend farther gingivally for the deeper gingival margin (Fig. 17-80).

Next, with the mirror lingual (or facial) to the tooth, position the reflecting surface to view the contour of the strip through the interproximal space (Fig. 17-81). Evaluate the band by viewing the proximal contour or contours of the band, and note the symmetry of the band and adjacent surface. The occlusogingival contour should be convex, with the height of contour at proper contact level and contacting the adjacent tooth. Next, observe the matrix from an occlusal aspect, and evaluate the position of the contact area in a faciolingual direction. It may be necessary to remove the retainer and reburnish the band for additional contouring. Minor alterations in contour and contact may be accomplished without removal from the tooth. The back side of the blade of the 15-8-14 spoon excavator (i.e., Black spoon) is an excellent instrument for improving both contour and contact (see Fig. 17-93). If a smaller burnishing instrument is used, use care not to create a grooved or

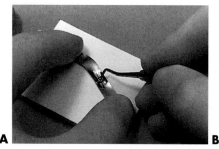
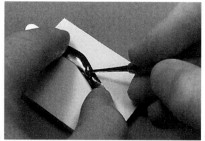
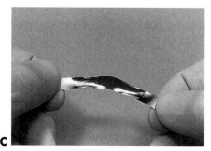

FIG. **17-78** Burnishing matrix band. **A,** With band on pad, use small burnisher to deform band. **B,** Use large burnisher to smooth band contour. **C,** Burnished matrix band for MOD tooth preparation.

FIG. **17-79** Positioning band in Universal retainer. **A,** Explorer pointing to locking vise. View is showing gingival side of vise. **B,** Pointed spindle is released from locking vise by turning small knurled nut counterclockwise. **C,** Fold band to form loop and position in retainer (occlusal edge of band first). **D,** Tighten spindle against band in locking vise.

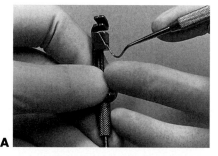
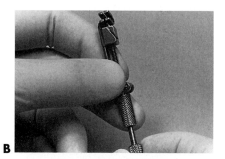
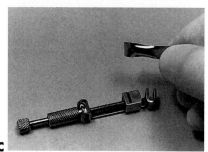
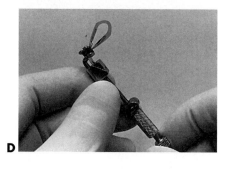

bumpy surface that will result in a restoration with an irregular proximal surface. Ideally the band should be positioned 1 mm apical to the gingival margin (or margins) or deep enough to be engaged by the wedge (whichever is less) and 1 to 2 mm above the adjacent marginal ridge or ridges.

A minor modification of the matrix may be indicated for restoring the proximal surface that is planned for a guide plane for a removable partial denture. Abutment teeth for a tooth-supported removable partial denture must provide amalgam contour to allow defining (by carving or [later] disking) a guide plane extending from the marginal ridge 2.5 mm gingivally (see Fig. 17-66, *B*). However, normal proximal contour, rather than overcontour, is usually sufficient and best for development of a guide plane. Guide plane development results in a gingival embrasure between the natural tooth and denture teeth that is less open and less likely to trap food (see Fig. 17-66, *B*).

Abutment teeth adjacent to the residual ridge for a tissue-supported (i.e., distal extension) removable partial denture are carved to provide normal morphology. Sufficient gingival embrasure should be provided to allow for the difference between the compression under load of the ridge soft tissues and that of the periodontal membrane (although a small area guide plane may be

provided). (Compare the embrasure in *D* to that in *B* in Fig. 17-66, *D*.)

After the matrix contour and extension are evaluated, place a wedge in the gingival embrasure or embrasures using the following technique. Break off approximately ½ inch (1.2 cm) of a round toothpick. Grasp the broken end of the wedge with the No. 110 pliers. Insert the pointed tip from the lingual or facial embrasure (whichever is larger), slightly gingival to the gingival margin. Wedge the band tightly against the tooth and margin (Fig. 17-82, *A*). If necessary, the gingival aspect of the wedge may be lightly wetted with lubricant to facilitate its placement. If the wedge is placed occlusal to the gingival margin, the band will be pressed into the preparation, creating an abnormal concavity in the proximal surface of the restoration (see Fig. 17-82, *B*). The wedge should not be so far apical to the gingival margin that the band will not be held tightly against the gingival margin. This improper wedge placement will result in gingival excess (i.e., "overhang") caused by the band moving slightly away from the margin during condensation of the amalgam. Such an overhang often goes undetected and may result in irritation of the gingiva or an area of plaque accumulation. To be effective, a wedge should be positioned as near to the gingival margin as possible without being occlusal to it. If the wedge is significantly apical of the gingival margin, a second (usually smaller) wedge may be placed on top of

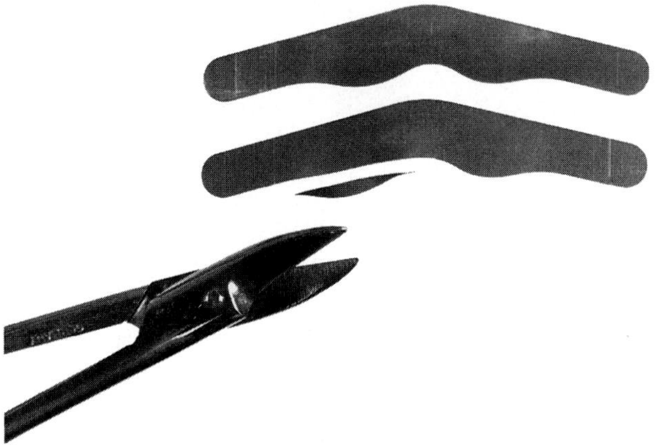

FIG. **17-80** Band may be trimmed for the shallower gingival margin, permitting matrix to extend farther gingivally for the deeper gingival margin on the other proximal surface.

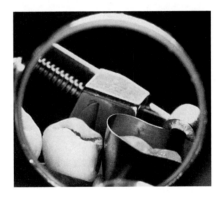

FIG. **17-81** Using mirror from facial or lingual position to evaluate proximal contour of matrix band.

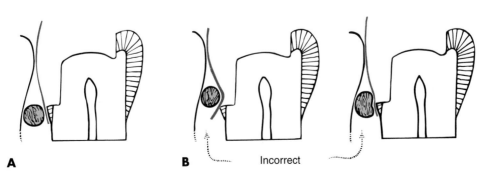

FIG. **17-82** **A,** Correct wedge position. **B,** Incorrect wedge positions.

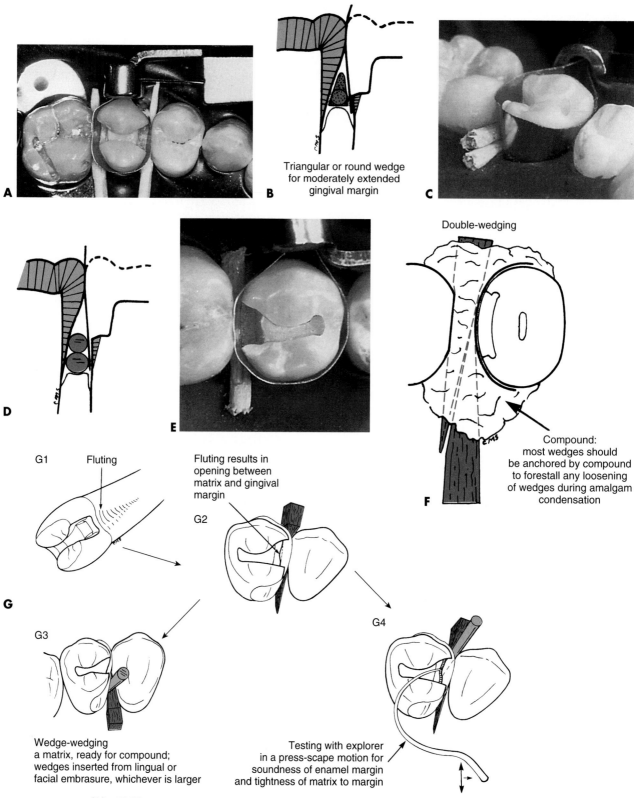

A and **B**

Triangular or round wedge
for moderately extended
gingival margin

C

D

E

Double-wedging

Compound:
most wedges should
be anchored by compound
to forestall any loosening
of wedges during amalgam
condensation

F

G1   Fluting

Fluting results in
opening between
matrix and gingival
margin

G2

G

G3

G4

Wedge-wedging
a matrix, ready for compound;
wedges inserted from lingual or
facial embrasure, whichever is larger

Testing with explorer
in a press-scape motion for
soundness of enamel margin
and tightness of matrix to margin

FIG. **17-83** Various double-wedging techniques. **A** and **B,** Proper wedging for matrix for typical
MOD preparation. **C** and **D,** Technique to allow wedging near gingival margin of preparation
when proximal box is shallow gingivally or interproximal tissue level has receded or both. **E** and
F, Double wedging may be used with faciolingually wide proximal boxes to provide maximal
closure of band along gingival margin. **G,** Another technique may be used on the mesial aspect
of maxillary first premolars to adapt the matrix to the fluted (i.e., concave) area of the gingival
margin *(G1,G2); G3,* second wedge inserted from lingual embrasure; *G4,* testing adaptation of
band after insertion of wedges from facial.

the first to wedge adequately the matrix against the margin (Fig. 17-83, *C* and *D*). This type of wedging is particularly useful for patients whose interproximal tissue level has receded.

The gingival wedge should be tight enough to prevent any possibility of an overhang of amalgam in at least the middle two thirds of the gingival margin (see Fig. 17-83, *A* and *B*). Occasionally, double wedging is permitted (if access allows), securing the matrix when the proximal box is wide faciolingually. Double wedging refers to using two wedges: one from the lingual embrasure and one from the facial embrasure (see Fig. 17-83, *E* and *F*). Two wedges help to ensure that the gingival corners of a wide proximal box can be properly condensed; they also help to minimize gingival excess. However, double wedging should be used only if the middle two thirds of the proximal margins can be adequately wedged. Because the facial and lingual corners are accessible to carving, proper wedging is important to prevent gingival excess of amalgam in the middle two thirds of the proximal box (see Fig. 17-83, *B*).

Occasionally, a concavity may be present on the proximal surface that is apparent in the gingival margin. This may occur on a surface with a fluted root, such as the mesial surface of the maxillary first premolar (see Fig. 17-83, *G1*). A gingival margin located in this area may be concave (see Fig. 17-83, *G2*). To wedge a matrix band tightly against such a margin, a second pointed wedge can be inserted between the first wedge and the band. (see Fig. 17-83, *G3* and *G4*).

The wedging action between the teeth should provide enough separation to compensate for the thickness of the matrix band. This will ensure a positive contact relationship after the matrix is removed (after the condensation and initial carving of the amalgam). If a Tofflemire retainer is used to restore a two-surface Class II preparation, the single wedge must provide enough separation to compensate for two thicknesses of band material. Test for tightness of the wedge by pressing the tip of an explorer firmly at several points along the middle two thirds of the gingival margin (against the matrix band) to verify that it cannot be moved away from the gingival margin (Fig. 17-84). While directing a gentle stream of air, press and drag the tip of the explorer along the gingival margin in both directions to ensure the removal of any remaining friable enamel. As an additional test, attempt to remove the wedge (using the explorer with moderate pressure) after first having set the explorer tip into the wood near the broken end. Moderate pulling should not cause dislodgement. Gingival overhangs of amalgam can inadvertently occur as a result of wedges becoming loose during amalgam condensation. Therefore the clinician must assess and carve this area carefully.

Often the rubber dam has a tendency to loosen the wedge. Rebounding of the dam stretched by the wedge

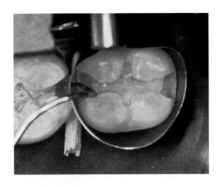

FIG. **17-84** Use explorer tip (with pressure) to ensure proper adaptation of the band to gingival margin. In addition, press and drag the tip along gingival margin in both directions to ensure removal of any friable enamel.

causes loosening. Stretching the interproximal dam septa before and during wedge placement in the direction opposite to the wedge (and lubricating the wedge) can prevent this. The stretched dam is released after the wedge is inserted.

Some situations may require a triangular-shaped wedge that can be modified (by knife or scalpel blade) to conform to the approximating tooth contours (Fig. 17-85). However, the round toothpick wedge is usually the wedge of choice with conservative proximal boxes because its wedging action is more occlusal (i.e., nearer the gingival margin) than with the triangular wedge (Fig. 17-86, *A* and *B*).

The triangular (i.e., anatomic) wedge is recommended for a preparation with a deep gingival margin. The triangular wedge is usually indicated with the Tofflemire MOD matrix band. The triangular wedge is positioned similarly to the round wedge, and the goal is the same. When the gingival margin is deep (cervically), the base of the triangular wedge will more readily engage the tooth gingival to the margin without causing excessive soft-tissue displacement. The anatomic wedge is preferred for deeply extended gingival margins because its greatest cross-sectional dimension is at its base (see Fig. 17-86, *C* and *D*).

To maintain gingival isolation attained by an anatomic wedge placed before the preparation of a deeply extended gingival margin, it may be appropriate to withdraw the wedge a small distance to allow passage of the band between the loosened wedge and the gingival margin. Tilting (i.e., canting) the matrix into place helps the gingival edge of the band slide between the loosened wedge and gingival margin. The band is then tightened and the same wedge is firmly reinserted.

Supporting the matrix material with the blade of a Hollenback carver during the insertion of the wedge for the difficult deep gingival restoration may be helpful.[51] The tip of the blade is placed between the matrix and gingival margin, and then the "heel" of the blade is leaned against the matrix and adjacent tooth (Fig. 17-87).

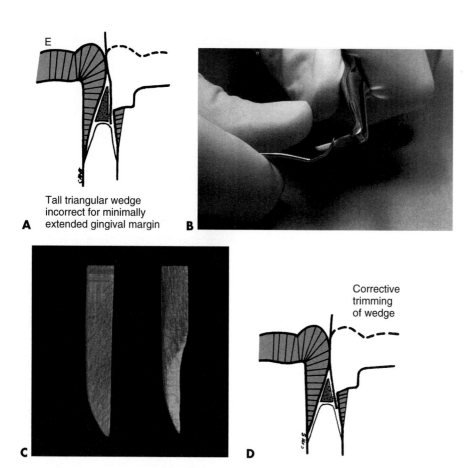

Tall triangular wedge incorrect for minimally extended gingival margin

Corrective trimming of wedge

FIG. **17-85** Modified triangular (i.e., anatomic) wedge. **A,** Depending on proximal convexity, triangular wedge may distort matrix contour. **B,** A sharp-bladed instrument may be used to modify the triangular steepness of the wedge. **C,** Modified and unmodified wedges compared. **D,** Properly modified triangular wedge prevents distortion of matrix contour.

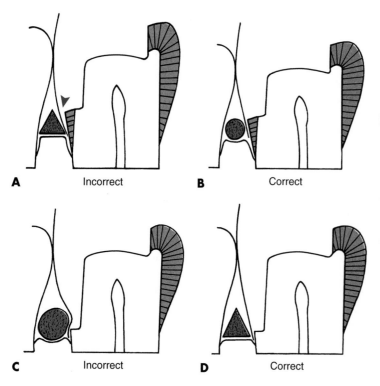

A   Incorrect

B   Correct

C   Incorrect

D   Correct

FIG. **17-86** Indications for round toothpick versus triangular (i.e., anatomic) wedges. **A,** As a rule, the triangular wedge will not firmly support the matrix band against the gingival margin in conservative Class II preparations (*arrow*). **B,** The round toothpick wedge is preferred with these preparations because its wedging action is nearer the gingival margin. **C,** In Class II preparations with deep gingival margins, the round toothpick wedge will crimp the matrix band contour if its diameter is above the gingival margin. **D,** The triangular wedge is preferred with these preparations because its greatest width is at its base.

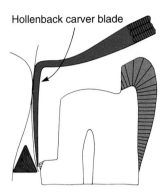

FIG. **17-87** Supporting matrix with blade of Hollenback carver during wedge insertion.

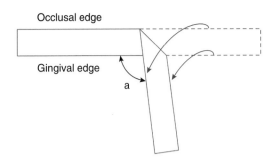

FIG. **17-88** Custom-made matrix strip is folded as indicated by arrows. The smaller angle (*a*) compared with angle of commercial strip increases difference between length of gingival and occlusal edges.

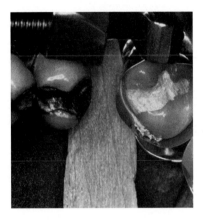

FIG. **17-89** Custom-made tongue blade wedge may be used when excessive space exists between adjacent teeth.

In this position the blade supports the matrix to help both in positioning the wedge sufficiently gingivally and preventing the wedge from pushing the matrix into the preparation. After the wedge is properly inserted, the blade is gently removed.

Assess all aspects of the band and make any desired corrections once the wedge is placed. Again, using a mirror, inspect the proximal aspects of the matrix band facially and lingually to verify that it contacts the adjacent tooth and that proper contour has been achieved. Reflected light must not be seen in the contact area between the band and the adjacent tooth (see Fig. 17-81). Carefully position the mirror to prevent a false impression of contact resulting from visual overlap of the band and the adjacent tooth. If the band does not reach the adjacent contact area or areas after contouring and wedging, release the tension of the band a small amount by turning the larger knurled nut of the Tofflemire retainer counterclockwise (many operators loosen the band one-quarter turn to ensure proximal contact). If loosening the loop of a Tofflemire band still does not allow for contact with an adjacent tooth, a custom-made band with a smaller angle can be used. Reducing the angle of the band increases the difference in length (i.e., circumferences) of the gingival and occlusal edges. To reduce the angle of the band, fold it as shown in Fig. 17-88. Next, burnish for appropriate occlusogingival contour (in the contact areas), and insert the band into the Tofflemire retainer. (To maximize the advantage of either this custom band or the loosened Tofflemire band, compound may be applied as described in the next section.)

A suitably trimmed tongue blade can wedge a matrix where the interproximal spacing between teeth is large (Fig. 17-89). Occasionally, however, it is impossible to use a wedge to secure the matrix band. In this case, the band must be sufficiently tight to minimize the gingival excess of amalgam. Because the band is not wedged, special care must be exercised by placing small amounts of amalgam in the gingival floor and condensing the first 1 mm of amalgam lightly, but thoroughly, in a gingival direction. Next, carefully continue condensation in a gingival direction using a larger condenser with firm pressure. Condensation against an unwedged matrix may cause the amalgam to extrude grossly beyond the gingival margin. (Obviously, without a wedge there will be some excess amalgam at the proximal margins that will be overcontoured, requiring correction by a suitable carver immediately after matrix removal.)

An advantage of amalgam over direct composite is that amalgam is condensed into place rather than packed or placed. Condensation strokes in a gingival direction help to ensure that no voids occur internally or along the margins. Condensation laterally helps to ensure that sufficient proximal contact and proximal contour are achieved. With direct composite, there is less potential to move the band laterally during packing or placement. Therefore proximal contact and contour must be ensured using the matrix band and wedge.

The matrix is removed after insertion of the amalgam, carving of the occlusal portion (including the occlusal embrasure or embrasures), and hardening of the amalgam to avoid fracture of the marginal ridge during band removal. Remove the retainer from the band after turning the small knurled nut counterclockwise to retract the pointed spindle. The end of the index finger may be placed on the occlusal surface of the tooth to stabilize the band as the retainer is removed. Next, remove any compound that was applied to support the matrix. Use the No. 110 pliers to tease the band free from one contact area at a time by pushing or pulling the band in a linguoocclusal (or facioocclusal) direction and, if possible, in the direction of wedge insertion (Fig. 17-90). Some operators prefer to leave the wedge or wedges in place

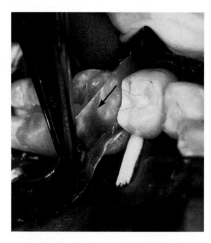

FIG. **17-90** Using No. 110 pliers, the matrix band should be removed in a linguoocclusal *(arrow)* or facioocclusal direction (not just in an occlusal direction).

to provide separation of the teeth while the matrix band is removed. By maintaining slight interdental separation, the wedge reduces the possibility of the amalgam fracturing. Avoid a straight occlusal direction during matrix removal to prevent breaking the marginal ridges. Remove the wedge or wedges, and complete the carving procedures (as described in a later section).

Compound-Supported Matrix. The compound-supported matrix is rarely used, but it is an alternative to the Universal matrix. A wedged matrix supported by compound provides most of the essential qualities of a good matrix, especially when used for two-surface proximal restorations.[88] It is more rigid than commercial matrices, provides better contact and contour, is virtually trouble-free during proper removal, requires very little proximal carving after the matrix removal, and only has one thickness of band material for which wedging must compensate.

Using $5/16$-inch (8-mm) wide, 0.002-inch (0.05-mm) thick stainless steel matrix material, cut a length sufficient to cover one third of the facial surface and extend through the prepared proximal surface to cover one third of the lingual surface. To prevent the matrix material from impinging on the facial and lingual gingiva, trim the gingival edge as shown in Fig. 17-91, *A.* Note that the remaining untrimmed gingival edge is longer

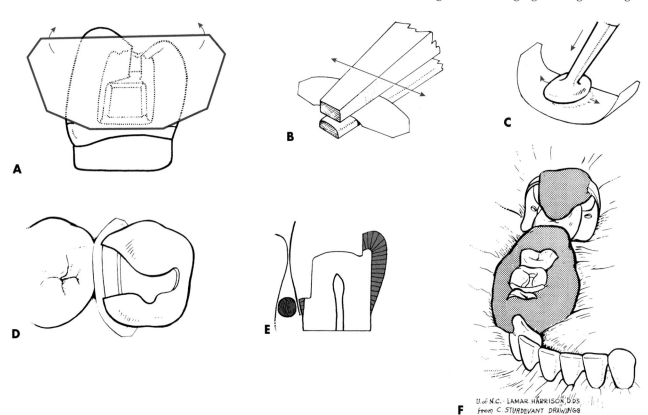

FIG. **17-91** Compound-supported matrix. **A,** Shape of stainless steel strip after trimming. **B,** Strip contoured to circumferential contour of tooth (fingers can be used). **C,** Burnishing the strip to produce occlusogingival contact contour (*left* and *right arrows* indicate short back-and-forth motion of burnisher). **D,** Contoured strip in position. **E,** Matrix strip properly wedged. **F,** Completed compound-supported matrix.

than the length of the gingival margin of the tooth preparation. With contouring pliers or fingers, contour the strip to conform to the circumferential contour of the tooth (see Fig. 17-91, *B* and *D*). When contouring with pliers, exercise care to produce a smoothly curved surface. Contour the strip occlusogingivally with the egg-shaped burnisher using a short back-and-forth motion (see *arrows*) (see Fig. 17-91, *C*). This is best accomplished with the strip laid on a resilient paper pad, which provides a yielding surface. Burnish with sufficient pressure to shape the steel strip to the desired contact contour. Contours vary both faciolingually and occlusogingivally because some teeth are more bulbous than others. Once the matrix band is in place and the contour verified, the appropriate interproximal wedge is inserted (see Fig. 17-91, *E*) and compound application is begun.

There are seven steps for applying low-fusing compound:

1. Soften a piece of low-fusing compound in a Bunsen flame.

2. Shape into a cone.
3. Slightly glaze the base by a quick pass through the edge of the flame.
4. Attach the base to the end of the appropriate gloved forefinger.
5. Glaze the tip of the cone by passing it through the side of the flame (Fig. 17-92, *A*).
6. Immediately press the softened tip into the facial (or lingual) embrasure formed by the matrix and adjacent tooth, forcing the compound into the gingival embrasure (into whichever side the wedge was inserted).
7. See that some of the compound is extended against the facial (lingual) surfaces of the operated tooth (past the edge of the matrix) and adjacent tooth (see Fig. 17-92, *B*).

These steps, except for the softening of the compound, should take only a few seconds. Now repeat this application of compound for the opposite side (i.e., the side showing the tip of the wedge) (see Fig. 17-92, *C*). Compound cones can be prepared in advance and stored for later use to save time during matrix application.

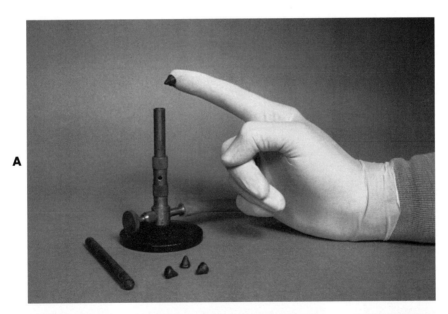

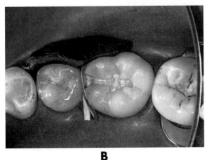

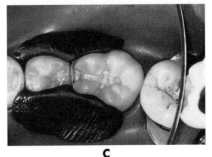

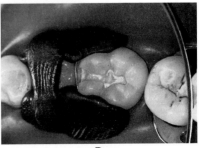

FIG. **17-92** Compound-supported matrix. **A,** Glazing tip of compound cone. **B,** Compound applied facially. **C,** Compound applied lingually. **D,** Stability of matrix ensured by uniting facial and lingual compound with additional compound over the occlusal surface of adjacent tooth.

With experience, making and placing compound cones requires very little time. When these compound cones are manipulated correctly, the consistency of the base portion (somewhat soft and moldable) forces the more fluid tip portion into the gingival embrasure and then out over half of the facial (or lingual) surfaces of the teeth. Practice is required to achieve the correct consistency and placement of the compound. An experienced operator may apply both facial and lingual cones simultaneously (i.e., one cone attached to the thumb and the other to the index finger). Compound softened and applied as described, will stick securely to clean, dry, tooth surfaces. However it is applied, the compound, if adapted properly to the facial and lingual tooth surfaces, enhances stability. Do not allow compound to encroach on the occlusal surface of the matrixed tooth or on the adjacent marginal ridge of the tooth that will be forming the proximal contact with the restoration. A common error is to apply too much compound, which results in a bulky matrix that is occasionally loosened by movements of the tongue or cheek or by the flexing of the rubber dam. Optionally, stability of the matrix may be by uniting the facial and lingual compound by adding compound over the occlusal surfaces of adjacent teeth (not over the adjacent marginal ridge) (see Figs. 17-91, *F*, and 17-92, *D*). Harden the compound by cooling with a stream of air.

If proper contact and contour are not established initially, they can be corrected. A unique property of the compound-supported matrix is its ability to respond to needed change in contour by the application of a warm burnishing instrument (i.e., the back of a 15-8-14 spoon excavator) pressed against the band from the preparation side (Fig. 17-93). This step should be routine to assure the operator that the compound has not moved the matrix away from the adjacent tooth. As warmth from the instrument is transferred readily through the metal strip to soften the compound immediately adjacent to the strip, a burnishing movement of the instrument with moderate pressure confirms (by tactile feel through the instrument) the contact of the strip against the adja-

cent tooth. A small amount of compound often exudes occlusal to the contact to reveal that compound was (but is no longer) between the strip and adjacent tooth. Do not release the pressure against the strip until the instrument, strip, and compound have been cooled with an air syringe. The shape of the matrix band against which the amalgam will be condensed determines the proximal contour. It is much easier, as well as more efficient and effective, to establish proper contours in the matrix before amalgam condensation rather than in the amalgam after matrix removal.

Two features of proximal surface contour should be considered. One feature is the normal slight convexity between the occlusal and middle thirds of the proximal surface when viewed from the lingual (or facial) aspect. Correct and incorrect contours are illustrated in Fig. 17-94, *A* through *C*. Proximal surface restorations often display an occlusogingival proximal contour that is too straight, whereupon the contact relationship is located too far occlusally (with little or no occlusal embrasure) (see Fig. 17-94, *C*). This condition allows food

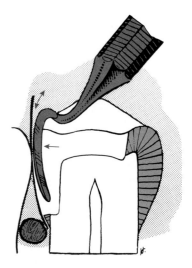

FIG. **17-93** Contour of compound-supported matrix may be altered by applying warm burnishing instrument against band from preparation side.

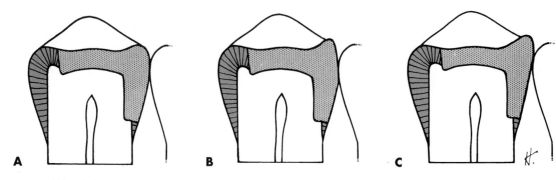

FIG. **17-94** Proximal contour. **A,** Correct proximal contour. **B,** Incorrect marginal ridge height and occlusal embrasure form. **C,** Occlusogingival proximal contour too straight, contact too high, and incorrect occlusal embrasure form.

impaction between the teeth with resultant injury to the interproximal gingiva and supporting tissues, and it invites caries.

The second feature of proximal surface contour is alteration of the matrix, when indicated, to provide the correct form to the proximofacial line angle region (Fig. 17-95). This feature can be provided to the matrix with a warm burnishing instrument. This contour feature may be present already if the first shaping of the matrix was correct before placement of the compound. If this contour is not present, the facial embrasure of the restoration will be too open, inviting food impaction and injury to underlying supporting tissues.

The matrix should be tight against the facial and lingual margins on the proximal surface so that the amalgam can be well condensed at the preparation margins. In addition, when the matrix is tight against the tooth, minimal carving is necessary on the proximal margins after the matrix is removed. However, it must be emphasized that a matrix, which is tight against the margins, requires thorough condensation of the amalgam into the matrix and tooth corners to prevent amalgam voids at the proximal margins.

As a last step before condensation, press and drag the tip of an explorer tine along the gingival margin in both directions to loosen and displace any weak portions of enamel (see Figs. 17-83, *G4*, and 17-84). Use the air syringe to clear all debris from the preparation, and recheck the matrix for correctness.

Removing the compound-supported matrix follows condensation of the amalgam and carving the occlusal surface, especially the occlusal embrasure (subjects described in a later section). First, break away the compound from the facial and lingual surfaces with a stiff explorer tine. Carefully loosen and remove any compound remaining in the gingival embrasure (Fig. 17-96). Assuming the wedge was inserted from the lingual, grasp (with No. 110 pliers) the facial edge of the matrix and remove it facially until free of the contact (Fig. 17-97). Otherwise, matrix removal is the same as described previously.

Precontoured Matrix Strips. Commercially available metal strips (e.g., Palodent Matrix System, Darway,

Inc., San Mateo, CA) are precontoured and ready for application to the tooth (Fig. 17-98). Palodent strips have limited application because of their very rounded contour. They usually are most suitable for mandibular first premolars and the distal surface of maxillary canines. The contact area of the adjacent tooth occasionally is too close to allow placement of the contoured Palodent strip without causing a dent in the strip's contact area, making it unusable.

As stated previously, position the steel strip (see Fig. 17-91, *D* and *E*), and carefully insert the gingival edge

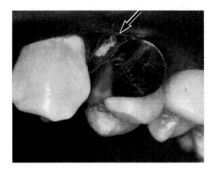

FIG. **17-96** Carefully remove any compound remaining in gingival embrasure (*arrow*) before matrix removal.

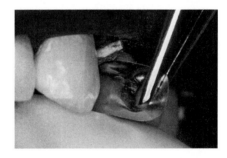

FIG. **17-97** Remove metal strip of compound-supported matrix by pulling it facially.

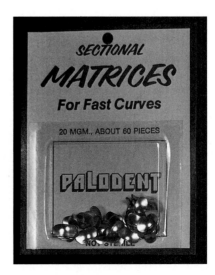

FIG. **17-98** Commercially manufactured, precontoured metal strips.

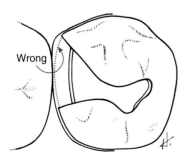

FIG. **17-95** Alteration of matrix contour to provide correct form to proximofacial line angle region.

Wrong

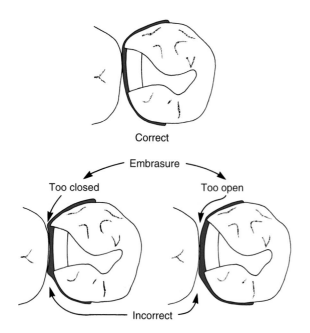

Correct

Embrasure

Too closed   Too open

Incorrect

FIG. **17-99** Correct or incorrect facial and lingual embrasure form is determined by the shape of the matrix strip.

into the gingival crevice about 1 mm apical to the gingival margin. The occlusal edge of the strip should extend 1 to 2 mm occlusal to the adjacent marginal ridge. Visually inspect the occlusogingival contour of the strip. Occasionally the strip cannot be properly evaluated until after placing the gingival wedge to stabilize it.

It may be necessary to remove the strip for reburnishing when the contour is incorrect. When the contour is appropriate, insert the strip, and (using a mirror) evaluate the matrix from the lingual (or facial) and occlusal embrasures for correctness. (Fig. 17-91, *E*, illustrates the correct occlusogingival contour.) The strip should be shaped so that proper facial and lingual embrasure form will be established after compound application (Fig. 17-99). If these embrasures are too open, food impaction and injury to underlying tissues may occur; if too closed with a broad contact, proper scouring by food movement or by the toothbrush is hindered.

Position the gingival wedge interproximally (see Fig. 17-91, *E*) to secure the band tightly at the gingival margin to prevent an excess of amalgam (i.e., "overhang"). The wedge also separates the teeth slightly to compensate for the thickness of the band material. Variations in wedge design and details on wedge placement, including tests for tightness, are the same as described previously. The application of compound is occasionally indicated with this matrix system to develop proper proximal contacts, proximal contours, embrasure form, and stability (i.e., rigidity) (see Figs. 17-91, *F*, and 17-92, *D*).

Automatrix. The Automatrix (Dentsply Caulk, Milford, Delaware) is a retainerless matrix system with four types of bands that are designed to fit all teeth, regard-

less of circumference (Fig. 17-100). The bands vary in height from $^{3}/_{16}$ to $^{5}/_{16}$ inch (4.7 to 7.9 mm) and are supplied in two thicknesses (0.0015 inch [0.038 mm] and 0.002 inch [0.05 mm]). The indicated use of this matrix is for extensive Class II preparations, especially those replacing two or more cusps. As with all matrix systems, it has advantages and disadvantages. One advantage is that the auto-lock loop can be positioned either on the facial or lingual surface with equal ease. A disadvantage is that the bands are not precontoured, and development of physiologic proximal contours is difficult. (For a more complete description of the Automatrix and its use, see Chapter 19.)

Inserting and Carving the Amalgam

Condensation. As stated previously, the principal objectives during insertion of amalgam are:

- Condensation to adapt the amalgam to the preparation walls and matrix and to produce a restoration free of voids
- Having as low as possible mercury content in the restoration to improve strength and decrease corrosion

Choose condensers that are best suited for use in each part of the tooth preparation and that can be used without binding. Remember that condensation of amalgam with spherical particles requires larger condensers than are commonly used for admixed amalgam, because spherical amalgam is initially easier to condense and admixed amalgam requires more condensation pressure.

Fill the amalgam carrier, and transfer into the proximal portion of the tooth preparation only the amount of amalgam that (when condensed) will fill the gingival 1 mm (approximately) of the proximal box. Condense the amalgam along the gingival floor with the previously selected condenser. Use the condenser in a gingival direction with sufficient force to adapt the amalgam to the gingival floor. Next, carefully condense the amalgam against the proximal margins of the preparation and into the proximal retention grooves. Firm, facially and lingually directed pressure (i.e., lateral condensation) of the condenser accomplishes this at the same time as exertion of gingivally directed force (Fig. 17-101). Also in the proximal box, condense mesially (or distally) to ensure proximal contact with the adjacent tooth. Lateral condensation should be a routine step for Class II amalgams.

Continue the procedure of adding amalgam and condensing until the amalgam reaches the level of the pulpal wall. Change condensers (usually to a larger one), if indicated, and condense amalgam in the remaining proximal portion of the preparation concurrently with the occlusal portion. It may be necessary to return to a smaller condenser when condensing in a narrow extension of the preparation or near the proximal margins. Remember that a smaller condenser face is more effec-

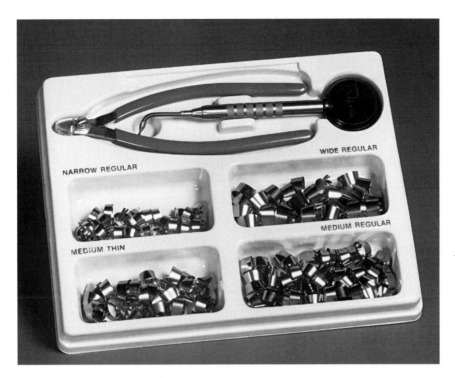

FIG. **17-100** Automatrix system.

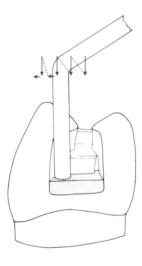

FIG. **17-101** Lateral and occlusogingival force is necessary to properly condense amalgam into proximal locks and into angles at junction of matrix band with margins of preparation.

tive at condensing as long as it does not significantly penetrate the amalgam. Because the area of a circular condenser face increases by the square of the diameter, doubling the diameter will require four times more force for the same pressure on a unit area.

When the occlusal margins are approached, exercise care not to injure the enamel margins. However, exert maximal pressure with the hand condenser as the occlusal margins are covered and overpacked by at least 1 mm. A slight rocking motion of the condenser may assist in condensation. Using a large condenser, make sure that the occlusal margins are well condensed.

Condensation should be completed within the working time for the alloy being used. Condensation should

be accomplished in 3 to 4 minutes (depending on the alloy). Otherwise, crystallization of the new amalgam matrix in the unused portion will be too advanced to permit:

- Proper coherence and homogeneity with minimal voids in the restoration
- Desired adaptation of the material to the walls of the preparation and matrix during condensation
- Development of the maximal strength and minimal flow (i.e., creep) in the completed restoration
- Proper intermingling of the adhesive and amalgam if a bonding system is used

Therefore, when inserting amalgam into large preparations and the mix is nearing 3 minutes old, a new mix should be made. While condensing, the operator should monitor the plasticity and wetness of the amalgam mass. To allow proper condensation, the mix should be neither wet (i.e., mercury rich) nor dry and crumbly (i.e., mercury poor).

Pneumatic, or mechanical, condensation may be used, but it has three distinct disadvantages. One disadvantage of the pneumatic condenser is the possibility of damaging the enamel margins with the condenser points. A second disadvantage is the risk of inadequate condensation in conservative tooth preparations.[18] A third disadvantage is patient objection to the constant pneumatic tamping. (Refer to Conservative Class I Amalgam Restorations for a discussion of mercury hygiene and amalgam selection and trituration.)

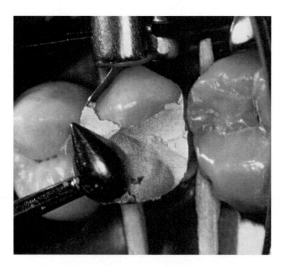

FIG. **17-102** Precarve burnish with large burnisher.

Carving the Occlusal Portion. Before carving procedures are initiated, precarve burnishing of the occlusal portion with a large egg-shaped or ball burnisher should be done (Fig. 17-102). As mentioned previously, precarve burnishing may be used as a form of condensation. (Refer to Conservative Class I Amalgam Restorations for a description of the technique.)

Use pressure similar to the force used when condensing the amalgam. Move the burnisher mesiodistally and faciolingually until it contacts the enamel surfaces external to the margins. Burnishing should not continue after this because some amalgam should remain for carving procedures. Precarve burnishing enhances the benefits of condensation.[54]

With the matrix band still in place, careful carving of the occlusal portion should begin immediately after condensation and burnishing. Sharp discoid instruments of suitable size are recommended carvers. Use the larger discoid first, followed by the smaller in regions not accessible to the larger instrument.

While the matrix is in place, carve the marginal ridge confluent with the tooth's anatomy and duplicate the height and shape of the adjacent marginal ridge (Fig. 17-103). Use an explorer or small Hollenback carver to carefully define (i.e., open) the occlusal embrasure. This step will significantly reduce the danger of marginal ridge fracture during matrix removal.

Recall that occlusal contacts were evaluated before tooth preparation. Remembering the pattern of occlusal contacts, observing the height of the adjacent marginal ridge, and knowing where the preparation cavosurface margins are located will aid the operator in completing carving of the occlusal surface, including the marginal ridge and occlusal embrasure.

If the restoration has extensive axial involvement of the tooth, the occlusal carving should be accomplished quickly. The objectives would be to develop the general occlusal contour but most importantly to develop the

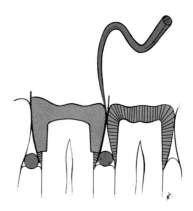

FIG. **17-103** Define marginal ridge and occlusal embrasure with explorer.

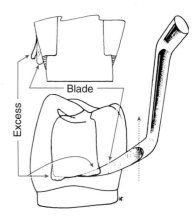

FIG. **17-104** Gingival excess may be removed with amalgam knives.

correct marginal ridge height and occlusal embrasure form (see Fig. 17-103). Then the matrix is removed and access gained to carve the axial portions of the restoration. This permits these areas (usually more inaccessible) to be carved while the amalgam is carvable. Once the axial carving is completed, the occlusal surface contouring is completed. Occasionally this may require the use of an abrasive stone or finishing bur if the amalgam has set.

Removal of the Matrix Band and Completion of Carving. As previously described, depending on the type of matrix used, remove the compound or the matrix retainer or both, and remove the matrix band (or strip) and any wedges. The proximal surface should be nearly completed, with proper contact evident and minimal carving required except to remove a possible small amount of excess amalgam at the proximal facial and lingual margins at the faciogingival and linguogingival corners and along the gingival margin. The amalgam knives (scalers, No. 34 and No. 35) (Fig. 17-104) are ideal for removing gingival excess preventing gingival overhangs. They are also ideal for refining embrasure form around the proximal contacts. Recall that the secondary (or "back") edges on the blades of the amalgam knives

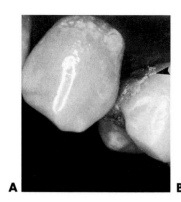
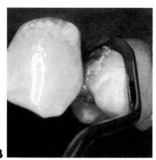
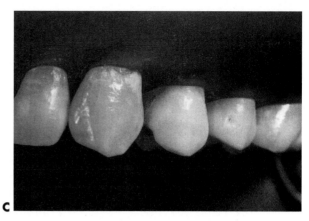

FIG. **17-105** Removal of gingival excess of amalgam. **A,** Excess of amalgam (*arrow*) at gingival corner of restoration. **B,** Use of amalgam knife for removal of gingival excess. **C,** Gingival corner of restoration with excess removed.

are occasionally helpful, using either a pull or push stroke. The Hollenback carver No. 3 or (occasionally) the side of the explorer may be suitable instruments for carving these areas. However, the explorer cannot refine the margins and contour as accurately as amalgam knives.

When carving the margins, the cutting surface of the carving instrument is held perpendicular to the margins. However, carving should be parallel to the margins using the tooth surface adjacent to the margin to guide the carver. If appreciable excess is present at the gingival margin or if the excess has set sufficiently, remove it with the amalgam knives (Fig. 17-105). Verify that the proximal contact exists by placing a mouth mirror lingual or facial to the contact and view it indirectly. It may be necessary to rotate the mirror slightly to ensure that the adjacent teeth are, in fact, in contact. No light should be seen between them.

If an amalgam adhesive was used, look for thin layers of set resin near the margin that formed between the matrix and the tooth. These are occasionally referred to as "barnacles" because they are very tenacious and difficult to remove even with amalgam knives. They are also difficult to see because they are often transparent. Barnacles, or adhesive excess, may be minimized by lightly applying adhesive to the tooth preparation before condensing the amalgam. Overapplication of amalgam adhesive increases the potential for barnacle formation. This is important because removing tenaciously bonded-and-set resin from a margin immediately adjacent to freshly carved amalgam that is relatively soft and carvable without damaging the amalgam is a challenge.

On the proximal surface where a guide plane is planned for a removable partial denture, do not overcarve the surface extending from the marginal ridge 2.5 mm gingivally. Development of normal tooth contour before defining the guide plane is usually the best procedure.

Once the carving is completed, the rubber dam is removed and the occlusion assessed. While removing the rubber dam, because of the possibility of fracturing the newly condensed restoration if the restoration is "high," advise the patient not to close until instructed to do so. Insert articulating paper over the quadrant of teeth in question, instruct the patient to close slowly and lightly and to stop closing when the teeth barely touch. Once the patient has reopened and the articulating paper is removed, look for two features of the occlusal relationship suggesting the restoration is high:

1. Cusp tips of the adjacent teeth are not in occlusal contact with certain mated areas, when it is known from the preoperative occlusal assessment that they should be touching.
2. A cusp that occludes with the new restoration contacts prematurely. For example, if a marginal ridge of the restoration is high, reduce the area contacting prematurely.

Observing the space (short of touching) between certain occlusally mated surfaces of nearby teeth indicates how much to reduce when carving. For example, if these opposing surfaces are 0.5 mm apart (estimating by eyesight), then reduce the high marginal ridge (or other area) by approximately that amount. This expedites occlusal adjustment, as compared with making an insufficient, shallower carving adjustment and then having to repeat closure and carving numerous times. After making the first occlusal adjustment, repeat the sequence of closure, observation, and carving until the appropriate surfaces of the opposing teeth are touching. When carving for occlusion, attempt to establish stable centric contacts of cusps (maximal intercuspation) to opposing surfaces that are perpendicular to occlusal forces. Occlusal contacts located on a cuspal incline or ridge slope are undesirable, because they cause a deflective force on the tooth and should be adjusted until the resulting contact is stable (i.e., the force vector of centric occlusal contacts should parallel the long axis of the tooth).

Until now the patient has been instructed to close only from a hinge and axis relationship (i.e., centric occlusion or maximal intercuspation). After placing the articulating paper over the tooth, now ask the patient to lightly close the teeth and to lightly slide them from side to side. After removing the paper, evaluate the occlusion and make any necessary adjustments (see Fig. 17-23). These should be small if the previous carving has been correct. Any contact area can be recognized on the amalgam by the depth of color imparted by the paper (and especially if the colored area has a silvery center). Reduce the deeper-colored or shiny-centered areas until all markings are uniformly of a light hue (and with no shiny centers) and contacts are noted on adjacent teeth. Guard against overcarving the restoration into infraocclusion, especially in the area of centric-holding contacts. Before the patient is dismissed, thin dental floss may be passed through the proximal contacts one time to remove any amalgam shavings on the proximal surface of the restoration and assess the gingival margin. Passing the floss through a contact more than once may weaken it. The floss is wrapped around the adjacent tooth when passed through the contact, minimizing the pressure exerted on the amalgam. Once positioned in the gingival embrasure, the floss is wrapped around the restored tooth and positioned apical to the gingival margin of the restoration. The floss is moved in a faciolingual direction while extended occlusally. The floss not only removes amalgam shaving, but it also smoothes the proximal amalgam and detects any amalgam gingival overhang. If an overhang is detected, further use of the amalgam knives is necessary.[71] Floss can

also be used to verify that the weight of the contact is similar to that of the neighboring teeth. When carving is completed, rinse and evacuate all debris from the mouth. Caution the patient not to use the new restoration for biting or chewing for a few hours.

Finishing and Polishing the Amalgam. Finishing of amalgam restorations may be necessary to correct a marginal discrepancy or improve the contour. However, evidence suggests that polishing of high-copper amalgams is unnecessary.[58] Although, they are less prone to corrosion and marginal deterioration than their low-copper predecessors, some operators still prefer to polish amalgam restorations. Finishing (and polishing) is usually delayed until all proposed restorations have been placed, rather than being done periodically during the course of treatment. Polishing an amalgam restoration is not attempted within 24 hours after insertion because crystallization is not complete.

Finishing and polishing the occlusal portion is similar to the procedures described for the Class I amalgam restoration (see Fig. 17-24). Finishing and polishing of the proximal surface is indicated where the proximal amalgam is accessible. This usually includes the facial and lingual margins and the amalgam occlusal to the contact. The remainder of the proximal surface is often inaccessible; however, the matrix band should have imparted sufficient smoothness to it.

If the amalgam along the facial and lingual proximal margins was slightly overcarved, the enamel margin can be felt as the explorer tip passes from amalgam across the margin onto the external enamel surface. When this occurs (and where the proximal amalgam is accessible), use sandpaper discs, rotating at slow speed, to smooth the enamel-and-amalgam margin. Sandpaper discs can also be used to smooth and contour the mar-

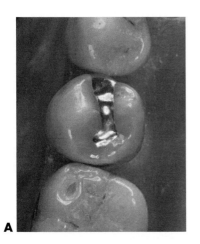
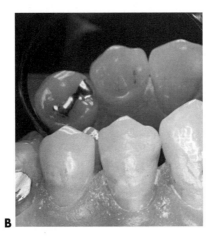
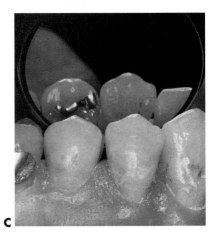

FIG. 17-106 Polished MO amalgam restoration. Note conservative extension. **A,** Occlusal view. **B,** Mesiofacial and occlusal views of mesiofacial margin. **C,** Facial and occlusal views of proximal surface contour and location of proximal contact.

ginal ridge. However, inappropriate use of sandpaper discs may "ledge" the restoration around the contact, resulting in inappropriate proximal contours.

In very conservative preparations the facial and lingual proximal margins are generally inaccessible for finishing and polishing. However, fine abrasive discs or the tip of sharpened rubber polishing points should be used to polish the proximal portion that is accessible. When proximal margins are inaccessible to finishing and polishing with discs or rubber polishing points and there is some excess amalgam (such as at the gingival corners and margins), the amalgam knives may occasionally be used to trim the amalgam back to the margin and to improve the contour. Such light surfacing can produce a smooth surface.

Some polishing techniques include the use of dental tape with a polishing agent on the proximal surface. With the polishing agent applied to the facial and lingual embrasures, pass dental tape through the contact. Then press and slide the tape sideways in both directions several times against the proximal surface gingival to the contact. Exercise care not to traumatize the soft tissue. Accessible facial and lingual proximal margins may also be polished using the edge of an abrasive rubber-polishing cup.

Final polishing of the occlusal surface and accessible areas of the proximal surface may be accomplished with a fine-grit rubber polishing point or by the rubber cup with flour of pumice followed by a high-luster agent, such as precipitated chalk. Fig. 17-106 illustrates examples of properly finished and polished amalgam restorations.

QUADRANT DENTISTRY

When several teeth are to be restored, experienced dentists usually treat them by quadrants rather than individually. Quadrant dentistry implies more efficiency for the dentist and less chair time for the patient. The use of the rubber dam is particularly important in quadrant dentistry. For maximal efficiency, when a quadrant of amalgam tooth preparations is planned, each rotary or hand instrument should be used on every tooth where it is needed before being exchanged.

When restoring a quadrant of Class II amalgam tooth preparations, it is permissible to apply matrix bands on alternate preparations in the quadrant and restore the teeth two at a time. Banding adjacent preparations requires excessive wedging to compensate for a double thickness of band material and makes the control of proximal contours and interproximal contacts very difficult. Extensive tooth preparations may need to be restored one at a time. If proximal boxes differ in size, teeth with smaller boxes should be restored first, because often the proximal margins are inaccessible to carving if the larger adjacent box is restored first. In addition, smaller boxes can be more quickly and accurately restored, because more tooth structure remains to guide the carver. If the larger proximal box is restored first, there is risk of damaging the gingival contour of the restoration when the wedge is inserted to secure the matrix band for the second, smaller restoration. If the adjacent proximal boxes are similar in size, start the banding of alternate preparations with a most posterior preparation, because this allows the patient to close slightly as subsequent restorations are inserted(Fig. 17-107).

Before restoring the second of two adjacent teeth, the operator should carefully establish the proximal contour of the first restoration (the first half of each interproximal contact). Its anatomy will serve as the guide to establish proper contact size and location of the second restoration; it will also serve as good embrasure form. If necessary, a finishing strip can be used to refine the contour of the first proximal amalgam contour (Fig. 17-108). However, the finishing strip is indicated only where the proximal contact is open. Using a finishing strip between contacting amalgam restorations may lighten or eliminate the proximal contact.

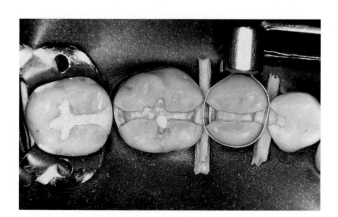

FIG. **17-107** Quadrant dentistry. Unless otherwise indicated, a quadrant of Class II preparations with similarly sized proximal boxes can be restored using two bands simultaneously if they are placed on every other prepared tooth. It is recommended to restore the most posterior tooth first.

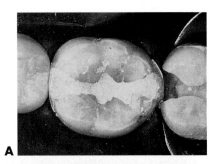

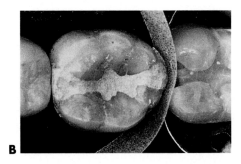

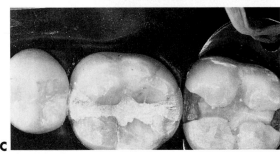

FIG. **17-108** When the first of two adjacent Class II preparations is restored, proper contour can be established using a finishing and contouring strip before restoring the second. **A,** Before using the strip. **B,** Applying the strip. **C,** Verification of proper contour can be achieved by viewing the restoration with a mirror from the occlusal, facial, and lingual positions. Proximal contour can also be evaluated after matrix placement by noting the symmetry between the restored surface and the burnished matrix band.

CLASS VI AMALGAM RESTORATIONS

The Class VI tooth preparation is used to restore the incisal edge of anterior teeth or the cusp tip regions of the posterior teeth. Such tooth preparations are frequently indicated where attrition (loss of tooth substance from the occluding of food, abrasives, and opposing teeth) has removed the enamel to expose the underlying dentin on those areas (Fig. 17-109, A). Such a wear pattern occurs more often in geriatric patients. Once the softer dentin is exposed, it wears faster than the surrounding enamel, resulting in "cupped-out" areas. As the dentin support is lost, the enamel begins to fracture away, exposing more dentin and often causing sensitivity. Sensitivity to hot and cold is a frequent complaint with Class VI lesions, and some patients are bothered by food impaction in the deeper depressions. Enamel edges may become jagged and sharp to the tongue, lips, or cheek. Lip, tongue, or cheek biting is occasionally a complaint. Rounding and smoothing such incisoaxial (or occlusoaxial) edges is an excellent service to the patient. Early recognition and restoration of these lesions is recommended to limit the loss of dentin and the subsequent loss of enamel supported by this dentin.

The Class VI tooth preparation also is indicated to restore the hypoplastic pit occasionally found on cusp tips (Fig. 17-110). Such developmental faults are vulnerable to caries, especially in high-risk patients, and should be restored as soon as they are detected. Rarely is caries found in the dentin where attritional wear has removed the overlying enamel.

Composite is generally used to restore Class VI preparations. Amalgam may be selected for posterior Class VI preparations because of its wear resistance and longevity. Moisture control for Class VI restorations is

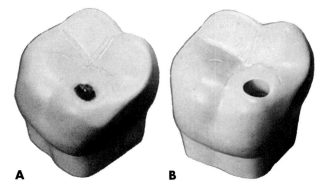

FIG. **17-109** Class VI preparation. **A,** Exposed dentin on mesiofacial cusp. **B,** Tooth preparation necessary to restore involved area.

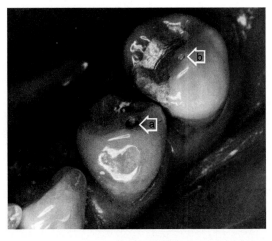

FIG. **17-110** Class VI lesions. Carious cusp tip fault on first premolar (*a*). Noncarious fault on second premolar (*b*).

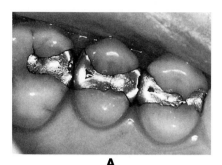
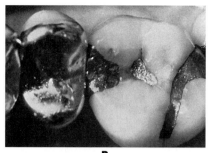
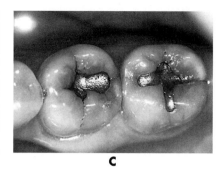

A   **B**   **C**

FIG. **17-111** Clinical examples of long-term amalgam restorations. **A,** 44-year-old amalgams. **B,** 58-year-old amalgams in the first molar. **C,** 65-year-old amalgams in molars. *(A and B, Courtesy of Drs. John Osborne and James Summitt.)*

usually achieved with cotton roll isolation. For Class VI amalgam preparations, enter the area with a small tapered fissure bur (e.g., No. 169L) and extend to a sufficient size to place the cavosurface margin on enamel that has sound dentin support (see Fig. 17-109, *B*). The preparation walls may need to diverge occlusally to ensure a 90-degree cavosurface margin. A depth of 1.5 mm is sufficient to provide bulk of material for strength. Retention of the restoration is ensured by the creation of small undercuts along the internal line angles. Be careful not to remove dentin that is immediately supporting the enamel. Conservative tooth preparation is particularly important with Class VI preparations because it is easy to undermine enamel on incisal edges and cusp tips. Inserting, carving, and polishing are similar to procedures described for Class I tooth preparations for amalgam.

Some older patients have excessive occlusal wear of most of the teeth in the form of large concave areas with much exposed dentin. Teeth with excessive wear may require indirect restorations.

SUMMARY

Class I and II amalgam restorations are still common procedures performed by general dentists. Class VI amalgam restorations are used infrequently. It is important for practitioners to understand the indications, advantages, techniques, and limitations of these restorations. When used correctly and in properly selected cases, they have demonstrated the potential to serve for many years (Fig. 17-111).

REFERENCES

1. Almquist TC, Cowan RD, Lambert RL: Conservative amalgam restorations, *J Prosthet Dent* 29(5):524, 1973.
2. Anusavice KJ, editor: *Phillips' science of dental materials*, ed 10, St Louis, 1996, Mosby.
3. Bader JD, Shugars DA: Variations in dentists' clinical decisions, *J Public Health Dent* 55(3):181, 1995.
4. Bauer JG: A study of procedures for burnishing amalgam restorations, *J Prosthet Dent* 57(6):669, 1987.
5. Ben-Amar A: Reduction of microleakage around new amalgam restorations, *J Am Dent Assoc* 119(6):725, 1989.
6. Berry TG, Laswell HR, Osborne JW, Gale EN: Width of isthmus and marginal failure of restorations of amalgam, *Oper Dent* 6(2):55, 1981.
7. Bjertness E, Sonju T: Survival analysis of amalgam restorations in long-term recall patients, *Acta Odontol Scand* 48(2):93, 1990.
8. Browning WD, Johnson WW, Gregory PN: Clinical performance of bonded amalgam restorations at 42 months, *J Am Dent Assoc* 131(5):607, 2000.
9. Burgess JO: Dental materials for the restorations of root surfaces caries, *Am J Dent* 8(6):342, 1995.
10. Collins CJ, Bryant RW: Finishing of amalgam restorations: a three-year clinical study, *J Dent* 20(4):202, 1992.
11. Council on Dental Materials, Instruments, and Equipment: Dental mercury hygiene: summary of recommendations in 1990, *J Am Dent Assoc* 122(8):112, 1991.
12. Crockett WD, Shepard FE, Moon PC, Creal AF: The influence of proximal retention grooves on the retention and resistance of class II preparations for amalgam, *J Am Dent Assoc* 91(5):1053, 1975.
13. de Morais PM, Rodrigues AL Jr, Pimenta LA: Quantitative microleakage evaluation around amalgam restorations with different treatments on cavity walls, *Oper Dent* 24(4):217, 1999.
14. Della Bona A, Summitt JB: The effect of amalgam bonding on resistance form of class II amalgam restorations, *Quintessence Int* 29(2):95, 1998.
15. Dilley DC et al: Time required for placement of composite versus amalgam restorations, *J Dent Child* 57(3):177, 1990.
16. Downer MC et al: How long do routine restorations last? A systematic review. *Br Dent J* 187(8):432, 1999.
17. Drummond JL et al: Surface roughness of polished amalgams, *Oper Dent* 17(4):129, 1992.
18. Duncalf WV, Wilson NHF: Adaptation and condensation of amalgam restorations in Class II preparations of conventional and conservative design, *Quintessence Int* 23(7):499, 1992.
19. Eakle WS, Staninec W: Retrospective study of bonded amalgam restorations, *J Dent Res* 78:445, 1999 (abstract).
20. Eakle WS, Staninec M, Lacy AM: Effect of bonded amalgam on the fracture resistance of teeth, *J Prosthet Dent* 68(2):257, 1992.
21. el-Badrawy WA: Cuspal deflection of maxillary premolars restored with bonded amalgam, *Oper Dent* 24(6):337, 1999.
22. Eliades G, Palaghias G: In-vitro characterization of visible-light-cured glass-ionomer liners, *Dent Mater* 9(3):198, 1993.

23. Fusayama T: Two layers of carious dentin: diagnosis and treatment, *Oper Dent* 4(2): 63, 1979.

24. Gilmore HW: Pulpal considerations for operative dentistry, *J Prosthet Dent* 14(4):752, 1964.

25. Gilmore HW: Restorative materials and tooth preparation design, *Dent Clin North Am* 15(1):99, 1971.

26. Goel VK et al: Effect of cavity depth on stresses in a restored tooth, *J Prosthet Dent* 67(2):174, 1992.

27. Goho C, Aaron GR: Enhancement of anti-microbial properties of cavity varnish: a preliminary report, *J Prosthet Dent* 68(4):623, 1992.

28. Görücü J, Tiritoglu M, Ozgünaltay G: Effects of preparation designs and adhesive systems on retention of class II amalgam restorations, *J Prosthet Dent* 78(3):250, 1997.

29. Gottlieb EW, Retief DH, Bradley EL: Microleakage of conventional and high-copper amalgam restorations, *J Prosthet Dent* 53(3):355, 1985.

30. Gwinnett AJ et al: Adhesive restorations with amalgam: guidelines for the clinician, *Quintessence Int* 25(10):687, 1994.

31. Hebling J, Giro EMA, Costa CAS: Human pulp response after an adhesive system application in deep cavities, *J Dent* 27(8):557, 1999.

32. Hilton TJ: Cavity sealers, liners, and bases: current philosophies and indications for use, *Oper Dent* 21(4):134, 1996.

33. Hilton TJ: Can modern restorative procedures and materials reliably seal cavities? In vitro investigations, *Trans Acad Dent Mater* 12:21, 1998.

34. Jokstad A, Mjor IA: The quality of routine class II cavity preparations for amalgam, *Acta Odontol Scand* 47(1):53, 1989.

35. Joynt RB et al: Fracture resistance of posterior teeth with glass ionomer-composite resin systems, *J Prosthet Dent* 62(1):28, 1989.

36. Kanai S: Structure studies of amalgam II. Effect of burnishing on the margins of occlusal amalgam fillings, *Acta Odontol Scand* 24(1):47, 1966.

37. Khera SC, Chan KC: Microleakage and enamel finish, *J Prosthet Dent* 39(4):414, 1978.

38. Korale ME, Meiers JC: Microleakage of dentin bonding systems used with spherical and admixed amalgams, *Am J Dent* 9(6):249, 1996.

39. Kreulen CM et al: Replacement risk of amalgam treatment modalities: 15-year results, *J Dent* 26(8):627, 1998.

40. Lagouvardos P, Sourai P, Douvitsas G: Coronal fractures in posterior teeth, *Oper Dent* 14(1):28, 1989.

41. Larson TD, Douglas WH, Geisfeld RE: Effect of prepared cavities on the strength of teeth, *Oper Dent* 6(1):2, 1981.

42. Leon AR: The periodontum and restorative procedures, a critical review, *J Oral Rehabil* 4(2):105, 1977.

43. Letzel H et al: The influence of the amalgam alloy on the survival of amalgam restorations: a secondary analysis of multiple controlled clinical trials, *J Dent Res* 76(11):1787, 1997.

44. Lindemuth JS, Hagge MS, Broome JS: Effect of restoration size on fracture resistance of bonded amalgam restorations, *Oper Dent* 25(3):177, 2000.

45. Loe H: Reactions of marginal periodontal tissues to restorative procedures, *Int Dent J* 18(4):759, 1968.

46. Lovadino JR, Ruhnke LA, Consani S: Influence of burnishing on amalgam adaptation to cavity walls, *J Prosthet Dent* 58(3):284, 1987.

47. Mahler DB: The amalgam-tooth interface, *Oper Dent* 21(6):230, 1996.

48. Mahler DB, Engle JH: Clinical evaluation of amalgam bonding in class I and II restorations, *J Am Dent Assoc* 131(1):43, 2000.

49. Mahler DB, Nelson LW: Sensitivity answers sought in amalgam alloy microleakage study, *J Am Dent Assoc* 125(3):282, 1994.

50. Mahler DB, Terkla LG: Analysis of stress in dental structures, *Dent Clin North Am* 2(11):789, 1958.

51. Markley MR: Restorations of silver amalgam, *J Am Dent Assoc* 43(2):133, 1951.

52. Maryniuk GA: In search of treatment longevity—a 30-year perspective, *J Am Dent Assoc* 109(5):739, 1984.

53. Maryniuk GA, Kaplan SH: Longevity of restorations: survey results of dentists' estimates and attitudes, *J Am Dent Assoc* 112(1):39, 1986.

54. May KN, Wilder AD, Leinfelder KF: Clinical evaluation of various burnishing techniques on high-copper amalgam, *J Prosthet Dent* 61:213, 1982 (abstract).

55. May KN, Wilder AD, Leinfelder KF: Burnished amalgam restorations: a two-year evaluation, *J Prosthet Dent* 49(2):193, 1983.

56. Mayhew RB, Schmeltzer LD, Pierson WP: Effect of polishing on the marginal integrity of high-copper amalgams, *Oper Dent* 11(1):8, 1986.

57. Mjor IA, Jokstad A, Qvist V: Longevity of posterior restorations, *Int Dent J* 40(1):11, 1990.

58. Moffa JP: The longevity and reasons for replacement of amalgam alloys, *J Dent Res* 68:188, 1989 (abstract).

59. Mondelli J et al: Influence of proximal retention on the fracture strength of Class II amalgam restorations, *J Prosthet Dent* 46(4):420, 1981.

60. Mondelli J et al: Fracture strength of amalgam restorations in modern Class II preparations with proximal retentive grooves, *J Prosthet Dent* 32(5):564, 1974.

61. Mondelli RF et al: Fracture strength of weakened human premolars restored with amalgam with and without cusp coverage, *Am J Dent* 11(4):181, 1998.

62. Moore DL: Retentive grooves for the Class 2 amalgam restoration: necessity or hazard? *Oper Dent* 17(1):29, 1992.

63. Neme AL, Evans DB, Maxson BB: Evaluation of dental adhesive systems with amalgam and resin composite restorations: comparison of microleakage and bond strengths results, *Oper Dent* 25(5):512, 2000.

64. Oliveira JP, Cochran MA, Moore BK: Influence of bonded amalgam restorations on the fracture strength of teeth, *Oper Dent* 21(3):110, 1996.

65. Osborne JW, Gale EN: Failure at the margin of amalgams as affected by cavity width, tooth position, and alloy selection, *J Dent Res* 60(3):682, 1981.

66. Osborne JW, Gale EN: Relationship of restoration width, tooth position and alloy to fracture at the margins of 13- to 14-year-old amalgams, *J Dent Res* 69(9):1599, 1990.

67. Osborne JW, Norman RD: 13-year clinical assessment of 10 amalgam alloys, *Dent Mater* 6(3):189, 1990.

68. Osborne JW et al: Two independent evaluations of ten amalgam alloys, *J Prosthet Dent* 43(6):622, 1980.

69. Osborne JW, Summitt JB: Extension for prevention: is it relevant today? *Am J Dent* 11(4):189, 1998.

70. Osborne JW, Norman RD, Gale EN: A 14-year clinical assessment of 12 amalgam alloys, *Quintessence Int* 22(11):857, 1991.

71. Pack AR: The amalgam overhang dilemma: a review of causes and effects, prevention, and removal, *N Z Dent J* 85(380):55, 1989.

72. *Restoration of tooth preparations with amalgam and tooth-colored materials: project ACCORDE student syllabus*, Washington, DC, 1974, US Department of Health, Education, and Welfare.

73. Robbins JW: The placement of bases beneath amalgam restorations: review of literature and recommendations for use, *J Am Dent Assoc* 113(6):910, 1986.

74. Rodda JC: Modern class II amalgam tooth preparations, *N Z Dent J* 68(312):132, 1972.

75. Schupbach P, Lutz F, Finger WJ: Closing of dentinal tubules by Gluma desensitizer, *Euro J Oral Sci* 105(5):414, 1997.

76. Setcos JC, Staninec M, Wilson NHF: Bonding of amalgam restorations: existing knowledge and future prospects, *Oper Dent* 25(2):121, 2000.

77. Smales RJ: Longevity of low- and high-copper amalgams analyzed by preparation class, tooth site, patient age, and operator, *Oper Dent* 16(5):162, 1991.

78. Smales RJ: Longevity of cusp-covered amalgams: survival after 15 years, *Oper Dent* 16(1):17, 1991.

79. Smales RJ, Wetherell JD: Review of bonded amalgam restorations and assessment in a general practice over five years, *Oper Dent* 25(5):374, 2000.

80. Sockwell CL: Dental handpieces and rotary cutting instruments, *Dent Clin North Am* 15(1):219, 1971.

81. Staninec M: Retention of amalgam restorations: undercuts versus bonding, *Quintessence Int* 20(5):347, 1989.

82. Straffon LH, Dennison JB, Asgar K: A clinical evaluation of polished and unpolished amalgams: 36-month results, *Pediatr Dent* 6(4):220, 1984.

83. Sturdevant JR et al: Conservative preparation designs for Class II amalgam restorations, *Dent Mater* 3(3):144, 1987.

84. Summitt JB et al: Effect of grooves on resistance form of conservative class 2 amalgams, *Oper Dent* 17(2):50, 1992.

85. Summitt JB, Osborne JW: Initial preparations for amalgam restorations: extending the longevity of the tooth-restoration unit, *J Am Dent Assoc* 123(11):67, 1992.

86. Summitt JB, Osborne JW, Burgess JO: Effect of grooves on resistance/retention form of Class 2 approximal slot amalgam restorations, *Oper Dent* 18(5):209, 1993.

87. Summitt JB et al: Effect of grooves on resistance form of Class 2 amalgams with wide occlusal preparations, *Oper Dent* 18(2):42, 1993.

88. Sweeney JT: Amalgam manipulation: manual vs. mechanical aids. II. Comparison of clinical applications, *J Am Dent Assoc* 27(12):1940, 1940.

89. Tangsgoolwatana J et al: Microleakage evaluation of bonded amalgam restorations: confocal microscopy versus radioisotope, *Quintessence Int* 28(7):467, 1997.

90. Vale WA: Tooth preparation and further thoughts on high speed, *Br Dent J* 107(11):333, 1959.

91. Vlietstra JR, Sidaway DA, Plant CG: Cavity cleansers, *Br Dent J* 149(10):293, 1980.

92. Waerhaug J: Histologic considerations which govern where the margins of restorations should be located in relation to the gingivae, *Dent Clin North Am* 4(3):161, 1960.

Classes III and V Amalgam Restorations

ALDRIDGE D. WILDER, JR.

THEODORE M. ROBERSON

ANDRÉ V. RITTER

KENNETH N. MAY, JR.*

*This author is inactive this edition. See the Acknowledgments.

CLASSES III AND V AMALGAM RESTORATIONS

This chapter presents information about Class III and Class V amalgam restorations. Class III restorations are indicated for defects located on the proximal surface of anterior teeth that do not affect the incisal edge. Part of the facial or the lingual surfaces may also be involved in Class III restorations. Class V restorations are indicated to restore defects on the facial or lingual cervical one third of any tooth.

The Class III amalgam restoration is used infrequently; its use has been supplanted by tooth-colored restorations (primarily composite) that have become increasingly wear resistant and color stable. However, because there are indications for Class III amalgam restorations, practitioners should be familiar with this restorative technique.

The Class V amalgam restoration can be especially technically sensitive because of location, extent of caries, and limited access and visibility. Cervical caries usually develops because the affected tooth surface is unclean and the patient has a caries-inducing diet. Patients with gingival recession have a predisposition to cervical caries, because dentin is more susceptible to demineralization than enamel. Patients with a reduced salivary flow caused by certain medical conditions (e.g., Sjögren's syndrome), medications, or head and neck radiation therapy also have a predisposition for cervical caries. These patients usually have less saliva to buffer the acids produced by oral bacteria. Cervical caries and root caries are terms often used interchangeably. However, the term *cervical caries* may be more accurate be-

cause Class V restorations, by definition, include the gingival one third (i.e., cervical area) of the facial and lingual surface of the tooth crown. However, root caries is also an accurate description of lesions that exist on the root surface of the tooth, although these may include the proximal surfaces as well.

Incipient, smooth-surface enamel caries appears as a chalky white line just occlusal or incisal to the crest of the marginal gingiva (usually on the facial surface) (Fig. 18-1). These areas are often overlooked in the oral examination unless the teeth are free of debris, isolated with cotton rolls, and dried gently with the air syringe. When incipient cervical caries has not decalcified the enamel sufficiently to result in cavitation (i.e., a break in the continuity of the surface), the lesion may be remineralized by appropriate techniques, including patient motivation for proper diet and hygiene. Occasionally, an enamel surface that is only slightly cavitated may be treated successfully by smoothing with sandpaper discs, polishing, and treating with a fluoride preparation or a dentin adhesive in an attempt to prevent further caries that may require a restoration. Obviously, this prophylactic, preventive treatment cannot be instituted if caries has progressed to decalcify and soften the enamel to an appreciable depth. In this instance, a Class V tooth preparation and restoration is indicated, particularly if caries has penetrated to the dentinoenamel junction (DEJ) (Fig. 18-2, *A*). When a large number of cervical lesions are present (see Fig. 18-2, *B*), a relatively high caries index is obvious. In addition to the restorative treatment, the patient should be instructed and encouraged to implement an aggressive prevention program to avoid recurrent decay.

PERTINENT MATERIAL QUALITIES AND PROPERTIES

Material qualities and properties important for Classes III and V amalgam restorations are strength, longevity, ease of use, and past success. (See Chapter 16 for a discussion of the pertinent material qualities and properties for amalgam.)

INDICATIONS

Class III. There are few indications for a Class III amalgam restoration. It is generally reserved for the distal surface of maxillary and mandibular canines if:

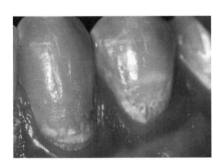

FIG. **18-1** Incipient carious lesions of enamel appear as white spots. The affected surface may be smooth (i.e., noncavitated). Carious white spots are more visible when dried.

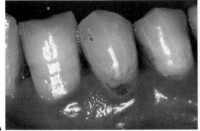
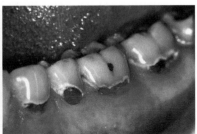

FIG. **18-2** Cervical caries. **A,** Cavitation involving both enamel and dentin. **B,** Relatively high caries index is obvious when large number of cervical lesions is present.

A   B

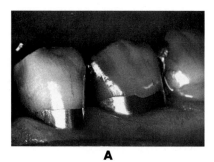
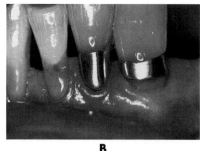
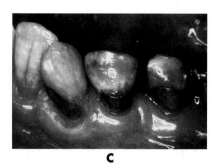

FIG. 18-3 **A,** 6-year-old cervical amalgam restoration. **B,** After 16 years some abrasion and erosion is evident at gingival margin of lateral incisor and canine restorations. **C,** 20-year-old cervical amalgam restorations.

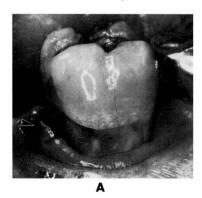
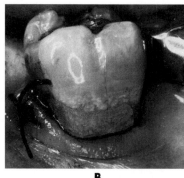
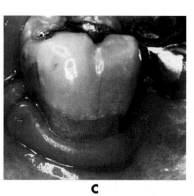

FIG. 18-4 Surgical access. **A,** Class V preparation requiring flap procedure with relaxing incision (*arrow*). **B,** Completed restoration with suture in place. **C,** 1-week postoperative with suture removed.

(1) the preparation is extensive with only minimal facial involvement, (2) the gingival margin involves primarily cementum, or (3) moisture control is difficult. For esthetic reasons, amalgam is rarely indicated for the proximal surfaces of incisors and the mesial surface of canines.

However, amalgam may be used for any Class III restoration that does not involve the facial surface or undermine the incisal corner. Access for the tooth preparation is generally from the lingual approach to conserve the enamel facial to the proximal contact. When the incisal corner is involved, a Class IV tooth preparation is necessary, and a composite is usually indicated for esthetics and retention.

Class V. Class V amalgam restorations may be used anywhere in the mouth. As with Class III amalgam restorations, they are generally reserved for nonesthetic areas, for areas where access and visibility are limited and where moisture control is difficult, and for areas that are significantly deep gingivally.

Because of limited access and visibility, many Class V restorations are difficult and present special problems during both the preparation and restorative procedures. Amalgam, composite, resin-modified glass ionomer, or compomer are most often used to treat cervical caries.

One measure of clinical success of cervical amalgam restorations is the length of time the restoration serves without failing (Fig. 18-3; see also Fig. 9-20, *B*). Many

properly placed Class V amalgams will be clinically acceptable for many years. However, some cervical amalgam restorations show evidence of failure even after a short period. Inattention to tooth preparation principles, improper manipulation of the material, and moisture contamination contribute to early failure. Extended service depends on the operator's care in following accepted treatment techniques, as well as proper care by the patient.

Amalgam may be preferred over esthetic restorative materials on partial denture abutment teeth, because amalgam is more resistant to wear as clasps move over the restoration. Furthermore, contours prepared in the restoration to provide rests and retentive areas for the clasp tips may be achieved more easily and maintained longer when an amalgam restoration is used.

Occasionally, amalgam is preferred when the carious lesion extends gingivally enough that a soft-tissue flap must be reflected for adequate access and visibility (Fig. 18-4). Proper surgical procedures must be followed, including sterile technique, careful soft-tissue management, and complete débridement of the operating site before wound closure.

CONTRAINDICATIONS

Classes III and V amalgam restorations are usually contraindicated in esthetically important areas because many patients object to metal restorations that are visi-

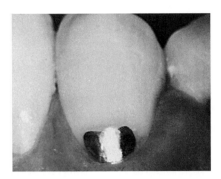

FIG. **18-5** Patients may object to metal restorations that are visible during conversation.

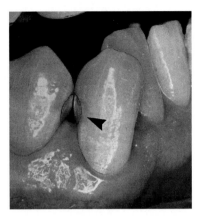

FIG. **18-6** Restoration for Class III tooth preparation using facial approach on mandibular canine. Restoration is 5 years old. *(Courtesy of Dr. C.L. Sockwell.)*

ble during conversation (Fig. 18-5). Generally, Class V amalgams placed on the facial surface of mandibular canines, premolars, and molars are not readily visible. However, those placed on maxillary premolars and first molars may be visible. Thus the patient's esthetic demands should be considered when planning treatment.

ADVANTAGES

Amalgam restorations are stronger than other Class III and V direct restorations. In addition, they are generally easier to place and may be less expensive to the patient. Because of its metallic color, amalgam is easily distinguished from the surrounding tooth structure. Therefore amalgam restorations are usually easier to finish and polish without damage to the adjacent surfaces.

DISADVANTAGES

The primary disadvantage of Class III and Class V amalgam restorations is that they are metallic and unesthetic. In addition, the preparation for an amalgam restoration typically requires 90-degree cavosurface margins, specific and uniform axial depths, and incorporation of secondary retentive features, all of which results in a less conservative preparation than that for most esthetic restorative materials. The potential for mercury contamination is another disadvantage.

CLINICAL TECHNIQUE FOR CLASS III AMALGAM RESTORATIONS

INITIAL PROCEDURES

After appropriate review of the patient's chart (including medical history), treatment plan, and radiographs, the gingival extension of the preparation should be anticipated. Anesthesia is frequently necessary when a vital tooth is to be restored. Additionally, prewedging in the gingival embrasure of the proximal site to be restored provides better (1) protection of the soft tissue and rubber dam, (2) access because of slight separation of teeth, and (3) reestablishment of the proximal contact. The use of a rubber dam is generally recommended (see Chapter 10); however, cotton roll isolation is acceptable if moisture can be adequately controlled.

TOOTH PREPARATION

Preparation for the Distal Surface of the Maxillary Canine. A lingual access preparation of the distal surface of the maxillary canine is recommended because the use of amalgam in that location is more likely. However, a facial approach for a mandibular canine may be indicated if the lesion is more facial than lingual. The mandibular restoration is often not visible at conversational distance (Fig. 18-6).

The outline form of the Class III amalgam preparation on a canine is similar to the conventional Class III composite preparation (see Chapter 12). However, there are differences. The amalgam preparation uses a bur instead of a diamond and incorporates no enamel bevels. In addition, it requires secondary retention features and a specific and uniform axial depth. Usually the outline form includes only the proximal surface; however, a lingual dovetail may be indicated if one existed previously or if additional retention is needed for a larger restoration.

Initial Tooth Preparation. Bur size selection depends on the anticipated size of the restoration. Usually a No. 2 bur is used for the entry cut on the distolingual marginal ridge. However, a No. 1/2 or No. 1 bur should be used when the tooth or carious lesion is small. The bur is positioned so that the entry cut will penetrate into the carious lesion, which is usually gingival to (and slightly into) the contact area. Ideally the bur is positioned so that its long axis is perpendicular to the lingual surface of the tooth but directed at a mesial angle as close to the adjacent tooth as possible. (The bur position may be described as perpendicular to the distolingual line angle of the tooth.) This conserves the marginal ridge enamel (Fig. 18-7, *A* through *C*). Penetration through the enamel positions the bur so that additional cutting will both isolate the proximal enamel affected by caries and remove some or all of the infected dentin. In addition, penetration should be at a limited initial axial depth (i.e., 0.5 to

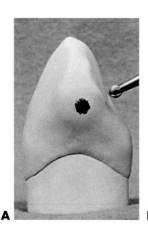
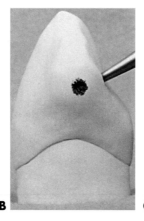
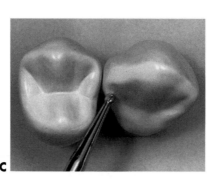
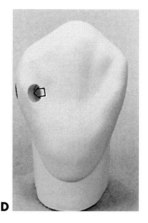

FIG. **18-7** Entry for Class III tooth preparation on maxillary canine. **A,** Bur position is perpendicular to enamel surface at point of entry. **B,** Initial penetration through enamel is directed toward cavitated, carious lesion. **C,** Initial entry should isolate proximal enamel, while preserving as much of the marginal ridge as possible. **D,** Initial cutting reveals DEJ (*arrow*).

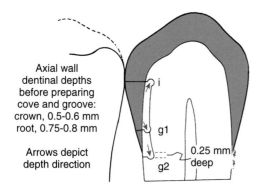

Axial wall dentinal depths before preparing cove and groove: crown, 0.5-0.6 mm root, 0.75-0.8 mm

Arrows depict depth direction

FIG. **18-8** Mesiodistal vertical section showing location, depth direction (*arrows*), and direction depth of retention form in Class III tooth preparations of different gingival depths. *i,* Incisal cove; *g1,* gingival groove, enamel margin; *g2,* gingival groove, root surface margin. Distance from outer aspect of *g2* groove to margin is approximately 0.3 mm; bur head diameter is 0.5 mm; direction depth of groove is half this diameter (or approximately 0.3 mm [0.25 mm]).

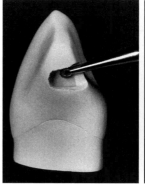
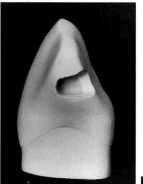

FIG. **18-9** Class III tooth preparation on maxillary canine. **A,** Round bur shaping incisal area. Note that incisal angle remains. **B,** Initial shape of preparation accomplished with round bur.

0.6 mm) inside the DEJ (see Fig. 18-7, *C* and *D*) or at a 0.75- to 0.8- mm axial depth when the gingival margin will be on the root surface (in cementum) (Fig. 18-8). This 0.75- mm axial depth on the root surface will allow a 0.25 mm distance (the diameter of the No. ¼ bur is 0.5 mm) between the retention groove (which will be placed later) and the gingival cavosurface margin. Infected dentin that is deeper than this limited initial axial depth is removed later during final tooth preparation.

For a small lesion, the facial margin is extended 0.2 to 0.3 mm into the facial embrasure (if necessary), with a curved outline from the incisal to the gingival margin (resulting in a less visible margin). The lingual outline blends with the incisal and gingival margins in a smooth curve, creating a preparation with little or no lingual wall. The cavosurface angle should be 90 degrees at all margins. The facial, incisal, and gingival walls should meet the axial wall at approximately right angles (although the lingual wall meets the axial wall at an obtuse angle or may be continuous with the axial wall) (Fig. 18-9). If a large, round bur is used, the internal angles will be more rounded. The axial wall should be uniformly deep into dentin and follow the faciolingual contour of the external tooth surface (Fig. 18-10). The initial axial wall depth may be in sound dentin (i.e., shallow lesion), in infected dentin (i.e., moderate to deep lesion), or in existing restorative material, if replacing a restoration.

Incisal extension to remove carious tooth structure may eliminate the proximal contact (Fig. 18-11). However, it is important to conserve as much tooth structure as possible at the distoincisal corner (i.e., canopy) to reduce the potential for subsequent fracture. When possible, it is best to leave the incisal margin in contact with the adjacent tooth.

When preparing a gingival wall that is near either the level of the rubber dam or apical to it, it is beneficial to

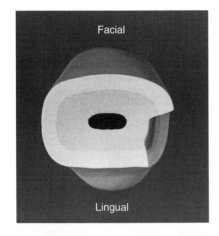

FIG. **18-10** Transverse section of mandibular lateral incisor illustrating that lingual wall of Class III tooth preparation may meet axial wall at an obtuse angle and that axial wall is a uniform depth into dentin and follows faciolingual contour of external tooth surface.

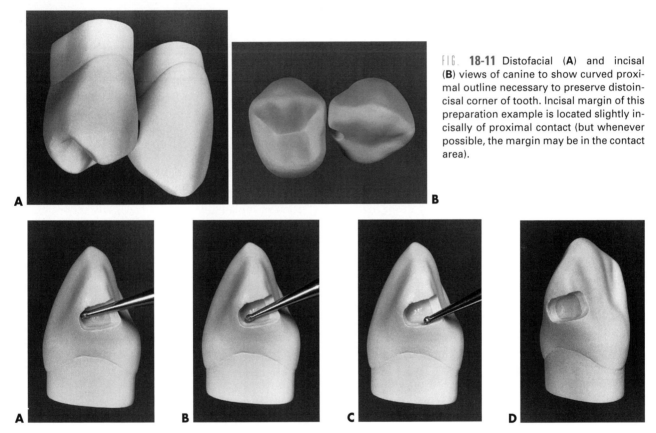

FIG. **18-11** Distofacial (**A**) and incisal (**B**) views of canine to show curved proximal outline necessary to preserve distoincisal corner of tooth. Incisal margin of this preparation example is located slightly incisally of proximal contact (but whenever possible, the margin may be in the contact area).

FIG. **18-12** Refining proximal portion. **A** through **C**, Small, round bur is used to shape preparation walls, define line angles, and initiate removal of any undermined enamel along gingival and facial margins. **D**, Tooth preparation completed except for final finishing of enamel margins and placing retention form.

have earlier placed a wedge in the gingival embrasure to depress and protect the soft tissue and rubber dam. As the bur is preparing the gingival wall, it may lightly shave the wedge. A triangular (i.e., anatomic) wedge, rather than a round wedge, is used for a deep gingival margin.

Complete the initial tooth preparation by using a No. ½ bur to accentuate the axial line angles (Fig. 18-12, *A* and *B*), particularly the axiogingival angle. This facilitates the subsequent placement of retention grooves

and leaves the internal line angles slightly rounded. Rounded internal preparation angles reduce stress concentration in the tooth, thereby reducing the potential of restoration fracture. In addition, they permit more complete condensation of the amalgam. The No. ½ bur may also be used to smooth any roughened, undermined enamel produced at the gingival and facial cavosurface margins (see Fig. 18-12, *C*). The incisal margin of the minimally extended preparation is often not accessible to the larger round bur without marring the adjacent

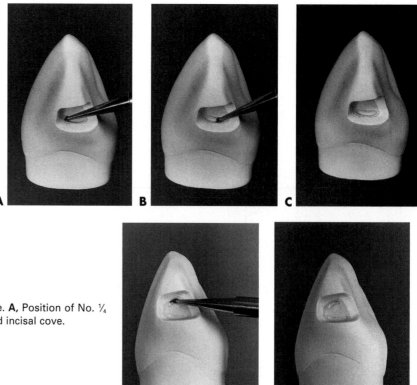

FIG. **18-13** Preparing gingival retention form. **A,** Position of No. ¼ bur in axiofaciogingival point angle. **B,** Advancing bur lingually to prepare groove along axiogingival line angle. (See Fig. 18-8 regarding location, depth direction, and direction depth of groove.) **C,** Completed gingival retention groove.

FIG. **18-14** Preparing incisal retention cove. **A,** Position of No. ¼ bur in axioincisal point angle. **B,** Completed incisal cove.

tooth (see Fig. 18-12, *D*). Further finishing of the incisal margin is presented later. At this point, the initial tooth preparation is completed.

Final Tooth Preparation. Final tooth preparation may involve removing any remaining infected dentin, protecting the pulp, developing secondary resistance and retention forms, finishing external walls, and the final procedures of cleaning, inspecting, and desensitizing or bonding. Remove any remaining infected carious dentin on the axial wall using a slowly revolving round bur (No. 2 or 4) or appropriate spoon excavators or both. (Refer to Chapters 6 and 11 for the indications and technique for placing a liner.)

For the Class III amalgam restoration, resistance form against postrestorative fracture is provided by: (1) cavosurface and amalgam margins of 90 degrees, (2) enamel walls supported by sound dentin, (3) sufficient bulk of amalgam (minimal 1-mm thickness), and (4) no sharp preparation internal angles. The boxlike preparation form provides primary retention form. Secondary retention form is provided by a gingival groove, an incisal cove, and, sometimes, a lingual dovetail.

Prepare the gingival retention groove by placing a No. ¼ bur (rotating at low speed) in the axiofaciogingival point angle. It is positioned in the dentin to maintain 0.2 mm of dentin between the groove and the DEJ. Move the bur lingually along the axiogingival line angle, with the angle of cutting generally bisecting the angle between the gingival and axial walls. Ideally, the direction of the gingival groove is slightly more gingival than axial (and the direction of an incisal [i.e., occlusal] groove would be slightly more incisal [i.e., occlusal] than axial) (Fig. 18-13; see also Fig. 18-8).

Alternatively, if less retention form is needed, two gingival coves may be used, as opposed to a continuous groove. One each may be placed in the axiogingivofacial and axiogingivolingual point angles. The diameter of the bur is 0.5 mm, and the depth of the groove should be half this diameter, or 0.25 mm. (See the location and depthwise direction of the groove, where the gingival wall is partially of enamel, in Fig. 8-18.) If the axiogingival line angle is ideally located, directing the groove depthwise (as described) should not undermine the enamel. When preparing a retention groove on the root surface, the angle of cutting is more gingival, resulting in the distance from the gingival cavosurface margin to the groove being approximately 0.3 mm (see Fig. 18-8). Careful technique is necessary in preparing the gingival retention groove. If the dentin that supports the gingival enamel is removed, the enamel is subject to fracture. In addition, if the groove is placed only in the axial wall, no effective retention form is developed and there is risk of pulpal involvement.

Prepare an incisal retention cove at the axiofacioincisal point angle with a No. ¼ bur in dentin, being careful not to undermine the enamel. It is directed similarly into the incisal point angle and prepared to one half the diameter of the bur (Fig. 18-14). Undermining the incisal

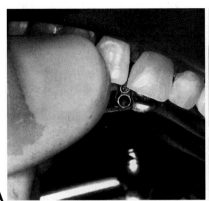

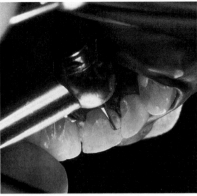

FIG. **18-15** Use of palm-and-thumb grasp to place incisal retention cove. **A,** Hand position showing thumb rest. **B,** Handpiece position for preparing incisal retention.

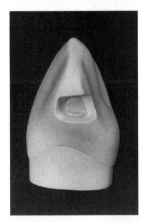

FIG. **18-16** Completed Class III tooth preparation for amalgam restoration.

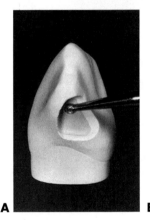

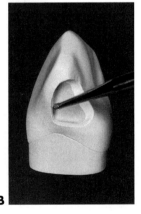

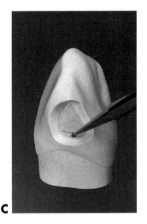

FIG. **18-17** Extensive Class III tooth preparation. **A,** Initial tooth preparation with No. 2 bur. **B,** Defining line angles and removing undermined enamel with No. ½ bur. **C,** Placing retention groove using No. ¼ bur. Note completed incisal cove.

enamel (or incisal canopy) should be avoided. For the maxillary canine, the palm-and-thumb grasp may be used to direct the bur incisally (Fig. 18-15). This completes the typical Class III amalgam tooth preparation (Fig. 18-16). (If the use of a bonding system is necessary, refer to Chapter 17 for a discussion of the technique.) As with Classes I and II amalgams, it is recommended that the clinician prepare mechanical retention (even if using an adhesive system).

A lingual dovetail is not required in small or moderately sized Class III amalgam restorations. It may be used in large preparations, especially those with excessive incisal extension in which additional retention form is needed. However, the dovetail may not be necessary

(even in large preparations) if incisal secondary retention form can be judiciously and effectively accomplished (Fig. 18-17).

If a lingual dovetail is needed, prepare it only after initial preparation of the proximal portion has been completed. Otherwise the tooth structure needed for the isthmus between the proximal portion and the dovetail may be removed when the proximal outline form is prepared. The lingual dovetail should be conservative, generally not extending beyond the mesiodistal midpoint of the lingual surface. This will vary according to the extent of the proximal caries. The axial depth of the dovetail should approximate 1 mm, and the axial wall should be parallel to the lingual surface of the tooth. This wall may or may not

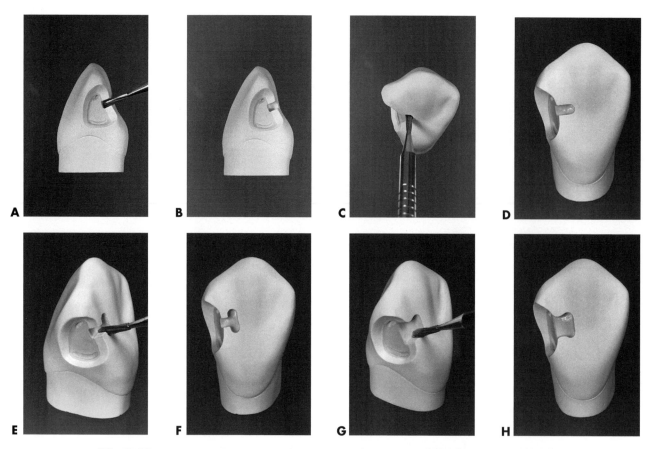

FIG. **18-18** Lingual dovetail providing additional retention for extensive amalgam restoration. **A,** Bur position at correct depth and angulation to begin cutting. **B,** Initial cut in beginning dovetail. **C,** Bur moved to most mesial extent of dovetail. **D,** If possible, cutting should not extend beyond midlingual position. **E,** Bur cutting gingival extension of dovetail. **F,** Incisal and gingival extensions of dovetail. **G,** Completing isthmus. Note that proximal and lingual portions are connected by incisal and gingival walls in smooth curves. **H,** Completed lingual dovetail.

be in dentin. Position the No. 245 bur in the proximal portion at the correct depth and angulation, and move the bur in a mesial direction (Fig. 18-18, *A* and *B*). The correct angulation places the long axis of the bur perpendicular to the lingual surface. Move the bur to the point that corresponds to the most mesial extent of the dovetail (see Fig. 18-18, *C* and *D*). Next, move the bur incisally and gingivally to create sufficient incisogingival dimension to the dovetail (approximately 2.5 mm) (see Fig. 18-18, *E* and *F*). Then, prepare the incisal and gingival walls of the isthmus in smooth curves connecting the dovetail to the proximal outline form (see Fig. 18-18, *G* and *H*).

The gingival margin trimmer may be used to bevel (or round) the axiopulpal line angle (i.e., the junction of the proximal and dovetail preparation). This increases the strength of the restoration at the junction of the proximal and lingual portions by providing bulk and reducing stress concentration. The lingual convergence of the dovetail's external walls (prepared with the No. 245 bur) usually provides sufficient retention form. However, retention coves, one in the incisal corner and one in the gingival corner (Fig. 18-19), may be placed in the dovetail to enhance retention if the axial wall of the

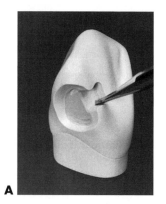
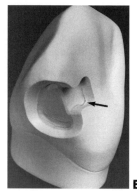

FIG. **18-19** Ensuring retention in lingual dovetail (often optional). **A,** Position of No. 33½ bur for cutting retention cove. **B,** Note that preparation of cove should not remove dentinal support of lingual enamel (*arrow*).

dovetail is in dentin. The coves are prepared with the No. 33½ bur in dentin that does not immediately support the lingual enamel. This may require deepening of the axial wall.

Remove any unsupported enamel, smooth enamel walls and margins, and refine the cavosurface angles

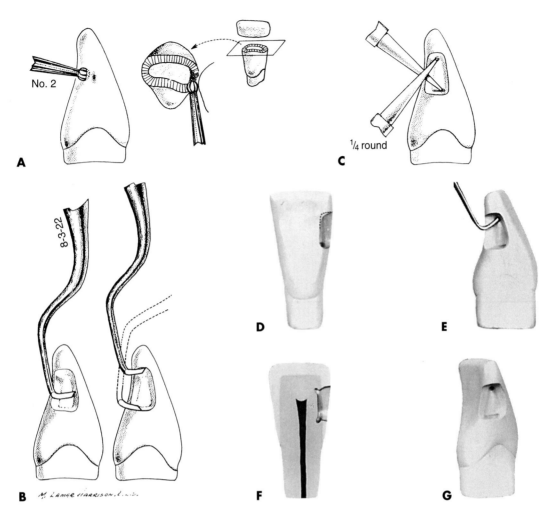

FIG. **18-20** Class III tooth preparation for amalgam restoration on mandibular incisor. **A,** Entering tooth from lingual approach. **B,** Finishing facial, incisal, and gingival enamel margins with an 8-3-22 triple angle hoe. Note how the reverse bevel blade is used on the gingival enamel. **C,** Placing incisal and gingival retention forms with No. ¼ bur. **D,** Dotted line indicates outline of additional extension sometimes necessary for access in placing incisal retention cove. **E,** Position of bibeveled hatchet 3-2-28 to place incisal retention cove. **F,** Axial wall forms convex surface over pulp. **G,** Completed tooth preparation. Note gingival retention groove.

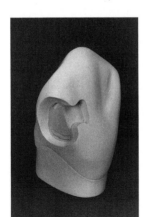

FIG. **18-21** Completed distolingual Class III tooth preparation for amalgam.

where indicated. The 8-3-22 hoe is recommended for finishing minimally extended margins (Fig. 18-20). If the gingival margin is in enamel, a slight bevel (approximately 20 degrees) is necessary to ensure full-length enamel rods forming the cavosurface margin. All the walls of the preparation should meet the external tooth surface to form a right angle (i.e., butt joint) (Fig. 18-21; see also Fig. 18-16). Various steps in a clinical procedure with the dovetail are shown in Fig. 18-22.

The completed tooth preparation should be carefully inspected and cleaned before restoration. Careful assessment should be made that all caries has been removed, depths are proper, margins provide for the correct amalgam and tooth preparation angles, and the tooth is cleaned of any residual debris. Desensitizers or bonding agents are used as part of the final preparation and restorative stages. (Refer to Chapters 16 and 17 for a discussion of bonded amalgam restorations.)

Preparation for the Mandibular Incisor. The use of a Class III amalgam restoration for a mandibular incisor is rare. If used, the preparation is similar to that for maxillary canines. Obviously for esthetic reasons, amalgam is best suited for the carious lesion that can be placed from lingual access rather than for the tooth

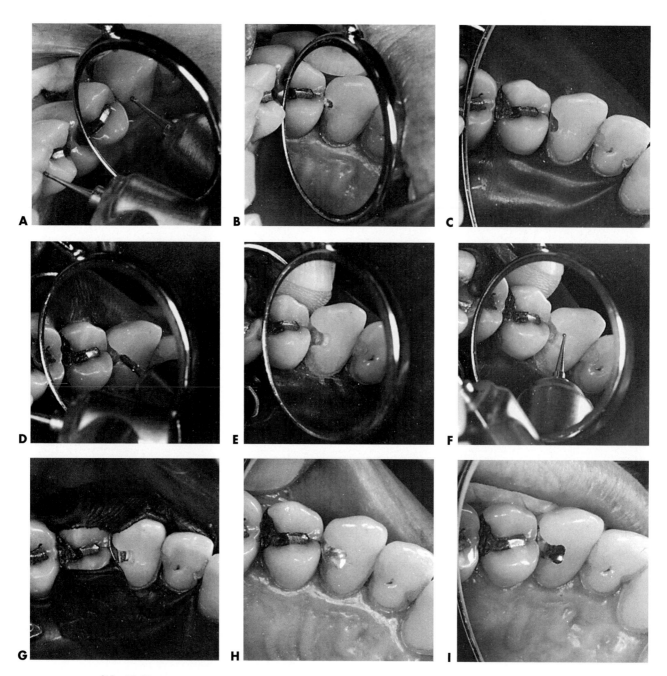

FIG. 18-22 Distolingual tooth preparation and restoration. **A,** Bur position for entry. **B,** Penetration made through lingual enamel to caries. **C,** Proximal portion completed except for retention form. **D,** Preparing dovetail. **E,** Completed preparation except for retention groove and coves. **F,** Bur position for incisal cove in dovetail. **G,** Compound matrix ready for insertion of amalgam. **H,** Carving completed and rubber dam removed. **I,** Polished restoration.

preparation that extends onto the facial surface. However, as with the distal surfaces of canines, amalgam can be used for mandibular incisors if: (1) access and visibility are limited, (2) the gingival margin in primarily in cementum, and (3) moisture control is difficult. Preliminary procedures for operating (e.g., anesthesia, isolation of the operating site, wedging) are the same as presented previously.

To prepare the outline form, enter the tooth from the lingual, when possible, or facial, when necessary. The choice of lingual or facial approach depends on the position of the tooth, the location of the carious lesion, and esthetics. (The initial and final tooth preparation technique is the same as described previously for the distal surface of a maxillary canine.)

RESTORATIVE TECHNIQUE

Sealer or Bonding Application. Adhesives are used occasionally for larger amalgam restorations where bonding may increase the resistance and retention

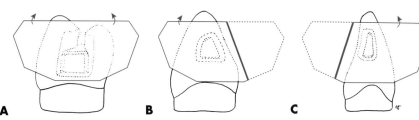

A   **B**   **C**

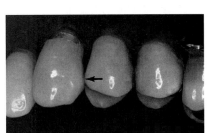

FIG. **18-23** Matrix strip design. **A,** Design required for compound-supported matrix for Class II tooth preparations. **B,** Alteration necessary for Class III preparation on maxillary canine. **C,** Alteration necessary for mandibular incisor. Note that strip material is cut to approximate slope of lingual surface.

forms (see Chapter 17 for adhesive application protocol). Smales and Wetherell were unable to demonstrate a significant difference between bonded and varnished amalgam restorations over five years.[5] However, Setcos et al concluded that bonded amalgam restorations may provide distinct advantages over nonbonded amalgam restorations, including decreased postoperative sensitivity, improved marginal adaptation, and a lower incidence of secondary caries.[4]

The use of a dentin desensitizer over the prepared tooth structure before placing a nonbonded amalgam is generally recommended as a sealer. Dentin desensitizer is rubbed onto the prepared tooth surface for 30 seconds and dried; then the amalgam is condensed into place. When using desensitizing agents, the etching and adhesive steps of typical adhesive systems are omitted. Berry et al reported that the primer component (i.e., dentin desensitizer) of several dentin bonding systems significantly reduced interfacial leakage of Class I amalgam restorations over 3 months compared with unlined and varnished groups.[2]

Matrix Placement. The wedged, compound-supported matrix may be used for the Class III amalgam restoration. Insertion of the amalgam into the Class III tooth preparation is usually from the lingual. Thus it is essential to trim the lingual portion of the strip matrix material correctly to avoid covering the preparation and blocking access for insertion of the amalgam. Using $\frac{5}{16}$ inch (8 mm) wide, 0.002 inch (0.05 mm) thick, (ribbon) stainless steel matrix material, cut a length that will cover one third of the facial surface and extend through the proximal to the lingual surface. Trim the lingual portion by cutting the strip at an angle that corresponds approximately to the slope of the lingual surface of the tooth (Fig. 18-23). Next, use fingers to contour the strip to approximate the circumferential contour of the tooth. Then, lay the strip on a resilient paper pad and burnish it using an egg-shaped burnisher, imparting the desired contact and contour form. Place the strip in position, and insert the wedge from the facial or lingual embrasure, whichever is greater. Now, stabilize the facial portion of the strip with low-fusing compound. A smaller amount of compound may be used lingually to position and stabilize the matrix material against the linguogingival corner (see Fig. 18-22, *G*). The experienced operator may coat the tip of the wedge with softened compound before the wedge is inserted and position the wedge and compound simultaneously. Precontoured

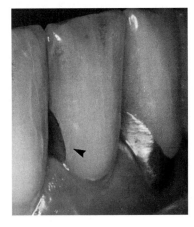

FIG. **18-24** Inconspicuous facial margin *(arrow)* of Class III amalgam restoration on maxillary canine.

FIG. **18-25** Class III amalgam restoration on mandibular incisor *(arrow)*.

metallic matrices may be used (instead of custom-made matrices) if the contour of the precontoured matrix coincides with that of the proximal surface being restored. If the preparation is small and the matrix is sufficiently rigid, compound may not be used.

Condensation and Carving. Insertion of the amalgam, initial carving, matrix removal, wedge removal, and final carving are similar to the techniques for posterior teeth (see Chapter 17). (If a dentin bonding system is to be used, refer to the section regarding bonded amalgam restorations in Chapter 17.) If necessary, the inserted restoration can be polished after a 24-hour delay. When properly placed, conservative restorations in incisors and canines are relatively inconspicuous (Fig. 18-24). Fig. 18-25 illustrates a Class III amalgam restoration in a mandibular incisor.

Finishing and Polishing. The finishing and polishing techniques and procedures are the same as presented in Chapters 16 and 17.

CLINICAL TECHNIQUE FOR CLASS V AMALGAM RESTORATIONS

INITIAL PROCEDURES

Proper isolation prevents moisture contamination of the operating site, enhances asepsis, and facilitates access and visibility. Moisture in the form of saliva, gingival sulcular fluid, or gingival hemorrhage must be excluded during caries removal, liner and adhesive application, if indicated, and insertion and carving of amalgam. Moisture impairs visual assessment, may contaminate the pulp during caries removal (especially with a pulpal exposure), and negatively affects the physical properties of restorative materials. The gingival margin of Class V tooth preparations is often apical to the gingival crest. Such a gingival margin necessitates retraction of the free gingiva with a retraction cord or appropriate rubber dam and retainer to protect it and to provide access, while also eliminating seepage of sulcular fluid into the tooth preparation or restorative materials.

These isolation objectives are met by local anesthesia and isolation by: (1) cotton roll (or rolls) and retraction

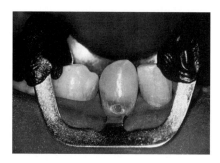

FIG. 18-26 The rubber dam and No. 212 retainer may be required to properly isolate carious area.

cord or (2) the rubber dam and suitable cervical retainer (Fig. 18-26) (see Chapter 10). Isolation by cotton roll (or rolls) and retraction cord is satisfactory when properly accomplished. This type of isolation is practical and probably the approach most often used.

The retraction cord should be placed in the sulcus before initial tooth preparation to reduce the possibility of cutting instruments damaging the free gingiva. The cord should produce a temporary, adequate, nontraumatic apical retraction and lateral deflection of the free gingiva. The cord may be treated with epinephrine. Epinephrine on abraded gingiva can be rapidly absorbed into the circulatory system, causing a rise in blood pressure, elevated heart rate, and possible dysrhythmia. Gentle placement of cord and absence of trauma to the free gingiva should preclude such systemic sequelae. Careful operative dentistry should generally not abrade the gingiva, even in tooth preparations extending subgingivally. Abrading the gingiva will open capillaries, which increases the absorption of epinephrine, causes bleeding, and limits visibility. Cords without epinephrine are available for patients at risk for cardiac problems.

Place the cotton roll (or rolls) and dry the area to be operated with the air syringe. Retraction cord may be braided, twisted, or woven. Cut retraction cord of suitable diameter to a length ¼ inch (6 mm) longer than the gingival margin. The diameter of the cord should be easily accommodated in the gingival sulcus. Some operators prefer to place the cord in a Dappen dish, wet it with a drop of styptic solution (e.g., Hemodent, Premier Dental Products, King of Prussia, PA), and then blot it with a 2 × 2 inch (5 × 5 cm) gauze to remove excess liquid. Next, the cord should be twisted tightly to remove

FIG. 18-27 Use of retraction cord for isolation of Class V lesion. **A,** Preoperative view. **B,** Cord placement initiated. **C,** Cord placement using a thin, flat-bladed instrument. **D,** Cord placement completed.

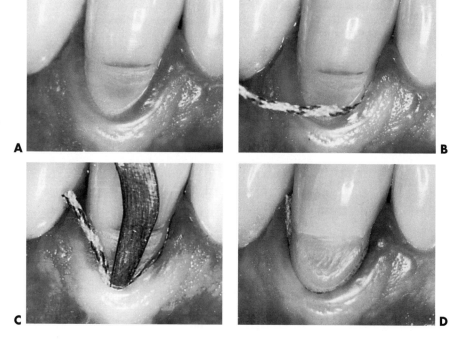

excess liquid and reduce the cord diameter. Braided or woven cord is usually easier to use because it will not unravel during placement. A larger cord can be inserted over the first cord, if the sulcus is large enough to accommodate two cords. Using a thin, blunt-edged instrument blade or the side of an explorer tine, gently insert the cord progressively to place. A slight backward direction of the instrument as it steps along the cord will help prevent dislodgment of previously inserted cord (Fig. 18-27). In addition, using a second instrument stepping along behind the first instrument can help prevent dislodgment of cord. Additionally, using the air syringe or cotton pellets to reduce or absorb the sulcular fluid in the cord already placed is helpful during the cord placement. The cord will result in adequate retraction in a short time. If significant blanching of the free gingiva is observed (or if too much pressure has to be applied to apply the cord), an oversized cord has been selected and should be exchanged with a cord of smaller diameter. The cord usually remains in place throughout tooth preparation and insertion and carving of amalgam. The cord can be moistened before or after placement with a styptic solution (e.g., Hemodent) if slight hemorrhage is anticipated or observed. Alternatively, the cord can be used dry.

As emphasized earlier, the size (i.e., diameter) of the cord should be selected according to the depth of the sulcus and the free gingiva characteristics. Usually insert the smallest diameter cord into the sulcus on the facial of anterior and premolar teeth because the free gingiva is thin, delicate, and tight. If necessary, a single strand of unbraided cord can be separated and twisted into a still smaller cord.

While carving amalgam at the gingival margin, the presence of the cord may cause difficulty in feeling the unprepared tooth surface gingival to the margin to prevent undercarving of the margin; this results in overcontour and marginal excess. In this instance, after carving gross excess the cord can be teased from place before completing the carving.

TOOTH PREPARATION

Proper outline form for Class V amalgam tooth preparations results in extending the cavosurface margins to sound tooth structure, while maintaining a limited axial depth of 0.5 mm inside the DEJ and 0.75 mm inside the

cementum (when on the root surface). The outline form for the Class V amalgam tooth preparation is primarily determined by the location and size of the caries or old restorative material. Historically, cervical amalgam restorations were made with preparation outlines that were overextended. Presently, a more conservative philosophy is used (resulting in smaller restorations with outline forms that are dictated primarily by the size of the defect). Clinical judgment determines final preparation outline, especially when the cavosurface margins approach or extend into areas of enamel decalcification. The operator must observe the prepared enamel wall to evaluate the depth of the decalcified enamel and to determine if cavitation exists peripheral to the wall. When no cavitation has occurred and when the decalcification does not extend appreciably into the enamel, extension of the outline form often should cease. In some cases, if all decalcification was included in the outline form, the preparation would extend into the proximal cervical areas (if not circumferentially around the tooth). Such a preparation would be difficult and perhaps unrestorable. A full-crown restoration should be considered for teeth with extensive cervical decalcification.

Initial Tooth Preparation. A Class V amalgam restoration is not often used in a mandibular canine, but it is presented here for illustration. The same general principles for tooth preparation apply for all other tooth locations. Using a tapered fissure bur of suitable size, enter the carious lesion (or existing restoration) to a limited initial axial depth of 0.5 mm inside the DEJ (Fig. 18-28). This depth is usually 1 to 1.25 mm total axial depth, depending on the incisogingival (i.e., occlusogingival) location. (The enamel is considerably thicker occlusally and incisally than cervically) However, if the preparation is on the root surface, the axial depth is approximately 0.75 mm. The end of the bur at the initial depth is in dentin, in infected carious dentin, or in old restorative material. Use the edge of the end of the bur to penetrate the area; this is more efficient than using the flat end of the bur, reducing the possibility of the bur's "crawling." Once the entry is made, the bur is maintained to ensure that all external walls are perpendicular to the external tooth surface and thereby parallel to the enamel rods (Fig. 18-29). Often this requires changing the orientation of the handpiece to accommodate the cervical mesiodistal and incisogingival (i.e.,

FIG. **18-28** Starting Class V tooth preparation. **A,** Bur positioned for entry into carious lesion. **B,** Entry cut is the beginning of outline form having a limited axial depth. (The end of bur in center of lesion may be in carious tooth structure or air.)

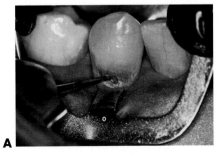
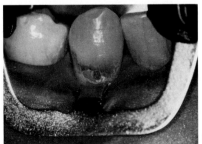

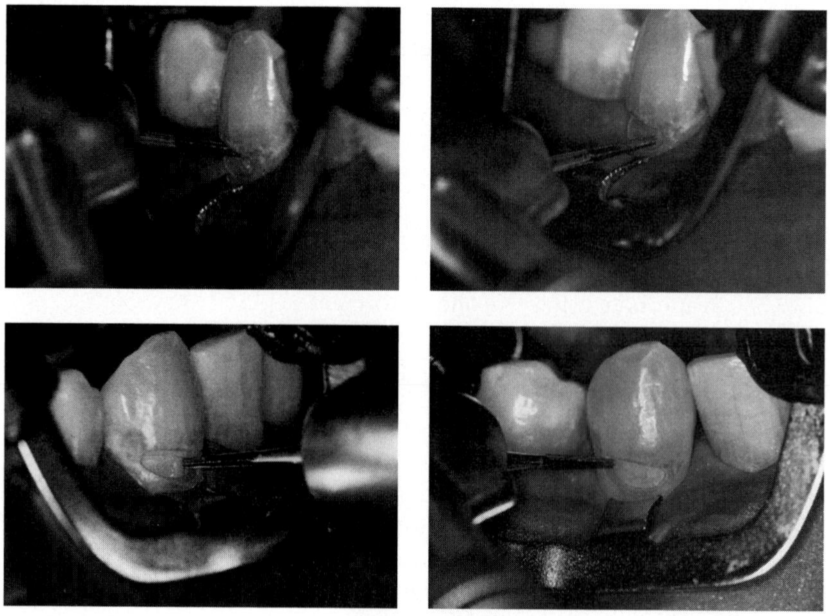

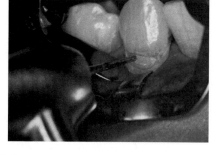

FIG. **18-29** When extending incisally (**A**), gingivally (**B**), mesially (**C**), and distally (**D**), position the bur to prepare these walls perpendicular to external tooth surface.

occlusogingival) convexity of the tooth. Extend the preparation incisally, gingivally, mesially, and distally until the cavosurface margins are positioned in sound tooth structure to establish an initial axial depth of 0.5 mm inside the DEJ (if on the root surface, the axial depth is 0.75 mm). When extending mesially and distally, it may be necessary to protect the rubber dam from the bur by placing a flat-bladed instrument over the dam (Fig. 18-30). The axial wall should be in sound dentin, unless there is remaining infected caries or old restorative material. Preparation of the axial wall depth 0.5 mm inside the DEJ results in a uniform depth for the entire preparation. Because the axial wall follows the mesiodistal and incisogingival (i.e., occlusogingival) contours of the facial surface of the tooth, it will usually be convex in both directions. In addition, the axial wall will usually be slightly deeper at the incisal wall, where there is more enamel (i.e., approximately 1 to 1.25 mm in depth) than at the gingival wall, where there may be little or no enamel (i.e., approximately 0.75 to 1 mm in depth). A depth of 0.5 mm inside the DEJ will permit placement of necessary retention grooves without undermining the enamel. This subtle difference in depth serves also to increase the thickness of the remaining dentin (between the axial wall and the pulp) in the gingival aspect of the preparation to aid in protecting the pulp. For the tooth preparation that is very extended incisogingivally, the axial wall should be more convex (because it follows the contour of the DEJ).

Alternatively, suitably sized, round carbide burs (usually a No. 2 or 4) may be used for the initial tooth preparation. In fact, round burs are indicated in areas inaccessible to a fissure bur that is held perpendicular to the tooth surface. If needed, smaller round burs may be used also to define internal angles in these preparations, enhancing proper placement of the retention grooves.

FIG. **18-30** Flat-bladed instrument protects rubber dam from bur.

Final Tooth Preparation. Final tooth preparation involves removal of any remaining infected dentin, pulp protection, retention form, finishing external walls, and final procedures of cleaning, inspecting, and desensitizing or bonding. Remove any remaining infected axial wall dentin with a No. 2 or No. 4 bur. Any old restorative material (including base and liner) remaining should not be removed if: (1) there is no clinical or radiographic evidence of recurrent caries, (2) the periphery of the base and liner is intact, and (3) the tooth is asymptomatic. With proper outline form, the axial line angles are already in sound dentin. If needed, apply an appropriate liner or base (see Chapter 16).

Because the mesial, distal, gingival, and incisal walls of the tooth preparation are perpendicular to the external tooth surface, they usually diverge facially. Consequently, this form provides no inherent retention, and retention form must be provided because the primary retention form for an amalgam restoration is macromechanical. Use a No. $\frac{1}{4}$ bur to prepare two retention grooves, one along the incisoaxial line angle and the other along the gingivoaxial line angle (Fig. 18-31). The handpiece is positioned so that the No. $\frac{1}{4}$ bur is directed generally to bisect the angle formed at the junction of

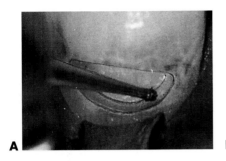

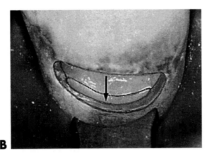

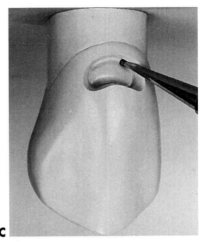

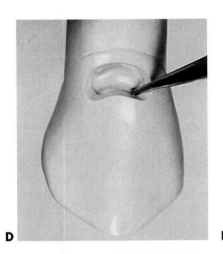

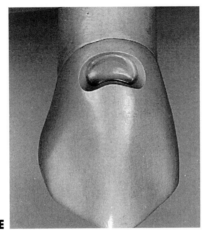

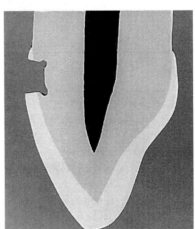

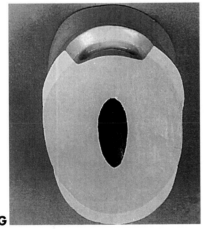

FIG. 18-31 Retention form. **A,** A No. ¼ bur positioned to prepare gingival retention groove. **B,** Gingival retention groove (*arrow*) prepared along gingivoaxial line angle generally to bisect the angle formed by the gingival and axial walls. Ideally, the direction of preparation is slightly more gingivally than pulpally. An incisal retention groove is prepared along incisoaxial line angle and directed similarly. **C** and **D,** Groove is placed with No. ¼ bur along gingivoaxial and incisoaxial line angles 0.2 mm inside DEJ and 0.25 mm deep. Note slight pulpal inclination of shank of No. ¼ bur. **E,** Facial view. **F,** Incisogingival section. Note that grooves depthwise are directed mostly incisally (gingivally) and slightly pulpally. **G,** Mesiodistal section.

the axial wall and the incisal or occlusal) wall. Ideally the direction of the incisal (i.e., occlusal) groove is slightly more incisal (i.e., occlusal) than axial, and the direction of the gingival groove is slightly more gingival than axial. Alternatively, four retention coves may be prepared, one in each of the four axial point angles of the preparation (Fig. 18-32).

Using four coves instead of two full-length grooves conserves dentin near the pulp, reducing the possibility of a mechanical pulp exposure. The depth of the grooves should approximate 0.25 mm, which is half the diameter of the bur. It is important that the retention grooves be adequate, because they provide the only retention form to the preparation. Regardless, the grooves should not remove dentin immediately supporting the enamel. In a large Class V amalgam preparation, extending the retention groove circumferentially around all the internal line angles of the tooth preparation may enhance retention form. Even if an amalgam bonding technique is used, mechanical retention is still recommended.

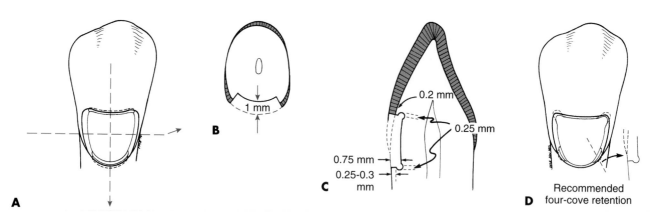

FIG. **18-32 A,** Extended Class V tooth preparation with axial wall following DEJ contour mesiodistally (**B**) and incisogingivally (**C**). Note axial wall pulpal depth of 1 mm in crown and 0.75 mm in root. In addition, note location and direction depth (0.25 mm) of retention grooves and dimension of gingival wall (0.25 mm) from root surface to retention groove. **D,** Large Class V preparation with retention coves prepared in the four axial point angles.

If access is inadequate for use of the No. ¼ bur, a 7-85-2½-6 angle former chisel may be used to prepare the retention form. In addition, a No. 33½ bur can be used. Both methods result in retention grooves that will be angular, but positioned in the same location and approximately to the same depth as when the No. ¼ bur is used. However, the rounded retention form placed with the No. ¼ bur is generally preferred, because amalgam can be condensed into rounded areas better than into sharp areas, resulting in better adaptation of the amalgam into the retention grooves. If necessary, use suitable hand instruments (e.g., chisels, margin trimmers) to plane the enamel margins, verifying soundness and 90-degree cavosurface angles.

Finally, clean the preparation using air-water spray and evacuation. Use the air syringe to remove visible moisture (do not desiccate tooth structure), and inspect the preparation for completeness. If the preparation is complete, either apply a desensitizer (for a nonbonded restoration) or begin the bonding procedures (for a bonded restoration). (See Sealer or Bonding Application, as well as Chapter 17, for specific information on amalgam bonding.)

Large Preparations That Include Line Angles. Caries on the facial (i.e., lingual) surface may extend beyond the line angles of the tooth. The maxillary molars, particularly the second molars, are most commonly affected by these extensive defects (Fig. 18-33, *A*). In this example, if the remainder of the distal surface is sound and the distal caries is accessible facially, the facial restoration should then extend around the line angle. This prevents the need for a Class II proximal restoration to restore the distal surface. Complete as much of the preparation as possible with a fissure bur. Then, using a round bur approximately the same diameter as the fissure bur, initiate the distal portion of the preparation (see Fig. 18-33, *B* and *C*). Use smaller round burs to ac-

centuate the distal portion's internal line angles. Preparing the facial portion first provides better access and visibility to the distal portion. Occasionally, hand instruments may be useful for completing the distal half of the preparation when space for the handpiece is limited (see Fig. 18-33, *D* through *F*).

Place retention grooves along the entire length of the occlusoaxial and gingivoaxial line angles to ensure retention of the restoration. Use the No. ¼ bur as previously described to prepare the retention grooves. A gingival margin trimmer or a 7-85-2½-6 angle former chisel can be used in the distal half of the preparation to provide retention form when access for the handpiece is limited (see Fig. 18-33, *G* and *H*).

Because of the proximity of the coronoid process, access to the facial surfaces of maxillary molars, particularly second molars, is often limited. Having the patient partially close and shift the mandible toward the tooth being operated will improve access and visibility (Fig. 18-34).

If the Class V outline form approaches an existing proximal restoration, it is better to extend slightly into the bulk of the proximal restoration, rather than to leave a thin section of tooth structure between the two restorations (Fig. 18-35). In this illustration, the previously placed amalgam served as the distal (i.e., mesial) wall of the preparation.

When proper treatment requires both Class II and Class V amalgam restorations on the same tooth, complete the Class II preparation and restoration before initiating the Class V. If the Class V were restored first, it may be damaged by the matrix band and wedge needed for the Class II restoration.

RESTORATIVE TECHNIQUE

Sealer or Bonding Application. The same considerations presented earlier in this chapter apply for the

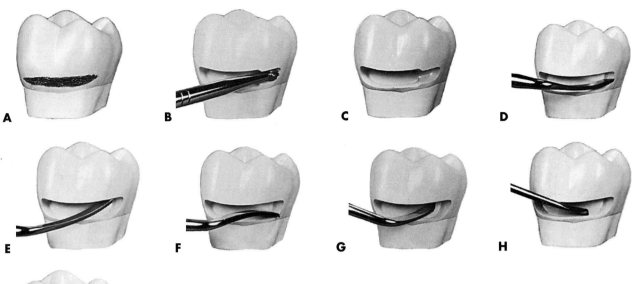

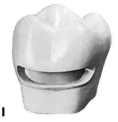

FIG. **18-33** Tooth preparation on maxillary molar. **A,** Caries extending around distofacial corner of tooth. **B** and **C,** Distal extension is accomplished with round bur. **D** through **F,** Gingival margin trimmer may be useful in completing distal half of preparation when handpiece access is limited. **G,** Gingival margin trimmer may be used to provide retention grooves. **H,** Angle former chisel may be used to prepare retention grooves in distal portion of preparation. **I,** Completed tooth preparation.

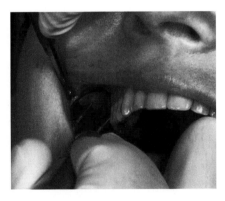

FIG. **18-34** Mandible shifted laterally for improved access and visibility.

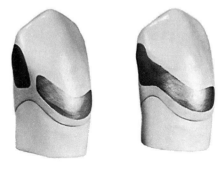

FIG. **18-35** When Class V outline form closely approaches an existing restoration, extend the preparation to remove remaining thin enamel wall, resulting in adjoining restorations.

Class V amalgam restoration. (Refer to Chapter 17 for a more complete review on the use of amalgam bonding techniques.) In vitro studies have shown that bonded Class V amalgam restorations initially exhibit significantly less leakage than varnish lined restorations. However, by 1 year there is no difference in the two groups.[1,3]

Matrix Placement. Most Class V amalgam restorations are placed without the use of any type of matrix. The most difficult condensation occurs in a tooth preparation with an axial wall that is very convex mesiodistally. Two alternative methods for insertion may be used. The preferred method is the application of a matrix that confines the amalgam in the mesial and distal portions of the preparation (Fig. 18-36). Short lengths of stainless steel matrix material, one each for the mesial and distal surfaces, are passed through the proximal contacts, carefully guided into the gingival sulcus, and wedged. The strips must be wide enough to extend occlusally through the respective proximal contacts and long enough to extend slightly past the facial (i.e., lingual) line angles. The strip usually requires compound support for stability and rigidity. It is often helpful to apply a small amount of softened compound on the tip of the wedge before wedge insertion. The strips offer resistance against condensing the mesial and distal portions, which provides support for condensing the center of the restoration. The gingival edge of the steel strip often must be trimmed to conform to the circumferential contour (level) of the base of the gingival sulcus to prevent soft-tissue damage. Rather than using two short pieces of steel strip, a longer length can be used that may be passed through one proximal contact, extended around the lingual (i.e., facial) surface, and passed through the other contact, forming a U-shaped matrix. Trimming the gingival edge to conform to the interproximal soft-tissue anatomy usually is more difficult with one matrix strip than when two strips are used.

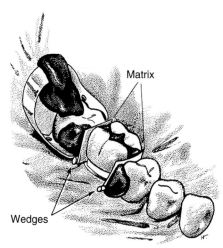

FIG. 18-36 Application of matrix to confine amalgam in mesial and distal extensions of preparation.

A conventional Tofflemire band and retainer may be used with a window cut into the band allowing access to the preparation for condensation (Fig. 18-37). Alternatively, the tooth may be prepared and restored in sections without using a matrix. Each successive section of the preparation should be extended slightly into the previously condensed portion to ensure caries removal. This procedure is time consuming but effective.

Condensation and Carving. Using the amalgam carrier, insert the mixed amalgam into the preparation in small increments (Fig. 18-38, *A*) and condense it into the retention areas first, with an appropriately sized condenser (see Fig. 18-38, *B*). Next, condense the amalgam against the mesial and distal walls of the preparation (see Fig. 18-38, *C*). Finally, provide sufficient bulk in the central portion to allow for carving the correct contour (see Fig. 18-38, *D*). As the surface of the restoration becomes more convex, condensation becomes increasingly difficult. The operator must guard against the amalgam's "land sliding" during over packing. A large condenser or plastic instrument held against the amalgam may help resist pressure applied elsewhere on the restoration (Fig. 18-39).

Carving may begin immediately after insertion of the amalgam (Fig. 18-40). All carving should be done using the side of the explorer tine or a Hollenback No. 3 carver

FIG. 18-37 Customized matrix band used to restore area of proximal root caries. **A,** Conventional Tofflemire matrix with window cut into band to allow access for condensation. **B,** Matrix in place around the tooth, allowing lingual access to preparation.

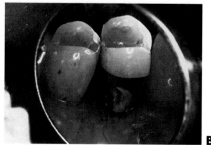

A

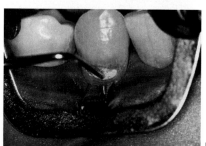

B

FIG. 18-38 Inserting amalgam. **A,** Place amalgam into preparation in small increments. **B,** Condense first into retention grooves with small condenser. **C,** Next condense against mesial and distal walls. **D,** Overfill and provide sufficient bulk to allow for carving.

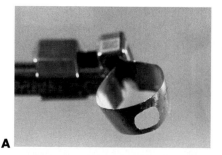

A

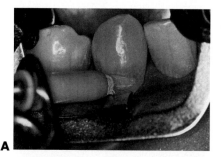

B

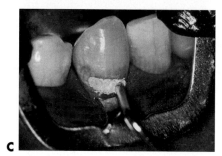

C

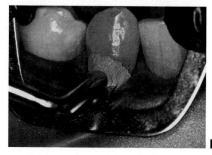

D

held parallel to the margins. In addition, the side of the carving instrument should always rest on unprepared tooth surface adjacent to the prepared cavosurface margin. This prevents overcarving. Begin the carving procedure by removing excess amalgam to expose the incisal (or occlusal) margin. Continue removing excess to expose the mesial and distal margins. Finally, carve away excess at the gingival margin. Carving the marginal areas should result in developing the desired convex contours in the completed restoration. Improper use of the carving instruments will result in a poorly contoured restoration. Note in Fig. 18-41 how carving instruments are positioned to provide the desired contours. There should be no amalgam excess at the margins, because it may either break away, creating a defect at the margin, or cause gingival irritation.

There are instances when it is appropriate to change facial contours because of altered soft-tissue levels (e.g., cervical lesions in periodontally treated patients). Facial contours may be increased (or relocated) only enough to prevent food impaction into the gingival sulcus and to provide access for the patient to clean the area. Over-

contouring must be avoided, because it will result in reduced stimulation and cleansing of the gingiva during mastication.

When a rubber dam and the No. 212 cervical retainer are used for isolation, clean the area well with an air-water syringe and explorer to remove any amalgam particles, particularly in the sulcus. Then, remove the No. 212 retainer using care to open the jaws of the retainer wide enough to prevent marring the surface of the restoration. Remove the rubber dam, and again clean the area well to ensure that no amalgam particles remain in the sulcus.

When retraction cord is used for isolation, it may interfere with carving any excess amalgam at the gingival margin. If so, carve away gross excess, carefully remove the cord, and then complete the final carving along the margin.

Finishing and Polishing. If carving procedures were performed correctly, no finishing of the restoration should be required. A slightly moistened cotton pellet held in the operative pliers may be used to further smooth the carved restoration. However, additional finishing and polishing of amalgam restorations may be necessary to correct a marginal discrepancy or improve the contour. Care is required when using stones or any rotating cutting instruments on margins positioned below the cementoenamel junction (CEJ). This is because of the possibility of removing cementum or notching the tooth structure gingival to the margin or both (Fig. 18-42). Fig. 18-43 illustrates reshaping a rubber abrasive point to allow optimal access to the gingival portion of a Class V amalgam restoration. *However, polishing restorations of high-copper amalgam is unnecessary, because high-copper amalgam is less prone to corrosion and marginal deterioration than its low-copper predecessor.* Nevertheless,

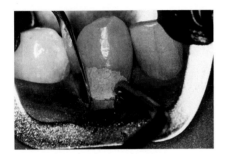

FIG. **18-39** Use large condenser or flat-bladed instrument to offer resistance to condensation pressure applied elsewhere on restoration.

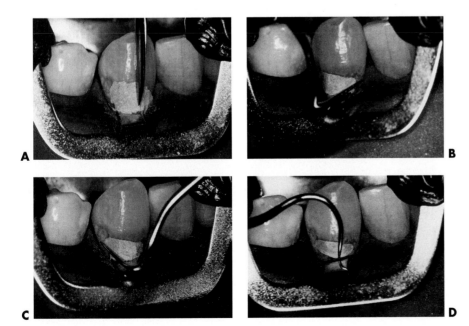

FIG. **18-40** Carving and contouring restoration. **A,** Begin carving procedure by removing excess and locating incisal margin. **B** and **C,** Explorer may be used to remove excess and locate mesial and distal margins. **D,** Finally, remove excess and locate gingival margin.

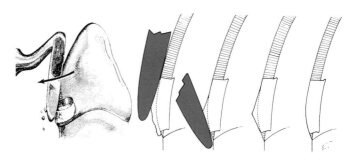

FIG. **18-41** Position of carving instrument to prevent over-carving amalgam and to develop desired gingival contours.

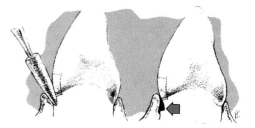

FIG. **18-42** Incorrect use of pointed stone at gingival margin results in removal of cementum or notching of tooth structure gingival to margin or both.

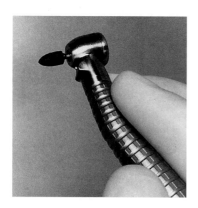
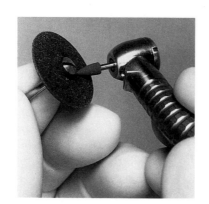
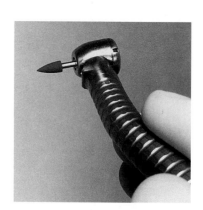

FIG. **18-43** Reshaping a rubber abrasive point against a mounted carborundum disk.

some operators prefer to polish all amalgam restorations to obtain a glossy surface. (The polishing technique is presented in Chapter 17.)

REFERENCES

1. Ben-Amar A, Liberman R, Rothkoff Z, Cardash HS: Long-term sealing properties of Amalgam bond under amalgam restorations, *Am J Dent* 7:141, 1994.
2. Berry FA et al: Microleakage of amalgam restorations using dentin-bonding system primers, *Am J Dent* 9:174, 1996.
3. Moore DS, Johnson WW, Kaplan I: A comparison of amalgam microleakage with a 4-META liner and copal varnish, *Int J Prosthodont* 8:461, 1995.
4. Setcos JC, Staninec M, Wilson NHF: Bonding of amalgam restorations: existing knowledge and future prospects, *Oper Dent* 25:121, 2000.
5. Smales RJ, Wetherell JD: Review of bonded amalgam restorations and assessment in a general practice over five years, *Oper Dent* 25:374, 2000.

19

Complex Amalgam Restorations

ALDRIDGE D. WILDER, JR.

ANDRÉ V. RITTER

THEODORE M. ROBERSON

KENNETH N. MAY, JR.*

*This author is inactive this edition. See the Acknowledgments.

INTRODUCTION

This chapter describes the use of amalgam for complex direct posterior restorations. Chapter 13 described the use of composite for complex posterior restorations. Complex posterior restorations are used to replace missing tooth structure of teeth that have fractured or are severely involved with caries or existing restorative material. These restorations usually involve the replacement of one or more missing cusps, and often, they utilize a bonding technique.

REVIEW OF PERTINENT MATERIAL QUALITIES AND PROPERTIES

The properties, advantages and limitations of amalgam are discussed in Chapters 4 and 16. Amalgam is easy to use and has a high compressive strength, excellent wear resistance, and a proven long-term clinical performance. However, it is metallic (unesthetic), requires a retentive tooth preparation, and does not seal or strengthen the tooth.

INDICATIONS

Complex posterior amalgam restorations should be considered when large amounts of tooth structure are missing, when one or more cusps need capping, and when increased resistance and retention forms are needed. They may be used as: (1) control restorations in teeth that have a questionable pulpal and/or periodontal prognosis, (2) control restorations in teeth with acute and severe caries, (3) definitive final restorations, or (4) foundations. When determining the appropriateness of a complex amalgam restoration, the factors discussed in the following sections must be considered.

Resistance and Retention Forms. In a tooth severely involved with caries or existing restorative material, any undermined enamel or weak tooth structure subject to fracture must be removed and restored. Usually, a weakened tooth is best restored with a properly designed indirect (usually cast) restoration that will prevent tooth fracture caused by mastication forces (see Chapter 20). However, in selected cases, preparations may be designed for amalgam that improve the resistance form of a tooth (Fig. 19-1).

When conventional retention features are not adequate because of insufficient remaining tooth structure, pins, slots, and amalgam bonding techniques may be used to enhance retention form. The retention features needed depend on the amount of tooth structure remaining and the tooth being restored. As more tooth structure is lost, more auxiliary retention is required. Pins, slots, and bonding also provide additional resistance form to the restoration.

Status and Prognosis of the Tooth. A tooth with severe caries that may require endodontic therapy or crown lengthening or that has an uncertain periodontal prognosis is often treated initially with a control restoration. A control restoration helps: (1) protect the pulp from the oral cavity (i.e., fluids, thermal stresses, pH changes, bacteria), (2) provide an anatomic contour against which the gingival tissue may be healthier, (3) facilitate control of caries and plaque, and (4) provide some resistance against tooth fracture (or propagation of an existing fracture). (Refer to Chapter 3 for caries control rationale and techniques.)

The status and prognosis of the tooth will determine the size, number, and placement of retention features. Larger restorations generally require more retention. However, the size, number, and location of retention features demand greater care in smaller teeth, in teeth that have been significantly excavated, and in symptomatic teeth. Carelessness can risk pulpal irritation or exposure.

Role of the Tooth in the Overall Treatment Plan. The restorative treatment choice for a tooth is influenced by its role in the overall treatment plan. Although complex amalgam restorations are used occasionally as an alternative to indirect restorations, they often are indicated for other purposes. Abutment teeth for fixed prostheses may utilize a complex restoration as a foundation. Extensive caries or previous restorations on abutment teeth for removable prostheses generally indicate a cast restoration for resistance and retention forms and for development of external surface contours for retention of the prosthesis. A tooth may be treated with a complex restoration if adequate resistance and retention forms can be provided. For periodontal and orthodontic patients, the complex restoration may be the restoration of choice until the final phase of treatment when cast restorations may be preferred.

Occlusion, Esthetics, and Economics. Complex amalgam restorations are sometimes indicated as interim restorations for teeth that require elaborate

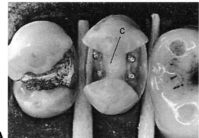
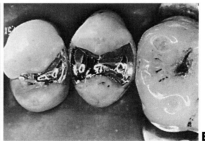

FIG. **19-1** Maxillary second premolar weakened both by extensive caries and by the small fracture line extending mesiodistally on the center of the excavated dentinal wall. **A,** Minikin pins placed in the gingival floor will improve resistance form after amalgam has been placed. Note that a calcium hydroxide liner has been placed (*c*). **B,** Restorations polished.

A   **B**

occlusal alterations ranging from vertical dimension changes to correcting occlusal plane discrepancies. When esthetics is a primary consideration, a complex amalgam restoration may not be the treatment of choice because of the display of metal. However, a more esthetic result may be obtained by inserting a composite veneer within the amalgam to mask some of the metallic appearance of the restoration (see Chapter 15).[57]

When cost of indirect restorations is a major factor for the patient, the complex direct amalgam restoration may be an appropriate treatment option, provided that adequate resistance and retention forms are included.

Age and Health of the Patient. For some geriatric and debilitated patients, the complex amalgam restoration may be the treatment of choice over the more expensive and time-consuming cast restoration.

CONTRAINDICATIONS

The complex amalgam restoration may be contraindicated if the patient has significant occlusal problems, or if the tooth cannot be properly restored with a direct restoration because of anatomic and/or functional considerations. The complex amalgam restoration also may be contraindicated if the area to be restored is esthetically important for the patient.

ADVANTAGES

Conserves Tooth Structure. The preparation for a complex amalgam restoration is usually more conservative than the preparation for an indirect restoration or a crown.

Appointment Time. The complex restoration can be completed in one appointment. The cast restoration requires at least two appointments.

Resistance and Retention Forms. Resistance and retention forms may be significantly increased by the use of pins, slots, and bonding (see Fig. 19-1).

Economics. Compared to an indirect restoration, the amalgam restoration is a relatively inexpensive restorative procedure. When cost is a factor, the complex amalgam restoration may provide the patient with the only alternative to extraction of the severely broken-down tooth. Martin and Bader[39] have published that 72% and 65% of four- and five-surface complex amalgams, respectively, are successful at 5 years compared with 84% of both gold and porcelain crowns. Smales[62] reported that 72% of amalgam restorations survived for 15 years, including those with cusp coverage.

DISADVANTAGES

Most of the disadvantages related to complex amalgam restorations refer to the use of pins used to provide retention for these restorations. However, some disadvantages apply to complex amalgam restorations in general.

Dentinal Microfractures. Preparing pinholes and placing pins may create craze lines or fractures, as well as internal stresses in the dentin.[5,66,72] Such craze lines and internal stress may have little or no clinical significance, but they may be important when minimal dentin is present.

Microleakage. In amalgam restorations using cavity varnish, microleakage around all types of pins has been demonstrated.[43] In vitro studies have demonstrated that microleakage of amalgam restorations using bonding systems is significantly reduced.[60,63] However, no clinically significant difference was found in conventional and bonded amalgams at ages ranging from 1 to 5 years.[19]

Decreased Strength of Amalgam. The tensile strength and horizontal strength of pin-retained amalgam restorations are significantly decreased.[27,73]

Resistance Form. Resistance form is more difficult to develop than when preparing a tooth for a cusp-capping onlay (skirting axial line angles of the tooth) or a full crown. The complex amalgam restoration does not protect the tooth from fracture as well as an extracoronal restoration. However, amalgam restorations with cusp coverage significantly increase the fracture resistance of weakened teeth as compared to amalgam restorations without cusp coverage.[44]

Penetration and Perforation. Pin retention increases the risk of penetrating into the pulp or perforating the external tooth surface.

Tooth Anatomy. Proper contours and occlusal contacts, and/or anatomy, are sometimes difficult to achieve with large complex restorations.

CLINICAL TECHNIQUE

In this chapter, the word *vertical* is used in lieu of the word *longitudinal* to describe tooth preparation walls and other preparation aspects that are approximately parallel to the long axis of the tooth. The word *horizontal* is used in lieu of the word *transverse* to describe the walls and other aspects that are approximately perpendicular to the long axis of the tooth.

INITIAL PROCEDURES SUMMARY

Treatment options should be discussed with the patient. Before the preparation for a complex amalgam restoration begins, an explanation of the procedure should be given to the patient. The limitations of the restoration itself and the possible complications that might occur during the procedure also should be presented. The initial procedures for each of the complex amalgam restoration types will be briefly discussed before the technique is presented. Usually, each type of complex amalgam restoration utilizes a bonding technique. If bonding is used, a precise technique and isolated operating field must be present.

Pin-Retained Amalgam Restorations. A pin-retained restoration may be defined as any restoration requiring the placement of one or more pins in the dentin to provide adequate resistance and retention

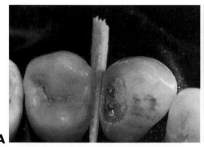
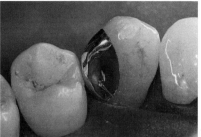

FIG. **19-2 A,** Maxillary canine with extensive loss of tooth structure using pins for additional retention form. **B,** Restoration polished.

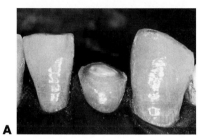
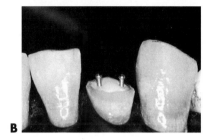
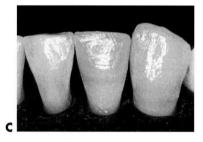

FIG. **19-3** Using light-cured composite to restore fractured mandibular lateral incisor. **A,** Cavosurface bevel prepared at 45 degrees to external enamel surface, and liner of calcium hydroxide applied. **B,** Minikin pins placed and enamel etched. **C,** Restoration completed.

forms. Pins are used whenever adequate resistance and retention forms cannot be established with slots, locks, or undercuts only. The pin-retained amalgam is an important adjunct in the restoration of teeth with extensive caries or fractures.[47] Amalgam restorations including pins have significantly greater retention than those using boxes only or those relying solely on bonding systems.[23]

Although this chapter focuses on large Class II restorations, pins have been used in other types of large restorations. The indication for pins in a Class IV restoration is rare. Because of the relatively small size of anterior teeth and the potential for enamel and dentin bonding, pins are used rarely in anterior teeth or with composite restorative materials. Occasionally, the use of pins may be considered for a large Class IV preparation on the distal surface of a canine that involves a significant amount of the distoincisal corner (Fig. 19-2), when this area is being restored with amalgam. Pins placed in the gingival portion may provide the needed retention for the restoration. However, use of a lingual dovetail as described in Chapter 18 is an alternative to pin retention, if enough lingual tooth structure is available for preparation of the dovetail.

Because of effective bonding to enamel and dentin, the need for pins in tooth preparations for direct composite restorations has virtually been eliminated. Proper use of bonding technique and selectively placed retention features usually provide adequate retention for composite restorations. The use of pins may be considered for a tooth that has insufficient enamel present for acid-etching, and/or insufficient remaining tooth structure for adequate retention features (Fig. 19-3). Ideally, such a tooth should be restored with an esthetic crown.

However, economics or time constraints may dictate the placement of a direct composite restoration. (Refer to Chapters 11, 12, and 13 for descriptions of composite restorations.)

The indication for pins in a Class V restoration is rare, if ever. Adequate retention can usually be achieved by the placement of a horizontal groove in the gingival and occlusal aspect of the preparation.

Slot-Retained Amalgam Restorations. For a complex restoration, a slot is a retention groove in dentin whose length is in a horizontal plane (Fig. 19-4). Slot retention may be used in conjunction with pin retention, or as an alternative to it. Because of the varying preparation forms of teeth requiring complex amalgam restorations, the operator should be familiar with both slot retention and pin retention.[58]

Fig. 19-5 illustrates the use of coves (placed with a No. ¼ bur) to provide additional retention form in a preparation that utilizes pins. Coves also may be used for preparations utilizing slots (see Fig. 19-4). Proximal locks, as described in Chapter 17, also are placed in the proximal box and in other locations where sufficient vertical tooth preparation permits (Figs. 19-6 and 19-7).

Some operators use slot retention and pin retention interchangeably. However, others more frequently use slot retention in preparations with vertical walls that allow retention locks to oppose one another. Pin retention is used more frequently in preparations with few or no vertical walls. Slots are particularly indicated in short clinical crowns and in cusps that have been reduced 2 to 3 mm for amalgam.[58] Compared with pin placement, more tooth structure is removed preparing slots. However, slots are less likely to create microfractures in the

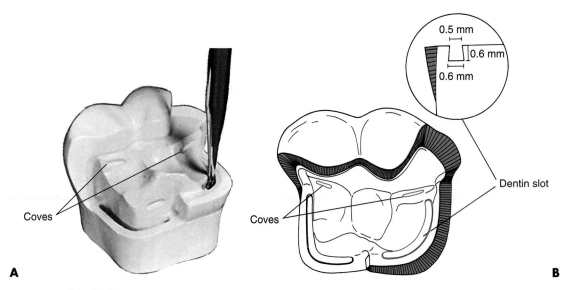

A   **B**

FIG. **19-4** Slots. **A** and **B,** With a No. 33½ bur, prepare dentinal slots approximately 0.6 mm deep and 0.5 to 1 mm inside dentinoenamel junction.

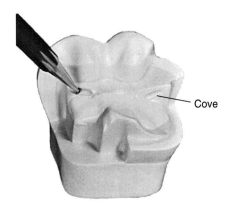

FIG. **19-5** Prepare coves in dentin with No. ¼ bur where appropriate.

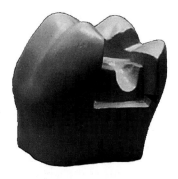

FIG. **19-6** A retention lock is a prepared groove whose length is in a vertical plane and which is in dentin.

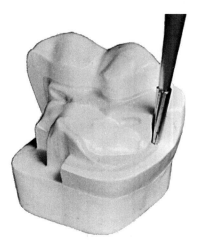

FIG. **19-7** Prepare vertical locks in dentin with a No. 169L bur where appropriate.

dentin and to perforate the tooth or penetrate into the pulp. Felton and others[22] reported that medium-sized self-threading pins elicited an inflammatory pulpal response if placed within 0.5 mm of the pulp. Slots placed in the same location did not.[22] Several authors found no significant difference in the retention provided by slots and pins in vitro [2,52,53] and in vivo.[25] In contrast, Pashley and associates[55] reported that the shear strength of pin retention was significantly stronger than slot retention.

Amalgam Foundations. A foundation is an initial restoration of a severely involved tooth. The tooth is restored so that the restorative material (amalgam, composite, or other) will serve in lieu of tooth structure to provide retention and resistance forms during the development of the subsequent final cast restoration. Thus a foundation is indicated for a tooth that is severely broken down and lacks the resistance and retention forms needed for an indirect restoration. The retention of the foundation material should not be compromised by tooth reduction during the final preparation for the indirect restoration. The foundation also should provide resistance form against forces that otherwise might fracture the remaining tooth structure.

Unlike a conventional amalgam restoration, an amalgam foundation may not depend primarily on remaining coronal tooth structure for support. Instead, it may rely mainly on secondary preparation retention features (pins, slots, coves, and proximal retention locks) and somewhat on bonding benefits. A temporary or caries control restoration may serve as a foundation, but only if the retention and resistance forms of the restoration are appropriate.

A temporary or caries control restoration is used to restore a tooth temporarily and/or to control caries in a tooth when definitive treatment is uncertain or when several teeth require immediate attention for control of caries. It also may be used when a tooth's prognosis is questionable. However, a temporary or control restoration may depend only on the remaining coronal tooth structure for support, using few auxiliary retention features. When preparing a tooth for either a foundation or temporary (control) restoration, remaining unsupported enamel may be left, except at the gingival, to aid in forming a matrix for amalgam condensation. In each case, remaining unsupported enamel is removed when the indirect restoration is placed. Occasionally, when providing a temporary or control restoration, the operator also may elect to provide sufficient retention and resistance forms to satisfy the requirements of a foundation.

As a rule, foundations are placed in preparation for a full crown, especially in endodontically treated teeth. However, not all teeth with foundations must be immediately restored with full coverage crowns. Smith and Schuman have reported that amalgam may be used as a definitive partial coverage restoration if only minimal coronal damage has occurred in endodontically treated teeth.[64] The greatest influence on fracture resistance is the amount of remaining tooth structure.[50]

The restorative materials used for foundations include amalgam, composite, and reinforced glass-ionomer cermets. Of the direct filling materials, amalgam is preferred because it is easy to use and stronger than composite or cermets. Threaded pins and slots can be used for retention in vital teeth, as described in later sections. Prefabricated posts and cast post and cores also may be used to provide additional retention for the foundation material in endodontically treated teeth receiving foundations. The use of prefabricated post and cast post and cores is limited to endodontically treated teeth, and is used generally on anterior teeth or single-canal premolars with little or no remaining coronal tooth structure. On endodontically treated molars the pulp chamber and/or canals typically provide retention for the foundation, and it is not necessary to use any form of intraradicular retention (see Tooth Preparation for Amalgam Foundations later in this chapter).

Before tooth preparation, evaluate occlusal factors, administer local anesthetic, and apply the rubber dam, if needed.

TOOTH PREPARATION

Tooth Preparation for Pin-Retained Amalgam Restorations

Initial Tooth Preparation. The general concept of the initial tooth preparation is presented in Chapter 17, and it applies for the pin-retained complex amalgam restorations described here.

When caries is extensive, reduction of one or more of the cusps for capping may be indicated (*capping cusps*). Robbins and Summit[59] and Smales[62] have documented the longevity of complex amalgam restorations involving one or more capped cusps. These authors report a survival rate of 72% after 15 years. In fact, Smales[62] did not find any difference in the survival rate of cusp-covered and non-cusp-covered amalgam restorations at 15 years, regardless of whether pins were used. When the facial or lingual extension exceeds two thirds the distance from a primary groove toward the cusp tip (or when the facial-lingual extension of the occlusal preparation exceeds two thirds the distance between the facial and lingual cusp tips), reduction of the cusp(s) for amalgam is usually required for the development of adequate resistance form (Fig. 19-8, *A*), as in preparations for cast metal restorations. Reduction should be accomplished during initial tooth preparation because it improves access and visibility for subsequent steps. If the cusp(s) to be capped is located at the correct occlusal height before preparation, depth cuts should be made on the remaining occlusal surface of each cusp to be capped, using the side of a carbide fissure bur or a suitable diamond instrument (see Fig. 19-8, *B*). The depth cuts should be 2 mm deep minimum for functional cusps and 1.5 mm deep minimum for nonfunctional cusps.[11] However, to correct an occlusal relationship, if the unreduced cusp(s) height is located less than the correct occlusal height, the depth cuts may be less. Likewise, if the unreduced cusp(s) height is located at more than the correct occlusal height, the depth cuts may be deeper. The goal is to ensure that the final restoration has restored cusps with a minimal thickness of 2 mm of amalgam for functional cusps and 1.5 mm of amalgam for nonfunctional cusps (see Fig. 19-8, *C*), while developing an appropriate occlusal relationship. Using the depth cuts as a guide, the reduction is completed to provide for a uniform reduction of tooth structure (see Fig. 19-8, *D*). The occlusal contour of the reduced cusp should be similar to the normal contour of the unreduced cusp. Any sharp internal corners of the tooth preparation formed at the junction of prepared surfaces should be rounded to reduce stress concentration in the amalgam and thus improve its resistance to fracture from occlusal forces (see Fig. 19-8, *E*). When reducing only one of two facial or lingual cusps, the cusp reduction should be extended just past the facial or lingual groove, creating a vertical wall against the adjacent unreduced cusp. Fig. 19-8, *F* and *G*, illustrate a final restoration. The procedure for capping the distolingual cusp of a maxillary first molar is illustrated in Fig. 17-70. Extending the facial or lingual wall of a proximal box to include the entire cusp is indicated only when necessary to include carious or unsupported tooth structure or existing restorative material. The typical extension of the proximal box for restoring an entire cusp is illustrated in Figs. 17-71 and 17-72, *B*.

When possible, opposing vertical walls should be formed to converge occlusally, to enhance primary retention form. Also, a facial or lingual groove may be extended arbitrarily to increase retention form. The pulpal and gingival walls should be relatively flat and perpendicular to the long axis of the tooth.

Final Tooth Preparation. After initial tooth preparation of a severely involved tooth, removal of any remaining infected carious dentin or removal of remaining old restorative material is usually necessary and is accomplished as described previously. A liner can be applied, if needed, and, if used, should not extend closer than 1 mm to a slot or a pin.

Pins placed into prepared pinholes (also referred to as pin channels) provide auxiliary resistance and retention forms. As described in Chapter 17, coves and retention locks should be prepared, when possible (Figs. 19-9, *A* and *C*, and 19-10). Coves are prepared in a horizontal plane and locks are prepared in a vertical plane. These locks and coves should be prepared before preparing pinholes and inserting pins. Cusp reduction significantly diminishes retention form by decreasing the height of the vertical walls. When additional retention is indicated, pins may be inserted in carefully positioned pinholes increasing retention. Slots may be prepared along the gingival floor, axial to the dentinoenamel

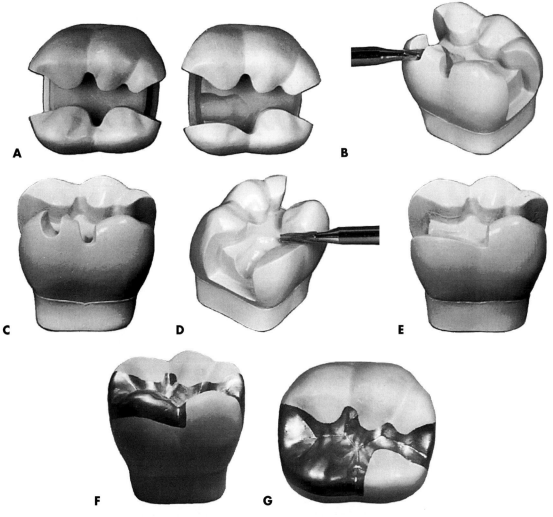

FIG. **19-8** Capping cusp with amalgam. **A,** Comparison of mesial aspects of normally extended (*left*) and extensive (*right*) mesiooocclusodistal tooth preparation. Note that the resistance form of the mesiolingual cusp of extensive preparation is compromised and indicated for capping with amalgam. **B,** Preparing depth cuts. **C,** Depth cuts prepared. **D,** Reducing cusp. **E,** Cusp reduced. **F** and **G,** Final restoration.

junction (DEJ) instead of, or in addition to, pinholes (see Fig. 19-9, *B*). Slot preparation is discussed later in this chapter.

Types of Pins. The most frequently used pin type is the small *self-threading pin*. Friction-locked and cemented pins, although still available, are rarely used (Fig. 19-11). The pin-retained amalgam restoration using self-threading pins was originally described by Going in 1966.[26] The diameter of the prepared pinhole is 0.0015 inch to 0.004 inch smaller than the diameter of the pin (Table 19-1). The threads engage the dentin as it is inserted, retaining the pin. The elasticity (resiliency) of the dentin permits insertion of a threaded pin into a hole of smaller diameter.[54] Although the threads of self-threading pins do not engage the dentin for their entire width, the self-threading pin is the most retentive of the

three types of pins (Fig. 19-12),[56] being three to six times more retentive than the cemented pin.[42,70] Vertical and horizontal stresses can be generated in the dentin when a self-threading pin is inserted. However, craze lines in the dentin are related to the size of the pin. Dilts et al[15] have reported that insertion of 0.031-inch self-threading pins produces more dentinal craze lines than insertion of either 0.021-inch self-threading pins or 0.022-inch friction-lock pins. However, Pameijer and Stallard[54] have shown that self-threading pins do not create dentinal crazing and that the crazing demonstrated in other studies may be caused by the technique used for preparation of the specimen. Pulpal stress is maximal when the self-threading pin is inserted perpendicular to the pulp.[68] The depth of the pinhole varies from 1.3 to 2 mm, depending on the diameter of the pin used.[16] However, a general guideline for pinhole depth is 2 mm. Several styles of self-threading pins also are available. Because of its: (1) versatility, (2) wide range of pin sizes, (3) color-coding system, (4) greater retentiveness,[21,30] and (5) gold-plated surface finish, which may eliminate the possibility of corrosion, the Thread Mate System (TMS) (Coltene/Whaledent Inc., Mahwah, New Jersey) is the most widely used self-threading pin.

In 1958 Markley[38] described a technique for restoring teeth with amalgam and *cemented pins* using threaded (or serrated) stainless steel pins. They are cemented into pinholes prepared 0.001 to 0.002 inch (0.025 to 0.05 mm) larger than the diameter of the pin. The cementing medium may be any standard dental luting agent.

In 1966, Goldstein[28] described a technique for the *friction-locked pin* in which the diameter of the prepared

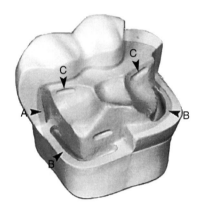

FIG. **19-9** Locks *(A)*, slots *(B)*, and coves *(C)*.

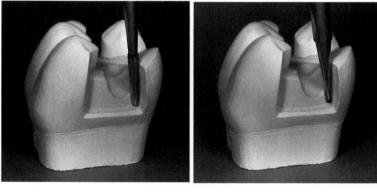

A　　　　　　　　　　　　　　　　　　　　　　　　**B**

FIG. **19-10** Placement of retention locks. **A,** Position of No. 169L bur to prepare retention lock. **B,** Lock prepared with No. ¼ bur.

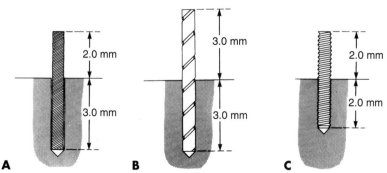

A　　　　　　**B**　　　　　　**C**

FIG. **19-11** Three types of pins. **A,** Cemented. **B,** Friction-locked. **C,** Self-threading.

pinhole is 0.001 inch (0.025 mm) smaller than the diameter of the pin. The pins are tapped into place, retained by the resiliency of the dentin, and are 2 to 3 times more retentive than cemented pins.[42]

Factors Affecting the Retention of the Pin in Dentin and Amalgam

Type. In the order of retentiveness in the dentin, the self-threading pin is the most retentive,[42] the friction-locked pin is intermediate, and the cemented pin is the least retentive.

Surface characteristics. The number and depth of the elevations (serrations or threads) on the pin influence retention of the pin in the amalgam restoration. The shape of the self-threading pin gives it the greatest retention value.

Orientation, number, and diameter. Placing pins in a nonparallel manner increases their retention. Bending pins to improve retention in amalgam is not desirable because bends may interfere with adequate condensation of amalgam around the pin and thereby decrease amalgam retention. Bending also may weaken the pin and risk fracturing the dentin. Pins should be bent only to provide for an adequate amount of amalgam (approximately 1 mm) between the pin and the external surface of the finished restoration (both on the tip of the pin and on its lateral surface). Only the specific bending tool should be used to bend a pin, not other hand instruments.

In general, increasing the number of pins increases the retention in dentin and amalgam. However, the benefits of increasing the number of pins must be compared to the potential problems created. As the number of pins increases: (1) the crazing of the dentin and the potential for fracture increase, (2) the amount of available dentin between the pins decreases,[34] and (3) the strength of the amalgam restoration decreases.[74]

Also generally, as the diameter of the pin increases, the retention in dentin and amalgam increases. However, as the number, depth, and diameter of pins increase, the danger of perforating into the pulp or the external tooth surface increases. A large number of long pins also can severely compromise condensation of the amalgam and the amalgam's adaptation to the pins. A pin technique should be used that permits optimal retention with minimal danger to the remaining tooth structure.[11]

Horizontal pins can be used for cross-splinting to provide effective reinforcement of weak remaining cusps.[7,36,45] However, horizontal pins are not generally recommended because of limited access for pin placement and for condensation once pins are placed.

Extension into dentin and amalgam. For self-threading pins, retention is not increased significantly when the depth of the pin into dentin exceeds 2 mm. A laboratory study demonstrated that a 0.024-inch (0.61 mm) self-threading pin fractures when removal from an embedment greater than 2 mm is attempted, while removal of the 0.031-inch (0.78 mm) self-threading

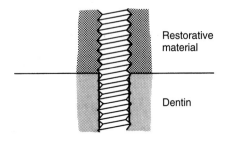

Restorative material

Dentin

FIG. 19-12 Complete width of threads of self-threading pins does not engage dentin.

TABLE 19-1 TMS Pins

NAME	ILLUSTRATION (NOT TO SCALE)	COLOR CODE	PIN DIAMETER (IN/MM)	DRILL DIAMETER (IN/MM)	TOTAL PIN LENGTH (MM)	PIN LENGTH EXTENDING FROM DENTIN (MM)
Regular (standard)		Gold	0.031/0.78	0.027/0.68	7.1	5.1
Regular (self-shearing)		Gold	0.031/0.78	0.027/0.68	8.2	3.2
Regular (two-in-one)		Gold	0.031/0.78	0.027/0.68	9.5	2.8
Minim (standard)		Silver	0.024/0.61	0.021/0.53	6.7	4.7
Minim (two-in-one)		Silver	0.024/0.61	0.021/0.53	9.5	2.8
Minikin (self-shearing)		Red	0.019/0.48	0.017/0.43	7.1	1.5
Minuta (self-shearing)		Pink	0.015/0.38	0.0135/0.34	6.2	1.0

1 mm = 0.03937 in.

pin results in fracture of the dentin.[42] Likewise, when the length of a 0.024-inch (0.61 mm) self-threading pin extends into the amalgam more than 2 mm and removal is attempted, the pin fractures. Removal of a 0.031-inch (0.78 mm) self-threading pin extending more than 2 mm into the amalgam results in fracture of the amalgam.[42] *Therefore pin extension into dentin and amalgam greater than 2 mm is unnecessary for pin retention and is contraindicated to preserve the strength of the dentin and the amalgam.*

Pin Placement Factors and Techniques

Pin size. Four sizes of pins are available (Fig. 19-13), each with a corresponding color-coded drill (see Table 19-1). Familiarity with drill sizes and their corresponding color is necessary to ensure the proper size pinhole is prepared for the desired pin. It is difficult to specify a particular size of pin that is always appropriate for a particular tooth. Two determining factors for selecting the appropriate size pin are the amount of dentin available to safely receive the pin and the amount of retention desired. In the Thread Mate System, the pins of choice for severely involved posterior teeth are the Minikin (0.019 inch [0.48 mm]) and, occasionally, the Minim (0.024 inch [0.61 mm]). The Minikin pins usually are selected to reduce the risk of dentin crazing, pulpal penetration, and potential perforation. The Minim pins usually are used as a backup in cases where the pinhole for the Minikin was overprepared or the pin threads stripped the dentin during placement and the Minikin pin lacks retention. Dilts et al reported that the larger diameter pins have the greatest retention.[13] Other studies showed that the Minuta pin is approximately half as retentive as the Minim and one third as retentive as the Minim pin.[21,30] Either the Minikin or Minim pins can be used in a given tooth, depending on the dentin available in the area where the pins are to be inserted. The Minuta (0.015 inch [0.38 mm]) pin is usually too small to provide adequate retention in posterior teeth. The Regular (0.031 inch [0.78 mm]) or largest diameter pin is rarely used because a significant amount of stress and crazing, or cracking, in the tooth (dentin and enamel) may be created during its insertion.[15,18] Of the four pin sizes, the Regular pin caused the highest incidence of dentinal cracking that communicated with the pulp chamber.[72]

Number of pins. Several factors must be considered when deciding how many pins are required: (1) the amount of missing tooth structure, (2) the amount of dentin available to receive pins safely, (3) the amount of retention required, and (4) the size of the pins. *As a rule, one pin per missing axial line angle should be used.* Certain factors may cause the operator to alter this rule. The fewest pins possible should be used to achieve the desired retention for a given restoration. When only 2 to 3 mm of the occlusogingival height of a cusp has been removed, no pin is required because enough tooth structure remains to use conventional retention features (Fig. 19-14; see also Fig. 19-8).

Remember that while the retention of the restoration increases as the number of pins increases, an excessive number of pins can fracture the tooth and significantly weaken the amalgam restoration.

Location. Several factors aid in determining pinhole locations: (1) knowledge of normal pulp anatomy and external tooth contours, (2) a current radiograph of the tooth, (3) a periodontal probe, and (4) the patient's age. Although the radiograph is only a two-dimensional picture of the tooth, it can give an indication of the position

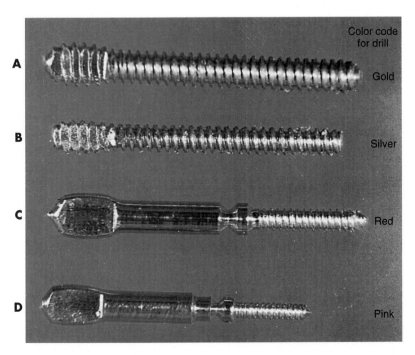

FIG. **19-13** Four sizes of TMS pins. **A,** Regular (0.031 inch [0.78 mm]). **B,** Minim (0.024 inch [0.61 mm]). **C,** Minikin (0.019 inch [0.48 mm]). **D,** Minuta (0.015 inch [0.38 mm]).

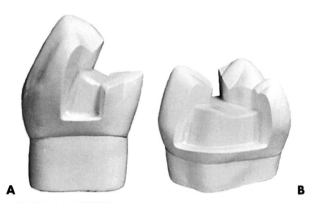

A   **B**

FIG. **19-14** Examples illustrating reduction of cusps without need for pin or pins. **A,** Mandibular first premolar with lingual cusp reduced for capping. **B,** Maxillary second molar prepared for restoration of mesial and distal surfaces and distofacial cusp.

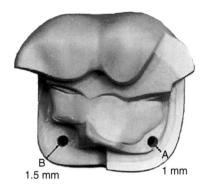

B   **A**
1.5 mm   1 mm

FIG. **19-15** Pinhole position. *A,* Position relative to DEJ. *B,* Position relative to external tooth surface.

of the pulp chamber, and the contour of the mesial and distal surfaces of the tooth. Consideration also must be given to the placement of pins in areas where the greatest bulk of amalgam will occur to minimize the weakening effect of the pins to tooth structure.[46] Areas of occlusal contacts on the restoration must be anticipated because a pin oriented vertically and positioned directly below an occlusal load weakens the amalgam significantly.[10] Occlusal clearance should be sufficient to provide 2 mm of amalgam over the pin.[14,17]

Several attempts have been made to identify the ideal location of the pinhole. Caputo and Standlee[8] state that, ideally, pinholes should be located halfway between the pulp and the DEJ or external surface of the tooth root. Standlee and others[66] have shown that there should be at least 1 mm of sound dentin around the circumference of the pinhole. Such location ensures the proper stress distribution of occlusal forces. Felton and associates[22] have demonstrated that pin placement providing at least 1 mm of remaining dentin thickness from the pulp elicits minimal pulpal inflammatory response.[22] Dilts and associates[15] have reported that pinholes should be placed at 0.5 mm inside the DEJ.

Because it is difficult to comply exactly with these conditions, the following philosophy may be more practical. *In the cervical one third of molars and premolars (where most pins are located), pinholes should be located near the line angles of the tooth, except as described later.*[11,29] *The pinhole should be positioned no closer than 0.5 to 1 mm to the DEJ or no closer than 1 to 1.5 mm to the external surface of the tooth, whichever distance is greater* (Fig. 19-15). Before the final decision is made about the location of the pinhole, the operator should carefully probe the gingival crevice to determine if any abnormal contours exist that would predispose the tooth to an external perforation. *As a rule, the pinhole should be parallel to the adjacent external surface of the tooth.*

The position of a pinhole must not result in the pin being so close to a vertical wall of tooth structure that condensation of amalgam against the pin or wall is jeopardized (Fig. 19-16, *A*). Therefore it may be necessary to prepare first a recess in the vertical wall with the No. 245 bur to permit proper pinhole preparation, as well as to provide a minimum of 0.5 mm clearance around the circumference of the pin for adequate condensation of amalgam (see Fig. 19-16, *B* and *C*).[71] If necessary, after a pin is inappropriately placed, the operator should provide clearance around the pin to provide sufficient space for the smallest condenser nib to ensure that amalgam can be condensed adequately around the pin. A No. 169L bur can be used, being careful not to damage, or weaken, the pin.

Pinholes should be prepared on a flat surface that is perpendicular to the proposed direction of the pinhole. Otherwise, the drill tip may slip or "crawl," and a depth-limiting drill (discussed later) cannot prepare the hole as deeply as intended (Fig. 19-17).

Whenever three or more pinholes are placed, they should be located at different vertical levels on the tooth, if possible. This will reduce stresses resulting from pin placement in the same horizontal plane of the tooth.

Spacing between pins, or the *interpin distance,* must be considered when two or more pinholes are prepared. The optimal interpin distance depends on the size of pin to be used. The minimal interpin distance is 3 mm for the Minikin (0.019 inch [0.48 mm]) pin and 5 mm for the Minim (0.024 inch [0.61 mm]) pin.[34] Maximal interpin distance results in lower levels of stress in dentin.[9]

Several posterior teeth have anatomic features that may preclude safe pinhole placement. Fluted and furcal areas should be avoided.[71] Specifically, external perforation may result from pinhole placement (1) over the prominent mesial concavity of the maxillary first premolar; (2) at the midlingual and midfacial bifurcations of the mandibular first and second molars; and (3) at the midfacial, midmesial, and middistal furcations of the maxillary first and second molars. Pulpal penetration may result from pin placement at the mesiofacial corner of the maxillary first molar and the mandibular first molar.

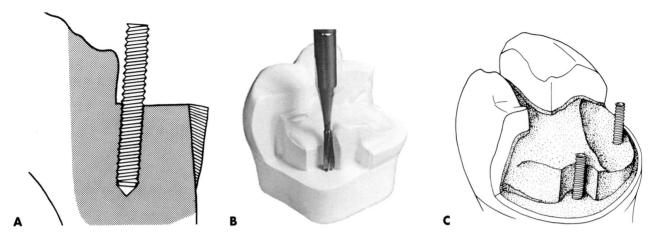

FIG. **19-16 A,** Pin placed too close to vertical wall such that adequate condensation of amalgam is jeopardized, **B** and **C,** Prepare recessed area in vertical wall of mandibular molar with No. 245 bur to provide adequate space for amalgam condensation around pin.

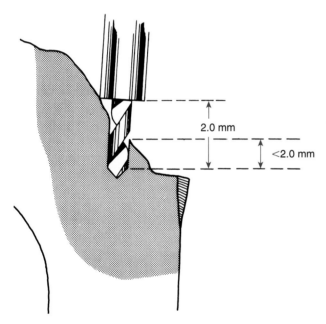

2.0 mm

<2.0 mm

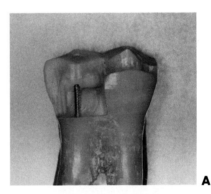

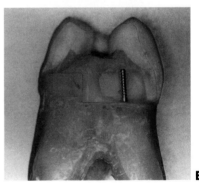

FIG. **19-17** Use of a depth-limiting drill to prepare a pinhole in surface that is not perpendicular to direction of pinhole will result in a pinhole of inadequate depth.

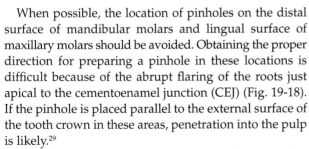

FIG. **19-18** Note distal flaring of mandibular molar (**A**) and palatal root flaring of maxillary molar (**B**). Root angulation should be considered before pinhole placement.

When possible, the location of pinholes on the distal surface of mandibular molars and lingual surface of maxillary molars should be avoided. Obtaining the proper direction for preparing a pinhole in these locations is difficult because of the abrupt flaring of the roots just apical to the cementoenamel junction (CEJ) (Fig. 19-18). If the pinhole is placed parallel to the external surface of the tooth crown in these areas, penetration into the pulp is likely.[29]

When the pinhole locations have been determined, a No. ¼ bur is first used to prepare a pilot hole (dimple) approximately one half the diameter of the bur at each location (Fig. 19-19). The purpose of this hole is to permit more accurate placement of the twist drill and to

prevent the drill from "crawling" once it has begun to rotate.

Pinhole preparation. The Kodex drill (a twist drill) should be used for preparing pinholes (Fig. 19-20). The drill is made of a high-speed tool steel that is swaged into an aluminum shank. The aluminum shank, which acts as a heat absorber, is color coded so that it can be easily matched with the appropriate pin size (Table 19-2; see also Table 19-1). The drill shanks for the Minuta and Minikin pins are tapered to provide a built-in "wobble"

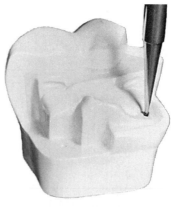

FIG. **19-19** Prepare pilot hole (dimple) with No. ¼ bur.

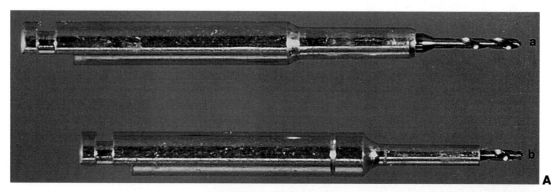

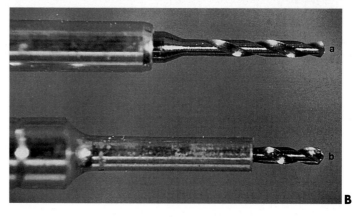

FIG. **19-20 A,** Two types of Kodex twist drills: standard (*a*) and depth-limiting (*b*). **B,** Drills enlarged: standard (*a*) and depth-limiting (*b*).

when placed in a latch-type contra-angle handpiece. This wobble allows the drill to be "free floating" and thus to align itself as the pinhole is prepared to minimize dentinal crazing or breakage of the small drills.

Because the optimal depth of the pinhole into the dentin is 2 mm (only 1.5 mm for the Minikin pin), a depth-limiting drill should be used to prepare the hole (see Fig. 19-20). Only when this type of drill prepares a hole on a flat surface that is perpendicular to the drill will it prepare the pinhole to the correct depth (see Fig. 19-17). When the location for starting a pinhole is neither flat nor perpendicular to the desired pinhole direction, either flatten the location area or use the standard twist drill (see Fig. 19-20), whose blades are 4 to 5 mm in length, to prepare a pinhole that has an effective depth. To minimize guessing when using the standard twist drill, the Omni-Depth gauge can be used to measure accurately the pinhole depth (Fig. 19-21).

With the drill in the latch-type contra-angle handpiece, place the drill in the gingival crevice beside the location for the pinhole, position it until it lies flat against the external surface of the tooth, and then, without changing the angulation obtained from the crevice position, move the handpiece occlusally and place the drill in the previously prepared pilot hole (Fig. 19-22, *A*). Now, view the drill from a 90-degree angle to the previous viewing position to ascertain that the drill is also correctly angled in this plane (see Fig. 19-22, *B*). Incorrect angulation of the drill may result in pulpal exposure or external perforation. Should the proximity of an adjacent tooth interfere with placement of the drill into the gingival crevice, place a flat, thin-bladed hand instrument into the crevice and against the external surface of the tooth to indicate the proper angulation for the drill.[12] *With the drill tip in its proper position and with the handpiece rotating at very low speed (300 to 500*

TABLE 19-2 TMS Link Series and Link Plus Pins

NAME	ILLUSTRATION (NOT TO SCALE)	COLOR CODE	PIN DIAMETER (IN/MM)*	DRILL DIAMETER (IN/MM)*	PIN LENGTH EXTENDING FROM SLEEVE (MM)	PIN LENGTH EXTENDING FROM DENTIN (MM)
LINK SERIES						
Regular (single shear)		Gold	0.031/0.78	0.027/0.68	5.5	3.2
Regular (double shear)		Gold	0.031/0.78	0.027/0.68	7.8	2.6
Minim (single shear)		Silver	0.024/0.61	0.021/0.53	5.4	3.2
Minim (double shear)		Silver	0.024/0.61	0.021/0.53	7.6	2.6
Minikin (single shear)		Red	0.019/0.48	0.017/0.43	6.9	1.5
Minuta (single shear)		Pink	0.015/0.38	0.0135/0.34	6.3	1.0
LINK PLUS						
Minim (double shear)		Silver	0.024/0.61	0.021/0.53	10.8	2.7

1 mm = 0.03937 in.

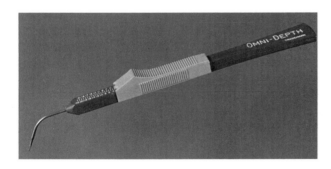

FIG. 19-21 Omni-Depth gauge is used to measure depth of pinhole(s).

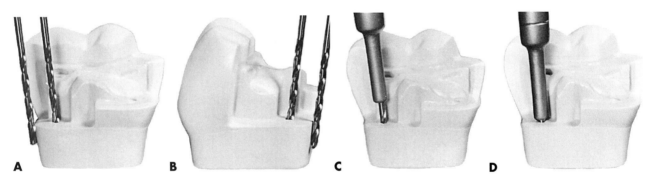

FIG. 19-22 Determining angulation for twist drill. **A,** Place drill in gingival crevice, and position it flat against tooth. Move it occlusally into position without changing angulation obtained. **B,** Repeat **A** while viewing drill from position 90 degrees left or right of that viewed in **A**. **C** and **D,** With twist drill at correct angulation, prepare pinhole in one or two thrusts until depth-limiting portion of drill is reached.

rpm), apply pressure to the drill, and prepare the pinhole in one or two movements until the depth-limiting portion of the drill is reached, and remove the drill from the pinhole (see Fig. 19-22, C and D). Using more than one or two movements, tilting the handpiece during the drilling procedure, or allowing the drill to rotate more than very briefly at the bottom of the pinhole will result in a pinhole that is too large. Although not usually recommended, a steady stream of air may be applied to the drill to dissipate heat. The drill should never stop rotating (from insertion to removal from the pinhole) to prevent the drill from breaking while in the pinhole.

Dull drills used to prepare pinholes can cause increased frictional heat and cracks in the dentin. Standlee et al have demonstrated that a twist drill becomes too dull for use after cutting 20 pinholes or less, and the signal for discarding the drill is the need for increased pressure on the handpiece.[67] Using a drill whose self-limiting shank shoulder has become rounded is contraindicated (Fig. 19-23). A worn and rounded shoulder may not properly limit pinhole depth and permit pins to be placed too deeply.

Certain clinical locations require extra care in determining pinhole angulation. The distal of mandibular molars and the lingual of maxillary molars have been mentioned previously as areas of potential problems because of the abrupt flaring of the roots just apical to the CEJ (see Fig. 19-18). Mandibular posterior teeth (with their lingual crown tilt), teeth that are rotated in the arch, and teeth that are abnormally tilted in the arch deserve careful attention before and during pinhole placement. For mandibular second molars that are severely tilted mesially, care must be exercised to orient properly the drill to prevent external perforation on the mesial surface and pulpal penetration on the distal surface

(Fig. 19-24). Because of limited interarch space, it is sometimes difficult to orient correctly the twist drill when placing pinholes at the distofacial or distolingual line angles of mandibular second and third molars (Fig. 19-25).

Pin design. For each of the four sizes of pins, several designs are available: standard, self-shearing, two-in-one, Link Series, and Link Plus (Fig. 19-26). The Link Series and Link Plus pins are recommended. TMS pins are available in titanium or stainless steel plated with gold.

The Link Series pin is contained in a color-coded plastic sleeve that fits a latch-type contra-angle handpiece or the specially designed plastic hand wrench (see Fig. 19-30, *D*). The pin is somewhat free floating in the plastic sleeve to allow it to align itself as it is threaded into the pinhole (Fig. 19-27). When the pin reaches the bottom of the hole, the top portion of the pin shears off, leaving a length of pin extending from the dentin. The plastic sleeve is then discarded. The Minuta, Minikin, Minim, and Regular pins are available in the Link Series. The Link Series pins are recommended because of their versatility, self-aligning ability, and retentiveness.[21]

The Link Plus pins are self-shearing and are available as a single or two-in-one pin contained in a color-coded plastic sleeve (Fig. 19-28). This design has a sharper thread, a shoulder stop at 2 mm, and a tapered tip to more readily fit the bottom of the pinhole as prepared by the twist drill. It also provides a 2.7-mm length of pin to extend out of the dentin, which usually needs to be shortened. Theoretically, and as suggested by Standlee et al[65] these innovations should reduce the stress created in the surrounding dentin as the pin is inserted and reduce the apical stress at the bottom of the pinhole. Kelsey et al have demonstrated for the two-in-one Link Plus pin that both the first and second pins seat completely into the pinhole before shearing.[33]

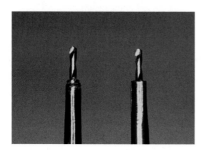

FIG. **19-23** Minikin self-limiting drill with worn shank shoulder (*left*) compared to a new drill with an unworn shoulder (*right*).

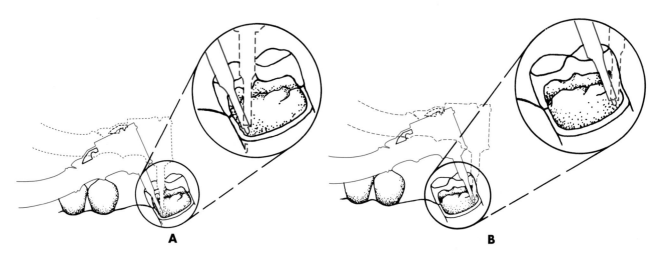

A   **B**

FIG. **19-24** Care must be exercised when preparing pinholes in mesially tilted molars to prevent external perforation on mesial surface (**A**) and pulpal penetration on the distal surface (**B**). Broken line is incorrect angulation of twist drill.

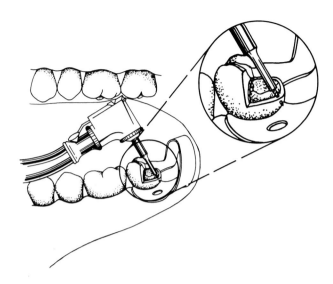

FIG. **19-25** When limited interarch space exists, care must be exercised when placing pinholes in molars to prevent external perforation on distal surface.

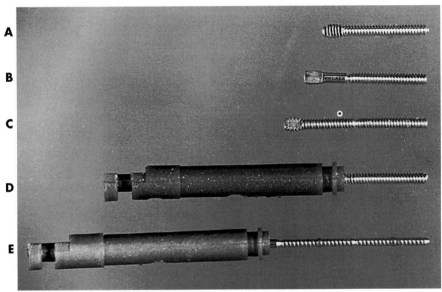

FIG. **19-26** Five designs of TMS pins. **A,** Standard. **B,** Self-shearing. **C,** Two-in-one. **D,** Link Series. **E,** Link Plus.

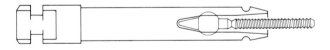

FIG. **19-27** Cross-sectional view of Link Series pin.

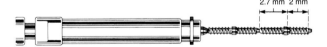

FIG. **19-28** Link Plus pin.

The standard pin is approximately 7 mm long with a flattened head to engage the hand wrench or the appropriate handpiece chuck, and is threaded to place until it reaches the bottom of the pinhole as judged by tactile sense. One advantage of the standard design pin is that it can be reversed one-quarter to one-half turn following insertion to full depth to reduce stress created at the apical end of the pinhole (Fig. 19-29).[31]

The self-shearing pin has a total length that varies according to the diameter of the pin (see Table 19-1). It also consists of a flattened head to engage the hand wrench

or the appropriate handpiece chuck for threading into the pinhole. When the pin approaches the bottom of the pinhole, the head of the pin shears off, leaving a length of pin extending from the dentin.

The two-in-one pin is actually two pins in one, with each one being shorter than the standard pin. The two-in-one pin is approximately 9.5 mm in length and also has a flattened head to aid in its insertion. When the pin reaches the bottom of the pinhole, it shears approximately in half, leaving a length of pin extending from the dentin with the other half remaining in the hand

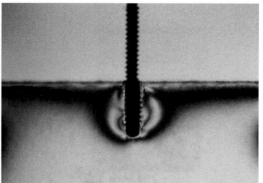

FIG. **19-29** Stress created by self-threading pin as illustrated in a photoelastic study. **A,** Pin fully seated in pinhole. **B,** Pin reversed one-quarter turn. *(Courtesy of Dr. Alan W. Irvin.)*

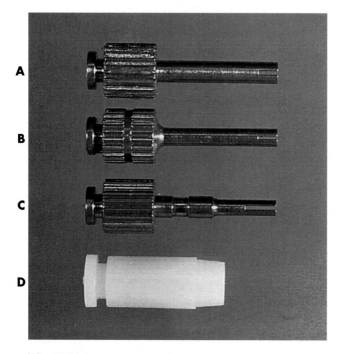

FIG. **19-30** Hand wrenches for TMS pins. **A,** Regular and Minikin. **B,** Minim. **C,** Minuta. **D,** Link Series and Link Plus.

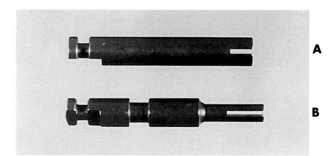

FIG. **19-31** Handpiece chucks for (**A**) TMS regular self-shearing and Minikin pins, and (**B**) TMS Minuta pins.

wrench or the handpiece chuck. This second pin may then be positioned in another pinhole and threaded to place in the same manner as the standard pin. The designs available with each size of pin are shown in Tables 19-1 and 19-2.

All of the pin designs can be inserted with an appropriate hand wrench (Fig. 19-30). A conventional latch-type contra-angle handpiece with the appropriate chuck (Fig. 19-31) also can be used to insert any of the pins except the standard design. A 10:1 reduction gear contra-angle handpiece also is available to insert the pins. It may aid the pin-insertion technique discussed later.

Selection of a particular pin design (see Tables 19-1 and 19-2) is influenced by the size of the pin being used, the amount of interarch space available, and operator preference. The Minuta and Minikin pins are available

only in the self-shearing and Link (also self-shearing) design. With minimal interarch space, the two-in-one design is undesirable because of its length. Studies have shown that the two-in-one pin and the self-shearing pin may sometimes fail to reach the bottom of the pinhole.[3,4,24] However, a study by May and Heymann[40] found that 93% of Link Series and Link Plus two-in-one pins extended to the optimal depth of 2 mm. Eames and Solly[21] demonstrated no significant difference between the retention of the self-shearing pin and the standard design pin. However, Newitter and Schlissel[49] have shown that more force is required to dislodge the standard design pin than the self-shearing pin.

Pin insertion. Two instruments for insertion of threaded pins are available: conventional latch-type contra-angle handpiece (Fig. 19-32), and TMS hand wrenches (see Fig. 19-30). Studies conflict as to which method of pin insertion produces the best results. The latch-type handpiece is recommended for the insertion of the Link Series and the Link Plus pins. The hand wrench is recommended for the insertion of standard pins.

When using the latch-type handpiece, insert a Link Series or a Link Plus pin into the handpiece and place the pin in the pinhole. Activate the handpiece at low speed until the plastic sleeve shears from the pin. Then, remove the sleeve and discard it. For low-speed handpieces with a low gear, the low gear should be used. Using low gear increases the torque and increases the tac-

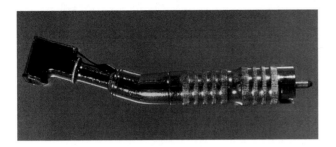

FIG. **19-32** Conventional latch-type contra-angle handpiece.

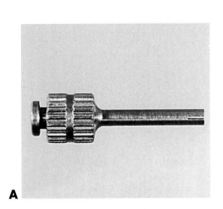
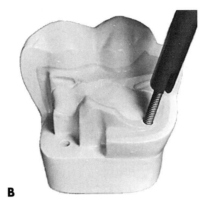
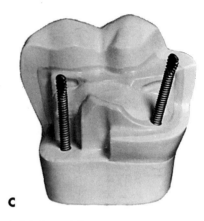

FIG. **19-33** **A,** Use of hand wrench to place pin. **B,** Thread pin to bottom of pinhole, and then reverse wrench one-quarter to one-half turn. **C,** Evaluate length of pin extending from dentin.

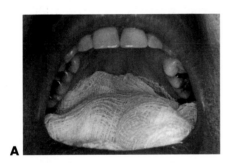
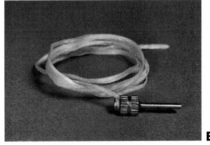

FIG. **19-34** Precautions must be taken if rubber dam is not used. **A,** Gauze throat shield. **B,** Hand wrench with 12 to 15 inches (30 to 38 cm) of dental tape attached.

tile sense of the operator. It also reduces the risk of stripping the threads in the dentin once the pin is in place.

A standard design pin is placed in the appropriate wrench (Fig. 19-33, A) and slowly threaded clockwise into the pinhole until a definite resistance is felt when the pin reaches the bottom of the hole (see Fig. 19-33, B). The pin should then be rotated one-quarter to one-half turn counterclockwise to reduce the dentinal stress created by the end of the pin pressing the dentin.[31] Carefully remove the hand wrench from the pin.

If the hand wrench is used without rubber dam isolation, a gauze throat shield must be in place, and a strand of dental tape approximately 12 to 15 inches (30 to 38 cm) in length should be securely tied to the end of the wrench (Fig. 19-34). These precautions will prevent the patient from swallowing or aspirating the hand wrench should it be dropped accidentally.

Once the pins are placed, evaluate their length (see Fig. 19-33, C). Any length of pin greater than 2 mm should be removed. As described before, 2 mm of pin length into amalgam is optimal. Also, whenever possible, it is desirable to have at least 2 mm thickness of amalgam occlusal to the end of the pin to prevent unnecessary weakening of the restoration. To remove the excess length of pin, use a sharp No. ¼, ½, or 169L bur at high speed and oriented perpendicular to the pin (Fig. 19-35, A). If oriented otherwise, the rotation of the bur may loosen the pin by rotating it counterclockwise. During removal of excess pin length, the assistant may apply a steady stream of air to the pin and have the evacuator tip positioned to remove the pin segment. Also during removal, the pin may be stabilized with a small hemostat or cotton pliers. After placement, the pin should be tight, immobile, and not easily withdrawn.

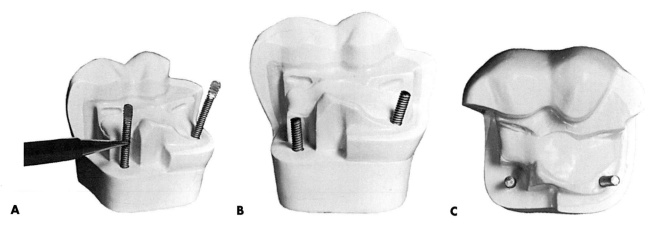

FIG. **19-35 A,** Use sharp No. ¼ bur held perpendicular to pin to shorten pin. **B** and **C,** Evaluate preparation to determine need for bending pins.

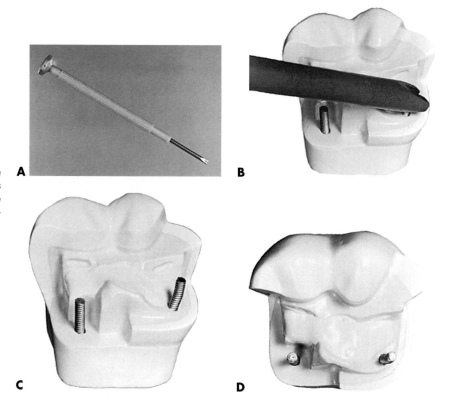

FIG. **19-36 A,** TMS bending tool. **B,** Use bending tool to bend pin. **C** and **D,** Pin is bent to position that provides adequate bulk of amalgam between pin and external surface of final restoration.

Using a mirror, view the preparation from all directions (particularly from the occlusal) to determine if any pins need to be bent to position them within the anticipated contour of the final restoration and to provide adequate bulk of amalgam between the pin and the external surface of the final restoration (see Fig. 19-35, B and C). Pins are not to be bent to make them parallel or to increase their retentiveness. However, occasionally, bending a pin may be necessary to allow for condensation of amalgam occlusogingivally. When pins require bending, the TMS bending tool (Fig. 19-36, A) must be used. The bending tool should be placed on the pin where the pin is to be bent, and with firm controlled

pressure, the bending tool should be rotated until the desired amount of bend is achieved (see Fig. 19-36, B through D). Use of the bending tool allows placement of the fulcrum at some point along the length of the exposed pin. A hand instrument such as an amalgam condenser or Black spoon excavator should not be used to bend a pin because the location of the fulcrum will be at the orifice of the pinhole. These hand instruments may cause crazing or fracture of the dentin, and the abrupt or sharp bend that usually results, increases the chance of breaking the pin (Fig. 19-37). Also, the operator has less control when pressure is applied with a hand instrument, and the chance of slipping is increased.

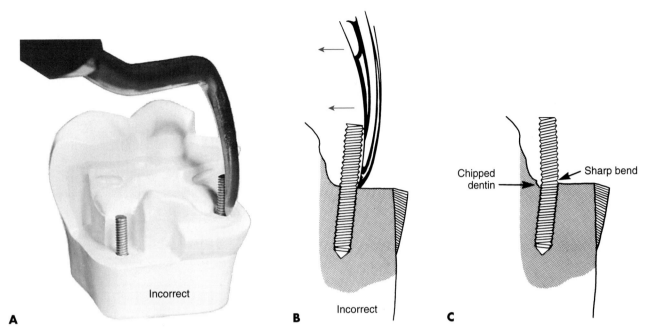

FIG. **19-37 A,** Do not use Black spoon excavator or other hand instrument to bend pin. **B** and **C,** Use of hand instruments may create sharp bend in pin and fracture dentin.

Cemented pins. Pinholes for cemented pins are prepared to a depth of 3 to 4 mm in dentin using a twist drill with a diameter of 0.027 inch (0.68 mm) or 0.021 inch (0.53 mm) (Fig. 19-38, *A*). Threaded stainless steel wire with a diameter of 0.025 inch (0.64 mm) is used for the 0.027-inch pinhole and 0.020-inch (0.51 mm) wire for the 0.021-inch pinhole (see Fig. 19-38, *B* through *F*). The pins are cemented into place with any suitable dental luting agent using a Lentulo spiral instrument (see Fig. 19-38, *G* and *H*).

Possible Problems With Pins

Failure of pin-retained restorations. The failure of pin-retained restorations might occur at any of five different locations (Fig. 19-39). Failure can occur: (1) within the restoration (restoration fracture), (2) at the interface between the pin and the restorative material (pin-restoration separation), (3) within the pin (pin fracture), (4) at the interface between the pin and the dentin (pin-dentin separation), and (5) within the dentin (dentin fracture). Failure is more likely to occur at the pin-dentin interface than at the pin-restoration interface. The operator must keep these areas of potential failure in mind at all times and apply the necessary principles to minimize the possibility of an inadequate restoration.

Broken drills and broken pins. Occasionally, a twist drill will break if it is stressed laterally or allowed to stop rotating before being removed from the pinhole. Use of sharp twist drills helps eliminate the possibility of drill breakage. The standard pin usually breaks if turned more than needed to reach the bottom of the pinhole. Pins also may break during bending, if care is not exercised. The treatment for both broken drills and broken pins is to choose an alternate location, at least 1.5 mm remote from the broken item, and prepare another pinhole. Removal of a broken pin or drill is difficult, if not impossible, and usually should not be attempted. The best solution for these two problems is prevention.

Loose pins. Self-threading pins sometimes do not properly engage the dentin because the pinhole was inadvertently prepared too large or a self-shearing pin failed to shear, resulting in stripped-out dentin. The pin should be removed from the tooth and the pinhole reprepared with the next largest size drill, and the appropriate pin inserted. Preparing another pinhole of the same size 1.5 mm from the original pinhole also is acceptable.

As described earlier, a properly placed pin can be loosened while being shortened with a bur, if the bur is not held perpendicularly to the pin and the pin is stabilized. If the pin is loose, remove it from the pinhole by holding a rotating bur parallel to the pin and lightly contacting the surface of the pin. This will cause the pin to rotate counterclockwise out of the pinhole. Try to insert another pin of the same size. If the second pin fails to engage the dentin tightly, prepare a larger hole, and insert the appropriate pin. Preparing another pinhole of the same size 1.5 mm from the original pinhole also is acceptable.

Penetration into the pulp and perforation of the external tooth surface. Either penetration into the pulp or perforation of the external surface of the tooth is obvious if there is hemorrhage in the pinhole following removal of the drill. Usually, the operator can tell when a penetration or perforation has occurred by an abrupt loss of resistance of the drill to hand pressure. Also, if a standard or Link Series pin continues to thread into the tooth beyond the 2 mm depth of the pinhole, this is an indication of a penetration or perforation. A pulpal penetration might be suspected if the patient is anesthetized and has had no sensitivity to tooth preparation until the pinhole is being completed or the pin is being placed. However, with profound anesthesia some patients may not feel pulpal penetration.

Radiographs can verify that a pulpal penetration has not occurred if the view shows dentin between the pulp and the pin. A radiograph projecting the pin in the same region as the pulp does not confirm a pulpal penetration because the pin and the pulp may be superimposed as a result of angulation. In contrast, a radiograph showing a pin projecting outside the tooth confirms external perforation. However, a radiograph showing the pin inside

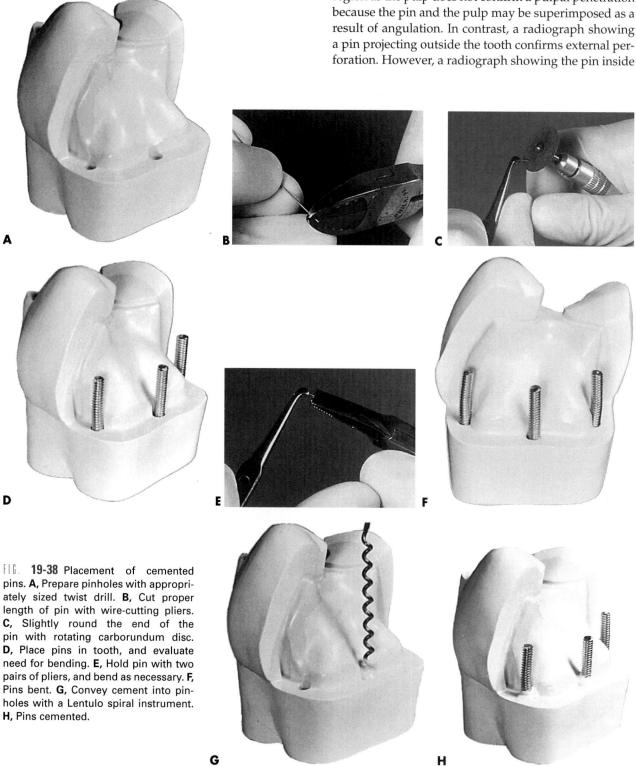

FIG. **19-38** Placement of cemented pins. **A,** Prepare pinholes with appropriately sized twist drill. **B,** Cut proper length of pin with wire-cutting pliers. **C,** Slightly round the end of the pin with rotating carborundum disc. **D,** Place pins in tooth, and evaluate need for bending. **E,** Hold pin with two pairs of pliers, and bend as necessary. **F,** Pins bent. **G,** Convey cement into pinholes with a Lentulo spiral instrument. **H,** Pins cemented.

the projected outline of the tooth does not exclude the possibility of an external perforation.

In an asymptomatic tooth, a pulpal penetration is treated as any other small mechanical exposure. If the exposure is discovered following preparation of the pinhole, control the hemorrhage, if any. Then, place a calcium hydroxide liner over the opening of the pinhole, and prepare another hole 1.5 to 2 mm away. If the exposure is discovered as the pin is being placed, remove the pin and control any hemorrhage. Place a calcium hydroxide liner over the pinhole, and prepare another hole 1.5 to 2 mm away. Although certain studies have shown that the pulp will tolerate pin penetration when placed in a relatively sterile environment,[1,17] it is not recommended that pins remain in place when a pulpal penetration has occurred. If the pin were left in the pulp, (1) the depth of the pin into pulpal tissue would be difficult to determine, (2) considerable postoperative sensitivity might ensue, and (3) the pin location might complicate subsequent endodontic therapy. *Regardless of the method of treatment rendered, the patient must be informed of the perforation or pulpal penetration at the completion of the appointment.* The affected tooth should be periodically evaluated using appropriate radiographs. The patient should be instructed to inform the dentist if any discomfort develops.

Because most teeth receiving pins have had extensive restorations and/or caries, the health of the pulp has probably already been compromised to some extent. Therefore the ideal treatment of a pulpal penetration for such a compromised tooth generally is endodontic therapy. Endodontic treatment should be strongly considered when such a tooth is to receive a cast restoration.

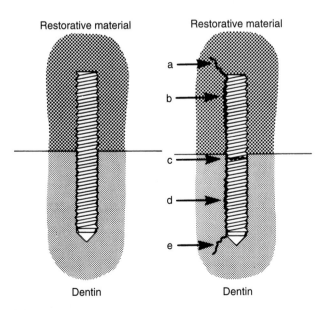

FIG. **19-39** Five possible locations of failure of pin-retained restorations. *a,* Fracture of restorative material; *b,* Separation of pin from restorative material; *c,* Fracture of pin; *d,* Separation of pin from dentin; *e,* Fracture of dentin.

An external perforation might be suspected if an unanesthetized patient senses pain when a pinhole is being prepared or a pin is being placed in a tooth that has had endodontic therapy. Observation of the angulation of the twist drill or the pin should indicate whether a pulpal penetration or external perforation has occurred.

Perforation of the external surface of the tooth can occur occlusal or apical to the gingival attachment. Careful probing and radiographic examination must accurately diagnose the location of a perforation. The method of treatment for a perforation often depends on the experience of the operator and the particular circumstances of the tooth being treated.

Three options are available for perforations that occur occlusal to the gingival attachment: (1) the pin can be cut off flush with the tooth surface and no further treatment rendered, (2) the pin can be cut off flush with the tooth surface and the preparation for a cast restoration extended gingivally beyond the perforation, or (3) the pin can be removed, if still present, and the external aspect of the pinhole enlarged slightly and restored with amalgam. Surgical reflection of the gingival tissue may be necessary to render adequate treatment. The location of perforations occlusal to the attachment often determines the option to be pursued.

Two options are available for perforations that occur apical to the attachment: (1) reflect the tissue surgically, remove the necessary bone, enlarge the pinhole slightly, and restore with amalgam, or (2) perform a crown-lengthening procedure, and place the margin of a cast restoration gingival to the perforation (Fig. 19-40). As with those perforations located occlusal to the gingival attachment, the gingivoapical location of the perforation and the design of the present or planned restoration determine which option to pursue. *As with pulpal penetration, the patient must be informed of the perforation and proposed treatment.* The prognosis of external perforations is favorable when they are recognized early and treated properly.

Having a thorough knowledge of pulpal and external anatomy of the teeth and an accurate representation of the tooth radiographically and following the techniques described in this chapter can substantially reduce the occurrence of pulpal penetrations and external perforations during the use of pins.

Finally, all concepts for tooth preparation for amalgam restorations presented in Chapters 16, 17, and 18 should be applied for a pin-retained amalgam restoration. The margins should be evaluated for soundness and a correct cavosurface angle of 90 degrees (or greater on the occlusal surface).

Tooth Preparation for Slot-Retained Amalgam Restorations. Slot length depends on the extent of the tooth preparation. Slots are usually placed on the facial, lingual, mesial, and distal aspects of the preparation.

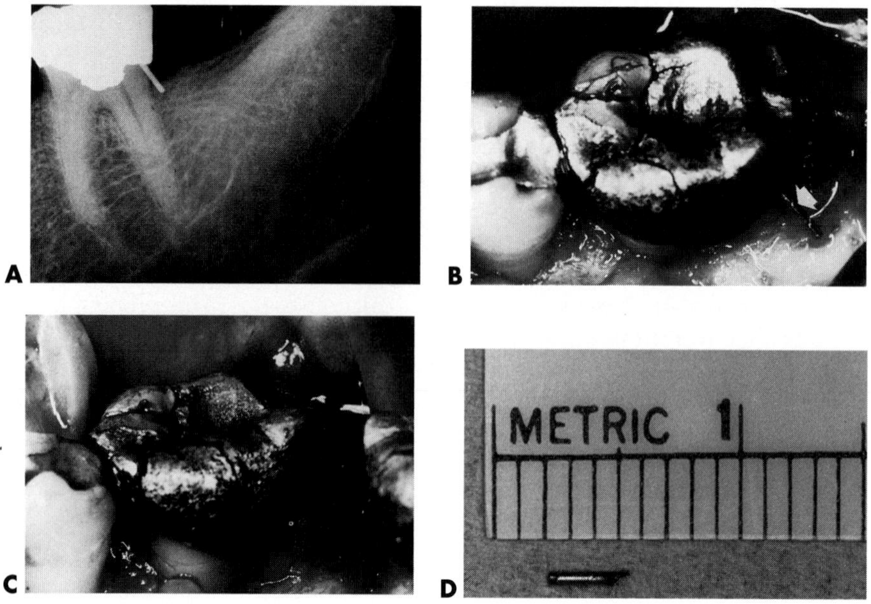

FIG. **19-40** External perforation of pin. **A,** Radiograph showing external perforation of pin. **B,** Surgical access to extruding pin (*arrow*). **C,** Pin cut flush with tooth structure and crown-lengthening procedure performed. **D,** Length of pin removed.

The slot may be continuous or segmented, depending on the amount of missing tooth structure and whether pins were used. McMaster[41] has shown that shorter slots provide as much resistance to horizontal force as do longer slots.

A No. 33½ bur is used to place a slot in the gingival floor 0.5 mm axial of the DEJ (see Fig. 19-4). The slot is at least 0.5 mm in depth and 1 mm or more in length, depending on the distance between the vertical walls. An alternative technique is to prepare the slot initially with a No. 169L bur. Then, ensure its convergence by refining it with a No. 33½ bur. Some operators find that this alternative technique provides more control because the No. 169L bur is less end-cutting than the No. 33½ bur. Alternatively, slots can be used in combination with pins to generate additional retention and resistance forms. No pins were used in this illustration.

Tooth Preparation for Amalgam Foundations. The technique of tooth preparation for a foundation depends on the type of retention that is selected—pin retention; slot retention; or, in the case of endodontically treated teeth, chamber retention. The techniques have in common the axial location of the retention. As stated previously, the retention for a foundation must be sufficiently deep axially so that final preparation for the subsequent indirect restoration does not compromise the resistance and retention forms of the foundation. The technique for each type of retention is discussed.

Pin Retention. Severely broken-down teeth with few or no vertical walls, where an indirect restoration is indicated, may require a pin-retained foundation. The main difference between the use of pins for foundations and the use of pins in definitive restorations is the distance of the pinholes from the external surface of the tooth.[35] For foundations: (1) the pinholes must be located farther from the external surface of the tooth (far-

ther internally from the DEJ), and (2) more bending of the pins may be necessary to allow for adequate axial reduction of the foundation without exposing the pins during the cast metal tooth preparation. Any removal of the restorative material from the circumference of the pin will compromise its retentive effect. If the material is removed from more than one half the diameter of the pin, any retentive effect of the pin has probably been eliminated.

The location of the pinhole from the external surface of the tooth for foundations depends on: (1) the occlusogingival location of the pin (external morphology of the tooth), (2) the type of restoration to be placed (a porcelain-fused-to-metal or all-ceramic preparation requires more reduction than a full gold crown), and (3) the type of margin to be prepared. Preparations with heavily chamfered margins at a normal occlusogingival location require pin (and slot) placement at a greater axial depth. Proximal retention locks should still be used wherever possible. The length of the pins also must be considered to permit adequate occlusal reduction without exposing the pins.

Slot Retention. Slots are placed in the gingival floor of a preparation with a No. 33½ bur (see Fig. 19-4). Foundation slots, as with pins, are placed slightly more axial (farther inside the DEJ) than indicated for conventional amalgam preparations. This more pulpal positioning depends on the type of preparation for a casting that is planned. The preparation for an indirect restoration should not eliminate or cut into the foundation's retentive features. The number of remaining vertical walls determines the indication for slots. Slots are used to oppose retention locks in vertical walls or to provide retention where no vertical walls remain. Retention locks are placed in remaining vertical walls with a No. 169L or ¼ bur as illustrated in Fig. 19-6. Slots are generally 0.5 to

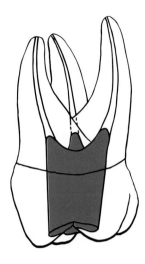

FIG. **19-41** Chamber retention with 2- to 4-mm extension of foundation into canal spaces

1 mm in depth and the width of the No. 33½ bur. Their length is usually 2 to 4 mm, depending on the distance between the remaining vertical walls.

Chamber Retention. For developing foundations in multirooted endodontically treated teeth, an alternative technique has been described by Nayyar et al.[48] This technique is recommended only when: (1) dimension to the pulp chamber is adequate to provide retention and bulk of amalgam, and (2) dentin thickness in the region of the pulp chamber is adequate to provide rigidity and strength to the tooth. Kane et al demonstrated that extension into the root canal space 2 to 4 mm is recommended when the pulp chamber height is 2 mm or less (Fig. 19-41). When the pulp chamber height is 4 to 6 mm, no advantage is gained from extension into the root canal space.[32] After matrix application, amalgam is then thoroughly condensed into the pulp canals, the pulp chamber, and the coronal portion of the tooth. Natural undercuts in the pulp chamber and the divergent canals provide necessary retention form. Resistance form against forces that otherwise may cause tooth fracture is improved by gingival extension of the crown preparation approximately 2 mm beyond the foundation onto sound tooth structure. This extension should have a total taper of opposing walls of less than 10 degrees.[61] If the pulp chamber height is less than 2 mm, the use of a prefabricated post, cast post and core, pins, or slots should be considered. Following placement of the foundation, the tooth may be prepared for the crown or onlay and the indirect restoration completed.

RESTORATIVE TECHNIQUE

Use of Desensitizer or Bonding System. Once the preparation is completed with the necessary resistance and retention forms incorporated, clean the preparation, if indicated, with air/water spray and remove visible moisture without desiccating the tooth. Inspect for detection and removal of any debris or unwanted liner. As discussed in Chapter 17, to reduce dentin permeability and seal the dentin, either a dentin desensitizer or dentin bonding system is used in lieu of varnish. Dentin bonding systems are usually recommended for extensive preparations, particularly with deep excavations, capped cusps, and in weak teeth.[6,69] If a dentin bonding system is used, care should be exercised to avoid pooling of the adhesive at the margins of the preparation and in retentive features such as slots, grooves, and undercuts. The technique for the use of dentin bonding systems for amalgam restorations is discussed in Chapter 17.

In contrast to the advantages of dentin bonding systems suggested by in vitro studies, a recent clinical review of bonded amalgam restorations in place over 5 years reported no difference in number of failures or marginal deterioration compared with restorations placed using cavity varnish.[63]

Matrix Placement. One of the most difficult steps in restoring a severely involved posterior tooth is development of a satisfactory matrix. Fulfilling the objectives of a matrix (as presented in Chapters 13, 16, and 17) is complicated by the possible gingival extensions, missing line angles, and capped cusps that are typical of these tooth preparations.

Universal Matrix. The Tofflemire retainer and band described in Chapter 17 can be used successfully for the majority of posterior amalgam restorations (Fig. 19-42). Use of the Tofflemire retainer requires sufficient tooth structure to retain the band after it is applied.

When the Tofflemire is placed appropriately but an opening remains next to prepared tooth structure, a closed system can be developed as illustrated in Fig. 19-43. Cut a strip of matrix material that is long enough to extend from the mesial to the distal corners of the tooth. The strip must extend into these corners sufficiently that the band, when tight, will hold the strip in position. Also, it must not extend into the proximal areas or a ledge will result in the restoration contour when the matrix is removed. Loosen the Tofflemire retainer one-half turn, and insert the strip of matrix material next to the opening, between the matrix band and the tooth. Tighten the retainer and complete the matrix as described previously in Chapter 17. Sometimes, it is helpful to condense a small amount of softened compound between the strip and open aspect of the band-retainer to stabilize and support the strip further (see Fig. 19-43, *G* and *H*).

When very little tooth structure remains and deep gingival margins are present, the Tofflemire matrix may not function successfully. In the following sections the Automatrix system (Dentsply Caulk, Milford, Delaware) (Figs. 19-44 and 19-45) and the compound-supported copper band (Fig. 19-46) are presented for use when minimal tooth structure is available.

Automatrix. The Automatrix (see Fig. 19-44) is a retainerless matrix system designed for any tooth regardless of its circumference and height. The Automatrix

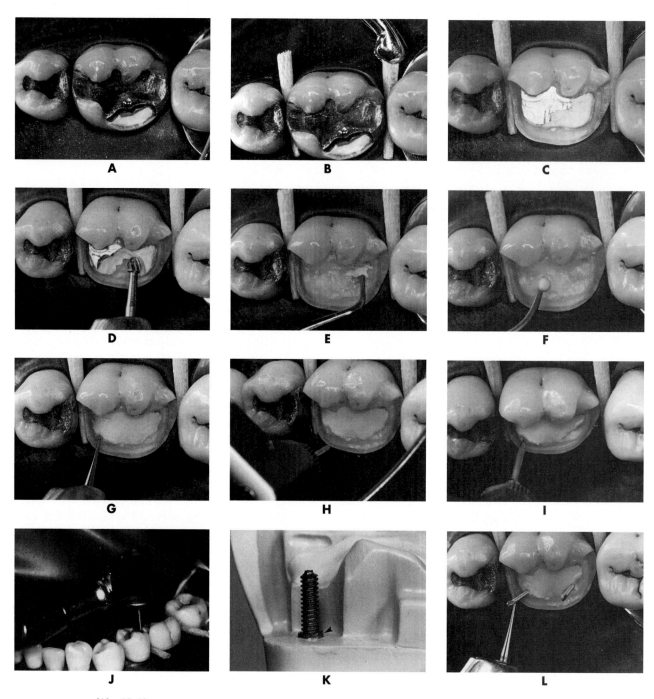

FIG. **19-42** **A,** Mandibular first molar with fractured distolingual cusp. **B,** Insert wedges. **C,** Initial tooth preparation. **D** and **E,** Excavate any infected dentin; if indicated, remove any remaining old restorative materials. **F,** Apply liner and base (if necessary). **G,** Prepare pilot holes. **H,** Align twist drill with external surface of tooth. **I,** Prepare pinholes. **J,** Insert Link pins with slow-speed handpiece. **K,** Note depth-limiting shoulder (*arrow*) of inserted Link Plus pin. **L,** Use No. ¼ bur to shorten pins.

bands are supplied in three widths: ³⁄₁₆, ¹⁄₄, and ⁵⁄₁₆ inch (4.8, 6.35, and 7.79 mm). The medium band is available in two thicknesses (0.0015 and 0.002 inch [0.038 and 0.05 mm]). The ³⁄₁₆- and ⁵⁄₁₆-inch band widths are available in the 0.002-inch thickness only. Advantages of this system include: (1) convenience, (2) improved visibility because

of absence of a retainer, (3) ability to place the autolock loop on the facial or lingual surface of the tooth, and (4) decreased time for application as compared to the copper band matrix. Disadvantages of this system are that: (1) the band is flat and difficult to burnish and is sometimes unstable even when wedges are in place, and (2)

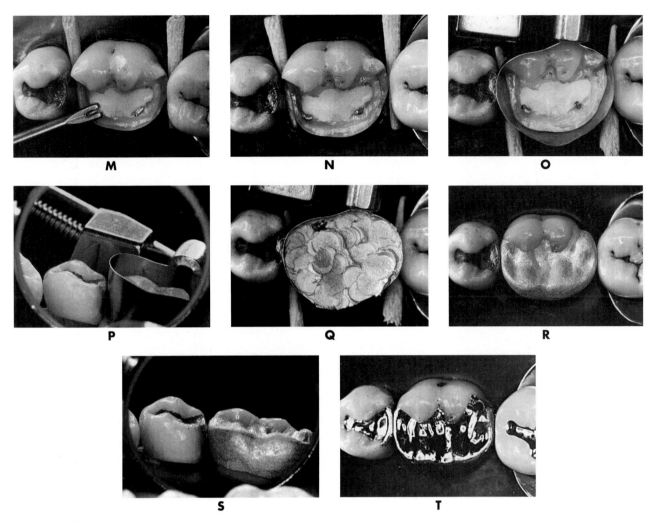

FIG. 19-42, cont'd M, Bend pins (if necessary) with bending tool. N, Final tooth preparation. O, Tofflemire retainer and matrix band applied to prepared tooth. P, Reflect light to evaluate proximal area of matrix band. Q, Preparation overfilled. R, Restoration carved. S, Reflect light to evaluate adequacy of proximal contact and contour. T, Restoration polished.

development of proper proximal contours and contacts can be difficult with the Automatrix bands. Use of the Automatrix system is illustrated in Fig. 19-45.

Compound-Supported Copper Band Matrix. The compound-supported copper band matrix also may be used when the Tofflemire matrix cannot be used successfully. Fabrication of the copper band matrix can be time consuming, but when done properly satisfies the requirements of a good matrix. Fig. 19-46 illustrates the fabrication of a compound-supported copper band matrix. A seamless, annealed copper band is used for the matrix. (Heating the band red-hot and then immediately immersing it in water can anneal the band.)

Select the smallest copper band that will fit over the circumference of the tooth, but still touch or nearly touch the proximal surfaces of the adjacent teeth. Before trying a band on the tooth, festoon the gingival end with curved crown and bridge scissors to correspond to the

level of the gingiva. Then, smooth any rough edges with a sandpaper disc or mounted rubber wheel, and contour the cut end with No. 114 contouring pliers (see Fig. 19-46, *B* through *F*). Slightly withdraw the wedges placed during preparation of the tooth. This will allow teasing the band between the wedges and gingival margin.

Continue to try-in the band and adjust the gingival end until the band extends approximately 1 mm past the gingival margins. No. 114 contouring pliers can be used to develop some contour to the proximal, facial, and lingual aspects of the band and to improve its gingival adaptation. With the band in place on the tooth, use a sharp explorer to scribe a line around the outer surface of the band to indicate the correct occlusal height (see Fig. 19-46, *G*). This line should be 1 to 2 mm above the marginal ridges of adjacent teeth and should provide adequate occlusal height on the facial and lingual surfaces to allow for restoration of reduced cusps.

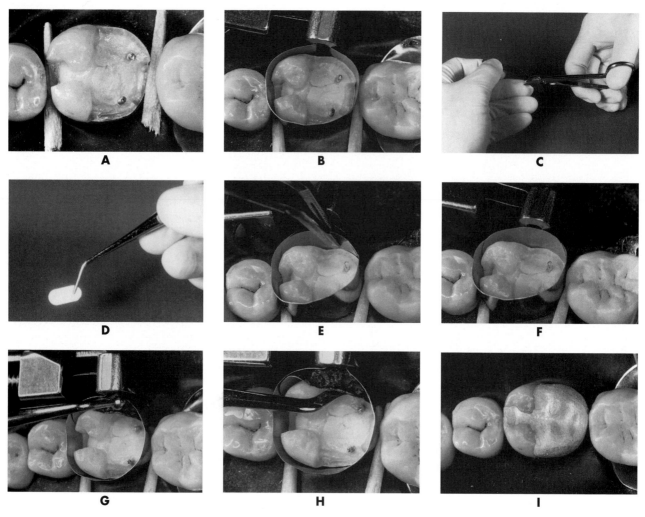

FIG. **19-43** Technique for closing open space of Tofflemire matrix system. **A,** Tooth preparation with wedges in place. **B,** Open aspect of matrix band next to prepared tooth structure. **C** and **D,** Cut appropriate length of matrix material. **E,** Insert strip of matrix material. **F,** Closed matrix system. **G** and **H,** Place compound between strip and matrix band, and contour if necessary. **I,** Restoration carved.

Remove the band, cut it with scissors along the scribed line, and smooth any rough edges with a sandpaper disc or mounted rubber wheel (see Fig. 19-46, *H* and *I*). To help ensure adequate proximal contact with the adjacent teeth, reduce the thickness of the band (but do not penetrate) by relieving the outer surface in the area of each proximal contact area using a rotating sandpaper disc or suitable mounted stone (see Fig. 19-46, *J*). Replace the band, and reinsert the wedges.

To further adapt the band to the tooth, crimp the facial surface in the gingival one third using No. 110 pliers (see Fig. 19-46, *L* and *M*). Evaluate proximal contacts and contour, making adjustments if indicated. Apply compound to stabilize the band and improve its adaptation to the tooth in the gingival aspect of the facial and lingual surfaces (see Fig. 19-46, *N,* and Chapter 17). Again, evaluate the matrix for adequate adaptation and con-

tour, and make corrections where indicated. Routinely burnish the preparation side of the matrix with a warmed, suitably shaped burnisher in the contact areas to ensure that no compound is between the band and the adjacent teeth (at the contacts). Assess tactilely that the band is touching the adjacent teeth (see Fig. 19-46, *O*).

Regardless of the type of matrix system used, the matrix must be stable. If the matrix for a complex amalgam restoration is not stable during condensation, a homogeneous restoration may not be developed. The restoration may be improperly condensed, weak, and may disintegrate when the matrix is removed, even if pins are used for retention. In addition to providing stability, the matrix should extend beyond the gingival margins of the preparation enough to provide support for the matrix and to permit appropriate wedge stabilization. *As a rule, the matrix should extend occlusally beyond the*

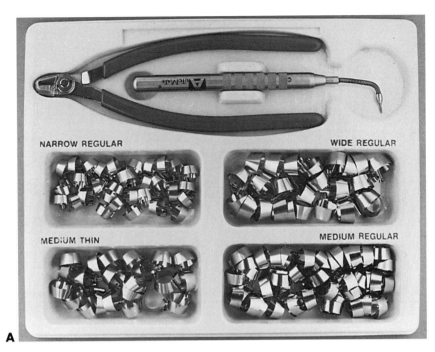

A

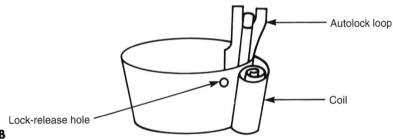

B

Autolock loop

Coil

Lock-release hole

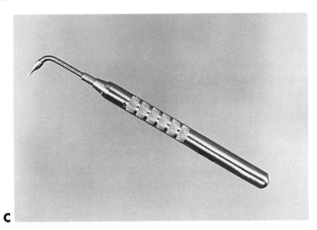

C

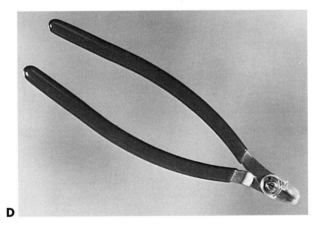

D

FIG. **19-44 A,** Automatrix retainerless matrix system. **B,** Automatrix band. **C,** Automate II tightening device. **D,** Shielded nippers. *(A, Courtesy of L.D. Caulk Company, Milford, Delaware.)*

marginal ridge of the adjacent tooth or teeth by 1 to 2 mm. Matrix stability during condensation is especially important for slot-retained amalgam restorations. If the matrix is not secure during condensation, it may slip out of position causing loss of the restoration. Assuming matrix stability, studies have shown that the retention provided by slots and by self-threading pins is comparable.[2,52] Therefore clinical experience will determine whether the slot-retained amalgam is more appropriate than the pin-retained amalgam.

Inserting the Amalgam. A high-copper alloy is strongly recommended for the complex amalgam restoration because of excellent clinical performance[37,51] and high early compressive strengths.[20] Spherical alloys have a higher early strength than the admixed alloys, and spherical alloys can be condensed quicker with less pressure to ensure good adaptation around the pins. However, proximal contacts may be easier to achieve with admixed alloys because of their condensability, and their extended working time may allow more ade-

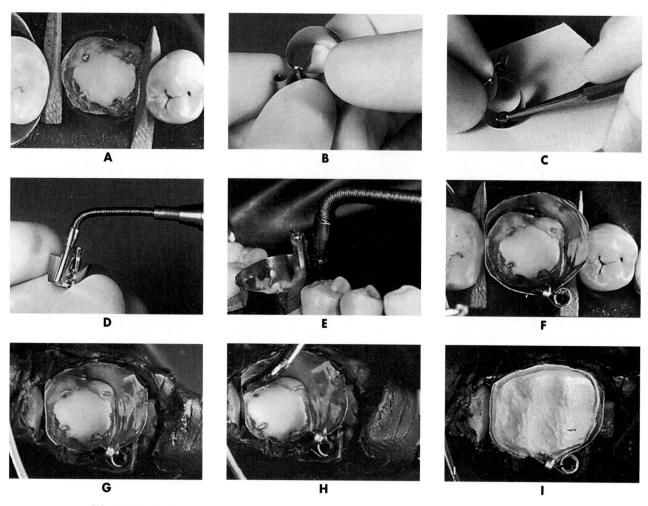

FIG. 19-45 Application of Automatrix for developing pin-retained "amalgam crown" on mandibular first molar. A, Tooth preparation with wedges in place. B, Enlarge circumference of band if necessary. C, Burnish band with egg-shaped burnisher. D through F, Place band around tooth, tighten with Automate II tightening device, and set wedges firmly to place. G, Apply green compound. H, Contour band with back of warm Black spoon excavator. I, Overfill preparation, and carve the occlusal aspect.

quate time for condensation, removal of the matrix band, and final carving. Because the complex amalgam restorations usually are very large, a slow or medium set amalgam may be selected to provide more time for the carving and adjustment of the restoration.

If the amalgam is to be bonded, the insertion of the amalgam must coincide with the placement of the bonding adhesive, as described in earlier chapters. Triturate a mix of amalgam according to the manufacturer's directions and with the amalgam carrier, transfer some of the amalgam to the gingival portion of the preparation. For very large restorations, some operators insert the entire triturated amalgam mass into the preparation. Using appropriately sized condensers, condense each increment of amalgam. Regardless of the insertion technique, care must be taken to condense the amalgam thoroughly in and around the retentive features of the preparation, such as slots, grooves and pins. If a mix of

amalgam becomes dry or crumbly, immediately triturate a new mix. Using only properly mixed amalgam can minimize layering, which weakens the restoration. Continue condensation until the preparation is overfilled.

With a complex (or any large) amalgam, carving time must be properly allocated. The operator must not spend too much time on occlusal carving without allowing adequate time for carving the more inaccessible gingival margins and proximal and axial contours. First, remove the bulk of excess amalgam on the occlusal surface and grossly develop the anatomy, especially the marginal ridge heights with a discoid carver. Then, define the occlusal embrasures running the tine of an explorer against the internal aspect of the matrix band. Accurately developed marginal ridge heights and embrasures reduce the potential of fracturing the marginal ridge(s) when the matrix is removed.

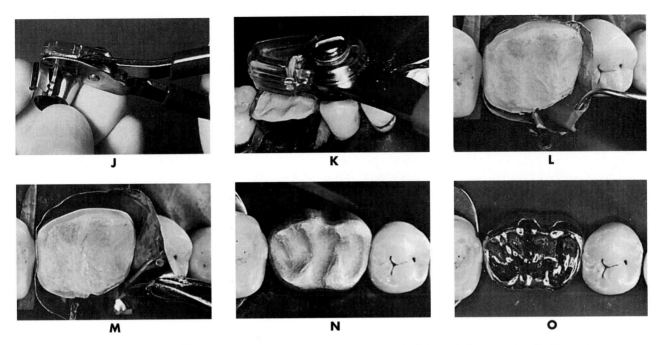

FIG. **19-45, cont'd J** and **K,** Use shielded nippers to cut autolock loop. **L,** Separate band with explorer. **M,** Remove band in oblique direction (facially with some occlusal vector). **N,** Restoration carved. **O,** Restoration polished.

Matrix removal is critical when placing complex amalgam restorations. Matrix removal is especially critical for slot-retained restorations.[58] If the matrix is removed prematurely, there is risk of amalgam fracture causing loss of the restoration. After condensation of the amalgam and initial carving of the occlusal aspect of the restoration (see Fig. 19-46, *P*), break away any compound (if used) with an explorer or Black spoon excavator. Tofflemire-retained matrices are removed first by loosening and removing the retainer, and then removing the matrix band with laterally oriented, short-range movements, as described later. Do not attempt to remove any matrix vertically because this will apply dislodging forces on the recently placed restoration. Automatrix bands are removed by using the system's instruments and, once the band is open, by the same technique described for the Tofflemire-retained matrices. To remove a copper band, carefully cut a groove occlusogingivally on the facial and lingual surfaces of the band with a No. 2 bur (see Fig. 19-46, *Q*). Tear the band apart along these grooves with an explorer, and remove the two sections in an oblique direction occlusolingually or occlusofacially (see Figs. 19-45, *M,* and 19-46, *R*). Complete the carving of the restoration (see Figs. 19-42, *R,* 19-45, *N,* and 19-46, *S*).

With the wedges still in place to maintain passive pressure on the band from the adjacent tooth, remove the Tofflemire retainer from the band, if one is being used. Leaving the wedges in place may help prevent fracturing the marginal ridge amalgam, even though some operators prefer to remove the wedges before matrix removal. Then, remove each end of the band by sliding it in an oblique direction (i.e., move the band facially or lingually while simultaneously moving it in an occlusal direction). Moving the band obliquely toward the occlusal surface minimizes the possibility of fracturing the marginal ridge. Preferably, the matrix band should be removed in the same direction as wedge placement to prevent dislodging the wedges. Next, remove the wedges and with an amalgam knife or an explorer remove any interproximal gingival excess. Develop facial and lingual contours with a Hollenback carver, amalgam knife, or an explorer to complete the carving (see Fig. 19-42, *R* and *S*). Remember that rotary instruments can be used to complete the occlusal carving if the amalgam has set to a hardness such that the force needed to carve with hand instruments might fracture portions of the restoration. Appropriate round and flame-shaped burs can be used to develop occlusal anatomy.

Evaluate the margins with an explorer and correct any discrepancy. Evaluate the adequacy of each proximal contact by using a mirror occlusally and lingually to ensure that no light can be reflected between the restoration and the adjacent tooth at the level of the proximal contact (see Fig. 19-42, *S*). When the proper proximal contour and/or contact cannot be achieved in the large, complex restoration, it may be possible to prepare a conservative two-surface tooth preparation within the initial amalgam to restore the proper proximal surface. The amalgam forming the walls of this "ideal" preparation must have sufficient bulk to prevent future fracture.

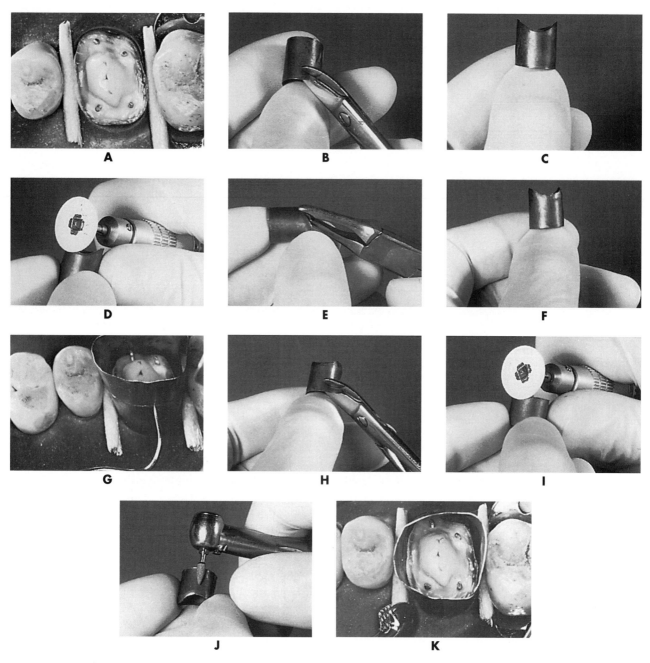

FIG. **19-46** Compound-supported copper band matrix for developing pin-retained "amalgam crown" on maxillary first molar. **A,** Tooth preparation with wedges in place. **B,** Festoon gingival end of band with curved crown and bridge scissors. **C,** Festooned band. **D,** Smooth any rough edges with rotating sandpaper disc. **E,** Contour gingival end of band with No. 114 contouring pliers. **F,** Contoured band. **G,** With band in place, use explorer to scribe a line around band at correct occlusal height. **H** and **I,** Remove band, trim at scribed line, and smooth any rough edges with rotating sandpaper disc. **J,** Thin the proximal contact areas with green stone. **K,** Place band around tooth, and set wedges firmly in place.

Remove the rubber dam and evaluate the occlusal contacts. Adjust the restoration as needed to maintain harmony with the remaining teeth. The procedure for obtaining desired occlusal contacts has been described in earlier chapters. Thin, unwaxed dental floss may be passed through the proximal contacts one time to help smooth the amalgam proximal surface and to remove any amalgam shavings on the proximal surface of the restoration. This should be accomplished by wrapping the floss around the proximal of the adjacent tooth when inserting the floss, thus reducing the force applied to the condensed amalgam. Once the floss is in the gingival embrasure, wrap it around the condensed amalgam and carefully move it occlusogingivally and facio-

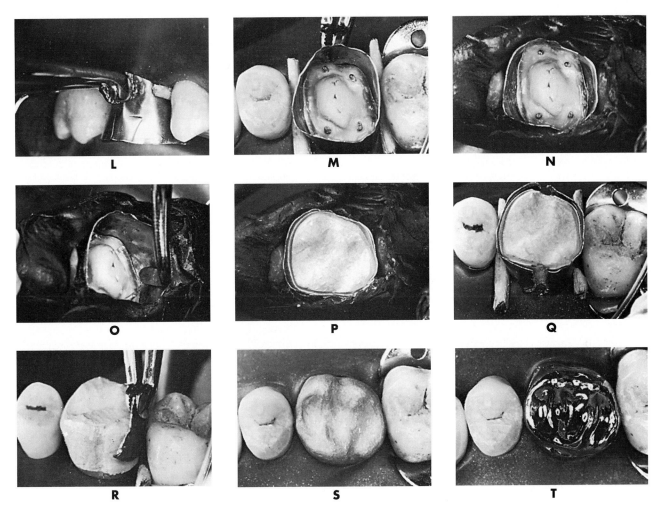

FIG. **19-46, cont'd** **L** and **M,** On facial surface use No. 110 pliers to crimp gingival aspect of band to further adapt it to tooth. **N,** Apply green compound. **O,** Contour band with back of warm Black spoon excavator. **P,** Overfill preparation, and carve occlusal aspect. **Q,** Break away compound, and section band occlusogingivally on facial and lingual surfaces. **R,** Remove sections in oblique direction (facially with some occlusal vector). **S,** Restoration carved. **T,** Restoration polished.

lingually to smooth the proximal amalgam surface while checking for amalgam excess. Passing the floss through a contact more than once may weaken a contact. The shavings should be removed to reduce the possibility of a rough proximal surface or embedment in the gingival sulcus. Caution the patient not to apply biting forces to the restoration for several hours.

When an amalgam foundation is being placed, if a fast-setting high-copper amalgam is used, the final crown or onlay preparation can be initiated within 30 to 45 minutes of insertion of the foundation. Composite or silver cermets might be the material of choice when an adequate matrix cannot be adapted to the tooth in the gingival aspect, such as a furcation area, assuming the area can be isolated from oral fluids. Note that oral fluids will interfere with the bonding of any material to tooth structure and with the setting of silver cermets. As

with amalgam, mechanical retention in addition to bonding may be necessary for composite foundations (see Chapter 13).

Contouring and Finishing the Amalgam. Finish and polish the amalgam restoration, if desired, according to procedures described in Chapters 16 and 17 (see Figs. 19-42, *T*, 19-45, *O*, and 19-46, *T*).

SUMMARY

Because of its history, the complex amalgam restoration may be the most frequently placed complex restoration. However, because of the increasing benefits of composites, the many types of auxiliary retention forms available, and the variations of tooth preparation required for complex restorations, the operator should be familiar with all of these techniques if he or she is to use these restorations on a regular basis.

REFERENCES

1. Abraham G, Baum L: Intentional implantation of pins into the dental pulp, *J South Cal Dent Assoc* 40(10):914-920, 1972.
2. Bailey JH: Retention design for amalgam restorations: pins versus slots, *J Prosthet Dent* 65(1):71-74, 1991.
3. Barkmeier WW, Cooley RL: Self-shearing retentive pins: a laboratory evaluation of pin channel penetration before shearing, *J Am Dent Assoc* 99(3):476-479, 1979.
4. Barkmeier WW, Frost DE, Cooley RL: The two-in-one, self-threading, self-shearing pin: efficacy of insertion technique, *J Am Dent Assoc* 97(1):51-53, 1978.
5. Boyde A, Lester KS: Scanning electron microscopy of self-threading pins in dentin, *Oper Dent* 4(2):56-62, 1979.
6. Browning WD, Johnson WW, Gregory PN: Clinical performance of bonded amalgam restorations at 42 months, *J Am Dent Assoc* 131(5):607-611, 2000.
7. Burgess JO: Horizontal pins: a study of tooth reinforcement, *J Prosthet Dent* 53(3):317-322, 1985.
8. Caputo AA, Standlee JP: Pins and posts—why, when, and how, *Dent Clin North Am* 20(2):299-311, 1976.
9. Caputo AA, Standlee JP, Collard EW: The mechanics of load transfer by retentive pins, *J Prosthet Dent* 29(4):442-449, 1973.
10. Cecconi BT, Asgar K: Pins in amalgam: a study of reinforcement, *J Prosthet Dent* 26(2):159-169, 1971.
11. Courtade GL, Timmermans JJ, editors: *Pins in restorative dentistry*, St Louis, 1971, Mosby.
12. Dilts WE, Coury TL: Conservative approach to the placement of retentive pins, *Dent Clin North Am* 20(2):397-402, 1976.
13. Dilts WE, Duncanson MG Jr, Collard EW et al: Retention of self-threading pins, *J Canad Dent Assoc* 47(2):119-120, 1981.
14. Dilts WE, Mullaney TP: Relationship of pinhole location and tooth morphology in pin-retained silver amalgam restorations, *J Am Dent Assoc* 76(5):1011-1015, 1968.
15. Dilts WE, Welk DA, Laswell HR et al: Crazing of tooth structure associated with placement of pins for amalgam restorations, *J Am Dent Assoc* 81(2):387-391, 1970.
16. Dilts WE, Welk DA, Stovall J: Retentive properties of pin materials in pin-retained silver amalgam restorations, *J Am Dent Assoc* 77(5):1085-1089, 1968.
17. Dolph R: Intentional implanting of pins into the dental pulp, *Dent Clin North Am* 14(1):73-80, 1970.
18. Durkowski JS et al: Effect of diameters of self-threading pins and channel locations on enamel crazing, *Oper Dent* 7(3):86-91, 1982.
19. Eakle WS, Staninec M: Restorative study of bonded amalgam restorations (abstract no. 2717), *J Dent Res* 78(special issue):445, 1999.
20. Eames WB, MacNamara JF: Eight high copper amalgam alloys and six conventional alloys compared, *Oper Dent* 1(3):98-107, 1976.
21. Eames WB, Solly MJ: Five threaded pins compared for insertion and retention, *Oper Dent* 5: 66-71, 1980.
22. Felton DA et al: Pulpal response to threaded pin and retentive slot techniques: a pilot investigation, *J Prosthet Dent* 66(5):597-602, 1991.
23. Fischer GM, Stewart GP, Panelli J: Amalgam retention using pins, boxes, and Amalgambond, *Am J Dent* 6(4):173-175, 1993.
24. Garman TA et al: Self-threading pin penetration into dentin, *J Prosthet Dent* 43(3):298-302, 1980.
25. Garman TA et al: A clinical comparison of dentinal slot retention with metallic pin retention, *J Am Dent Assoc* 107(5):762-763, 1983.
26. Going RE: Pin-retained amalgam, *J Am Dent Assoc* 73(3):619-624, 1966.
27. Going RE et al: The strength of dental amalgam as influenced by pins, *J Am Dent Assoc* 77(6):1331-1334, 1968.
28. Goldstein PM: Retention pins are friction-locked without use of cement, *J Am Dent Assoc* 73(5):1103-1106, 1966.
29. Gourley JV: Favorable locations for pins in molars, *Oper Dent* 5(1):2-6, 1980.
30. Hembree JH: Dentinal retention of pin-retained devices, *Gen Dent* 29(5):420-422, 1981.
31. Irvin AW et al: Photoelastic analysis of stress induced from insertion of self-threading retentive pins, *J Prosthet Dent* 53(3):311-316, 1985.
32. Kane JJ, Burgess JO, Summitt JB: Fracture resistance of amalgam coronal-radicular restorations, *J Prosthet Dent* 63(6):607-613, 1990.
33. Kelsey WP III, Blankenau RJ, Cavel WT: Depth of seating of pins of the Link Series and Link Plus Series, *Oper Dent* 8(1):18-22, 1983.
34. Khera SC, Chan KC, Rittman BR: Dentinal crazing and inter-pin distance, *J Prosthet Dent* 40(5):538-543, 1978.
35. Lambert RL, Goldfogel MH: Pin amalgam restoration and pin amalgam foundation, *J Prosthet Dent* 54(1):10-2, 1985.
36. Lambert RL, Robinson FB, Lindemuth JS: Coronal reinforcement with cross-splinted pin-amalgam restorations, *J Prosthet Dent* 54(3):346-349, 1985.
37. Leinfelder KF: Clinical performance of amalgams with high content of copper, *Gen Dent* 29(1):52-55, 1981.
38. Markley MR: Pin reinforcement and retention of amalgam foundations and restorations, *J Am Dent Assoc* 56(5):675-679, 1958.
39. Martin JA, Bader JD: Five-year treatment outcomes for teeth with large amalgams and crowns, *Oper Dent* 22(2):72-78, 1997.
40. May KN, Heymann HO: Depth of penetration of Link Series and Link Plus pins, *Gen Dent* 34(5):359-361, 1986.
41. McMaster DR et al: The effect of slot preparation length on the horizontal strength of slot-retained restorations, *J Prosthet Dent* 67(4):472-477, 1992.
42. Moffa JP, Razzano MR, Doyle MG: Pins—a comparison of their retentive properties, *J Am Dent Assoc* 78(3):529-535, 1969.
43. Moffa JP, Razzano MR, Folio J: Influence of cavity varnish on microleakage and retention of various pin-retaining devices, *J Prosthet Dent* 20(6):541-551, 1968.
44. Mondelli RF, Barbosa WF, Mondelli J et al: Fracture strength of weakened human premolars restored with amalgam with and without cusp coverage, *Am J Dent* 11(4):181-184, 1998.
45. Mondelli J, Ishikiriama A, Pereira JC et al: Cross-splinting a weakened tooth with a horizontal pin: a new method, *J Prosthet Dent* 57(4):442-445, 1987.
46. Mondelli J, Vieira DF: The strength of Class II amalgam restorations with and without pins, *J Prosthet Dent* 28(2):179-188, 1972.
47. Mozer JE, Watson RW: The pin-retained amalgam, *Oper Dent* 4(4):149-155, 1979.
48. Nayyar A, Walton RE, Leonard LA: An amalgam coronal-radicular dowel and core technique for endodontically treated posterior teeth, *J Prosthet Dent* 43(5):511-515, 1980.
49. Newitter DA, Schlissel ER: Evaluation of four instruments for inserting self-threading pins, *Oper Dent* 5(4):142-145, 1980.
50. Oliveira F de C, Denehy GE, Boyer DB: Fracture resistance of endodontically prepared teeth using various restorative materials, *J Am Dent Assoc* 115(1):57-60, 1987.

51. Osborne JW, Binon PP, Gale EN: Dental amalgam: clinical behavior up to eight years, *Oper Dent* 5(4):24-25, 1980.

52. Outhwaite WC, Garman TA, Pashley DH: Pin vs. slot retention in extensive amalgam restorations, *J Prosthet Dent* 41(4):396-400, 1979.

53. Outhwaite WC et al: Slots vs. pins: a comparison of retention under simulated chewing stresses, *J Dent Res* 61(2):400-402, 1982.

54. Pameijer CH, Stallard RE: Effect of self-threading pins, *J Am Dent Assoc* 85(4):895-899, 1972.

55. Pashley EL et al: Amalgam buildups: shear strength and dentin sealing properties, *Oper Dent* 16(3):82-89, 1991.

56. Perez E, Schoeneck G, Yanahara H: The adaptation of noncemented pins, *J Prosthet Dent* 26(6):631-639, 1971.

57. Plasmans PJ, Reukers EA: Esthetic veneering of amalgam restorations with composite resins—combining the best of both worlds?, *Oper Dent* 18(2):66-71, 1993.

58. Robbins JW, Burgess JO, Summitt JB: Retention and resistance features for complex amalgam restorations, *J Am Dent Assoc* 118(4):437-442, 1989.

59. Robbins JW, Summitt JB: Longevity of complex amalgam restorations, *Oper Dent* 13(2):54-57, 1988.

60. Setcos JC, Staninec M, Wilson NH: The development of resin-bonding for amalgam restorations, *Brit Dent J* 186(7):328-332, 1999.

61. Shillingburg HT Jr, editor: *Fundamentals of fixed prosthodontics*, ed 3, Chicago, 1997, Quintessence.

62. Smales RJ: Longevity of cusp-covered amalgams: survivals after 15 years, *Oper Dent* 16(1):17-20, 1991.

63. Smales RJ, Wetherell JD: Review of bonded amalgam restorations, and assessment in a general practice over five years, *Oper Dent* 25(5):374-381, 2000.

64. Smith CT, Schuman N: Restoration of endodontically treated teeth: a guide for the restorative dentist, *Quintessence Int* 28(7):457-462, 1997.

65. Standlee JP, Caputo AA, Collard EW: Retentive pin installation stresses, *Dent Pract Dent Rec* 21(12):417-422, 1971.

66. Standlee JP, Caputo AA, Collard EW et al: Analysis of stress distribution by endodontic posts, *Oral Surg* 33(6):952-960, 1972.

67. Standlee JP, Collard EW, Caputo AA: Dentinal defects caused by some twist drills and retentive pins, *J Prosthet Dent* 24(2):185-192, 1970.

68. Trabert KC, Caputo AA, Collard EW et al: Stress transfer to the dental pulp by retentive pins, *J Prosthet Dent* 30(5):808-815, 1973.

69. Uyehara MY, Davis RD, Overton JD: Cuspal reinforcement in endodontically treated molars, *Oper Dent* 24(6):364-370, 1999.

70. Vitsentzos SI: Study of the retention of pins, *J Prosthet Dent* 60(4):447-451, 1988.

71. Wacker DR, Baum L: Retentive pins: their use and misuse, *Dent Clin North Am* 29(2):327-340, 1985.

72. Webb EL, Straka WF, Phillips CL: Tooth crazing associated with threaded pins: a three-dimensional model, *J Prosthet Dent* 61(5):624-628, 1989.

73. Welk DA, Dilts WE: Influence of pins on the compressive and horizontal strength of dental amalgam and retention of pins in amalgam, *J Am Dent Assoc* 78(1):101-104, 1969.

74. Wing G: Pin retention amalgam restorations, *Aust Dent J* 10(1):6-10, 1965.

Class II Cast Metal Restorations

JOHN R. STURDEVANT

CLIFFORD M. STURDEVANT*

*This author is inactive this edition. See the Acknowldgements.

INTRODUCTION

The *cast metal restoration* is versatile and is especially applicable to Class II onlay preparations. To be satisfactory, the restoration procedure requires meticulous care both in preparation and in proper manipulation of dental materials, and the dentist and the laboratory technician must be devoted to perfection. The high degree of satisfaction and service derived from a properly made cast metal restoration is a reward for the painstaking application required.

The Class II *inlay* involves the occlusal and proximal surfaces of a posterior tooth and may cap one or more, but not all of the cusps. The Class II *onlay* involves the proximal surfaces of a posterior tooth, and caps all of the cusps.

The procedure requires two appointments: the first for preparing the tooth and making an impression, and the second for delivering the restoration to the patient. The fabrication process is referred to as an *indirect procedure* because the casting is made on a replica of the prepared tooth in a dental laboratory.

MATERIAL QUALITIES

Cast metal restorations can be made from a variety of casting alloys. Although the physical properties of these alloys vary, their major advantages are high compressive and tensile strengths. These high strengths are especially valuable in restorations that rebuild most or the entire occlusal surface.

The American Dental Association (ADA) Specification No. 5 for Inlay Casting Gold requires a minimum total gold-plus-platinum-metals-content of 75 weight percent. Such traditional high-gold alloys are quite unreactive in the oral environment and are some of the most biocompatible materials available to the restorative dentist.[14]

At the present time, *four distinct groups of alloys* are in use for cast restorations: the traditional high-gold alloys, low-gold alloys, palladium-silver alloys, and base metal alloys. Each of the alternatives to high-gold alloys has required some modification of technique or acceptance of reduced performance, most commonly in regard to decreased tarnish resistance and decreased burnishability.[13] Also, they have been associated with higher incidences of postrestorative allergy, most often demonstrated by irritated soft tissues adjacent to the restoration.[14]

INDICATIONS

Large Restorations. The cast metal inlay is an alternative to amalgam or composite when the *higher strength* of a casting alloy is needed or when the *superior control of contours and contacts* that the indirect procedure provides is desired. The cast metal onlay is often an excellent alternative to a crown for teeth that have been greatly weakened by caries or by large, failing restora-

tion(s), but the facial and lingual tooth surfaces are relatively unaffected by disease or injury. For such weakened teeth, the superior physical properties of a casting alloy are desirable to withstand occlusal loads placed on the restoration; also, the onlay can be *designed to distribute occlusal loads* over the tooth in a manner that decreases the chance of tooth fracture in the future. *Moreover, preserving intact facial and lingual enamel (or cementum) is conducive to maintaining the health of contiguous soft tissues.*

When proximal surface caries is extensive, favorable consideration should be given to the cast inlay or onlay. The indirect procedure used to develop the cast restoration allows more control of contours and contacts (both proximal and occlusal).

Endodontically Treated Teeth. A molar or premolar with endodontic treatment can be restored with a cast metal onlay providing the onlay has been thoughtfully designed to strengthen the remaining tooth.

Teeth at Risk for Fracture. Fracture lines in enamel and dentin, especially in teeth having extensive restorations, should be recognized as cleavage planes for possible future fracture of the tooth. Restoring these teeth with a restoration that braces the tooth against fracture injury may sometimes be warranted. Such restorations are cast onlays (with skirting) and crowns.

Dental Rehabilitation with Cast Metal Alloys. When cast metal restorations have been used to restore adjacent or opposing teeth, the continued use of the same material may be considered to eliminate electrical and corrosive activity that sometimes occurs between dissimilar metals in the mouth, particularly when they contact each other.

Diastema Closure and Occlusal Plane Correction. Often the cast inlay or onlay is indicated when extension of the mesiodistal dimension of the tooth is necessary to form a contact with an adjacent tooth. Cast onlays also can be used to correct the occlusal plane of a slightly tilted tooth.

Removable Prosthodontic Abutment. Teeth that are to serve as abutments for a removable partial denture can be restored with a cast metal restoration. The major advantages of a cast restoration are: (1) the superior physical properties of the cast metal alloy allow it to better withstand the forces imparted by the partial denture, and (2) the rest seats, guiding planes, and other aspects of contour relating to the partial denture are better controlled when the indirect technique is used.

CONTRAINDICATIONS

High Caries Rate. Facial and lingual (especially lingual) smooth-surface caries is indicative of a high caries activity that should be brought under control before expensive cast metal restorations are used. If caries or previous restorations are present on the facial and lingual surfaces in addition to the occlusal and proximal surfaces, full crown restorations are usually indicated to restore all the lesions with one casting.

Young Patients. With younger patients amalgam or composite is usually the restorative material of choice for Class I and Class II restorations unless the tooth is severely broken down or endodontically treated. Often younger patients will neglect oral hygiene, which may result in additional caries.

Esthetics. The dentist must consider the esthetic impact (display of metal) of the cast metal restoration. This factor often limits the use of cast metal restorations to tooth surfaces that are not visible at a conversational distance. Composite and porcelain restorations are alternatives in esthetically sensitive areas.

Small Restorations. Because of the success of both amalgam and composite, few cast metal inlays are done in small Class I and II restorations.

ADVANTAGES

Strength. The inherent strength of dental casting alloys allows them to restore large damaged or missing areas and be used in ways that protect the tooth from future fracture injury. Such restorations include onlays and crowns.

Biocompatibility. As previously mentioned, high gold dental casting alloys are quite unreactive in the oral environment. This can be helpful for many patients who have allergies or sensitivities to other restorative materials.

Low Wear. Although individual casting alloys vary in their wear resistance, castings are able to withstand occlusal loads with minimal changes. This is especially important in large restorations that restore a large percentage of occlusal contacts.

Control of Contours and Contacts. Through the use of the indirect technique, the dentist has great control over contours and contacts. This becomes especially important when the restoration is larger and more complex.

DISADVANTAGES

Number of Appointments and Higher Chair Time. The cast inlay or onlay requires at least two appointments and much more time than a direct restoration, such as amalgam or composite.

Temporary. Patients must have temporary restorations between the preparation and delivery appointments. Temporaries occasionally loosen and or break, requiring additional visits.

Cost. In some instances, cost to the patient becomes a major consideration in the decision to restore teeth with cast metal restorations. The cost of materials, laboratory bills, and the time involved make indirect cast restorations more expensive than direct restorations.

Technique Sensitive. Every step of the indirect procedure requires diligence and attention to detail. Errors at any part of the long, multistep process tends to be compounded, resulting in a less-than-optimal restoration.

Splitting Forces. Small inlays may produce a wedging effect on facial and/or lingual tooth structure, and thereby increase the potential for splitting the tooth.

INITIAL PROCEDURES

Occlusion. Before an anesthetic is administered and before preparation of any tooth, evaluate the occlusal contacts of the teeth. As part of this evaluation, decide if the existing occlusal relationships can be improved with the cast metal restoration. An evaluation should include: (1) the occlusal contacts in maximum intercuspation (MI) where the teeth are brought into full interdigitation, and (2) the occlusal contacts that occur during mandibular movements (Fig. 20-1). The pattern of occlusal contacts influences the preparation design, the selection of interocclusal records, and type of articulator or cast development needed.

Anesthesia. Local anesthesia of the tooth to be operated on, as well as the adjacent soft tissues, usually is advocated. Anesthetizing these tissues eliminates pain and reduces salivation, resulting in a more pleasant operation for both the patient and the operator.

Considerations for Temporary Restorations. Before preparation of the tooth, consideration must be given to the method that will be used to fabricate the temporary restoration. Most temporary restoration techniques require the use of a preoperative impression to reproduce the occlusal, facial, and lingual surfaces of the temporary restoration to the preoperative contours.

The technique involves making a preoperative impression with an elastic impression material. Alginate impression material is a common choice because it sets quickly and is relatively inexpensive. If the tooth to be restored has any large defects, such as a missing cusp, either of two methods may be used to reproduce the missing cusp in the temporary. First, a hand instrument can be used to remove impression material in the area of the missing cusp or tooth structure, to simulate the desired form for the temporary. Secondly, wax can be added to the tooth before the impression as follows. Dry the tooth, and fill the large defects with utility wax. Smooth the wax, and make an impression using a quadrant tray if no more than two teeth are to be prepared (Fig. 20-2, *A*). A full-arch tray may be used for greater stability. Seat the tray filled with impression material (see Fig. 20-2, *B*). After the impression has set, remove the impression and examine it for completeness (see Fig. 20-2, *C*). Alginate impressions can distort quickly if they are allowed to gain or lose moisture, so wrap the impression in wet paper towels to serve as a humidor (see Fig. 20-2, *D*). The preoperative impression may be made with a polyvinyl siloxane impression material if additional accuracy, stability, and durability are required (such as when making multiple temporaries over an ex-

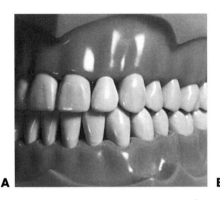
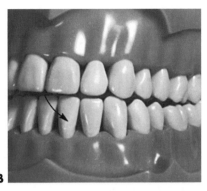
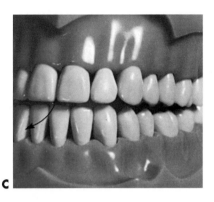

FIG. **20-1** Evaluate occlusal relationships in MI (**A**), and during mandibular movements (**B** and **C**). Be alert for problems with tooth alignment and contact position. Note the amount of posterior separation provided by the guidance of anterior teeth (working side) and articular eminence (nonworking side).

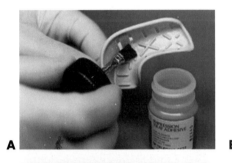
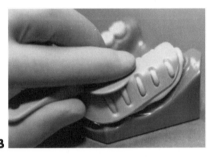
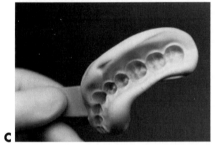
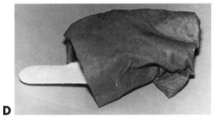

FIG. **20-2 A,** Applying tray adhesive to stock quadrant tray. **B,** Making preoperative impression. **C,** Inspecting preoperative impression for completeness. **D,** When using alginate, wrap impression with wet paper towels to serve as a humidor.

tended period of time). The preoperative impression is set aside for later use in forming the temporary

TOOTH PREPARATIONS FOR CLASS II CAST METAL RESTORATIONS

A small distal, cavitated, carious lesion in the maxillary right first premolar is used to illustrate the classic two-surface preparation for an inlay (Fig. 20-3, *A*). Treatment principals for other defects are presented later in this section. As indicated previously, few small one- or two-surface inlays are done. However, because the description of a small tooth preparation presents the basic concepts, it is used to illustrate the technique. More extensive tooth preparations are presented later in the chapter.

TOOTH PREPARATION FOR CLASS II CAST METAL INLAYS

Initial Preparation. Carbide burs used to develop the vertical internal walls of the preparation for cast metal inlays and onlays are plane cut, tapered fissure burs. These burs are plane cut so the vertical walls will be smooth. The side and end surfaces of the bur should be straight to aid in the development of uniformly tapered walls and smooth pulpal and gingival walls. Recommended dimensions and configurations of the burs to be used are shown in Fig. 20-3, *B*. Suggested burs are the No. 271 and the No. 169L (Brassler USA, Inc., Savannah, Georgia). The operator is cautioned to verify the measurements of unfamiliar burs before they are used to judge depth into the tooth during preparation. Note that the sides and end surface of the No. 271 bur meet in a slightly rounded manner so that sharp, stress-inducing

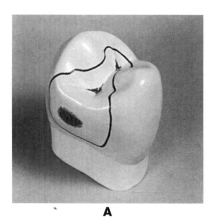

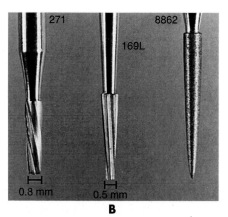

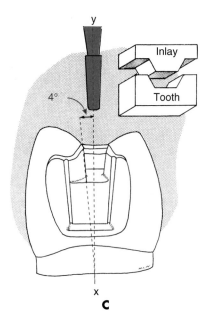

FIG. **20-3 A,** Proposed outline form for DO preparation. **B,** Dimensions and configuration of No. 271, No. 169L, and No. 8862 instruments. **C,** Conventional 4-degree divergence from line of draw (line *xy*).

internal angles will not be formed in the preparation.[7] The marginal bevels are placed with a slender, fine-grit, flame shaped diamond instrument, such as the No. 8862 (Brassler USA, Inc., Savannah, Georgia).

Throughout preparation for a cast inlay, the cutting instruments used to develop the vertical walls are oriented to a single "draw" path, usually the long axis of the tooth crown, so that the completed preparation will have draft (no undercuts) (see Fig. 20-3, C). The gingival-to-occlusal divergence of these preparation walls may range from 2 to 5 degrees per wall from the line of draw. If the vertical walls are unusually short, a maximum of 2 degrees occlusal divergence is desirable to increase retention potential. As the occlusogingival height increases, the occlusal divergence should increase because lengthy preparations with minimal divergence (more parallel) may present difficulties during pattern withdrawal, trial seating and withdrawal of the casting, and cementing.

Occlusal Step. With the No. 271 carbide bur held parallel to the long axis of the tooth crown, enter the fossa/pit closest to the involved marginal ridge, using a punch cut to a depth of 1.5 mm to establish the depth of the pulpal wall (Fig. 20-4, A and B). In initial preparation do not exceed this specified depth, regardless of whether the bur end is in dentin, caries, old restorative material, or air. The bur should be rotating at high speed (with air-water spray) before application to the tooth and should not stop rotating until it is removed. This minimizes perceptible vibration and prevents breakage or chipping of the bur blades. *A general rule is to maintain the long axis of the bur parallel to the long axis of the tooth crown at all times* (see Fig. 20-4, B and C). For mandibular molars and second premolars whose crowns tilt slightly lingually, this rule dictates that the bur should tilt slightly (5 to 10 degrees) lingually to conserve the strength of the lingual cusps (see Fig. 20-4, D). It is em-

phasized that when the operator is cutting at high speeds, a properly directed air-water spray is used to provide the necessary cooling and cleansing effects.[1]

Maintaining the 1.5-mm initial depth and the same bur orientation, extend the preparation outline mesially along the central groove/fissure to include the mesial fossa/pit (see Fig. 20-4, E and F). Ideally the faciolingual dimension of this cut should be minimal. Exercise care to keep the mesial marginal ridge strong by not removing the dentin support of the ridge (see Fig. 20-4, F and H). The use of light intermittent pressure will minimize heat production on the tooth surface and reduce the incidence of enamel crazing ahead of the bur. Occasionally a fissure extends onto the mesial marginal ridge. This defect, if shallow, may be treated with enameloplasty, or it may be included in the outline form with the cavosurface bevel, which is applied in a later step in the tooth preparation (see Fig. 20-4, G).

Enameloplasty, as presented in earlier chapters, will occasionally reduce extension along the fissures, thereby conserving tooth structure vital for pulp protection and strength of the remaining tooth crown. The extent to which enameloplasty can be used usually cannot be determined until the operator is in the process of extending the preparation wall, when the depth of the fissure in the enamel wall can be observed (Fig. 20-5). When enameloplasty proves a fissure in a marginal ridge to be deeper than one third the thickness of the enamel, then utilize the procedures described in the later section.

Extend to include faulty facial and lingual fissures radiating from the mesial pit. During this extension cutting, the operator is cautioned again not to remove the dentin support of the proximal marginal ridge. To conserve tooth structure and the strength of the remaining tooth, the final extension up these fissures can be ac-

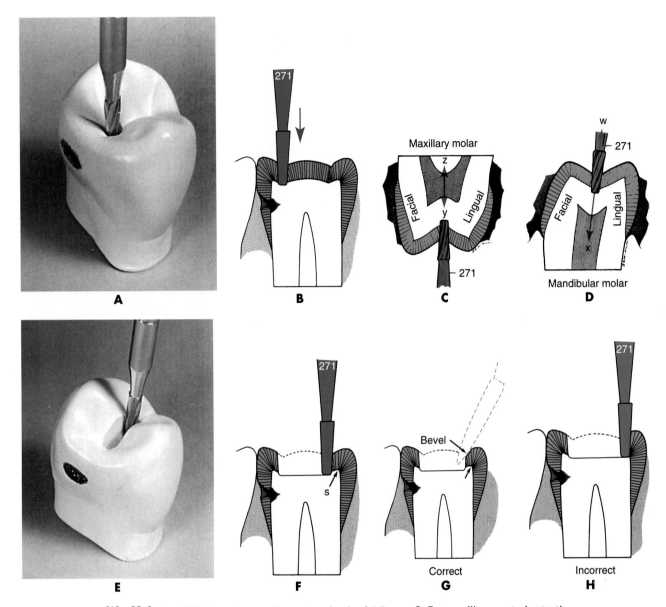

FIG. 20-4 **A** and **B,** Bur after punch cut to a depth of 1.5 mm. **C,** For maxillary posterior teeth, long axis of bur should parallel long axis of tooth crown (line *yz*). **D,** For molar and second premolar teeth of mandibular dentition, long axis of bur should tilt slightly lingually to parallel long axis of tooth crown (line *wx*). **E** and **F,** Extending mesial wall, taking care to conserve dentin that supports marginal ridge *(s).* **G,** Marginal bevel can provide additional extension. **H,** Improper extension that has weakened the marginal ridge.

complished with the slender No. 169L carbide bur (Fig. 20-6, *A*). Tooth structure and strength can be further conserved by remembering that: (1) enameloplasty of the fissure ends should be employed when possible and (2) the marginal bevel of the final preparation often can be used to include (eliminate) the terminal ends of these fissures in the outline form. The facial and lingual extension in the mesial pit region should provide the desired *dovetail retention form,* which resists distal displacement of the inlay (see Fig. 20-6, *B*). When these facial and lingual grooves are not faulty, sufficient facial extension in the mesial pit region should be made, nevertheless, to provide this dovetail retention form against

distal displacement. Minor extension in the transverse ridge area to include remaining facial or lingual caries may necessitate additional facial or lingual extension in the mesial pit to provide this dovetail feature. (Recall the principle that during such facial or lingual extensions to sound tooth structure, the bur depth is maintained at 1.5 mm.) If major facial or lingual extension is required to remove undermined occlusal enamel, capping the weak remaining cuspal structure may be indicated, as well as additional features in the preparation to provide adequate retention and resistance forms. These considerations are discussed in the subsequent sections.

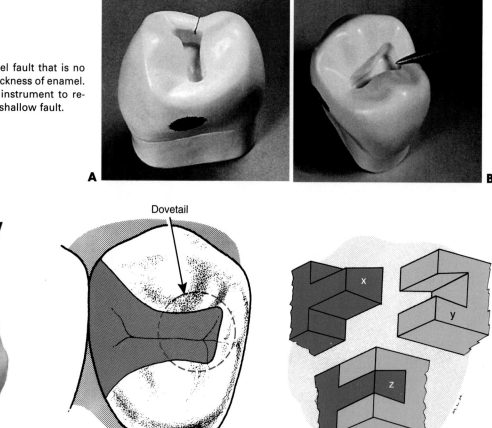

FIG. 20-5 A, Shallow enamel fault that is no deeper than one third the thickness of enamel. B, Using fine-grit diamond instrument to remove enamel that contains shallow fault.

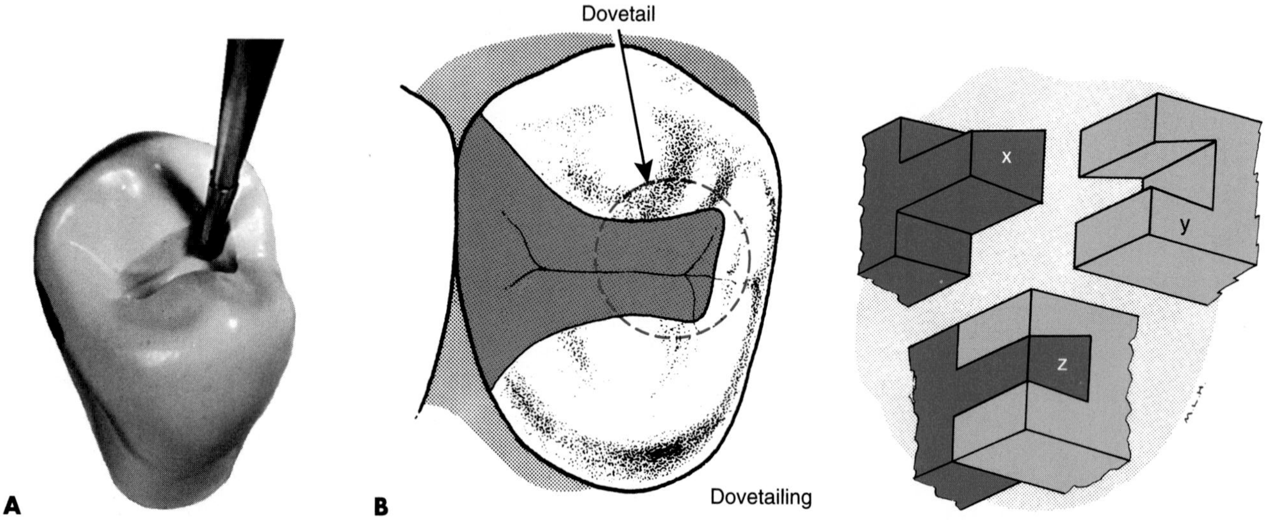

FIG. 20-6 A, Extending up the mesiofacial triangular groove using slender No. 169L bur. B, Dovetail retention form is created by extension shown in A. As x fits into y only in one direction resulting in z, similarly dovetail portion of inlay fits into dovetail portion of preparation only in an occlusal-to-gingival direction.

Continuing at the initial depth, extend the occlusal step distally into the distal marginal ridge sufficiently to expose the junction of the proximal enamel and the dentin (Fig. 20-7, A and B). While extending distally, progressively widen the preparation to the desired faciolingual width in anticipation for the proximal box preparation. The increased faciolingual width enables the facial and lingual walls of the box to project (visually) perpendicularly to the proximal surface at positions that will clear the adjacent tooth by 0.2 to 0.5 mm (see Fig. 20-7, F). The facial and lingual walls of the occlusal step should go around the cusps in graceful curves, and the prepared isthmus in the transverse ridge ideally should be only slightly wider than the bur, thus conserving dentinal protection for the pulp and maintaining strength of the cusps. If the occlusal step has been prepared correctly, any caries on the pulpal floor should be uncovered by facial and lingual extension to sound enamel (supported by dentin).

Proximal Box. Continuing with the No. 271 carbide bur, isolate the distal enamel by cutting a proximal ditch (see Fig. 20-7, C to F). Allow the harder enamel to guide the bur. Slight pressure toward the enamel is necessary to prevent the bur from cutting only dentin. If the bur is allowed to cut only dentin, the resulting axial wall will be too deep. The mesiodistal width of the ditch should be 0.8 mm (the tip diameter of the bur) and prepared approximately two thirds (0.5 mm) at the expense of dentin and one third (0.3 mm) at the expense of enamel. The gingival extension of this cut may be checked with the length of the bur by first measuring the depth from the height of the marginal ridge and then removing the bur and holding it beside the tooth. A periodontal probe also may be used for this measurement. While penetrating gingivally, extend the proximal ditch facially and lingually beyond the caries to the desired position of the facioaxial and linguoaxial line angles. If the carious lesion is minimal, the ideal extension facially and lingually will be as previously described (see Fig. 20-7, F). Ideal extension gingivally of a minimal, cavitated lesion will eliminate caries on the gingival floor and provide 0.5-mm clearance of the unbeveled gingival margin

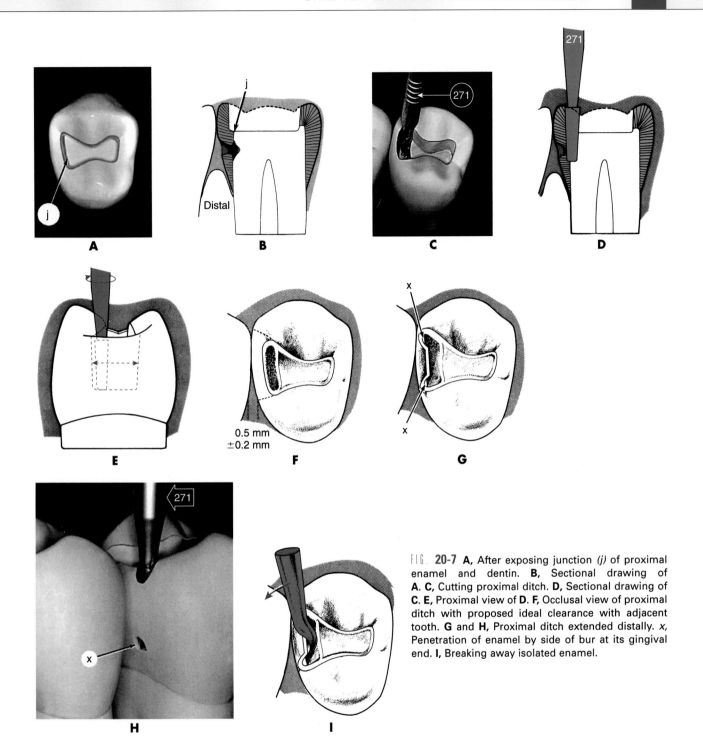

FIG. **20-7 A,** After exposing junction *(j)* of proximal enamel and dentin. **B,** Sectional drawing of A. **C,** Cutting proximal ditch. **D,** Sectional drawing of C. **E,** Proximal view of D. **F,** Occlusal view of proximal ditch with proposed ideal clearance with adjacent tooth. **G** and **H,** Proximal ditch extended distally. *x,* Penetration of enamel by side of bur at its gingival end. **I,** Breaking away isolated enamel.

with the adjacent tooth. Moderate-to-extensive caries on the proximal surface dictates continued extension of the proximal ditch to the extent of the caries at the denti-noenamel junction (DEJ), but *not pulpally* (see Fig. 20-11, *D*). *When preparing the proximal portion of the preparation, maintain the side of the bur at the specified axial wall depth regardless of whether it is in dentin, caries, old restorative material, or air.* Guard against overcutting the facial, lingual, and gingival walls, which would not conserve tooth structure and could result in: (1) overextension of the margins in the completed preparation, (2) a weakened tooth, and (3) possible injury of the soft tissue. Be-

cause the proximal enamel diminishes in thickness from the occlusal to gingival level, the end of the bur will be closer to the external tooth surface as the cutting progresses gingivally. The axial wall should follow the contour of the tooth faciolingually. *Any carious dentin on the axial wall should not be removed at this stage of preparation.*

Then with the No. 271 carbide bur, make two cuts, one at the facial limit of the proximal ditch and the other at the lingual limit, extending from the ditch perpendicularly toward the enamel surface (in the direction of the enamel rods) (see Fig. 20-7, *G*). Extend these cuts until the bur is nearly through the marginal ridge enamel (the side of the bur may emerge slightly through the surface at the level of the gingival floor) as shown in Fig. 20-7, *H*. This weakens the enamel by which the remaining isolated portion is held. Also, confirm the level of the gingival floor by observing where the end of the bur emerged through the proximal surface. If indicated, additional gingival extension can be accomplished while the remaining enamel still serves to guide the bur and prevent it from marring the proximal surface of the adjacent tooth. At this time, however, the remaining wall of enamel often breaks away during cutting, especially when high speeds are employed. If the isolated wall of enamel is still present, it can be fractured out with a spoon excavator (see Fig. 20-7, *I*). At this stage, the ragged enamel edges left from breaking away the proximal surface may be touching the adjacent tooth.

Planing the distofacial, distolingual, and gingival walls by hand instruments to remove all undermined enamel may be indicated if minimal extension is needed to fulfill an esthetic objective. Depending on access, use a No. 15 (width) straight chisel, binangle chisel (Fig. 20-8), or enamel hatchet. For a right-handed operator, the distal beveled binangle chisel is used on the distofacial wall of a distoocclusal (DO) preparation for the maxillary right premolar. Plane the wall by holding the instrument in the modified palm-and-thumb grasp, and use a chisel-like motion in an occlusal-to-gingival direction (see Fig. 20-8, *A* and *B*). Plane the gingival wall by using the same instrument as a hoe, scraping in a lingual-to-facial direction (see Fig. 20-8, *C*). In this latter action the axial wall may be planed with the side edge (secondary edge) of the blade. The distolingual wall is planed smooth by using the binangle chisel with the mesial bevel (see Fig. 20-8, *D*). When proximal caries is minimal, ideal facial and lingual extension at this step in the preparation results in margins that clear the adjacent tooth by 0.2 to 0.5 mm.

The experienced operator usually does not use chisel hand instruments during preparation for inlays, inasmuch as the narrow, flame-shaped, fine-grit diamond instrument, when artfully used, will remove ragged, weak enamel during application of the cavosurface bevel and flares and will cause the patient to be less apprehensive (see Figs. 20-12 and 20-13). If the diamond instrument is to be used exclusively in finishing the enamel walls and margins, this procedure is postponed until after the removal of any remaining infected dentin and/or old restorative material, and the application of any necessary base. This prevents any hemorrhage (which occasionally follows the beveling of the gingival margin) from hindering: (1) the suitable removal of remaining infected dentin and old restorative material and (2) the proper application of a necessary base. Hand instruments are more useful on the mesiofacial surfaces of the maxillary premolars and first molars, where min-

imal extension is desired to prevent an unsightly display of metal.

Shallow (0.3 mm deep) *retention grooves* may be cut in the facioaxial and linguoaxial line-angles with the No. 169L carbide bur (see Fig. 20-8, *E* to *I*). These grooves are indicated especially when the prepared tooth is short. When properly positioned, the grooves are in sound dentin, near but not contacting, the DEJ. The long axis of the bur must be held parallel to the line of draw. Preparing these grooves may be postponed until after any required bases are applied during final preparation.

Final Preparation

Removal of Infected Carious Dentin and Pulp Protection. After the initial preparation has been completed, evaluate the internal walls of the preparation visually and tactilely (with an explorer) for indications of remaining carious dentin. If carious dentin remains, and if it is judged to be infected, but shallow or moderate (1 mm or more of remaining dentin between the caries and the pulp), satisfactory *isolation* for removal of such caries and the application of any necessary base may be attained by the reduction in salivation resulting from anesthesia and the use of cotton rolls, a saliva ejector, and gingival retraction cord. The retraction cord also serves to widen the gingival sulcus and slightly retract the gingiva in preparation for beveling and flaring the proximal margins (Fig. 20-9; see also Fig. 20-12, *A* and *B*). For insertion of the cord refer to the later sections, Bevels and Flares and Tissue Retraction. The removal of the remaining caries and placement of a necessary base can be accomplished during the time required for the full effect of the inserted cord. Use a slowly revolving round bur (No. 2 or No. 4) or spoon excavator to remove the carious infected dentin (see Fig. 20-9, *F* and *G*). If the bur is used, improve visibility by using air alone. This excavation is done just above stall-out speed with light, intermittent cutting. Take care not to unnecessarily desiccate the exposed dentin during this procedure.

Light-cured glass-ionomer cement may be mixed and applied with a suitable applicator to these shallow (or moderately deep) excavated regions to the depth and form of the ideally prepared surface. Placing a base takes very little time and should be considered because it results in working dies (subsequently in the laboratory phase) that have preparation walls with no undercuts, as well as "ideal" position and contour. Also, applying a base at this time minimizes additional irritation of the pulp during subsequent procedures necessary for the completion of the restoration. The light-cured glass ionomer adheres to tooth structure and does not require retentive undercuts when the base is small to moderate. The material is applied by conveying small portions on the end of a periodontal probe and is light-cured when the correct form has been achieved (see Fig. 20-9, *H* and *I*). Any excess cement can be trimmed back to ideal form

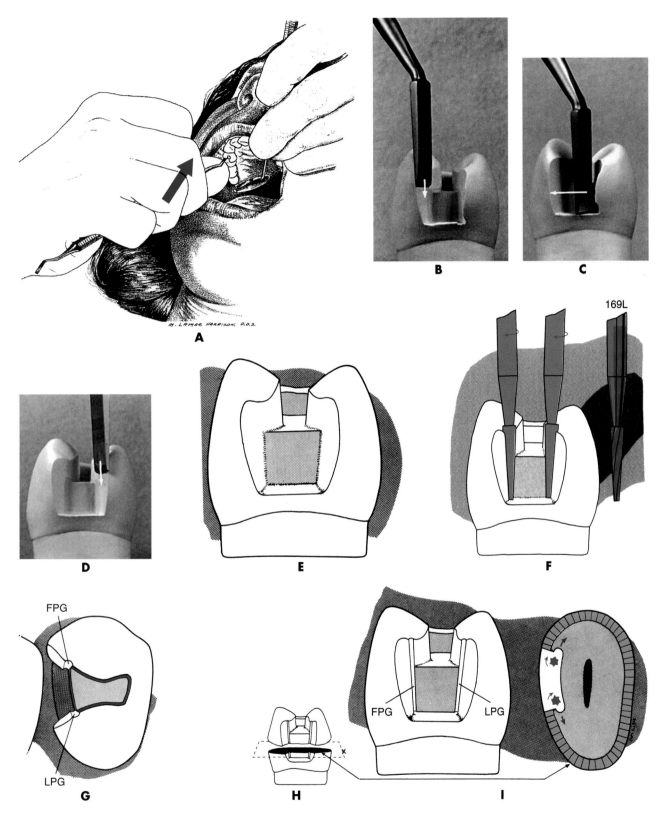

FIG. 20-8 Using modified palm-and-thumb grasp (A) to plane distofacial and distolingual walls (B and D) and to scrape gingival wall (C). E, Before cutting retention grooves. F, Cutting retention grooves. G and H, *FPG*, facial proximal groove; *LPG*, lingual proximal groove. I, Section in plane *x*. Larger arrows depict direction of translation of rotating bur.

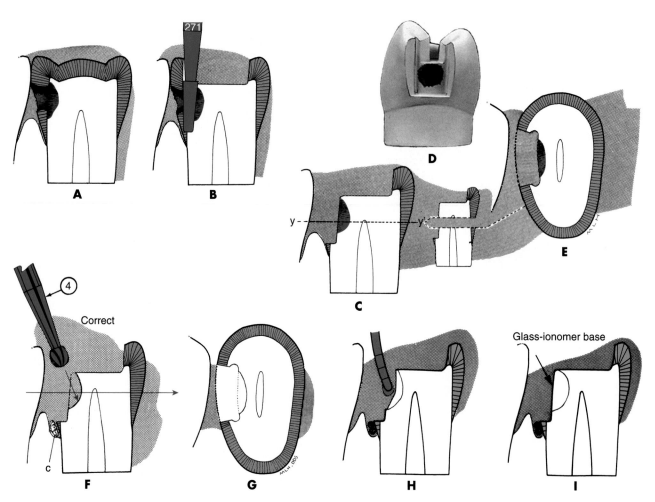

FIG. **20-9** Moderately deep caries. Extending proximal ditch gingivally (**B**) to a sound floor free from caries (**C**). **D,** Remaining caries on axial wall. **E,** Section of **C** in plane *yy`*. **F,** Removing remaining infected dentin. *c,* Inserted retraction cord. **G,** Section of **F**. **H,** Inserting glass-ionomer base with periodontal probe. **I,** Completed base.

with the No. 271 carbide bur after the cement has hardened.

If the carious lesion is judged to closely approach the pulp, a rubber dam should be applied before the removal of infected dentin. This provides the optimal environment for successfully treating a pulp exposure should it occur. When excavating extensive caries, attempt to remove only the infected dentin and not the affected dentin, since +removal of the latter might expose a healthy pulp. Ideally, caries removal should continue until the remaining dentin is as hard as normal dentin; however, heavy pressure should not be applied with an explorer tip (or any other instrument) on dentin next to the pulp, lest an unnecessary pulpal exposure be created. If removal of soft, infected dentin leads directly to a pulpal exposure (carious pulpal exposure), then root canal treatment should be accomplished before completing the cast metal restoration.

If the pulp is inadvertently exposed as a result of operator error or misjudgment (mechanical pulpal expo-

sure), then it must be decided whether to proceed with root canal treatment or to attempt a direct pulp capping procedure. A clinical evaluation should be made regarding health of the pulp. A favorable prognosis for the pulp after direct pulp capping may be expected if the following criteria are met:

- The exposure is small (less than 0.5 mm in diameter).
- The tooth has been asymptomatic, showing no signs of pulpitis.
- Any hemorrhage from the exposure site is easily controlled.
- The invasion of the pulp chamber was relatively atraumatic with little physical irritation to the pulp tissue.
- A clean, uncontaminated operating field is maintained (i.e., a rubber dam).

If the excavation closely approaches the pulp or if a direct pulp cap is indicated, first apply a lining of *calcium*

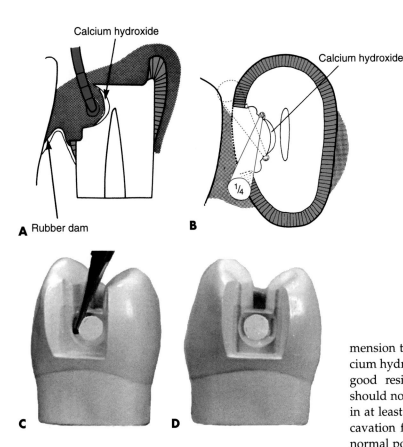

FIG. **20-10 A,** Deep caries excavations near the pulp are first lined with calcium hydroxide. Note rubber dam. **B** to **D,** Cutting retention coves for retaining glass-ionomer cement.

hydroxide using a flow technique (without pressure). This calcium hydroxide liner should cover and protect any possible near or actual exposure and also extend over a major portion of the excavated dentin surface (Fig. 20-10, *A*). Although undetected, there may be an exposed recessional tract of a pulp horn in any deep excavation. Calcium hydroxide treatment of an exposed, healthy pulp promotes the formation of a dentin bridge, which would close the exposure.[12] Leave the peripheral 0.5 to 1 mm of the dentin excavation available for bonding the light-cured glass-ionomer cement base subsequently applied.

Although the light-cured glass-ionomer cement is adhesive to dentin, large cement bases can be subjected to considerable stresses during fabrication of the temporary, and try-in/cementation of the cast metal restoration. Also, if a calcium hydroxide liner has been applied, less dentin is available for adhesive bonding. In these circumstances, small mechanical undercuts can increase the retention of the glass-ionomer base. If suitable undercuts are not present after removal of infected dentin, retention coves are placed with the No. ¼ carbide bur (see Fig. 20-10, *B* through *D*). These coves are placed in the peripheral dentin of the excavation and are as remote from the pulp as possible. The light-cured glass-ionomer cement should be applied without pressure. It should completely cover the calcium hydroxide lining and some peripheral dentin for good adhesion (Fig. 20-11). The cement base should be sufficiently thick in di-

mension to protect the thin underlying dentin and calcium hydroxide liner from subsequent stresses. Usually, good resistance form dictates that the pulpal wall should not be formed entirely by a cement base; rather, in at least two regions, one diametrically across the excavation from the other, the pulpal wall should be in normal position, flat, and formed by sound dentin (see region *s* in Fig. 20-11, *E,* depicting basing in a mandibular molar). One should consider the addition of other retention features, such as proximal grooves, if a major portion of a proximal axial wall is composed mostly of cement base because this base should not be relied on for contributing to retention of the cast restoration (see Fig. 20-8, *F*).

Remaining old restorative material on the internal walls should be removed if any of the following conditions are present: (1) the old material is judged to be thin and/or nonretentive, (2) there is radiographic evidence of caries under the old material, (3) the pulp was symptomatic preoperatively, or (4) the periphery of the remaining restorative material is not intact, (i.e., there is some breach in the junction of the material with the adjacent tooth structure that may indicate caries under the material). If none of these conditions is present, the operator may elect to leave the remaining restorative material to serve as a base, rather than risk unnecessary removal of sound dentin or irritation or exposure of the pulp. The same isolation conditions described previously for removal of infected dentin also apply for the removal of old restorative material.

After the cement has hardened, spread a thin coat of petroleum jelly over the base with a small cotton pellet. This serves to prevent the adherence of subsequently applied unpolymerized materials such as the material used for the temporary restoration and the final impression material.

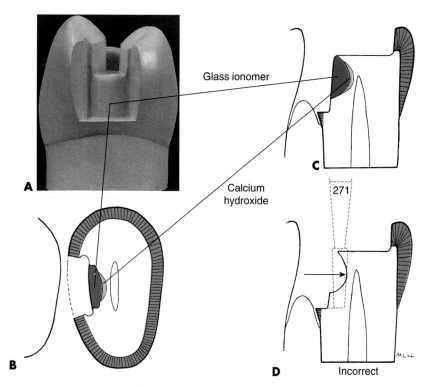

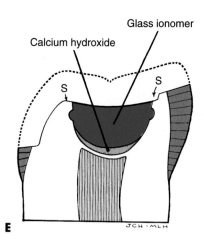

FIG. 20-11 **A** to **C,** Completed base for treatment of deep caries. **D,** Never deepen entire axial wall with side of fissure bur to remove caries because pulp will be greatly irritated from resulting closeness of gingivoaxial region of preparation. **E,** Cement base placed in deep excavation on mandibular molar. Note flat seats in sound dentin (*S*) that are required for adequate resistance form.

The future need of root canal therapy is a possibility for any tooth treated for deep caries that approximates or exposes the pulp. When treating a tooth that has had such extensive caries, consider (1) reducing all cusps to cover the occlusal surface with metal, for better distribution of occlusal loads and (2) adding skirts to the preparation to augment resistance form because teeth are more prone to fracture after root canal therapy.

Preparation of Bevels and Flares. After the cement base (where indicated) is completed, the slender, flame-shaped, fine-grit diamond instrument is used to bevel the occlusal and gingival margins and to apply the secondary flare on the distolingual and distofacial walls. This should result in 30- to 40-degree marginal metal on the inlay (Figs. 20-12, *H,* 20-13, *J,* and 20-14, *B*). This cavosurface design helps seal and protect the margins and results in a strong enamel margin with an angle of 140 to 150 degrees. A cavosurface enamel angle of more than 150 degrees is incorrect because it results in a less defined enamel margin (finish line), and the marginal cast metal alloy is too thin and weak if its angle is less than 30 degrees. Conversely, if the enamel margin is 140 degrees or less, the metal is too bulky and difficult to burnish when its angle is greater than 40 degrees (see Fig. 20-14, *F*).

Usually it is helpful to insert a gingival retraction cord of suitable diameter into the gingival sulcus adjacent to the gingival margin, and leave it in place for several minutes just before the use of the flame-shaped diamond instrument on the proximal margins (see Fig. 20-12, *A* through *C*). The cord should be small enough in di-

ameter to permit relatively easy insertion and to preclude excessive pressure against the gingival tissue, yet it should be large enough to widen the sulcus to about 0.5 mm. Immediately before the flame-shaped diamond instrument is used, the cord may be removed, resulting in an open sulcus that improves visibility for beveling the gingival margin and helps prevent injury and subsequent hemorrhage of the gingival tissue. However, some operators prefer to leave the cord in the sulcus while placing the gingival bevel.

Using the flame-shaped diamond instrument, rotating at high speed, prepare the lingual secondary flare (see Figs. 20-12, *D* through *F,* and 20-13, *A*). Approach from the lingual embrasure, as shown in Fig. 20-12, *F,* moving the instrument mesiofacially. Compare the direction of the distolingual wall and the position of the distolingual margin before and after this extension (see Figs. 20-8, *G,* and 20-13, *A*). Notice in Fig. 20-13, *A,* that the distolingual wall extends from the linguoaxial line angle into the lingual embrasure in two planes. The first is termed the lingual *primary flare;* the second is named the lingual *secondary flare.* During this (secondary) flaring operation, the long axis of the instrument is held nearly parallel to the line of draw, with only a slight tilting mesially and lingually for assurance of draft (see Fig. 20-12, *D* and *E*), and the direction of translation of the instrument is that which results in a marginal metal angle of 40 degrees (see Figs. 20-12, *F,* and 20-13, *J*).

Bevel the gingival margin by moving the instrument facially along the gingival margin (see Figs. 20-12, *G,* and 20-13, *A*). While cutting the *gingival bevel,* reduce the

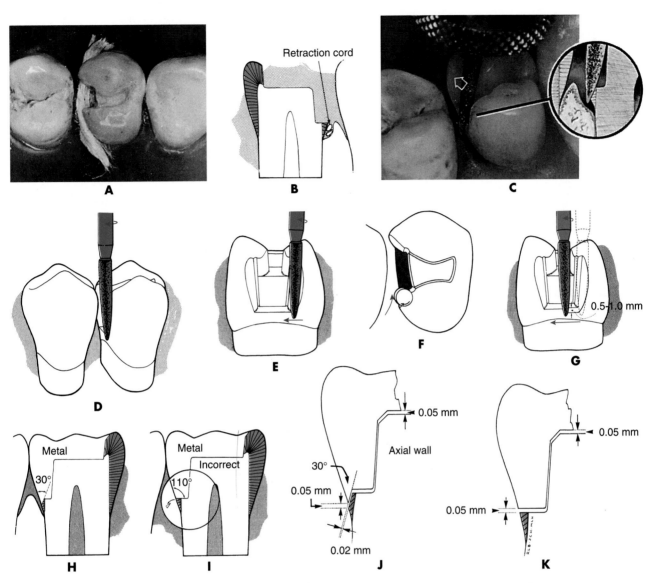

FIG. 20-12 A and B, Retraction cord is inserted in gingival sulcus and left for several minutes. C, "Open" gingival sulcus after cord shown in A is removed facilitates beveling gingival margin with diamond instrument. D to F, Diamond instrument preparing lingual secondary flare. Large arrow in F depicts direction of translation. G, Beveling gingival margin. Note in C the mesial tilting of diamond instrument to produce a bevel properly directed to result in 30-degree marginal metal as shown in H. H, Properly directed gingival bevel resulting in 30-degree marginal metal. I, Failing to bevel gingival margin results in weak margin formed by undermined rods (note easily displaced wedge of enamel) and 110-degree marginal metal, an angular design unsuitable for burnishing. J, Lap, sliding fit of prescribed bevel metal decreases 50-μm error of seating to 20 μm. K, A 50-μm error of seating will produce an equal cement line of 50 μm along unbeveled gingival margin.

rotational speed to increase the sense of touch; otherwise overbeveling may result. The instrument should be tilted slightly mesially to produce a gingival bevel with the correct steepness to result in 30-degree marginal metal (see Fig. 20-12, *C, H,* and *J*). If the instrument is not tilted in this manner, the bevel will be too steep, resulting in gingival bevel metal that is too thin (less than 30-degree metal) and thus too weak. Although the instrument is tilted mesially, its long axis must not tilt fa-

cially or lingually (see Fig. 20-12, *G*). The *gingival bevel should be 0.5 to 1 mm wide* and should blend with the lingual secondary flare.

Complete the gingival bevel, and then prepare the facial secondary flare (see Fig. 20-13, *A* through *F*). The long axis of the instrument during this secondary flare is again returned nearly to the line of draw with only a small tilting mesially and facially, and the direction of translation of the instrument is that which results in

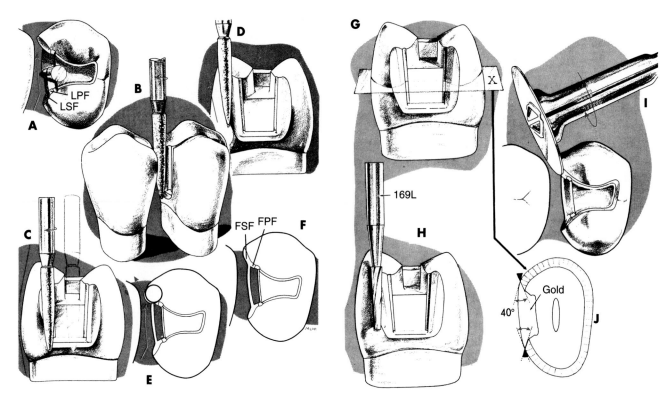

FIG. 20-13 **A,** Occlusal view of Fig. 20-12, *G. LSF* and *LPF* designate lingual secondary and lingual primary flares. **B** to **D,** Preparing facial secondary flare. Large arrows in **B, D,** and **E** depict direction of translation. **F,** Completed facial secondary flare. *FSF* and *FPF* designate facial secondary and facial primary flares. **G,** Distal view of **F.** *x,* Plane of cross-section shown in **J.** Preparing secondary flare with the No. 169L carbide bur **(H)** or with paper disc **(I). J,** Secondary flares are directed to result in 40-degree marginal metal and 140-degree marginal enamel.

40-degree marginal metal (see Fig. 20-13, *E* and *J*). When the adjacent proximal surface (mesial of the second premolar) is not being prepared, care must be exercised neither to abrade the adjacent tooth nor to overextend the distofacial margin. To help in preventing such abrasion or overextension, the instrument may be raised occlusally (thus using the narrower portion at its tip end) to complete the most facial portion of the wall and margin (see Fig. 20-13, *D*). Also, the more slender No. 169L carbide bur may be used rather than the flame-shaped diamond instrument (see Fig. 20-13, *H*). Moreover, the No. 169L bur produces an extremely smooth surface to the secondary flare and a smooth, straight distofacial margin. When access permits, a fine-grit sandpaper disc may be used on the facial and lingual walls and margins of the proximal preparation, especially when minimal extension of the facial margin is desired (see Fig. 20-13, *I*). This produces smooth walls and helps create respective margins that are straight (not ragged) and sound.

In the flaring and beveling of the proximal margins, as described in the previous paragraphs, the procedure

began at the lingual surface and proceeded to the facial surface; however, the direction may be reversed, starting at the facial surface and moving toward the lingual surface. On the mesiofacial surface of maxillary premolars and first molars where extension of the facial margin should be minimal, it is usually desirable to use the lingual-to-facial direction.

The gingival bevel serves the following purposes:

- *Weak enamel is removed.* If the gingival margin is in the enamel, it would be weak if not beveled because of the gingival declination of the enamel rods (see Fig. 20-12, *I*).
- *The bevel results in 30-degree metal that is burnishable* (on the die) because of its angular design (see Fig. 20-12, *H*). Bulky 110-degree metal along an unbeveled margin is not burnishable (see Fig. 20-12, *I*).
- *A lap, sliding fit is produced at the gingival margin* (see Fig. 20-12, *J*). This helps improve the fit of the casting in this region. With the prescribed gingival bevel, if the inlay fails to seat by 50 μm, the void between the bevel metal and the gingival bevel on

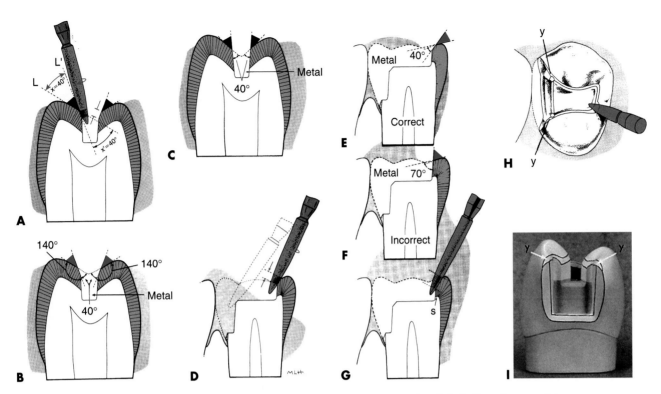

FIG. 20-14 A, Diamond instrument beveling occlusal margin when it is indicated to result in 40-degree marginal metal as shown in B. Angles x and x' are equal because opposite angles are equal when two lines (L and L') intersect. Therefore diamond instrument is always directed so that an angle of 40 degrees is made by side of instrument and external enamel surface. B, Occlusal marginal metal is approximately 40 degrees in cross-section, thus making enamel angle 140 degrees. C, When cuspal inclines are steep, no beveling is indicated inasmuch as 40-degree metal will result without beveling. D, Beveling mesial margin and axiopulpal line angle. E, Mesial bevel is directed correctly to result in 40-degree marginal metal. F, Unbeveled mesial margin is incorrect because it results both in weak enamel margin and unburnishable marginal metal. G, To conserve dentin support (s), occlusal defects on marginal ridge are included in outline form by applying cavosurface bevel, which may be wider than usual, when necessary. H, Occlusal view of G. Preparing 140-degree cavosurface enamel angle at regions labeled y usually dictates that occlusal bevel be extended over marginal ridges into secondary flares. I, Distal view of H.

the tooth may be as small as 20 μm; however, failure to apply such a bevel would result in a void (and a cement line) as great as the failure to seat (see Fig. 20-12, K).

Uninterrupted blending of the gingival bevel into the secondary flares of the distolingual and distofacial walls results in the distolingual and distofacial margins joining the gingival margin in a desirable arc of a small circle; also, the gingivofacial and gingivolingual line angles no longer extend to the marginal outline. *If such line angles are allowed to extend to the preparation outline, early failure may follow because of an "open" margin, dissolution of exposed cement, and eventual leakage, all potentially resulting in caries.*

The secondary flare is necessary for several reasons: (1) The secondary flaring of the proximal walls extends the margins into the embrasures, making these margins more self-cleansing and more accessible to finishing procedures during the inlay insertion appointment, and does so with conservation of the dentin. (2) The direction of the flare results in 40-degree marginal metal (see Fig. 20-13, J). Metal with this angular design is burnishable; however, metal shaped at a larger angle is unsatisfactory for burnishing; metal with an angle less than 30 degrees is too thin and weak, with a corresponding enamel margin that is too indefinite and ragged. (3) A more blunted and stronger enamel margin is produced because of the secondary flare.

In a later section, the secondary flare is omitted for esthetic reasons on the mesiofacial proximal wall of preparations on premolars and first molars of the maxillary dentition. In this location the wall is completed

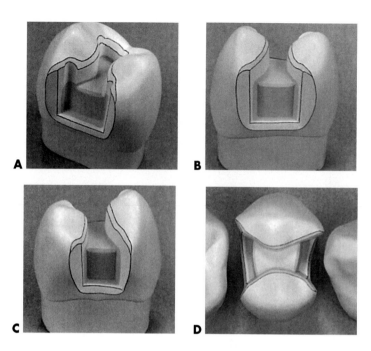

FIG. **20-15 A,** Completed DO preparation for inlay. **B,** MOD preparation for inlay on maxillary right first premolar, DO view. **C,** Same preparation as in **B,** MO view. **D,** Same preparation as in **B,** occlusal view. Note absence, for esthetic reasons, of secondary flare on mesiofacial aspect and minimal extension of mesiofacial margin.

with minimal extension by using either hand instruments (straight or binangle chisel) followed by a fine-grit sandpaper disc or very thin rotary instruments.

The flame-shaped, fine-grit diamond instrument also is used for *occlusal bevels.* The width of the cavosurface bevel on the occlusal margin should be approximately one fourth the depth of the respective wall (see Fig. 20-14, *A* and *B*). The exception to the rule is when a wider bevel is desired to include an enamel defect (see Fig. 20-14, *G* and *H*). The resulting occlusal marginal metal of the inlay should be 40-degree metal; thus the occlusal marginal enamel is 140-degree enamel (see Fig. 20-14, *B* and *E*). Beveling the occlusal margins in this manner increases the strength of the marginal enamel and helps seal and protect the margins. While beveling the occlusal margins, a guide to diamond positioning is to maintain an approximate 40-degree angle between the side of the instrument and the external enamel surface. This also indicates when an occlusal bevel is necessary (see Fig. 20-14, *A*). For example, if the cusp inclines are so steep that the diamond instrument, when positioned at a 40-degree angle to the external enamel surface is parallel with the enamel preparation wall, then no bevel is indicated (see Fig. 20-14, *C*). Using this technique demonstrates that margins on the proximal marginal ridges always require a cavosurface bevel (see Fig. 20-14, *D* and *I*). Failure to apply a bevel in these regions leaves the enamel margin weak and subject to injury by fracture, both before the inlay insertion appointment and during the try-in of the inlay when burnishing the marginal metal. Also, the failure to bevel margins on the marginal ridges results in metal alloy that is difficult to burnish because it is too bulky (see Fig. 20-14, *F*). Similarly, the importance of extending the occlusal bevel to include those portions of the occlusal margin that cross

over the marginal ridge cannot be overemphasized (see Fig. 20-14, *H* and *I*). These margins are beveled to result in 40-degree marginal metal. Otherwise fracture of the enamel margin in such stress-vulnerable regions may occur in the interim between the preparation and the cementation appointment.

The diamond instrument also is used to lightly bevel the axiopulpal line angle (see Fig. 20-14, *D*). Such a bevel provides a thicker and therefore stronger wax pattern at this critical region.

Thus the desirable metal angle at the margins of inlays is 40 degrees, except at the gingival margins, where the metal angle should be 30 degrees. The completed preparation is illustrated in Fig. 20-15, *A.*

Modifications in Inlay Tooth Preparations. Again, realizing that the indications for small inlays are rare, the following sections provide procedural information that may promote better understanding of their applications in more complex and larger inlay or onlay restorations.

Mesioocclusodistal Preparation. If a marginal ridge is severely weakened because of excessive extension, the preparation outline often should be altered to include the proximal surface. For example, the DO preparation illustrated in the previous section would be extended to a mesioocclusodistal (MOD) preparation (Fig. 20-16, *A* through *C*; see also Fig. 20-15, *B* through *D*). The decision to extend the preparation in this manner calls for clinical judgment as to whether the remaining marginal ridge will withstand occlusal forces without fracture. A fortunate factor in favor of not extending the preparation is that such ridge enamel is usually composed of *gnarled enamel* and thus is stronger than it appears.

Obviously, caries present on both proximal surfaces will result in a MOD preparation and restoration. The

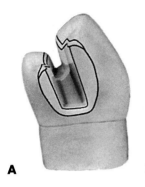 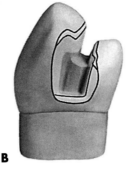 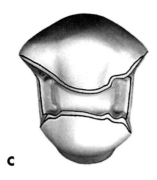

FIG. **20-16** Mandibular first premolar prepared for MOD inlay, distal view (**A**), mesial view (**B**), and occlusal view (**C**).

only difference in technique as described previously is the inclusion of the other proximal surface.

Modifications of Class II Preparation for Esthetics. For esthetic reasons, minimal flare is desired for the mesiofacial proximal wall in the maxillary premolars and first molars in Class II cast metal preparations (see Fig. 20-15, *D*). The mesiofacial margin is minimally extended facially of contact to such a position that the margin is barely visible from a facial viewing position. To accomplish this, the secondary flare is omitted, and the wall and margin are developed with either (1) a chisel or enamel hatchet and final smoothing with a fine-grit paper disc, or (2) a narrow diamond or bur when access permits.

Facial or Lingual Surface Groove Extension. Sometimes a faulty facial groove (fissure) on the occlusal surface is continuous with a faulty facial surface groove (mandibular molars), or a faulty distal oblique groove on the occlusal surface is continuous with a faulty lingual surface groove (maxillary molar). This requires extension of the preparation outline to include the fissure to its termination (Fig. 20-17; see also Fig. 20-19, *C*). Occasionally the operator may extend further gingivally than the fissure length to improve retention form. Such groove extensions, when sufficiently long, are very effective for increasing retention. Likewise, this extension may be indicated to provide sufficient retention form even though the facial or lingual surface grooves are not fissured.

For extension onto the facial surface, use the No. 271 carbide bur held parallel to the line of draw, and extend through the facial ridge (see Fig. 20-17, *A* and *B*). The depth of the cut should be 1.5 mm. The floor (pulpal wall) should be continuous with the pulpal wall of the occlusal portion of the preparation (see Fig. 20-17, *D*).

With the bur still aligned with the path of draw, use the side of the bur to cut the facial surface portion of this extension (see Fig. 20-17, *C*). The diameter of the bur serves as a depth gauge for the axial wall, which is in dentin. The blade portion of the No. 271 bur is 0.8 mm in diameter at its tip end and 1 mm at the neck; the axial wall depth should approximate 1 mm or slightly more. The bur should be tilted lingually as it is drawn occlusally, to develop the uniform depth of the axial

wall (see Fig. 20-17, *D*). The same principles apply for extension of a lingual surface groove.

When a facial or lingual groove is included, it also must be beveled. With the flame-shaped, fine-grit diamond instrument, bevel the gingival margin (using no more than one third the depth of the gingival floor) to provide for 30-degree marginal metal (see Fig. 20-17, *E*). Apply a light bevel on the mesial and distal margins that will be continuous with the occlusal and gingival bevels and will result in 40-degree metal at these margins (see Fig. 20-17, *F* and *G*). The bevel width around the extended groove will be approximately 0.5 mm.

Class II Preparation for Abutment Teeth and Extension Gingivally to Include Root-Surface Lesions. Extending the facial, lingual, and gingival margins may be indicated on the proximal surfaces of abutments for removable partial dentures to increase the surface area for development of guiding planes. In addition, the occlusal outline form must be wide enough faciolingually to accommodate any contemplated rest preparation(s) without involving the margins of the restoration. These extensions may be accomplished by simply increasing the width of the bevels.

The following modified preparation is recommended when further gingival extension is indicated to include a root lesion on the proximal surface. The gingival extension should be accomplished primarily by lengthening the gingival bevel, especially when preparing a tooth that has a longer clinical crown than normal as a result of gingival recession. It is necessary to only slightly extend (gingivally) the gingival floor, and although the axial wall consequently must be moved pulpally, this should be minimal. If additional extension of the gingival floor is necessary, it should not be as wide pulpally as when the floor level is at a normal position (Fig. 20-18, *A*). These considerations are necessary because of the draft requirement and because the tooth is smaller apically. Extending the preparation gingivally without these modifications would result in a dangerous encroachment of the axial wall on the pulp (see Fig. 20-18, *B*).

Maxillary First Molar with Unaffected, Strong Oblique Ridge. When a maxillary first molar is to be restored, consideration should be given to preserving the

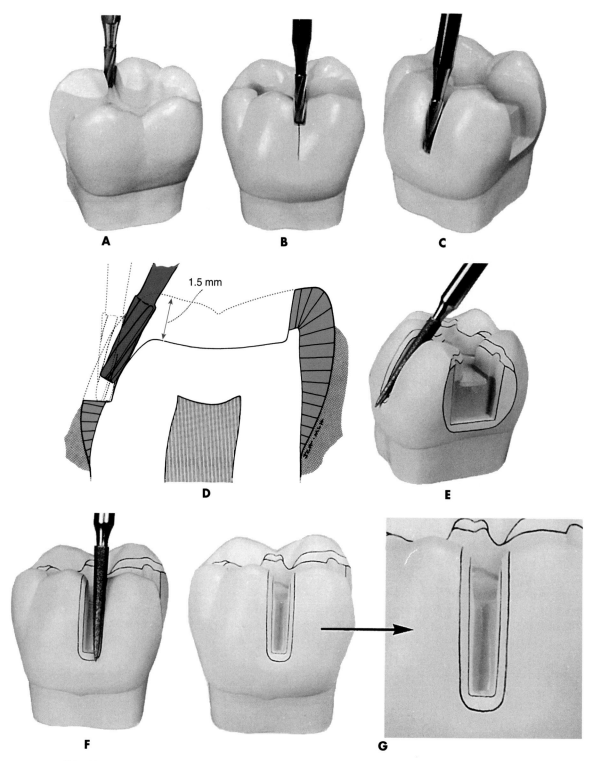

FIG. 20-17 A to C, Extending to include occlusal fissure that is continuous with facial fissure on facial surface. D, Section of C. Beveling gingival margin (E) and mesial and distal margins (F) of fissure extension. G, Beveling completed.

Correct   Incorrect

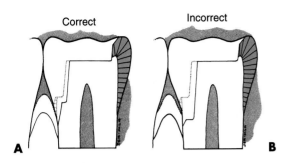

A   **B**

FIG. **20-18** Modifications of preparation when extending to include proximal root-surface lesions after moderate gingival recession. **A,** Correct. **B,** Incorrect. Note decreased dentinal protection of pulp, compared with management depicted in **A.**

oblique ridge if it is strong and unaffected, especially if only one proximal surface is carious. A mesioocclusal (MO) preparation for an inlay is illustrated in Fig. 20-19, *A* and *B.*

If a distal surface lesion appears subsequently to the insertion of a MO restoration, the tooth may be prepared for a distoocclusolingual inlay (see Fig. 20-19, *H* and *I*). The distoocclusolingual restoration that caps the distolingual cusp is preferable to the DO restoration because it protects the miniature distolingual cusp from subsequent fracture. The distoocclusolingual preparation requires diligent application to develop satisfactory retention and resistance forms. Retention form is attained by: (1) creating a maximum of 2-degree occlusal divergence of the vertical walls, (2) accentuating some line angles, and (3) extending the lingual surface groove to create an axial wall height in this extension of at least 2.5 mm occlusogingivally. Proper resistance form dictates: (1) routine capping of the distolingual cusp and (2) maintaining sound tooth structure between the lingual surface groove extension and the distolingual wall of the proximal boxing.

To prepare the distoocclusolingual preparation, first reduce the distolingual cusp with the side of the No. 271 carbide bur. The cusp should be reduced a uniform 1.5 mm. Next prepare the remaining occlusal step of the preparation with the No. 271 carbide bur. Then prepare the proximal box portion of the preparation. Prepare the lingual groove extension only after the position of the distolingual wall of the proximal boxing is established. This permits the operator to judge the best position of the lingual surface groove extension to maintain a minimum of 3 mm of sound tooth structure between this extension and the distolingual wall. If this is not possible because of extensive caries, then a more extensive type of preparation may be indicated (one that crosses the oblique ridge). Use the side of the No. 271 carbide bur to produce the lingual surface groove extension (see Fig. 20-19, *C*). The diameter of the bur is the gauge for the depth (pulpally) of the axial wall in this extension, and the occlusogingival dimension of this axial wall is a minimum of 2.5 mm. With the end of this bur, also es-

tablish a 2-mm depth to that portion of the pulpal floor that connects the proximal boxing to the lingual surface groove extension. This additional depth to the pulpal floor helps strengthen the wax pattern and casting in later steps of fabrication. This should create a definite 0.5-mm step from the reduced distolingual cusp to the pulpal floor.

Using the No. 169L carbide bur, increase retention form in the distoocclusolingual preparation by: (1) creating mesioaxial and distoaxial grooves in the lingual surface groove extension (see Fig. 20-19, *D*) and (2) preparing facial and lingual retention grooves in the distal boxing (see Fig. 20-19, *E*).

Use the flame-shaped, fine-grit diamond instrument to bevel the proximal gingival margin and to prepare the secondary flares on the proximal enamel walls, as well as to bevel the lingual margins. A lingual *counterbevel* is prepared on the distolingual cusp that is generous in width and results in 30-degree metal at the margin (see Fig. 20-19, *F*). Occlusion should be checked at this point because the counterbevel should be sufficiently wide to extend beyond any occlusal contacts, either in MI or during mandibular movements. The bevel on the gingival margin of the lingual extension should be 0.5 mm wide and should provide for a 30-degree metal angle. The bevels on the mesial and distal margins of the lingual extension are also approximately 0.5 mm wide and result in 40-degree marginal metal.

Fissures in the Facial and Lingual Cusp Ridges or Marginal Ridges. In the preparation of Class II preparations for inlays, facial and lingual occlusal fissures may extend nearly to, or through, the respective facial and lingual cusp ridges, but not onto the facial or lingual surface. Proper outline form dictates that the preparation margin should not cross such fissures, but should be extended to include them. For example, when preparing the occlusal step portion of the preparation, initially extend along the lingual fissure with the No. 271 carbide bur until only 2 mm of tooth structure remains between the bur and the lingual surface of the tooth. Additional lingual extension at this time is incorrect because it may remove the supporting dentin unnecessarily (Fig. 20-20, *A* and *B*). If this extension almost includes the length of the fissure, remember that additional extension is achieved later by virtue of the occlusal bevel; moreover, this bevel may be wider than conventional if the remaining fissure can be eliminated by such a wider bevel (see Fig. 20-20, *C*). Also recall that enameloplasty sometimes may eliminate the end portion of the fissure and provide a smooth enamel surface where once there was a fault, thus reducing the extent of the required extension (see Fig. 20-20, *D*). Therefore if possible, include the fissure in the preparation outline without extending the margin to the height of the ridge. If, however, the occlusal bevel places the margin on the height of the ridge, then the marginal enamel likely is

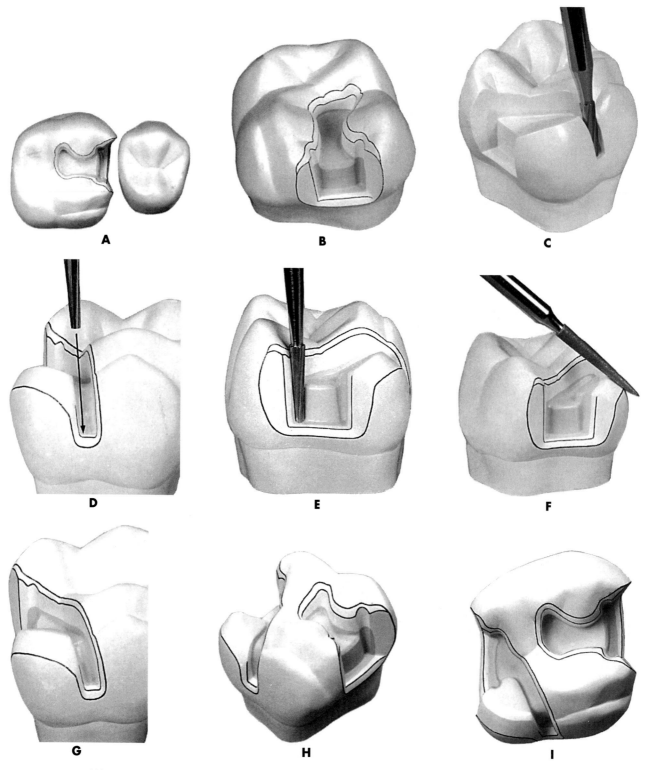

FIG. 20-19 **A** and **B,** MO preparation on maxillary molar having unaffected oblique ridge. **C,** Preparing lingual groove' extension of distoocclusolingual preparation. Cutting retention grooves in lingual surface extension (**D**) and distal box (**E**). **F** and **G,** Completed distoocclusolingual preparation on maxillary molar having unaffected oblique ridge. **H** and **I,** Preparations for treating both proximal surfaces of maxillary molar having strong, unaffected oblique ridge.

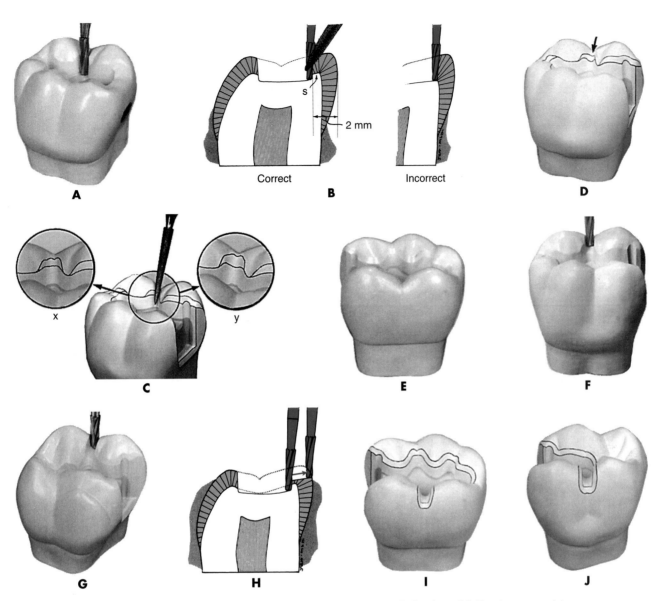

FIG. 20-20 **A,** Extending to include lingual (occlusal) fissure. **B,** Section of **A.** Dentin support (*s*) of lingual cusp ridge should not be removed. Bevel can provide additional extension to include fissure that does not extend to crest of ridge. **C,** Completed preparations with standard width bevel (*x*) and with wider bevel to include groove defect that nearly extends to ridge height (*y*). **D,** Completed preparation illustrating enameloplasty for elimination of shallow fissure extending to or through lingual ridge height. (Compare smooth, saucer-shaped lingual ridge contour with **C,** where no enameloplasty has been performed.) **E,** Fissure remaining through lingual ridge following unsuccessful enameloplasty. *This indicates procedures subsequently illustrated.* Extending preparation if enameloplasty has not eliminated fissure in lingual ridge (**F**) or facial ridge (**G**). **H,** Section of **F.** Completed preparations after beveling margins of extensions through lingual ridge (**I**) and facial ridge (**J**).

weak because of both its sharpness and the inclination of the enamel rods in this region. Therefore the preparation outline should be extended just onto the facial or lingual surface (see Fig. 20-20, *I* and *J*). Such extension onto the facial or lingual surface would also be indicated if the fissure still remains through the ridge after enameloplasty (see Fig. 20-20, *E*).

When necessary, extension through a cusp ridge is accomplished by cutting through the ridge at a depth of

1 mm with the No. 271 carbide bur (see Fig. 20-20, *F* and *G*). Bevel the margins of the extension with the flame shaped, fine-grit diamond instrument to provide for the desired 40-degree marginal metal on the occlusal, mesial, and distal margins and for 30-degree marginal metal on the gingival margin (see Fig. 20-20, *C, D, I,* and *J*).

In the same manner, manage the fissures that may extend into or through a proximal marginal ridge, assuming that the proximal surface otherwise was not to be

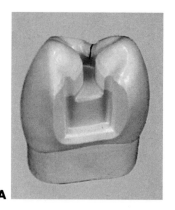
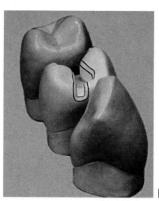

A

B

FIG. **20-21** Fissure that remains on mesial marginal ridge after unsuccessful enameloplasty (**A**) is treated (**B**) in same manner as lingual or facial ridge fissures (see Fig. 20-20, *I* and *J*).

included in the outline form and that such fissure management does not extend the preparation outline near the adjacent tooth contact. This treatment particularly applies to a mesial fissure of the maxillary first premolar (Fig. 20-21). If this procedure extends the margin near or into the contact, the outline form on the affected proximal surface must be extended to include the contact, as for a conventional proximal surface preparation.

Capping Cusps. The facial and lingual margins on the occlusal surface frequently must be extended toward the cusp tips to the extent of existing restorative materials and to uncover caries (Fig. 20-22, *B* and *C*). Undermined occlusal enamel should be removed because it is weak; moreover, removing such enamel provides access for proper excavation of caries. When the occlusal outline is extended up the cusp slopes more than half the distance from any primary occlusal groove (central, facial, or lingual) to the cusp tip, capping the cusp should be considered. If the preparation outline is extended two thirds of this distance or more, capping the cusp is usually necessary to: (1) protect the weak, underlying cuspal structure from fracture caused by masticatory force and (2) remove the occlusal margin from a region subjected to heavy stress and wear (see Fig. 20-22, *A* and *B*). At this point in preparation the pulpal floor, depth can be increased from 1.5 mm to 2 mm. This additional pulpal depth ensures sufficient reduction in an area that is often underreduced, and will result in greater strength and rigidity to the wax pattern and cast restoration. The following section describes the technique for capping less than all of the cusps of a posterior tooth.

Reduce the Cusps for Capping as Soon as the Indication for Such Capping Is Determined Because This Improves Access and Visibility for Subsequent Steps in Preparation. If a cusp is in infraocclusion of the desired occlusal plane before reduction, then the amount of cusp reduction is less and needs only to be that which provides the required *clearance* with the desired occlusal plane. Before reducing the surface, prepare *depth gauge grooves (depth cuts)* with the side of the No. 271 carbide bur (see Fig. 20-22, *D*). Such depth cuts should help to prevent thin spots in the restoration.

With the depth cuts serving as guides, complete the cusp reduction with the side of the carbide bur (see Fig. 20-22, *E*). The reduction should provide for a uniform 1.5 mm of metal thickness over the reduced cusp. On maxillary premolars and first molars, the reduction should be minimal (i.e., 0.75 to 1 mm) on the facial cusp ridge to decrease the display of metal. This reduction should increase progressively to 1.5 mm toward the center of the tooth to help provide rigidity to the capping metal (Fig. 20-23, *A* and *C*).

If only one of the two lingual cusps of a molar is reduced for capping, the reduction must extend to just include the lingual groove between the reduced and unreduced cusps. This reduction should terminate with a distinct vertical wall that has a height that is the same as the prescribed cusp reduction. Applying the bur vertically, as shown in Fig. 20-22, *F*, should help establish a vertical wall of proper depth and direction. Similar principles apply when only one of the facial cusps is to be reduced (see Figs. 20-22, *L*, and 20-23, *B*).

A bevel of generous width is prepared on the facial (lingual) margin of a reduced cusp with the flame-shaped, fine-grit diamond instrument (with the exception of esthetically prominent areas). This bevel is referred to as a *reverse bevel* or *counterbevel*. The width varies because it usually should extend beyond any occlusal contact with the opponent teeth, either in MI or during mandibular movements (see Fig. 20-26, *C*). It should be at an angle that results in 30-degree marginal metal (see Fig. 20-22, *G* and *H*). The exception is the facial margin on maxillary premolars and the first molar where esthetic requirements dictate only a blunting and smoothing of the enamel margin (a *stub margin*) by the light application of a fine-grit sandpaper disc or the fine-grit diamond instrument (flame-shaped) held at a right angle to the facial surface (see Fig. 20-23, *C*). Slightly round any sharp external corners to strengthen them and reduce the problems they may generate in future steps (see Fig. 20-22, *J* and *K*).

Cusp reduction appreciably decreases retention form because of decreasing the height of the vertical walls; consequently, proximal retention grooves usually are recommended (see Fig. 20-22, *I*). It may be necessary to

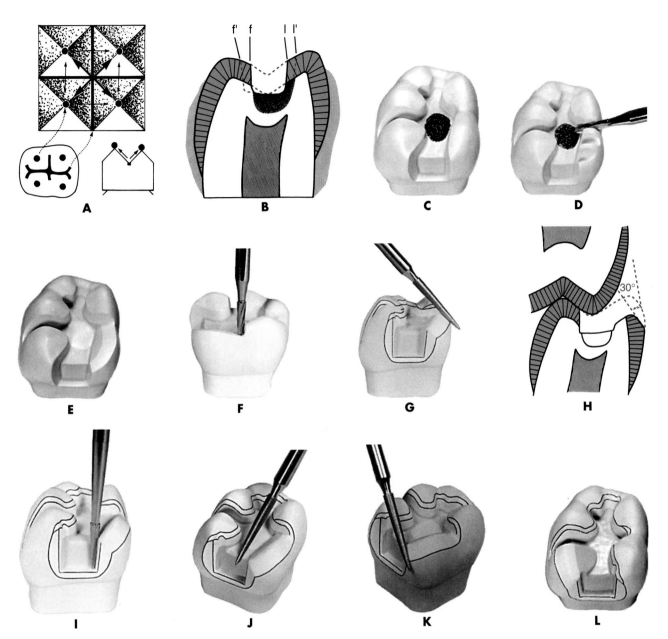

FIG. **20-22** **A,** When extension of occlusal margin is one half the distance from any point on primary grooves (*cross*) toward cusp tip (*dot*), capping the cusp should be considered; when this distance is two thirds or more, capping the cusp is usually indicated. **B,** *l'* is midway between central groove and lingual cusp tip. *f'* is midway between central groove and facial cusp tip. When enamel at *l* and *f* is undermined by caries, respective walls must be extended to dotted lines *l'* and *f'* for caries to be uncovered. Then cusps should be reduced for capping. **C,** Extension to uncover caries indicates that mesiolingual cusp should be reduced for capping. **D,** Depth cuts. **E,** Reduced mesiolingual cusp. Note that caries has been removed and cement base has been placed. **F,** Applying bur vertically helps establish vertical wall that barely includes lingual groove. **G,** Counterbeveling reduced cusp. **H,** Section of counterbevel. **I,** Improving retention form by cutting proximal retention grooves. Preparation is complete except for rounding axiopulpal line angle (**J**) and rounding junction of counterbevel and secondary flare (**K**). Facial surface groove extension improves both retention and resistance forms. **L,** Preparation when reducing one of two facial cusps on mandibular molar.

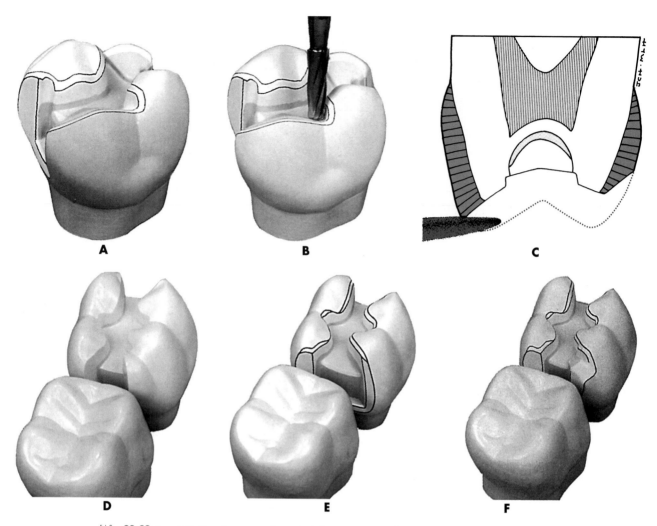

FIG. **20-23 A** and **B,** Capping one of two facial cusps on maxillary molar. **C,** Blunting margin of reduced cusp when esthetics is major consideration. **D** to **F,** Margin shown crossing distal cusp in **D** indicates treatment illustrated in either **E** or **F.**

increase retention form by extending facial and lingual groove regions of the respective surfaces, or by *collar* and *skirt* features presented in the later section. These additional retention features also provide the desired resistance form against forces tending to split the tooth (see Fig. 20-22, *K*; see also Fig. 20-28).

The principles stated in the preceding paragraphs may be applied in the treatment of the distal cusp of the mandibular first molar when preparing a MOD preparation (see Fig. 20-23, *D*). Proper extension of the distofacial margin usually places the occlusal margin in a region subjected to heavy masticatory forces and wear. Satisfactory treatment usually dictates either (1) extending the distofacial margin (and wall) slightly mesial of the distofacial groove (see Fig. 20-23, *E*) or (2) capping the remaining portion of the distal cusp (see Fig. 20-23, *F*).

After cusp reduction, visually verify that the occlusal clearances are sufficient. A wax interocclusal record is helpful when checking occlusal clearances, especially in areas difficult to visualize, such as in the central groove/lingual cusp regions. To make a wax "bite," first dry the

preparation(s) free of visible moisture; do not, however, desiccate the dentin (Fig. 20-24, *A*). Next lightly press a portion of softened, low-fusing inlay wax over the *prepared* tooth (teeth); then immediately request the patient to close into the soft wax and slide the teeth in all directions (see Fig. 20-24, *B* through *F*). During the mandibular movements, observe to verify that (1) the patient moves in right lateral, left lateral, and protrusive movements; (2) the adjacent unprepared teeth are in contact with the opposing teeth; (3) the wax in the preparation is stable (not loose and rocking); and (4) the wax is not in infraocclusion. Now cool and carefully remove the wax. Hold it up to a light, and note the degree of light transmitted. With experience, this is a good indicator of the thickness of the wax. An alternative method is to use wax calipers, or to section the wax to verify its thickness. Insufficient thickness calls for more reduction in the indicated area before proceeding.

Including Portions of the Facial and Lingual Smooth Surfaces Affected by Caries or Other Injury. When portions of both a facial (lingual) smooth surface

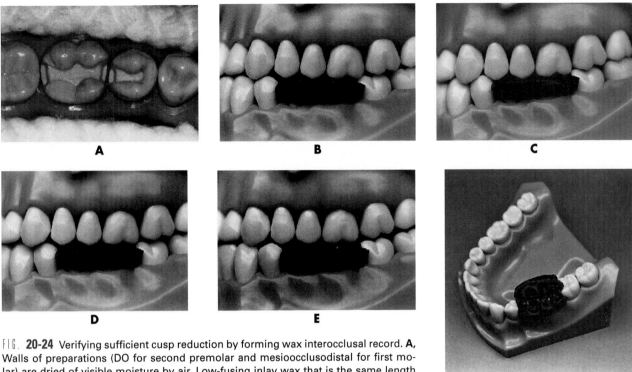

FIG. **20-24** Verifying sufficient cusp reduction by forming wax interocclusal record. **A,** Walls of preparations (DO for second premolar and mesioocclusodistal for first molar) are dried of visible moisture by air. Low-fusing inlay wax that is the same length as mesiodistal length of inlay preparations is softened and pressed over prepared teeth. Patient moves mandible into all occlusal positions, left lateral (**B**), through MI (**C**), to right lateral (**D**) and protrusive (**E**). **F,** Completed interocclusal record.

and a proximal surface are affected by caries or some other factor (e.g., fracture) (Fig. 20-25, *A* and *I*), the treatment may be a large inlay, an onlay, a three-quarter crown, a full crown, or multiple amalgam or composite restorations. Generally, if carious portions are extensive, the choice between the previously listed cast metal restorations is determined by the degree of tooth circumference involved. A full crown is indicated if both the lingual and facial smooth surfaces are defective, especially if the tooth is a second or third molar. When only a portion of the facial smooth surface is carious and the lingual surfaces of the teeth are conspicuously free of caries, an MODFL inlay or onlay with a lingual groove extension is chosen over the crown because the former is more favorable to the health of the gingival tissues and more conservative in the removal of tooth structure. Often this is the treatment choice for the maxillary second molar, which may exhibit caries or decalcification on the distofacial surface as a result of poor oral hygiene (due to poor access) in this region (see Fig. 20-25).

In the preparation of the maxillary molar referred to in the preceding paragraph, usually the mesiofacial and distolingual cusps, as well as the distofacial cusp, are reduced for capping. If the distofacial cusp defect is primarily shallow decalcification, the flame-shaped diamond instrument is used to both reduce the involved facial surface and distofacial corner approximately the depth of the enamel and to establish the gingival mar-

gin of this reduction apical to the affected area (see Fig. 20-25, *D*). This instrument also is used to terminate the facial surface reduction in a definite facial margin running gingivoocclusally and in a manner to provide for 40-degree metal at this margin (see Fig. 20-25, *E*).

If the distofacial defect is more extensive and deeper into the tooth (see Fig. 20-25, *I*), thereby eliminating the opportunity for an effective distal box or groove (no facial wall possible), then the No. 271 carbide bur should be used to cut a gingival shoulder extending from the distal gingival floor around to include the affected facial surface. This *shoulder* partially provides the desired resistance form. (A gingival floor, perpendicular to occlusal force, has been provided in lieu of the missing pulpal wall in the distofacial cusp region.) Use the No. 271 bur to also create a nearly vertical wall in the remaining facial enamel (see Fig. 20-25, *J*). The width of the shoulder should be the diameter of the end of the cutting instrument. The vertical walls should have the appropriate degree of draft to contribute to retention form. Then the faciogingival and facial margins are beveled with the flame-shaped, fine-grit diamond instrument to provide 30-degree metal at the gingival margin (see Fig. 20-25, *K*) and 40-degree metal along the facial margin (see Fig. 20-25, *L*). These two bevels should blend together (see *x* in Fig. 20-25, *M*), and the faciogingival bevel should be continuous with the gingival bevel on the distal surface. Additional retention and resistance form is indicated for this preparation and can be developed by an arbitrary lingual groove extension (see Fig. 20-25, *N*), or a distolingual skirt extension (see Fig. 20-25, *O* and *P*). These preparation features resist forces normally opposed by the missing distofacial wall and help protect the restored tooth from fracture injury.

TOOTH PREPARATION FOR CAST METAL ONLAYS

The preceding sections have presented basic tooth preparation principles and techniques for small, simple cast metal inlays. This section presents the tooth preparation principles and techniques for larger, more complex cast metal onlay restorations. Onlay and larger inlay restorations have many clinical applications and may be desirable by many patients. Although not esthetic, these restorations have a well-deserved reputation for providing the finest dental treatment.

The cast metal onlay restoration spans the gap between the inlay, which is primarily an intracoronal restoration, and the full crown, which is a totally extracoronal restoration. *The cast metal onlay by definition caps all of the cusps of a posterior tooth and can be designed to help strengthen a tooth that has been weakened by caries or previous restorative experiences.* It can be designed to distribute occlusal loads over the tooth in a manner that greatly decreases the chance of future fracture.[5,7] It is more conservative of tooth structure than the full crown preparation and its supragingival margins, when possible, are less irritating to the gingiva. Usually an onlay diagnosis is made preoperatively because of the tooth's status. However, sometimes the diagnosis is deferred until extension of the occlusal step of an inlay preparation facially and lingually to the limits of the carious lesion demonstrates that cusp reduction is mandatory.

The mandibular first molar is used to illustrate one MOD preparation for a cast metal onlay; other onlay preparations are presented subsequently.

Initial Preparation

Occlusal Reduction. As soon as the decision is made to restore the tooth with a cast metal onlay, the cusps should be reduced because this improves both the access and the visibility for subsequent steps in tooth preparation. With the cusps reduced, the efficiency of both the cutting instrument and the air-water cooling spray is improved. Also, once the cusps are reduced, it is easier to assess the height of the remaining clinical crown of the tooth, which determines the degree of occlusal divergence necessary for adequate retention form. Using the No. 271 carbide bur held parallel to the long axis of the tooth crown, prepare a 2-mm deep pulpal floor along the central groove (Fig. 20-26, *A*). To verify the preoperative diagnosis for cusp reduction, this occlusal preparation may be extended facially and lingually just beyond the caries to sound tooth structure (see Fig. 20-26, *B*). However, the groove should not be extended farther than two thirds the distance from the central groove to the cusp tips because the need for cusp reduction is verified at this point. With the side of the No. 271 carbide bur, prepare uniform 1.5 mm deep *depth cuts* on the remaining occlusal surface (see Fig. 20-26, *C* and *D*). The depth cuts are usually placed on the crest of the triangular ridges and in the facial and lingual groove regions. These depth cuts will help prevent thin spots in the final restoration. It should be remembered that if a cusp is in infraocclusion of the desired occlusal plane before reduction, then the amount of cusp reduction is less and needs only that which provides the required clearance with the desired occlusal plane. *Caries and old restorative material that is deeper in the tooth than the desired clearance is not removed at this step in preparation.*

With the depth cuts serving as guides for the amount of reduction, complete the cusp reduction with the side of the No. 271 bur. This reduction, when completed, should reflect the general topography of the original occlusal surface (see Fig. 20-26, *E*). Do not attempt to completely reduce the mesial and distal marginal ridges at this time to avoid possibly hitting an adjacent tooth. The remainder of the ridges will be reduced in a later step when the proximal boxes are prepared.

Throughout the next steps in initial preparation, the cutting instruments used to develop the vertical walls are oriented continually to a single "draw" path, usually the long axis of the tooth crown, so that the completed preparation will have draft (i.e., no undercuts). For mandibular molars and second premolars whose crowns tilt slightly lingually, the bur should tilt slightly (5 to 10 degrees) lingually to help preserve the strength of the lingual cusps (see Fig. 20-4, *D*). The gingival-to-occlusal divergence of these preparation walls may range from 2 to 5 degrees from the line of draw, depending on their height. If the vertical walls are unusually short, a minimum of 2 degrees occlusal divergence is desirable for retentive purposes. Cusp reduction appreciably decreases retention form because of decreasing the height of the vertical walls, so this minimal amount of divergence is often indicated in the preparation of a tooth for a cast metal onlay. As the gingivoocclusal height of the vertical walls increases, the occlusal divergence should increase, allowing as much as 5 degrees in the preparation of greatest gingivoocclusal length. The latter preparations present difficulties during pattern withdrawal, trial seating and withdrawal of the casting, and cementing unless this maximal divergence is provided.

Occlusal Step. After cusp reduction there should be a 0.5 mm deep occlusal step in the central groove region between the reduced cuspal inclines and the pulpal floor. Maintaining the pulpal depth (0.5 mm) of the step, extend it facially and lingually just beyond any carious areas, to sound tooth structure (or to sound base/restorative material if certain conditions, discussed subsequently, have been met). Extend mesially and distally far enough to expose the proximal DEJ (see Fig. 20-26, *F*).

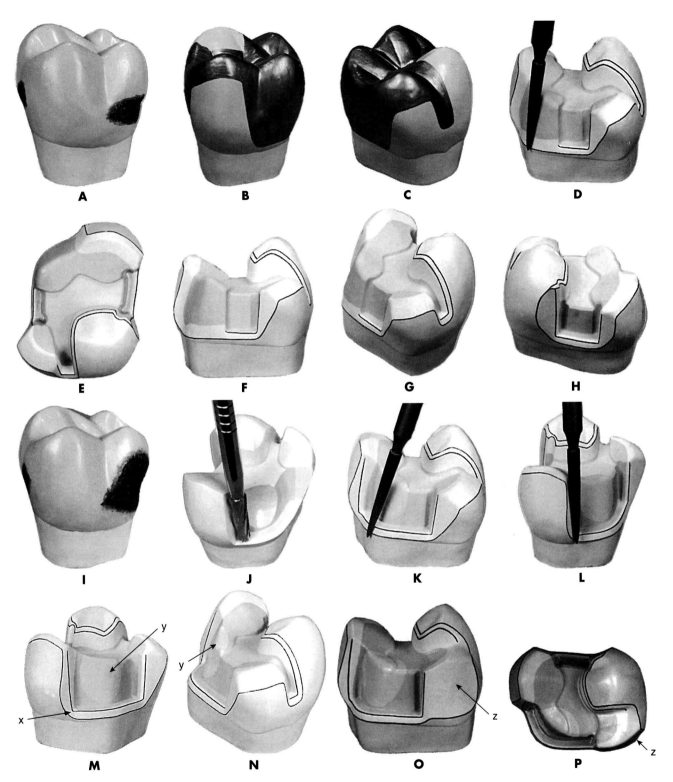

F I G. **20-25 A,** Maxillary molar with caries on both distofacial corner and mesial surface. Completed MODFL inlay for treating caries shown in **A**, faciooocclusal view (**B**) and distolinguoocclusal view (**C**). Preparation for treating caries illustrated in **A**, DO view with diamond instrument being applied (**D**); occlusal view (**E**); distal view (**F**); distolinguoocclusal view (**G**); MO view (**H**). **I,** Maxillary molar with deeper caries on distofacial corner and with mesial caries. **J,** Preparation (minus bevels and flares) for MODFL inlay to restore carious molar shown in **I**. No. 271 carbide bur is used to prepare gingival shoulder and vertical wall. **K** and **L,** Beveling margins. **M** and **N,** Completed preparation for treating caries shown in **I**. Gingival and facial bevels blend at *x*, and *y* is cement base. **O** and **P,** When lingual surface groove has not been prepared and when facial wall of proximal boxing is mostly or totally missing, forces directed to displace inlay facially can be opposed by lingual skirt extension (*z*).

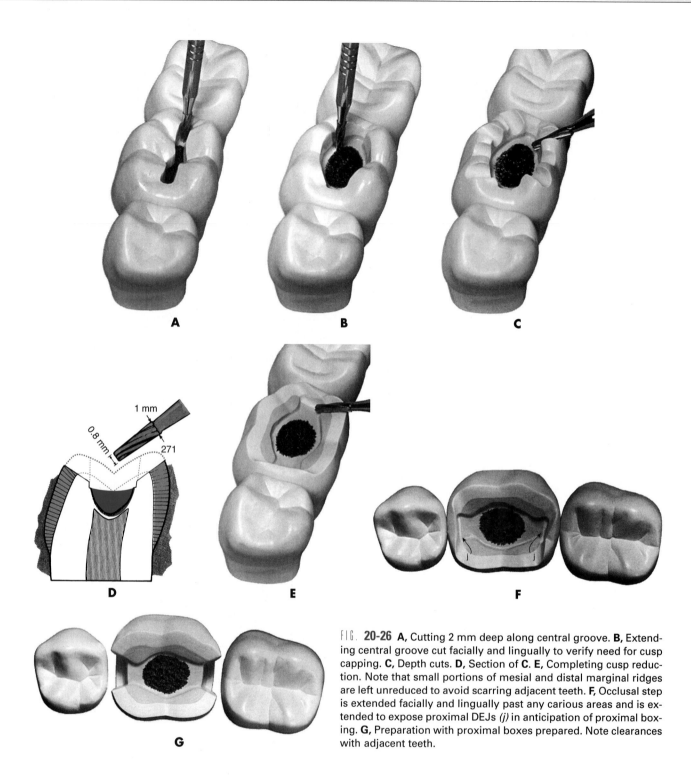

FIG. **20-26 A,** Cutting 2 mm deep along central groove. **B,** Extending central groove cut facially and lingually to verify need for cusp capping. **C,** Depth cuts. **D,** Section of **C. E,** Completing cusp reduction. Note that small portions of mesial and distal marginal ridges are left unreduced to avoid scarring adjacent teeth. **F,** Occlusal step is extended facially and lingually past any carious areas and is extended to expose proximal DEJs *(j)* in anticipation of proximal boxing. **G,** Preparation with proximal boxes prepared. Note clearances with adjacent teeth.

Extend the step along any remaining facial (and lingual) occlusal fissures as far as they are faulty (fissured). The facial and lingual walls of the occlusal step should go around the cusps in graceful curves, and the isthmus should only be as wide as necessary to be in sound tooth structure or sound base/restorative material. Old restorative material or caries that is deeper pulpally than this 0.5-mm step is not removed at this stage of tooth preparation.

As the occlusal step approaches the mesial and distal surfaces, it should widen faciolingually in anticipation for the proximal box extensions (see Fig. 20-26, *F*). This 0.5-mm occlusal step will contribute to the retention of the restoration[11] and will provide the wax pattern and cast metal onlay with additional bulk for rigidity.

Proximal Box. Continuing with the No. 271 carbide bur held parallel to the long axis of the tooth crown, prepare the proximal boxes as described in the inlay section. Fig. 20-26, *G,* illustrates the preparation after the proximal boxes are prepared.

Final Preparation

Removal of Infected Carious Dentin and Defective Restorative Materials and Pulp Protection. If the occlusal step and the proximal boxes have been extended properly, any caries or previous restorative materials remaining on the pulpal and axial walls should be visible. Remove them as described previously.

Preparation of Bevels and Flares. After the cement base (when indicated) is completed (Fig. 20-27, *A),* use the slender, flame-shaped, fine-grit diamond instrument to place *counterbevels* on the reduced cusps, to apply the *gingival bevels,* and to create *secondary flares* on the facial and lingual walls of the proximal boxes. First insert a gingival *retraction cord* as described in the previous inlay section. During the few minutes required for the cord's effect on the gingival tissues, use the diamond instrument for preparing the counterbevels on the facial and lingual margins of the reduced cusps. The bevel should be of generous width and should result in 30-degree marginal metal. The best way to judge this is to always maintain a 30-degree angle between the side of the instrument and the external enamel surface beyond the counterbevel (see Fig. 20-27, *B* and *C*). The counterbevel should usually be wide enough so that the cavosurface margin is beyond (gingival to) any contact with the opposing dentition.

If a facial (lingual) surface fissure extends slightly beyond the normal position of the counterbevel, it may be included (removed) by deepening the counterbevel in the region of the fissure (see Fig. 20-27, *D*). However, if the fissure extends gingivally more than 0.5 mm, then manage the fissure as described later.

A counterbevel is not placed on the facial cusps of maxillary premolars and first molars where esthetic considerations may dictate using a stubbed margin by blunting and smoothing of the enamel margin by either the light application of a fine-grit sandpaper disc or the fine-grit diamond instrument (flame-shaped) held at a right angle to the facial surface (see Fig. 20-23, *C*). The surface created by this blunting should be approximately 0.5 mm in width.

For beveling the gingival margins and flaring (secondary) the proximal enamel walls, refer to the inlay section.

After beveling and flaring, slightly round any sharp junctions between the counterbevels and the secondary flares (see Fig. 20-27, *E*). The fine-grit diamond instrument also is used to lightly bevel the axiopulpal line angles (see Fig. 20-27, *F*). Such a bevel produces a stronger wax pattern at this critical region by increasing its thickness. Slightly round any sharp projecting corners in the preparation because these projections are difficult to reproduce without voids when developing the working cast and often cause difficulties when seating the casting. The desirable metal angle at the margins of onlays

is 40 degrees, except at the gingivally directed margins, where the metal angle should be 30 degrees.

When deemed necessary, shallow (0.3 mm deep) retention grooves may be cut in the facioaxial and the linguoaxial line angles with the No. 169L carbide bur (see Fig. 20-27, *G*). These grooves are especially important for retention when the prepared tooth is short, which is often the case after reducing all the cusps. When properly positioned, the grooves are entirely in dentin near the DEJ and therefore do not undermine the enamel. The direction of cutting (translation of the bur) is parallel to the DEJ. The long axis of the No. 169L bur must be held parallel to the line of draw and the tip of the bur positioned in the gingival box internal point angles. However, if the axial walls are deeper than ideal, the correct reference for placing retention grooves is just inside the DEJ to minimize pulpal impacts yet avoid undermining enamel.

The model showing the completed preparation is illustrated in Fig. 20-27, *H.*

Modifications in Onlay Tooth Preparations

Facial or Lingual Surface Groove Extension. A facial surface fissure (mandibular molar) or a lingual surface fissure (maxillary molar) is included in the outline in the same manner as described in the inlay section. *This extension is sometimes indicated to provide additional retention form even though the groove is not faulty.* A completed MODF onlay preparation on a mandibular first molar is illustrated in Fig. 20-27, *I.*

Inclusion of Portions of the Facial and Lingual Smooth Surfaces Affected by Caries, Fractured Cusps, or Other Injury. For inclusion of shallow to moderate lesions on the facial and lingual smooth surfaces, refer to the inlay section.

A mandibular molar with a fractured mesiolingual cusp is used to illustrate the treatment of a fractured cusp of a molar (Fig. 20-28, *A*). Use a No. 271 carbide bur to cut a shoulder perpendicular to occlusal force by extending the proximal gingival floor (adjacent to the fracture) to include the affected surface. This shoulder partially provides the desired resistance form by being perpendicular to gingivally directed occlusal force. Use this instrument also to create a vertical wall in the remaining lingual enamel (see Fig. 20-28, *B*). The width of the gingival floor should be the diameter of the end of the cutting instrument. The vertical walls should have the degree of draft necessary for retention form. If the clinical crown of the tooth is short, it is advisable to cut proximal grooves for additional retention with the No. 169L bur. The linguogingival and lingual margins are beveled with the flame-shaped, fine-grit diamond instrument to provide 30-degree metal at the gingival margin (see Fig. 20-28, *C*) and 40-degree metal along the lingual margin (see Fig. 20-28, *D*). These two bevels should blend together (*x* in Fig. 20-28, *E*), and the linguogingival bevel is continuous with the gingival bevel

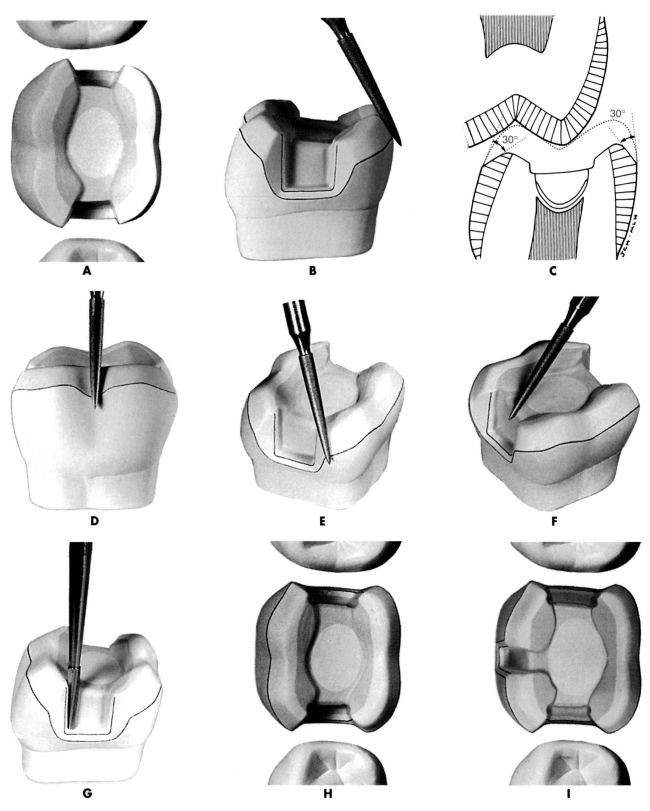

FIG. **20-27** **A,** Caries has been removed, and cement base has been inserted. **B,** Counterbeveling facial and lingual margins of reduced cusps. **C,** Section of **B**. **D,** Fissure that extends slightly gingival to normal position of counterbevel may be included by slightly deepening counterbevel in fissured area. **E,** Slightly round the junctions between counterbevels and secondary flares. **F,** Lightly bevel axiopulpal line angle. **G,** Improving retention form by cutting proximal grooves. **H,** Completed MOD onlay preparation. **I,** Completed MODF onlay preparation showing extension to include facial surface groove/fissure.

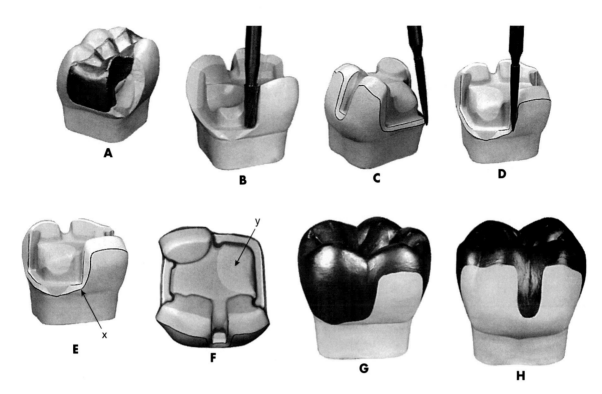

FIG. **20-28 A,** Mandibular first molar with large MOD amalgam and fractured mesiolingual cusp. **B,** Preparation (minus bevels and flares) for MODFL onlay to restore fractured molar shown in **A.** No. 271 carbide bur is used to prepare gingival shoulder and vertical lingual wall. Reducing cusps for capping and extending out facial groove improve retention and resistance forms. **C** and **D,** Beveling margins. **E** and **F,** Completed preparation. Gingival and lingual bevels blend at *x,* and *y* is cement base. **G** and **H,** Completed onlay.

on the mesial surface. Additional features to improve retention and resistance forms are indicated and can be developed by a mesiofacial skirt extension or by a facial groove extension. These preparation features, discussed in the following section: (1) improve retention form and (2) resist forces normally opposed by the missing mesiolingual wall, and (3) help protect the restored tooth from further fracture injury.

Enhancement of Resistance and Retention Forms. When the tooth crown is short (which is often the case when all cusps are reduced), the operator must strive to maximize *retention form* in the preparation. Retention features that have already been presented include:

1. Minimal amount of taper (2 degrees per wall) on the vertical walls of the preparation
2. Addition of proximal retention grooves
3. Preparation of facial (or lingual) surface groove extensions

In the preparation of a tooth that has been grossly weakened by caries or previous filling material and is judged to be prone to fracture under occlusal loads, the resistance form that cusp capping provides should be augmented by the use of skirts, collars, or facial (lin-

gual) surface groove extensions. When properly placed, these features result in onlays that will distribute occlusal forces over most or all of the tooth and not just a portion of it, thus reducing the likelihood of fractures of the teeth, as depicted in Fig. 20-29, *A* and *B.* The lingual "skirt" extension(s) (see Fig. 20-29, *C* through *E*), the lingual "collar" preparation (see Fig. 20-29, *F*), or the lingual surface groove extension on a maxillary molar protect the facial cusps from fracture. The facial skirt extension(s), the facial collar preparation, or the facial surface groove extension on a mandibular molar protect the lingual cusp(s) from fracture.

Skirt preparation. Skirts are thin extensions of the facial or lingual proximal margins of the cast metal onlay that extend from the primary flare to a termination just past the transitional line angle of the tooth. A skirt extension is a conservative method of improving both the retention form and the resistance form of the preparation. It is relatively atraumatic to the health of the tooth because it involves removing very little (if any) dentin. Usually the skirt extensions are prepared entirely in enamel.

When the proximal portion of a Class II preparation for an onlay is being prepared and the lingual wall is partially or totally missing, retention form normally

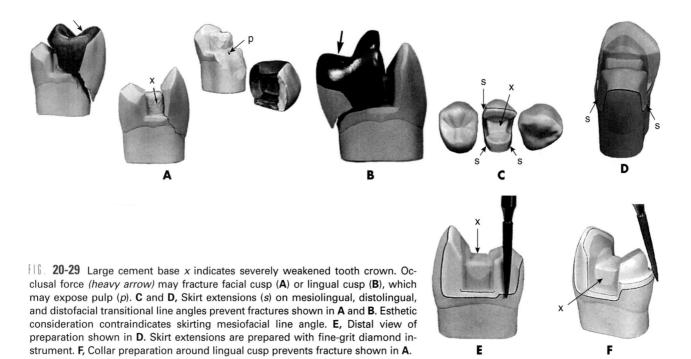

FIG. 20-29 Large cement base *x* indicates severely weakened tooth crown. Occlusal force *(heavy arrow)* may fracture facial cusp (**A**) or lingual cusp (**B**), which may expose pulp (*p*). **C** and **D,** Skirt extensions (*s*) on mesiolingual, distolingual, and distofacial transitional line angles prevent fractures shown in **A** and **B**. Esthetic consideration contraindicates skirting mesiofacial line angle. **E,** Distal view of preparation shown in **D**. Skirt extensions are prepared with fine-grit diamond instrument. **F,** Collar preparation around lingual cusp prevents fracture shown in **A**.

provided by this wall can be developed with a skirt extension of the facial margin (Fig. 20-30, *A* through *C*). Similarly, if the facial wall is not retentive, a skirt extension of the lingual margin will supply the desired retention form (see Fig. 20-25, *O* and *P*). When both the lingual and facial walls of a proximal boxing are inadequate, skirt extensions on both the respective lingual and facial margins can satisfy retention and resistance form requirements. *The addition of properly prepared skirts to three of four line angles of the tooth virtually eliminates the chance of postrestorative fracture of the tooth because the skirting onlay is primarily an extracoronal restoration that encompasses and braces the tooth against forces that might otherwise split the tooth.* The skirting onlay is often used successfully for many teeth that exhibit the split-tooth syndrome.

The addition of skirt extensions also is recommended when the proximal surface contour and contact are to be extended more than the normal dimension to develop a proximal contact. Extending these proximal margins onto the respective facial and lingual surfaces aids in recontouring the proximal surface to this increased dimension. Also, when improving the occlusal plane of a mesially tilted molar by a cusp capping onlay, reshaping the mesial surface to a satisfactory contour and contact is aided when the mesiofacial and mesiolingual margins are extended generously.

Skirting also is recommended when splinting posterior teeth together with onlays. The added retention and resistance form is very desirable because of the increased stress on each unit. Because the facial and lingual proximal margins are extended generously, the

ease of soldering the connector(s) and finishing of the proximal margins is increased.

A disadvantage of skirting is that it increases the display of metal on the facial and lingual surfaces of the tooth. For this reason, skirts are not placed on the mesiofacial margin of maxillary premolars and first molars. Skirting the remaining three line angles of the tooth provides ample retention and resistance form.

The preparation of a skirt is done entirely with the slender, flame-shaped, fine-grit diamond instrument. Skirt preparations follow the completion of the proximal gingival bevel and primary flares. However, experienced operators will often prepare the skirt extensions at the same time that the gingival bevel is placed, working from the lingual toward the facial or vice versa. Maintaining the long axis of the instrument parallel to the line of draw, translate the rotating instrument into the tooth to create a definite vertical margin, just beyond the line angle of the tooth, providing at the same time a 140-degree cavosurface enamel angle (40-degree metal angle) (see Fig. 20-30, *D* through *F*). The occlusogingival length of this entrance cut varies, depending on the length of the clinical crown and the amount of extracoronal retention and resistance forms desired. *Extending into the gingival third of the anatomic crown is usually necessary for effective resistance form.* Note that in most instances, the gingival margin of the skirt extension is occlusal to the position of the gingival bevel of the proximal box (see Fig. 20-30, *H* and *L*).

Use less than one half the tip diameter of the flame-shaped diamond instrument to avoid creating a ledge at

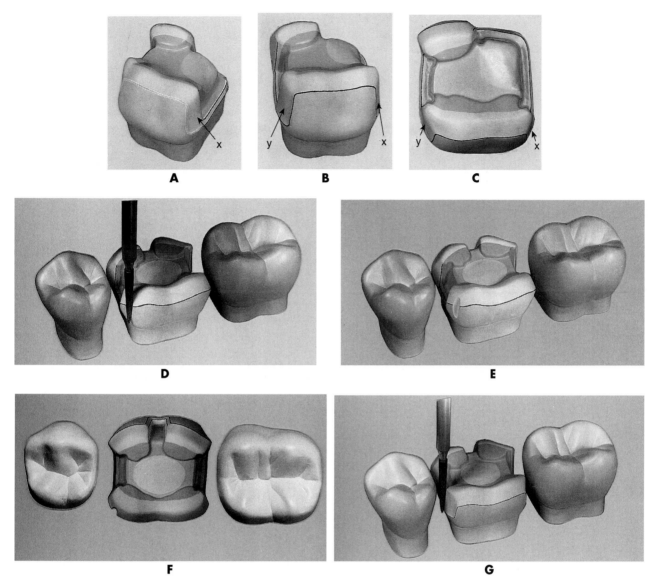

FIG. 20-30 **A,** When lingual wall of proximal boxing is inadequate or missing, retention form can be improved by facial skirt extension (*x*). **B,** Facioocclusal view of **A.** Maximal resistance form is developed by skirting distofacial (*y*) and mesiofacial (*x*) transitional line angles. **C,** Occlusal view of **B. D** through **F,** Initial cut for skirt is placed just past transitional line angle of tooth. **G** and **H,** Blending skirt into primary flare.   *Continued*

the gingival margin of the skirt extension. Using high speed and maintaining the long axis of the diamond instrument parallel with the line of draw, translate the instrument from the entrance cut toward the proximal box to blend the skirt into the primary flare and the proximal gingival margin (see Fig. 20-30, *G* and *H*). *Be sure not to overreduce the line angle of the tooth when preparing skirt extensions* (see *x* in Fig. 20-30, *I* and *K*). If the line angle of the tooth is overreduced, the bracing effect of the skirt will be diminished.

Holding the diamond instrument at the same angle that was used for preparing the counterbevel, round the junction between the skirt and the counterbevel (see Fig.

20-30, *J*). Be sure to slightly round any sharp angles that remain after preparation of the skirt because these often lead to difficulties in subsequent steps of completing the restoration.

Collar preparation. To increase the retention and resistance forms when preparing a weakened tooth for a MOD onlay capping all cusps, a facial or lingual "collar," or both, may be provided (Fig. 20-31). To reduce the display of metal, however, facial surfaces of maxillary premolars and first molars are not usually prepared for a collar.

Use a No. 271 carbide bur at high speed parallel to the line of draw to prepare a 0.8-mm deep shoulder (equivalent

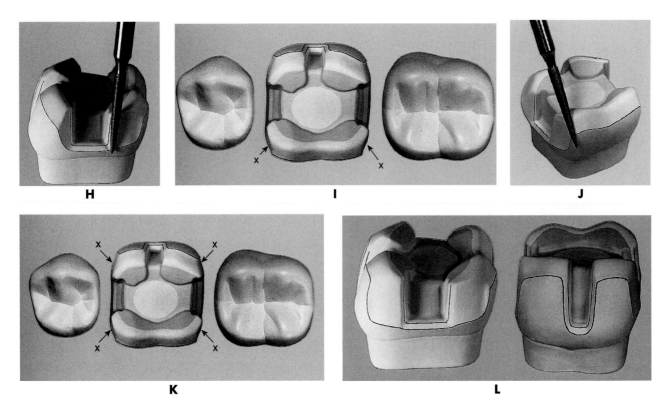

FIG. 20-30, cont'd G and H, Blending skirt into primary flare. I, Occlusal view showing mesi-olingual and distolingual skirts. Caution is exercised to prevent overreduction of transitional line angles (*x*). Facial surface groove extension also improves both retention and resistance forms. J, Slightly round the junction of skirt and counterbevel. K, Skirting all four transitional line angles of tooth further enhances retention and resistance forms. Again, caution is exercised to prevent overreduction of transitional line angles (*x*). L, Mesial and facial views of preparation shown in K.

FIG. 20-31 A, First position of bur in preparing for lingual collar on weakened maxillary premolar. Section drawings of first position of bur (B) and second and third positions (C). D, Beveling lingual margin. Note distofacial skirt extension. E, Completed preparation. F, Completed onlay.

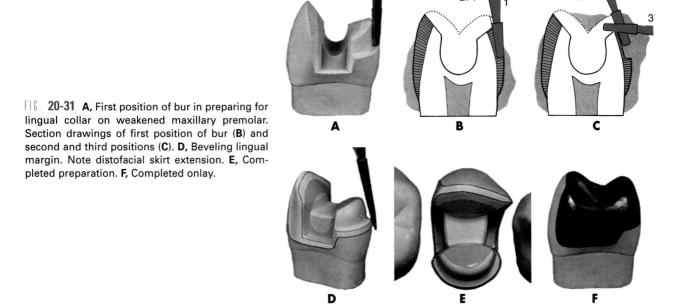

to the diameter of the tip end of the bur) around the lingual (or facial) surface to provide for a collar about 2 to 3 mm high occlusogingivally (see Fig. 20-31, *A* and *B*). To provide for a uniform thickness of metal, the occlusal 1 mm of this reduction should be prepared to follow the original contour of the tooth (see Fig. 20-31, *C*) and should round any undesirable sharp line angle formed by the union of the prepared lingual and occlusal surfaces. Complete this aspect of the preparation by lightly beveling the gingival margin of the shoulder with the flame-shaped, fine-grit diamond instrument to result in a 30-degree metal angle at the margin (see Fig. 20-31, *D*).

Slot preparation. Occasionally the use of a slot in the dentin is helpful to provide the necessary retention form. An example is the mandibular second molar that has no molar posterior to it and requires a MO onlay restoration capping all of the cusps (Fig. 20-32, *A* through *C*). The distal, facial, and lingual surfaces are free of caries or other injury, and these surfaces also are judged not to be prone to caries. After cusp reduction, the vertical walls of the occlusal step portion of the preparation have been reduced so as to provide very little retention form. The necessary retention can be achieved by cutting a distal slot. Such a slot is preferred over preparing a box in the distal surface because: (1) the former is more conserving of tooth structure and of strength of the tooth crown and (2) the linear extent of marginal outline is less.

To form this slot, use a No. 169L carbide bur whose long axis should parallel the line of draw (this must be reasonably close to a line parallel with the long axis of the tooth) (see Fig. 20-32, *A*). The slot is cut in dentin so that if it were to be extended gingivally, it would pass midway between the pulp and the DEJ (see Fig. 20-32, *C*). Such a position and direction of the slot averts: (1) exposure of the pulp, (2) removal of the dentin supporting the distal enamel, and (3) perforation of the distal surface of the tooth at the gingival termination of the slot. The slot should have the following approximate dimensions: (1) mesiodistally, the width (diameter) of the bur; (2) faciolingually, 2 mm; and (3) depth, 2 mm gingival of the normally positioned pulpal wall. To be effective, the mesial wall of the slot must be in sound dentin; otherwise insufficient retention form will be obtained.

A comparable situation occasionally occurs in which the maxillary first premolar requires a DO onlay restoration capping the cusps, and the mesial surface is noncarious and judged not prone to caries (see Fig. 20-32, *D* through *F*). To reduce metal display and to conserve tooth structure, a slot similar to that described in the preceding paragraph, except that it is mesially positioned and 1.5 mm wide faciolingually, may be used for the production of adequate retention. The mesial occlusal marginal outline in this preparation should be distal of the height of the mesial marginal ridge.

Modifications for Esthetics on Maxillary Premolars and First Molars. To minimize the display of metal on maxillary premolars and first molars, several modifications for esthetics are made to the basic onlay preparation. On the facial cusps of maxillary premolars and on the mesiofacial cusp of the maxillary first molar, the occlusal reduction should only be 0.75 to 1 mm on the facial cusp ridge to decrease the display of metal. This thickness should increase progressively to 1.5 mm

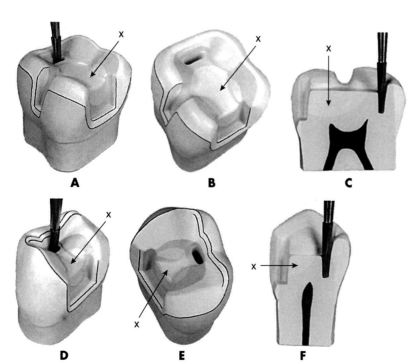

FIG. **20-32 A** and **B,** Cutting distal slot for retention for MO onlay to treat terminal molar having large cement base (*x*) resulting from extensive occlusal and mesial caries. **C,** Section of **A. D** and **E,** Preparing mesial slot for retention for DO onlay to treat maxillary first premolar that has large cement base (*x*). **F,** Section of **D.**

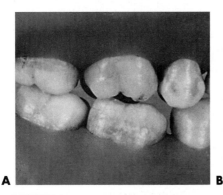 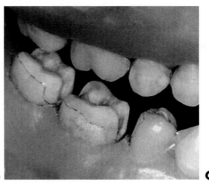 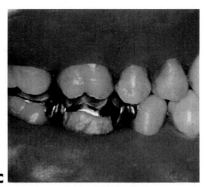

A   **B**   **C**

FIG. **20-33** **A,** Mandibular second and third molars tilted mesially, often the result of failure to replace lost first molar by bridgework. Note poor contact relationship between molars and between molar and second premolar. **B,** Second premolar is prepared for inlay, and molars are prepared for onlays. Margins of preparations are well extended on facial and lingual surfaces to aid in recontouring teeth to improve occlusal relationship and to improve proximal contours and contacts. **C,** Completed restorations. Note improvement both in occlusal plane and in proximal contacts.

toward the center of the tooth to help provide rigidity to the capping metal. Furthermore, these cusps do not receive a counterbevel but are "stubbed" or blunted by the application of a sandpaper disc or the fine-grit diamond instrument held at a right angle to the facial surface (see Fig. 20-23, C). The surface created by this blunting should be approximately 0.5 mm in width.

To further decrease the display of metal on maxillary premolars and first molars, the mesiofacial margin is minimally extended facially of contact to such a position that the margin is barely visible from a facial viewing position. To accomplish this, the secondary flare is omitted, and the wall and margin are developed with a chisel or enamel hatchet. Final smoothing with the fine-grit paper disc is recommended when access permits. The cavosurface margin should result in a gold angle of 40 to 50 degrees, if possible.

When more than ideal extension of the mesiofacial margin is necessary because of caries or previous restorations and when the esthetic desires of the patient dictate, the operator may choose to place a composite insert at this margin. This is a more conservative option than preparing the tooth to receive a porcelain-veneered metal crown. When preparing the mesiofacial margin, no attempt is made to develop a straight mesiofacial wall past the point of ideal extension. After caries excavation a glass-ionomer cement base is inserted to temporarily form the missing portion of the wall. The cement is contoured to ideal form, and the preparation can continue, terminating the mesiofacial onlay margin in ideal position in the cement. Following cementation, remove (with small round burs) the glass-ionomer cement to a depth of 1 mm for a composite insert. Small undercuts should be prepared in the wall formed by the cast metal onlay (see Fig. 20-68, A). (It is best to carve the undercut in the wall formed by the onlay during the wax pattern stage.) After beveling the enamel cavosurface margin and

preparing a gingival retention groove where, and if, enamel is thin or missing, insert the composite veneer (see Fig. 20-71, A).

Endodontically Treated Teeth. Routinely, teeth that have had endodontic treatment are weak and subject to fracture from occlusal forces. These teeth require restorations designed to provide protection from this injury (see Fig. 20-30, K and L). This particularly applies to the posterior teeth, which receive greater stress. The need for such protection is accentuated when much of the strength of the tooth has been lost because of extensive caries or previous restorations. When the facial and lingual surfaces of an endodontically treated tooth are sound, it is more conservative for the health of the facial and lingual gingival tissues not to prepare the tooth for a full crown but for a MOD onlay that has been designed with adequate resistance form to prevent future tooth fracture. Such features include skirt extensions and collar preparations. These features make the onlay more of an extracoronal restoration that encompasses the tooth, such that the tooth is better able to resist lateral forces that might otherwise fracture the tooth.

Before starting the preparation of an endodontically treated molar, the pulp chamber should be excavated to the chamber floor and sometimes into the canals (1 to 2 mm), and an amalgam foundation placed. This will give the onlay a firm base on which to rest. In the preparation of an endodontically treated premolar for an onlay, the canal is usually prepared for a metal post, which is placed in the canal before the onlay preparation is completed. This post will help the tooth resist forces that might otherwise cause a horizontal fracture of the entire tooth crown from the root. The post should extend roughly two thirds the length of the root and should terminate, leaving at least 3 mm of the root canal filling material at the apical portion of the root.

Restoring the Occlusal Plane of a Tilted Molar. An onlay is excellent for restoring the occlusal plane of a mesially tilted molar (Fig. 20-33). When the unprepared occlusal surface (mesial portion) is less than the desired occlusal plane, a corresponding decrease in occlusal surface reduction is indicated. To facilitate increasing the height of the tooth and yet maintaining both the desirable faciolingual dimension of the restored occlusal surface and good contour of the facial and lingual surfaces, the counterbevels on the latter surfaces often should be extended gingivally more than usual (see Fig. 20-33, *B*).

Furthermore, often the mesiofacial and mesiolingual margins (on the "submerged" proximal surface) should be well extended onto the respective facial and lingual surfaces to help in recontouring the mesial surface to desirable proximal surface contour and contact. This extension can be accomplished with a minimal loss of tooth structure by preparing facial and lingual skirt extensions on the respective proximal margins, which improves retention and resistance forms. In comparison, achieving extension by preparing the mesiofacial and mesiolingual walls facially and lingually, respectively, does not improve retention or resistance forms and is less conservative of tooth structure.

Verification of appropriate cusp reduction is the same as presented for the inlay tooth preparation and is illustrated in Fig. 20-24.

RESTORATIVE TECHNIQUES FOR CAST METAL RESTORATIONS
INTEROCCLUSAL RECORDS

Before preparation of the tooth, the occlusal contacts in MI and in all lateral and protrusive movements should have been carefully evaluated.

If the patient has sufficient canine guidance to provide disocclusion of the posterior teeth, then the necessary registration of the opposing teeth can be obtained by (1) making a *MI interocclusal record* with commercially available bite registration pastes or (2) making full-arch impressions and mounting the casts made from these impressions on a simple hinge articulator. The interocclusal record works well when preparing one tooth; the full-arch casts are preferred when more than two prepared teeth are involved.

The MI interocclusal record can be made from one of several commercially available bite registration pastes with or without a disposable gauze-covered bite frame (Fig. 20-34, *A*). The most commonly used bite registration pastes are composed of heavily filled silicone or polyether impression materials. Several materials are available in cartridge systems that automatically mix the base and accelerator pastes together as they are expressed through a special disposable mixing tip. The mixed impression material may be applied to both sides of a gauze-covered bite frame (see Fig. 20-34, *B*). Usually

a layer 2 mm thick on both sides of the frame is sufficient. The frame is positioned over the maxillary teeth so that no portion of the frame will interfere with closure, and then the patient closes completely (see Fig. 20-34, *C*). Observe teeth not covered by the bite registration paste to verify that the teeth are in MI. Once the material has set, remove the interocclusal record from the teeth and inspect it for completeness (see Fig. 20-34, *D*). When held up to a light, there should be areas where the adjacent unprepared teeth have penetrated through the material. With some systems, the gauze frame is optional. The bite impression material can be dispensed directly onto the prepared teeth as well as their opponents, and then have the patient close into MI. The interocclusal record is set aside for later use in the laboratory.

The MI interocclusal records described in the previous paragraph provide information on the shape and position of the opposing teeth in MI. Such records give the laboratory technician some information on how to form the occlusal surface and position occlusal contacts on the restoration, but supply no data on how these structures and contacts might function during mandibular movements. This is also true when full-arch casts are mounted on a simple hinge articulator. Cast metal restorations made with these simple bite registration techniques often require adjustments in the mouth to alleviate interferences during mandibular movements.

If information is desired in the laboratory about the pathways of cusps during mandibular movements (such as when the tooth is to be restored in group function), an excellent technique involves making full-arch impressions and mounting casts made from these impressions on a properly adjusted semiadjustable articulator (Fig. 20-35).

The use of full-arch casts mounted on a semiadjustable articulator is recommended when restoring a large portion of the patient's posterior occlusion with cast metal restorations. It involves very little extra chair time and gives the laboratory technician much more information about the general occlusal scheme, pathways of cusps, opposing cusp steepness and groove direction, and the anatomy of the other teeth in the mouth. The technique uses a full-arch tray when making the final impression, which requires mixing more material, especially when using stock trays. The opposing arch is impressed with alginate impression material, and the appropriate mandibular movement and face-bow transfer records are made. The reader is referred to Chapter 2 for principles regarding the use of the semiadjustable articulator in developing proper occlusal relationships for cast metal restorations.

TEMPORARY RESTORATION

Between the time the tooth is prepared and the cast metal restoration is delivered, it is important that the patient be comfortable and the tooth be protected and stabilized with an adequate temporary restoration. The temporary restoration should satisfy the following requirements:

1. It should be nonirritating and protect the prepared tooth from injury.
2. It should protect and maintain the health of the periodontium.
3. It should maintain the position of the prepared, adjacent, and opposing teeth.
4. It should provide for esthetic, phonetic, and masticatory function as indicated.
5. It should have adequate strength and retention to withstand the forces to which it will be subjected.

When properly made, the custom temporary can satisfy the above requirements and is the preferred temporary restoration. Temporaries can be fabricated intraorally directly on the prepared teeth (*direct technique*) or

outside of the mouth using a postoperative cast of the prepared teeth (*indirect technique*). The indirect technique is not as popular because of increased number of steps and complexity; however, it is useful when making temporaries that might become "locked on" (e.g., intracoronal inlays) when using the direct technique.

Technique for Indirect Temporary. The indirect temporary technique has the following advantages:

1. At one time it was shown that the marginal accuracy of indirect resin temporaries was significantly better than that of temporaries made by the direct technique.[4] However, current direct techniques and materials provide acceptable marginal accuracy and are much faster. Accurate marginal fit is desirable to prevent cement washout and pulpal irritation due to penetration of oral fluids and bacteria. Good marginal fit also promotes good oral hygiene and periodontal health.

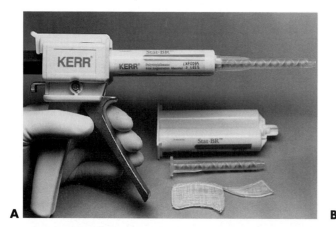

A

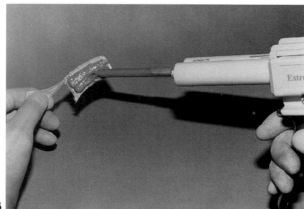

B

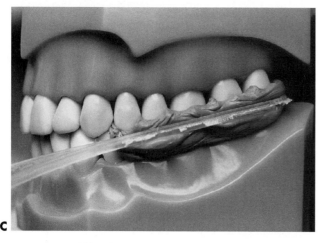

C

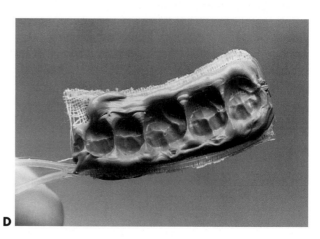

D

FIG. **20-34** MI interocclusal record made with polyvinyl siloxane bite registration paste. **A,** One of many commercially available bite registration pastes and gauze-covered bite frame used in this technique. **B,** Using cartridge dispenser and disposable automixing tip, the base and accelerator pastes are automatically mixed and applied to both sides of bite frame (2 mm thick on each side). **C,** Seeing that no portion of bite frame interferes with closure, have patient close into MI position. Be sure that adjacent, unprepared teeth are touching in their normal relationships. **D,** Remove MI interocclusal record carefully after it has set, and inspect it for completeness. There should be areas where adjacent, unprepared teeth have penetrated through paste.

2. The indirect technique avoids the possibility of "locking on" the set temporary material into undercuts on the prepared tooth or the adjacent teeth.
3. The indirect technique avoids placing polymerizing temporary material directly on freshly prepared dentin and investing soft tissue, thus reducing potential irritation to these tissues.[6,8,10]
4. The postoperative cast made in the indirect technique affords an opportunity to evaluate the preparation (before the final impression) and serves as an excellent guide when trimming and contouring the temporary.
5. Fabrication of the temporary can be delegated to a well-trained dental auxiliary.

To form the indirect temporary, first make an impression of the prepared tooth (teeth) with fast-setting impression material. Use a stock, plastic impression tray that has been painted with tray adhesive (Fig. 20-36, A). If using alginate, be sure that the teeth are slightly moist with saliva, then apply some alginate over and into the preparation(s) with a fingertip to avoid or minimize trapping air (see Fig. 20-36, B); then seat the tray over the region (see Fig. 20-36, C). After the material has become elastic, remove the impression with a quick pull in the direction of draw of the preparation and inspect it for completeness (see Fig. 20-36, D). Pour this impression with fast-setting plaster or stone (see Fig. 20-36, E).

As soon as the postoperative cast has been recovered from the impression, inspect the cast for any negative or positive defects (see Fig. 20-36, F). Small voids on the cast may be filled in with utility wax. Large voids indicate repouring the impression. Positives (blebs) on the cast should be carefully removed with a suitable instrument.

Seat the postoperative cast into the preoperative impression (Fig. 20-37, A through D). If using alginate, recall that the preoperative impression has been wrapped

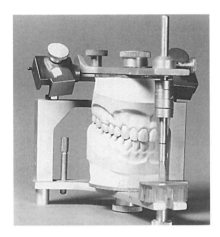

FIG. 20-35 Full-arch casts mounted via a facebow transfer on a semiadjustable articulator provide maximal information in the laboratory on how to position cusps to prevent undesirable contacts.

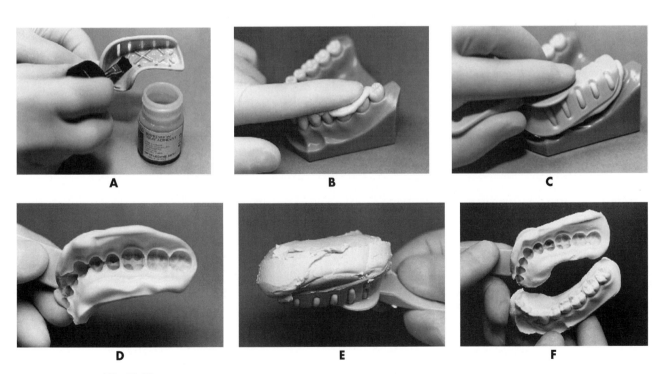

A   B   C

D   E   F

FIG. 20-36 Making a postoperative plaster cast for indirectly forming a temporary. A, Interior of tray is coated with alginate tray adhesive. B, Apply some alginate over and into preparations with fingertip to avoid trapping air. C, Alginate-filled tray in place. D, Alginate impression. E, Alginate impression is poured with fast-setting plaster. F, Plaster cast of preparations shown in Fig. 20-24, A.

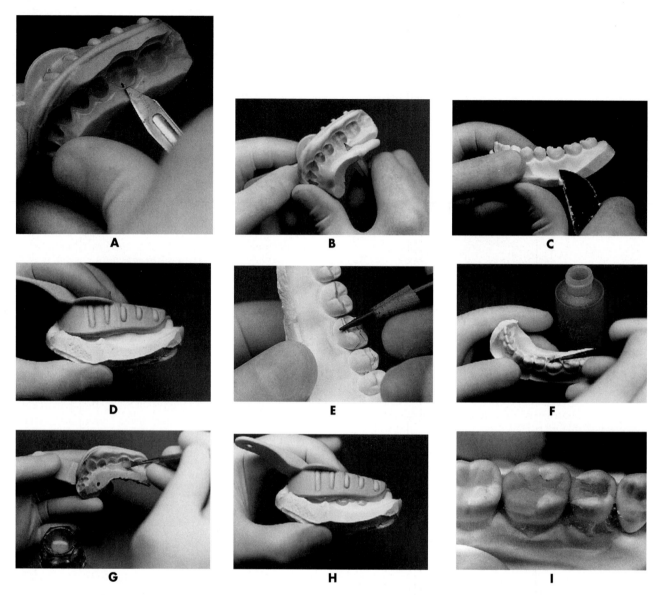

FIG. **20-37** Forming indirect temporaries for preparations initially shown in Fig. 20-24, A. **A,** Cut away thin edges of preoperative impression material that record gingival sulcus because these are apt to tear when seating postoperative cast in impression. **B** and **C,** Trimming away much of the soft tissue areas recorded by impression and cast also facilitates seating. **D,** Trial seating the postoperative cast into preoperative impression. **E,** Marking margins with red pencil. **F,** Applying release agent to cast. **G,** Fill preoperative impression with temporary material in area of tooth preparation. **H,** Seating cast into impression, taking care not to overseat or tilt cast. **I,** Formed temporary.

in wet paper towels from the time it was made (see Fig. 20-2, *D*). Cut away the thin edges of the postoperative alginate impression material that record the gingival sulcus (see Fig. 20-37, *A*). If these thin edges are not removed, they may tear off and keep the postoperative cast from seating completely in the impression. Trial-seat the postoperative cast into the preoperative impression to verify that it seats completely. Soft tissue areas around the perimeter of the impression and/or the cast may have to be relieved to allow full seating (see Fig. 20-37, *B* and *C*).

Once satisfied that the gypsum cast seats completely in the preoperative impression (see Fig. 20-37, *D*), remove the cast, and mark the margins of the preparations on the cast with a red pencil to facilitate trimming (see Fig. 20-37, *E*). Brush a release agent on the preparations and adjacent teeth (see Fig. 20-37, *F*). Mix tooth-colored temporary material (following the manufacturer's instructions) and flow into the preoperative impression in the area of the prepared teeth (see Fig. 20-37, *G*). When adjacent teeth are prepared, the temporary material is continuous from one tooth to the next. Seat the cast into

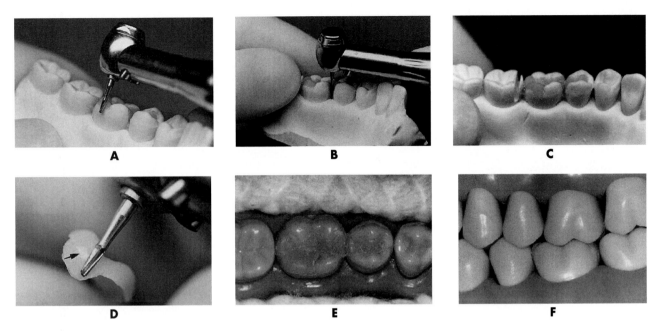

FIG. **20-38** Trimming and adjusting indirect temporaries. **A,** Trim excess material back to accessible facial and lingual margins (marked by red line on plaster cast). **B,** On multiple-unit temporaries, a slender bur or diamond instrument can be used to refine interproximal embrasure form. **C,** On cast, cut away any tooth adjacent to temporary. **D,** Trimming proximal surface of temporary to proper contour. Take care not to remove proximal contact (*c*). **E** and **F,** After final impression is made, temporary is cemented with temporary cement. Note anatomic contour and fit (**E**) and functional occlusion of temporary restoration (**F**).

the preoperative impression, making sure it seats completely (see Fig. 20-37, *H*). Do not apply too much pressure on the cast, or the temporary will be distorted and too thin in some areas. When the cast is seated, wrap the cast and the impression passively with a rubber band (too much pressure from the rubber band can distort the temporary), and submerge the assembly in hot water to accelerate the setting reaction. The formed temporary is shown in Fig. 20-37, *I*.

With suitable burs (No. 271, small acrylic bur, or diamond), begin trimming away excess temporary material along the facial and lingual margins. The red line previously placed will help, especially if an auxiliary is trimming the temporary (Fig. 20-38, *A*). On multiple-unit temporaries, a thin diamond instrument or the slender 169L bur or diamond can be used to refine interproximal embrasures (see Fig. 20-38, *B*). After the excess temporary material has been removed from the facial and lingual embrasures, cut through the adjacent unprepared tooth (teeth) 1 mm away from the proximal contact(s) (see Fig. 20-38, *C*). Insert a knife into the cut, and pry off the temporary from the cast. Now improve the contour of the proximal surface that will contact the adjacent, unprepared tooth (see Fig. 20-38, *D*). Do not disturb the contact area on the temporary that was accurately formed on the gypsum cast.

Try the temporary on the teeth (see Fig. 20-38, *E*). It should fit well, make desirable contact with the adjacent teeth, and meet occlusal requirements with minimal ad-

justments (see Fig. 20-38, *F*). If occlusal adjustments are indicated, alternately mark the prematurities with articulating paper and reduce these with an appropriate rotary instrument. After correcting the occlusion, smooth any roughness or undesirable sharp edges with a rubber point or wheel. Remove the temporary from the mouth, and lay it aside for cementation with temporary cement after the final impression has been made.

Technique for Direct Temporary. The direct temporary technique involves forming the temporary restoration directly on the prepared tooth (teeth) and has the following advantages (Fig. 20-39): (1) The direct technique involves fewer steps and materials because no postoperative impression and gypsum cast are required. (2) It is much faster than the indirect technique.

The main disadvantages of the direct temporary technique include the following: (1) there is a chance of locking hardened temporary materials into small undercuts on the prepared tooth and the adjacent teeth, (2) the marginal fit may be slightly inferior to the indirect technique,[2] and (3) it is more difficult to contour the temporary without the guidelines offered by the postoperative cast.

Forming the temporary directly on the prepared tooth requires the preoperative impression (see Fig. 20-2, *C*). Trial seat the preoperative impression onto the teeth to verify that it seats completely.

Because there is a potential for locking the temporary on the tooth, it is necessary to eliminate undercuts in the

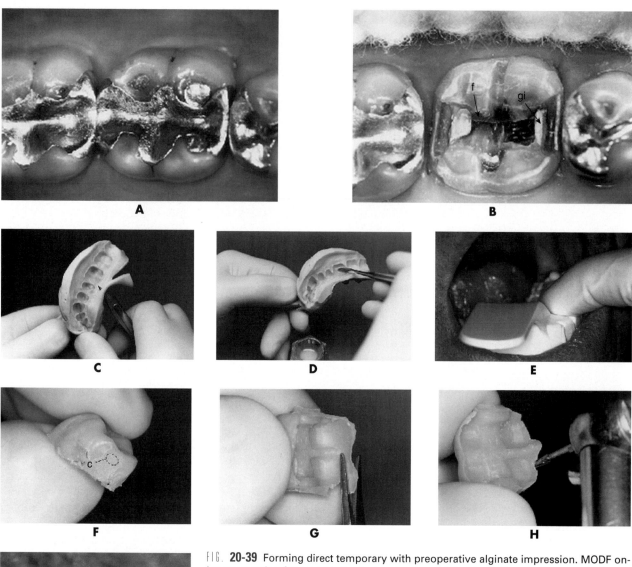

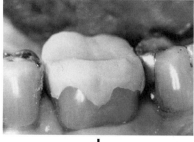

FIG. **20-39** Forming direct temporary with preoperative alginate impression. MODF onlay preparation for mandibular first molar is used for illustration. **A,** Preoperatively, patient had symptoms indicating incomplete fracture of vital tooth. **B,** After preparation for onlay, incomplete fracture *(f)* of dentin seen extending mesiodistally along pulpal floor. To maximize retention and resistance forms, all cusps are reduced for capping, a facial surface groove extension is prepared, and all four transitional line angles have skirt extensions. Glass-ionomer cement bases were inserted into excavations on axial walls *(gi)*. Cement bases should have light coat of water-soluble lubricant to prevent adhesion. **C,** Trim away much of the border of preoperative alginate impression to facilitate seating. Trial seating of preoperative impression helps identify areas that interfere with seating. **D,** Flow mixed temporary material into preoperative impression of prepared tooth. **E,** Seat preoperative impression with temporary material onto prepared tooth. **F,** Formed temporary is removed from preparation (note contact area, *c,* which must not be removed during trimming). **G,** Thin excess can be removed with scissors. **H,** Internal surface of temporary has record of cavosurface margin that is used as guide for final trimming. **I,** After final impression is made, temporary is cemented with temporary cement. Temporary material over skirt extensions is left slightly overcontoured for additional strength.

preparation and occasionally in the proximal areas. Undercuts in the preparation should be "blocked out" using a light-cured glass-ionomer cement base (see Fig. 20-39, *B*). A light film of petroleum jelly over any exposed base prevents adherence and facilitates removal.

When using the direct technique with inlay and onlay preparations (preparations that gain their retention primarily through internal retention features), it is helpful to select temporary material systems that become elastic before final set, thus allowing removal from undercuts without permanent distortion. Mix the temporary material following the manufacturer's instructions. Place the material into the preoperative impression in the area of the prepared tooth, taking care not to entrap air (see Fig. 20-39, *D*). Place the impression on the teeth, making sure it seats completely (see Fig. 20-39, *E*). Follow the manufacturer's instructions for gauging the setting time. Most temporary systems recommend monitoring the setting by rolling some excess material into a small ball and holding it between two fingers. When the temporary material has set to a firm stage, remove the impression. The formed temporary should remain on the prepared tooth. Test the temporary by pressing on the occlusal surface slightly, and when the material is sufficiently strong, remove it from the tooth using a Black spoon excavator (see Fig. 20-39, *F*). Trim away the excess material (see Fig. 20-39, *G*). The cavosurface margins of the preparation can be seen inside the temporary and are used as a guide for trimming the critical external areas near the margins (see Fig. 20-39, *H*). The techniques for try-in, adjustment, and finishing the direct temporary are identical to those described in the previous section (see Fig. 20-39, *I*).

FINAL IMPRESSION

The indirect technique for making cast metal restorations is accurate and dependable. Fabrication of the cast metal restoration takes place in the laboratory, using a gypsum cast made from an impression of the prepared and adjacent unprepared teeth. The impression material used for the final impression should have the following qualities:

1. It must become *elastic* after placement in the mouth because it must be withdrawn from *undercut* regions that usually exist on the prepared and adjacent teeth. Note the shaded portions in Fig. 20-40, which are undercut areas with regard to the line of draw of the preparation. A satisfactory impression must register some of this undercut surface to sharply delineate the margin and to signify the desirable contour of the restoration in regions near the margin.
2. It must have adequate strength to resist breaking or tearing on removal from the mouth.
3. It must have adequate dimensional accuracy, stability, and reproduction of detail so that it is an exact negative imprint of the prepared and adjacent unprepared teeth.
4. It must have handling and setting characteristics that meet clinical requirements.
5. It must be free of toxic or irritating components.
6. It must be able to be disinfected without distortion.

In addition to the previously mentioned absolute requirements, the choice of impression material is usually made by comparisons of *cost; ease of use; working time; shelf life; and pleasantness of odor, taste, and color.* The most

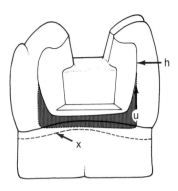

FIG. **20-40** Shaded area on prepared tooth is undercut in relation to line of withdrawal of impression. Impression material that is in position of greatest undercut (*u*) must be withdrawn in direction of *vertical arrow* and flexed over greatest heights of contour (*h*). Position of gingival attachment is indicated by *x*.

common impression materials used for the indirect casting technique are the *polyvinyl siloxanes* (addition reaction silicones). The technique for the use of this material is discussed in detail in the following sections.

Tissue Retraction. Final impression materials will only make accurate impressions of tooth surfaces that are visible, clean, and dry. Therefore when margins are subgingival, it is necessary to use *retraction cord* to temporarily displace the free gingiva away from the tooth and to control the flow of any gingival hemorrhage and sulcular fluids. The objective of gingival retraction is to widen the gingival sulcus to provide access for the impression material to reach the subgingival margins in adequate bulk to resist tearing during impression withdrawal (see Fig. 20-40). The objective of hemorrhage and moisture control is met by the use of retraction cord impregnated with appropriate *styptics* (such as aluminum chloride) and/or *vasoconstrictors* (such as epinephrine). *The use of vasoconstrictors in retraction cord is contraindicated in some patients,* especially those who have cardiac arrhythmias, severe cardiovascular disease, uncontrolled hyperthyroidism, diabetes, and those receiving drugs such as β-blockers, monoamine oxidase inhibitors, or tricyclic antidepressants.[9]

All sensory nerves to the region should be anesthetized, cotton rolls applied, and the saliva ejector inserted. *Profound local anesthesia substantially reduces salivation to facilitate a dry field and allows tissue retraction without patient discomfort.* Select and cut a retraction cord of suitable diameter that is slightly longer than the length of the gingival margin. The cord may be cut long enough to extend from one gingival margin to another if they are on the same tooth or on adjacent teeth. Note in Fig. 20-41, *A* and *B,* that the cord is inserted into the gingival sulcus only in areas where the cavosurface margin is prepared subgingivally. Using the edge of a paddle-tipped instrument or the side of an explorer, gently place one end of the cord into the sulcus, about

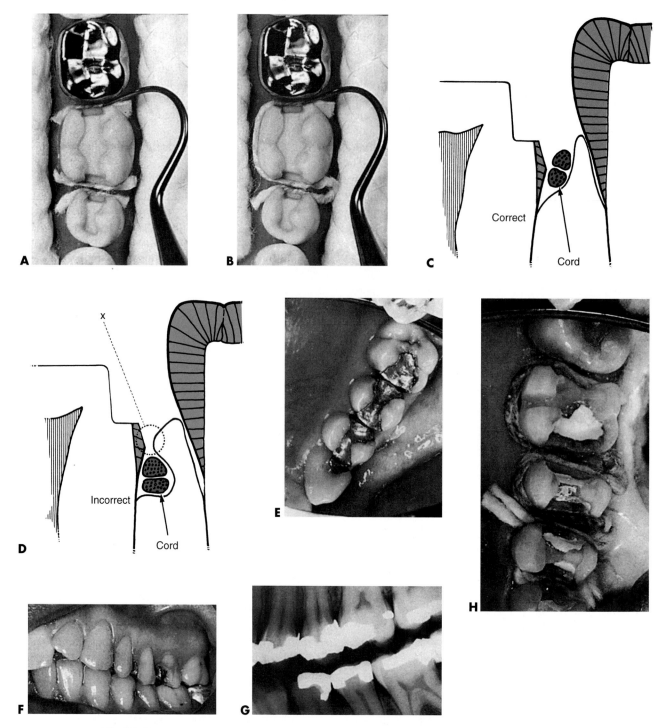

FIG. 20-41 A and B, Inserting retraction cord to widen gingival sulcus for exposing gingival margin. Separate lengths of cord can be inserted (one for each gingival margin) (A), or a cord long enough to run from one gingival margin to another can be inserted (B). Where margin is not subgingival, as on lingual surface of molar, cord should not be in sulcus. C, Correct application of retraction cord. D, Incorrect application of retraction cord causing impression material to tear at x. E, Maxillary quadrant before preparing teeth for onlays. Note fracture of mesiofacial cusp of molar. F, Facial view of E. G, Bitewing radiograph of E. H, Teeth prepared for onlays and ready for making final impression. Lingual and distofacial transitional line angles of premolars are prepared for skirting.

2 mm facial to the point where the facial margin passes under the free gingiva. Then progressively place the cord into the remainder of the sulcus, leaving the end of the cord exposed, to grasp with tweezers later in the technique (see Fig. 20-41, *A* to *C* and *H*). *It is emphasized that the cord is placed to widen the sulcus and not to depress soft tissue gingivally* (although some temporary retraction does occur apically).

Occasionally, when the gingival margin is deep, it is helpful to insert a second cord of the same or larger diameter over the first. *When the free gingiva is thin and the sulcus is narrow (e.g., facial surface of the maxillary or mandibular canine), a cord of very small diameter must be selected to prevent undue trauma to the tissue.* In instances when a small diameter cord is used, layering a second cord on top of the first may be necessary to keep the sulcus from narrowing at the gingival crest.

In Fig. 20-41, *D*, the cord is incorrectly placed because it is tucked too deeply into a sulcus whose depth permitted such positioning. When the cord is withdrawn before the injection of the impression material, the sulcus will be wide at the bottom but narrow at the top. If impression material is successfully injected into such a sulcus, the material is likely to tear in the region of *x* during the removal of the impression from the mouth. Correct application of the retraction cord is shown in Fig. 20-41, *C*.

Occasionally the retraction cord becomes displaced from the sulcus during its insertion if there is slight hemorrhage or seepage, but this can be controlled if an assistant repeatedly touches the cord with dry cotton pellets or dries the area with a gentle stream of air. When excessive hemorrhage from the interproximal tissue occurs, first wet a cotton pellet with aqueous aluminum chloride solution, and then wedge the pellet in between the teeth so that it presses on the bleeding tissue. Leave this pellet for several minutes before removing it and inserting the cord. Recall that the widening or opening of the gingival sulcus by the previous insertion of retraction cord before the beveling of the gingival margin also should minimize or eliminate hemorrhage of the gingiva.

For retracting a large mass of tissue, first make a suitably shaped, large-diameter cotton pack by rolling cotton fibers between the fingertips; then wet the pack with a drop or two of aqueous aluminum chloride, and insert it into the sulcus.

The cords remain in place for several minutes. When hemorrhage or excessive tissue is present, more time is recommended. The region must remain free of saliva during this interval, and the patient should be cautioned not to close or allow the tongue to wet the teeth. Placing cotton rolls over the teeth and having the patient close lightly to relax while the teeth remain isolated is sometimes helpful.

Caution: Some brands of latex gloves and some hemostatic agents contain chemicals that can inhibit the setting of *polyvinyl siloxane impression materials. Judicious cleaning of the teeth and the retraction cord to remove any chemicals that could prevent the setting of the impression material may be necessary. After cleaning, do not excessively dry the prepared teeth with compressed air. Have the patient close lightly on cotton rolls until the impression material is ready to be applied.*

Polyvinyl Siloxane Impression. The polyvinyl siloxane impression is discussed in detail because it is widely used, and the technique for its use can be readily applied to most other impression materials. Polyvinyl siloxane impression materials have many advantages over other impression materials used for final impressions. They have excellent reproduction of detail and excellent dimensional stability over time. They are user-friendly because they are easy to mix and have no unpleasant odor or taste. Polyvinyl siloxane impressions can withstand disinfection routines without significant distortion. Some silicone impression materials come in the form of two pastes (base and catalyst) that are mixed before application to the teeth (Fig. 20-42, *A*). For even more convenience, most of these materials are available in disposable, automix, cartridge dispensing systems. These automix systems provide excellent mixing of the accelerator and base pastes as they are dispensed through a disposable injection tip (see Fig. 20-42, *B*).

Tray Selection and Preparation. The impression tray must be sufficiently rigid to avoid deformation during the impression technique. If the tray bends or flexes at any time, the accuracy of the impression may be affected. Two types of trays, commercial stock and custom made, are suitable. The convenience and time saved with the use of stock, plastic trays is noteworthy. The custom resin tray made over a 2- to 3-mm wax spacer on the study cast is an excellent tray. A thickness of impression material greater than 3 mm increases shrinkage and the chance of voids; a thickness less than 2 mm may lead either to distortion or tear of the impression material, or to breakage of narrow or isolated teeth on the cast during withdrawal from the impression. Adequate bonding of impression material to the tray is accomplished with the application of a special adhesive to the tray (see Fig. 20-42, *C*).

Impression Technique. Most dental manufacturers offer their polyvinyl siloxane impression materials in automix dispensing systems. The automixing systems have many advantages, including (1) speed, (2) consistent and complete mixing of accelerator and base pastes, and (3) the incorporation of very few air voids during mixing and delivery to the teeth. The technique requires two viscosities of impression material, a light-bodied material to inject around the preparation and a heavy-bodied material to fill the tray. Two dispensing guns are needed (Fig. 20-43, *A*). The dispensers are loaded with cartridges that contain the accelerator and base pastes (see Fig. 20-43, *B*). A disposable automixing tip fits onto

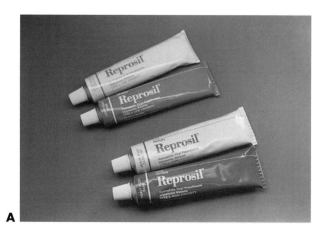

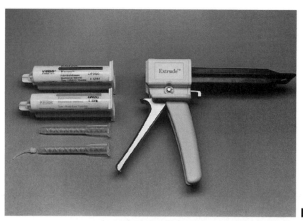

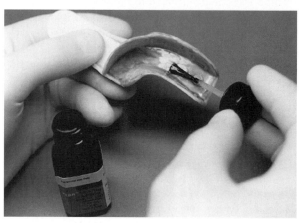

FIG. **20-42 A,** Light-bodied (syringe-type) and heavy-bodied (tray-type) polyvinyl siloxane impression materials. **B,** Automixing system for polyvinyl siloxane impression materials. **C,** Painting adhesive on stock tray.

the end of each cartridge (see Fig. 20-43, C). The light-bodied mixing tip has an accessory curved tip that is small enough to gain access to the smallest, most remote areas of the preparation (see Fig. 20-43, D).

Use the first dispenser to mix and fill the impression tray with the heavy-bodied impression material (see Fig. 20-43, E). Keep the dispensing tip embedded in the impression material as it is expressed into the tray, to decrease the chances of trapping air. Now use the second dispenser to mix and inject the light-bodied impression material on the prepared teeth (see Fig. 20-43, F). Examine the teeth to be sure the field is still clean and dry. Remove any visible moisture on the teeth with compressed air. Gently remove the retraction cord with operative pliers. *All preparation surfaces should be clean, dry, and exposed to view.* Next, deliberately and progressively (moving from distal to mesial) fill the opened gingival sulci and preparations over and beyond the margins with material from the syringe. To avoid trapping air, keep the tip directly on the gingival and pulpal walls, thereby filling the preparations from gingival to occlusal, and regulate the flow so that material will not be extruded too fast ahead of the tip. Light-bodied material also is injected on the occlusal surfaces of the unprepared adjacent teeth to eliminate the trapping of air on the occlusal grooves.

After filling and covering the teeth with material from the syringe, immediately remove the cotton rolls, and

seat the loaded tray over the region. Follow the product instructions for how long to let the material set before removal. As an additional safeguard, test the set of the impression material wherever it is accessible at the periphery of the tray. When it recovers elastically from an indentation made by the tips of the operative pliers, it is ready for removal.

Removing and Inspecting the Impression. After the polyvinyl siloxane impression has properly polymerized, remove it from the mouth by a quick, firm pull that is directed as much as possible in line with the draw of the preparation. Removal is aided by inserting a fingertip at the junction of the facial border of the impression and the vestibule fornix, disrupting the vacuum that occasionally occurs during withdrawal, especially with full-arch impressions. Inspect the impression carefully with good lighting and magnification. It should register every detail of the teeth and preparation(s) (Fig. 20-44).

WORKING CASTS AND DIES

The *working cast* is an accurate replica of the prepared and adjacent unprepared teeth that allows the cast metal restoration to be fabricated in the laboratory. During this fabrication procedure, it is most helpful if the replicas of prepared and adjacent unprepared teeth, called *dies,* are individually removable. The most used methods for creating a working cast with removable

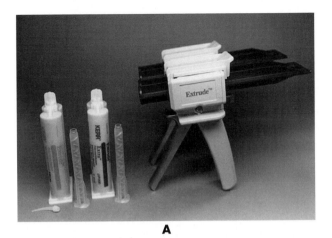

A

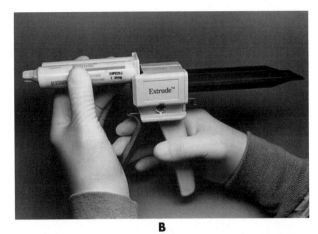

B

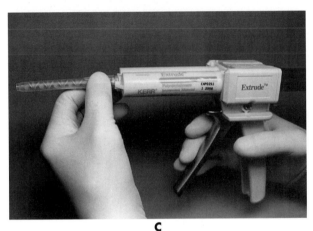

C

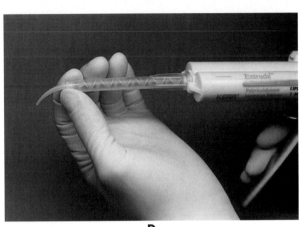

D

FIG. **20-43 A,** Dispensers, cartridges, and mixing tips for automixing polyvinyl siloxane impression materials. **B,** One dispenser is loaded with light-bodied impression material, while other dispenser is loaded with heavy-bodied impression material. **C,** Disposable automixing tip fits onto end of cartridge. **D,** Accessory curved tip is added to end of automixing tip for the light-bodied material.   *Continued*

dies from an elastic impression require two pours. The first pour is made to produce the removable dies, and the second pour is made to establish intra-arch relationships. Working casts made in this manner are called *split casts.*

Several satisfactory methods are available for making a split cast with removable dies. The Pindex system (Coltene/Whaledent Inc., Mahwah, New Jersey) is illustrated because it offers many advantages, including:

1. The first pour becomes the die segment and can be made quickly and easily.
2. Dowel pins can be positioned precisely where needed.
3. Dowel pins are automatically positioned parallel, which facilitates die removal.

Pouring the Final Impression. Make a mix of high-strength die stone using a vacuum mechanical mixer and pour the dies with the aid of a vibrator and a No. 7 spatula. *Apply the first increments in small amounts, allowing the material to flow into the remote corners and an-*

gles of the preparation without trapping air. Surface tension–reducing agents are available that allow the stone to more readily flow into the deep, internal corners of the impression. The impression should be sufficiently filled so that the dies will be approximately 15 to 20 mm tall occlusogingivally after trimming. This may require surrounding the impression with boxing wax before pouring. After the die stone has set, remove the cast from the impression and inspect it for completeness (Fig. 20-45). This first pour (die segment) will become the removable dies.

Completing the Working Cast. Trim the base of the die segment flat on a model trimmer (Fig. 20-46, *A*). This trimming will be approximately parallel to the occlusal surfaces of the teeth. Be careful while doing this not to allow any grinding slurry to splash onto the dies. Remember that you want the dies to be approximately 15 mm occlusogingivally. Once the base of the die segment is flat, trim the sides closer to the facial and lingual of the teeth (see Fig. 20-46, *B*). Remove deep scratches left by the model trimmer by wet sanding the base of the die segment with 220-grit wet/dry sandpaper.

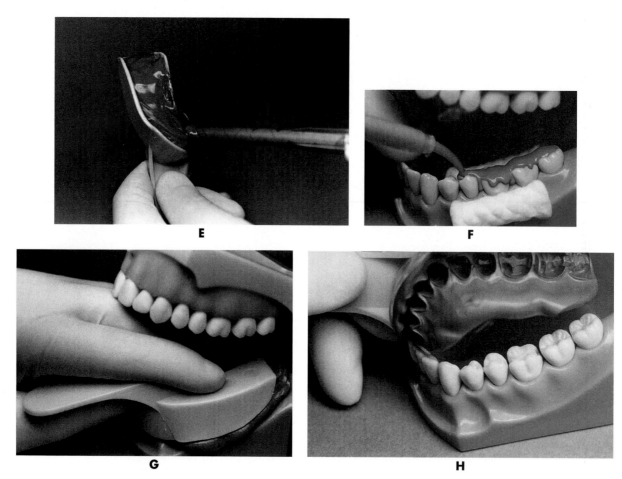

FIG. 20-43, cont'd E, Impression tray is filled with heavy-bodied material. F, Remove retraction cord and progressively fill opened sulci and preparations over and beyond cavosurface margins without trapping air. Note that occlusal surfaces of adjacent unprepared teeth are covered by light-bodied impression material. G, Remove cotton rolls and seat impression tray. H, Completed automixed polyvinyl siloxane impression.

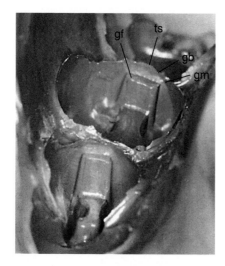

FIG. 20-44 Close-up view of impression shows sharp detail of record of gingival floor (gf), gingival bevel (gb) and margin (gm), and a small amount of unprepared tooth surface (ts) beyond the margin.

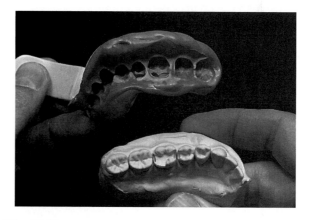

FIG. 20-45 Cast poured from die stone is inspected for completeness.

General rule: The teeth to be removable are the prepared teeth with proximal gingival margins and any unprepared teeth adjacent to prepared proximal surfaces.

There are two main advantages to making removable dies of unprepared teeth adjacent to prepared proximal

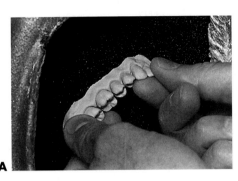
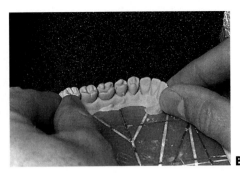

FIG. 20-46 **A,** Base of die segment is trimmed flat and approximately parallel to the occlusal surfaces with a model trimmer. Dies should be approximately 15 mm tall occlusogingivally. **B,** Die segment is trimmed on the facial and lingual surfaces to reduce need for trimming in later steps.

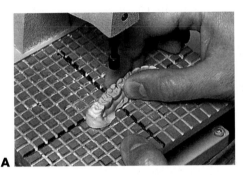
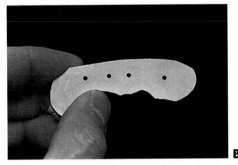

FIG. 20-47 **A,** Die segment on Pindex machine, ready to drill hole for first molar die. A small red dot of light helps position the cast. **B,** Holes drilled for removable dies.

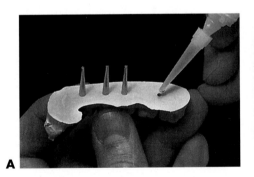
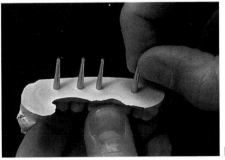

FIG. 20-48 **A,** Flow a drop of cyanoacrylate glue into each hole. The cast must be dry for the glue to adhere. **B,** Immediately insert a dowel pin into the hole, being sure it is fully seated.

surfaces: (1) The adjacent tooth will not interfere with removing the die that has the preparation, as occasionally may happen otherwise. (2) Adjusting the contacts is easier and more accurate when waxing and finishing the castings.

Usually place one dowel pin in each prepared tooth and each adjacent tooth. When long sections of teeth are to be removable, you may wish to place more than one pin to increase stability and prevent rotation of the die. Place the cast on the Pindex drilling machine and drill one hole into the die base precisely in the middle of each tooth that is to be removable (Fig. 20-47, *A* and *B*). A small light beam helps position the cast correctly. Once

all the holes are drilled, a small drop of cyanoacrylate glue is placed in each hole, and a dowel pin is inserted (Fig. 20-48, *A* and *B*). The cast must be dry before cementing the pins, or the cement may not adhere. Remove any excess glue and be sure the dowel pins are parallel to one another (Fig. 20-49, *A*). To prevent rotation of the dies on the model base, small dimples may be placed just facial and lingual to each dowel pin with one third the diameter of a No. 6 round bur (see Fig. 20-49, *B*). Place a bead of rope wax around the die segment level with the base of the dies (Fig. 20-50, *A*). Now add boxing wax around this to form a container for the base pour (see Fig. 20-50, *B*). Apply a separating medium on

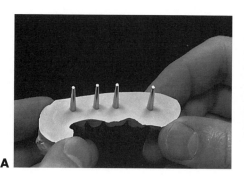
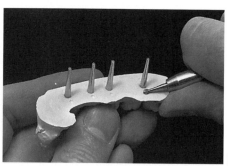

FIG. **20-49 A,** Be sure the dowel pins are parallel to one another, fully seated, and there is no excess glue. **B,** To aid in indexing, cut small dimples in the base of the dies, using one third the diameter of a large (No. 6) round bur. Typically these are positioned facial and lingual to the dowel pin.

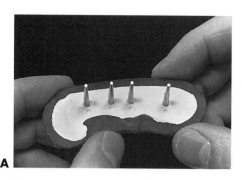
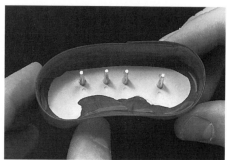

FIG. **20-50 A,** Place rope wax around the cast, flush with the die bases. **B,** Place boxing wax around the rope wax to create a container for the base pour. A separating agent must be painted on die bases to prevent adherence with base pour.

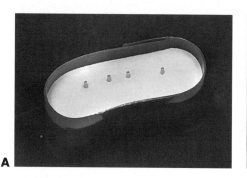
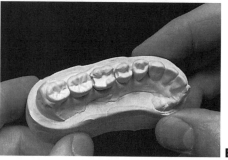

FIG. **20-51 A,** Base pour completed. Leave at least 1 mm of the dowel pin protruding. **B,** Cast after removing boxing and rope wax.

the die segment, and vibrate a mix of dental stone into the boxing wax container (Fig. 20-51, *A*). Allow at least 1 mm of the ends of the dowel pins to protrude. To provide adequate strength, the base of the cast should not be less than 10 mm thick.

After the stone has hardened, remove the boxing and rope wax. Remove the cast from the impression (see Fig. 20-51, *B*). Tap the end of each dowel pin *lightly* with the end of an instrument handle until a different sound is heard; this indicates that the die segment has moved slightly from its seating (Fig. 20-52, *A*). Next, carefully push the ends of the pins conjointly, causing the die segment to move equally away from its seating (see

Fig. 20-52, *B*). After the die segment is removed in this manner, the teeth that are to be individually removable must be cut apart from one another (Fig. 20-53). This requires the use of a saw, bur, or disk. To aid in carving the wax pattern and polishing the casting, carefully trim the gingival aspect of the dies to properly expose the gingival margins (Fig 20-54, *A* to *C*). The trimmed dies should have a positive and complete seating in the base portion of the cast (Fig. 20-55, *A* and *B*).

Caution: Do not allow any debris between the die portion and base or the accuracy will be compromised. This is especially true for the walls of the dowel pin holes. A small bit of wax or gypsum can be carelessly pressed onto the

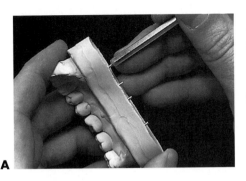
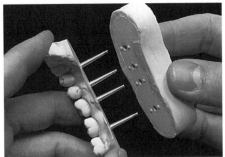

FIG. **20-52 A,** Tap on the end of each dowel pin until the die segment moves. **B,** Removing die segment from base.

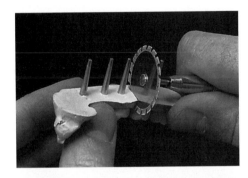

FIG. **20-53** Carefully cut the dies apart using a saw, bur, or thin diamond abrasive disk. Eye protection and dust collection are essential.

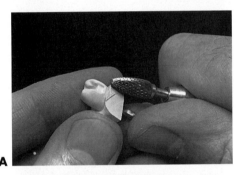
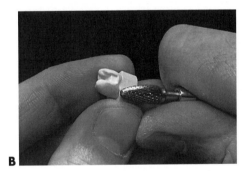

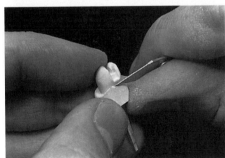

FIG. **20-54 A,** Excess die stone around gingival margins usually prevents good access for later steps in fabrication. **B,** Removing the excess die stone with a large crosscut carbide bur in slow speed handpiece. Trimming across slightly gingival of recorded gingival contour of tooth weakens the excess, causing it to fall away. **C,** Final trimming is completed with a sharp scalpel.

wall and prevent complete seating of the pin. Such debris is difficult to detect and remove to regain accuracy.

Use of the Interocclusal Records. A MI interocclusal record was made before making the final impression. From this interocclusal record, a gypsum cast of the opposing teeth is made that can be accurately related to the working cast, when forming the occlusal surface of the wax pattern. This step can be omitted if full-arch casts are to be used in waxing. (See Chapter 2 for the

principles of developing occlusion when using full-arch casts.)

When using this type of interocclusal record, the working cast is mounted on a simple hinge articulator. Attach the working cast to one member of the articulator with fast-setting plaster. Carefully fit the interocclusal record on the dies of the working cast (Fig. 20-56, *A* and *B*). The interocclusal record should and must seat completely without rocking. Interocclusal bite records

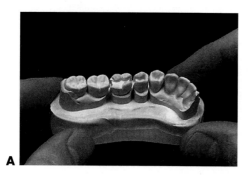
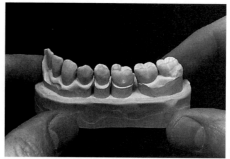

FIG. 20-55 A, Cast completed, lingual view. Note how each prepared tooth is removable, as well as the adjacent unprepared teeth. B, Cast completed, facial view. Note full seating of dies.

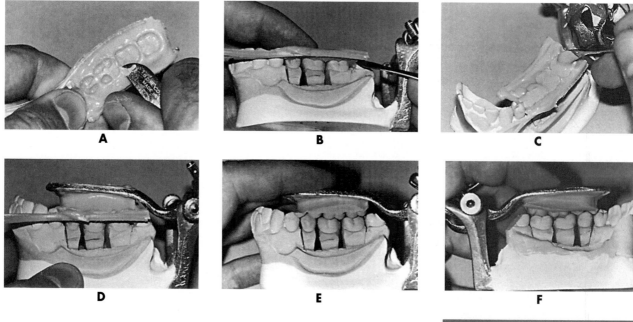

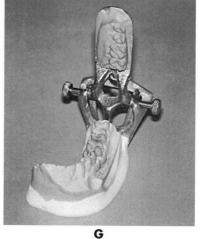

FIG. 20-56 Pouring interocclusal record made with bite registration paste. A, Trimming away some of the interocclusal record (on preparation side) with sharp knife is often necessary to allow complete seating on working cast. B, Fastening seated interocclusal record to working cast of preparations first shown in Fig. 20-33, A, with small amounts of sticky wax. C, Pouring stone into interocclusal record. D, Attaching gypsum to upper member of hinge articulator. E through G, Three views of completed mounting.

must never touch registrations of soft tissue areas on the cast because these contacts usually interfere with complete seating. Such areas of contact on the interocclusal record can be easily trimmed away with a sharp knife. After ensuring that the interocclusal record is completely seated, lute the record to adjacent unprepared teeth with sticky wax to prevent dislodgment when dental stone is poured into the record. Then pour dental stone into the record (see Fig. 20-56, C). Now attach this gypsum to the opposite arm of the hinge articulator (see Fig. 20-56, D), let this set, and remove the interocclusal record (see Fig. 20-56, E through G).

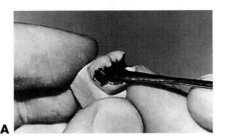
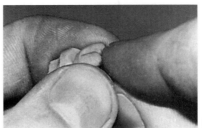

FIG. **20-57** To ensure optimal wax adaptation to preparation walls, first flow on a thin layer of wax (**A**), and then apply finger pressure for several seconds while wax cools (**B**).

WAX PATTERNS

Forming the Pattern Base. Lubricate the die and incrementally add liquid wax from a No. 7 wax spatula by the "flow and press" method to form the proximal, facial, and lingual surface aspects of the pattern. Then add a thin layer of wax on the occlusal surface (Fig. 20-57, *A*). Wax shrinks as it cools and hardens and therefore tends to pull away from the die. This effect can be minimized and pattern adaptation thus improved, by applying finger pressure for at least several seconds on each increment of wax soon after surface solidification and before any subsequent wax additions (see Fig. 20-57, *B*). In this incremental technique, the wax that is flowed on the previously applied wax must be hot enough, or else voids will be formed.

Forming the Proximal Contour and Contact. The proximal contour and contact of the pattern are now formed upon the pattern base (Figs. 20-58 and 20-59). The normal proximal contact relationship between teeth is that of two curved surfaces touching one another. Therefore the contact on each curved proximal surface is a point inside a small area of near approach. However, it must be realized that soon after eruption and the establishment of proximal contact, wear of the contact point due to physiologic movement of teeth will create a contact surface. Lack of a proximal contact is usually undesirable because it opens the possibility of proximal drifting of teeth, shifting occlusion, food impaction, and damage to the supporting tissues. Total lack of a proximal contact is often referred to as an *open contact* and is to be avoided.

Drawings of two maxillary premolars (see Fig. 20-59) are used to illustrate forms of contact and mesiodistal widths of interproximal spaces. Fig. 20-59, *A* through *C*, represent normal conditions. In Fig. 20-59, *A*, the position of the contact is marked with an *x*, the area of near approach of the two surfaces is indicated with a broken line and the position of the crest of the gingiva with a continuous line. Fig. 20-59, *B*, is a mesiodistal section through the teeth at the point of contact and Fig. 20-59, *C*, is an occlusal view.

A broad contact faciolingually is illustrated in Fig. 20-59, *D* through *F*. In the proximal view, Fig. 20-59, *D*, the position of a normal contact is marked *x*, while the con-

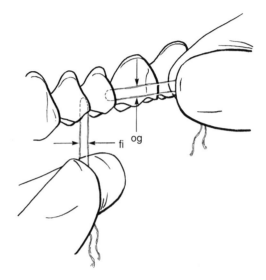

FIG. **20-58** Measuring diameters of proximal contact faciolingually *(fl)* and occlusogingivally *(og)* with dental floss. Two parallel strands should not be more than 1 to 2 mm apart. *(Modified from Black GV: Operative dentistry, ed 8, vol 2, Woodstock, Ill, 1947, Medico-Dental.)*

tact of this tooth is the outlined oblong area; the area of near approach is the broken line. As a rule, the crest of the gingiva is less arched, being almost horizontal along the area of near approach. Viewed from the facial in the mesiodistal section, Fig. 20-59, *E*, the contact appears to be the same as in Fig. 20-59, *B*, but a comparison of the occlusal views Fig. 20-59, *F* and *C*, shows the extra breadth of this contact at the expense of the lingual embrasure. Fig. 20-59, *H*, shows a contact that is too far to the gingival. Its position in comparison with normal is shown by the relation of the circle to the *x* in Fig. 20-59, *G*. The problem with such a contact is in the inclinations of the proximal surfaces from the occlusal marginal ridges to the contact. Stringy food is likely to become packed into this space and the contact may impinge on the interproximal tissue.

Fig. 20-59, *I* and *J*, illustrate a contact too close to the occlusal. This form is frequently observed in restorations (especially amalgams), seldom in the virgin teeth. Such a contact allows food to fill the gingival embrasure and invites proximal caries.

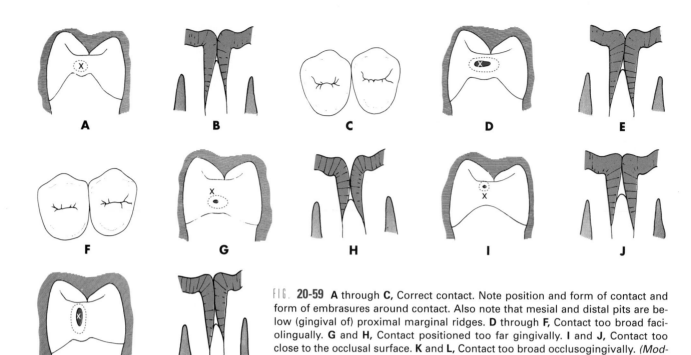

FIG. **20-59** **A** through **C**, Correct contact. Note position and form of contact and form of embrasures around contact. Also note that mesial and distal pits are below (gingival of) proximal marginal ridges. **D** through **F**, Contact too broad faciolingually. **G** and **H**, Contact positioned too far gingivally. **I** and **J**, Contact too close to the occlusal surface. **K** and **L**, Contact too broad occlusogingivally. *(Modified from Black GV:* Operative dentistry, *ed 8, vol 2, Woodstock, Ill, 1947, Medico-Dental.)*

Fig. 20-59, *K* and *L*, illustrate a contact that is too broad in the occlusogingival direction but narrow faciolingually. The principal objections to this form of contact are that stringy foods are likely to be caught and held; also, if proximal recurrent caries occurs, it will be farther to the gingival, requiring a tooth preparation very close to the CEJ.

In cases of excessive proximal wear of the teeth, the condition of the contact areas is similar to the combination of the areas illustrated in Fig. 20-59, *D* and *K*, resulting in a facet of considerable dimensions.

Forming the Occlusal Surface. Payne[11] developed the fundamental principles in the following method of waxing. The technique is particularly applicable when capping cusps. With practice, it has proved to be faster than the old method of building up wax, cutting away, building up again, and so on. The amount of wax desired is added in steps until the occlusal surface of the pattern is completed (Fig. 20-60).

To obtain the faciolingual position of the cusp tips, divide the faciolingual width of the tooth in quarters. Facial cusps are located on the first facial quarter line. Lingual cusps will fall on the first lingual quarter line (see Fig. 20-60, *B*). To obtain the mesiodistal position of the cusp tips, note the regions in the opposing tooth that should receive the cusp tips. Now wax to the pattern small cones of inlay wax to establish the cusp tips one at a time (see Fig. 20-60, *C* and *D*).

Now wax the inner and outer aspects of each cusp, being careful not to generate premature occlusal contacts (see Fig. 20-60, *D* to *F*). Again it is suggested to wax only one aspect of each cusp into occlusion at a time. For ex-

ample, on the maxillary molar illustrated in Fig. 20-60, *D*, where all cusps are being restored, there are nine aspects, each one to be waxed separately before waxing another. Follow the proper angle on the inner and outer aspects as shown in Fig. 20-60, *E*.

Next, wax the distal slopes of the cusps (one at a time) into occlusal relation with the opposing teeth. Then wax the mesial slopes of the cusps (again, one at a time) (see Fig. 20-60, *G*). After the cusps are formed, wax in the proximal marginal ridge areas (see Fig. 20-60, *H*). Develop the same level to adjacent proximal marginal ridges, even though occasionally this may sacrifice a contact on one of the two ridges. Restoring marginal ridges to the same level avoids a "food trap" that otherwise would be created. The mesial and distal pit regions also should be carved enough to have them deeper than the respective marginal ridges. This will provide appropriate spillways for the removal of food from the occlusal table and help prevent food impaction in the occlusal embrasure area of the proximal surface.

To complete the occlusal wax-up, add wax (where appropriate) to the fossae until they contact the opposing centric holding cusps (see Fig. 20-60, *I*). Establish spillways for the movement of food by carving appropriately placed grooves. Flat-plane occlusal relationships are not desired.

This technique is a systematic and practical method of waxing the occlusal aspect of the pattern into proper occlusion. Forming one small portion at a time results in waxing each portion into proper occlusion before adding another, thus simplifying the procedure. Moreover, building the occlusal aspect by such small increments should

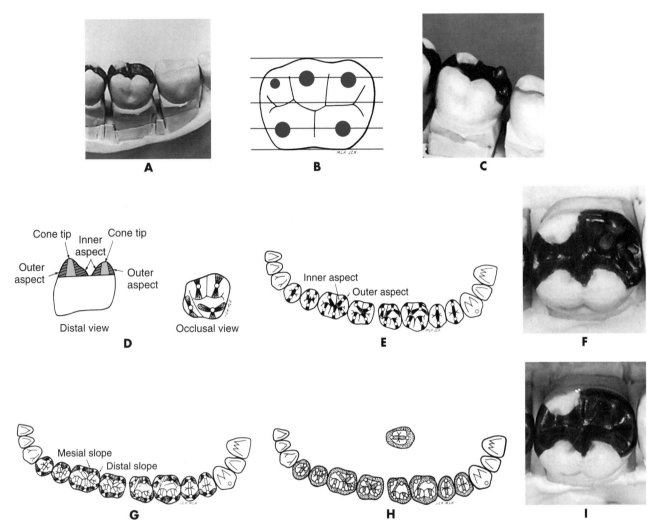

FIG. **20-60** **A,** Pattern base is completed and ready for waxing two reduced cusps (distolingual and distal) into occlusion by using Payne's waxing technique. **B,** Facial cusps are located on first facial quarter line, and lingual cusps will fall on first lingual quarter line. **C,** Distolingual and distal cusp tips are waxed into occlusion in the form of small cones. **D,** Cone tips and inner and outer aspects. **E,** Cone tips and inner and outer aspects of cusps of teeth. **F,** Inner and outer aspects of distolingual and distal cusps have been added to pattern base. **G,** Mesial and distal slopes of cusps of teeth. **H,** Marginal ridges of teeth. **I,** After marginal ridge is added to pattern base, fossae are waxed in, and grooves are carved to complete wax pattern. *(Modified from Payne E: Ney Tech Bull 1[9], 1961.)*

help develop a pattern with minimal stress and distortion. Whenever a large portion of wax is added, there is potential for pattern distortion caused by the large shrinkage of such an addition.

For establishing stable occlusal relationships, take care to place cusp tips against flat plateaus or into fossae on the stone cast of the opposing teeth. In other areas, the wax is shaped to simulate normal tooth contours, using adjacent teeth for references. Some relief between opposing cusp inclines should be provided because these incline contacts often interfere during mandibular movements. Remember, the MI record only provides information regarding the position of opposing teeth in MI. Therefore some adjustment to the cast-

ing may be necessary in the mouth to eliminate interferences during mandibular movements. The reader is referred to Chapter 2 for the principles of cusp and fossa placement when using full-arch casts mounted on a semiadjustable articulator.

Finishing the Wax Pattern. Careful attention to good technique is required for waxing the margins of the wax pattern. There must be a continuous adaptation of wax to the margins, with no voids, folds, or faults. If adaptation is questionable, remelt the marginal wax to a distance into the pattern of approximately 2 mm. Apply finger pressure immediately after surface solidification and before subsequent cooling of the wax, maintaining this pressure for at least 4 seconds. This finger pressure helps develop close adaptation to the die by offsetting the cooling shrinkage of the wax. Additional wax should be added during the remelting procedure to ensure a slight excess of contour and extension beyond the margin.

Wax that is along the margins is now carved back to the cavosurface outline with a warmed No. 7 wax spatula (Fig. 20-61, *A* through *E*). This warming of the spatula permits carving the marginal wax with light pressure so that the stone margins will not be damaged. A little practice will help the user determine how much to heat the instrument to result in easy and effective carving. It must be emphasized that the No. 7 spatula should not have sharp edges; thus when it lightly touches the die, it will not abrade or injure the die surface. Use the die surface just beyond the cavosurface margin to guide the position and direction of the carving instrument. *The direction of the instrument movement is not dictated by the margin but by the contour of the unprepared tooth (die) surface just beyond the margin.* Hold the instrument blade parallel to this surface, thus using it as a guide for the contour of the pattern near the margin. This should result in a continuity of contour across the margin. This principle of carving is too often neglected, resulting in the contour errors depicted in *x* in Fig. 20-61, *B* through *D;* correct application of the carving instrument results in correct contours, exemplified by *y*. The completed patterns are shown in Fig. 20-61, *F* through *I.*

On accessible surfaces of the carved pattern, satisfactory smoothness can be imparted by a few strokes with the end of a finger if surfaces have been carefully carved with the No. 7 spatula. Rubbing with cotton that has been twisted onto a round toothpick may smooth less accessible surfaces, such as grooves.

Initially Withdrawing and Reseating the Wax Pattern. Care must be exercised when initially withdrawing the wax pattern from the die. The wax can be dislodged by holding the die and pattern as shown in Fig. 20-62. Once the pattern has been dislodged, gently remove it from the preparation. Inspect the preparation side of the pattern to see if there are any wrinkles or holes. Such voids indicate poor wax adaptation and should be corrected if: (1) such voids are in critical regions of the preparation designed to provide retention form, (2) if they are numerous, or (3) if they are closer than 1 mm to the margin. To eliminate these voids, first relubricate the die and reseat the pattern on the die. Then pass a hot instrument through the wax to the unadapted area. This usually results in the air (void) rising through the liquid wax to the pattern's surface as the wax takes the place of the air. A consequence of this correcting procedure on the occlusal surface is the obliteration of the occlusal carving in the affected region, thus requiring the addition of wax, recarving, and rechecking the occlusion.

SPRUING, INVESTING, AND CASTING

If there is a delay of several hours or more between the forming of the wax pattern and the investing procedure, the pattern should remain on the die, and the margins should be inspected carefully, once again, before spruing and investing. When such a delay is contemplated, it is suggested to add the sprue to the pattern before the delay period. If the addition of the sprue caused the induction of enough stress to produce pattern distortion, such a condition is more evident after the rest period, and corrective waxing can be instituted before investing. The reader is referred to textbooks on dental materials for the principles and techniques of spruing, investing, casting, and cleaning the casting. Be certain that all investment is removed from the casting and that it is properly pickled.

SEATING, ADJUSTING, AND POLISHING THE CASTING

It is critical to closely examine the casting, preferably under magnification, before testing the fit on the die. Closely examine the internal and external surfaces with good lighting, being alert for any traces of investment, any positive defects (blebs), or any negative defects (voids). Voids in critical areas indicate rejection of the casting, unless they can be corrected by soldering. Carefully remove any small positive defects on the internal surface with an appropriately sized round bur in the high-speed handpiece.

Try the casting on the die before removing the sprue and sprue button, which serve as a handle to remove the casting, if removal is necessary. The casting should seat with little or no pressure (Fig. 20-63, *A*). Ideally it should have the same feel when being placed on the die as the feel of the wax pattern when it was seated on the die. If the casting fails to seat completely, remove it and inspect the die surface for small scratches to see where it is binding. Usually failure to seat is caused by small positive defects not seen on the first inspection. Attempts at forcing the casting to place will cause irreparable damage to the die and difficulties when trial-seating the casting in the mouth.

Once satisfied with the accuracy of the casting, separate the casting from the sprue, as close to the inlay as possible, using a carborundum separating disc. Make the cut twice as wide as the thickness of the disc to prevent binding, and do not cut completely through the sprue (leave a small uncut portion) (see Fig. 20-63, *B*). If the cut is made completely through, control of the disc is sometimes lost, often resulting in damage to the casting or to the operator's fingers. The uncut portion should be so small that bending with the fingers will break it with very little effort (see Fig. 20-63, *C*).

Having seated the casting on the die, hand *burnish* the marginal metal using a ball or beavertail burnisher (see

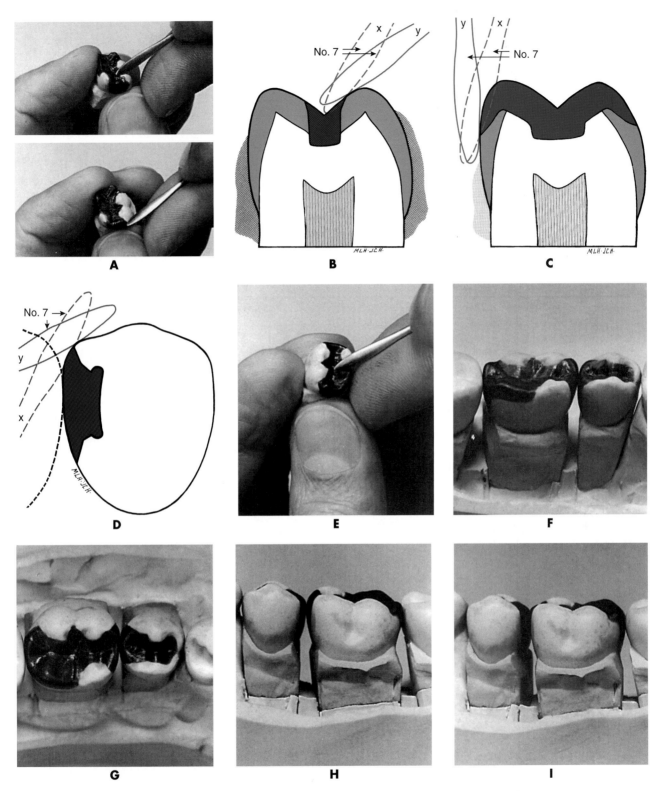

FIG. 20-61 A, Wax is carved to margins with warm No. 7 spatula. B through D, Incorrect application of No. 7 spatula to carve contour of marginal wax is shown by *x;* correct manner is labeled *y.* E, Carving occlusal groove and pit anatomy. F, Adjacent marginal ridges should be on same level as much as possible. G, Occlusal view of completed patterns. Note shape of facial and lingual embrasures and position of contact. H and I, Facial view of completed patterns. Note gingival and occlusal embrasures and position of contact.

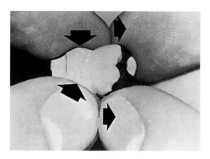

FIG. **20-62** Removing wax pattern by indirect finger pressure. (*Arrows* indicate direction of pressure.) Care must be used not to squeeze and distort wax pattern as it is initially withdrawn.

Fig. 20-63, *D*). Burnish an area approximately 1 mm in width, using strokes that increasingly approach the marginal metal and are directed parallel to the margin. Burnishing improves marginal adaptation and begins the smoothing process, almost imparting a polish to this rubbed surface. While burnishing, continually assess the adaptation of the casting along the margin, using magnification as needed to see any marginal opening as small as 0.05 mm. Moderate pressure during burnishing is indicated during closure of small marginal gaps. Once the casting is well adapted, pressure is reduced to a gentle rubbing for continued smoothing of the metal surface. At this stage, marginal openings and irregularities should not be detectable even under (×1.5 or ×2) magnification (see Fig. 20-63, *E* and *F*). Care must be taken not to overburnish the metal because this can crush and destroy the underlying die surface. Such overburnished metal will prevent complete seating of the casting on the prepared tooth. Proper burnishing usually improves the retention of the casting on the die, so that the casting does not come loose during subsequent polishing steps. *A casting must not be loose on the die if the inlay is to be properly polished.*

Carefully remove the remaining sprue metal with a heatless stone or a carborundum disc (see Fig. 20-63, *G* and *H*). Accentuate the grooves by lightly applying a somewhat dull No. 1 round bur (see Fig. 20-63, *I*) or other appropriate rotary instrument. Next, use a knife-edge rubber polishing wheel on accessible surfaces (see Fig. 20-63, *J*) (Burlew disc, J.F. Jelenko & Co., Armonk, New York). Guard against the polishing wheel touching the margins or die because they can be unknowingly and quickly polished away, resulting in "short" margins on the tooth. Also, at this time, adjust the proximal contacts one at a time. For example, if the distal surface of a MOD casting on the first molar is being adjusted, only the first and second molar dies are on the cast. *Remember that proximal contacts are correct when they are the correct size, correctly positioned, and passive.* If a temporary restoration was properly made, these contact relationships will be the same in the mouth as on the cast. Thus chair time can be conserved by carefully finishing the contacts on the cast.

Now check the occlusion of the castings by marking the occlusal contacts with articulating paper. Correct any premature contacts and refine their locations by selective grinding. Often prematurities occur where the sprue was attached and insufficient sprue metal was removed. Now apply a smaller, rubber, knife-edge wheel, which should reach some of the remaining areas not accessible to the larger disc (Fig. 20-64, *A* and *B*). The grooves, pits, and other most inaccessible regions are smoothed by rubber, abrasive points (Browne and Greenie rubber points, Shofu Dental Corp., Menlo Park, California) (see Fig. 20-64, *C*). Exercise care when using the rubber discs and points not to touch the die surface and not to destroy anatomic contours by overpolishing. When finished with the rubber abrasives, the surface of the casting should have a smooth, satin finish. Be sure that the contact relationships with the adjacent and opposing teeth have the correct size, position, and intensity.

Now brush the occlusal surface of the casting with a soft bristle disc and tripoli (or buffing bar compound [BBC]) (BBC Buffing Bar Compound, J.F. Jelenko & Co., Armonk, New York) polishing compound, running the disc parallel with the grooves (see Fig. 20-64, *D*). Use a small felt wheel with polishing compound on the proximal and other accessible surfaces (see Fig. 20-64, *E*). The metal should be so smooth before this application of polishing compound that a beautiful luster should develop in a few seconds. A high sheen may be imparted, if desired, with a felt or chamois wheel and rouge (see Fig. 20-64, *F* and *G*). Again, as in the application of tripoli/BBC, only a few seconds of rouge application should be required. If more time were expended in the application of these polishing compounds, overpolishing (polishing away) of the margins and die would result. Also, such overuse of polishing compounds is often an unsuccessful attempt to mask the fact that the preliminary stages of polishing were not thoroughly completed.

Clean the polished casting of polishing compounds by immersing the die with its inlay in a suitable solvent for a minute or two or by scrubbing with a soft brush and soap and water. Rinse, and then remove the casting from the die. *No polishing compounds should be found on the preparation side of the casting or on the preparation walls of the die.* The presence of such materials on these surfaces indicates that marginal adaptation on the die is not as good as it should be.

TRYING-IN THE CASTING

Preparing the Mouth. Local anesthesia of the tooth may be necessary before removal of the temporary and the try-in of the casting on the tooth. This blocks stimuli from inducing pain and salivation, neither of which are conducive to the best results, particularly in cementation. However, when the teeth are not particularly sensitive, an option is to delay or eliminate administering

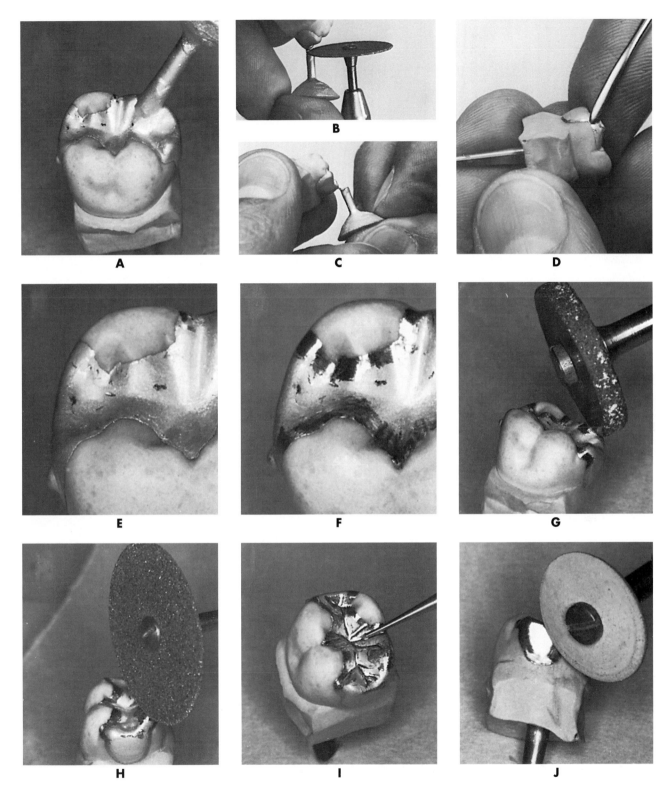

FIG. **20-63 A,** Try cleaned casting on die to determine if it has a satisfactory fit. To remove sprue, first make a cut that is not quite complete and twice the width of the disc (**B**), and then bend-break the slim, uncut portion (**C**). **D,** Inlay is burnished with No. 2 burnisher along 1-mm path that is parallel with and adjacent to margin. **E,** Magnified view of casting before burnishing. **F,** Magnified view of same marginal region shown in **E** after burnishing. Removing remaining sprue metal with heatless stone (**G**) or with carborundum disc (**H**). **I,** Accentuating grooves with dull No. 1 round bur. **J,** Smoothing surfaces accessible to rubber polishing wheel.

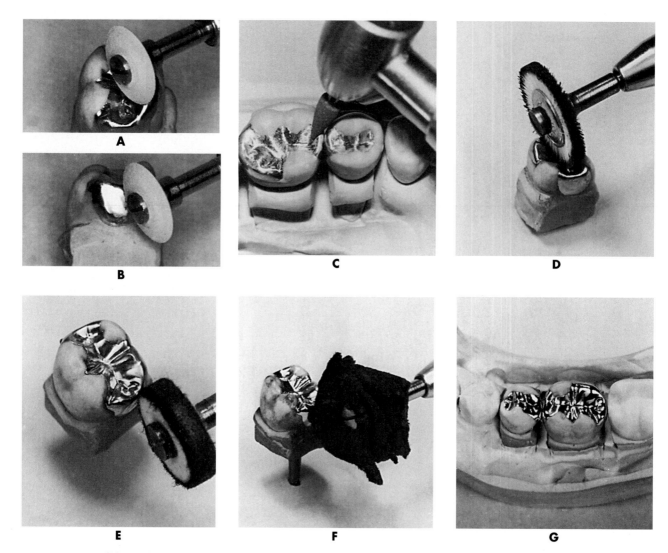

FIG. 20-64 Using a small knife-edge rubber disc on areas of the occlusal surface that are accessible to this wheel (**A**) and on proximal surfaces (**B**). **C,** Polishing grooves and other relatively inaccessible areas with rubber point. **D,** Applying tripoli/BBC to occlusal surface using bristle disc. **E,** Applying tripoli/BBC to proximal surfaces using felt wheel. **F,** Imparting luster using chamois wheel and rouge. **G,** Polished castings.

the anesthesia because the patient can better tell if the proximal contacts are tight or if the occlusion is high.

Remove the temporary restoration, making sure that all the temporary cement has been dislodged from the preparation walls and cleared away. To improve vision, isolate the region with cotton rolls. Then remove saliva from the tooth and adjacent teeth with the air syringe.

Seating the Casting and Adjusting Proximal Contacts. Now confirm the fit of the casting on the tooth. A 3 × 3 inch (7.5 × 7.5 cm) gauge sponge should be placed as a "throat screen" to catch the casting if it is accidentally dropped (see Fig. 20-69, *A*). Try the casting on the tooth, using light pressure. *Do not force the casting on the tooth.* If the casting does not seat completely, the most likely cause is an overcontoured proximal surface. Using the mouth mirror where needed, view into the

embrasures from the facial, lingual, and occlusal aspects. Judge where the proximal contour needs adjustment to allow final seating of the casting, producing at the same time the correct position and form to the contact. Passing dental floss through the contact(s) will indicate the tightness and position, thus signifying to the trained operator the degree of excess contact and its location. Apply the floss at an angle and with secure finger-bracing to pass it gently through the contact and not with a snap that is likely to injure the interproximal soft tissues. If the floss will not enter or tears on entering, the contact is excessive. *Caution: When adjusting a MOD restoration, adjust only one excess contact at a time (the stronger one) before trying again on the tooth and evaluating, unless both contacts feel equally strong.* This is done because one excessively strong contact can cause the other

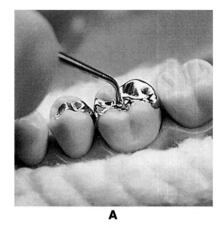

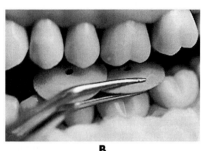

A

B

F I G . **20-65 A,** Use hand pressure to initially seat casting on tooth by applying ball burnisher in pit anatomy. **B,** If casting fits to within 0.2 mm of seating, ensure complete seating using masticatory pressure by having patient close on Burlew wheel interposed between casting and opponent tooth (teeth). **C,** Inspect marginal fit of tried-in inlay. Do not use cotton roll (**D**) or piece of wood (**E**) in lieu of Burlew wheel method (**B**).

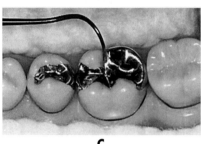

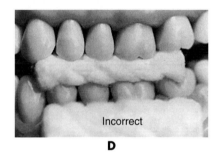

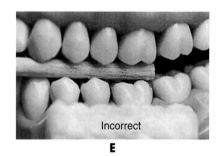

C

Incorrect

D

Incorrect

E

to feel strong, when in actuality, the latter contact may be correct or even found to be weak (short of contact) after the excessively strong contact is properly adjusted.

Use the Burlew rubber wheel to adjust the proximal contour and to correct the contact relationship. This often requires several trials on the tooth, but it is best not to remove too much at a time. After each trial and removal, the position of contact is visible in the form of a bright spot on the satiny surface left on the casting from previous surfacing by the rubber wheel. By noting the position of this bright spot in conjunction with observation in the mouth of the contact relationship, judgment can be rendered regarding the contact position and form and whether additional adjustment should be made to alter this position and form. (For removing the casting after each trial on the tooth, see Removing the Casting.)

Often the patient is able to indicate whether the contact is strong, particularly when an anesthetic has not been given. The patient should not be aware of pressure between the teeth after the final adjustment of contacts.

Remember that proper proximal contact occurs when a visual inspection verifies that the adjacent proximal surfaces are touching, and the position and form of the contact relationship are correct; the correct "tightness" of the contacts is best judged with dental floss. This contact should be passive because any pressure between the teeth would soon resolve and disappear in undesirable tooth movement.

If the contact is open (short of touching the adjacent tooth), a new contact area must be soldered to the casting. An open contact is best detected by visual inspec-

tion with the aid of the mouth mirror. The region must be isolated with cotton rolls and dried with the air syringe. Selection of the proper horizontal viewing angle usually discloses the space between the teeth. Such an open contact permits the passage of food, which will affect and irritate the interproximal gingiva.

When satisfied that the proximal contacts are correct and when hand pressure first positions the casting to within 0.2 mm of seating (Fig. 20-65, *A*), remove the 3 × 3 inch (7.5 × 7.5 cm) gauze sponge and make sure the casting completely seats on the tooth by the application of masticatory pressure. This use of masticatory pressure should be a routine procedure. It is accomplished by positioning a Burlew disc (unmounted) on the occlusal of the restoration and requesting the patient to bite firmly; also request the patient to move the jaw slightly from side to side while maintaining this firm pressure (see Fig. 20-65, *B*). At this time, the operator must judge whether the restoration is satisfactory or should be rejected and another casting made. When evaluating the fit (seating) of the casting, view particularly the margins that are horizontally directed (i.e., those that are perpendicular to the line of draw). Along at least half of the marginal outline, the tip of the explorer tine should move from tooth onto the metal, and vice versa, with barely a catch or a bump (see Figs. 20-65, *C*, and 20-66). Some operators advocate the use of a cotton roll or a piece of wood for the patient to bite on for seating pressure (see Fig. 20-65, *D* and *E*). However, the cotton roll may be too large and soft to be effective for seating inlays, and the piece of wood may not properly distribute the pressure, thus resulting in less effective seating or

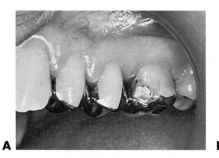
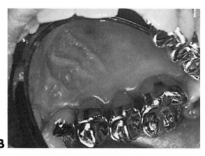
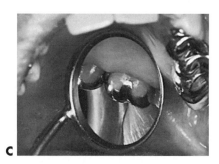

FIG. 20-66 A through **C,** Castings tried on teeth. Photographs were taken immediately after restorations were first seated on teeth before any dressing down or burnishing of margins. Neither occlusal adjustment nor contact adjustment was required. Extension of mesiofacial margin of second premolar was necessary because of extension of a previous amalgam restoration; extension of distofacial margins of premolars is caused by skirting (or bracing), which provides maximal resistance form to these weak teeth. Note area on mesiofacial margin of first molar that is to have composite insert placed after cementation.

tooth fracture. Fig. 20-66 shows the castings tried on the teeth that were first shown in Fig. 20-41, *H*.

Occluding the Casting. When the proximal contacts have been adjusted and the casting is satisfactorily seated on the tooth, have the patient close into MI, and inspect the unprepared adjacent teeth to see if there is any space between opposing wear facets. Usually the patient can indicate correctly if the casting needs occlusal adjustment; however, the dentist should verify the occlusal relationship objectively. After drying the teeth of saliva, insert a strip of articulating paper and request the patient to close and tap the teeth together (in MI) several times. Remove the paper, and examine it by holding it up toward the light for evidence of any areas of penetration caused by the restoration. Any holes can be matched with heavy markings on the casting, and there will be shiny, metal-colored spots in the center of the marks (Fig. 20-67, *A*). Such heavy contacts should be reduced with suitable abrasive stones while carefully observing the following fundamental concepts for equilibration of occlusion. The space observed between opposing wear facets of adjacent unprepared teeth (when the teeth are "closed") is an indication of the maximal amount of vertical reduction of the casting required. Often the "high" occlusal contacts are too broad and extend onto cusp or ridge slopes. When this occurs, *grind away the most incorrect portion of the incline contact (a deflective contact), leaving the most correct portion intact* (see Fig. 20-67, *B*). *Occlusal contacts in MI should be composed of supporting cusp tips placed against flat or smoothly concave surfaces (or into fossae) for stability. The force vector of occlusal contacts should be one that parallels the long axis of the tooth* (see Fig. 20-67, *C*). *Contacts on inclines tend to deflect the tooth and are less stable* (see Fig. 20-67, *D*). The use of articulating paper and the stone is continued until: (1) the heavy markings are no longer produced, (2) the contacts on the restoration have optimal position and form, and (3) there is an even distribution of con-

tacts on the casting and the adjacent teeth. Visual inspection should verify that the adjacent unprepared teeth are absolutely touching.

Care must be used not to overreduce occlusal contacts. In the final phase of equilibration, the strength of occlusal contacts can be tested by using thin plastic shim stock (Artus Corp., Englewood Cliffs, New Jersey) [0.0005 inch thick (0.013 mm)] as a "feeler gauge." Test the intensity of the occlusal contacts of the casting and the adjacent unprepared teeth to see if they hold the shim stock equally (see Fig. 20-67, *E*). It may be helpful to test the occlusal contacts of the adjacent unprepared teeth with the casting out of the mouth for comparison.

Once the occlusal contacts have been adjusted in MI, check the casting for contacts that occur during lateral mandibular movements. Lateral *working (functional) contacts* on the casting are marked by: (1) inserting a strip of articulator paper over the quadrant with the casting, (2) having the patient close into MI, and (3) then "sliding" the teeth toward the side of the mouth where the casting is located. Contacts between the lingual inclines of the maxillary lingual cusps and facial inclines of the mandibular lingual cusps are considered unusually stressful and should be eliminated (see Fig. 20-67, *F*). Contacts between the lingual inclines of the maxillary facial cusps and the facial inclines of the mandibular facial cusps should remain only if they are passive and a group function pattern of occlusion is desired.

Insert a strip of articulating paper over the teeth with the castings, have the patient close into MI, and then slide the teeth laterally toward the opposite side. This will mark any lateral *nonworking (nonfunctional) contacts* on the restoration. In a normal arrangement of teeth, contacts that might occur during the nonworking pathway are positioned on the facial inclines of the maxillary lingual cusps and the lingual inclines of the mandibular facial cusps. These nonworking contacts must be removed with a suitable stone (Fig. 20-67, *G*). Complete

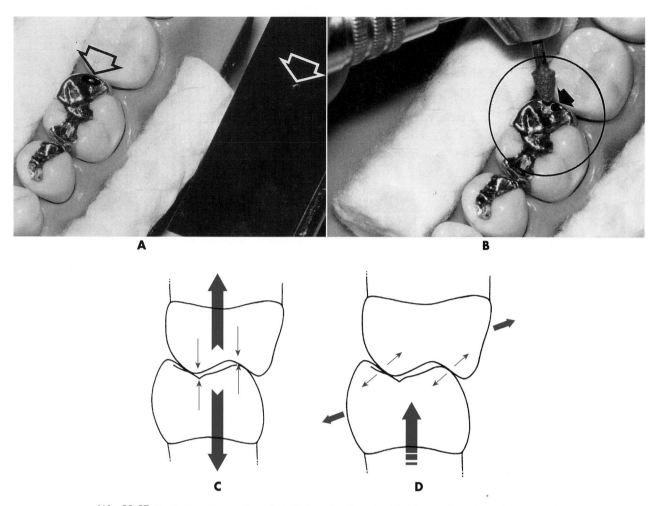

FIG. **20-67** Occluding the casting. **A,** Initial occlusal contact is high and produces heavy mark with metal-colored center. Note corresponding perforation in articulating paper. **B,** When adjusting occlusal contacts, remove most incorrect portion of contact, leaving most correct portion intact. **C,** Proper occlusal contacts in MI are composed of cusp tips placed against flat or smoothly concave surfaces (or fossae) for stability. **D,** Incline contacts are less stable and tend to deflect tooth. *Continued*

elimination of nonworking contacts can be verified by using the plastic shim stock. Insert a strip of shim stock over the casting, and have the patient bite together firmly. As soon as the patient begins sliding the mandible toward the opposite side, the shim stock should slip out from between the teeth.

Now examine the casting for interferences in *protrusive mandibular movements* using the shim stock and articulating paper. The areas that may have to be adjusted to prevent contact are the distal inclines of the maxillary teeth and the mesial inclines of the mandibular teeth.

Finally, interferences that occur on the casting between centric occlusion (CO) and MI are identified and removed. Most patients have a small discrepancy between centric occlusion and MI. Such a "skid" is considered normal for most patients, but the operator should be sure that the casting does not have premature contact at any point between CO and MI. The preferred technique for manipulating the mandible into centric relation (CR) and making the teeth touch in CO is credited to Dawson.[3] Once the teeth have been marked in CO, observe the teeth to be sure the casting does not have premature contacts in CO and that it does not exacerbate any CO-MI skid. If it does, the mesial inclines of maxillary restorations and the distal inclines of mandibular restorations are the areas that may need adjustment.

Improving Marginal Adaptation. The next step is to "dress down" the margins, that is, to adapt the metal as closely as possible to the margins of the tooth. Regardless of how accurately a casting may seat in the preparation, the fit usually can be improved by using the following procedures.

With a ball or beaver-tail burnisher, improve marginal adaptation by burnishing the marginal metal with strokes that parallel the margin, the gingival margin ex-

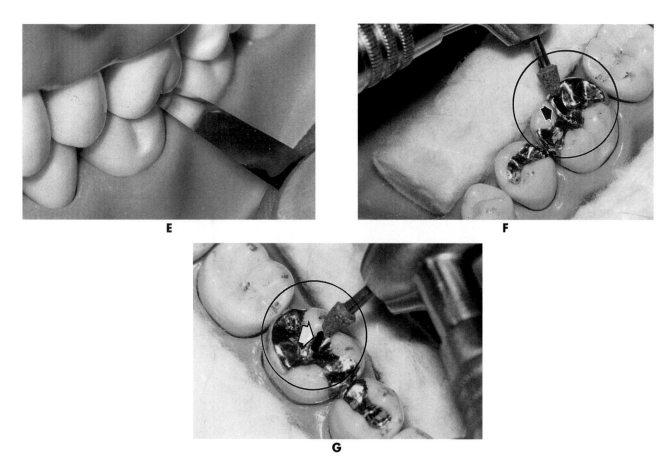

FIG. **20-67, cont'd** Occluding the casting. **E,** Testing intensity of occlusal contacts with thin (0.0005 inch [0.013 mm] thick) shim stock used as a "feeler gauge." **F,** Removing undesirable contact (lingual range) that may occur on working side during lateral mandibular movement. **G,** Removing undesirable contact that may occur on nonworking side during lateral mandibular movement.

cepted (Fig. 20-68, *A*). If the margin is inaccessible to the ball or beaver-tail burnisher (as sometimes occurs at the termination of the casting in groove regions where possibly more enameloplasty or extension could have been employed), the edge of the discoid-type hand instrument serves well as a burnisher. The discoid is held perpendicular to the margin and is moved parallel with the margin (see Fig. 20-68, *B*). The sharp edges of the discoid also will trim away any slight excess of metal at the margin. Continue with the discoid on other portions of accessible margins where a slight excess of metal is present. When burnishing the casting on the tooth, be certain the casting is fully seated. Otherwise, burnishing may bend the marginal metal, keep the casting from seating, and result in rejection of the casting.

If necessary, the marginal adaptation and continuity can be further improved by the application of a pointed, fine-grit carborundum stone, especially where the marginal enamel is slightly "high" and should be reduced or where more than just a slight amount of excess metal should be removed (see Fig. 20-68, *C*). This stone should

be used at low speed with light pressure and should rotate either parallel with the margin or from metal to tooth across the margin (never from tooth to metal). After this procedure, again burnish the margins to enhance marginal adaptation and to smooth the marginal metal.

Another instrument that can be used to improve marginal fit in accessible areas (such as the occlusal two-thirds of the proximal margins) is a fine-grit paper disk. Wherever possible, the disc should be revolved in a direction from the metal toward the tooth (see Fig. 20-68, *D*). Sometimes these margins are inaccessible to the disc, and a gingival margin trimmer, a gold file, or a cleoid instrument may be helpful to remove a slight excess of metal (see Fig. 20-68, *E*). It is moved in a scraping motion parallel to the margin and will burnish and trim the metal.

The experienced operator, if properly using the elastic impression material, with care can produce restoration margins that require very little or no burnishing or dressing down. Certainly one of the significant advan-

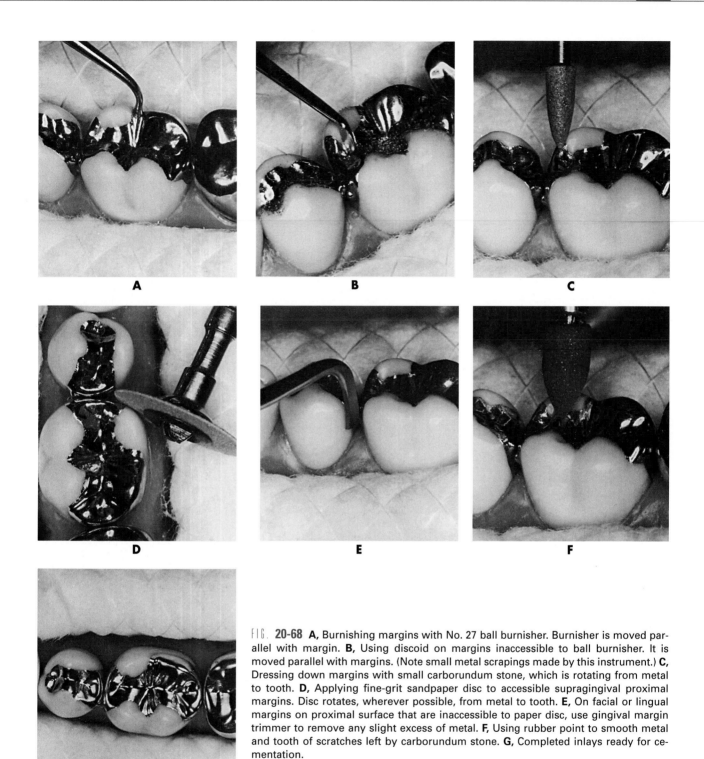

FIG. **20-68** **A,** Burnishing margins with No. 27 ball burnisher. Burnisher is moved parallel with margin. **B,** Using discoid on margins inaccessible to ball burnisher. It is moved parallel with margins. (Note small metal scrapings made by this instrument.) **C,** Dressing down margins with small carborundum stone, which is rotating from metal to tooth. **D,** Applying fine-grit sandpaper disc to accessible supragingival proximal margins. Disc rotates, wherever possible, from metal to tooth. **E,** On facial or lingual margins on proximal surface that are inaccessible to paper disc, use gingival margin trimmer to remove any slight excess of metal. **F,** Using rubber point to smooth metal and tooth of scratches left by carborundum stone. **G,** Completed inlays ready for cementation.

tages of the indirect procedure, when correctly applied, is the high degree of accuracy of the gingival margin adaptation.

Now the margins should be such that the explorer tip can pass across the margins smoothly without jumping or catching. Use rubber polishing points of increasing fineness at low speed to smooth and polish the accessible areas of roughness left from adjusting procedures (see Fig. 20-68, *F* and *G*). Attempt to preserve anatomic contour and detail. Take care to use light, intermittent

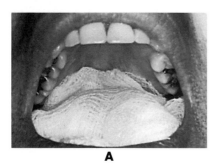
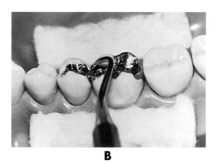
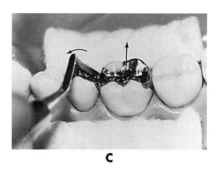

A   **B**   **C**

FIG. **20-69** Initiating removal of inlay before cementation. **A,** Place 3 × 3 inch (7.5 × 7.5 cm) gauze throat screen to prevent swallowing or aspiration of casting should it be accidentally mishandled. **B,** Tip of sharp Black spoon (15-8-14) is first inserted as deep as possible in occlusal embrasure with back of spoon against adjacent marginal ridge. **C,** Spoon is then pivoted in direction of arrow using adjacent tooth as a fulcrum. Note that casting has lifted from its seating. After only slight unseating, apply similar procedure to distal aspect.

pressure when using rubber points to prevent overheating the tooth. Clean and dry the casting surface to verify that it is smooth and free of scratches.

Removing the Casting. When preparing to remove a casting from a tooth, first place a 3 × 3 inch (7.5 × 7.5 cm) gauze sponge throat screen to prevent the patient from swallowing or aspirating the casting in the event that it is accidentally mishandled (Fig. 20-69, *A*). If the casting is very retentive, first initiate removal with the aid of a sharp Black spoon (15-8-14). The tip of the spoon is inserted as deep as possible in the occlusal embrasure with the back of the spoon resting against the marginal ridge of the adjacent tooth (see Fig. 20-69, *B*). With the tip of the spoon firmly seated against the metal casting, pivot the spoon using the adjacent tooth as a fulcrum (see Fig. 20-69, *C*). Repeat this procedure on the other occlusal embrasure if the casting is a MOD restoration. This should initiate the displacement of the casting, making complete removal thereafter easy.

CEMENTATION

Cement Selection. The selection of cement for permanent cementation is very important to the success of the final restoration. The advantages and disadvantages of each cement are discussed in detail in Chapter 4. No cement is without shortcomings. Each product has specific requirements in regard to tooth surface conditioning, casting surface conditioning, and manipulation techniques. *To obtain optimal performance from the cement, carefully follow the manufacturer's instructions for dispensing, mixing, and application.*

Cementation Technique. Before cementing the casting, isolate the tooth from saliva with the aid of cotton rolls (and saliva ejector if necessary) (Fig. 20-70, *A*). With the air syringe, dry the preparation walls, but do not desiccate them. This air should eliminate visible moisture from the walls, except possibly on the gingival bevel. Now mix the cement following the manufacturer's instructions. With the cement mix applied generously to the preparation side of the casting (see Fig. 20-

70, *B*), start the casting to place with the fingers or with operative pliers. Next, place the ball burnisher in the pit areas (first one and then another), exerting firm pressure to seat the casting (see Fig. 20-70, *C*). Then place a Burlew disc over the casting, remove the saliva ejector, and request the patient to close and exert biting force (see Fig. 20-70, *D* and *E*). Ask the patient also to move the mandible slightly from side-to-side, while continuing to exert pressure. Several seconds of this pressure is sufficient. When the disc is removed, much of the occlusal area should be clean of the cement mix and therefore easier to inspect and verify complete seating of the casting. When the cusps are capped, complete seating of the casting is verified by inspection of the facial and lingual margins after wiping the excess cement away (see Fig. 20-70, *F*). Now while the cement is still soft, burnish all accessible margins. The saliva ejector is replaced in the mouth and the *region is kept dry during the setting of the cement.* Excess moisture during this setting reaction can weaken many types of cement.

After the cement has hardened, excess is cleaned off with an explorer and air-water spray. Dental floss should be passed through the contact, carried into the interproximal gingival embrasures and sulci, and pulled facially and lingually to help in the removal of cement in this region (see Fig. 20-70, *G*). Tying a small knot in the floss will help dislodge small bits of interproximal cement. Finally, directing a stream of air into the gingival sulcus will open it and reveal any remaining small pieces of cement, which then should be removed. When cementing has been properly accomplished, a cement line should not be a visible at the margins (see Fig. 20-70, *H*). A quadrant of inlays after cementation is illustrated in Fig. 20-71.

REPAIR

The weak link of most cast metal inlays and onlays is the cement seal. At times you will find discrepancies at margins that require replacement or repair. If the restoration is intact and retentive, and if the defective

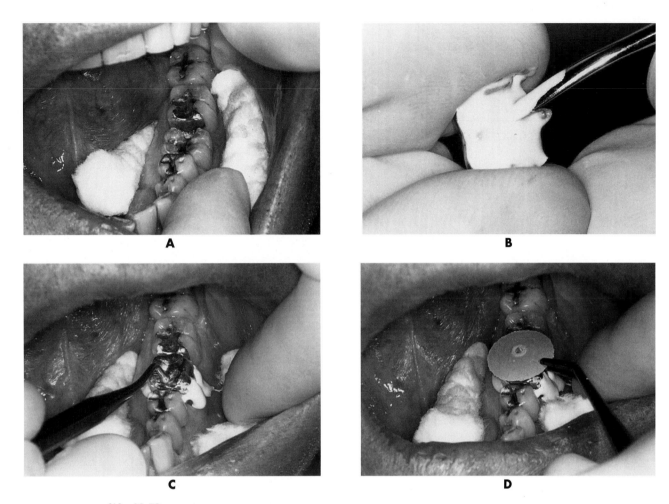

FIG. **20-70** Cementing cast metal onlay on preparation initially shown in Fig. 20-39, *B.* **A,** Isolate tooth from saliva with cotton rolls. **B,** Applying cement with No. 2 beaver-tail burnisher to preparation side of onlay. **C,** Seating onlay with ball burnisher and hand pressure. **D,** Placing Burlew disc over onlay. *Continued*

margin area is small and accessible, then small repairs can be attempted with amalgam or composite. However, if cement loss is found in one area of the restoration, other areas are usually suspect. The most common procedure once defects are found is to remove the defective restoration and replace it.

SUMMARY

Cast metal inlays and onlays offer excellent restorations that may be underutilized in dentistry. The technique requires multiple patient visits and excellent laboratory support, but the resulting restorations are durable and long lasting. High noble alloys are desirable for patients concerned with allergy or sensitivity to other restorative materials. Cast metal onlays in particular, can be designed to strengthen the restored tooth while conserving more tooth structure than a full crown. Disadvantages such as high cost and esthetics limit their use, but when indicated they provide a restorative option that is

less damaging to pulpal and periodontal tissues than a full crown.

REFERENCES

1. Carson J et al: A thermographic study of heat distribution during ultra-speed cavity preparation, *J Dent Res* 58(7):1681-1684, 1979.
2. Crispin BL et al: The marginal accuracy of treatment restorations: a comparative analysis, *J Prosthet Dent* 44:283-290, 1980.
3. Dawson PE: A classification system for occlusions that relates maximal intercuspation to the position and condition of the temporomandibular joints, *J Prosthet Dent* 75(1):60-66, 1996.
4. Fisher DW et al: Indirect temporary restorations, *J Am Dent Assoc* 82:160-163, 1971.
5. Fisher DW et al: Photoelastic analysis of inlay and onlay preparations, *J Prosthet Dent* 33(1):47-53, 1975.
6. Grajower R et al: Temperature rise in pulp chamber during fabrication of temporary self-curing resin crowns, *J Prosthet Dent* 41(5):535-540, 1979.

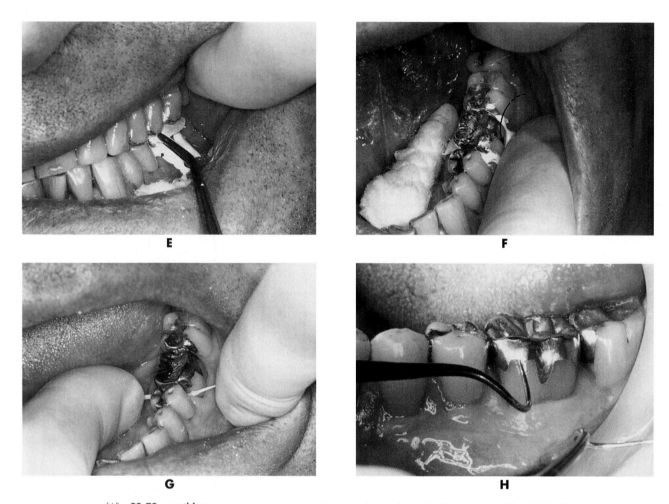

FIG. **20-70, cont'd** Cementing cast metal onlay on preparation initially shown in Fig. 20-39, *B*. **E,** Patient is instructed to apply masticatory pressure, while at the same time slightly moving the jaw from side to side. **F,** When disc is lifted from casting, much of occlusal is free from cement. With a sweeping, rolling motion of forefinger, clean any accessible facial surface margin of excess cement to permit visual inspection for verification of proper seating of onlay. Similarly clean any accessible lingual margin of excess cement. Full seating also should be verified tactilely with explorer tine. **G,** Remove excess set cement with explorer and air-water spray. Use dental tape with small knot to dislodge small pieces of interproximal cement. **H,** Onlay after cementation.

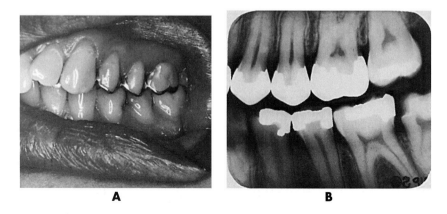

FIG. **20-71 A,** Cemented castings on teeth first shown in Fig. 20-41, *E*. Photo was taken immediately after cementation and insertion of composite insert on molar. **B,** Bitewing radiograph of restored quadrant shown in **A.** Note fit of inlays at gingival margins and contour of proximal surfaces.

7. Hood JA: Biomechanics of the intact, prepared and restored tooth: some clinical implications, *Int Dent J* 41(1):25-32, 1991.

8. Hume WR: A new technique for screening chemical toxicity to the pulp from dental restorative materials and procedures, *J Dent Res* 64(11):1322-1325, 1985.

9. Malamed SF: *Handbook of local anesthesia*, ed. 4, St Louis, 1997, Mosby.

10. Moulding MB, Loney RW: The effect of cooling techniques on intrapulpal temperature during direct fabrication of provisional restorations, *Int J Prosthodont* 4(4):332-336, 1991.

11. Payne E: Reproduction of tooth form, *Ney Tech Bull* 1(9), 1961.

12. Stanley HR: Effects of dental restorative materials: local and systemic responses reviewed, *J Am Dent Assoc* 124(10):76-80, 1993.

13. Sturdevant JR et al: The 8-year clinical performance of 15 low-gold casting alloys, *Dent Mater* 3(6):347-352, 1987.

14. Wataha JC: Biocompatibility of dental casting alloys: a review, *J Prosthet Dent* 83(2):223-234, 2000.

21

Direct Gold Restorations

GREGORY E. SMITH

DIRECT GOLDS AND PRINCIPLES OF MANIPULATION

Several types of dental restorative materials are currently available. Generally they are grouped into categories such as amalgam materials, cast golds, tooth-colored materials, dental porcelains, porcelains fused to metal, and direct golds. *Direct golds* are those gold restorative materials that are manufactured for compaction directly into prepared cavities. Two types of direct golds are manufactured for dental use: gold foil and powdered gold; they differ in their metallurgic structure.

Pure gold has been in use in dentistry in the United States for well over 100 years.[3,5,9,11,16,18] A variety of techniques have been advanced for its use in the restoration of teeth. It is generally agreed that this noble metal is a superior restorative material for treatment of many small lesions and defects in teeth, given sound pulpal and periodontal health. Success is achieved with direct gold restorations if meticulous care is given to an exacting technique in tooth-preparation design and material manipulation. Direct gold restorations can last for a lifetime if attention is paid to details of restorative technique and to proper homecare. The longevity of direct gold restorations is a result of both the superb biocompatibility of gold with the oral environment and its excellent marginal integrity.

It is the purpose of this chapter to discuss the various forms of direct gold presently available and explain the principles required for their manipulation. The principles of tooth preparation are reviewed as they are applied to direct gold restorations, and a detailed consideration is given to Class I, Class V, and Class III preparations and their restoration.

MATERIALS AND MANUFACTURE

There have been several physical types of direct-filling golds produced.[10] All are "compactable" in that they are inserted into tooth preparations under force and compacted or condensed into preparation line and point angles and against preparation walls.

Gold foil is manufactured by beating pure gold into thin sheets. The gold foil is cut into 4 × 4 inch (10 × 10 cm) sheets and sold in books of sheets, separated by pages of thin paper. The books contain $\frac{1}{10}$ or $\frac{1}{20}$ oz of gold. The sheets of foil that weigh 4 gr each are termed No. 4 foil; the sheets weighing 3 gr are termed No. 3 foil; and the sheets weighing 2 gr are termed No. 2 foil. Because the 4 × 4 inch sheets of foil are too large to use in restorative procedures, they are rolled into cylinders or pellets before insertion into tooth preparations. (The gold foil referred to in the restorative sections of this chapter is in pellet form.)

Pellets of gold foil are generally rolled from $\frac{1}{32}$-, $\frac{1}{43}$-, $\frac{1}{64}$-, or $\frac{1}{128}$-inch sections cut from a No. 4 sheet of foil. The book of foil is marked and cut into squares or rectangles (Fig. 21-1, *A*). Each piece is placed on clean fingertips, and the corners are tucked into the center (see Fig. 21-1, *B* and *C*); then it is lightly rolled into pellet form (see Fig. 21-1, *D*). In addition, cylinders of gold foil may be rolled from segments of a sheet (see Fig. 21-1, *A*). After pellets of gold are rolled, they may be conveniently stored in a *gold foil box* (Fig. 21-2), which is divided into labeled sections for various sizes of pellets. Cylinders of foil and selected sizes of other types of gold may also be stored in the box. Preferential contamination is suggested by placing a damp cotton pellet dipped into 18% ammonia into each section of the box.

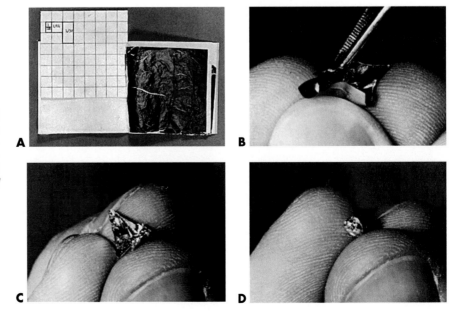

FIG. **21-1 A,** 4 × 4 inch book of foil marked for cutting and rolling into pellets of various sizes. **B** and **C,** Corners of foil piece are tucked into center. **D,** Foil is rolled into a completed pellet. **(A,** *Courtesy of Terkla and Cantwell.)*

This will serve to prevent deleterious oxides from forming on the gold until it is used.

Powdered gold is made by a combination of chemical precipitation and atomization, with an average particle size of 15 mm[12] (see Fig 21-3, *A*). The atomized particles are mixed together in wax, cut into pieces, and wrapped in No. 4 or No. 3 foil (see Fig 21-3, *B*). Several sizes of these pellets are available. This product is marketed as Williams E-Z Gold.

COHESION AND DEGASSING

Direct golds are inserted into tooth preparations under force. The purpose of the force is to weld the gold into restorations containing minimal porosity or internal void spaces.[6,7,14] Welding occurs because pure gold with an absolutely clean surface will cohere as a result of metallic bonding. As the gold is forced and compressed into a tooth preparation, succeeding increments cohere to those previously placed. For successful welding to occur during restoration, *the gold must be in a cohesive state before compaction, and a suitable, biologically compatible compacting force must be delivered.*

Direct gold may be either *cohesive* or *noncohesive*. It is noncohesive if surface impurities or wax are present that prevent one increment of gold from cohering to another. The manufacturer supplies books of gold foil or prerolled cylinders in a cohesive or noncohesive state. E-Z Gold pellets are supplied with a wax coating that must be burned off before compaction.

Because gold attracts gases that render it noncohesive, such gases must be removed from the surface of the gold before dental compaction. This process is usually referred to as *degassing* or *annealing* and is accomplished by application of heat. Degassing is the preferred term, because the desired result is to remove residual surface contamination (although further annealing, resulting in additional internal stress relief or recrystallization, may also occur in this process). All direct-filling gold products are degassed immediately before use, except when noncohesive foil is specifically desired. Underheating during degassing is to be avoided, because it fails to render the gold surface pure. Overheating is also to be avoided, because it may cause the gold to become brittle or melt and render it unusable. Degassing is accomplished by heating the gold foil on a mica tray over a flame or on an electric annealer or by heating each piece of gold over a pure ethanol flame (Fig. 21-4).

The advantage of the technique involving use of the pure ethanol flame is that each piece of gold is selected and heated just before insertion, and waste of gold is avoided. A careful technique is needed to correctly degas an increment of gold in the flame. The gold is passed into the blue inner core of the flame on the tip of a foil passing instrument and held just until the gold becomes dull red; then the instrument is withdrawn from the flame. After a few seconds are allowed for cooling, the gold is placed in the preparation.

Although any of the three degassing procedures is satisfactory for gold foil, this is not the case for E-Z Gold. The E-Z Gold pellet must be heated ½ to 1 inches above the ethanol flame until a bright flame occurs (caused by ignition of the wax) and the pellet becomes dull red for 2 to 3 seconds; then it is withdrawn from above the flame.

PRINCIPLES OF COMPACTION

Direct-filling golds must be compacted during insertion into tooth preparations.[2] With the exception of E-Z Gold, the *compaction* takes the form of malleting forces that are delivered either by a hand mallet used by the

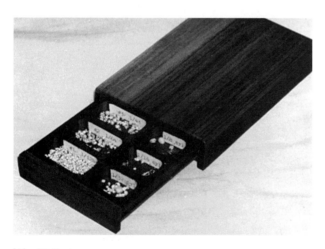

FIG. **21-2** Gold foil box. Compartments are labeled to show pellet size.

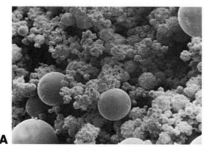
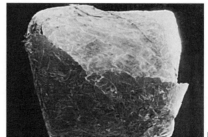

FIG. **21-3** Scanning electron photomicrographs of direct-filling golds. **A,** Spheres of E-Z Gold, **B,** Wrapped E-Z pellet that contains spheres. *(Courtesy of Ivoclar-Williams Company, Inc.)*

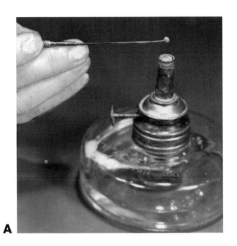
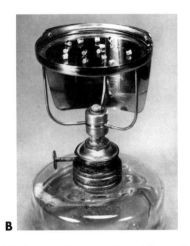
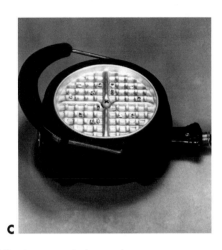

A   B   C

FIG. 21-4 **A,** Pellet of gold foil is degassed in *pure* ethanol flame. **B,** Mica tray mounted over alcohol lamp for degassing several increments of gold simultaneously. **C,** Gold foil degassed on an electric annealer. *(Courtesy of Terkla and Cantwell.)*

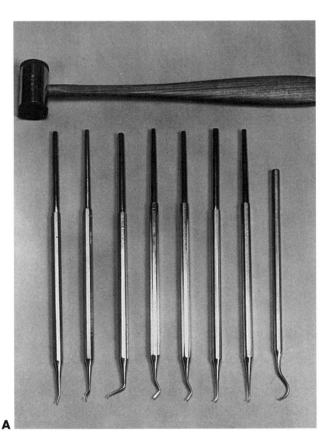

FIG. 21-5 **A,** Hand mallet and condensers used for hand mallet compaction of direct gold. **B,** A selection of variously shaped nibs. *Left to right:* Three round-faced nibs, oblique-faced nib, foot condenser, and rounded rectangular nib. *(A, Courtesy of Terkla and Cantwell.)*

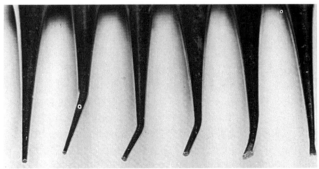

A   B

assistant or by an Electro-Mallet or a pneumatic mallet used by the dentist. E-Z Gold, because of its powdered form, may be compacted by heavy hand pressure delivered in a rocking motion with specially designed hand condensers.[1,19] Successful malleting of the gold foil may be achieved with any of the currently available equipment. Some operators prefer the Electro-Mallet or pneumatic mallet because a dental assistant is not required for the procedure.

A technique preferred by many clinicians uses a hand mallet to deliver light blows to a condenser held by the dentist (Fig. 21-5, *A*). This technique allows great control of malleting forces when variations are called for, and it allows for rapid change in condenser nibs, or tips, when a multitude of condensers is required. In any case a suitable condenser must be stepped over the gold systematically to achieve a dense, well-compacted restoration (see Fig. 21-8).

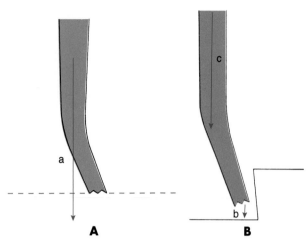

FIG. 21-6 **A,** Oblique-faced condenser with nib face established perpendicular to long axis of handle and perpendicular to line of force (*a*). **B,** Conventional monangle condenser; nib face is not perpendicular to line of force (*b*); condenser nib face is established perpendicular to end portion of shank rather than perpendicular to handle (*c*).

Condensers are designed to deliver forces of compaction to direct golds. Condensers used in the handpieces of the Electro-Mallet or pneumatic mallet consist of a *nib,* or working tip, and a short *shank* (approximately 1 inch [2.5 cm] in length) that fits into the malleting handpiece. Condensers used with the hand mallet are longer (approximately 6 inches [15 cm]) and have a blunt-ended *handle* that receives light blows from the hand mallet.

Condenser *nibs* are available in several shapes and sizes (see Fig. 21-5, *B*). All have pyramidal serrations on the nib faces to prevent slipping on the gold. Those described in this chapter are: (1) the round condensers, 0.4 to 0.55 mm in diameter; (2) the Varney foot condenser, which has a rectangular face that is approximately 1 to 1.3 mm, and (3) the parallelogram condensers, which are used only for hand pressure compaction and have nib faces that measure approximately 0.5 to 1 mm.

Condenser *shanks* may be straight, monangled, or offset, and their *nib faces* may be cut perpendicular to the long axis of the handle or perpendicular to the end portion of the shank (Fig. 21-6). The smaller the nib face size (i.e., area), the greater the pounds per square inch delivered (given a constant malleting force). For example, if the nib diameter is reduced by half, the effective compaction force in pounds per square inch is four times greater (because the area of a circle is proportional to the square of the diameter). For most gold, the 0.4- to 0.55-mm diameter nibs are suitable. Smaller condensers tend to punch holes in the gold, whereas larger ones are less effective in forcing the gold into angles in the tooth preparation.

Two fundamental principles involved in compaction of cohesive gold are to: (1) weld the gold into a cohesive mass and (2) wedge as much gold as possible into the

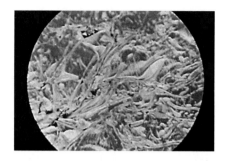

FIG. 21-7 Compacted gold foil. Linear channels are evident between creases in the foil pellet. Dark spots are void spaces in the compacted mass.

tooth preparation.[13] Welding takes place primarily as a result of the coherence of a noble metal to itself. Wedging results from careful compacting technique. Regardless of the technique used, some *bridging* will occur, resulting in void spaces not only in the compacted gold but also along the preparation walls. Success depends on minimizing these voids, particularly on the surface of the restoration and at the cavosurface interface where leakage to the internal aspects of the restoration may begin.

Gold foil compacts readily because of its thin form and produces a mass with isolated linear channels of microporosity (Fig. 21-7). Because the thin folds of the gold pellet weld to each other, the remaining channels of microporosity do not appear to be entirely confluent with one another.

It is recommended that compaction of E-Z Gold be done by hand pressure. As compaction is performed, the bag of atomized gold is opened and the spheres of gold powder move over one another and against the preparation walls. Heavy and methodic hand pressure with the condensers is required to compact this form of gold effectively.

COMPACTION TECHNIQUE FOR GOLD FOIL

Compaction begins when a piece of gold is placed in a tooth preparation. The gold is first pressed to place by hand; then a condenser of suitable size is used to begin malleting in the center of the mass (often this is done while this first increment is held in position with a holding instrument). Each succeeding step of the condenser overlaps (by half) the previous one as the condenser is moved toward the periphery (Fig. 21-8). The gold moves under the nib face of the condenser, effecting compaction as malleting proceeds.

The most efficient compaction occurs directly under the nib face.[13] Some compaction also occurs by lateral movement of the gold against surrounding preparation walls. The result of compaction is to remove most of the void space from within each increment of gold, to compact the gold into line and point angles and against walls, and to attach it to any previously placed gold via the process of cohesion.[8]

The line of force is important when any gold is compacted. The line of force is that direction through which the force is delivered (i.e., the direction in which the condenser is aimed) (Fig 21-9). Specific instructions regarding line of force are given in subsequent sections of this chapter as they relate to the restorations.

Research has shown that a biologically acceptable pulpal response occurs after proper direct gold procedures.[17] Care is required when condensing forces are applied to preclude pulpal irritation. The Electro-Mallet is an acceptable condenser if the manufacturer's instructions for mallet intensity are followed. Correct hand-malleting technique requires a light, bouncing application of the mallet to the condenser, rather than the delivery of heavy blows.

COMPACTION TECHNIQUE FOR E-Z GOLD

Using an amalgam condenser or a gold foil condenser, the first pellet of E-Z Gold is pressed into the depth of the tooth preparation and tamped into position. A small condenser is then selected to thrust and wedge the gold into opposing line angles and against opposing walls, to secure the mass in the preparation. Additional pellets are added (one at a time, banking against the preparation walls) until the entire preparation is filled. To avoid creation of large void spaces in the restoration, a dense, fully condensed surface is obtained with each pellet before subsequent pellets are added.

PRINCIPLES OF TOOTH PREPARATION FOR DIRECT GOLD RESTORATIONS

FUNDAMENTALS OF TOOTH PREPARATION

The principles of tooth preparation for all direct gold restorations demand meticulous attention to detail for success. Failure to give attention to outline form may result in an unsightly restoration or, at the least, one in which cavosurface deficiencies are immediately obvious. Poor resistance form can result in tooth fracture; inadequate retention form may result in a loose restoration that is frustrating to the dentist. Lack of detailed convenience form may render an otherwise excellent tooth preparation unrestorable. The preparation must be smoothed and débrided to permit the first increments of gold to be stabilized.

The margins in *outline form* must not be ragged. They are established on sound areas of the tooth that can be finished and polished. The outline must include all structural defects associated with the lesion. The marginal outline must be designed to be esthetically pleasing, because the final restoration may be visible.

Resistance form is established by orienting preparation walls to support the integrity of the tooth, such as a pulpal wall that is flat and perpendicular to occlusal forces. All enamel must be supported by sound dentin. Opti-

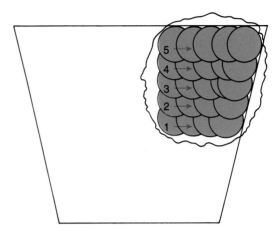

FIG. **21-8** Diagrammatic order of compaction for increment of direct-filling gold. Condensers are moved across surface of gold in an orderly stepping motion. Each succeeding step of the nib overlaps the previous one by at least half of the nib face diameter. Condensation begins at position *1* and moves to the right, then resumes at *2* and repeats movement to the right. Finally, it continues in rows *3*, *4*, and *5*.

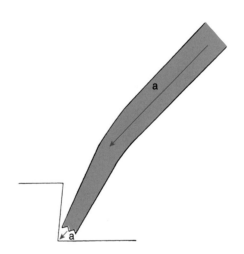

FIG. **21-9** Line of force (*a*) remains parallel with shaft or handle of condenser, regardless of any angles in shank of instrument.

mally placed axial or pulpal walls promote the integrity of the restored tooth, thus providing a suitable thickness of remaining dentin.

The *retention form* is established by parallelism of some walls and by strategically placed converging walls (as will be described in detail for each tooth preparation). In addition, walls must be smooth and flat where possible (to provide resistance to loosening of the gold during compaction), and internal line angles must be sharp (to resist movement). Internal form includes an initial depth into dentin, ranging from 0.5 mm from the dentinoenamel junction (DEJ) in Class I preparations to 0.75 mm from the cementum in Class V preparations.

Optimal *convenience form* requires suitable access and a dry field provided by the rubber dam. Access may additionally require the use of a gingival retractor for

Class V restorations or a separator to provide a minimal amount of separation (0.5 mm maximum) between anterior teeth for Class III restorations. Sharp internal line and point angles are created in dentin to allow convenient "starting" gold foil as compaction begins. Rounded form is permitted when E-Z Gold is used to begin the restorative phase.

Removal of remaining carious dentin, final planing of cavosurface margins, and débridement complete the tooth preparation for direct gold.

INDICATIONS AND CONTRAINDICATIONS

Class I direct gold restorations are one option for the treatment of small carious lesions in pits and fissures of most posterior teeth and the lingual surfaces of anterior teeth. Direct gold is also indicated for treatment of small, cavitated Class V carious lesions or for the restoration, when indicated, of abraded, eroded, or abfraction areas on the facial surfaces of teeth (although access to the molars is a limiting factor). Class III direct gold restorations can be used on the proximal surfaces of anterior teeth where the lesions are small enough to be treated with esthetically pleasing results. Class II direct gold restorations are an option for restoration of small cavitated proximal surface carious lesions in posterior teeth in which marginal ridges are not subjected to heavy occlusal forces (e.g., the mesial or distal surfaces of mandibular first premolars and the mesial surface of some maxillary premolars). Class VI direct gold restorations may be used on incisal edges or cusp tips. A defective margin of an otherwise acceptable cast gold restoration also may be repaired with direct golds.

Direct gold restorations are contraindicated in some teeth with very large pulp chambers, in severely periodontally weakened teeth with questionable prognosis, when economics is a severely limiting factor, and in handicapped patients who are unable to sit for the long dental appointments required for this procedure. Root canal filled teeth are generally not restored with direct gold because these teeth are brittle, although in some cases gold may be the material of choice to close access preparations (for root canal therapy) in cast gold restorations.

TOOTH PREPARATIONS AND RESTORATIONS

The following section presents the preparation and the restoration of Classes I, V, and III lesions. The preparations described may be restored entirely with pellets of gold foil, or E-Z Gold may be used. If powdered gold is selected, heavy hand pressure compaction may be substituted for hand mallet or automatic mallet techniques. Classes I and V E-Z Gold restorations may be veneered with gold foil pellets, if desired. (The Class III tooth preparation discussed in this chapter is recommended by Ferrier, and only pellets of gold foil are used for the restoration.)

All tooth preparations and restorative procedures are accomplished after a suitable field of operation has been achieved (usually by application of the rubber dam).

CLASS I TOOTH PREPARATION AND RESTORATION

Tooth Preparation Design. The marginal *outline form* for the Class I tooth preparation for compacted gold is extended to include the lesion on the tooth surface treated, as well as any fissured enamel. The preparation outline may be a simple circular design for a pit defect, or it may be oblong, triangular, or a more extensive form (if needed to treat a defective fissure) (Fig. 21-10, *A*). Preparation margins are placed beyond the extent of pits and fissures. All noncoalesced enamel and structural defects are removed; the outline is kept as small as possible, consistent with provision of suitable access for instrumentation and for manipulation of gold.

For Class I tooth preparations, the external walls of the preparation are parallel to each other. However, in extensive occlusal preparations, the mesial or distal wall or walls (or both) may diverge slightly occlusally to avoid undermining and weakening marginal ridges.

FIG. **21-10 A,** Typical Class I occlusal marginal outlines for pit restorations with direct gold. **B,** Cross-section of model of lingual Class I preparation on maxillary incisor. Undercuts (*a* and *b*) are placed in dentin incisally and gingivally for additional retention.

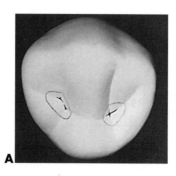

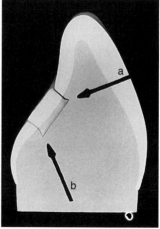

The pulpal wall is of uniform depth, parallel with the plane of the surface treated, and established at 0.5 mm into the dentin. The pulpal wall meets the external walls at a slightly rounded angle created by the shape of the bur. Small undercuts may be placed in the dentin if additional retentive features are required to provide convenience form in beginning the compaction of gold (see Fig. 21-10, B). Undercuts, when desired, are placed facially and lingually in posterior teeth (or incisally and gingivally on the lingual surface of incisors) at the level of the ideal pulpal floor position. These undercut line angles must not undermine marginal ridges. A very slight cavosurface bevel may be placed to: (1) create a 30- to 40-degree metal margin for ease in finishing the gold and (2) remove remaining rough enamel. The bevel is not greater than 0.2 mm in width and is placed with a white rotary stone or suitable finishing bur.

Instrumentation. For description and illustration, the preparation of a carious pit on the mandibular first premolar is presented (Fig. 21-11, A). By use of a high-speed handpiece with air-water spray, the No. 330 or No. 329 bur is aligned and the outline form (which includes the limited initial depth) is established (see Fig. 21-11, B). When the preparation is extensive because of including fissured enamel, a small hoe, 6½-2½-9, may be used to complete the desired degree of flatness of the pulpal wall. Using the No. 33½ bur at low speed, small retentive undercuts are prepared into the dentin portion of the external walls at the initial pulpal wall depth; these also may be prepared using a 6½-(90)-2½-9 angle-former chisel. Round burs of suitable size are used to remove any infected carious dentin that remains on the pulpal wall. The preparation is completed by finishing the cavosurface with an angle former, a small

finishing bur (e.g., No. 7802), or a flame-shaped white stone (see Fig. 21-11, C through E).

Restoration. The restorative phase begins with insertion of a pellet of E-Z Gold or gold foil. The gold is first degassed in the alcohol flame, cooled momentarily in air, and inserted into the preparation with the passing instrument. The gold is pressed to place with the nib of a small round condenser. In larger preparations, a pair of condensers is used for this initial stabilization of the gold. Next, compaction of the gold begins with a line of force directed against the pulpal wall (Fig. 21-12, A). Hand pressure is used for E-Z Gold; malleting is used for gold foil. The gold is compacted into the pulpal line angles and against the external walls, and the line of force is changed to a 45-degree angle to the pulpal and respective external walls (to best compact the gold against the internal walls) (see Fig. 21-12, B). Additional increments of gold are added, and the procedure is repeated until the preparation is about three-quarters full of compacted gold. If E-Z Gold is to be the final restoration surface, compaction is continued until the restoration is slightly overfilled.

If gold foil is selected to veneer this restoration, then pellets of suitable size are selected; in larger preparations large pellets are convenient, whereas for small pit preparations the operator should begin with 1/64-size pellets (Fig. 21-13). The pellet is degassed and carried to the preparation. First, hand pressure compaction is used to secure the pellet against the compacted E-Z Gold and spread it over the surface; then mallet compaction is used. Likewise each succeeding pellet is hand compacted and then mallet compacted. The condenser point is systematically stepped over the gold twice as malleting proceeds. Generally the line of force is perpendicu-

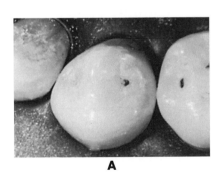
A

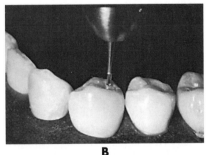
B

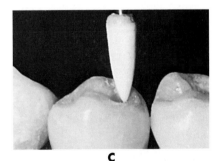
C

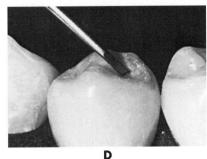
D

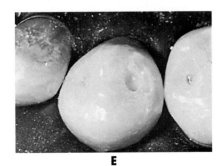
E

FIG. **21-11** Class I preparation for direct gold. **A,** Preoperative view of pit lesion. **B,** A No. 330 bur is aligned properly for occlusal preparation. **C,** Occlusal cavosurface bevel is prepared with white stone. **D,** The bevel may be placed with an angle former. **E,** Completed tooth preparation.

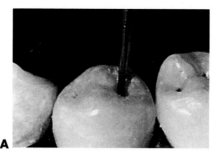
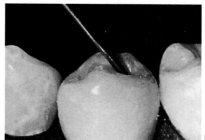

FIG. **21-12 A,** Compaction forces are delivered by condenser held at 90-degree angle to pulpal wall. **B,** Gold is condensed against external preparation walls.

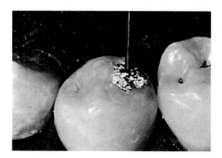

FIG. **21-13** Placement of pellet of gold foil and compaction into tooth preparation.

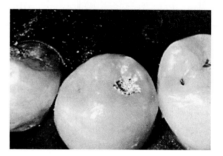

FIG. **21-14** Compaction of gold foil has proceeded sufficiently to cover all cavosurface margins.

lar to the pulpal floor in the center of the mass and at a 45-degree angle to the pulpal floor as the external walls are reached. At this stage and during all building of the restoration, the compacted surface should be saucer shaped, with the compaction of gold on the external walls slightly ahead of the center. The surface should never be convex in the center, because this may result in voids in the gold and poor adaptation of the gold along the external walls when the condenser nib is "crowded out" along the wall by the center convexity. Continue building the restoration until the cavosurface margin is covered with foil (Fig. 21-14). *Exercise extreme care that gold is always present between the condenser face and the cavosurface margin;* otherwise the condenser may injure (i.e., fracture) the enamel margin. Now fill in the central area of the restoration's surface to the desired level. Tooth surface contour of the gold is created to simulate the final anatomic form, and a slight excess of gold is compacted on the surface to allow for the finishing and polishing procedures.

The first step in the finishing procedure is to burnish the gold (Fig. 21-15, *A*). A flat beaver-tail burnisher is used with heavy hand pressure to harden the surface gold. A cleoid-discoid carver is used to continue the burnishing process and remove excess gold on the cavosurface margin. The cleoid, always directed so that a portion of the working edge is over or resting on enamel adjacent to or near the margins, is pulled from gold to tooth across the surface. This is done to smooth the surface and trim away excess gold (see Fig. 21-15, *B*). If considerable excess gold has been compacted, a green stone may be necessary to remove the excess in Class I

restorations. Care must be taken at this stage to avoid abrading the surface enamel. After use of the cleoid-discoid, a small round finishing bur (No. 9004) is used to begin polishing (see Fig. 21-15, *C*). It is followed by the application of flour of pumice and tin oxide or white rouge (see Fig. 21-15, *D*). These powdered abrasives are applied dry, with a webless, soft-rubber cup in a low-speed handpiece. Care is taken to use light pressure. Gentle blasts of air cool the surface during polishing. The completed restoration is illustrated in Figure 21-16.

CLASS V TOOTH PREPARATION AND RESTORATION

The Operating Field. As with all direct gold restorations, the rubber dam must be in place to provide a suitable, dry field for a Class V restoration. Furthermore, for lesions near the gingiva or that extend into the gingival sulcus, it is necessary to provide appropriate access to the lesion by placing a No. 212 retainer or gingival retractor. The punching of the rubber dam is modified to provide ample rubber between the teeth and to provide enough rubber for coverage and retraction of the soft tissue on the facial side of the tooth. The hole for the tooth to be treated is punched 1 mm facial of its normal position, and an extra 1 mm of dam is left between the hole for the treated tooth and the holes for the immediately adjacent teeth.

Several modifications may be made to the No. 212 retainer to facilitate its use. If the notches that are engaged by the retainer forceps are shallow, they may be deepened slightly with a large, carbide fissure bur to provide a more secure lock for the forceps (Fig. 21-17, *A*). If the

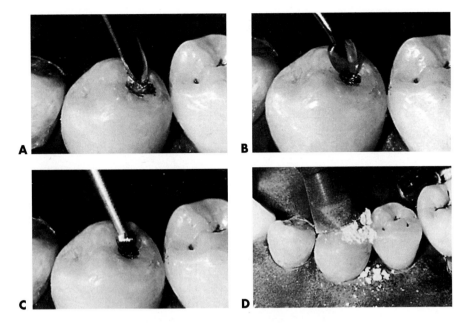

FIG. **21-15** Steps in finishing Class I direct gold restoration. **A,** Burnisher work hardens the surface gold. **B,** Cleoid-discoid removes excess gold from cavosurface margins. **C,** A No. 9004 bur is used to begin polishing phase. **D,** Polishing abrasives are applied with rubber cup.

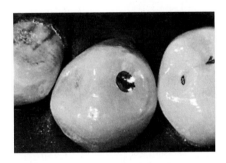

FIG. **21-16** Completed restoration.

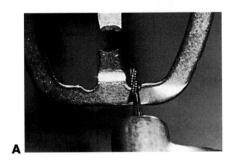
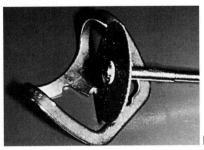

FIG. **21-17 A,** Notches are deepened for secure holding of the No. 212 retainer. **B,** Jaws may be modified with a disc to facilitate retainer placement on rotated teeth.

tips of the retainer jaws are very sharp, they may be slightly rounded with a garnet disc and then polished to avoid scratching cementum during placement. For application to narrow teeth (e.g., mandibular incisors), the facial and lingual jaws may be narrowed by grinding with a heatless stone or carborundum disc, after which they are polished with a rubber wheel. To expedite placement on rotated teeth, the jaws may be modified by grinding suitable contour to the tip edge (see Fig. 21-17, *B*). The jaws may be bent for use on teeth where gingival access to lesions is difficult. This is done by heating the jaws to a cherry red color in a flame, then grasping the entire facial jaw with suitable pliers and slightly bending the jaw apically. The procedure is repeated for the lingual jaw, bending it slightly occlusally (Fig. 21-18).

The No. 212 retainer must be carefully applied to avoid damage to the soft or hard tissue. The retainer is secured in the retainer forceps and carried to the mouth after the rubber dam has been placed. The lingual jaw is positioned just apical to the lingual height of contour, and the index finger is placed against the jaw to prevent its movement. The retainer is rotated faciogingivally with the forceps, while the thumb retracts the dam; then the facial jaw is set against the tooth (Fig. 21-19, *A*). Next a ball burnisher is placed into one of the retainer notches and used to move the facial jaw gingivally (without scraping the jaw against the tooth) to the final position

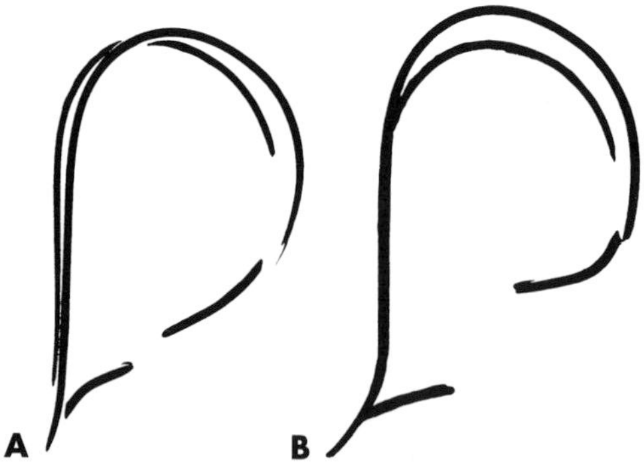

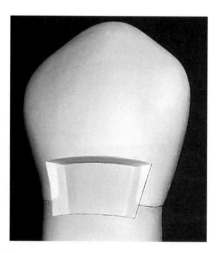

FIG. 21-18 **A,** Drawing of a No. 212 retainer as received from the manufacturer. **B,** Modified facial and lingual jaws.

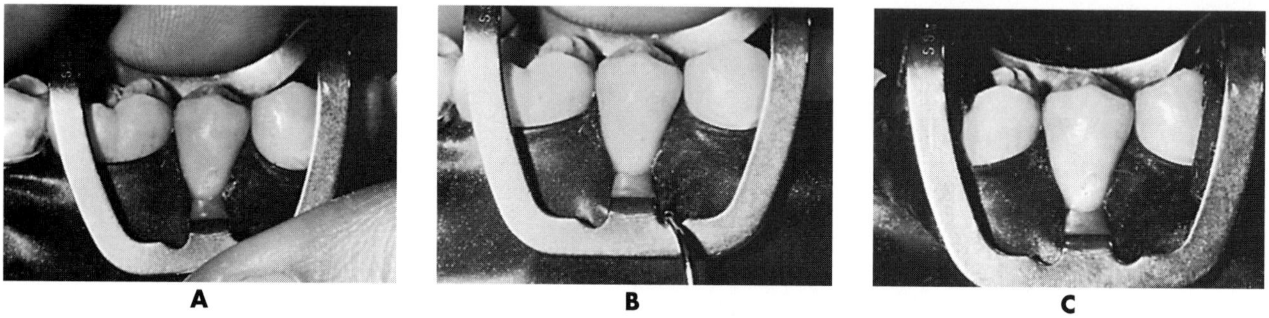

FIG. 21-19 Placement of No. 212 retainer. **A,** Initial placement of facial jaw after first placing lingual jaw. **B,** Use of ball burnisher to carry facial jaw to final position. **C,** Retainer stabilized with compound to distribute compaction forces, prevent tipping, and prevent either apical or occlusal movement of retainer.

FIG. 21-20 Facial view of Class V tooth preparation for direct gold. Occlusal and gingival margins are straight, parallel with each other, and extend mesially and distally to respective mesiofacial and distofacial tooth crown line angles. Mesial and distal walls diverge facially and form obtuse angles with axial wall. Line angles and point angles are sharp (see Fig. 21-22, *B*).

(i.e., 0.5 to 1 mm apical of the expected gingival margin) (see Fig. 21-19, *B*). Gentle pressure is used to position the facial jaw so that only the free gingiva is retracted and the epithelial attachment is not harmed. The retainer is supported and locked into this desired position with compound, which is softened, molded by the fin-

gers, and placed between the bows and the gingival embrasures (see Fig. 21-19, *C*). The compound also serves to distribute compaction forces among all the teeth included in the retainer application. (Also see application of the No. 212 retainer in Chapters 10, 12, and 18.)

Tooth Preparation Design. The typical Class V tooth preparation for restoration with direct gold is trapezoidal (Figs. 21-20, 21-21, and 21-22). This outline form is created to satisfy both esthetic needs and requirements for retention and convenience forms in the treatment of lesions in the gingival third of the clinical crowns of teeth. The straight occlusal margin improves the esthetic result, and by virtue of its straight design, excess gold is readily discerned and removed in the final stages of the restorative process. The gingival outline is shorter than the occlusal, because the tooth narrows in the gingival area. In addition, it is prepared parallel with the occlusal margin for easy identification in finishing phases. The mesial and distal margins connect the gingival margin to the occlusal margin.

The occlusal margin is straight and parallel with the occlusal plane of the teeth in the arch (see Figs. 21-20 and 21-21); it is extended occlusally to include the lesion. (When several adjacent teeth are restored, some additional extension is permissible to create a uniform level that may be more esthetically pleasing.) Often the mesiodistal extension to the line angles of the tooth will place the junction of the occlusal and mesial and distal

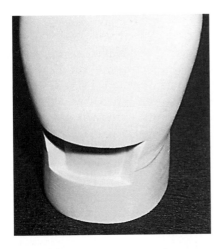

FIG. **21-21** Faciooclusal view of design of gingival wall in Class V preparation for direct gold. Axiogingival line angle is acute and was prepared at expense of gingival wall. This gingival margin is on cementum. If on enamel, the gingival cavosurface would be beveled slightly (see Fig. 21-26, *E*).

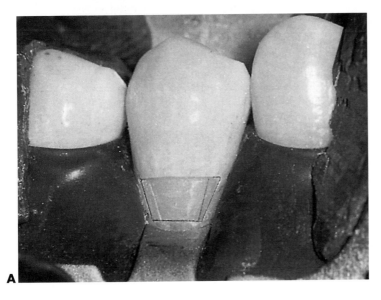

A

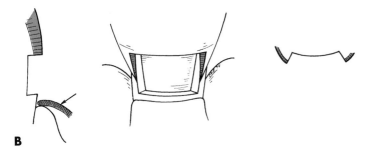

B

FIG. **21-22 A,** Clinical Class V tooth preparation. Note proper isolation of operating field. This gingival margin is on cementum. **B,** Longitudinal section, faciooclusal view, and cross-section. Line and point angles are sharp.

margins gingival to the crest of the free gingiva, rendering the most esthetic result. The gingival margin is also straight, parallel with the occlusal margin, placed only far enough apically to include the lesion, and extends mesiodistally to the line angles of the tooth.

The mesial and distal margins are parallel to the proximal line angles of the tooth (see Fig. 21-22, *A*) and usually are positioned sufficiently mesially and distally (respectively) to be covered by the free gingiva. The mesial and distal margins are straight lines that meet the occlusal margin in sharp, acute angles and meet the gingi-

val margin in sharp, obtuse angles, both of which complete the trapezoidal form.

The depth of the axial wall varies with the position of the preparation on the tooth. The axial wall is approximately 1 mm deep in the occlusal half of the preparation. As the outline approaches the cervical line, the axial wall depth may decrease from 1 to 0.75 mm. The axial wall must be established in dentin, and occlusogingivally it should be relatively flat and parallel (approximately) with the facial surface of the tooth (see Fig. 21-22, *B*). Mesiodistally, the axial wall is also prepared approximately parallel with the surface contour of the tooth. This contour may create a slight mesiodistal curvature in the axial wall in both convex contoured teeth and where the preparation is extensive proximally. Mesiodistal curvature of the axial wall prevents encroachment of the tooth preparation on the pulp. Excessive axial curvature results in a preparation that is either too shallow in the center or too deep at the proximal extensions, and it further complicates restoration by failing to provide a reasonably flat wall against which to begin compaction. A subaxial wall may be created within the axial wall to remove infected caries that has progressed deeper than the ideal axial wall placement.

The occlusoaxial internal line angle is a sharp right angle. The occlusal wall also forms a right angle with the external enamel surface, thus precluding undermining of the enamel. The gingivoaxial internal line angle is a sharp, acute angle, created at the expense of the gingival wall (see Fig. 21-22, *B*). The mesioaxial and distoaxial internal line angles are sharp, obtuse angles. These obtuse line angles are created to prevent the undermining of the mesial and distal enamel, although still providing some resistance to movement of the gold during compaction. They must never be acute angles.

The mesial and distal prepared walls are flat and straight. They meet the occlusal wall in a sharp, acute line angle and meet the gingival wall in a sharp, obtuse line angle. The mesial and distal walls provide resistance for gold compaction, but they provide no retention.

The orientation of the gingival wall is the key to the retention form of the preparation. It is straight mesiodistally, meeting the mesial and distal walls in sharp line angles. Retention is provided by sloping the gingival wall internally to meet the axial wall in a sharply defined acute line angle. Retention is thereby provided by the facial convergence of the occlusal and gingival walls. Gold wedged between these two walls is locked into the tooth.

If the gingival margin is established on enamel, the cavosurface is beveled slightly to remove the unsupported enamel (see Fig. 21-26, *E*). When placed on cementum, the gingival cavosurface is not beveled (see Fig. 21-24, *B*).

The outline of the preparation may be modified. In those clinical situations demanding reduced display of gold, such as in anterior teeth, the incisal outline may be curved to follow the contour of the soft tissue mesiodistally (Fig. 21-23). This modification is made only when required, because preparation instrumentation and finishing of gold are more difficult than when a straight marginal outline is created. A similar modification may be made in the occlusal outline when caries extends more occlusally as the proximal extensions are reached. Also the mesiodistal extension (i.e., dimension) of a preparation may be limited when caries is minimal, thus conserving intact tooth structure. When access requires, the gingival wall may be modified to also curve mesiodistally to include the gingival extent of advanced caries. The entire axial wall should not be extended pulpally to the depth of the lesion when deep cervical abrasion, abfraction, or erosion is treated; rather the axial wall is positioned normally, leaving a remaining V notch at its center to be restored with gold. When failing restorations are removed and restored with direct gold, the preparation outline is partially dictated by the previous restoration (Fig. 21-24).

Instrumentation. The No. 33½ bur is used to establish the general *outline form* of the preparation. The end of the bur establishes the distal wall (Fig. 21-25, *A*); the side establishes the axial depth and the occlusal, gingival, and the mesial walls (see Fig. 21-25, *B*). When access permits, the end of the bur may be used to establish the mesial and gingival walls (see Fig. 21-25, *C* and *D*). The

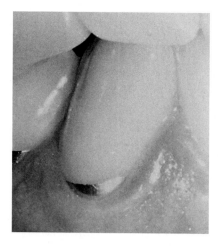

FIG. **21-23** Completed Class V gold restoration. Incisal margin curved to follow contour of gingival tissue for best esthetic result.

FIG. **21-24 A,** Failing Class V amalgam restoration. **B,** Replacement direct gold restoration.

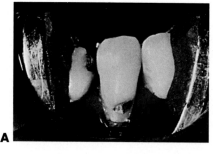

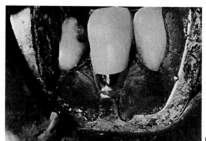

A

B

gingival and mesial walls may be prepared with the side of the bur if access so dictates (see Fig. 21-25, *E* and *F).* The end of the bur is used to place the axial wall in dentin (see Fig. 21-25, *G).*

The 6½-2½-9 hoe or the larger 10-4-8 hoe is useful for planing preparation walls, establishing sharp internal line angles (Fig. 21-26, *A),* and finishing margins. The Wedelstaedt chisel is used to finish the occlusal cavosurface margin (see Fig. 21-26, *B)* and also may be used to plane the axial wall.

The acute axiogingival angle is established with the 6½-2½-9 hoe, cutting from the cavosurface to the axial wall in a push-cut stroke (see Fig. 21-26, *C).* The chips of dentin produced at the axiogingival angle may be removed with the tip of an explorer (see Fig. 21-26, *D)* or the point of a 6½-(90)-2½-9 small angle former. Care must be taken not to gouge the axial wall. When its use is indicated, the gingival bevel is prepared with the Wedelstaedt chisel or a hoe (Fig. 21-26, *E).*

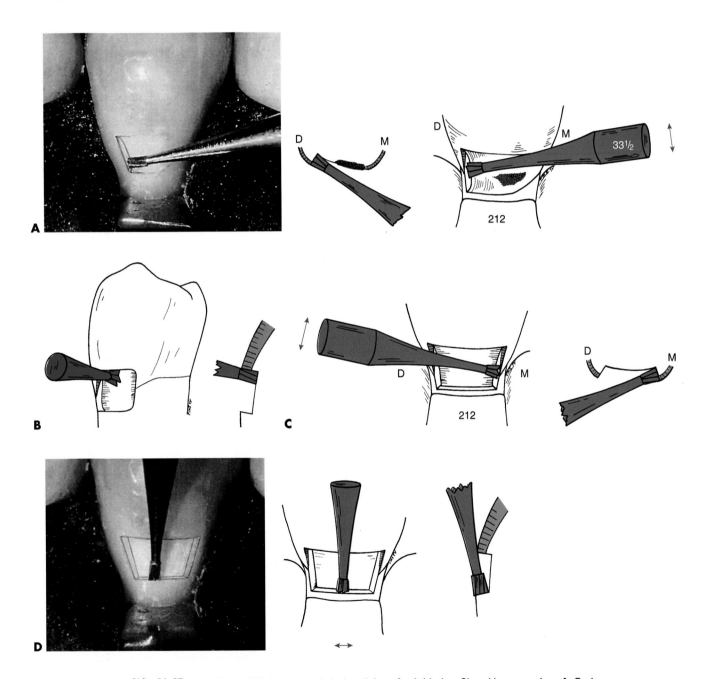

FIG. **21-25** Use of No. 33½ bur in straight handpiece for initiating Class V preparation. **A,** End of bur is used to establish distal wall. **B,** Side of bur is used to establish occlusal wall. **C,** End of bur prepares mesial wall if access permits. **D,** End of bur is used to establish gingival wall if access permits. *Continued*

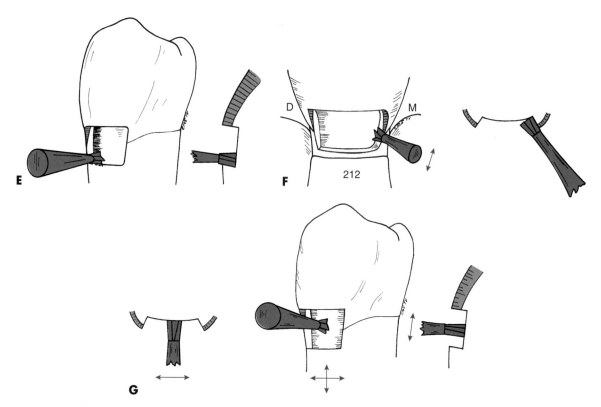

FIG. **21-25, cont'd** **E,** Preparation of gingival wall with side of bur. **F,** Preparation of mesial wall with side of bur. **G,** The end of bur may be used to establish initial axial wall depth in dentin.

Restoration. Restoration of the Class V preparation begins with application of cavity varnish (if desired), after which a piece of degassed E-Z Gold is placed into the preparation. The gold is first degassed in the alcohol flame and then carried to place in the preparation with the passing instrument. Parallelogram foil condensers or other suitable serrated condensers are used to firmly force the gold against the axial wall and to wedge it into the line angles. Then one instrument may be put aside (and the other is used as a holding instrument to prevent movement of the entire piece of gold), and compaction can begin by delivering heavy compacting forces to the gold.

Once stabilized, completion of compaction of the initial mass of gold begins in the center of the mass with a 0.5-mm diameter, round, serrated condenser nib. Careful, methodic stepping of the gold proceeds outward toward the external walls (to wedge the gold in the tooth and remove internal voids). As soon as the gold is stabilized, a holding instrument is unnecessary. As the walls are reached, a line of force of 45 degrees to the axial wall is used to drive the gold into the line angles and against the external walls. The entire surface of the gold is condensed twice to complete compaction of the gold. Additional increments of E-Z Gold are added until the prepa-

ration is filled to at least half its depth. E-Z Gold pellets are then used to complete the restoration covering the margins first, and then to complete compacting in the center of the facial surface. Pellets of gold foil may also be used to complete the outer one half of the restoration (Fig. 21-27).

If gold foil is used for the outer one half of the restoration, compaction proceeds with medium-sized pellets at the mesioocclusal or distoocclusal line angle and then across the occlusal wall. The entire wall and occlusal cavosurface margin are covered with compacted gold foil (see Fig. 21-27, *A*). To ensure that gold protects the margin from blows of the condenser face, care should be exercised when the condenser approaches any enamel margin. Next the gingival, mesial, and distal walls are covered, which leaves the restoration concave (see Fig. 21-27, *B*). It is essential that all cavosurface margins be covered at this time, before the final convex surface of the restoration is formed.

Medium and large pellets (sizes $\frac{1}{43}$ and $\frac{1}{32}$) are then compacted in the center of the restoration to complete the formation of the appropriate contour. A slight excess contour is developed and is removed later when the gold is finished and polished. Any small remaining deficiencies in the surface contour are filled with small pellets. A Varney foot condenser (or other large condenser)

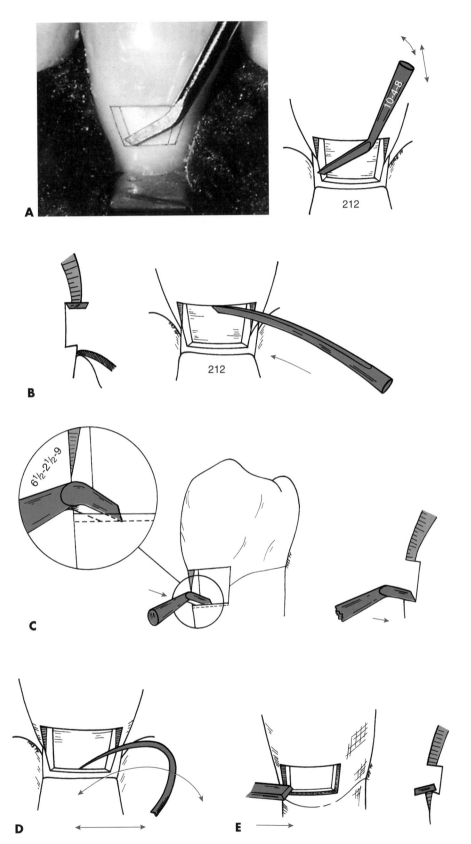

FIG. 21-26 Use of hand instruments in Class V tooth preparation. **A,** Small hoe planes preparation walls. **B,** Wedelstaedt chisel refines occlusal wall and margin. **C,** Small hoe creates acute axiogingival line angle in dentin. **D,** Explorer is used to remove debris from completed preparation. **E,** Chisel blade bevels gingival cavosuface margin when indicated. *(**E,** From Howard WC, Moller RC: Atlas of operative dentistry, St Louis, 1981, Mosby.)*

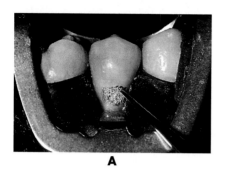
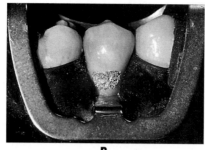
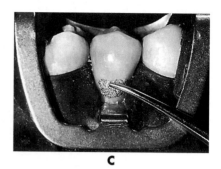

A   B   C

FIG. **21-27** Completion of compaction where gold foil is used to overlay the E-Z Gold. **A,** Condensation of foil proceeds to cover cavosurface margins. A slight excess of gold has been condensed over mesial half of occlusal cavosurface margin. **B,** All cavosurface margins are covered with a slight excess of gold. Restoration at this stage of insertion is concave. **C,** After additional foil pellets are compacted in central area to form convex restoration surface with slight excess, a foot condenser is used to confirm condensation.

FIG. **21-28** Finishing the Class V restoration. **A,** Burnisher work hardens surface. **B,** Small, fine garnet disc removes excess gold contour. **C,** Gold knife's secondary edge used with push-stroke *(arrow)* removes excess gold from gingival margin. **D,** After final surfacing with cuttle discs, any remaining marginal excess is removed with cleoid carver.

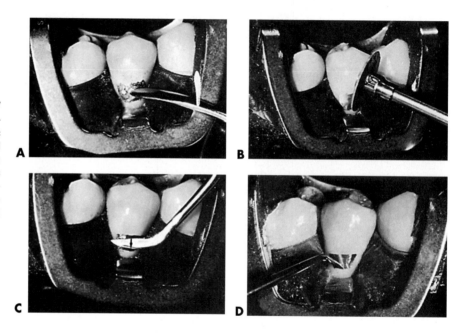

A   B

C   D

is malleted over the entire surface to make it smooth and assist in detection of any poorly compacted areas (see Fig. 21-27, *C*).

Finishing begins with application of a beaver-tail burnisher to work harden and smooth the surface (Fig. 21-28, *A*). Petroleum jelly may be applied to the dam to avoid abrasion from discs; it also may be applied to the discs. Gross excess contour, if any, is removed with a fine garnet disc applied with a Sproule or other suitable mandrel in a low-speed handpiece (see Fig. 21-28, *B*). Excess gold is removed from the cavosurface margins with the cleoid-discoid instrument (using pull-cut strokes) or the gold knife (using only push-and-cut strokes from gold to tooth) (see Fig. 21-28, *C* and *D*). *When removing excess gold over the gingival margin, care is exercised not to remove cementum or "ditch" the root surface (especially when using rotary instruments).*

Once final contour has been obtained, cuttle discs may be used in decreasing abrasiveness (i.e., coarse to

medium to fine) to ready the surface for final polishing. These discs and the cleoid are helpful in removing very fine fins of gold from margins. Polishing is performed with fine pumice followed by tin oxide or white rouge (applied with a soft, webless rubber cup). *Care is also required at this stage to avoid ditching the cementum with the polishing abrasive.* Therefore the abrasives are used dry so that the field may be kept clean and the exact position of the rubber cup can be seen at all times (Fig. 21-29).

After polishing, the No. 212 retainer and rubber dam are removed. Removal of the retainer is best accomplished with the forceps firmly locked into the notches on the retainer. The retainer jaws are opened from the tooth with the forceps and carefully removed occlusally (without scratching the restoration or the surface enamel of the tooth). The gingival sulcus is rinsed and examined to ascertain that it is free of debris. The soft tissue is massaged gently before the patient is dismissed.

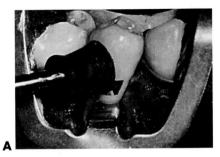

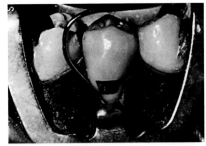

FIG. **21-29 A,** Soft-rubber cup is used to apply polishing abrasives. **B,** Explorer is used to remove any remaining polishing powder from site of completed restoration.

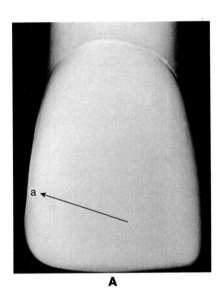

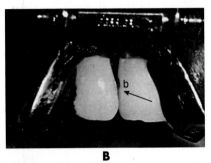

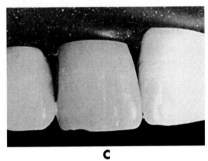

FIG. **21-30** Class III direct gold restoration. **A,** Model of preparation demonstrates esthetic marginal outline (*a*). **B,** Central incisor (*b*) before distal preparation. **C,** Completed Class III restoration.

CLASS III TOOTH PREPARATION AND RESTORATION

Many styles of Class III preparations are advocated for use with direct gold. Some preparations are based on the lingual approach and are restored with E-Z Gold. Others may be instrumented from either the facial or lingual surface and use gold foil as the restorative material. The outline form selected must provide adequate access for placing the restoration, as well as developing an acceptable esthetic result. Although the preparation design presented in subsequent sections was first described by Ferrier in the early years of the twentieth century,[4] it is still used today. It has the advantage not only of conserving tooth structure, but also of providing access for compaction of gold foil directly against all preparation walls and cavosurface margins. This results in a dense, esthetically pleasing result (if careful attention is given to management of the outline design). This preparation is instrumented primarily from a facial approach, although lingual instrumentation may be used in maxillary teeth. The preparation may be modified for mandibular anterior teeth, the distal surface of maxillary canines, and the distal surface of some lateral incisors.

Tooth Preparation Design for Maxillary Incisors. The *marginal outline* is most important. From a facial view the gingival four fifths of the facial margin is straight and (generally) parallel with the contour of the tooth (Fig. 21-30). The facial margin forms a gentle curve in its incisal one fifth to blend with the incisal margin. When viewed from a proximofacial aspect, the facial outline follows the general contour of the adjacent tooth (Fig. 21-31) and meets the gingival outline in a slightly obtuse angle. This juncture may be curved very slightly to enhance esthetics.

The gingival margin is critical to the entire preparation. Its faciolingual length dictates the remainder of the preparation. Where possible, the gingival margin is established just apical to the crest of the free gingiva to enhance the esthetic result. It is straight faciolingually and is approximately at a right angle to the long axis of the tooth. It meets the facial margin in a sharply defined obtuse angle that may be rounded slightly (as previously described), and it meets the lingual margin in a sharply defined acute angle.

Viewed from the lingual, the lingual margin generally parallels the long axis of the tooth (Fig. 21-32). However, it may diverge slightly proximally from the long axis to

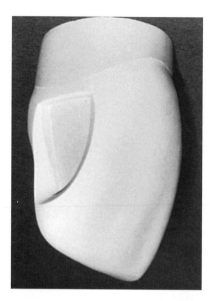

FIG. **21-31** Proximofacial view of Class III preparation.

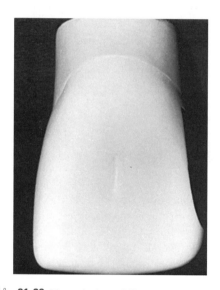

FIG. **21-32** Lingual view of Class III preparation.

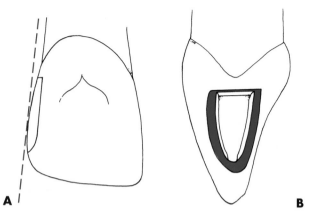

FIG. **21-33** Lingual marginal outline of Class III preparation. **A,** View of lingual outline. Note sharp linguogingival angle. **B,** Proximal view of preparation. Note linguogingival angle is sharp and acute in this view. **(A,** *From Stibbs GD: Direct golds in dental restorative therapy,* Oper Dent *5[3]:107, 1980.)*

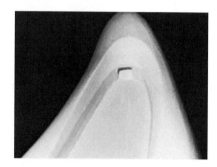

FIG. **21-34** View of incisal retention in Class III preparation. Undercut is placed in dentin but does not undermine enamel.

more nearly parallel the proximal contour. It meets the gingival margin in a sharply defined angle that is nearly 90 degrees when viewed from the lingual (Fig. 21-33), but it is acute when viewed from the proximal. The lingual margin is straight in its gingival two thirds, but then it curves abruptly to meet the incisal margin.

The incisal margin is placed incisally to the contact area to provide access to the preparation; however, it is not extended enough to weaken the incisal angle of the tooth. It forms a smooth curve that connects the facial and the lingual margins of the preparation.

To provide suitable resistance form, the internal aspects of the preparation are precisely instrumented. The gingival wall is flat faciolingually. The axial wall is flat faciolingually and incisogingivally, and it is established

0.5 mm into the dentin. Resistance form is also created by establishing sharp, obtuse axiofacial and axiolingual line angles in dentin. The facial and lingual walls diverge only enough to remove undermined enamel, yet they provide firm, flat walls against which the gold can be compacted.

As in the Class V restoration, retention form is provided only between the gingival and incisal walls. In the Class III preparation the dentinal portion of the gingival wall (as in the Class V gingival wall) slopes apically inward to create an acute axiogingival line angle. However, in the Class III preparation the incisal portion is undercut (Fig. 21-34). This undercut is placed in dentin, facioincisally, to create a mechanical lock between the incisal and gingival walls. This increased retention form in the Class III preparation is required because of the length of the preparation incisogingivally and because of the difficulty of access in compacting the gold.

Provision for *convenience form* is made by the abrupt incisolingual curve (which permits introduction of a condenser directed toward the gingival wall), by adequate clearance of all margins from the adjacent tooth, and by placement of sharp internal point angles suitable for beginning compaction of gold. The facioaxiogingival

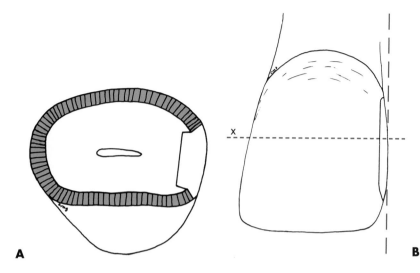

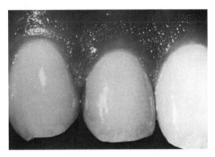

FIG. **21-35** Class III preparation internal form and facial marginal outline. **A,** Incisal view of cross-section of preparation in plane *x* shown in *B*. Facial and lingual cavo-surface bevels are shown placed in enamel. **B,** Facial view of facial marginal outline of preparation. *(From Stibbs GD: Direct golds in dental restorative therapy,* Oper Dent *5[3]:107, 1980.)*

A

B

and linguoaxiogingival point angles may be enlarged slightly to assist in initial stages of foil compaction, if desired.[15]

The *finishing of enamel walls* requires placement of a facial, incisal, and lingual cavosurface bevel, which determines the final marginal outline. This bevel is made with hand instruments and is established totally in enamel. It is designed to create maximum convenience form, to remove all surface irregularities and any unsupported enamel, and to establish a more esthetically pleasing result (Fig. 21-35; see also Fig. 21-30).

Modifications of Class III Preparations. The distal surface of maxillary canines may require a modification in preparation design for convenience in gold compaction. Because a highly convex surface is generally present, it is often desirable to create a "straight-line preparation" in which the facial outline appears as a slice. This modification provides clearance from the mesial marginal ridge of the first premolar and provides considerable convenience form to allow compaction of gold on the gingival wall directly from an incisal position. This type of preparation is also appropriate for the distal surface of highly contoured lateral incisors (Fig. 21-36).

The mandibular incisors require a modified Class III preparation because of their small size and because access from a lingual position may be exceptionally difficult. The lingual wall is created in one plane, and extension of both the lingual and incisal walls is limited. The axiolingual line angle will be a right or slightly obtuse angle. Care is taken to avoid lingual overextension of the lingual wall, because this can result in removal of dentin support for the lingual enamel; thereby rendering the preparation unrestorable by direct gold. Outline form is extended lingually only far enough to include the lesion and to allow access for finishing of the gold. Incisal extension is restricted because the proximal contact area between mandibular incisors is often near the incisal angle. Extension incisally past the contact may

FIG. **21-36** Direct gold restoration of a clinical Class III preparation of straight line design on distal portion of maxillary lateral incisor.

weaken this critical area of the tooth; thus a mechanical separator may be necessary to obtain clearance between the teeth. This provides access for both tooth preparation and gold compaction. Facial extension is similar to the maxillary preparation (Fig. 21-37).

Internally the incisal retentive angle for the mandibular Class III preparation is placed directly incisally, rather than facioincisally as in maxillary teeth. This modification is made to conserve the thickness of the tooth structure at the facioincisal angle, where wear of mandibular anterior teeth frequently occurs.

Lingual approach Class III restorations may be made using E-Z Gold. In such cases the lingual "slot" type of preparation is made with rounded internal line angles.

Separation of Teeth. Separation of teeth is frequently needed for instrumentation or finishing procedures performed on Class III direct gold restorations. The Ferrier separator is a convenient instrument for accomplishing this separation. It is applied and stabilized with compound (similar to stabilization of a No. 212 retainer) (Fig. 21-38). The jackscrews of the separator are activated with the separator wrench to slightly draw the teeth apart, thus creating a maximum space of 0.25 to 0.5 mm. It is desirable to provide only this minimum separation and to remove the separator as soon as possible (preventing damage to periodontal structures).

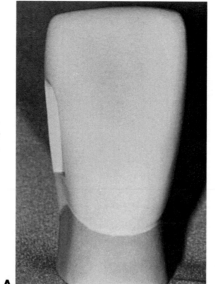
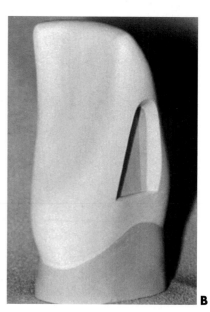

FIG. 21-37 Mandibular Class III preparation. **A,** Facial view. Facial margin is similar to that in maxillary preparation. **B,** Linguoproximal view.

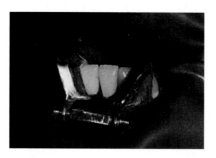

FIG. 21-38 Separator placed before clinical Class III preparation for mandibular incisor.

Instrumentation. The No. 33½ bur (or a suitable Wedelstaedt chisel) is used to begin the preparation (Fig. 21-39). The bur is angled from the facial to position the gingival outline and the facial wall. A Wedelstaedt chisel establishes the lingual extension, and the No. 33½ bur then defines the linguogingival line angle (Fig. 21-40) and completes the gingival floor preparation. The outline form is then completed by beveling the cavosurface areas with a Wedelstaedt chisel. The dentinal part of the gingival, lingual, facial, and incisal walls are next planed. A small hoe (i.e., 6½-2½-9) is used for the lingual and gingival walls (Fig. 21-41). An angle former is used to plane the facial dentinal wall (Fig. 21-42). An axial plane (i.e., 8-1-23) smoothes the axial wall, and a bibeveled hatchet (i.e., 3-2-28) establishes the incisal retentive angle with a chopping motion (Fig. 21-43). Small angle formers are used to complete the sharp facioaxiogingival and linguoaxiogingival point angles, as well as the slightly acute axiogingival angle (Fig. 21-44). The point angles may be further enlarged with the No. 33S bur (i.e., end-cutting bur) for additional convenience form. The Wedelstaedt chisel may be used again to complete the final planing of the cavosurface margins (Fig. 21-45).

Restoration. The separator is used to obtain a separation of 0.25 to 0.5 mm. Compaction of gold foil begins at the linguoaxiogingival point angle (Fig. 21-46). A small (i.e., 0.4 mm) monangle condenser is used to compact the gold, which is held by a small holding instrument. Pellets size $\frac{1}{64}$ or $\frac{1}{128}$ are used in the beginning of the restorative phase. The line of force is directed over the facial surface of the adjacent tooth and into the linguoaxiogingival point angle (see Fig. 21-46, *B*). As soon as ample gold has been compacted into the linguogingival area to cover the linguogingival shoulder, compaction continues across the gingival wall (Fig. 21-47) and into the faciogingival angle. The offset condenser (with a faciogingival line of force) is used to fill the facioaxiogingival point angle (Fig. 21-48). Compaction of gold at the linguogingival area is next confirmed with the oblique-faced monangle condenser (i.e., 0.5 mm) from the linguoincisal position (Fig. 21-49). Failure to provide dense gold in this linguogingival area at this stage may result in a void at the linguogingival angle, and subsequently, may lead to restoration failure.

The bulk of the restoration is now compacted with $\frac{1}{43}$- or $\frac{1}{32}$-sized pellets, mainly from a facial (occasionally from a lingual) direction (Fig. 21-50).

The line of force is maintained in an axiogingival direction with the 0.5-mm monangle or oblique-faced monangle condenser (see Fig. 21-50, *B*). This requires that the incisal surface of the growing restoration always slopes apically, with the gold on the axial wall ahead of the proximal surface of the restoration. During the compaction procedure, the vector of the line of force should always be toward the internal portion of the preparation to prevent dislodgment of the restoration.

The next step is the restoration of the incisal portion of the preparation, referred to as "making the turn." It is *Text continued on p. 897*

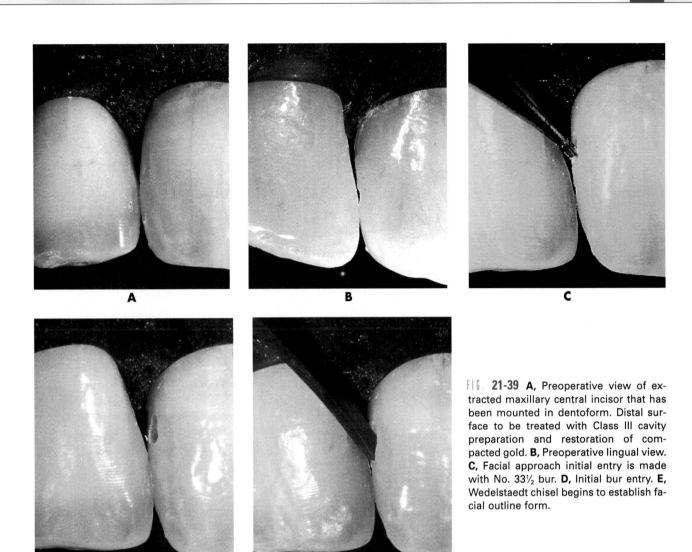

FIG. 21-39 A, Preoperative view of extracted maxillary central incisor that has been mounted in dentoform. Distal surface to be treated with Class III cavity preparation and restoration of compacted gold. B, Preoperative lingual view. C, Facial approach initial entry is made with No. 33½ bur. D, Initial bur entry. E, Wedelstaedt chisel begins to establish facial outline form.

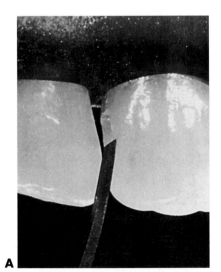
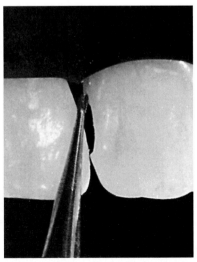

FIG. 21-40 Lingual view of preparation instrumentation. A, Wedelstaedt chisel planing lingual enamel wall. B, Inverted cone bur is used to establish sharp linguogingival shoulder.

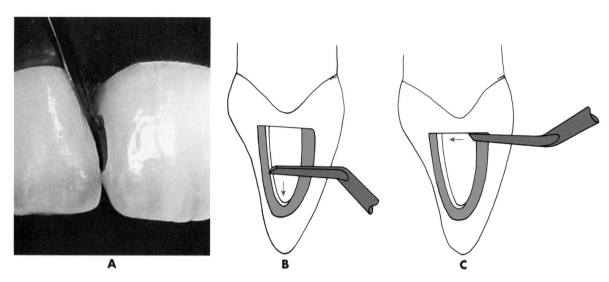

FIG. **21-41** Use of small hoe facial approach in tooth preparation. **A,** Hoe planes lingual dentinal wall from incisal to gingival aspect. **B,** Hoe also planes this wall from gingival to incisal aspect (*arrow*). **C,** Hoe planes gingival cavosurface (*arrow*). See Fig. 21-44, *D,* for direction of enamel portion of gingival wall for strong margin (full-length enamel rods).

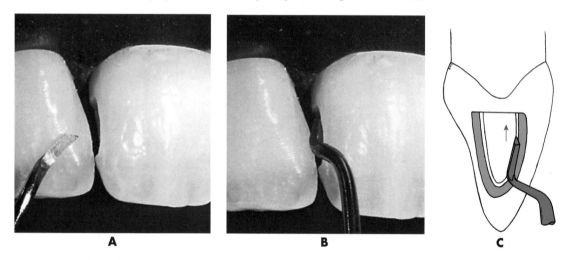

FIG. **21-42** Use of angle former to plane facial dentinal wall. **A,** Angle former before placement in preparation. **B,** Angle former in preparation. **C,** Angle former is directed apically (*arrow*) to plane facial dentinal wall.

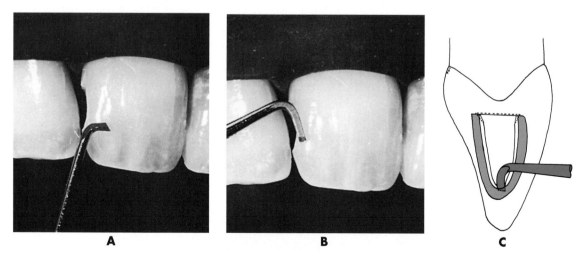

FIG. **21-43** **A,** Axial plane before placement in preparation. **B,** Bibeveled hatchet before placement in preparation. **C,** Bibeveled hatchet is used to establish incisal retentive angle.

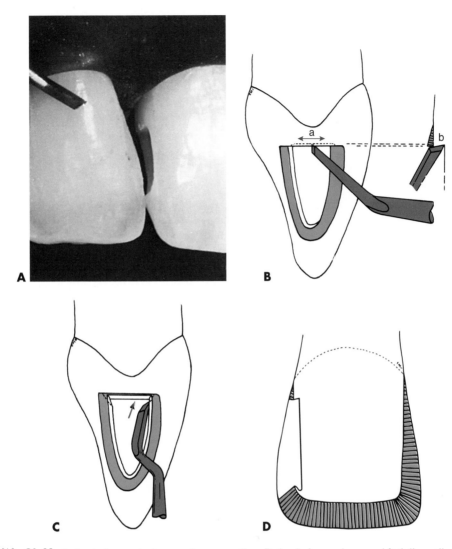

FIG. 21-44 A, Angle former before use in preparation. B, Angle former is moved faciolingually (*a*) to establish acute axiogingival line angle (*b*). C, Offset angle former thrust faciogingivally establishes acute facioaxiogingival point angle. D, Completed incisal and gingivoaxial retention form. (*D, From Stibbs GD: Direct golds in dental restorative therapy, Oper Dent 5[3]:107, 1980.*)

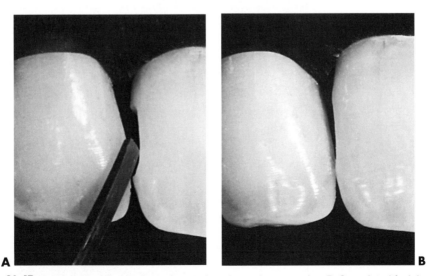

FIG. 21-45 A, Wedelstaedt chisel may be used again to plane margins. B, Completed facial margin of Class III tooth preparation viewed from facial position.

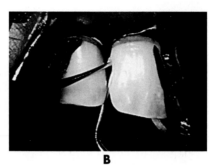

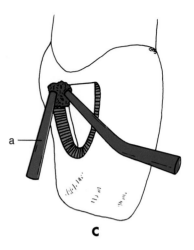

FIG. 21-46 A, First pellet of gold foil is placed from facial aspect into preparation. Note separation of teeth by 0.25 to 0.5 mm. B, Compaction of pellet into linguoaxiogingival point angle. Line of force is directed linguoaxiogingivally while holding instrument is placed from lingual position. C, Holding instrument (a) prevents dislodgment of foil during compaction.

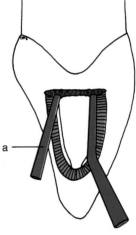

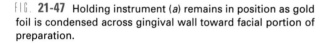

FIG. 21-47 Holding instrument (a) remains in position as gold foil is condensed across gingival wall toward facial portion of preparation.

FIG. 21-48 A, Offset condenser before placement in cavity preparation. B, Compacted gold foil covering gingival wall and cavosurface.

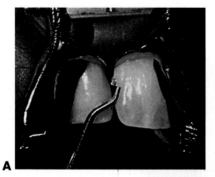

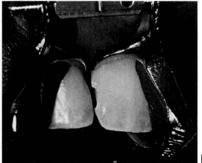

FIG. 21-49 Lingual view. Monangle condenser confirms compaction of gold at linguogingival aspect of restoration.

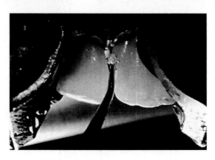

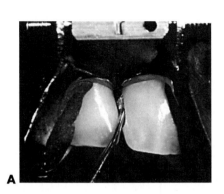

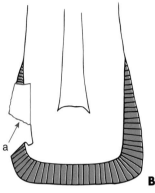

FIG. **21-50 A,** Monangle condenser is used to build bulk of gold in gingival half of preparation. **B,** Gingival half of restoration in longitudinal section. Line of force *(a)* is directed axiogingivally during compaction of gold to prevent dislodgment of restoration.

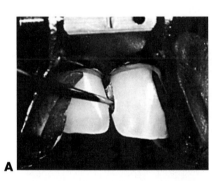

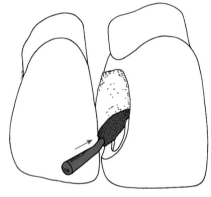

FIG. **21-51 A,** Condenser is directed over facial surface of adjacent tooth, while gold is built toward incisal aspect. **B,** Gold is compacted from facioincisal aspect to cover lingual cavosurface; however, compaction direction must continue to have a major vector *(arrow)* toward axial wall to prevent dislodgment. Therefore (at this stage) the compacted foil on axial wall must be well ahead (incisally) of the "growing" proximal surface.

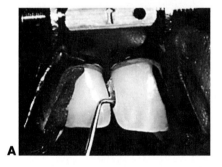

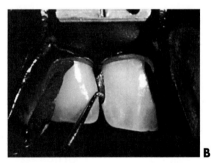

FIG. **21-52 A,** Right-angle hand condenser begins to press gold into incisal retention. **B,** This condenser forces gold deeply into incisal retentive undercut.

accomplished in three phases. First, sufficient gold is built up on the lingual wall so that the gold is very near the incisal angle (Fig. 21-51). Second, the incisal area is filled by compacting $\frac{1}{128}$-size pellets with the right-angle hand condenser (Fig. 21-52). Third, pellets of foil are compacted into the incisolingual and incisal areas with the offset condenser. This fills the incisal portion, making a complete turn from lingual to facial (Fig. 21-53, *A*). The entire incisal cavosurface is covered with gold (Fig. 21-53, *B*).

Additional gold compaction finishes the facial one third of the restoration, then the Varney foot condenser is used to "after-condense" over the contour of the restoration. More separation is generated by slight activation of the separator, before finishing and polishing the restoration. A sharp, gold foil knife is used to remove excess in the contact area, permitting a fine finish-

ing strip or steel matrix strip to pass through. A pull-cut Shooshan file or gold knife may facilitate removal of excess gold facially (Fig. 21-54). Initial contouring of the contact area is performed with long, extra-narrow, extra-fine cuttle finishing strips, to gain access to the proximal surface. Next, a wide, medium cuttle strip may be used for rapid removal of excess gold. Final contouring continues with the medium and fine, narrow strips. Finishing is performed with the extra-narrow, extra-fine cuttle strip (Fig. 21-55). Care is taken to only finish the facial or lingual areas with the strip and to avoid flattening the contact area. The gold knife or cleoid-discoid can be used to remove final excess gold from cavosurface margins. The separator is then removed.

Final polishing is accomplished with a worn, extra-fine cuttle strip. Polishing powder may be used. However, omitting this step results in a satin finish that is

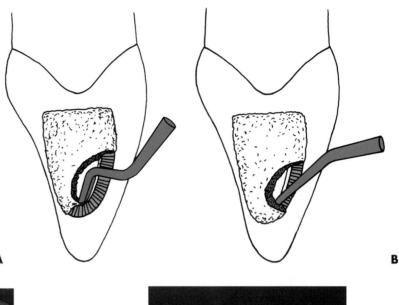

FIG. **21-53** Completing the compaction of gold into incisal region of preparation. **A,** Offset bayonet condenser condenses gold into incisal retention with mallet compaction. **B,** Incisal cavosurface is restored with gold foil condensed with small monangle condenser.

A

B

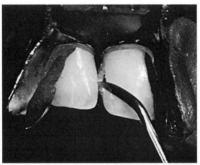

FIG. **21-54** A sharp, thin-bladed gold knife removes excess gold from facial surface.

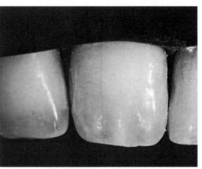

FIG. **21-56** Completed maxillary Class III gold foil restoration.

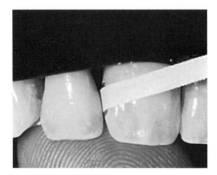

FIG. **21-55** Fine cuttle finishing strips polish proximal surface of gold foil restoration.

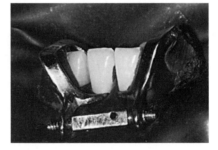

FIG. **21-57** Completed mandibular Class III gold foil restoration of lesion in Fig. 21-38.

less reflective of light and, therefore, perhaps more esthetic (Fig. 21-56).

SUMMARY

Direct-filling golds are useful in restorative dentistry. If carefully manipulated by a dentist, these restorative materials may provide lifetime service to patients and promote their oral health (Fig. 21-57). Direct-filling golds contribute to both the art and science of restorative dentistry.

ACKNOWLEDGMENTS

Pure gold materials used for photography in this chapter were provided courtesy of Ivoclar-Williams Company, Inc., Amherst, NY.

REFERENCES

1. Baum L: Gold foil (filling golds) in dental practice, *Dent Clin North Am,* 199, 1965.
2. Black GV: The nature of blows and the relation of size of plugger points force as used in filling teeth, *Dent Rev* 21:499, 1907.

3. Dwinelle WH: Crystalline gold, its varieties, properties, and use, *Am J Dent* 5:249, 1855.

4. Ferrier WI: Treatment of proximal cavities in anterior teeth with gold foil, *J Am Dent Assoc* 21:571, 1934.

5. Ferrier WI: The use of gold foil in general practice, *J Am Dent Assoc* 28:691, 1941.

6. Hodson JT: Compaction properties of various pure gold restorative materials, *J Am Acad Gold Foil Oper* 12:52, Sept 1969.

7. Hodson JT: Structure and properties of gold foil and mat gold, *J Dent Res* 42:575, 1963.

8. Hodson JT, Stibbs GD: Structural density of compacted gold foil and mat gold, *J Dent Res* 41:339, 1962.

9. Hollenback GM: There is no substitute for gold foil in restorative dentistry, *J South Calif Dent Assoc* 33:275, 1965.

10. Ingersol CE: Personal communication, 1982.

11. Lambert RL: A survey of the teaching of compacted gold, *Oper Dent* 5(1):20, 1980.

12. Lund MR, Baum L: Powdered gold as a restorative material, *J Prosthet Dent* 13:1151, 1963.

13. Smith GE: Condenser selection for pure gold compaction, *J Am Acad Gold Foil Oper* 15:53, Sept 1972.

14. Smith GE: *The effect of condenser design and lines of force on the dental compaction of cohesive gold* (Master's thesis), Seattle, 1970, University of Washington.

15. Smith GE, Hodson JT, Stibbs GD: A study of the degree of adaptation possible in retention holes, convenience points and point angles in Class III cavity preparations, *J Am Acad Gold Foil Oper* 15(1):13, 1972.

16. Stibbs GD: Direct golds in dental restorative therapy, *Oper Dent* 5(3):107, 1980.

17. Thomas JJ, Stanley HR, Gilman HW: Effects of gold foil condensation on human dental pulp, *J Am Dent Assoc* 78:788, 1969.

18. Trueman WH: An essay upon the relative advantage of crystallized gold and gold foil as a material for filling teeth, *Dent Cosmos* 10:128, 1868.

19. Williams (Ivoclar-Williams Company): *E-Z Gold instructional brochure*, Amherst, NY, Ivoclar-Williams.